# The Physiological Basis of Rehabilitation Medicine

**Second Edition**

# The Physiological Basis of Rehabilitation Medicine

## Second Edition

Edited by

## John A. Downey, M.D., D.Phil. (Oxon)

Simon Baruch Professor of Rehabilitation Medicine
College of Physicians and Surgeons
Columbia University
Attending Physician
The Presbyterian Hospital in the City of New York
New York, New York

## Stanley J. Myers, M.D.

A. David Gurewitsch Professor of Clinical Rehabilitation Medicine
College of Physicians and Surgeons
Columbia University
Attending Physician
The Presbyterian Hospital in the City of New York
New York, New York

## Erwin G. Gonzalez, M.D.

Professor of Rehabilitation Medicine
Mount Sinai School of Medicine
City University of New York
Director, Department of Physical Medicine and Rehabilitation
Beth Israel Medical Center
New York, New York

## James S. Lieberman, M.D.

H. K. Corning Professor of Rehabilitation Medicine Research
Chairman, Department of Rehabilitation Medicine
College of Physicians and Surgeons
Columbia University
Director, Rehabilitation Medicine Service
The Presbyterian Hospital in the City of New York
New York, New York

With 43 contributing authors.

## Butterworth-Heinemann

Boston   London   Oxford   Singapore   Sydney   Toronto   Wellington

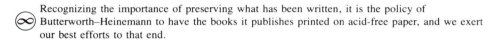
**Library of Congress Cataloging-in-Publication Data**
The Physiological basis of rehabilitation medicine / edited by John A.
  Downey . . . [et al.]. —2nd ed.
    p.    cm.
  Includes bibliographical references and index.
  ISBN 1-56372-080-9 (alk. paper)
  1. Medical rehabilitation. 2. Human physiology. I. Downey, John
A., 1930–
  [DNLM: 1. Physiology. 2. Pathology. 3. Rehabilitation. QZ 140
P578 1994]
RM930.P48   1994
612'.0024617—dc20
DNLM/DLC
for Library of Congress                                                       93-37020
                                                                                    CIP

**British Library Cataloging-in-Publication Data.**
A catalogue record for this book is available from the British Library.

Butterworth–Heinemann
313 Washington Street
Newton, MA 02158–1626

10  9  8  7  6  5  4  3  2

Printed in the United States of America

To Robert C. Darling, the first Simon Baruch Professor of Rehabilitation Medicine at Columbia University's College of Physicians and Surgeons and founder of its Department of Rehabilitation Medicine.

Dr. Darling graduated from Harvard College and Harvard Medical School with high honors. After medical residency at The Presbyterian Hospital he became a distinguished colleague of Nobel prize winners Doctors Andre Cournand and Dickinson Richards, during which time he contributed much to the elucidation of pulmonary and cardiovascular function. He later continued his work in exercise and environmental physiology at the Harvard Fatigue Laboratory, whence came much of the foundation of these fields in modern medicine. He rose to become director of that laboratory before returning to Columbia-Presbyterian Medical Center, where he was asked to develop and found the Department of Rehabilitation Medicine at Columbia University. His work in academics, medicine, and science exemplifies the ideal for the future direction of rehabilitation medicine.

# Contents

# Contributing Authors

**Jose A. Alonso, M.D.**
Assistant Professor of Clinical Rehabilitation
Medicine
College of Physicians and Surgeons
Columbia University
Assistant Attending Physician
The Presbyterian Hospital in the City of New
York
New York, New York

**Jerry G. Blaivas, M.D.**
Department of Urology
New York Hospital/Cornell Medical Center
New York, New York

**Joanne Borg-Stein, M.D.**
Assistant Professor of Rehabilitation Medicine
Tufts University School of Medicine
Medical Director
Spaulding and Newton Wellesley Hospital
Rehabilitation Center
Spaulding Rehabilitation Hospital
Boston, Massachusetts
Associate Chief, Physical Medicine and
Rehabilitation
Newton Wellesley Hospital
Newton, Massachusetts

**Richard Borkow, M.D.**
Assistant Professor
Department of Rehabilitation Medicine
Albert Einstein College of Medicine
Bronx, New York

**Anne Breuer, M.D.**
Clinical Assistant Professor of Orthopaedics and
Rehabilitation
University of Miami School of Medicine
Miami, Florida

**John C.M. Brust, M.D.**
Professor of Clinical Neurology
College of Physicians and Surgeons
Columbia University
Director
Department of Neurology
Harlem Hospital Center
New York, New York

**Elsworth R. Buskirk, Ph.D.**
Professor of Applied Physiology, Emeritus
Noll Laboratory for Human Performance
Research
The Pennsylvania State University
University Park, Pennsylvania

**Malcolm B. Carpenter, M.D.**
Professor and Chairman Emeritus
Department of Anatomy
Uniformed Services University
Bethesda, Maryland

**Arminius Cassvan, M.D.**
Associate Professor of Clinical Rehabilitation
Medicine
State University of New York, Stony Brook
Stony Brook, New York
Chief, Rehabilitation Medicine
Franklin Hospital Medical Center
Valley Stream, New York
Director, Rehabilitation Medicine
Hempstead General Hospital Medical Center
Hempstead, New York

**Yasoma Challenor, M.D.**
Clinical Professor of Rehabilitation Medicine
College of Physicians and Surgeons
Columbia University
New York, New York
Director
Department of Rehabilitation Medicine
Blythedale Children's Hospital
Valhalla, New York

**W. Crawford Clark**
Associate Professor of Medical Psychology
College of Physicians and Surgeons
Columbia University
Research Scientist VI
Department of Biopsychology
New York State Psychiatric Institute
New York, New York

**Paul J. Corcoran, M.D.**
Visiting Professor and Interim Director
Division of Physical Medicine and Rehabilitation
Harvard Medical School
Clinical Director
Department of Rehabilitation Medicine
Spaulding Rehabilitation Hospital
Boston, Massachusetts

**Felicia Cosman, M.D.**
Assistant Professor of Medicine
Regional Bone Center
College of Physicians and Surgeons
Columbia University
New York, New York
Regional Bone Center
Helen Hayes Hospital
West Haverstraw, New York

**Lucien J. Cote, M.D.**
Associate Professor
Department of Neurology
College of Physicians and Surgeons
Columbia University
New York, New York

**John A. Downey, M.D., D.Phil. (Oxon)**
Simon Baruch Professor of Rehabilitation
Medicine
College of Physicians and Surgeons
Columbia University
Attending Physician
The Presbyterian Hospital in the City of New
York
New York, New York

**Robert J. Downey, M.D.**
Fellow, Cardiothoracic Surgery
College of Physicians and Surgeons
Columbia University
New York, New York

**Erwin G. Gonzalez, M.D.**
Professor of Rehabilitation Medicine
Mount Sinai School of Medicine
City University of New York
Director, Department of Physical Medicine and
Rehabilitation
Beth Israel Medical Center
New York, New York

**James Gordon, Ed.D., P.T.**
Assistant Professor
Program in Physical Therapy
Research Scientist
Center for Neurobiology and Behavior
College of Physicians and Surgeons
Columbia University
New York, New York

**Leonard C. Harber, M.D.**
Rhodebeck Professor of Dermatology
College of Physicians and Surgeons
Columbia University
Attending Physician
The Presbyterian Hospital in the City of New
York
New York, New York

**Martha E. Heath, Ph.D.**
Department of Environmental Medicine
Navy Medical Research Institute
Bethesda, Maryland
Associate Research Scientist
Department of Rehabilitation Medicine
College of Physicians and Surgeons
Columbia University
New York, New York

**Mazher M. Jaweed, Ph.D.**
Clinical Associate Professor
Department of Physical Medicine and
Rehabilitation
Baylor College of Medicine
Houston, Texas

**E. Ralph Johnson, M.D.**
Associate Professor and Acting Chairman
Physical Medicine and Rehabilitation
University of California, Davis, School of
Medicine
Davis, California
Attending Physician
Physical Medicine and Rehabilitation
University of California, Davis, Medical Center
Sacramento, California

**Steven A. Kaplan, M.D.**
Assistant Professor of Urology
College of Physicians and Surgeons
Columbia University
Director, Neuro-Urology and Prostate Center
The Presbyterian Hospital in the City of New
York
New York, New York

**David D. Kilmer, M.D.**
Assistant Professor of Physical Medicine and
Rehabilitation
University of California, Davis, School of
Medicine
Davis, California

**Fredi Kronenberg, Ph.D.**
Assistant Professor of Rehabilitation Medicine
College of Physicians and Surgeons
Columbia University
New York, New York

**Daniel E. Lemons, Ph.D.**
Associate Professor of Biology
City College of the City University of New York
New York, New York

**James S. Lieberman, M.D.**
H.K. Corning Professor of Rehabilitation
Medicine Research
Chairman, Department of Rehabilitation
Medicine
College of Physicians and Surgeons
Columbia University
Director, Rehabilitation Medicine Service
The Presbyterian Hospital in the City of New
York
New York, New York

**Cynthia Lien, M.D.**
Assistant Professor of Anesthesiology
Cornell University Medical College
Associate Attending Anesthesiologist
The New York Hospital
New York, New York

**Robert Lindsay, M.B.Ch.B., Ph.D., F.R.C.P.**
Professor of Medicine
College of Physicians and Surgeons
Columbia University
Chief, Department of Internal Medicine
Helen Hayes Hospital
New York, New York

**Robert E. Lovelace, M.D., F.R.C.P. (Lond)**
Professor of Neurology
College of Physicians and Surgeons
Columbia University
New York, New York

**Brenda S. Mallory**
Assistant Professor of Rehabilitation
College of Physicians and Surgeons
Columbia University
Assistant Attending Physician
The Presbyterian Hospital in the City of New
York
New York, New York

**J.P. Mohr, M.D.**
Sciarra Professor of Clinical Neurology
College of Physicians and Surgeons
Columbia University
New York, New York

**Jonathan R. Moldover, M.D.**
Associate Clinical Professor of Rehabilitation
Medicine
College of Physicians and Surgeons
Columbia University
New York, New York
Chief, Rehabilitation Medicine
Helen Hayes Hospital
West Haverstraw, New York

**Van C. Mow, Ph.D., B.A.E.**
Professor of Mechanical Engineering and
Orthopaedic Bioengineering
Director, Orthopaedic Research Laboratory
College of Physicians and Surgeons
Columbia University
New York, New York

**Stanley J. Myers, M.D.**
A. David Gurewitsch Professor of Clinical
Rehabilitation Medicine
College of Physicians and Surgeons
Columbia University
Attending Physician
The Presbyterian Hospital in the City of New
York
New York, New York

**Janet H. Prystowsky, M.D., Ph.D.**
Irving Assistant Professor of Dermatology
Columbia University
Assistant Attending Physician
Department of Dermatology
The Presbyterian Hospital in the City of New
York
New York, New York

**Kristjan T. Ragnarsson, M.D.**
Dr. Lucy G. Moses Professor and Chairman
Department of Rehabilitation Medicine
Mount Sinai School of Medicine
City University of New York
New York, New York

**Joel Stein, M.D.**
Instructor in Medicine
Division of Physical Medicine and Rehabilitation
Harvard Medical School
Attending Physician
Physical Medicine and Rehabilitation
Spaulding Rehabilitation Hospital
Boston, Massachusetts

**N. Venketasubramanian, M.D.**
Post-doctoral Fellow
Department of Neurology
College of Physicians and Surgeons
Columbia University
New York, New York
Tan Tok Seng Hospital
Singapore

**Charles Weissman, M.D.**
Associate Professor of Clinical Anesthesiology
and Clinical Medicine
College of Physicians and Surgeons
Columbia University
New York, New York

**Steven L. Wolf, Ph.D., F.A.P.T.A.**
Professor and Director of Research
Department of Rehabilitation Medicine
Professor
Department of Medicine
Associate Professor
Department of Anatomy and Cell Biology
Emory University School of Medicine
Atlanta, Georgia

**William L. Young, M.D.**
Associate Professor of Anesthesiology
College of Physicians and Surgeons
Columbia University
New York, New York

**Jerald R. Zimmerman, M.D.**
Assistant Professor of Physical Medicine and
Rehabilitation
UMDNJ—New Jersey Medical School
Newark, New Jersey
Clinical Chief of Orthopaedic Rehabilitation
Kessler Institute for Rehabilitation
West Orange, New Jersey

# Preface

Rehabilitation medicine is the area of specialty concerned with the management of patients with impairments of function due to disease or trauma. A careful distinction should be made between impairments, which are the physical losses themselves, and disabilities, which are the effects of impairments on overall function of the individual. Understanding and utilization of this distinction require knowledge of the manner in which the human body adapts to and compensates for the peculiar forms of stress which the original injury has produced. In this way, physiology is the parent basic science in this area of medicine.

This book is a compilation of essays on selected physiologic topics most pertinent to adaptation and compensatory adjustments in patients with neurological, musculoskeletal and circulatory impairments. In some instances these physiologic topics address reduction of the impairments themselves, but more often they relate to the principles of compensatory adaptations that can reduce the resulting disability. The chapters are not designed to be directly applicable to immediate practice; they are compendia of background knowledge on which the practitioner can build.

The range of topics has been chosen by criteria not wholly logical or comprehensive. An encyclopedic approach obviously would have been impossible in a single volume of modest dimensions. There is an insufficient body of basic knowledge in some topics of importance to justify a chapter. For other topics on which there may be sufficient knowledge in scattered sources, the editors could not discover an appropriate author. Selectivity also resulted from the editors' bias, which favors the areas of their personal experiences. We have chosen, when possible, topics on which there is important new evidence and data, but we have avoided areas in which the evidence is so recent that it is likely to be modified or possibly disproved in the near future. In this way, we may have missed some exciting and useful frontiers of knowledge, we hope our book will have more than fleeting validity.

In this volume physiology is interpreted broadly. Where structure and functions are closely linked, as in studies of the central nervous system, we have considered neuroanatomy as a physiologic topic. Where function is not associated with any local definite structure as in psychology, we have still considered human motivation as a physiologic subject, as long as it is based on sound observation, in a system in which stimulus leads to a predictable response.

The contributors were asked to cover thoroughly their assigned areas and not to oversimplify. Yet the result of their efforts, and of the efforts of the editors, is a presentation of material that is easily understandable to physicians and other health professionals with a scientific background. References listed at the conclusion of each chapter are designed to allow any student or practitioner who so desires to explore the topic in greater depth.

Another reason for a book on physiology for practitioners in rehabilitation medicine lies in the nature of therapy in this area of medicine. Treatment by drugs and diet lends itself to controlled therapeutic trials with carefully constructed controls. Treatment by exercise devices, physical agents, and environmental manipulation, since these require active participation and knowledge on the part of the patient, presents greater difficulties to construction of controls. although efforts along these lines are being made and should continue. Rehabilitation medicine depends heavily for its scientific base on knowledge of normal responses to physiologic stimuli and deduction therefrom as to the likely response of patients. Various efforts are needed to reduce empiricism, to discard traditions not in accord with modern scientific fact,

and to build up a body of validated knowledge peculiar to this growing area of medical need.

The preceding paragraphs, modified from the first edition, set forth the goal shared by the current editors, who are professors of rehabilitation medicine: to continue the physiologic approach to the teaching of medical students and young physicians. To solidify this interest and emphasis, many of the chapters in this edition, as in the first, are authored or coauthored by specialists currently or formerly of this department and by others who were trained in this tradition.

JOHN A. DOWNEY

# Acknowledgments

The editors wish to acknowledge their indebtedness to many former colleagues and students. JAD wishes particularly to mention Dr. John B. Armstrong, FRCP(C), and the late Professors E. C. Eppinger, Sir George Pickering, FRS, and R. F. Loeb and to acknowledge that much of his contribution to this edition was developed and produced during a sabbatical spent as Visiting Professor at the International Center for the Disabled in New York City. This institution was the first comprehensive medical and vocational rehabilitation facility, and it remains one of the foremost in the United States. There, Dr. Downey received much of his earliest training, and it afforded the ideal atmosphere for academic and intellectual pursuits. SJM wishes to acknowledge the late Dr. A. David Gurewitsch for his example of what a clinician should be. Though not a scientist, he set an example of the practice of the "art" of medicine, which is the end result of this book. EGG would like to acknowledge all former residents trained by him during the 12 years he directed the rehabilitation medicine residency program at Columbia-Presbyterian, whose constant quest for "scientific rationale" served as inspiration to update the book; Dr. Robert Newman, President of Beth Israel Medical Center for allowing the time needed to complete the work; and Agustin Hernandez for his literary assistance. JSL would like to acknowledge his mentors, Professors Gilbert H. Glaser, Sid Gilman, and William M. Fowler, Jr., who were instrumental in developing his interest in and knowledge of the physiology of the nervous system and of muscle.

The editors wish to acknowledge their appreciation to Mr. Peter F. Skinner of the International Center for the Disabled for his incisive and expert editorial contributions, and to Ms. Rosemary Bleha of The Presbyterian Hospital for her organizational and administrative assistance.

JOHN A. DOWNEY, M.D.
STANLEY J. MYERS, M.D.
ERWIN G. GONZALEZ, M.D.
JAMES S. LIEBERMAN, M.D.

# Chapter 1

# Upper and Lower Motor Neurons

MALCOLM B. CARPENTER

Loss of motor function in parts of the body owing to a neural lesion is a distressing and fearful event for anyone. A lesion involving the motor systems is evidenced by loss of voluntary movement, muscle weakness, loss of muscle tone, loss or alteration of reflex activity, abnormal postures, and ultimately substitution of inferior and awkward motor activity. Evaluation of loss or disturbances of motor function should begin by determining the site of the lesion. The location of the lesion frequently provides clues to its nature and insights into the specific pathology. Because disturbances of voluntary motor function may involve either the upper or lower motor neuron, the first step is to distinguish which is involved. This relatively simple, yet frequently puzzling, distinction is one of the cornerstones of clinical neurology.

## The Lower Motor Neuron

Anterior horn cells and their peripheral processes (axons), which innervate striated muscle, constitute anatomic and physiologic units referred to as the *final common motor pathway,* or the lower motor neuron. The concept of the lower motor neuron is not limited to spinal cord. Motor cranial nerve nuclei, which innervate muscles in the head and neck, also are classified as lower motor neurons.

*Anterior horn cells,* the prototype for all motor neurons, lie in cell columns in the anterior gray horn of the spinal cord. Several distinct cell columns are evident in the anterior horn. A medial cell column extending throughout the length of the spinal cord, divisible into cell groups, innervates the long and short axial muscles. The lateral cell column innervates the remaining body musculature. In the thoracic region the lateral cell column is small and innervates the intercostal and anterolateral trunk musculature. In the cervical and lumbosacral enlargements the lateral cell column enlarges and consists of several large subgroups. Cell groups of the lateral cell column in the cord enlargements innervate the muscles of the extremities. Cells of the lateral column, located anteriorly and peripherally, innervate extensor and abductor muscle groups; cells located dorsal and central to these innervate flexor and adductor muscle groups (Figure 1-1). The spinal gray matter has cytoarchitectural lamination that divides it into separate zones.[1,2] Anterior horn cells lie with Rexed's lamina IX, characterized by large motor neurons, 30 to 100 $\mu$ in diameter (Figure 1-2). These large multipolar neurons have coarse Nissl granules, large central nuclei, and multiple dendrites that extend beyond the limits of lamina IX. Axons of these cells emerge via the ventral root and become mixed with dorsal root fibers distal to the dorsal root ganglion. Spinal nerves containing both motor and sensory fibers are referred to as *mixed spinal nerves.* Fibers of the mixed spinal nerve divide into dorsal and ventral primary rami (Figure 1-3). In the spinal enlargements the primary rami par-

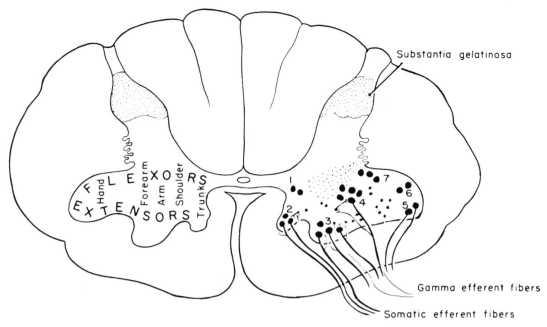

**Figure 1-1.** Diagram of the motor nuclei of the anterior gray horn in a lower cervical spinal segment. On the left, the approximate locations of neurons innervating different muscle groups are shown. On the right, groups of motor neurons are indicated by numbers. Both alpha and gamma fibers are shown emerging from the anterior horn. (From Carpenter MB. Core Text of Neuroanatomy, ed 3. Baltimore: Williams & Wilkins, 1985.)

ticipate in plexus formation, resulting in the formation of the brachial and lumbosacral plexuses. Nerves given off from these plexuses provide innervation for the muscles of the upper and lower extremities.

Not all cells in the anterior gray horn innervate striated muscle. Some, usually smaller than motor neurons, have processes confined to the spinal cord. These cells, referred to as internuncial neurons, have axons that project to other segments,

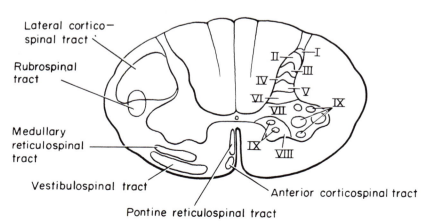

**Figure 1-2.** Drawing of a transverse section of the spinal cord at C-8 with the laminae of Rexed on the right and the position of the principal descending tracts indicated on the left.

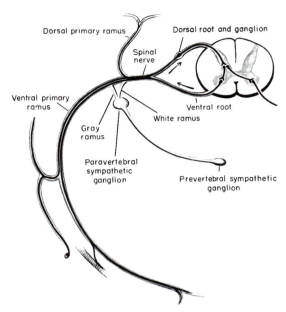

**Figure 1-3.** Schematic diagram of a thoracic spinal nerve showing peripheral branches and central connections. (From Noback CR, Demarest RJ. The Human Nervous System, ed 3. New York: McGraw-Hill, 1981.)

to the opposite side of the spinal cord, or to motor neurons. Cells whose axons emerge from the spinal cord are known as *root cells;* these cells subserve effector functions. Root cells of the anterior horn are of two types: (1) *alpha (α) motor neurons* give rise to large fibers that innervate striatal (extrafusal) muscle and (2) *gamma (γ) motor neurons* innervate muscle spindles (intrafusal; Figures 1-2 and 1-4). The spectrum of myelinated fibers in the ventral roots indicates two groups of fibers. Approximately 70% of the fibers are between 8 and 13 μm in diameter and are classified as alpha fibers; the remaining 30% of the fibers, 3 to 8 μm in diameter, are designated gamma fibers. In addition, the ventral roots in thoracic and upper lumbar spinal segments contain unmyelinated or poorly myelinated preganglionic sympathetic fibers. Sacral ventral roots (S-2, S-3, and S-4) contain similar poorly myelinated preganglionic parasympathetic fibers. These preganglionic fibers project to various autonomic ganglia.

Alpha motor neurons are cholinergic and terminate upon skeletal muscle fibers in small, flattened expansions known as *motor end-plates,* which constitute the so-called *myoneural junction.* Electrical stimulation of a motor nerve causes quanta of acetylcholine (ACh) to be liberated at the myoneural junction, which produces contractions of muscle fibers. Following the contractions, acetylcholinesterase (AChE) hydrolyzes the ACh. Stimulation of a muscle nerve with graded shocks results in twitches of the muscle related directly to the strength of the stimulus, until the alpha spike reaches its full potential. Increasing the size of the stimulus does not produce a stronger contraction, even though gamma fibers may be discharged. Thus, impulses conducted by alpha motor fibers are related to the contractile elements of striated muscle and gamma motor neurons do not contribute directly to muscle contraction. Gamma fibers are distributed to the polar (contractile) portions of the muscle spindles. Contraction of the polar portions of the muscle spindle may be sufficient to cause the discharge of muscle spindle afferent fibers (group IA), but these contractions do not directly alter muscle tension or length. Impulses conducted by group IA enter the spinal cord via the dorsal root and distribute collaterals directly on alpha motor neurons. This two neuron linkage (one sensory neuron in the dorsal root ganglion and one motor neuron in the ventral horn) establishes part of the so-called *gamma loop.* The loop is closed by gamma efferent fibers, which arise from cells in the anterior horn and pass directly to polar parts of the muscle spindle (see Figure 1-4). Thus, impulses conveyed by gamma motor neurons can indirectly excite alpha motor neurons by causing the muscle spindle to fire. Part of this mechanism forms the basis for the *myotatic (or stretch) reflex.* Only part of the afferents from the muscle spindle pass to the anterior horn; a large part of the afferent volley ascends via relays in the spinal cord to the cerebellum.

The *myotatic or deep tendon reflex* is a monosynaptic reflex dependent on two neurons: one neuron in the dorsal root ganglion that receives afferent impulses from the muscle spindle and the alpha motor neuron that innervates the striated muscle containing the muscle spindles. Sudden, abrupt stretching of a muscle produced by sharply tapping the tendon of the muscle, causes stretching of the muscle spindle and discharge of the group IA fibers. The IA fibers make synaptic contact with the alpha motor neurons in the anterior horn, and after a brief delay impulses pass peripherally via the ventral root back to the same muscle and cause it to contract (see Figure 1-4). The myotatic

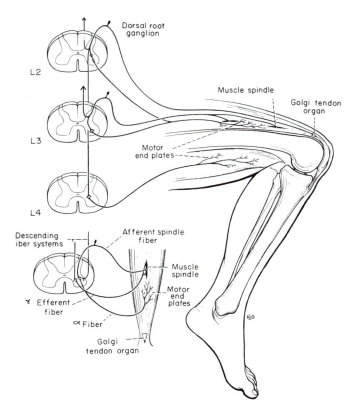

**Figure 1-4.** Schematic diagram of the sensory and motor elements involved in the patellar tendon reflex. Muscle spindle afferents are shown entering only the L-3 spinal segment; Golgi tendon organ afferents are shown entering only the L-2 segment. In this monosynaptic reflex afferent fibers enter L-2, L-3, and L-4 spinal segments and efferent fibers from the anterior horn cells at these same levels project to the extrafusal muscle fibers of the quadriceps femoris. Efferent fibers from L-4 projecting to the hamstrings represent part of the pathway involved in reciprocal inhibition. The small diagram on the left illustrates the gamma loop. Contractions of the polar parts of the muscle spindle initiate an afferent volley conducted centrally to alpha motor neurons. Discharge of the alpha motor neuron is conveyed to the motor end-plate of the same muscle. The gamma efferent fiber controls the sensitivity of the muscle spindle. (From Carpenter MB. Core Text of Neuroanatomy, ed 3. Baltimore: Williams & Wilkins, 1985.)

reflex is a segmental, monosynaptic reflex that usually involves two or three spinal segments, because most muscles are innervated by fibers arising from several adjacent spinal segments. The segment of a muscle innervated by afferent fibers from a single spinal segment constitutes a *myotome.* This unit is similar to a *dermatome,* the *cutaneous* area innervated by fibers that arise from a single dorsal root ganglion. Both myotomes and dermatomes have considerable overlap of innervation provided by nerve fibers arising from adjacent spinal segments.

Afferent fibers derived from dorsal root ganglia constitute one of the major sources of input to the lower motor neuron (Figure 1-5). Input via the dorsal root conveys impulses from a variety of different receptors, both superficial and deep. Impulses conveyed by group IB fibers from the Golgi tendon organ end upon internuncial neurons, rather than upon alpha motor neurons. Group IB fibers establish a disynaptic relationship with anterior horn cells (see Figure 1-4). Golgi tendon organs are stretch receptors, as the muscle spindles are,

but they exhibit a much higher threshold and unlike the muscle spindle have no known efferent innervation. These stretch receptors, unlike the muscle spindles, can be caused to discharge by either contracting or stretching the muscle. The Golgi tendon organ has been conceived as being "in series" with striated muscle fibers, whereas the muscle spindle appears to be arranged "in parallel."[3] Impulses conveyed by group IB fibers have a disynaptic inhibitory influence on alpha motor neurons; group IA fibers have a monosynaptic excitatory action on these neurons. The inhibitory influence of the Golgi tendon organ on spinal motor neurons is of clinical importance for understanding the melting away of resistance to passive movement in spasticity.

Impulses from receptors concerned with painful or noxious stimuli also enter the spinal cord via the dorsal root (see Figure 1-5). Many of these fibers, considered to have substance P as their neurotransmitter, terminate in Rexed's lamina I.[4,5] Even though opiate-binding sites are distributed in parts of laminae I and II and the central nervous

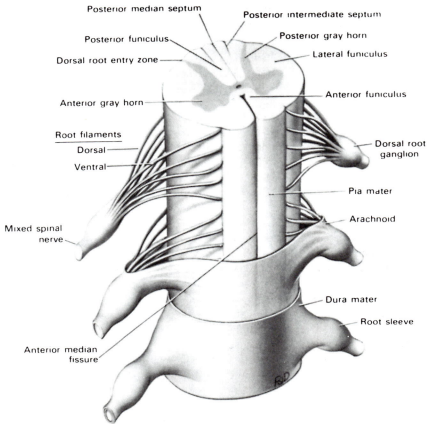

**Figure 1-5.** Drawing of a segment of the spinal cord shows nerve roots, ganglia, and meninges. (From Carpenter MB. Core Text of Neuroanatomy, ed 3. Baltimore: Williams & Wilkins, 1985.)

system contains endogenous opiods such as enkephalin,[6] some afferents from these receptors reach the lower motor neuron. Noxious and painful stimuli produce powerful contractions of flexor muscle groups, which effect withdrawal from the offending stimulus. The *flexion reflex* produces powerful contractions of ipsilateral flexor muscles and relaxation of ipsilateral extensor muscles in a reciprocal fashion, so that an entire limb may be withdrawn. Afferent input in the flexor reflex arises from broad receptive fields, is conveyed by small fibers (secondary muscle spindle and cutaneous afferents), and involves multisynaptic articulations with both flexor and extensor motor neurons. This reflex is characterized by longer synaptic delays and diffuseness of efferent discharge. There is sustained firing of motor units,

which may outlast the stimulus. Noxious stimuli applied to a peripheral part of a limb result in powerful flexor responses in all parts of the extremity.

The *crossed extensor reflex* is regarded as part of the flexor reflex.[7] Collateral fibers involved in the flexor reflex cross in the spinal cord and establish reciprocal connections opposite to those that prevail ipsilaterally. Contralateral excitation involves extensor muscles; inhibition prevails upon flexor motor neurons. In the case of the lower extremity, the crossed extensor response serves to support the body when the ipsilateral lower limb is flexed. Segmental input to the lower motor neuron is profuse, direct and indirect, and largely, but not exclusively, ipsilateral. Muscle spindle afferents (group IA) project directly to the lower motor neuron, whereas most other receptors, including the Golgi tendon organ (group IB), influence lower motor neurons indirectly via internuncial neurons. Group IA and IB fibers influence ipsilateral cell groups of the spinal cord, whereas other sensory receptors are distributed by multisynaptic circuits to both sides of the spinal cord. The lower motor neuron also is under powerful suprasegmental control via descending systems. These systems are discussed in conjunction with upper motor neuron.

## Lesions of the Lower Motor Neuron

Lesions selectively involving the lower motor neuron result in weakness or paralysis, loss of muscle tone, loss of reflexes, and muscle atrophy. All of these changes are confined to the affected muscles. Weakness or paralysis, occurring in the affected muscles, has a direct relationship to the extent and severity of the lesion. Because anterior horn cells that innervate a single muscle extend longitudinally through several spine segments, and because several such cell columns exist at each level, a lesion confined to one spinal segment causes some weakness, but not complete paralysis, in the several muscles that it innervates. Complete paralysis of a muscle occurs only when the lesions involve the column of cells in several segments that innervate a particular muscle, or ventral root fibers from these cells. Because most appendicular muscles are innervated by fibers arising from three spinal segments, complete paralysis of a muscle resulting from a spinal lesion in the anterior horn indicates involvement of several segments. Neighboring cell columns are likely to be involved at each level, resulting in paralysis of a group of muscles rather than an individual one.

Because the lower motor neuron consists of the anterior horn cells and their axons, which emerge via the ventral root, it is sometimes necessary to distinguish motor deficits that occur as a consequence of lesions in spinal segments from those that involve the ventral root, spinal nerves, and peripheral nerves (see Figures 1-3 and 1-5). Lesions of the ventral root usually produce the same motor deficits as destruction of the corresponding anterior horn cells. These two types of lesions are not the same in certain spinal regions (thoracolumbar and sacral), because in these regions preganglionic autonomic fibers arise from cell groups in the lateral horn but exit via the ventral root. Thus, a lesion involving the ventral root at T-1 produces Horner's syndrome (miosis, pseudoptosis, apparent enopthalmos, and dryness of the skin over the face) in addition to some weakness in the small muscles of the hand. These autonomic disturbances might not occur with a spinal lesion confined to the anterior horn at T-1. Section of a single ventral root, for example C-5, would produce weakness in the supraspinatus, infraspinatus, subscapularis, biceps brachii, and brachioradialis muscles, but not complete paralysis of any of these muscles. This pattern of distribution is unique to C-5 ventral root fibers and different from that of any single peripheral nerve.

Lesions of mixed spinal nerves produce motor and sensory deficits that correspond to those of combined dorsal and ventral root lesions (see Figure 1-3). The motor deficits correspond almost exactly to those resulting from lesions of the ventral root, but the sensory disturbances follow a dermatomal distribution and tend to be less extensive because of the characteristic overlapping nature of dermatomes. A lesion involving a single dorsal root such as C-5 would not result in detectable sensory loss, because dorsal root fibers from C-4 and C-6 "cover" most of the C-5 area.[8,9]

These observations are in sharp contrast with the motor and sensory deficits resulting from a peripheral nerve lesion (Figure 1-3), deficits that correspond to the peripheral distribution of the particular nerve distal to the injury. An ulnar nerve injury near the wrist would produce paralysis of the adductor pollicis, the deep head of the flexor pollicis brevis, the interossei, the inner lumbrical muscles, and the muscles of the hypothenar eminence, along with loss of sensation in all of the little finger, the ulnar half of the ring finger, and corresponding portions of the dorsal and volar surfaces of the hand.

Loss of muscle tone, *hypotonia,* is a characteristic and constant finding in lower motor neuron lesions. The muscle is flaccid, soft and offers no resistance to passive movement. The reduction in muscle tone results from the withdrawal of streams of efferent impulses that are normally transmitted to the muscle which maintain its tone. The gamma loop, which helps to maintain tone, has been broken. Reflexes in the affected muscles are greatly diminished, and usually lost (*areflexia*), in lower motor neuron lesions because the reflex arc is interrupted. In this type of lesion the effector limb of the reflex arc has been destroyed.

Although paralysis, hypotonia, and areflexia occur almost immediately following a lower motor neuron lesion, *atrophy,* or muscle wasting, does not become evident for a week or two. Atrophy occurs gradually and in time is obvious on inspection. Why muscles undergo atrophy is not fully understood, but it seems likely that the morphological and functional properties of muscle are dependent on the transmitter substance (ACh) liberated at the motor end-plates. Some degree of muscle wasting occurs when muscles are not used (*disuse atrophy*). This type of muscle atrophy is seen in limbs immobolized for a time in a plaster cast, in muscles whose tendons have been cut, and in upper motor neuron paralysis of long duration.

In some diseases involving the lower motor neuron the muscles supplied by these neurons exhibit small, localized, spontaneous contractions known as *fasciculations*. These small muscle twitches, visible beneath the skin, represent the discharge of groups of muscle fibers. Fasciculations occur asynchronously in parts of different muscles and are thought to be due to triggering mechanisms within the motor neuron. It is possible that these small contractions may be due to "leakage" of small quanta of acetylcholine at the motor end-plates of a diseased neuron. Fasciculations commonly are seen in amyotrophic lateral sclerosis and sometimes in acute inflammatory lesions of peripheral nerves, but usually they are not seen when anterior horn cells are rapidly destroyed, as in poliomyelitis. The term *fibrillation,* misused as the equivalent of fasciculation, refers to the small (10 to 200-$\mu$V) potentials of 1 to 2 msec duration that occur irregularly and asynchronously in electromyograms of denervated muscle. These potentials represent spontaneous activation of single muscle fibers and produce no detectable shortening of muscles.

From this discussion it is apparent that the lower motor neuron exerts important trophic, metabolic, chemical, and electrical influences on striated muscle. One of the most striking effects of muscle denervation is the supersensitivity that develops to acetylcholine (ACh).

## The Upper Motor Neuron

All of the descending fibers systems that can influence or modify activities of the lower motor neuron constitute the upper motor neuron. This is a more inclusive definition than that used by most clinicians who equate the upper motor neuron solely with the corticospinal tract. The narrower concept has developed because the corticospinal tract is so large and the functional roles of other descending systems have not been clearly defined. Increasing information on non-pyramidal systems makes it necessary to consider the upper motor neuron in the broadest sense. Descending influences transmitted to spinal levels by a group of heterogeneous spinal tracts are concerned mainly with (1) voluntary motor control, (2) modification of muscle tone, (3) maintenance of posture and equilibrium, (4) suprasegmental control of reflexes, (5) innervation of viscera and autonomic structures, and (6) modification of sensory signals transmitted centrally. With one exception, all descending spinal tracts arise from the three most caudal segments of the brain stem. The exception is the corticospinal tract.

### Corticospinal System

The corticospinal system consists of all fibers that originate from cells in the cerebral cortex, pass through the medullary pyramids, and enter the spinal cord (Figure 1-6). This massive fiber system constitutes the largest and most important descending system in the neuraxis. Each medullary pyramid in humans contains approximately 1 million fibers, which project to spinal levels via three separate tracts. The largest number of fibers, approximately 90%, cross in the corticospinal decussation and descend contralaterally as the *lateral corticospinal tract*. A smaller bundle of fibers (8%) descends directly into the anterior funiculus, where it forms the *anterior corticospinal tract*. These fibers cross in small fascicles within cervical spinal segments (see Figure 1-2). Remaining fibers in the

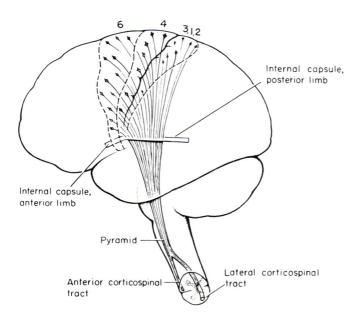

**Figure 1-6.** Schematic drawing of the lateral surface of the brain, indicating the origin and course of the corticospinal tract.

medullary pyramids descend uncrossed into the lateral funiculus of the spinal cord as the *antero-lateral corticospinal tract*. Fibers of the corticospinal tract originate from pyramidal cells in layer V of the primary motor area (area 4), the premotor area (area 6), and from somatosensory regions of the parietal lobe.[10,11] Pyramidal cells contributing to the tract show great variation in size and occur in clusters; the largest cells, found in area 4, are referred to as the *giantopyramidal cells of Betz*. Giant pyramidal cells in the human brain are not distributed uniformly; the largest number is found superiorly in the leg area and the smallest number inferiorly in the face area. Though the primary motor cortex appears somatotopically organized in that electrical stimulation of specific regions gives rise to localized movements on the opposite side of the body, anatomically this tract is not somatotopically organized. Movements elicited by electrical stimulation of the motor cortex in patients under local anesthesia, interpreted as ''voluntary'' movements, usually involve groups of muscles. Fibers of the corticospinal tract largely descend in the dorsal part of the lateral funiculus and enter the spinal gray matter in the intermediate zone (lamina VII), from which site they are distributed to laminae IV, V, VII and parts of lamina IX (see Figure 1-2).[12,13] Fibers projecting directly to lamina IX, which contains large motor neurons, ap-

pear greatest in the cord enlargements and are most abundant in dorsolateral regions, which innervate distal musculature. Corticospinal fibers projecting to laminae in the dorsal horn arise predominantly from sensory cortical areas.[14]

A recent finding of much importance concerning the CST is that virtually all corticospinal neurons have multiple collateral branches that terminate at several levels of the spinal cord.[15,16] This observation explains why tracers injected at one spinal level retrogradely label cortical neurons scattered over a wide area. It also explains why a microlesion in one region of the motor cortex produces degeneration distributed over as many as nine spinal segments. These data clearly indicate that the CST is not somatotopically organized and the tract does not consist of private lines from cortical neurons to spinal motor neurons. Cortical motor neurons exert multiple influences on different groups of motor neurons in widely separate spinal segments via axonal collaterals.

Phylogenetically, the corticospinal tract is a relatively recent development in the central nervous system that is found only in mammals. In humans at birth the tract is immature and unmyelinated. It takes approximately 2 years for the tract to become fully developed and myelinated. It is during this period of postnatal development that the infant learns to stand and walk and acquires fine motor skills.[17] Signals conveyed by the CST are thought to be concerned with discrete movements of parts of the body that display an almost unlimited range and versatility. The tract has the largest number of fibers concerned with motor function, extends the length of the neuraxis, and passes through or near every major division of the central nervous system except the cerebellum. It is for these reasons that the corticospinal tract is frequently involved by a variety of pathologic processes. Lesions involving the corticospinal tract almost invariably involve adjacent structures and produce varying degrees of paralysis, alterations of muscle tone, and modifications of reflexes. Involvement of adjacent structures often helps to localize the site of a lesion involving this long pathway.

In comparison to the corticospinal system the nonpyramidal descending tracts are small. These tracts arise from nuclei in the midbrain (red nucleus), pons, and medulla (vestibular nuclei and reticular formation).

### Rubrospinal Tract

This tract arises from an oval collection of neurons that occupies the central part of the midbrain tegmentum (Figure 1-7). Large cells in caudal parts of the nucleus give rise to fibers that cross the midline immediately and descend to spinal levels in the lateral funiculus. These fibers are partially intermingled with those of the corticospinal fibers (Figure 1-2). The rubrospinal tract has been considered to be somatotopically organized in the sense that cells in dorsal parts of the nucleus project to cervical spinal segments whereas those in ventral regions terminate in lumbosacral segments.[18] Fibers of the tract enter the intermediate zone of the spinal gray and are distributed within Rexed's laminae IV, V, VI, and VII.[19,20] Terminations are on internuncial neurons. The somatotopic features of this tract have been somewhat blurred by the observation that some cells in the red nucleus have axonal collaterals projecting to several spinal segments.[20]

The red nucleus receives input from two sources, the cerebral cortex and some of the deep cerebellar nuclei. Corticorubral fibers from the motor cortex descend ipsilaterally and are somatotopically organized.[21] Thus, corticorubral and rub-

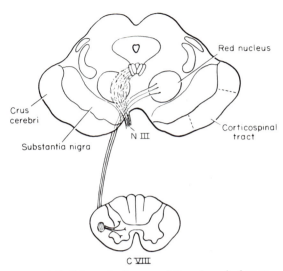

**Figure 1-7.** Schematic diagram of the rubrospinal tract.

rospinal fibers together constitute a somatotopically organized nonpyramidal linkage from the motor cortex to spinal levels that exert effects contralaterally, because the rubrospinal tract is crossed. A second input to the red nucleus arises from the emboliform and globose nuclei of the cerebellum; these fibers are crossed and link portions of the opposite cerebellar cortex (i.e., paravermal) with the red nucleus.[22] Cerebellar influences on cells of the red nucleus are expressed ipsilaterally because cerebellar efferent fibers and rubrospinal fibers are both crossed.

The most important function of the rubrospinal tract is maintaining muscle tone, particularly contralateral flexor muscle tone. Stimulation of the red nucleus produces flexion in the contralateral limbs.[23,24] Microelectrode studies indicate excitatory postsynaptic potential in contralateral flexor alpha motor neurons and inhibitory postsynaptic potentials in extensor alpha motor neurons.[25] Both of these effects on contralateral alpha motor neurons are mediated by internuncial neurons, as fibers of the rubrospinal tract do not terminate directly on motor neurons.

### Vestibulospinal Tract

The vestibular nuclei constitute a complex in the lateral part of the floor of the fourth ventricle of

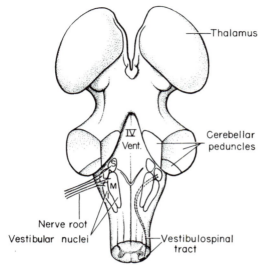

**Figure 1-8.** Schematic drawing of the brain stem and cervical spinal cord showing the locations of the vestibular nuclei in the floor of the fourth ventricle and the course of the vestibulospinal tract. S, L, M, and I indicate the superior, lateral, medial, and inferior vestibular nuclei, respectively.

the pons and medulla (Figure 1-8). The four major nuclei of this complex receive afferents from the vestibular apparatus (semicircular ducts and the otoliths) concerned with maintenance of equilibrium, posture, and orientation in three-dimensional space. In addition, parts of these nuclei receive input from portions of the cerebellar cortex and the most medial deep cerebellar nucleus (fastigial nucleus). The vestibulospinal tract arises mainly from the giant cells of the lateral vestibular nucleus and descends in the ventral part of the lateral funiculus of the spinal cord (see Figures 1-2 and 1-8). This tract has been regarded as somatotopically organized and is present in all spinal segments.[26] Fibers of the tract enter the medial part of the anterior horn and are distributed to Rexed's laminae VII, VIII, and parts of IX.[27–29] The somatotopic features of the vestibulospinal tract now appear less precise than as originally conceived, because some fibers appear to originate from other vestibular nuclei, and axons descending in the spinal cord give collaterals to multiple spinal segments.[29–31] There is evidence that vestibulospinal fibers terminate directly upon the somata and dendrites of large extensor motor neurons and have a threefold to fourfold greater influence on cervical and lumbosacral spinal segments. Impulses conveyed by the VST produce increases in ipsilateral extensor muscle tone.

Vestibular ganglion cells, which innervate the macula of the utricle, appear to project exclusively to the ventral part of the lateral vestibular nucleus.[32] This suggests that stimuli that excite the utricle, such as head tilt, gravity, and linear acceleration, must play an important role in maintaining extensor muscle tone. Direct input to dorsal regions of the lateral vestibular nucleus is derived from Purkinje cells in the anterior lobe vermis of the cerebellum.[33] This pathway exerts inhibitory influences on cells of the lateral vestibular nucleus mediated by the neurotransmitter γ-aminobutyric acid.[34] The fastigial nucleus of the cerebellum projects crossed and uncrossed fibers fairly symmetrically to ventral parts of both lateral vestibular nuclei and appears to have excitatory influences mediated by glutamic acid.[35,36] Thus, the excitatory influences of the vestibular end-organ can be modulated directly by cerebellar inputs. Lesions of the anterior lobe of the cerebellum in experimental animals produce increases in extensor muscle tone that resembles decerebrate rigidity.

### Reticulospinal Tracts

Anatomically, the term *reticular formation* is used to designate the core of the brain stem characterized by aggregations of cells of various sizes enmeshed in a fiber network. The matrix that forms the reticular formation is phylogenetically the oldest part of the brain stem and is surrounded by newer pathways concerned with specific functions. Development of the reticular formation parallels the process of encephalization. For many years the organization of the reticular formation was considered to be diffuse and nonspecific. In the late 1950s it became apparent that the reticular formation could be divided into regions that possessed a specific cytoarchitecture, distinctive fiber connections, and unique internal features.[37,38] The reticular formation can be regarded as the principal integrator of motor, sensory, and visceral activities in the brain stem. Basically, the reticular formation can be divided into four main subdivisions: (1) a lateral sensory part, (2) a medial effector or motor part, (3) a paramedian part related largely to the cerebellum, and (4) the raphe nuclei, which contain a variety of different neurotransmitters.

Spinal projections arise from the medial zone of the pontine and medullary reticular formation. *Medullary reticulospinal fibers* arise from a large collection of cells in the medial two thirds of the reticular formation, dorsal to the inferior olivary complex, and project largely uncrossed to all levels of the spinal cord (Figure 1-9). Fibers from this tract descend in the anterior part of the lateral funiculus and terminate largely on internuncial neurons in lamina VII, although some end upon processes of cells in lamina IX (see Figure 1-2). *Pontine reticulospinal fibers* arise from a corresponding larger medial regions of the pontine reticular formation. Virtually all fibers of the pontine reticulospinal tracts are uncrossed, descend in the ventral funiculus near the midline, and end on internuncial neurons in laminae VII and VIII (see

Figures 1-2 and 1-9). Unlike some fibers of the rubrospinal and vestibulospinal tracts, none of the reticulospinal fibers are somatotopically organized.

One of the characteristic features of the reticular formation is that it receives signals from multiple sources, which include virtually all types of receptors, the cerebellum, and the cerebral cortex. Sensory input to the reticular formation loses its identification with specific stimuli. Functions of the reticular formation are multiple, but some can be related to specific subdivisions. The reticular formation can (1) facilitate or inhibit voluntary motor activity, (2) modify muscle tone and reflex activity, (3) exert a variety of different autonomic responses, and (4) facilitate or inhibit central transmission of sensory signals. Major inhibitory functions appear to be related to the medullary reticular formation. Inhibition concerns most forms of motor activity, including myotatic and flexor reflexes and muscle tone. Reductions in muscle tone and deep tendon reflexes appear to be mediated by

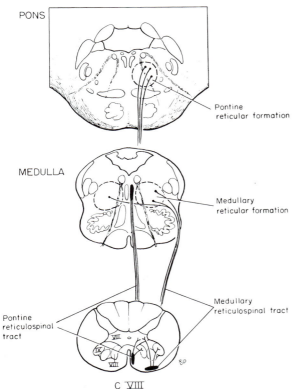

**Figure 1-9.** Schematic diagram of sections of the lower brain stem indicating the origin, course, and regions of termination of the reticulospinal tracts.

medullary reticulospinal fibers that inhibit gamma motor neurons, which influence the muscle spindle and alpha motor neurons via the gamma loop.

A far larger region of the brain stem reticular formation facilitates motor responses, muscle tone, and somatic spinal reflexes. The facilitatory region includes most of the pontine reticular formation and extends into the caudal midbrain. The facilitatory region of the reticular formation includes neurons that do not project directly to spinal cord; thus, effects from these regions must involve polysynaptic pathways. Most of the effects from the facilitatory region appear to involve internuncial neurons at various spinal levels. Not all of the influences of the reticular formation are directed toward modification of spinal neuronal activities. Large regions of both the medullary and pontine reticular formation exert powerful ascending influences that control the electrical excitability of broad regions of the cerebral cortex and affect the state of alertness and behavioral arousal.

### Descending Autonomic Pathways

It has been difficult to distinguish reticular neurons concerned exclusively with autonomic functions, but modern axoplasmic transport methods and immunocytochemical techniques have yielded important information. The principal nuclei giving rise to descending autonomic fibers are (1) several regions of the hypothalamus, (2) portions of the parasympathetic nuclei of the oculomotor nuclear complex, (3) the locus ceruleus, (4) parts of the nucleus solitarius, and (5) collections of catecholamine neurons in the ventrolateral lower brain stem. In addition, the raphe nuclei, which contain cells rich in serotonin, project bilaterally to spinal levels and modulate pain mechanisms.[39] Large cells in the paraventricular and posterior regions of the hypothalamus project directly to spinal levels, where some of these fibers end on autonomic neurons.[40] Some parasympathetic neurons in the oculomotor nucleus project to spinal levels and end in parts of laminae I and V.[40,41] The locus ceruleus, recognized as a principal source of noradrenergic fibers widely distributed in the neuraxis, projects to parts of the anterior and posterior horns and the intermediolateral cell column, which gives rise to preganglionic sympathetic fibers.[42]

Descending fibers from the nucleus solitarius project fibers to neurons of the phrenic nerve nucleus and to anterior horn cells in the thoracic region; these crossed projections are concerned with excitation of inspiratory motor neurons.[43] Ventrolateral noradrenergic neurons located near the facial nucleus project bilaterally to the intermediolateral cell column in thoracic and upper lumbar spinal segments.[44] Very few lesions in the brain stem and spinal cord fail to involve the descending autonomic fiber system.

### Upper Motor Neuron Lesions

Lesions involving the upper motor neuron at a variety of locations produce paralysis, alterations of muscle tone, and changes in reflex activity. These lesions are rarely selective, are usually incomplete, and frequently involve adjacent structures. The degree of paresis or paralysis is not always directly related to the size of the lesions or the extent of involvement of the corticospinal tract.[45] Lesions of the upper motor neuron may result from vascular disease, trauma, neoplasms, or infectious and degenerative disease. Unilateral lesions in the cerebral hemisphere or brain stem produce contralateral paralysis, usually hemiplegia. Spinal lesions, most commonly the result of trauma, usually are bilateral and cause paraplegia.

The most common lesion involving the upper motor neuron is the so-called *cerebrovascular accident*. Thrombosis of a major cerebral artery, commonly the middle cerebral artery or the main trunk of the internal carotid artery, deprives regions of the brain of blood and oxygen, causing necrosis. Tissues surrounding the infarcted area become congested and edematous. In the majority of patients the onset is sudden. Initial symptoms are both focal and general. Generalized symptoms include headache, nausea, vomiting, convulsions, and coma. Focal symptoms, such as paralysis, sensory loss, and disturbances of speech, usually are related to the site of the lesion. Immediately after the vascular lesion, usually called a *stroke,* the paralyzed limbs are completely flaccid and the myotatic reflexes are depressed or absent. The plantar response, elicited by stroking the sole of the foot, shows extension of the great toe and fanning of the other toes (i.e., the *Babinski re-*

*sponse).* Although the Babinski response is of great clinical importance, the physiologic mechanism is not understood.

After a variable period of time, muscle tone gradually returns to the affected limb and ultimately exceeds that of the normal side. This exaggeration of muscle tone is not seen in all muscles. The increase in muscle tone develops in the antigravity muscles. In the upper extremity tone is increased in the adductors and internal rotators of the shoulder, in the flexors and pronators of the forearm, and in the flexors of the wrist and digits. In the lower extremity it is seen in the adductors of the hip, the extensors of the hip and knee, and in the plantar flexors. This increase in antigravity muscle tone is referred to as *spasticity.* Spasticity is characterized by (1) increased resistance to passive movement, (2) hyperactive deep tendon reflexes (low threshold, large amplitude and a forceful brisk nature), and (3) the presence of clonus. *Clonus* represents an extreme exaggeration of the myotatic reflex in which a stretch of the muscle initiates a self-perpetuating stretch reflex in an antagonistic muscle group. Paralysis tends to become less severe with time. Paralysis that initially involved both upper and lower extremities equally may now appear less severe in one limb. Some voluntary motor function begins to return. The motor functions most affected are those associated with fine, skilled movements. Gross movements that involve the whole limb often show considerable restitution. Many hemiplegics show appreciable recovery of motor function and become ambulatory. The hemiplegic gait is characteristic: the partially paralyzed leg is circumducted en bloc at the hip and swung forward because of difficulty flexing the knee. The foot is in plantar flexion, and the toe of the shoe is dragged in a circular fashion. The arm on the affected side is flexed at the elbow and wrist, the forearm is pronated, and the digits are flexed.

Upper motor neuron syndromes due to lesions of the brain stem are much less common than those involving deep structures of the cerebral hemisphere. Motor disturbances resulting from relatively small lesions are similar, except that cranial nerves and ascending sensory pathways are commonly involved. Large lesions of the brain stem usually are not compatible with survival and often are associated with protracted coma.

Spinal cord transection immediately produces, below the level of the lesion (1) loss of all motor function, (2) loss of all somatic sensation, (3) loss of visceral sensation, (4) loss of muscle tone, and (5) loss of all reflex activity. Initially there is no evidence of neural activity in the isolated spinal cord caudal to the lesion (i.e., spinal shock). *Spinal shock* occurs in all animals following transection of the spinal cord and is considered to be due to the sudden, abrupt interruption of all descending excitatory influences. The duration of spinal shock varies in different animals; in humans it averages about 3 weeks. The termination of the period of spinal shock is heralded by the appearance of the Babinski sign. A fairly orderly sequence of recovery of function follows, with some variations. The phases of recovery of some functions in the isolated portion of the spinal cord have been carefully documented.[46] Recovery phases and their approximate duration are as follows: (1) period of minimal reflex activity (3 to 6 weeks), (2) period of flexor muscle spasms (6 to 16 weeks), (3) period of alternate flexor and extensor spasms (after 4 months), and (4) period of extensor muscle spasms (after 6 months). The period of minimal reflex activity is characterized by weak flexor responses to nociceptive stimuli, noted first in distal muscle groups, flaccid muscles, absence of deep tendon reflexes, and the Babinski sign. The phase of flexor muscle spasms is associated with increasing tone in the flexor muscles and stronger responses to painful stimuli. It is during this phase that the *triple flexion response* is seen, which involves simultaneous flexion at the hip, knee, and ankle in response to a mild nociceptive stimulus. The most exaggerated form of this reflex is the *mass reflex* provoked by trivial stimuli and resulting in bilateral powerful triple flexion responses. In the mass reflex, afferent impulses spread bilaterally over many spinal cord segments and cause repeated discharge of flexor motor units. This powerful reflex is distressing to the patient, who is unable to prevent it. The mass reflex tends to diminish as extensor muscle tone begins to increase. Extensor muscle tone ultimately predominates, and some patients can momentarily support their weight in a standing position.[46] Examination of the patient 1 year after spinal cord transection reveals no change with respect to voluntary motor function or sensory perception. There is marked extensor muscle tone below the level of the lesion, hyperactive deep tendon reflexes, clonus, and bilateral Babinski's signs. Loss of bowel and bladder control present a continuing major problem.

## Analysis of the Upper Motor Neuron

It has been presumed for some time that the upper motor neuron syndrome was due solely to interruption of fibers of the corticospinal tract in their trajectory through the neuraxis. This concept was based on the thesis that this system directly and indirectly conveyed excitatory input to lower motor neurons and was responsible for voluntary movement. This thesis considered the intact corticospinal system to be associated with voluntary skilled movement and the damaged system to be associated with paralysis, or paresis, and residual spasticity expressed as exaggerated muscle tone in the antigravity muscles. It is difficult to understand how a lesion in this system could produce both paresis and spasticity. The assumption has been that lesions of the corticospinal tract in some way removed inhibitory influences, which resulted in the spasticity. Lesions of the corticospinal system almost invariably involve other neural structures or pathways. The only pure corticospinal lesion is one that destroys the medullary pyramid in the medulla, which is very rare. Experimental lesions of the medullary pyramids of monkeys and chimpanzees produce a condition best characterized as hypotonic paresis.[47–49] There is no complete paralysis, in the sense that no part of the body is rendered useless, but there is grave and general poverty of movement. In long-term experiments, a wide range of gross movements show some recovery, but voluntary movement was stripped of the qualities that endow it with precision and versatility. There is persistent slowness of movement, loss of individual finger movement, and the ability to fractionate movements. In chimpanzees paresis is more prominent than hypotonia, the deep tendon reflexes are brisk and of large amplitude, and the Babinski sign is evident. If some fibers of the corticospinal tract are preserved, return of motor function, dexterity, and discrete finger movements are more pronounced than with a total lesion. These studies suggest that residual motor functions

evident following bilateral section of the medullary pyramids must be the expression of activity in subcorticospinal systems that arise from brain stem nuclei. These subcorticospinal systems collectively are capable of initiating and guiding a limited range of motor activities. Thus, nonpyramidal descending systems make important contributions to total motor function, which in normal persons appear to form a basic mechanism upon which the corticospinal system is superimposed. Studies of the nonpyramidal descending systems suggest they are especially concerned with maintenance of erect posture, integration of body and limb movements, and with directing progression movements.[50]

Though these basic studies provide some insights into the contributions made by various components of the upper motor neuron, they provide little information concerning the mechanism of spasticity. Spasticity is not associated with relatively pure lesions of the corticospinal system or with lesions of the individual descending systems from the brain stem. Although spasticity is a regularly occurring phenomenon with most upper motor neuron lesions, its nature has eluded the most meticulous analysis. The possibility is raised that spasticity might be due to involvement of a system not considered in this analysis. Some evidence supports this suggestion, but it offers only a partial solution.

Humans and monkeys have an additional motor representation on the medial aspect of the hemisphere, known as the *supplementary motor area* (Figure 1-10).[51–54] This motor area (referred to as MII) is somatotopically organized in a sequential fashion, somewhat similar to the primary motor area (MI). Focal stimulation of MI produces localized movements contralaterally, whereas stronger and more prolonged stimulation of MII elicits complex synergistic patterned movements bilaterally. MII has been considered to be involved in (1) control of posture, (2) somatosensory integration passed on to MI, and (3) programming of motor activities.[54] Only a small percentage of MII neurons can be activated by input from peripheral receptors, though about 80% of MI neurons are activated by such stimuli. One of the major sources of input to MII is derived from the ventral lateral nucleus of the thalamus, which receives afferents from the basal ganglia.[55] Although MII has exten-

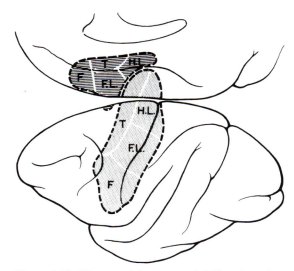

**Figure 1-10.** Diagram of the precentral (MI) and supplementary (MII) motor areas in the monkey. MI on the lateral convexity of the hemisphere (*stippled*) includes the region hidden in the depths of the central sulcus (represented posterior to the central sulcus). MII is on the medial surface of the hemisphere (shown above as a lined area). Abbreviations indicate the somatotopic features: F, face and head; T, trunk; FL, forelimb; HL, hindlimb. (From Carpenter MB. Core Text of Neuroanatomy, ed 3. Baltimore: Williams & Wilkins, 1985.)

sive connections with MI and with multiple subcortical structures, it is now clear that a small number of fibers (5%) project directly to spinal levels, probably via the corticospinal tract.[11,54,56]

Lesion studies of MII in primates have focused attention on its possible role in the control of muscle tone. Bilateral ablation of MII has been reported to produce disturbances of posture and muscle tone without paresis.[57] Gradually developing hypertonus in flexor muscle groups ultimately re-

sulted in contractures. This observation has been questioned,[58] but there is good agreement that lesions of the MI and MII in the same hemisphere result in contralateral spastic hemiparesis.[57,59] Lesions of MI alone produce flaccid contralateral hemiparesis. Though the role of the supplementary motor area remains unclear, there is evidence that its projections probably play some role in alterations of muscle tone and in programming skilled learned movements.

## References

1. Rexed B. The cytoarchitectonic organization of the spinal cord in the cat. J Comp Neurol 1952; 96:415–495.
2. Rexed B. A cytoarchitectonic atlas of the spinal cord in the cat. J Comp Neurol 1954; 100:297–379.
3. Fulton JF, Pi-Suñer J. A note concerning the probable function of various end-organs in skeletal muscle. Am J Physiol 1928; 83:554–562.
4. Hökfelt T, Kellerth J-O, Nilsson G, et al. Experimental immunohistochemical studies on the localization and distribution of substance P in cat primary sensory neurons. Brain Res 1975; 100:235–252.
5. Jessell TM, Iversen LL. Opiate analgesics inhibit substance P release from rat trigeminal nucleus. Nature 1977; 268:549–551.
6. LaMotte CC, Pert CB, Snyder SH. Opiate receptor binding in primate spinal cord: Distribution and changes after dorsal root section. Brain Res 1976; 112:407–412.
7. Patton HD. Reflex regulation of movement and posture. In: Ruch TC, Patton HD, eds. *Physiology and Biophysics,* ed 19. Philadelphia: WB Saunders, 1965; 181–206.
8. Mott FW, Sherington CS. Experiments upon the influence of sensory nerves upon movement and nutrition of the limbs. Proc R Soc Lond 1895; 57:481–488.
9. Haymaker W. Bing's Local Diagnosis in Neurological Diseases. St. Louis: CV Mosby, 1956; 57–62, 105–112.
10. Coulter JD, Ewing L, Carter C. Origin of primary sensorimotor cortical projections to lumbar spinal cord of cat and monkey. Brain Res 1976; 103:366–372.
11. Jones EG, Wise SP. Size, laminar and columnar distribution of efferent cells in the sensory-motor cortex of monkeys. J Comp Neurol 1977; 175:391–438.

This work was supported by research grants CO7005 from the Department of Defense, Uniformed Services University of the Health Sciences, and NS-26658 from the National Institutes of Health, Bethesda, Maryland. The opinions and assertions contained herein are the private ones of the author and are not to be construed as official or reflecting the views of the Department of Defense or the Uniformed Services University of the Health Sciences. Experiments reported herein were conducted according to the principles set forth in the "Guide for the Care and Use of Laboratory Animals," Institute of Laboratory Animal Resources, National Research Council, NIH Pub. No. 80-23.

12. Liu CN, Chambers WW. An experimental study of the corticospinal system in the monkey (*Macaca mulatta*). The spinal pathways and preterminal distribution of degenerated fibers following discrete lesions of the pre- and postcentral gyri and the bulbar pyramid. J Comp Neurol 1964; 123:257–283.

13. Kuypers HGJM, Brinkman J. Precentral projections to different parts of the spinal cord intermediate zone in the rhesus monkey. Brain Res 1970; 24:29–48.

14. Coulter JD, Jones EG. Differential distribution of corticospinal projections from individual cytoarchitectonic fields in the monkey. Brain Res 1977; 129:335–340.

15. Shinoda Y, Zarzecki P, Asanuma H. Spinal branching of pyramidal tract neurons in the monkey. Exp Brain Res 1979; 34:59–72.

16. Shinoda Y, Yamaguchi T, Futami T. Multiple axon collaterals of single corticospinal axons in the cat spinal cord. J Neurophysiol 1986; 55:425–448.

17. Porter R. Corticomotoneuronal projections: Synaptic events related to skilled movement. Proc R Soc Lond 1987; B231:147–168.

18. Pompeiano O, Brodal A. Experimental demonstration of a somatotopical origin of rubrospinal fibers in the cat. J Comp Neurol 1957; 108:225–251.

19. Nyberg-Hansen R, Brodal A. Sites and mode of termination of rubrospinal fibres in the cat. An experimental study with silver impregnation methods. J Anat 1964; 98:235–253.

20. Shinoda Y, Ghez C, Arnold A. Spinal branching of rubrospinal axons in the cat. Exp Brain Res. 1977; 30:203–218.

21. Hartmann-von Monakow K, Akert K, Kunzle H. Projections of precentral and premotor cortex to the red nucleus and other midbrain areas in *Macaca fascicularis*. Exp Brain Res 1979; 34:91–105.

22. Courville J. Somatotopical organization of the projection from the nucleus interpositus anterior of the cerebellum to the red nucleus. An experimental study in the cat with silver impregnation methods. Exp Brain Res. 1966; 2:191–215.

23. Pompeiano O. Sulle riposte posturali alla stimolazione elettrica del nucleo rosso nel gatto decerebrato. Boll Soc Ital Biol Sper 1956; 32:1450–1451.

24. Pompeiano O. Analisi degli effetti della stimolazione elettrica del nucleo rosso nel gatto decerebrato. Rend Accad Naz Lincei Rend Cl Sci Fis Mat Nat 1957; 22:100–103.

25. Massion J. The mammalian red nucleus. Physiol Rev 1967; 47:383–436.

26. Pompeiano O, Brodal A. The origin of vestibulospinal fibres in the cat. An experimental anatomical study, with comments on the descending medial longitudinal fasciculus. Arch Ital Biol 1957; 95:166–195.

27. Nyberg-Hansen R, Mascitti TA. Sites and mode of termination of fibers of the vestibulospinal tract in the cat. An experimental study with silver impregnation methods. J Comp Neurol 1964; 122:369–387.

28. Grillner S, Hongo T, Lund S. The vestibulospinal tract. Effects on alphamotoneurons in the lumbosacral spinal cord in the cat. Exp Brain Res 1970; 10:94–120.

29. Shinoda Y, Ohgaki T, Futami T. The morphology of single lateral vestibulospinal tract axons in the lower cervical spinal cord of the cat. J Comp Neurol 1986; 249:226–241.

30. Abzug C, Maeda M, Peterson BW, et al. Cervical branching of lumbar vestibulospinal axons. J Physiol Lond 1974; 243:499–522.

31. Akaike T. Neuronal organization of the vestibulospinal system in the cat. Brain Res 1983; 259:217–227.

32. Siegborn J, Grant G. Brainstem projections of different branches of the vestibular nerve. An experimental study by transganglionic transport of horseradish peroxidase in the cat. I. The horizontal ampullar and utricular nerves. Arch Ital Biol 1983; 121:237–248.

33. Walberg F, Pompeiano O, Brodal A, et al. The fastigiovestibular projection in the cat. An experimental study with silver impregnation methods. J Comp Neurol 1962; 118:49–75.

34. Houser CR, Barber RP, Vaughn JE. Immunocytochemical localization of glutamic acid decarboxylase in the dorsal lateral vestibular nucleus: Evidence for an intrinsic and extrinsic GABAergic innervation. Neurosci Lett 1984; 47:213–220.

35. Carpenter MB, Batton RR III. Connections of the fastigial nuclei in the cat and monkey. Exp Brain Res Suppl 1982; 6:250–295.

36. Monaghan PL, Beitz AJ, Larson AA, et al. Immunocytochemical localization of glutamate-, glutaminase-, and aspartate aminotransferase-like immunoreactivity in the rat deep cerebellar nuclei. Brain Res 1986; 363:364–370.

37. Brodal A. The Reticular Formation of the Brain Stem: Anatomical Aspects and Functional Correlations. Springfield, Ill: Charles C Thomas, 1957.

38. Scheibel ME, Scheibel AN. Structural substrates for integrative patterns in the brain stem reticular core. In: Reticular Formation of the Brain, Boston: Little, Brown, 1958; 31–55.

39. Basbaum AL, Ralston DD, Ralston HJ III. Bulbospinal projections in the primate: A light and

electron microscopic study of a pain modulating system. J Comp Neurol 1986; 250:311–323.

40. Saper CB, Loewy AD, Swanson LW, et al. Direct hypothalamo-autonomic connections. Brain Res 1976; 117:305–312.

41. Loewy AD, Saper CB. Edinger-Westphal nucleus: Projections to brain stem and spinal cord in the cat. Brain Res 1978; 150:1–27.

42. Westlund KN, Bowker BM, Ziegler MG, et al. Origins and terminations of descending noradrenergic projections to spinal cord of monkey. Brain Res 1984; 292:1–16.

43. Loewy AD, Burton H. Nuclei of the solitary tract: Efferent projections to lower brain stem and spinal cord in the cat. J Comp Neurol 1978; 181:421–450.

44. Loewy AD, McKellar S, Saper CB. Direct projections from the A5 catecholamine cell group to the intermediolateral cell column. Brain Res 1979; 174:309–314.

45. Lassek AM. The Pyramidal Tract:Its Status in Medicine. Springfield: Charles C Thomas, 1954.

46. Kuhn RA. Functional capacity of the isolated human spinal cord. Brain 1950; 75:1–51.

47. Tower SS. Pyramidal lesion in the monkey. Brain 1940; 63:36–60.

48. Tower SS. Pyramidal tract. In: Bucy PC, ed. The Precentral Motor Cortex, ed 2. Urbana: University of Illinois Press, 1948; 149–172.

49. Lawrence DG, Kuypers HGJM. The functional organization of the motor system in the monkey. I. The effects of bilateral pyramidal lesions. Brain 1968; 91:1–14.

50. Lawrence DG, Kuypers HGJM. The functional organization of the motor system in the monkey. II. The effects of lesions of the descending brain-stem pathways. Brain 1968; 91:15–36.

51. Penfield W, Rasmussen T. The Cerebral Cortex of Man: A Clinical Study of Localization of Function. New York: Macmillan, 1950.

52. Woolsey CN. Organization of somatic and motor areas of the cerebral cortex. In: Harlow HF, Woolsey CN eds. Biological and Biochemical Bases of Behavior, Madison: University of Wisconsin Press, 1958; 63–81.

53. Wise SP, Tanji J. Supplementary and precentral motor cortex: Contrast in responsiveness to peripheral input in the hindlimb area of the unanesthetized monkey. J Comp Neurol 1981; 195:433–451.

54. Brinkman C, Porter R. Supplementary motor area and premotor area of monkey cerebral cortex: Functional organization and activities of single neurons during performance of a learned movement. In: Desmedt JE, ed. Motor Control Mechanisms in Health and Disease, New York: Raven Press, 1983; 393–420.

55. Jürgens U. The efferent and afferent connections of the supplementary motor area. Brain Res 1981; 300:63–81.

56. Bertrand G. Spinal efferent pathways from the supplementary motor area. Brain 1956; 79:461–473.

57. Travis AM. Neurological deficiencies following supplementary motor area lesions in *Macaca mulatta*. Brain 1955; 78:174–198.

58. Coxe WS, Landau WM. Observations upon the effects of supplementary motor cortex ablation in the monkey. Brain 1965; 88:763–772.

59. Denny-Brown D, Botterell EH. The motor function of the agranular frontal cortex. Res Publ Assoc Res Nerv Ment Dis 1948; 27:235–345.

60. Carpenter MB. Core Text of Neuroanatomy, ed 3. Baltimore: Williams & Wilkins, 1985.

61. Noback CR, Demarest RJ. The Human Nervous System, ed 3. New York: McGraw-Hill, 1981.

# Chapter 2

# Anatomy and Physiology of the Vascular Supply to the Brain

N VENKETASUBRAMANIAN
J P MOHR
WILLIAM L YOUNG
CYNTHIA LIEN
ANN BREUER

## Brain Anatomy

The brain is divided into two major areas, the large cerebral convexities connected by the white matter pathways known as the corpus callosum, and the brain stem, which has the form of a narrow stalk expanding upward from below and links the brain above with the spinal cord below.

### Convexities

The surface of the brain is a continuous structure with numerous folds providing a large surface area in a compact space (Figures 2-1 and 2-2). Major clefts such as the *longitudinal fissure* separating the two halves of the brain are readily identifiable. In each half hemisphere of the brain the major clefts or fissures serve as anatomic landmarks. The most prominent is the fissure of Sylvius (*sylvian fissure*), which runs from the inferior frontal surface on the side of the brain, broadly separating the upper, frontal lobe from the lower, temporal lobe. Opening up this large fissure exposes the island (insula) of Reil. Another large sulcus, the fissure of Rolando (*rolandic fissure*), passes up the side of the brain, above the Sylvian fissure. This structure is of interest because of its relative constancy of position and because the major motor

(forward of the fissure) and sensory (behind the fissure) systems straddle it.

In front of the rolandic fissure, in the *frontal lobe* of the brain, are fissures that separate the numerous convolutions. The resulting lobules are usually sufficiently distinctly positioned to be described as the inferior, middle, and superior lobules of the frontal lobe. The frontal lobe is heavily involved in motor activity. The large portion of brain behind the rolandic fissure is known as the *parietal lobe* (wall portion). Its upper and lower halves, usually slightly divided by the long, curving intraparietal fissure, contain the main sensory functions of the brain. The back portion of the parietal lobe is so convoluted as to preclude descriptive labeling; however, some convolutions have names that roughly reflect their shape or position: the angular gyrus, postparietal gyrus, and inferior parietal gyrus, among others. On the lower side of the brain is the *temporal lobe,* so named because it governs the sense of time and sleep; its functions also include memory and hearing. This long lobe runs the length of the lower side of the brain, bounded in its anterior half from above by the sylvian fissure and in its posterior half by the parietal lobe. The temporal lobe has three undistinguished minor sulci, the first, second, and third temporal gyri. The temporal lobe blends with the back end of the brain, the *occipital lobe*. This

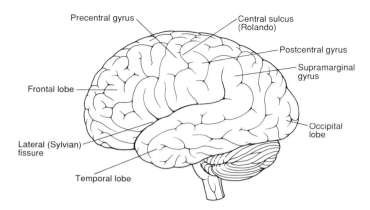

**Figure 2-1.** Lateral view of the brain. Labels show main lobes and gyri.

lobe, much of which is on the under and inner aspects of the brain, is involved with vision. A large mass of fibers, the corpus callosum, binds the two halves of the brain together.

### Depths

Each half of the brain contains large collections of cells clustered in formations known as kernels, nuclear groups, or ganglia. In these masses of nerve cells are arranged complex activities, such as coordination among various motor and sensory pathways. A large collection of nuclear groups arranged in the very center of the brain, forming the extreme upper end of the brain stem and supporting much of the brain above, is known as the *thalamus* (Greek for *inner chamber*). Through this structure are routed many of the pathways that connect the brain above with the brain stem and

spinal cord below. To either side of the thalamus are the basal ganglia, which process motor movements. The nerve cell bodies are anatomically similar, whether on the crest of a fold (convolution or gyrus) or down in a cleft between folds (fissure or sulcus).

### Brain Stem

The brain stem, which is the upward extension of the spinal cord, carries sensory and motor information to and from the brain by means of long bundles of fibers known as tracts or pathways. Embedded in the brain stem and differentiating it from spinal cord functions are a variety of specialized regions that control breathing, heart rate, blood pressure, and similar functions; movement of the face, mouth, and throat; and sleep and wakefulness.

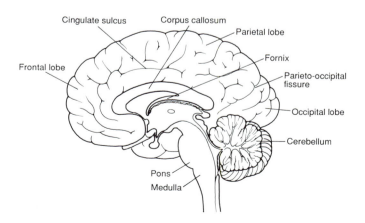

**Figure 2-2.** Medial view of the saggital section of the brain. Labels show main lobes and gyri.

## Cerebellum

Attached to the back of the brain stem is the *cerebellum* (little brain), a structure which sits astride the brain stem like a small roof. It forms the bulge at the lower back of the head.

The cerebellum contains nerve cells important for fine coordination.

## Study of Brain Vascular Physiology

A number of techniques are used to study the blood flow and anatomy of the brain in health and disease: ultrasonography and Doppler devices to measure blood flow in vessels; angiography, which requires injection of contrast agents directly into the circulation to demonstrate the anatomy of the vessels (Figure 2-3); and computed tomography, (CT) and magnetic resonance imaging (MRI) to visualize alterations in tissues directly.

### Magnetic Resonance Imaging

MRI (formerly known as NMR, for nuclear magnetic resonance) is among the most modern techniques for diagnosing stroke due to hemorrhage or occlusion. This technique is based on the interaction between magnetically induced radio waves and nuclei of the element hydrogen in the presence of a powerful magnetic field. The strong magnetic field makes the body parts being scanned susceptible to excitation by a radiofrequency pulse. Once excitation occurs, the energy absorbed from the radiotransmission is released at a rate that can be measured, and the measurements can be displayed as images. Because bone gives little in the way of an MR signal, MRI offers an imaging advantage over CT for infarcts in the brain stem.

When the tissue being scanned has completely reemitted the absorbed energy, it has undergone complete relaxation. During the process of relaxation, two tissue-specific relaxation constants, known as T1 and T2, are measured and images are reconstructed from the signals obtained. In clinical practice, three types of images are generated: in the favored T2-dependent ones spinal fluid has increased or lighter signal intensity than the brain; in T1-dependent images spinal fluid has decreased or darker signal intensity than the brain, and fat has increased signal intensity; and in "balanced" images the signals from brain and spinal fluid are comparable. Images of brain tissue are obtained in "slices."

To diagnose and date hemorrhage, pulse sequences known as T2 and T1 are necessary, whereas to diagnose small infarcts, a long-interval T2 image is preferred. The changes in tissue water accompanying infarction are easily documented by MRI, making it a useful technique to follow the evolution of cerebral infarction (Figures 2-4 and 2-5).

Since no signal is obtained from flowing blood, which moves out of a plane of section before giving up its signal, information on the patency of arteries can also be obtained, and practical MR angiography is already widely available (Figure 2-6).

Paramagnetic agents, especially gadolinium, enhance MR imaging through blood-brain barrier disruption. With improvement in magnet design and in computer programming, images are emerging whose resolution was beyond imagination only a few years ago.

### Computed Tomography

Using computers that measure the tissue absorption of x-rays, it is possible from among the tiny differences in absorption values to magnify and

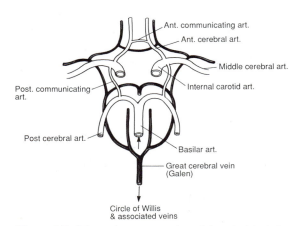

**Figure 2-3.** Schematic representation of the arterial circle of Willis and accompanying veins.

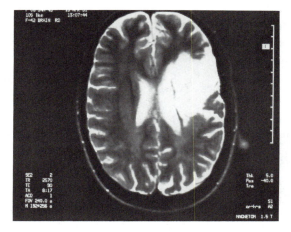

A

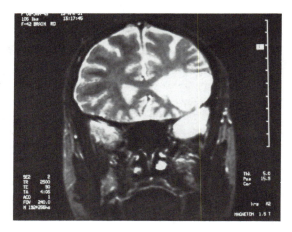

B

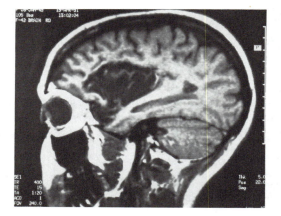

C

**Figure 2-4.** MRI shows a large left cerebral infarct: (*A*) T2-weighted transverse view, (*B*) T2-weighted coronal view, (*C*) T1-weighted saggital view.

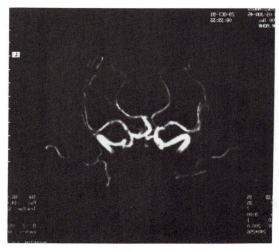

**Figure 2-5.** T2-weighted MRI shows a right brain stem infarct.

separate x-ray attenuations of tissues and display the images of air, fluid, brain, and bone as separate shades of gray. To achieve this result, a fan beam of x-rays is emitted from a single source, passes through the patient's body, and is received by an array of detectors. The x-ray source rotates around the body, and the attenuated x-ray beams are measured by each of the detectors along various lines through the plane of section, divided into compartments called *pixels*.

**Figure 2-6.** A normal MR angiogram of the distal internal carotid arteries, middle cerebral arteries and anterior cerebral arteries.

Modern CT imaging permits differentiation of white and gray matter, the main divisions of the basal ganglia and the thalamus. Injection of certain chemicals into the blood results in enhanced contrast in a CT scan, increasing the image intensity of the signals from acutely damaged brain tissue, from normal or chronically damaged tissue, and from air, fat, soft tissue, and calcification. Even the major arteries can be imaged. Because of the thick bone and small size of the brain tissue, images from the posterior fossa are still not satisfactory.

CT is a reliable means of displaying and measuring the size of intracranial hemorrhages in the first week, when they exhibit their characteristic high density (Figure 2-7). The high signal of fresh blood is lost over days to weeks, owing to chemical changes in the blood. Consequently the CT appearance evolves from initial hyperdensity through an isodense (subacute) phase to hypodensity in the chronic state. During the subacute phase, contrast administration may result in ring enchancement around the hemorrhage. In the chronic state, a hematoma is usually reduced to a slitlike cavity and may disappear entirely. Subarachnoid hemorrhage is even more transient and may not appear on the CT scan at all unless it is particularly dense.

With infarction, the CT may be normal for the first 4 days; if the collateral blood supply to the region is large, CT findings are usually positive within 24 hours, showing reduced density of the image due to the fluid accumulation (edema; Figures 2-8 and 2-9) or high-density zones when hemorrhagic transformation has occurred.[1] Infarcts with little collateral supply or edema may remain isodense for days or weeks, later appearing only as focal atrophy. Contrast enhancement of infarction usually occurs within a week and may persist 2 weeks to 2 months. Standard CT techniques do not image the extent of ischemia separate from infarction.

### Angiography

Angiography involves the injection of contrast agents directly into the arteries to demonstrate the anatomy of the vessels using either conventional radiographic or digital subtraction techniques. It remains unsurpassed in demonstrating occlusion

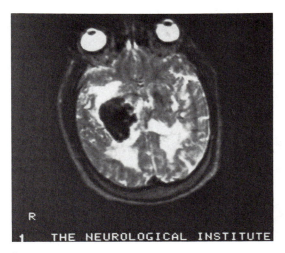

A

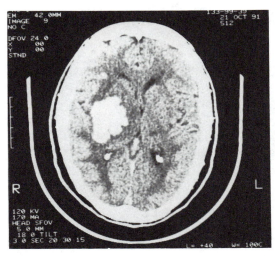

B

**Figure 2-7.** MRI (*A*) and CT (*B*) images show a large right basal ganglia hemorrhage.

(Figure 2-10), ulceration and injuries to the large arteries, and stenosis of small arteries. It is relied on for detection of aneurysms and arteriovenous malformations. Angiography fails to reliably image vessels smaller than 0.5 mm in diameter and so is not usually helpful in diagnosing the cause of deep infarctions due to occlusion of tiny vessels. Before direct brain imaging methods were devised, angiography was much relied on to outline intra- and extraaxial hematomas, evaluate vasospasm after ruptured aneurysms, and estimate the degree of extracranial arterial stenosis. Many of these

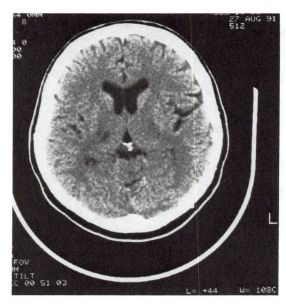

A

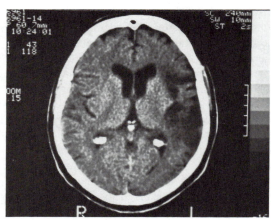

**Figure 2-9.** CT image of a large left middle cerebral arteries territory infarct.

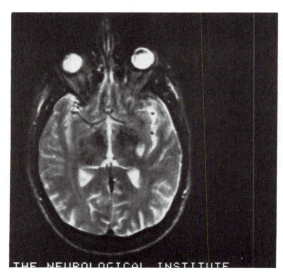

B

**Figure 2-8.** (*A*) CT image shows a small, deep infarct in the posterior limb of the right internal capsule. (*B*) MR image of a similar infarct in the left internal capsule.

conditions are now subject to diagnosis by non-invasive methods.

Angiography is uncomfortable and carries a small risk. At present it is used when alternative noninvasive imaging modalities fail to conclu-sively diagnose the cause of a stroke. Thus, it requires appropriate forethought to maximize the information to be gained. For a diagnosis of embolism, angiography should be undertaken within hours of the ictus, as the embolic particle may fragment early, changing the appearance of the affected vessel from occlusion to one indistin-guishable from arterial stenosis or arteritis, and may subsequently appear patent with a normal lumen. Where atheromatous stenosis of large arteries is suspected, preangiographic Doppler insonation helps to focus the angiographic study, allowing the angiographer to concentrate on the major territories thought to be diseased.

### Doppler Insonation and Imaging

The simplest Doppler devices pass a high-frequency continuous-wave sound signal over the vessels in the neck, receive the signals reflected from moving blood in the arteries and veins, and feed them through a small acoustic speaker. The examiner detects flow by the changing pitch of the sound waves.

*Duplex Doppler* devices have two crystals, one atop the other (duplex), in a single probe head, one crystal insonating the vessel for evidence of flow, the other analyzing the reflected sound waves to create an image of the vessel wall (B-mode imaging). Improvements in crystal design are steadily reducing the size of the probe, but its size still makes it difficult to image and insonate the carotid artery high up under the mandible. The crystal in modern Doppler units has an "adjustable range gate" to permit analysis of flow signals from specified depths in the tissues, from a fraction of a millimeter up. This gating eliminates conflicting signals where arteries and veins overlie one another. Some devices have two range gates, allowing an adjustable "volume" or "window" to insonate the moving column of blood in an artery in volumes as small as 0.6 mm, the size of the tightest stenosis. The capacity to interrogate the flow pattern from wall to wall across the lumen makes this technique a sensitive tool for detecting, measuring, and monitoring degrees of vascular stenosis.

Because the duplex Doppler unit is sensitive to cross-sectional area and not to wall anatomy, its use before angiography often warns the angiographer to seek stenoses that might not otherwise be noticed. The sonographic images of the vessels are relatively insensitive to most minor ulcerations, which are better seen by conventional angiography. Duplex Doppler methods, although developed to insonate the carotid arteries, can also be used to study the extracranial vertebral artery passing through the intervertebral foramina.

*Transcranial Doppler*

Using a probe with great tissue penetration properties, it is possible to insonate the major vessels of the circle of Willis, and the vertebral and basilar arteries. Transcranial Doppler devices are range gated but not (yet) duplex, so they document the direction and velocity of the arterial flow, and spectrum analysis of the signal allows estimation of the degree of stenosis. Extracranial stenosis severe enough to restrict flow (hemodynamically significant) has been shown to damp the waveform in the ipsilateral arteries distal to the stenosis, allowing the effect of the extracranial disease to be measured and followed over time. All these techniques are demanding; patience and skill are required to detect the signal to detect the signal and then to find the best angle for insonation at a given depth. Minor anatomic variations can cause otherwise misleading changes in signal strength; however, as the procedure is fast and safe and uses a probe and microprocessor of tabletop size, the

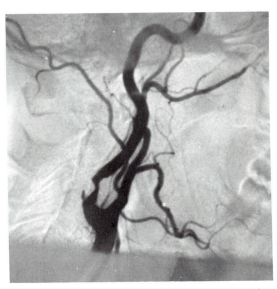

**Figure 2-10.** Digital subtraction angiogram shows tight stenosis at the origin of the right interior carotid arteries.

device can be taken to the bedside, even in an intensive care unit. There it can be used to diagnose developing vasospasm, collateral flow above occlusions, recanalization of an embolized artery, and the presence of important basilar or cerebral artery stenoses. When combined with high-field magnetic resonance imaging (MRI), it is possible to diagnose basilar and middle cerebral artery stem stenoses entirely noninvasively.

## Methods of Assessing Cerebral Blood Flow

### Regional Cerebral Blood Flow

The techniques of cerebral blood flow (CBF) determination in humans relies on wash-in or washout of (ideally) freely diffusable and inert indicators (tracers), where the rate of change in brain concentration is proportional to flow. The basic principles of tracer kinetics are generally applicable to newer CBF methodologics such as positron emission tomography (PET) and single-photon emission computed tomography (SPECT).

Kety and Schmidt[2] originally described a 10- to 15-minute period of inhalation of 15% nitrous oxide ($N_2O$). The tracer reaches equilibration between arterial and venous (and therefore tissue) concentrations, and samples are taken intermittently from a peripheral artery and the jugular bulb for determination of tracer concentration. The amount of tracer taken up by the brain over a period of time must equal the amount of tracer delivered to the brain via the arterial blood minus that recovered by the cerebral venous blood in the same amount of time. Assuming that the brain concentration is proportional to venous concentration, CBF can be determined with knowledge of the blood-brain partition coefficient of the tracer used. Lassen and Ingvar[3,4] offered significant progress in measurement of human cerebral perfusion. The technique involves injecting a radioactive tracer (krypton 85 or xenon 133) as a bolus directly into a carotid artery. Following the cerebral washout with external scintillation counting over the skull allows determination of *regional* CBF.

Modern noninvasive methods were developed primarily by Obrist[5] and later modified by Prohovnik.[6] A 1-minute period of inhalation of $^{133}$Xe is followed by a 10-minute period of washout, which is similar to that achieved with intraarterial concentration. The input of tracer to the brain is not instantaneous but is smeared, owing to mixing of the tracer in the heart and lungs. The slow compartment (corresponding to white matter flow for the intra-carotid method) is contaminated by extracranial clearance, making the noninvasive method suitable principally for assessing gray matter flow.

Serial studies are easily done and are limited only by cumulative radiation exposure, which is minimal. CBF may be measured over both hemispheres and in the posterior fossa with a fair degree of spatial (two-dimensional) resolution, because the isotope is delivered to all areas of the brain.

### Single-Photon Emission Computed Tomography

In one technique of brain imaging, a camera sensitive to radioactivity (gamma camera) is used to count the density of signals emitted from an injected agent minutes after it is given intravenously. The injected agent circulates through the vasculature and is concentrated where the vessels are open and the flow is greatest. In addition to tracers, which are trapped in tissue in proportion to CBF, $^{133}$Xe washout may be used for imaging with SPECT cameras. The emitted signals are assigned

to pixels and displayed in slice form, like CT images. The technique is inexpensive, shows regional flow abnormalities from occlusions of individual branches, and is a sensitive test of perfusion disturbances that are larger than the areas of tissue damage.

### Positron Emission Tomography

PET also generates axial images using a technique similar to MRI, but the agents that are injected or inhaled are short-lived isotopes. Regional brain metabolic activity is reflected in the emitted metabolic end products of such important substrates as oxygen and glucose. The images obtained are still poorly focused and fuzzy, but PET remains the only currently practical technique for imaging chemical reactions in the living brain.

### Cold Xenon Computed Tomography

The cold xenon method uses a standard CT scanner. The patient breathes a relatively high concentration of nonradioactive xenon (30%). The change in x-ray transmission through the brain with wash-in and washout of the gas can be quantified in a manner analogous to the quantification of radioactive xenon with a gamma camera. This method generates tomographic CBF information similar to that generated by SPECT and PET. Unfortunately, high concentrations of xenon are not physiologically inert and may have mild anesthetic effects.

### Magnetic Resonance Imaging of Cerebral Perfusion

Although it is still experimental, progress is being made in developing paramagnetic tracers that will allow wash-in and washout determinations using standard MRI equipment. This will be a major advance in clinical imaging of cerebral physiologic function.

## Determinants of Cerebral Blood Flow

### Cerebral Blood Flow Autoregulation

Autoregulation entails matching of metabolic demand with the blood supply–bearing substrate.

The metabolic demand of the brain is totally dependent on the oxidative metabolism of blood-borne glucose, which fuels all cellular processes. A large part of basal metabolism is devoted to the maintenance of the normal transmembrane ion gradients, the most important being maintenance of intracellular potassium and extracellular sodium. The remainder of basal metabolism is concerned with protein and neurotransmitter synthesis and other basic cellular functions.

Two different factors seem to be involved in autoregulation: local metabolic factors and myogenic responses. The exact mechanism by which local metabolic factors are related to CBF is unclear; probably many factors play a role. At one time it was thought that increased hydrogen ion concentration alone controlled vascular resistance, but this is doubtful now. Although extracellular hydrogen ion can increase CBF, it is not required for cerebrovascular dilatation. Extracellular potassium and calcium appear to have minor roles in the control of local CBF. Recent evidence suggests that endothelium-derived nitric oxide is the predominant metabolic "messenger" between cerebral function and a tightly regulated continuous supply of oxygen, as borne by CBF. Other cellular metabolites that may serve as messengers for regulation of vascular tone include cyclooxygenase products of phospholipid membrane metabolism and adenosine. Autonomic nerves do not appear to be necessary for this autoregulatory response, but they may modify it.

### Hemodynamic Autoregulation

Vascular autoregulation refers to the intrinsic capacity of the cerebral vasculature to maintain constant blood flow in the face of varying cerebral perfusion pressure. CBF remains constant between mean arterial pressures of 50 and 150 mm Hg in normotensive persons by virtue of active vasomotion at the arteriolar level.[7] Autoregulation may be affected by either disease or concomitant drug therapy. If mean arterial pressure decreases to less than 50 mm Hg, the resistive beds of the cerebral vasculature become maximally dilated. CBF decreases with a further fall in mean arterial pressure (MAP). When MAP is greater than 150 mm Hg, the cerebral vasculature becomes maximally constricted; CBF increases passively as perfusion

pressure further increases. In chronic arterial hypertension, the autoregulatory curve is displaced to the right. Because of this adaptation to higher pressure with vessel wall hypertrophy, marked increases in blood pressure may not result in CBF increases; however, a blood pressure reduction that would be of no consequence in normotensive persons could result in a significant reduction in cerebral perfusion that may be poorly tolerated by the hypertensive patient.[8] There is evidence that, with antihypertensive medication and gradual normalization of blood pressure, the autoregulatory curve shifts back toward the left (toward normal) and tolerance of hypotension is improved.

CBF normally is not altered by small changes in central venous pressure (CVP), but, with severe right-sided heart failure, CVP is greatly increased and cerebral perfusion pressure may be significantly lowered.[9]

Arterial oxygen and carbon dioxide concentrations also determine CBF. Oxygen tension exerts its predominant effect at the extremes of oxygen concentration. Moderate changes in arterial oxygen concentration near the physiologic range do not influence CBF, though hypoxemia is a most potent stimulus for increasing CBF.

Cerebrovascular resistance is exquisitely sensitive to changes in carbon dioxide tension. The greatest responsiveness to carbon dioxide changes occurs when the $pCO_2$ is in the physiological range of 20 to 60 mm Hg. CBF changes by $PaCO_2$ are influenced by the arteriolar tone set by the systemic arterial pressure. Moderate hypotension blunts the ability of the cerebral circulation to respond to changes in $PaCO_2$, and severe hypotension abolishes it altogether.[10]

The mechanism by which carbon dioxide exerts its effect on cerebrovascular resistance is not known. Current evidence suggests that cerebrovascular resistance is varied by interstitial pH rather than $PaCO_2$ directly. Carbon dioxide, as a product of oxidation, provides a feedback loop for vasomotor control. With an increase in metabolic rate, carbon dioxide production is increased, causing vasodilatation and increased CBF. The increased blood flow provides a more plentiful supply of nutrients and clearance of lactic and hydrogen ions from the extracellular space, decreasing the amplitude of local pH changes.

In the face of continuing hyper- or hypocapnia,

CBF tends to return toward normal levels. This occurs through a process of pH normalization brought about by varying cerebrospinal fluid bicarbonate concentrations. As a clinical corollary, artificial hyperventilation to reduce intracranial pressure by decreasing CBF is not effective for indefinite periods, and, as these changes in bicarbonate require 24 to 36 hours to fully evolve, chronic hypo- or hypercapnia should not be rapidly corrected.

## Vascular Anatomy and Ischemic Syndromes

Arterial occlusions from thrombosis or embolism produce syndromes that have distinguishing characteristics for each arterial territory. Many classical syndromes are now recognized, though the effect of collateral circulation can alter the size and shape of the infarct. Thus the syndromes encountered may be different from those expected.[11] In the following section I review the anatomy of each vessel and the syndrome most commonly associated with ischemia in its territory.[12]

### Carotid Artery System

#### Common Carotid Artery

Occlusion of the common carotid artery may not produce any neurologic deficit because of extensive collateral flow between the carotid and vertebrobasilar circulation, both intracranially and extracranially, and between the left and right carotid arteries.

The most frequent collateralization develops between the vertebral and the external carotid vessels. The extracranial vertebral artery can form an anastomosis with the occipital (scalp) branch of the external carotid artery at the skull base, through which retrograde flow reaches the external carotid artery and the common carotid bifurcation and proceeds anterograde up the internal carotid artery to the brain.

#### Internal Carotid Artery

A common location for atherosclerosis is the origin of the internal carotid artery at the bifurcation of the common carotid artery. Collateral circulation available to the internal carotid artery is limited, and intracranial symptoms are often produced.[13]

The external carotid artery forms anastomoses extracranially with the internal carotid artery via the vessels of the orbit, most often through the ophthalmic artery. Intracranially, collaterals may develop across the anterior or posterior branches of the circle of Willis or over the convexity of the brain by way of border zone vessels that link the distal ends of each major hemispheral arterial territory with the others.

The internal carotid artery supplies the ipsilateral eye (by means of the middle and anterior cerebral artery), the entire frontal lobe, and almost all of the temporal and parietal lobes. Ipsilateral blindness from occlusion of the ophthalmic artery is rare, owing to the excellent collateral system from the external carotid artery. The intracranial symptoms of carotid artery occlusion reflect the loss of function of that cerebral hemisphere and include contralateral hemiparesis with an associated sensory loss. Aphasia occurs when the dominant hemisphere is infarcted. Disturbance in awareness of the neurologic deficit occurs when the infarct involves the non-dominant hemisphere. Homonymous hemianopia is infrequent, but a temporary hemineglect for the contralateral visual field is common. Coma is rare, since some degree of collateral circulation usually spares the anterior cerebral artery and parts of the middle cerebral artery.

### Middle Cerebral Artery

The blood supply to the surface of the cerebrum is composed of some 12 to 15 individual branches, which are usually grouped into an upper, or anterior, division and a lower, or posterior, division. The upper division supplies the entire insula, most of the frontal lobe, and almost all of the convex surface of the anterior half of the parietal lobe. The lower division branches at the posterior end of the sylvian fissure, supplying almost all of the temporal lobe, the posterior half of the parietal lobe, and the adjacent lateral occipital region. The stem of the middle cerebral artery gives off the dozen or so small lenticulostriate arteries that penetrate deep into the brain to supply the caudate nucleus, anterior limb, genu, and posterior limb of the internal capsule, putamen, external capsule, and claustrum.

The middle cerebral artery and its branches are occluded more frequently by embolism than is any other intracranial vessel, though the stem is occasionally blocked by atherosclerosis.

Occlusion of the main trunk causes softening of the basal ganglia, internal capsule, and a large portion of the cerebral hemisphere, resulting in contralateral hemiplegia, hemianesthesia, and hemianopia.[14] Total or global aphasia or impaired awareness of the stroke also occurs, depending on which hemisphere is affected. When the infarct is large, the hemianopia may be due to involvement of the visual radiations deep in the brain. More often, the hemianopia is part of a syndrome of hemineglect for the opposite side of space and is accompanied by failure to turn toward the side affected by the hemiplegia in response to stimuli from that side.[15]

When the occlusion involves only the upper division of the middle cerebral artery, the sensorimotor syndrome is similar to that of occlusion of the stem. When the hemiparesis involves the face and arm more than the leg, the picture is the opposite of that seen in anterior cerebral artery disease. Isolated weakness of the face, arm, or leg is rare and is seen only with the smallest focal infarcts. Aphasia, when it occurs, is most often of the motor type (Broca's aphasia) because the occlusions usually affect the anterior branches of the upper division, but a syndrome of literal paraphasias (the misuse of spoken words or combination of words) occurs if the disease is limited to the posterior (anterior parietal) branches of the upper division. Pure aphasia (Wernicke's aphasia) without hemiparesis occurs in lower division obstruction in dominant hemisphere infarction, while the nondominant behavioral disturbances may appear alone when the opposite side is involved. When the involvement is limited to the territory of a small penetrating artery branch of the main stem, a small, deep infarct (lacuna) may occur, affecting the internal capsule, producing a syndrome of pure hemiparesis, without sensory, visual, language, or behavior disturbances.

*Anterior Cerebral Artery*

The stem of the anterior cerebral artery gives rise to small branches that penetrate into the brain to supply the anterior limb of the internal capsule, the head of the caudate nucleus, and the anterior putamen. The anterior cerebral artery distal to the trunk courses forward, upward, and then backward over the corpus callosum, which it supplies, to reach its major territory, the frontal lobe/pole, upper portion of the anterolateral frontal lobe, and the medial surface of the cerebral hemisphere including the paracentral lobule. The paracentral lobule provides motor and sensory control for the legs and genitalia.

Occlusion of the proximal portion of the anterior cerebral artery is rare. Obstruction of one or more of its surface branches produces paralysis and sensory loss chiefly affecting the leg of the opposite side. Occlusion of the anterior cerebral artery serving the dominant hemisphere may precipitate profound changes in behavior, producing a severe reduction in the rate and complexity of language and speech responses. This syndrome is known as abulia, or, if very severe, as akinetic mutism. Involvement of the medial surface of the frontal lobe, and perhaps of the corpus callosum, may lead to ideomotor dyspraxia, which is disruption in the ability of the limbs served by the nondominant hemisphere to respond correctly to verbal commands.

*Posterior Cerebral Artery*

The area supplied by the posterior cerebral artery includes the inferomedial portions of the temporal and occipital lobes, including the calcarine cortex. This artery usually arises from the basilar artery but is a branch of the internal carotid in 10% of cases. It supplies the midbrain and thalamus via small, deep-penetrating branches arising from the trunk. Thalamic infarction can give rise to delayed development of contralateral, agonizing, burning pain (Dejerine-Roussy syndrome).

More often, the infarction involves the cortical territory of the posterior cerebral artery beyond the brain stem. When infarction is confined to the calcarine cortex, contralateral homonymous hemianopia occurs, unaccompanied by other deficits. Commonly, collateral flow from the anterior cerebral artery across the cuneus spares the upper bank of the calcarine cortex; in such cases, the infarct may be confined to the lower bank and may present only as contralateral upper quadrantic homonymous hemianopia. Small infarcts anterior to the calcarine cortex and posterior to the callosum may cause isolated disturbances in spatial orientation. Larger infarcts involving the lingual and fusiform gyri produce disturbances in discrimination and naming of colors and in reading the half of words in the contralateral visual field, a syndrome more obvious when the dominant hemisphere is involved. Still larger infarcts affecting the dominant hemisphere may result in total alexia and disturbances in the recall of names for a wide variety of items (amnestic aphasia). The hippocampus is usually affected only by the largest infarcts, but when it is involved as part of a dominant hemisphere infarct, a severe amnestic state occurs, which usually fades over a period of months.

### Vertebrobasilar System

#### Vertebral Arteries

The two vertebral arteries supply muscles of the neck in their extracranial course and form anastomoses with the occipital scalp branches of the external carotid artery. The vertebral arteries also supply branches to the spinal cord via the anterior and posterior spinal arteries. After entering the cranium through the foramen magnum, the vertebral arteries pass across the anterior surface of the medulla oblongata and fuse together at the pontomedullary junction to form the basilar artery.

Occlusion of a vertebral artery at its origin from the subclavian is usually asymptomatic, since collateral flow develops via the ipsilateral occipital branch of the external carotid artery. Occlusion intracranially may result in lateral medullary infarction. If the infarct also affects the cerebellum, owing to involvement of the posterior inferior cerebellar artery (which comes off the vertebral artery near its termination), the edema associated with the cerebellar infarct may produce life-threatening brain stem compression within days, a result that often develops with little warning. Finally, in the few cases where one vertebral artery provides essentially the entire supply to the basilar artery, its occlusion leads to a full basilar artery syndrome.

#### Basilar Artery

The basilar artery is formed by the junction of the two vertebral arteries and supplies blood to the pons, midbrain, and cerebellum. It usually forms

the two posterior cerebral arteries but may terminate at the level of the superior cerebellar arteries and be connected to the posterior cerebral arteries only by a small trunk.

Occlusion of the basilar artery can produce a wide spectrum of syndromes. Which one occurs depends on the site of the occlusion and the efficiency of the collateral circulation.[16] In most instances, the basilar artery is occluded by the process of thrombosis, and the syndrome is usually preceded by transient ischemic attacks (TIAs). These attacks commonly consist of fragments of the subsequent infarct syndrome. The symptoms most often encountered in vertebrobasilar TIAs are dizziness, diplopia, dysarthria, circumoral numbness, ataxia, and hemiparesis or hemisensory disturbances on one or both sides of the body. When thrombosis occludes the basilar artery, collateral flow is often efficient, often limiting the symptoms of basilar occlusion to the region supplied by the small branches at the actual site of the occlusion.

Each side of the brain stem can be divided into two areas: the paramedian and the lateral. The paramedian area is nourished by short, perforating arteries that arise from the basilar or vertebral arteries. The lateral area is supplied by surface conducting arteries that travel some distance from their point of origin before entering the brain stem.

Occlusions of paramedian vessels result in paresis of the arm and leg on the contralateral side and involvement of one or more cranial nerves on the same side as the lesion. The usual presentation is ipsilateral ophthalmoplegia from involvement of the third nerve nucleus and pathways; less often it is contralateral hemiparesis from damage to the cerebral peduncle. The majority of symptomatic paramedian branch occlusions involve the pons. Because the bulk of the ventromedial portion of the pons controls motor movements, occlusions result in some form of partial or complete contralateral hemiparesis or ataxia, either alone or as a prominent part of the syndrome. Depending on how deep the band of infarction penetrates, a number of cranial nerves may be involved ipsilaterally: infarction of the seventh nerve as it hooks around the sixth nucleus paralyzes the face; infarction of the nucleus of the sixth nerve makes the eye on the side of the lesion deviate inward because of paralysis of the abducting muscles; if the lesion is a little larger, paralysis of conjugate gaze occurs to the side of the lesion, owing to involvement of the medial longitudinal fasciculus and related pathways. Rhythmic contractions of the palate (palatal myoclonus) may occur with damage to the olivodentatorubral connections. The occlusion of paramedian branches supplying the medulla oblongata, a rare event, causes softening of the pyramid, the nucleus of the twelfth nerve, the medial lemniscus, and the medial portion of the olive. The result is paralysis and atrophy of the homolateral half of the tongue, paralysis of the opposite arm and leg, and impairment of the tactile sensation in the trunk and extremities on the paralyzed side.

The circumferential arteries, which arise from the basilar artery, supply the dorsolateral areas of the brain stem and the cerebellum. Occlusion of these vessels disrupts cerebellar projections and the nuclei and tracts in the lateral portion of the brain stem. The important structures in this area of the brain stem are the sensory nuclei of the fifth and eighth cranial nerves, the descending sympathetic pathways, and the ascending spinal lemniscus. The superior cerebellar artery, which arises immediately below the termination of the basilar artery, supplies the lateral area of the midbrain. Its involvement produces a syndrome of cerebellar dysfunction that can be so mild that only slight ataxia is encountered even when the infarct is large; palatal myoclonus is rare, and impairment of pain and temperature of the entire contralateral half of the body occurs only occasionally. The anterior inferior cerebellar artery supplies the lateral area of the pons. Its occlusion produces ipsilateral cerebellar ataxia (brachium conjunctivum), deafness (eighth nerve nucleus), facial paralysis (fifth nerve nucleus), and loss of touch sensibility in the face with contralateral impairment of pain and temperature (lateral spinothalamic tract).

Infarction of the lateral area of the medulla usually results from occlusion of the intracranial portion of the vertebral artery, producing Wallenberg's syndrome, manifested by dysphagia and dysarthria; ipsilateral Horner's syndrome of miosis, ptosis, and diminished sweating of the face, neck, and axilla; ipsilateral impairment of pain and temperature on the face; ipsilateral cerebellar ataxia; and contralateral impairment of pain and temperature on the body. Hiccups usually occur, but the lesion site is uncertain. This remarkable syndrome produces little long-term disability

itself, but when the cerebellum is infarcted edema may be voluminous enough to produce fatal brain stem compression.

## References

1. Fishman R. Brain edema. N Engl J Med 1975; 293:706–711.
2. Kety SS, Schmidt CF. Nitrous oxide method for the quantitative determination of cerebral blood flow in man: Theory, procedure and normal values. J Clin Invest 1948; 27:475–483.
3. Ingvar DD, Lassen NA, Quantitative determination of regional cerebral blood flow in man. Lancet 61; 11:806–807.
4. Lassen N, Ingvar DH, Skinhoj E. Brain function and blood flow. Changes in the amount of blood flowing in areas of human cerebral cortex, reflecting changes in the activity of those areas, are graphically revealed with the aid of radioactive isotope. Sci Amer 1978; 239:62.
5. Obrist WD, Thompson HK, Wang KS, et al. Regional cerebral blood flow estimated by 133-xenon inhalation. Stroke 1975; 6:245–256.
6. Prohovnik I, Knudsen E, Risberg J. Accuracy models and algorithms for determination of fast compartment flow by non-invasive $^{133}$Xe clearance. In: Magistretti P, ed. Functional Radionuclide Imaging of the Brain. New York: Raven Press, 1983; 87–115.
7. Aatru AA, Merriman HG. Hypocapnia added to hypertension to reverse EEG changes during carotid endarterectomy. Anesthesiology 1989; 70:1016–1018.
8. Solomon RA, Fink ME, Lennihan L. Early aneurysm surgery and prophylactic hypervolemic hypertensive therapy for the treatment of aneurysmal subarachnoid hemorrhage. Neurosurgery 1988; 23:699–704.
9. Young WL, Prohovnik I, Ornstein E, et al. Monitoring of intraoperative cerebral hemodynamics before and after arteriovenous malformation resection. Anesth Analg 1988; 67:1011–1014.
10. Young WL, Solomon RA, Prohovnik I, et al. $^{133}$Xe blood flow monitoring during arteriovenous malformation resection: A case of intraoperative hyperperfusion with subsequent brain swelling. Neurosurgery 1988; 22:765–769.
11. Mohr JP. Clinical worsening in acute stroke. In: Battistini, et al., eds. Acute Brain Ischemia: Medical and Surgical Therapy. New York: Raven Press, 1986; 173–178.
12. Mohr JP, et al. The Harvard cooperative stroke registry. Neurology 1978; 28:754.

13. Castaigne P, et al. Internal carotid artery occlusion: A study of 61 instances in 50 patients with post-mortem data. Brain 1970; 93:231.

14. Foix C, Levy M. Les ramollissements sylviens. Rev Neurol 1927; 11:1.

15. Caplan LR, et al. Right middle cerebral artery inferior division infarcts: The mirror image of Wernicke's aphasia. Neurology 1985; 35:121.

16. Caplan LR. "Top of the basilar" syndrome. Neurology 1980; 30:72.

# Chapter 3

# Cerebellum and Basal Ganglia

MALCOLM B. CARPENTER

Two large nuclear complexes derived from separate parts of the embryonic neural tube play major roles in the control of motor function. These structures are the cerebellum and the basal ganglia. Much is known about them and the disturbances associated with pathologic processes involving them. In spite of this knowledge, a complete understanding of their neural mechanisms still eludes both basic scientists and clinicians. Both structures influence brain stem nuclei, but their major effects are exerted on different motor regions of the cerebral cortex via thalamic relays. Influences on motor activity are indirect and involve circuits that modify neural activity at segmental levels. Both structures play major roles in suprasegmental control of motor function.

## The Cerebellum

The cerebellum is derived from the rhombic lip, a thickening along the superior margins of the fourth ventricle. This region of the embryonic neural tube is regarded as sensory in nature. Though the cerebellum receives sensory inputs from virtually all receptors, it is not concerned with conscious sensory perception. Sensory information transmitted to the cerebellum is utilized in the automatic coordination and control of somatic motor function. The cerebellum is a prime example of the importance of sensory integration in motor function.

Structurally the cerebellum consists of a median portion, the cerebellar vermis, and two lateral lobes, the cerebellar hemispheres. The cerebellum is composed of (1) a superficial gray cellular mantle, the cerebellar cortex, (2) an internal white matter, composed of fibers, and (3) four pairs of intrinsic nuclei deep within the white matter. The cerebellar cortex, unlike the cerebral cortex, is thrown into narrow leaf–like laminae known as *folia,* most of which are oriented in the transverse plane. Three paired cerebellar peduncles connect the cerebellum with the three most caudad segments of the brain stem—the medulla (inferior cerebellar peduncle), the pons (middle cerebellar peduncle), and the midbrain (superior cerebellar peduncle). Three distinctive parts of the cerebellum are recognized based upon embryonic and hodologic considerations (Figure 3-1). The phylogenetically oldest part, the *archicerebellum,* consists of the nodulus and paired appendages known as the flocculi. This small part of the cerebellum has connections mainly with the vestibular end-organ and the vestibular nuclei and is concerned with maintenance of equilibrium and orientation in three-dimensional space. All parts of the cerebellum rostrad to the primary fissure constitute the *paleocerebellum,* also known as the anterior lobe. This division of the cerebellum receives input from most stretch receptors (muscle spindles and Golgi tendon organs) and from cutaneous receptors. The anterior lobe of the cerebellum plays an important role in automatic regulation of muscle tone. The newest and largest

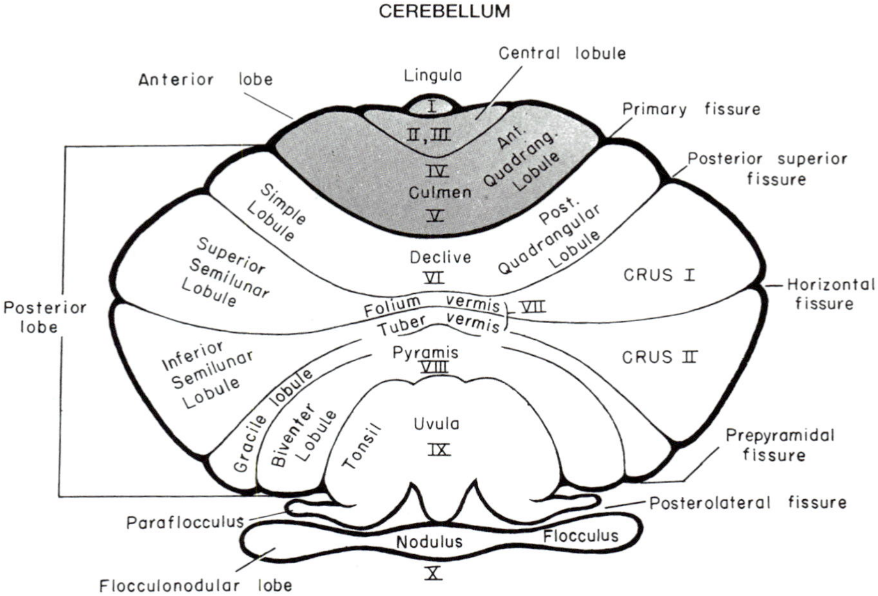

CEREBELLUM

**Figure 3-1.** Schematic diagram of the fissure and lobules of the cerebellum spread out in a single plane. Portions of the cerebellum caudal to the posterolateral fissure represent the flocculonodular lobule, also known as the archicerebellum. The anterior lobe of the cerebellum lies rostrad to the primary fissure and constitutes the paleocerebellum. The neocerebellum lies between the primary and posterolateral fissures. (From Carpenter MB. Core Text of Neuroanatomy, ed 3. Baltimore: Williams & Wilkins, 1985, with permission.)

part of the cerebellum, the *neocerebellum*, forms the posterior lobe. Input to the posterior lobe of the cerebellum arises from broad regions of the contralateral cerebral cortex and is relayed to the cerebellar cortex via the pontine nuclei. The posterior lobe of the cerebellum is concerned with coordination of skilled motor activities initiated at cortical levels.

### Cerebellar Cortex

The cerebellar cortex is uniform throughout and consists of three well-defined layers (Figure 3-2). Cells and their processes have specific geometric relationships that are constant and uniform. The three cellular layers of the cerebellar cortex are (1) a superficial molecular layer, (2) a deep granular layer composed of enormous numbers of small cells, and between these, (3) a ganglionic layer of large flask-shaped Purkinje cells. The granular layer, composed of closely packed chromatic nuclei with little cytoplasm, contains a number of larger inhibitory Golgi cells and relatively clear

spaces that contain synaptic complexes known as cerebellar glomeruli. This layer receives the principal inputs to the cerebellar cortex and can be regarded as the receptive layer. The Purkinje cell layer is the discharge layer and gives rise to the only output system from the cortex. The molecular layer contains a small number of cells and an enormous number of myelinated fibers, a large part of which synapse upon Purkinje cell dendrites. The molecular layer contains axons of granule cells, which divide in a T-shaped formation and extend transversely to synapse on the dendrites of a number of Purkinje cells. Granule cells are excitatory and have as their neurotransmitter glutamate.[1,2] All other neuron types in the cerebellar cortex appear positive for γ-aminobutyric acid (GABA), an inhibitory neurotransmitter. Golgi cells appear to be the most powerful "GABA-ergic" neurons in the cerebellar cortex. There is some chemical heterogeneity in Purkinje cells: though most contain GABA, some have both GABA and motilin.[3]

All afferent fibers entering the cerebellar cortex lose their myelin sheath and terminate as either mossy fibers or climbing fibers. The most abun-

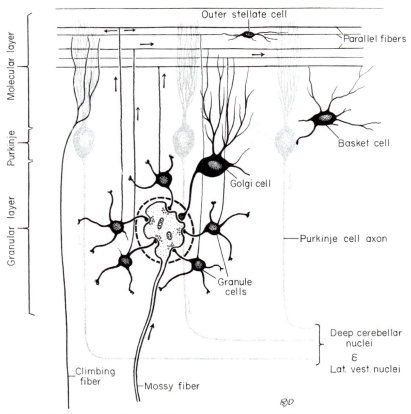

**Figure 3-2.** Schematic diagram of the structural elements of the cerebellar cortex as seen in a plane parallel to the long axis of a folium. Layers of the cerebellar cortex are indicated on the left. Excitatory inputs to the cerebellar cortex are conveyed by mossy and climbing fibers. The broken line represents a single glial lamella surrounding a cerebellar glomerulus. Granule cell axons ascend to the molecular layer, bifurcate in a T-shape and form synapses with the dendrites of a number of Purkinje cells across the width of the cerebellum. Climbing fibers that originate from the inferior olivary complex, ascend through all layers and climb the dendrites of a single Purkinje cell. Outer stellate, basket, and Golgi cells are all inhibitory. Output from the cerebellar cortex is conveyed by Purkinje cell axons; these cells are "GABA-ergic" and inhibit the deep cerebellar nuclei and cells in dorsal regions of the lateral vestibular nucleus. (From Carpenter MB. Core Text of Neuroanatomy, ed 3. Baltimore: Williams & Wilkins, 1985, with permission.)

dant afferents are mossy fibers, which end in the granular layer by breaking up into numerous terminals known as *mossy fiber rosettes*. A single mossy fiber rosette forms the core of a cerebellar glomerulus, a synaptic complex that also contains Golgi cell axons and numerous granule cell dendrites. This synaptic complex controls a major part of the input to the cerebellar cortex because it can inhibit the input to granule cells, which have an excitatory action on Purkinje cells.[4] Climbing fibers, which originate from the inferior olivary nu-

clear complex, are unique because they pass through the white matter, the granular layer and climb the dendrites of Purkinje cells (see Figure 3-2). These excitatory fibers, considered to use glutamate as their neurotransmitter, produce "all-or-none" responses in Purkinje cells.[5,6]

Although the cerebellar cortex seems relatively simple and has been regarded in one sense as the "Rosetta stone" of the central nervous system, it has an elaborate structural and functional organization in which multiple interactions influence

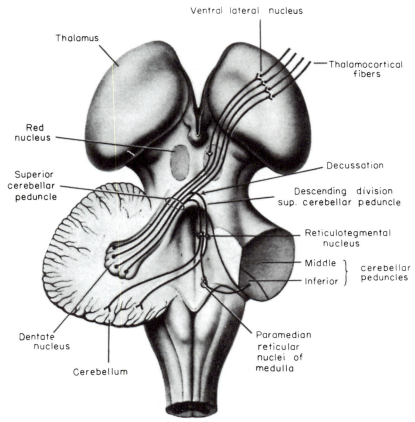

**Figure 3-3.** Diagram of the cerebellum and brain stem shows the cerebellar peduncles and the projections of the superior cerebellar peduncle. Ascending projections from the dentate nucleus project to the rostral third of the opposite red nucleus and to the cell-sparse zone of the thalamus, which includes the ventral posterolateral (VPLo, pars oralis) and the ventral lateral (VLc, pars caudalis) nuclei. (From Carpenter MB. Core Text of Neuroanatomy, ed 3. Baltimore: Williams & Wilkins, 1985, with permission.)

conduction of impulses, synaptic articulations, and output, which passes via Purkinje cell axons to the deep cerebellar nuclei and portions of the lateral vestibular nucleus. The most puzzling feature of the cerebellar cortex is that all excitatory input via mossy and climbing fibers is converted to inhibition.[4]

### Afferent Fibers

Cerebellar afferents are nearly three times more numerous than efferents[7] and, with some exceptions, terminate mainly in the cerebellar cortex. These pathways convey impulses from peripheral receptors and from relay nuclei in the brain stem and spinal cord. Afferents enter the cerebellum largely via the inferior and middle cerebellar peduncles (Figure 3-3).

The *inferior cerebellar peduncle* conveys input from spinal cord and cerebellar relay nuclei in the medulla. These fibers include the posterior spinocerebellar tract, the cuneocerebellar tract, reticulocerebellar fibers, and olivocerebellar fibers, which numerically form the largest constitutent of this bundle. Both the posterior spinocerebellar and the cuneocerebellar tracts convey impulses from stretch receptors (i.e., Ia and Ib fibers) to the anterior lobe of the cerebellum, where they end, topographically.[8]

The *middle cerebellar peduncle* is the final link in the pathway between the cortex of one cerebral hemisphere and the posterior lobe of the contralateral cerebellum. Corticopontine fibers project to the ipsilateral pontine nuclei, and fibers from pontine nuclei cross in the basilar portion of the pons to enter the cerebellum via the middle cerebellar peduncle. Fibers that form this system are massive and interrelate virtually all regions of the cerebral cortex—including motor, somesthetic, auditory, visual, and associations areas—with parts of the posterior lobe of the cerebellum.

### Deep Cerebellar Nuclei

Within the medullary core (white matter) of the cerebellum are four paired nuclear masses, the *deep cerebellar nuclei* (Figure 3-4). The most lateral and largest is the dentate nucleus, which in section appears as a crumpled bag with the hilus directed medially. This nucleus receives most of its input from Purkinje cells in the hemisphere. Medial to the dentate nucleus are two smaller nuclei, the emboliform and globose nuclei, which receive inputs from Purkinje cells in paravermal regions of the cerebellar cortex. The most medial, and second largest of the deep cerebellar nuclei, the fastigial nucleus, receives Purkinje projections from all regions of the cerebellar vermis that converge in a fan-shaped array. The principle efferent

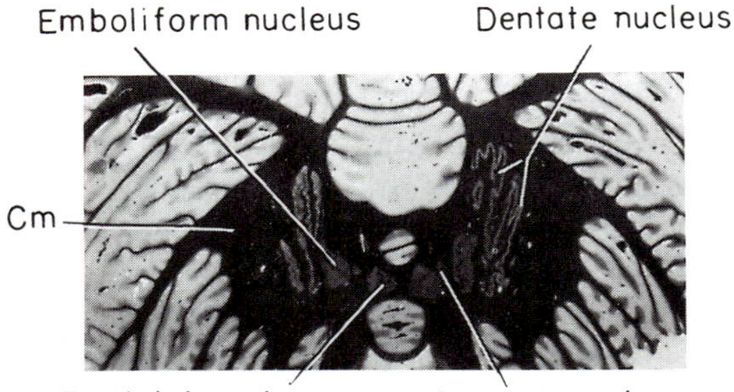

Figure 3-4. Section through the cerebellum shows parts of the deep cerebellar nuclei that lie within the white matter of the cerebellum. (From Carpenter MB. Core Text of Neuroanatomy, ed 3. Baltimore: Williams & Wilkins, 1985, with permission.)

fibers from the cerebellum arise from the deep cerebellar nuclei, are excitatory in nature, and are considered to use glutamate as their neurotransmitter.[2] Some direct excitatory influences on the deep cerebellar nuclei arise from extracerebellar sources, such as the red nucleus and the inferior olivary complex. Cortical inhibition of the deep cerebellar nuclei is intermittent and localized.

### Efferent Fibers

Two separate cerebellar efferent systems arise from the deep cerebellar nuclei. The largest and most important bundle, the *superior cerebellar peduncle,* arises from the dentate, emboliform, and globose nuclei, sweeps ventromediad in the caudal midbrain tegmentum, and decussates completely (Figures 3-3 and 3-5). Large numbers of fibers in the emboliform and globose nuclei project fibers and collaterals somatotopically upon cells in the caudal two thirds of the contralateral red nucleus.[9] Fewer fibers from these nuclei project rostrad to terminations in the contralateral thalamic nuclei.[10,11] Fibers from the dentate nucleus contained in the superior cerebellar peduncle project collaterals to the rostral third of the opposite red nucleus, and more profusely to terminations in the contralateral thalamus. Projections of these three cerebellar nuclei to the thalamus terminate in parts of the ventral lateral nuclei (VLc, pars caudalis) and the ventral posterolateral (VPLo, pars oralis) nuclei, which have been characterized as the "cell-sparse" zone.[11-13] Fibers from the individual deep cerebellar nuclei terminate in an interdigitating fashion without apparent overlap. Although evidence for a somatotopic representation in the deep cerebellar nuclei is not compelling, the pattern of efferent fiber terminations in the thalamus appears somatotopic: rostral parts of the body are represented medial in thalamus and anterior body parts (i.e., extremities) ventrally.[11] One of the most important features of the so-called cell-sparse zone of the thalamus is that it projects directly on the primary motor cortex.[10,14-16] This anatomic circuitry provides a means by which the major output of the deep cerebellar nuclei can influence somatic motor activity.

Fibers and collaterals from the emboliform and globose nuclei projecting somatotopically to the

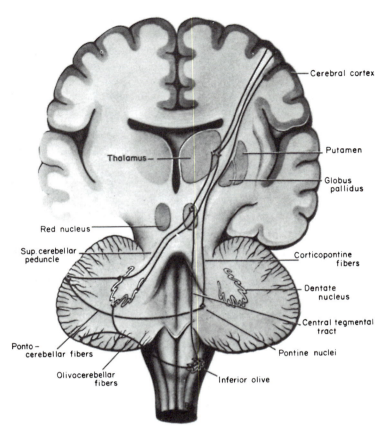

**Figure 3-5.** Schematic diagram of some afferent and efferent cerebellar pathways. Projections from all areas of the cortex pass to the pontine nuclei, which in turn give rise to fibers that pass via the middle cerebellar peduncle to the contralateral half of the cerebellum. Cortical efferents also project to parts of the ipsilateral inferior olivary nucleus, which project crossed climbing fibers to the cerebellar cortex of the opposite side. Purkinje cell axons project to the deep cerebellar nuclei, which in turn form the superior cerebellar peduncle. Fibers of the superior cerebellar peduncle cross in the midbrain, give collaterals and terminals to the red nucleus, and project to the cell-sparse zone in the ventral lateral thalamus. These thalamocortical fibers are considered to project somatotopically upon the primary motor cortex. (From Carpenter MB. Core Text of Neuroanatomy, ed 3. Baltimore: Williams & Wilkins, 1985, with permission.)

opposite red nucleus can influence ipsilateral flexor muscle tone via the rubrospinal tract (crossed).

Fastigial efferent fibers do not emerge from the cerebellum via the superior cerebellar peduncle. These fibers partially cross within the cerebellum and emerge via the uncinate fasciculus (crossed) and the juxtarestiform body (uncrossed) (Figure 3-6). In the brain stem fastigial efferent fibers are distributed fairly symmetrically in ventral parts of the lateral and inferior vestibular nuclei and in parts of the reticular formation.[17] Smaller numbers of ascending fibers project bilaterally to portions of the cell-sparse zone of the thalamus.[11] Fastigial projections to the lateral vestibular nucleus appear organized to facilitate extensor muscle tone via the vestibulospinal tract (uncrossed).

Although most of the cerebellar efferent fibers orginate from the deep cerebellar nuclei, regions of the vermal cortex project directly to the lateral vestibular nucleus.[18] Purkinje cell axons in the vermal cortex project selectively upon dorsal re-

gions of the ipsilateral lateral vestibular nucleus.[19,20] This connection means that GABA-ergic Purkinje cells can directly inhibit extensor muscle tone via their action upon cells of the lateral vestibular nucleus.

### Cerebellar Functions

Although the cerebellum receives a large part of its input from sensory systems, the cerebellum is not concerned with conscious sensory perception, but rather with the complex reciprocal innervations that underlie coordinated motor function. The cerebellum automatically regulates muscle tone and plays an integral part in virtually all simple and complex motor activity. One of the best ways of demonstrating the important regulatory role of the cerebellum is to describe the disturbances that occur with cerebellar lesions. Several general principles apply to cerebellar lesions: (1) distur-

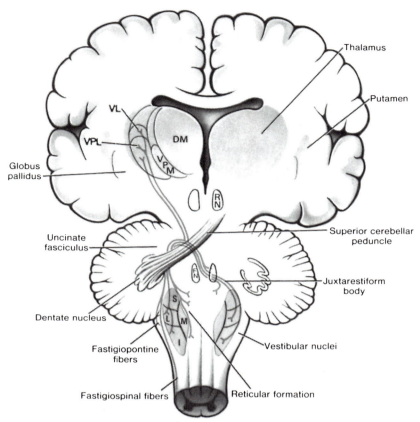

**Figure 3-6.** In a schematic diagram of fastigial efferent fibers, the fastigial nuclei lie in the cerebellar vermis, medial to the other deep cerebellar nuclei. They give rise to fibers that partially cross within the cerebellum (uncinate fasciculus) and ispsilateral fibers that leave the cerebellum via the juxtarestiform body. Crossed and uncrossed fastigial efferent fibers terminate fairly symmetrically in parts of the vestibular nuclei and the reticular formation. Ascending fastigial efferents project bilaterally (not shown), but in smaller numbers, to the cell-sparse zone of the thalamus. (From Carpenter MB. Core Text of Neuroanatomy, ed 3. Baltimore: Williams & Wilkins, 1985, with permission.)

bances occur ipsilateral the lesion, (2) disturbances usually occur as a constellation of related phenomena, (3) disturbances due to nonprogressive causes undergo attenuation with time, and (4) disturbances are viewed as the physiologic expression of the activity of intact structures deprived of the controlling and regulating influences of the cerebellum.

Three distinct cerebellar syndromes are recognized. The most common is the *neocerebellar syndrome,* associated with lesions of the lateral lobe of the cerebellum involving the dentate nucleus or the superior cerebellar peduncle. This syndrome is characterized by hypotonia and asynergic disturbances. Muscles on the side of the lesion show diminished resistance to passive movement, are soft, and tire easily with minimal activity. The tendon reflexes often are difficult to obtain and frequently exhibit a pendular quality. Asynergic disturbances are expressed by inappropriate force, direction, and range of muscle contractions. Impairment of ability to gauge distances in the finger-to-nose test is striking. Asynergia underlies the impaired ability to perform rapid successive movements (e.g., alternately pronating and supinating the forearm), the breaking up of complex movements into successive simple movements (e.g., decompensation of movement), and impaired ability to maintain certain positions and postures. The most dramatic asynergic disturbances are tremor and ataxia.

*Tremor* associated with neocerebellar lesions classically occurs during voluntary and associated movement, has a coarse quality, and is irregular in both frequency and amplitude. This tremor is referred to as *intention tremor,* but it is an involuntary motor activity that cannot be controlled by the patient, except by stopping all voluntary and associated movements. Cerebellar tremor frequently is contrasted with the tremor associated with Parkinson's disease (paralysis agitans), which classically occurs in the absence of voluntary motor activity.

*Ataxia* is a form of asynergic disturbance that results in bizzare gross and forceful distortions of basic movement patterns. This disturbance involves the large axial muscles and muscles of the shoulder and pelvic girdles that result in wild distortions of gait. The gait is broad based and unsteady; the patient lurches and stumbles; and there is a tendency to overstep and veer to one side.

Speech disturbances, common to neocerebellar lesions, are characterized by unnatural separation of syllables, uttered in a slurred and explosive manner. Nystagmus is common with these lesions and is most pronounced on the lesion side.

Lesions involving the posterior vermis (i.e., nodulus and uvula) produce the *archicerebellar syndrome.* Such lesions particularly affect axial musculature involved in maintenance of equilibrium and in locomotion. This syndrome, seen mainly in children with a midline cerebellar tumor (medulloblastoma), is characterized by unsteadiness in standing, a tendency to fall backward, and ataxic gait. Muscle tone is little affected and tremor usually is absent.

Though there is no paleocerebellar syndrome in humans, evidence from animal studies indicates that lesions in the anterior lobe of the cerebellum result in severe disturbances of posture and muscle tone. Animals with such lesions exhibit opisthotonus, hyperactive reflexes, increased positive supporting mechanisms, and periodic tonic seizures.[21]

Similar tonic seizures occur in humans as a consequence of brain stem compression. Classic studies of Sherrington[22] and Dow and Moruzzi[23] clearly indicate that ablations of the anterior lobe of the cerebellum cause exaggeration of decerebrate rigidity. Exaggeration of muscle tone following ablations of the anterior lobe appears to be due to the removal of inhibitory influences of Purkinje cells acting on brain stem nuclei that influence extensor muscle tone.

## The Basal Ganglia

The basal ganglia are large subcortical masses derived largely, but not exclusively, from the telencephalon or forebrain. The corpus striatum, consisting of the putamen, caudate nucleus, and globus pallidus, has long been regarded as an integrator of somatic motor functions. The oldest part of the basal ganglia, the amygdala, receives olfactory inputs and visceral afferents from brain stem nuclei. The amygdala has reciprocal connections with the hypothalamus and widely disseminated connections with the neocortex.[24] Because the amygdala is concerned primarily with visceral, behavioral, and endocrine functions it is regarded as an important component in the limbic system. In this discussion I focus on the corpus striatum and related nuclei that serve somatic motor functions. These structures are of great clinical interest because pathologic processes involving the corpus striatum and related nuclei are associated with a variety of syndromes characterized by forms of abnormal involuntary movement (referred to collectively as *dyskinesias*), disturbances of muscle tone, and sometimes impairment of other motor functions. Many of the syndromes involving the corpus striatum are progressive, and some are the result of genetic defects.

### Striatum

The caudate nucleus and the putamen together constitute the neostriatum, or striatum, the largest part of the corpus striatum. Both of these nuclear masses are derived from the telencephalon. The putamen lies lateral to the globus pallidus and deep to the insular cortex (Figure 3-7). The caudate

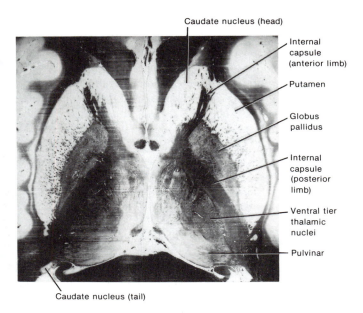

Caudate nucleus (head)

Internal capsule (anterior limb)

Putamen

Globus pallidus

Internal capsule (posterior limb)

Ventral tier thalamic nuclei

Pulvinar

Caudate nucleus (tail)

**Figure 3-7.** Horizontal section through the brain shows the relationships of the corpus striatum (caudate nucleus, putamen, and globus pallidus) to the internal capsule and thalamus.

nucleus has a C-shaped configuration that follows the curvature of the lateral ventricle (Figure 3-8). Rostrally and ventrally the caudate nucleus and the putamen are continuous. Cytologically the caudate nucleus and the putamen appear identical, and both are composed of enormous numbers of primarily small and medium-sized cells. Two classes of striatal neurons have been identified: those with spiny dendrites and those with smooth dendrities.[25,26] Spiny striatal neurons give rise to seven or eight primary dendrites radiating from the somata and one long axon projecting beyond the striatum (Figure 3-9). Dendrites of these neurons receive all striatal afferents. Axons of these cells provide all efferents. Immunocytochemically, spiny striatal neurons have at least three neurotransmitters, GABA, enkephalin (ENK), and substance P (SP).[27–30] Although GABA is the major neurotransmitter, in most cells it appears to coexist with ENK or SP.[30]

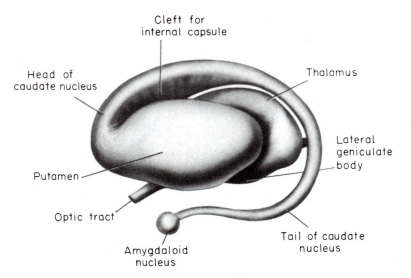

Cleft for internal capsule

Head of caudate nucleus

Putamen

Optic tract

Amygdaloid nucleus

Thalamus

Lateral geniculate body

Tail of caudate nucleus

**Figure 3-8.** Schematic drawing of the isolated neostriatum (caudate nucleus and putamen). The caudate nucleus and putamen are in continuity rostrally and ventrally. The caudate nucleus has a C shape that follows the curvature of the lateral ventricle. The tail of the caudate nucleus lies in the roof of the inferior horn of the lateral ventricle and extends rostrally to the amygdaloid nucleus. (From Carpenter MB. Core Text of Neuroanatomy, ed 3. Baltimore: Williams & Wilkins, 1985, with permission.)

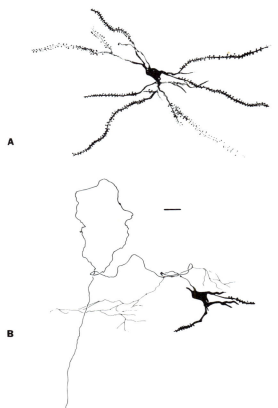

**A**

**B**

ceives massive inputs originating from diverse sources and each input has a different neurotransmitter. All known striatal inputs terminate upon dendrites of spiny neurons. Afferents to the striatum originate from (1) broad regions of the cerebral cortex (corticostriate), (2) thalamic nuclei (thalamostriate), (3) the pars compacta of the substantia nigra (SNC; nigrostriatal), (4) the dorsal nucleus of the raphe, (5) portions of the amygdala, and (6) cells of the substantia innominata (Figure 3-10).

### Corticostriate Fibers

Corticostriate fibers originate from broad areas of the cerebral cortex and terminate in "mosiac" patterns.[35–37] The primary motor area projects bilaterally and somatotopically upon the putamen in a patchy fashion.[38] Because corticostriate fibers originate from virtually all cortical areas, some of which have no demonstrated motor function, it seems likely that the striatum, or parts of it, may have other functions.[39,40] Corticostriate fibers

**Figure 3-9.** Drawings of a single spiny striatal neuron. All striatal inputs form synapses on dendritic spines of these cells and all axons of these cells project to either the globus pallidus or the substantia nigra. Immunocytochemical studies indicated that these cells have GABA, substance P, and enkephalin as their neurotransmitters; GABA is the dominant neurotransmitter. (A) Reconstruction of soma and dendrites; (B) reconstruction of soma and projecting axon. Calibration in B is 20 μm. (From Carpenter MB. Core Text of Neuroanatomy, ed 3. Baltimore: Williams & Wilkins, 1985, with permission.)

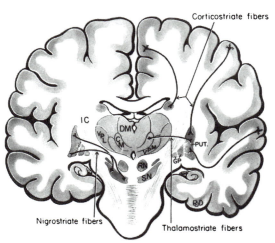

**Figure 3-10.** In a schematic diagram of striatal afferent systems, corticostriate fibers arise from broad areas of the cerebral cortex and terminate in a patchy fashion. Thalamostriate fibers arise from the centromedian (CM) and parafascicular (not shown) nuclei. Nigrostriate fibers convey dopamine to cells in the caudate nucleus and putamen. Not shown in this schematic are projections from the dorsal nucleus of the raphe, which convey serotonin to ventral parts of the putamen. (From Carpenter MB. Core Text of Neuroanatomy, ed 3. Baltimore: Williams & Wilkins, 1985, with permission.)

Three different short-axoned Golgi type II striatal neurons have no dendritic spines (i.e., "aspiny" neurons). These short-axoned cells are intrinsic striatal neurons. The most prevalent type (type I) uses GABA as its neurotransmitter, whereas the giant cells of type II are cholinergic.[31–34]

### Striatal Afferents

The neostriatum can be regarded as the receptive component of the corpus striatum because it re-probably use the excitatory neurotransmitter glutamate.[1,41]

### Thalamostriate Fibers

The intralaminar thalamic nuclei have long been identified as a source of input to the striatum.[42] Recent studies indicate that the centromedian nucleus projects to the putamen and the parafascicular nucleus to the caudate nucleus; very few cells in this complex project to both nuclei.[43] The neurotransmitter utilized by these fibers has not been identified.

### Nigrostriatal Fibers

Fluorescence histochemical studies first revealed the extensive nature of the dopaminergic projection system from the pars compacta of the substantia nigra (SNC) to the striatum.[44,45] Terminal dopamine varicosities form a fine matrix about virtually all striatal neurons; however, clusters of cells within the SNC project to either the putamen or the caudate nucleus, but not to both.[46,47] Pathologic processes that impair the synthesis and transmission of dopamine to the striatum constitute a major feature of Parkinson's disease. Dopamine is regarded as having an inhibitory action on striated neurons, but its effect is modulated by two different receptors.[48]

### Amygdalostriate Fibers

Though the amygdala and the corpus striatum have been considered to have different functions, these structures are in part related by a projection from the amygdala to both the caudate nucleus and the putamen.[49,50] Regions of the striatum that receive afferents from the amygdala are referred to as the *limbic striatum*. In addition, in monkeys about 10% of the cells of the substantia innominata (nucleus basalis) project to the caudate nucleus.[51]

### Other Striatal Afferents

Other afferents are minor in comparison to those already discussed. They arise from the dorsal nucleus of the raphe (DNR), the pedunculopontine nucleus (PPN), the locus ceruleus, and the subthalamic nucleus. Serotoninergic neurons in the DNR project to ventrocaudal regions of the putamen and provide collaterals to the substantia nigra.[52-54] The large cells of PPN are cholinergic and appear to project widely to thalamic nuclei.[55,56] A noncholinergic cell group central to PPN is considered to have projections to the striatum, globus pallidus, substantia nigra, and subthalamic nucleus.[57] The region of PPN is considered to be involved with locomotor functions.[58]

## Globus Pallidus

The globus pallidus lies medial to the putamen and consists of two distinct segments separated by thin medullary laminae (Figure 3-11). Unlike the striatum, the globus pallidus is a diencephalic derivative formed from hypothalamic neurons that have migrated lateral to the internal capsule.[59,60] Pallidal neurons are large, ovoid cells with smooth dendrites that ramify in discoid arrays parallel to the medullary laminae.[61,62] Virtually all pallidal neurons appear to use GABA as their neurotransmitter.[1,63,64]

Although the cells in the two segments of the globus pallidus appear morphologically and cytochemically identical, their afferent and efferent connections are different. The medial segment of the globus pallidus (MPS) gives rise to a major part of the output system for the entire corpus; the larger lateral pallidal segment (LPS) projects mainly to the subthalamic nucleus.[65] Surgical attempts to ameliorate dyskinesia in Parkinson's disease have been directed at interruption of pallidothalamic fibers originating in the MPS.

### Pallidal Afferent Systems

Major afferent fibers to the segments of the globus pallidus arise from the striatum and the subthalamic nucleus. Unlike the striatum, the globus pallidus does not receive inputs from the cerebral cortex, the thalamus, or the substantia nigra. The most massive inputs arise from spiny striatal neurons and project to both pallidal segments in an organized manner.[66-68]

*Striatopallidal fibers* traverse the discoid dendritic arbors of pallidal neurons making multiple synaptic contacts. GABA is the major neurotransmitter of striatopallidal fibers to both pallidal seg-

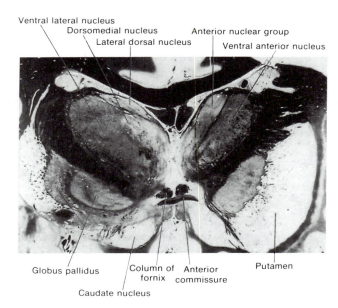

Ventral lateral nucleus
Dorsomedial nucleus
Lateral dorsal nucleus
Anterior nuclear group
Ventral anterior nucleus

Globus pallidus
Column of fornix
Anterior commissure
Putamen
Caudate nucleus

**Figure 3-11** Asymmetric transverse section through the thalamus, internal capsule, and corpus striatum. On the left segments of the globus pallidus are well-defined by medullary lamina. (From Carpenter MB. Core Text of Neuroanatomy, ed 3. Baltimore: Williams & Wilkins, 1985, with permission.)

ments,[69] but some of these fibers also contain SP and ENK. ENK fibers terminate selectively in the LPS; fibers containing SP end mainly in the MPS.[70,71]

*Subthalamopallidal fibers* arise from the subthalamic nucleus and project in arrays to both pallidal segments.[72,83] The neurotransmitter of subthalamic nucleus neurons is unknown.

### Pallidal Efferent Systems

Cells in each pallidal segment project to different brain stem nuclei (Figure 3-12). Fibers arising from the MPS project to thalamic nuclei that have access to regions of the motor cortex and in addition have a small descending projection to PPN. Cells in the LPS project almost exclusively to the subthalamic nucleus.[73]

*Pallidothalamic fibers* arising from the MPS must cross through, or go around, the internal capsule to reach the thalamus. These fibers follow both courses. Fibers that loop ventrally around the internal capsule form the *ansa lenticularis;* those that pass through the internal capsule form the *lenticular fasciculus* (Figure 3-12). Both of these fiber bundles merge and project to the rostral ventral tier thalamic nuclei. Pallidothalamic fibers terminate in the ventral lateral (VLo, pars oralis) and ventral anterior (VApc, pars principalis) nuclei of

the thalamus and give off collaterals to the centromedian nucleus.[74,75] Pallidothalamic projections have thalamic terminations distinct and separate from those that originate in the deep cerebellar nuclei.[10,12,15] Thalamic nuclei receiving fibers from the MPS project to the supplementary motor area (located on the medial aspect of the hemisphere) and to the lateral premotor area.[10,16] Thus, the major influences of the corpus striatum, mediated by striatopallidal, pallidothalamic, and thalamocortical fibers, are upon a motor cortical region considered to be concerned with programming of motor activities and known to influence motor function bilaterally.[76] Cells of the MPS have been demonstrated to project collaterals to both the thalamus and the pedunculopontine nucleus at isthmus levels of the brain stem.[77]

### Substantia Nigra

The substantia nigra, the largest single mesencephalic nucleus, lies dorsal to the crus cerebri and extends the length of this brain stem segment (Figure 3-13). The nucleus has two divisions: (1) The pars compacta (SNC), which lies dorsally, contains pigmented (melanin) cells that synthesize dopamine.[44,78] (2) The pars reticulata (SNR), close to the crus cerebri, is composed of less densely

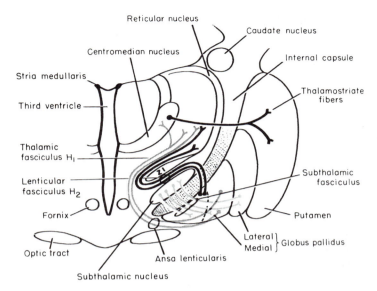

Reticular nucleus
Caudate nucleus
Centromedian nucleus
Internal capsule
Stria medullaris
Internal capsule
Thalamostriate
fibers
Third ventricle
Thalamic
fasciculus H₁
Lenticular
fasciculus H₂
Subthalamic
fasciculus
Fornix
Putamen
Optic tract
Lateral
Medial } Globus pallidus
Ansa lenticularis
Subthalamic nucleus

**Figure 3-12.** In a schematic diagram of projection fibers from the globus pallidus, pallidal efferent fibers from the medial segment project to rostral ventral tier thalamic nuclei (VApc and VLo) and the centromedian nucleus via the ansa lenticularis and the lenticular fasciculus. These fibers constitute the principal output of the corpus striatum. Fibers from the lateral pallidal segment project mainly to the subthalamic nucleus. The subthalamic nucleus projects mainly to both segments of the globus pallidus but also has a projection to the substantia nigra. (From Carpenter MB. Core Text of Neuroanatomy, ed 3. Baltimore: Williams & Wilkins, 1985, with permission.)

packed neurons containing the neurotransmitter GABA.[63] In Golgi preparations of the substantia nigra, cells of the SNC have dendrities oriented dorsoventrally whereas dendrities of cells in the SNR have a rostrocaudal orientation.[79] Cytologically distinct parts of the substantia nigra have different inputs and outputs. Cells of the SNC constitute the principal source of striatal dopamine, and cells of the SNR form part of the output system from the corpus striatum (i.e., striatonigral and nigrothalamic fibers).

*Nigral Afferents*

Afferents arise from the striatum, the subthalamic nucleus, the midbrain raphe, and the pedunculopontine nucleus. Each projection has a different neurotransmitter.

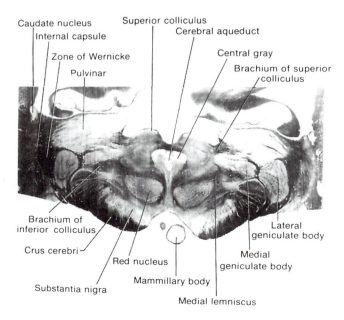

Caudate nucleus
Internal capsule
Superior colliculus
Cerebral aqueduct
Zone of Wernicke
Central gray
Pulvinar
Brachium of superior
colliculus
Brachium of
inferior colliculus
Lateral
geniculate body
Crus cerebri
Medial
geniculate body
Red nucleus
Substantia nigra
Mammillary body
Medial lemniscus

**Figure 3-13.** Transverse section of the midbrain through the substantia nigra. (From Carpenter MB. Core Text of Neuroanatomy, ed 3. Baltimore: Williams & Wilkins, 1985, with permission.)

*Striatonigral fibers* form the most massive input to the SNR. Like striatal afferents to the segments of the globus pallidus, these fibers use GABA, SP, and ENK as neurotransmitters. Terminals with different neurotransmitters are segregated in the SNR. GABA is the dominant neurotransmitter.[30]

The neurotransmitter of *subthalamonigral fibers* projecting to the SNR is as yet unidentified. A single population of subthalamic nucleus (STN) neurons has been shown to project to both the globus pallidus and the SNR. In rats, virtually all STN neurons project to both sites[80]; in monkeys only about 10% of the cells project to both the globus pallidus and the substantia nigra.[81]

*Midbrain Nigral Afferents* arise from the dorsal nucleus of the raphe (DNR) and from the pedunculopontine nucleus (PPN). Cells of the DNR use serotonin as their neurotransmitter and project to the SNR.[82,83] It is suspected that this projection has an inhibitory influence. Noncholinergic neurons from the midbrain locomotor center near PPN are considered to project to SNR, but their function is unknown.[57]

### Nigral Efferent Fibers

Efferent fibers from the two divisions of the substantia nigra project to different nuclei and have different neurotransmitters.

*Nigrostriatal fibers* arise from the cells of the SNC, have dopamine as their neurotransmitter, and terminate in a fine fiber matrix about all types of striatal neurons. Collections of cells in the SNC project to either the putamen or the caudate nucleus, but not to both.[47] The basic pathologic process in Parkinson's disease involves degeneration of dopaminergic neurons in the SNC, which reduces the synthesis and transmission of dopamine to the striatum. Dramatic improvements result from L-dopa therapy, which raises the level of dopamine in the striatum. L-Dopa, a precursor of dopamine, is given because dopamine does not pass the blood-brain barrier.

*Nigrothalamic fibers* represent the principal projection from cells of the SNR, which are known to be GABA-ergic. These fibers project to thalamic nuclei rostral to those that receive fibers from the MPS. In the thalamus they terminate in the ventral anterior (VAmc, pars magnocellularis), the ventromedial (VM, pars lateralis), and the paralaminar part of the dorsomedial (DMpl) nuclei.[84,85] These

thalamic nuclei are considered to relay signals to the premotor and prefrontal cortex.[86] Fibers that pass to the frontal eye field seem particularly important, as cells in SNR also project large numbers of collaterals to the superior colliculus.[47,87] Though the full significance of the nigrothalamic projection remains unknown, it forms a significant part of the output system of the corpus striatum.

### Subthalamic Nucleus

The STN is a small lens-shaped nucleus medial to the fibers of the posterior limb of the internal capsule immediately rostrad to the substantia nigra (Figure 3-14). Like the globus pallidus it is a derivative of the lateral cell column of the hypothalamus. Interest in this nucleus centers around the observation that small lesions in it produce the most violent known form of dyskinesia, hemiballism.[88] Discrete lesions in the STN of monkeys produce a similar form of dyskinesia, the only dyskinesia that can be produced in an animal by a small localized lesion.[89,90]

Neurons of the STN in humans and primates exhibit a wide range of sizes and shapes, have six or seven stem dendrites, and all have long axons. Evolved differences in dendritic development confer upon primates the potential for more specific organization.[91,92] Some labeled STN neurons of rats reveal dichotomizing axons with branches that project to both the globus pallidus and the SNR.[93]

### Subthalamic Afferents

Projections to the subthalamic nucleus (STN) arise mainly from the motor cortex and the lateral pallidal segment. *Corticosubthalamic fibers* project ipsilaterally and somatotopically upon lateral parts of the STN[94] and are considered to monosynaptically excite STN neurons.[95] The most massive input to the STN arises from the lateral pallidal segment, to form the *pallidosubthalamic projection*.[72,73,75,83] It is inhibitory and has GABA as its neurotransmitter.[64,96]

### Subthalamic Efferents

Cells of the STN project profusely to both segments of the globus pallidus, and about 10% pro-

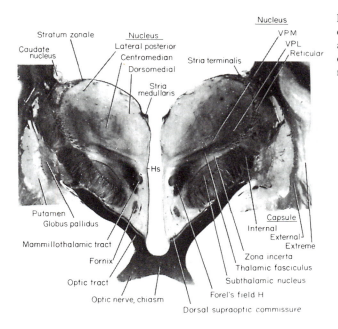

Figure 3-14. Transverse section through the diencephalon and corpus striatum showing the subthalamic nucleus on the medial border of the internal
capsule. (From Carpenter MB. Core Text of Neuroanatomy, ed 3. Baltimore: Williams & Wilkins,
1985, with permission.)

ject to both globus pallidus and SNR.[81] The neurotransmitter of STN neurons remains unknown.[97]
Claims that it might be GABA[98,99] have not been
substantiated by immunocytochemical methods. It
has been suggested that the STN may have excitatory influences on pallidal neurons.[100] Though
STN neurons have no projection to thalamic nuclei, these cells appear organized to modulate the
output systems from the MPS and the SNR that
have access to thalamic neurons that can influence
activity of cortical neurons.

*Functional Considerations*

Though considerable progress has been made in
understanding the anatomical organization of the
corpus striatum and related nuclei, the physiological mechanisms and the neurotransmitters that effect and modulate these activities are just beginning to be understood. The principal thrust of
current research is to define anatomical pathways
and the respective neurotransmitters. Such information not only provides a key to physiological
mechanisms but in some instances leads to specific
therapy.

Most of the diseases of the corpus striatum are
associated with relatively widespread pathological
processes, but for many syndromes it has been
possible to focus on key elements. This has been
most successful in Parkinson's disease, which is
characterized by *tremor at rest* (in the absences of
voluntary movement), *rigidity, bradykinesia*
(slowness of movement), and certain autonomic
disturbances. The tremor is a rhythmical, alternating activity of relative regular frequency and amplitude that commonly involves the digits (pill rolling) and the lips. Rigidity, which is progressive
and involves virtually all muscles, is the most
disabling disturbance. Rigidity can easily be demonstrated by passively flexing and extending the
limbs or by passively rotating the the hand at the
wrist in a circular fashion. These movements are
interrupted by a series of jerks, referred to as
*"cog-wheel"* *phenomena.* In addition to these
"positive" features, Parkinsonism is characterized
by what have been called "negative" features.
Negative features actually are neural deficits expressed in impairment of locomotion, postural fixation, phonation, or speech. Patients with the par-
kinsonian syndrome exhibit a masklike face, blink
infrequently, and have a stooped posture with characteristic flexion of the neck, trunk, and knees.
The gait is slow and shuffling and the steps are
small. There is a loss of associated movements
(swing of the arms when walking), and speech is
slow and dysarthric. Many of these patients show
amelioration of these disturbances after L-dopa
therapy, which supplies the needed striatal dopa-

mine. While this therapy brings dramatic improvement initially, it often appears to be less effective over time, probably because the basic progressive pathologic process is not arrested by this drug.

The accidental observation that a clandestinely synthesized cocaine contained a meperdine analogue (1, methyl-4-phenyl-4-1,2,56-tetrahydropyridine, MPTP) that produced a severe and chronic form of parkinsonism, provided additional evidence implicating the cells of the substantia nigra in this syndrome.[101] With this meperdine analogue it has been possible to produce a Parkinson's-like syndrome in monkeys associated with degeneration in the substantia nigra.[102] This animal model provides opportunities for studies that cannot be done on humans.

The term *athetosis* is used to describe a form of dyskinesia characterized by slow, writhing, vermicular movements involving the extremities, cervical muscles, and face. Athetosis gives the appearance of a mobile spasm. *Dystonia,* considered a form of athetosis, involves the axial muscles. Involuntary contractions of the axial muscles results in bizzare distortions and twisting of the trunk. Athetosis and dystonia often occur together.[103] This type of dyskinesia frequently is part of the cerebral palsy syndrome that involves both the cerebral cortex and large parts of the corpus striatum. Paresis and spasticity often are severe. The slow, writhing quality of the dyskinesia appears in part to be related to the paresis and spasticity.

*Chorea* is the term applied to a variety of dyskinesias characterized by involuntary movements that have a brisk, graceful quality and resemble fragments of purposeful movements. Choreoid activity most commonly is seen in the muscles of the hands, face, and tongue. Moderate degrees of hypotonus occur in this syndrome. Choreoid activity occurs as a consequence of a number of disease processes, but it is most commonly associated with Huntington's disease,[104] a hereditary disorder associated with an autosomal dominant gene localized on chromosome 4. Symptoms are progressive and reflect both behavioral and motor disturbances. The cerebral cortex and the corpus striatum bear the brunt of the pathologic process, but changes are not confined to these structures. Brains of patients who died from Huntington's disease demonstrate that striatal neurons have reduced concentrations of GABA and choline acetyltransferase; in these same patients tyrosine hydroxylase and dopamine appeared nearly normal in the striatum.[105] It is well known that large doses of L-dopa given to patients with Parkinson's syndrome may cause choreiform activity to appear. In addition, L-dopa tends to exacerbate choreoid activity in Huntington's disease. It would seem logical to try to increase striatal GABA in this syndrome. Such attempts have met with little success, because GABA does not pass the blood-brain barrier and because GABA-ergic and cholinergic receptors may be damaged and/or reduced in number.

*Ballism* or *hemiballism* is the term used to describe the violent, forceful, flinging movements, primarily of the proximal appendicular musculature. This form of dyskinesia usually appears suddenly in elderly patients with hypertension as a consequence of a small vascular lesion in the subthalamic nucleus.[88] The violence of the dyskinesia is exhausting, and without treatment most patients succumb from secondary medical problems. This is the only syndrome of this group that can be produced in monkeys by a small, discrete lesion.[89] These animals exhibit marked hypotonus and ballistic activity contralateral to the lesion. Ballistic activity in monkeys shows some attenution with time but is still recognizable a year after the lesion was produced. This form of dyskinesia can be ameliorated and abolished by lesions of the medial pallidal segment or ventral lateral thalamic nuclei that convey signals to the thalamus and the cerebral cortex.[89] Lesions of these types do not produce paresis. The original working hypothesis in this unique form of dyskinesia was that destruction of at least 20% of the cells in the STN, which project to the globus pallidus, resulted in removal of inhibitory influences on the cells of the medial pallidal segment. The removal of this inhibition (i.e., release phenomenon) was considered to be expressed by the appearance of ballistic activity on the opposite side of the body.

Additional information on the physiologic activities of the subthalamic nucleus and globus pallidus suggest that the neural mechanism may be much more complex. Determination of the neurotransmitter for subthalamic nucleus neurons seems to be crucial to a complete understanding of this form of dyskinesia, and to the development of specific therapy.

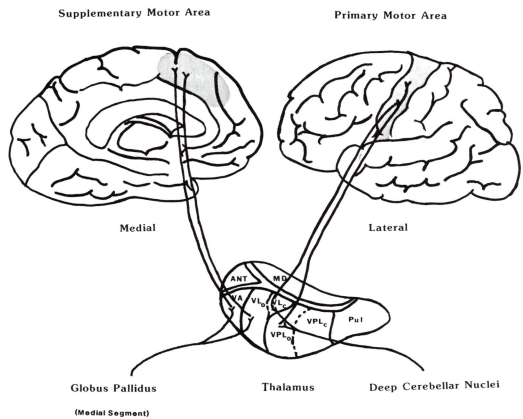

**Supplementary Motor Area**

**Primary Motor Area**

Medial

Lateral

**Globus Pallidus**          **Thalamus**          **Deep Cerebellar Nuclei**

**(Medial Segment)**

**Figure 3-15.** Schematic diagram comparing the thalamic and cortical projections of the globus pallidus and the deep cerebellar nuclei. Fibers from the medial pallidal segment project ipsilaterally to the ventral anterior (VApc) and ventral lateral (VLo) thalamic nuclei. These nuclei project upon the supplementary motor area located on the medial aspect of the hemisphere. Ascending projections from the deep cerebellar nuclei cross in the midbrain and terminate in the so-called cell-sparse zone of the thalamus (VLc and VPLo). Cells in the cell-sparse zone of the thalamus project directly to the primary motor cortex. Key: Ant, anterior nuclei of the thalamus; MD, mediodorsal nucleus; Pul, pulvinar; VPLc, ventral posterolateral nucleus, pars caudalis.

Comparisons of cerebellar and basal ganglia dyskinesia reveal certain common features in their neural mechanisms, even though these structures are widely separate and have different neurotransmitters. Both the cerebellar cortex and the corpus striatum have massive input systems that convey highly varied information. Both output systems have major influences on thalamic nuclei, but each system has descending components that modify activities of brain stem nuclei. Thalamic nuclei, which receive the outputs of the cerebellum and the corpus striatum (from the medial globus pallidus and the pars reticulata of the substantia ni-

gra), are entirely separate and without overlap. These separate thalamic relay nuclei exert their influences on related but different regions of the motor cortex (Figure 3-15). Cerebellar influences are exerted on the primary motor cortex; influences of the corpus striatum complex act upon the supplementary motor area, a region that in part appears to operate through the primary motor area. The primary motor area, associated with skilled, voluntary motor function, acts almost exclusively on contralateral segmental motor neurons. The supplementary motor area is a bilateral system involved in programming motor functions at cortical levels and appears to be involved in most motor activities.

## References

1. Ottersen OP, Storm-Mathisen J. Glutamate- and GABA-containing neurons in the mouse and rat brain, as demonstrated with a new immunocyto-chemical technique. J Comp Neurol 1984; 229:374–392.
2. Monaghan PL, Beitz AJ, Larson AA, et al. Immunocytochemical localization of glutamate- glu-taminase- and aspartate aminotransferase-like immunoreactivity in the rat deep cerebellur nuclei. Brain Res 1986; 363:364–370.
3. Chan-Palay V, Nilaver G, Palay S, et al. Chemical heterogeneity in cerebellar Purkinje cells: Existence and coexistence of glutamic acid decarbox-ylase-like and motlin-like immunoreactivities. Proc Natl Acad Sci USA 1981; 78:7787–7791.
4. Eccles JC, Ito M, Szentagothai J. The Cerebellum as a Neuronal Machine. New York: Springer Verlag, 1967.
5. Hudson DB, Valcana T, Bean G, et al. Glutamic acid: A strong candidate as the neurotransmitter of the cerebellar granule cell. Neurochem Res 1976; 1:73–81.
6. Wiklund L, Toggenburger G, Cuenod M. Selective retrograde labeling of the rat olivocerebellar climbing fiber system with D-[³H] aspartate. Neuroscience 1984; 13:441–468.
7. Snider RS. Recent contributions to the anatomy and physiology of the cerebellum. Arch Neurol Psychiatry 1950; 64:196–219.
8. Carpenter MB. Core Text of Neuroanatomy, ed 3. Baltimore: Williams & Wilkins, 1985.
9. Courville J. Somatotopical organization of the projection from the nucleus interpositus anterior of the cerebellum to the red nucleus: An experimental study in the cat with silver impregnation methods. Exp Brain Res 1966; 2:191–215.
10. Asanuma C, Thach WT, Jones EG. Distribution of cerebellar terminations and their relation to other afferent terminations in the ventral lateral thalamic region of the monkey. Brain Res Rev 1983; 5:237–265.
11. Asanuma C, Thach WT, Jones EG. Anatomical evidence for segregated focal groupings of efferent cells and their terminal ramifications in the cere-bellothalamic pathway of the monkey. Brain Res Rev 1983; 5:267–297.
12. Percheron G. The thalamic territory of cerebellar afferents and the lateral region of the thalamus of the macaque in stereotaxic ventricular coordinates. J Hirnforsch 1977; 18:375–400.
13. Thach WT, Jones EG. The cerebellar dentatothalamic connection: Terminal field, lamellar, rods and somatotopy. Brain Res 1979; 169:168–172.
14. Jones EG, Wise SP, and Coulter JD. Differential thalamic relationships of sensory-motor and parietal cortical fields in monkeys. J Comp Neurol 1979; 183:833–881.
15. Tracey DJ, Asanuma C, Jones EG, et al. Thalamic relay to motor cortex: Afferent pathways from brain stem, cerebellum and spinal cord in monkeys. J Neurophysiol 1980; 44:532–554.
16. Schell GR, Strick PL. The origin of thalamic inputs to the arcuate premotor and supplementary motor areas. J Neurosci 1984; 4:539–560.
17. Carpenter MB, Batton RR III. Connections of the fastigial nucleus in the cat and monkey. Exp Brain Res 1982; 6 (suppl):250–295.
18. Carleton SC, Carpenter MB. Afferent and efferent connections of the medical, inferior and lateral vestibular nuclei in the cat and monkey. Brain Res 1983; 278:29–51.
19. Walberg F, Jansen J. Cerebellovestibular fibers in the cat. Exp Neurol 1961; 3:32–52.
20. Houser CR, Barber RP, Vaughn JE. Immuno-ctyochemical localization of glutamic acid decarboxylase in the dorsal lateral vestibular nucleus: Evidence for an intrinsic and extrinsic GABA-ergic innervation. Neurosci Lett 1984; 47:213–220.
21. Fulton JF. Functional Localization in the Frontal Lobes and Cerebellum. Oxford: Clarendon Press, 1949.
22. Sherrington CS. Decerebrate rigidity and reflex coordination of movements. J Physiol 1898; 22:319–332.
23. Dow RS, Moruzzi G. Albation experiments. In: Dow RS, Moruzzi G, eds. The Physiology and Pathology of the Cerebellum. Minneapolis: University of Minnesota Press, 1958; 8–102.
24. Amaral DG, Price JL. Amygdalo-cortical projec-

This work was supported by research grants CO7005 from the Department of Defense, Uniformed Services University of the Health Sciences, and NS-26658 from the National Institutes of Health, Bethesda, Maryland. The opinions and assertions contained herein are the private ones of the author and are not to be construed as official or reflecting the views of the Department of Defense or the Uniformed Services University of the Health Sciences. Experiments reported herein were conducted according to the principles set forth in the *Guide for the Care and Use of Laboratory Animals,* Institute of Laboratory Animal Resources, National Research Council, NIH Pub. No. 80-23.

tions in the monkey (Macaca fascicularis). J Comp Neurol 1984; 230:465–496.

25. DiFiglia M, Pasik P, Pasik T. A Golgi study of neuronal types in the neostriatum of monkeys. Brain Res 1976; 114:245–256.

26. Pasik P, Pasik T, DiFiglia M. The internal organization of the neostriatum in mammals. In: Divac I, ed. The Neostriatum. Oxford: Pergamon Press, 1979; 5–36.

27. Jessell TM, Emson PC, Paxinos G, et al. Topographical projections of substance P and GABA pathways in the striato- and pallido-nigral system: A biochemical and immunohistochemical study. Brain Res 1978; 152:487–498.

28. Ribak CE. The GABAergic neurons of the extrapyramidal system as revealed by immunocytochemistry. In: DiChiara G, Gessa GL, eds. GABA and the Basal Ganglia, New York: Raven Press, 1981; 23–36.

29. DiFiglia M, Aronin N, Martin JB. Light and electron microscopic localization of immunoreactive Leu-enkephalin in the monkey basal ganglia. J Neurosci 1982; 2:303–320.

30. Penny GR, Afsharpour S, Kitai ST. The glutamic acid decarboxylase- , leucine- , enkephalin- , methionine enkephalin- , and substance P-immunoreactive neurons in the neostriatum of the rat and cat: Evidence for partial population overlap. Neuroscience 1986; 17:1011–1045.

31. Ribak CE, Vaughn JE, Roberts E. The GABA neurons and their axon terminals in the rat corpus striatum as demonstrated by GAD immunocytochemistry. J Comp Neurol 1979; 187:261–284.

32. Kimura H, McGeer RL, Pong JH, et al. The central cholinergic system studied by choline acetyltransferase immunohistochemistry in the cat. J Comp Neurol 1980; 200:151–201.

33. Parent A, Csonka C, Etienne P. The occurrence of large acetylcholinesterase-containing neurons in human neostriatum as disclosed in normal and Alzheimer's disease brains. Brain Res 1984; 291:154–158.

34. Pasik P, Pasik T, Holstein GR, et al. GABAergic elements in the neuronal circuits of the monkey neostriatum: A light and electron microscopic immunocytochemical study. J Comp Neurol 1988; 270:157–170.

35. Goldman PS, Nauta WJH. An intricately patterned prefrontocaudate projection in the rhesus monkey. J Comp Neurol 1977; 171:369–386.

36. Jones EG, Coulter JD, Burton H, et al. Cells of origin and terminal distribution of efferent cells in the sensory-motor cortex of monkeys. J Comp Neurol 1977; 175:391–438.

37. Künzle H. An autoradiographic analysis of the efferent connections from premotor and adjacent prefrontal regions (areas 6 and 9) in Macaca fascicularis. Brain Behav Evol 1978; 15:185–234.

38. Künzle H. Bilateral projections from precentral motor cortex to the putamen and other parts of the basal ganglia. Brain Res 1975; 88:195–210.

39. Divac I. Neostriatum and functions of prefrontal cortex. Acta Neurobiol Exp 1972; 32:461–477.

40. Rolls ET, Williams GV. Neuronal activity in the ventral striatum of primates. In: Carpenter MB, Jayaraman A, eds. Basal Ganglia II Structure and Function—Current Concepts. New York: Plenum Press, 1987; 349–356.

41. Fonnum F, Storm-Mathison J, Divac I. Biochemical evidence for glutamate as neurotransmitter in corticostriate and corticothalamic fibres in rat brain. Neuroscience 1981; 6:863–873.

42. Powell TPS, Cowan WM. A study of thalamostriate relations in the monkey. Brain 1956; 79:364–390.

43. Smith Y, Parent A. Differential connections of caudate nucleus and putamen in the squirrel monkey (Saimiri sciureus), Neuroscience 1986; 18:347–371.

44. Dahlström A, Fuxe K. Evidence for the existence of monamine containing neurons in the central nervous system. I. Demonstration of monoamines in the cell bodies of brain stem neurons. Acta Physiol Scand 1964; 62:1–55.

45. Andén N-E, Dahlström A, Fuxe K, et al. Ascending monoamine neurons to the telencephalon and diencephalon. Acta Physiol Scand 1966; 67:313–326.

46. Parent A, Mackey A, DeBellefeuille L. The subcortical afferents to caudate nucleus and putamen in primate: A fluorescence retrograde double labeling study. Neuroscience 1983; 10:1137–1150.

47. Parent A, Mackey A, Smith Y, et al. The output organization of the substantia nigra in primate as revealed by a retrograde double labeling method. Brain Res Bull 1983; 10:529–537.

48. Calabresi P, Mercuri N, Stanzione P, et al. Role of D1 and D2 dopamine receptors in the mammalian striatum: Electrophysiological studies and functional implications. In: Carpenter MB, Jayaraman A, eds. The Basal Ganglia II Stucture and Function—Current Concepts. New York: Plenum Press, 1987; 145–148.

49. Kelley AE, Domesick VB, Nauta WJH. The amygdalostriatal projection in the rat. An anatomical study by anterograde and retrograde tracing methods. Neuroscience 1982; 7:615–630.

50. Russchen FT, Price JL. Amygdalostriatal projec-

tions in rat. Topographical organization and fiber morphology shown using lectin PHA-L as an anterograde tracer. Neurosci Lett 1984; 47:15–22.

51. Arikuni T, Kubota K. Substantia innominata projection to caudate nucleus in macaque monkeys. Brain Res 1984; 302:184–189.

52. Dray A. The physiology and pharmacology of mammalian basal ganglia. Prog Neurol 1980; 14:221–335.

53. van der Kooy D, Hattori T. Dorsal raphe cells with collateral projections to the caudate-putamen and substantia nigra: A fluorescent retrograde double labeling study in the rat. Brain Res 1980; 186:1–7.

54. Parent A, Descarries L, Beaudet A. Organization of ascending serotonin systems in the adult rat brain. A radioautographic study after intraventricular administration of [$^3$H] 5-hydroxytryptamine. Neuroscience 1981; 6:115–138.

55. Sugimoto T, Hattori T. Organization and efferent projections of nucleus tegmenti pedunculopontinus pars compacta with special reference to its cholinergic aspects. Neuroscience 1984; 11:931–946.

56. Hallanger AE, Levey AI, Lee HJ, et al. The origins of cholinergic and other subcortical afferents to the thalamus in the rat. J Comp Neurol 1987; 262:105–124.

57. Lee HJ, Rye DB, Hallanger AE, et al. Cholinergic versus noncholinergic efferents from the mesopontine tegmentum to the extrapyramidal motor system nuclei. J Comp Neurol 1988; 275:469–492.

58. Garcia-Rill E. The basal ganglia and the locomotor regions. Brain Res Rev 1986; 11:46–63.

59. Kuhlenbeck H, Haymaker W. The derivatives of the hypothalamus in the human brain; their relation to the extrapyramidal and autonomic systems. Milit Surgeon 1949; 105:26–52.

60. Richter E. Die Entwicklung des Globus Pallidus und des Corpus Subthalamicum. Berlin: Springer-Verlag, 1965.

61. Francois C, Percheron G, Yelnik J, et al. A Golgi analysis of the primate globus pallidus. I. Inconstant processes of large neurons, other neuronal types and afferent axons. J Comp Neurol 1984; 227:182–199.

62. Yelnik J, Percheron G, Francois C. A Golgi analysis of the primate globus pallidus. II. Quantitative morphology and spatial orientation of dendritic arborizations. J Comp Neurol 1984; 227:200–213.

63. Mugnaini E, Oertel WH. An atlas of the distribution of GABAergic neurons and terminals in the rat CNS as revealed by GAD immunohistochemistry. In: Björklund A, Hökfelt T, eds. Handbook of Chemical Neuroanatomy, GABA and Neuro-

peptides in the CNS. Amsterdam: Elsevier, 1985; 436–595.

64. Smith Y, Parent A, Seguela P, et al. Distribution of GABA-immunoreactive neurons in the basal ganglia of the squirrel monkey (*Saimiri sciureus*). J Comp Neurol 1987; 259: 50–64.

65. Carpenter MB. Anatomy of the basal ganglia. In: Vinken P, Bruyn GW, Klawans H, eds. Handbook of Clinical Neurology. Amsterdam: Elsevier, 1987; 1–18.

66. Szabo J. Topical distribution of striatal efferents in the monkey. Exp Neurol 1962; 5:21–36.

67. Szabo J. The efferent projections of the putamen in the monkey. Exp Neurol 1967; 19:463–476.

68. Szabo J. Projections from the body of the caudate nucleus in the rhesus monkey. Exp Neurol 1970; 27:1–15.

69. Fonnum F, Gottesfeld Z, Grofova I. Distribution of glutamate decarboxylase, choline acetyltransferase and aromatic amino acid decarboxylase in the basal ganglia of normal and operated rats. Evidence for striatopallidal, striatoentopeduncular and striatonigral GABAergic fibers. Brain Res 1978; 153:370–374.

70. Haber SN, and Elde RP. Correlation between metenkephalin and substance P immunoreactivity in the primate globus pallidus. Neuroscience 1981; 6:1291–1297.

71. Haber SN, Elde RP. The distribution of enkephalin immunoreactive fibers and terminals in the monkey central nervous system: an immunohistochemical study. Neuroscience 1982; 7:1049–1095.

72. Carpenter MB, Batton RR III, Carleton SC, et al. Interconnections and organization of pallidal and subthalamic nucleus neurons in the monkey. J Comp Neurol 1981; 197:579–603.

73. Carpenter MB, Fraser RAR, Shriver J. The organization of the pallidosubthalamic fibers in the monkey. Brain Res 1968; 11:522–559.

74. Kuo JS, Carpenter MB. Organization of pallidothalamic projections in the rhesus monkey. J Comp Neurol 1973; 151:201–236.

75. Kim R, Nakano K, Jayaraman A, et al. Projections of the globus pallidus and adjacent structures: An autoradiographic study in the monkey. J Comp Neurol 1976; 169:263–289.

76. Porter R. Corticomotorneuronal projections: Synaptic events related to skilled movement. Proc R Soc Lond 1987; B231:147–168.

77. Parent A, DeBellefeuille L. Organization of efferent projections from the internal segment of the globus pallidus in primate as revealed by fluorescence retrograde labeling method. Brain Res 1982; 245:201–213.

78. Hökfelt T, Ungerstedt U. Electron and fluores-

cence microscopical studies on the nucleus caudatus putamen of the rat after unilateral lesions of ascending nigro-neostriatal dopamine neurons. Acta Physiol Scand 1969; 76:415–426.

79. Rinvik E, Grofová I. Observations on the fine structure of the substantia nigra in the cat. Exp Brain Res 1970; 11:229–248.

80. van der Kooy D, Hattori T. Single subthalamic nucleus neurons project to both globus pallidus and substantia nigra in rat. J Comp Neurol 1980; 192:751–768.

81. Parent A, Smith Y. Organization of efferent projections of the subthalamic nucleus of the squirrel monkey as revealed by retrograde labeling method. Brain Res 1987; 436:296–310.

82. Kanazawa I, Marshall GR, Kelly JS. Afferents to the rat substantia nigra studied with horseradish peroxidase, with special reference to fibres from the subthalamic nucleus. Brain Res 1976; 115:485–491.

83. Carpenter MB, Carleton SC, Keller JT, et al. Connections of the subthalamic nucleus in the monkey. Brain Res 1981; 224:1–29.

84. Carpenter MB, Peter P. Nigrostriatal and nigrothalamic fibers in the rhesus monkey. J Comp Neurol 1972; 144:93–116.

85. Carpenter MB, Nakano K, Kim R. Nigrothalamic projections in the monkey demonstrated by autoradiographic technics. J Comp Neurol 1976; 144:93–116.

86. Ilinsky IA, Jouandet ML, Goldman-Rakic PS. Organization of the nigrothalamocortical system in the rhesus monkey. J Comp Neurol 1985; 236:315–330.

87. Anderson ME, Yoshida M. Axonal branching patterns and location of nigrothalamic and nigrocollicular neurons in the cat. J Neurophysiol 1980; 43:883–895.

88. Whittier, JR. Ballism and the subthalamic nucleus (nucleus hypothalamicus; corpus luysi). Arch Neurol Psychiatry 1947; 58:672–692.

89. Carpenter MB, Whittier JR, Mettler FA. Analysis of choreoid hyperkinesia in the rhesus monkey: Surgical and pharmacological analysis of hyperkinesia resulting from lesions in the subthalamic nucleus of Luys. J Comp Neurol 1950; 92:293–331.

90. Carpenter MB. Brain stem and infratentorial neuraxis in experimental dyskinesia. Arch Neurol 1961; 5:504–524.

91. Yelnik J, Percheron G. Subthalamic neurons in primates: A quantitative and comparative analysis. Neuroscience 1979; 4:1717–1743.

92. Hammond C, Yelnik J. Intracellular labeling of rat subthalamic neurones with horseradish peroxidase: Computer analysis of dendrites and characterization of axon arborization. Neuroscience 1983; 8:781–790.

93. Kita H, Chang HT, Kitai ST. The morphology of intracellularly labeled rat subthalamic neurons: A light microscopic analysis. J Comp Neurol 1983; 215:245–257.

94. Hartmann-von Monakow K, Akert K, Künzle H. Projections of the precentral motor cortex and other cortical areas of the frontal lobe to the subthalamic nucleus in the monkey. Exp Brain Res 1978; 33:395–403.

95. Kitai ST, Deniau JM. Cortical inputs to the subthalamus, intracellular analysis. Brain Res 1981; 214:411–415.

96. Tsubokawa T, Sutin J. Pallidal and tegmental inhibition of oscillatory slow waves and unit activity in the subthalamic nucleus. Brain Res 1972; 41:101–118.

97. Kita H, Chang HT, Kitai ST. Pallidal inputs to subthalamus: Intracellular analysis. Brain Res 1983; 264:255–265.

98. Nauta HJW, Cuenod M. Perikaryal cell labeling in the subthalamic nucleus following the injection of [$^3$H]-γ-aminobutyric acid into the pallidal complex: An autoradiographic study in cat. Neuroscience 1982; 7:2725–2734.

99. Crossman AR, Sambrook MA, Jackson A. Experimental hemichorea/hemiballismus in the monkey: Studies on the intracerebral site of action in a drug induced dyskinesia. Brain 1984; 107:579–596.

100. Kitai ST, Kita H. Anatomy and physiology of the basal ganglia [Abstr]. Proc Int Union Physiol Sci 1986; 16:516.

101. Langston JW, Ballard P, Tetrud JW, et al. Chronic parkinsonism in humans due to a product of meperidine synthesis. Science 1983; 249:979–980.

102. Kolata G. Monkey model of Parkinson's disease. A contaminant of illicit drugs has caused Parkinson's disease in humans and monkeys. Science 1983; 230:705.

103. Carpenter MB. Athetosis and the basal ganglia. Arch Neurol Psychiatry 1950; 63:875–901.

104. Gusella JF, Wexler NS, Conneally PM. A polymorphic DNA marker genetically linked to Huntington's disease. Nature 1983; 306:234–238.

105. Bird ED, Iversen LL. Huntington's chorea: Postmortem measurements of glutamic acid decarboxylase, choline acetyltransferase and dopamine in basal ganglia. Brain 1974; 97:457–472.

# Chapter 4

# The Autonomic Nervous System

MARTHA E. HEATH

The autonomic nervous system (ANS) regulates the action of smooth muscle and glands. Its efferent nerves supply all tissues except skeletal muscle and are involved in the regulation of heart contraction, blood vessel diameter, sweating, saliva secretion, pupil diameter, intestinal secretions and movement, kidney function, piloerection, urination, sexual function, and lipolysis. Thus, it is responsible for orchestrating much of the automatic life-sustaining processes of circulation (heart rate, cardiac output, blood flow, blood pressure), temperature regulation, metabolism, digestion, fluid balance, and adrenergic function. These processes are discussed in detail in other chapters. In this chapter I focus on the organization and function of the autonomic nervous system.

## Terminology

The terms *autonomic nervous system,*[1–3] *involuntary nervous system,*[4] and *vegetative nervous system*[5] are synonymous. Two subdivisions of the ANS have long been recognized, but the popularization of three different sets of terminology, which are not completely interchangeable, can cause some confusion. The terms *sympathetic* (which has its origin in the 16th century) and *parasympathetic* were coined as labels for two subdivisions that often have opposite effects on these same smooth muscles or glands. A second classification assigns anatomic names to the same subdivisions, according to the site of origin of the efferent paths from the central nervous system (CNS). *Thoracolumbar* includes the nerves arising from the thoracic and upper lumbar regions of the vertebral column. *Craniosacral* nerves include efferent fibers arising from the cranial region and the sacral vertebrae. A third, pharmacologic, classification differentiates fibers as *adrenergic* if their nerve terminals release the catecholamine norepinephrine, or *cholinergic* if the terminals release acetylcholine. Parasympathetic is synonymous with *craniosacral* and *cholinergic*. Sympathetic is synonymous with *thoracolumbar*. This latter subdivision contains predominatly adrenergic fibers (called *sympathetic adrenergic*) but also some cholinergic fibers (called *sympathetic cholinergic*), specifically those responsible for active vasodilation[6] and those that innervate sweat glands in humans.[7]

Langley[8] designated a third subdivision of the ANS, the *enteric nervous system* (ENS). The ENS comprises the intrinsic (enteric) neurons of the gastrointestinal tract, the sensory fibers that serve these tissues, and the sympathetic and parasympathetic efferent projections to the gut tissues. The ENS is a complex neural network with about as many neurons as the spinal cord,[9] and it can perform many functions independent of extrinsic inputs from the CNS. Though until now the ENS received little attention, it is now being rigorously investigated.

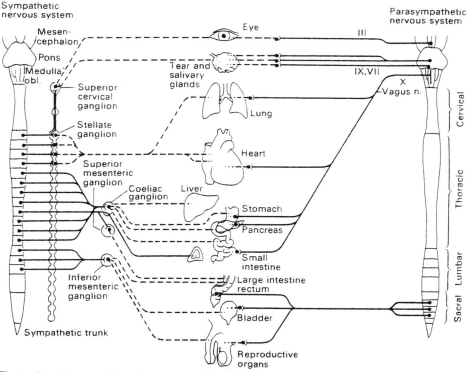

**Figure 4-1.** Schematic illustration of the peripheral ANS, including neural pathways and ganglia for specific organs or tissues. Sympathetic innervation of the sweat glands, piloerector muscles, and peripheral vasculature is omitted. (From Brain RL. Clinical Neurology, ed 6. Oxford: Oxford University Press, 1985; 124–125, with permission.)

## Anatomic Organization (Figure 4-1)

The neural networks that serve as control systems in the ANS comprise three types of neurons: (1) sensory or transducing elements (e.g., temperature, pressure, stretch, pain) and their associated *afferent* neurons; (2) *interneurons* within the CNS, which have neither transducing elements nor smooth muscle targets but connect one neuron to others and serve to integrate afferent signals and direct regulating stimuli to appropriate effector neurons; and (3) *efferent* or effector neurons, which are the end of the pathway and direct the appropriate stimuli to target smooth muscle or glands. Also important to any discussion of the ANS are sites of multiple synaptic interconnections, which occur both peripherally and centrally. These are peripheral *ganglia* and the *CNS centers of autonomic function.*

Neurons in the ANS are predominantly nonmyelinated, in contrast to neurons in the somatic motor system, which are myelinated. A second marked difference is the location of the last synaptic junction. In the somatic motor system all interneurons and their connections occur within the CNS. In the ANS the last interneuron actually traverses either an anterior (ventral) root or a cranial nerve and forms a synapse with one or more efferent fibers in an ANS ganglion outside the CNS. Thus, every ANS efferent neuron has its origin in an ANS ganglion. The ANS interneurons that terminate in the ganglion and form synapses with efferent neurons are called *preganglionic neurons,* and ANS effector neurons are called *postganglionic neurons.*

### Afferents

Afferent fibers are usually nonmyelinated and reach the CNS via the vagus, pelvis splanchnic, and other autonomic and somatic nerves. In the vagus nerves, for example, most of the fibers are afferent rather that efferent. There are no clear differences between afferents involved in somatic and autonomic function, and there may be significant overlap. The cell bodies of autonomic afferent fibers are in dorsal root ganglia of spinal nerves and in corresponding ganglia of cranial nerves. Sensory elements or transducers, which are located throughout the viscera, blood vessels, skin, and skeletal muscle and respond to mechanical and chemical stimuli, heat, intraluminal pH, glucose, and amino acids, have been identified.[10]

Sensory nerves in the ENS are very important, as they afford it the ability to function independently of the CNS. Some of these sensory nerves transmit information to the CNS, but the majority are intrinsic, running either to prevertebral ganglia or directly to other target enteric nerves without connections to the CNS. The pathways of pelvic afferents have been clearly defined by deGroat.[11,12]

### Central Regions Involved in Autonomic Function

Several specific regions or centers integrate autonomic functions, but there is also enormous overlap or autonomic and somatic centers in the CNS. Most autonomic reflexes can be stimulated at the level of the spinal cord—sweating, blood pressure changes, vasomotor responses, micturition, defecation, and erection and ejaculation among them. These spinal reflexes are largely controlled voluntarily in the conscious state via higher centers in the CNS located in the medulla, pons, and hypothalamus. Regions of the medulla involved in the regulation of blood pressure and respiratory movements occur in the nucleus tractus solitarius, paramedian nucleus, nucleus ambiguus, and retroambigualis. Supraspinal centers for the control of micturition and respiratory movements also occur in the inferior colliculus and rostral regions of the pons, respectively. The hypothalamus is a region of extensive integration of neurons involved in autonomic function, and specifically involved in regulation of body temperature, fluid balance, carbohydrate and fat metabolism, blood pressure, sexual function, sleep, and emotional states. The cerebral cortex provides a further level of involvement in autonomic integration. This is the highest level of integration for gastrointestinal, cardiovascular, and other autonomic functions. It is of much importance to the integration of both sensory and effector components of voluntary and involuntary neural functions.

### Efferent Divisions

#### Thoracolumbar (Sympathetic) Division

The preganglionic somata of the thoracolumbar division occur in the lateral horns of the spinal cord (intermediolateral cell column, Figure 4-2) from the eighth cervical or first thoracic to the second or third lumbar segment. The axons of the preganglionic neurons leave the spinal cord via the anterior nerve roots and terminate in one of three types of ganglion: *paravertebral* (sympathetic chain) ganglia, *prevertebral* (collateral) ganglia, or *terminal* (peripheral) ganglia on the organs innervated. Distal to the anterior root the preganglionic fibers traverse the *white ramus communicans* and enter the paravertebral ganglia of the sympathetic chain. Some of the fibers synapse with postganglionic fibers there; others continue on to one of the other types of ganglion.

**Paravertebral (sympathetic chain) ganglia.** A series of 22 pairs of ganglia lie on both sides and close to the vertebral segments and are interconnected by ascending and descending fibers in these two nodular cords. These are the *sympathetic chains,* which extend from the base of the skull to the ventral surface of the coccyx. They are normally called *cervical, thoracic, lumbar,* and sacral ganglia, according to the spinal segments they serve.

**There are three cervical ganglia.** The *superior cervical ganglion* occurs at the base of the skull. Its preganglionic fibers originate from the lower cervical or upper thoracic segments, and its postganglionic fibers innervate the blood vessels, smooth muscles, and glands of the head and neck.

The preganglionic fibers of the *middle cervical ganglion* also originate from the upper thoracic segments. Its postganglionic fibers follow three paths: (1) along the fifth and sixth cervical nerves to innervate the blood vessels, sweat glands, and cutaneous muscles in the region served by complementary sensory fibers in these same nerves;

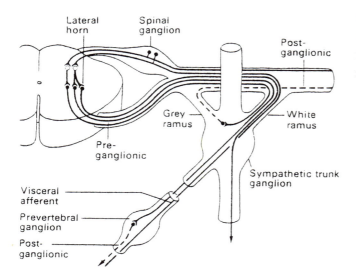

**Figure 4-2.** Schematic diagram of the autonomic reflex arch, including afferents and sympathetic nerve paths and ganglia at the level of the spinal cord. (From Brain RL. Clinical Neurology, ed 6. Oxford: Oxford University Press, 1985; 124–125, with permission.)

(2) along the middle cardiac nerve to the cardiac plexuses; and (3) along the thyroid artery to innervate the thyroid and parathyroid glands.

In humans, the *inferior cervical ganglion* is also called the *stellate ganglion* when it incorporates the first (and sometimes the second) thoracic ganglion and the seventh and eighth cervical ganglia. Its postganglionic fibers travel along the seventh and eighth (and sometimes the sixth) cervical and the first and second thoracic nerves, the inferior cardiac nerve, and the subclavian artery and branches from it. The fibers innervate the blood vessels and sweat glands served by the appropriate spinal nerves, the cardiac plexuses, and the vertebral, axillary, and proximal portion of the brachial arteries.

There are 10 to 12 pairs of *thoracic ganglia* (the number depends on whether the first and second thoracic ganglia are part of the stellate ganglion). The preganglionic fibers originate in the corresponding vertebral segments. Postganglionic nerves traverse corresponding or adjacent spinal nerves to serve peripheral blood vessels and sweat glands or join the *greater* or *lesser splanchnic* nerves, which innervate the stomach, small intestine, adrenal medulla, and large intestine.

Four *lumbar ganglia* innervate the large intestine and bladder, and four or five *sacral ganglia* likewise innervate the colon and bladder.

**Prevertebral (Collateral) Ganglia.** *Collateral ganglia* are those that occur near major arteries—

the *celiac ganglion* (also called *solar* or *semilunar ganglion*) lying at the origin of the celiac artery, and the *superior mesenteric ganglion* lying just below the superior mesenteric artery.

**Terminal Ganglia.** Terminal ganglia occur near or at innervated tissues. Several occur in the pelvic region, on or near the bladder and colon.

*Craniosacral (Parasympathetic) Division*

The preganglionic somata of the craniosacral division occur in four nuclei in the brain stem: (1) the *Edinger-Westphal nucleus* (or *accessory oculomotor nucleus*), which is part of the oculomotor nucleus in the midbrain, (2) the *superior* and (3) the *inferior salivatory nucleus* in the base of the pons, and (4) the *dorsal vagal nucleus* in the medulla. The preganglionic fibers from these nuclei leave the CNS through the skull via cranial nerves III, VII, IX, and X, respectively, though the preganglionic fibers comprise only a small portion of the total fibers in these nerves. In the sacral region additional preganglionic somata occur in the intermediate columns of the second, third, and fourth segments of the sacral spinal cord and emerge from the CNS via sacral spinal nerves S2–4S (see Figure 4-1).

The preganglionic fibers in cranial nerve III (oculomotor nerve) enter the orbit via the superior orbital fissure and form synapses with postganglionic fibers in the *ciliary ganglion*. The postganglionic neurons are short and terminate in the sphincter pupillae of the iris, which are responsible for reducing the size of the pupil and controlling the amount of light entering the eye, and the ciliary muscles of the eyes, which allow the lens to increase its curvature to focus on nearby objects.

The preganglionic fibers in the seventh (facial) nerve follow two paths, both of which begin by passing through the *geniculate ganglion*. Some fibers follow the facial nerve through the facial canal. Within the canal the parasympathetic fibers form their own nerve, the *chorda tympani,* then branch and traverse their own canal to the middle ear and pass between the malleus and the incus. The chorda tympani leaves the skull through the petrotympanic fissure and follows a branch of the lingual nerve to the floor of the mouth. Its fibers form synapses with postganglionic fibers in the *submandibular ganglion* that innervate submandibular and sublingual glands and mucous membranes of the mouth. Other postganglionic fibers from the submandibular ganglion join the petrosal nerve, reenter the cranium, and innervate the middle meningeal artery and its branches. Some fibers leave the facial nerve just after passing through the geniculate ganglion. They follow the greater (superficial) petrosal nerve, which passes through a bony canal, emerging through the foramen lacerum, and traversing the pterygoid canal to reach the *pterygopalatine ganglion*. There, the fibers synapse with postganglionic fibers that innervate the lacrimal gland and mucous membranes of the soft palate, nasopharynx, and pharynx. The greater petrosal nerve is joined in the pterygoid canal by the deep petrosal nerve, which contains postganglionic sympathetic fibers derived from the superior cervical ganglia and somata along the internal carotid artery. The sympathetic fibers pass through the pterygopalatine ganglion without forming synapses.

The preganglionic fibers in the ninth cranial (glossopharyngeal) nerve branch from it between its two ganglia, and, with sensory fibers, form the *tympanic nerve*. The tympanic nerve enters the middle ear, where the sensory fibers ramify to form the *tympanic plexus*. Its parasympathetic fibers merely traverse the plexus and form the lesser (deep) petrosal nerve, which exits the skull at the foramen ovale and forms synapses in the *otic gan-*

*glion*. The postganglionic fibers travel with a branch of the mandibular nerve and innervate the parotid gland, the mucous membrane of the tympanic cavity, the mastoid air-cells, the auditory tube, and the internal ear.

The preganglionic fibers in the tenth (vagus) nerve follow various branches to thoracic and abdominal tissues that they serve, including heart, bronchi, esophagus, stomach, and intestine, and terminate in ganglia within those tissues, called *intramural ganglia*. Thus, the preganglionic fibers serving the heart terminate at ganglion cells in the cardiac tissues. Preganglionic fibers serving the bronchi form synapses with postganglionic cells in the intrinsic plexus in the wall of bronchi. Preganglionic fibers serving the esophagus, stomach, and intestine form synapses with postganglionic fibers in the *myenteric plexus of Auerbach* and the *submucous plexus of Meissner*.

The preganglionic fibers of the sacral region leave the CNS via the anterior roots (just as the sympathetic fibers do), traverse the spinal nerves, but then separate from the spinal nerves and proceed peripherally as the *pelvic nerve* (or *nervus erigens*) as part of the pelvic plexus. The ganglia where pre- and postganglionic fibers form synapses are on or near the organs that they serve. The postganglionic fibers include some motor units that innervate the walls of the descending colon, rectum, and bladder; others that inhibit internal anal and visceral sphincters and uterine tissue; and some of vasodilation function that innervate the vessel walls of the bladder, rectum, and genitalia.

### Enteric Nervous System

#### Intrinsic Nerves

The intrinsic (enteric) nerves in the ENS include two plexuses within the gut wall that extend from the esophagus to the anal sphincters. The *submucous plexus of Meissner,* a network of ganglion cells in the submucous layers, has two anatomically differentiated subdivisions. *Henle's plexus* lies along the inner surface of the circular muscles of the gut. *Meissner's plexus* is closer to the gut mucosa. The *myenteric plexus of Auerbach* is a network of ganglia that lie between the circular and longitudinal muscle layers of the gut. The plexuses are comprised of ganglion cells interconnected by unmyelinated fibers. The submucosal and myenteric plexuses are interconnected, and together they serve the mucosal cells, muscles, and blood vessels that supply these cells. Thus, the subdivisions of the ENS are purely anatomic, and no functional differences are yet known. The intrinsic nerves are predominantly cholinergic.

Studies of the ultrastructure of the enteric plexus revealed large numbers of unmyelinated axons, dendrites, and supporting cells. The latter have some features in common with Schwann cells and others in common with astroglial cells in the CNS. In contrast to other peripheral ganglia, where collagen cells are interspersed among the nerve cells, the enertic plexus ganglia lack collagen. The myenteric plexus is isolated from the extracellular space and capillaries by the basal lamina and supporting glial cells, which form a sheath around it.

*Extrinsic Nerves*

Whereas the normal function of the esophagus and stomach depends on intact extrinsic innervation, the small and large intestines continue to function normally in the absence of extrinsic input from the CNS. Lesions involving the intrinsic nerves can, however, lead to significant bowel dysfunction. The parasympathetic innervation of the enteric plexus occurs via the vagus and sacral nerves, with the vagal innervation extending from the esophagus to the transverse portion of the large intestine. The distal portion of the colon is innervated via the pelvic nerves, which originate from the second, third, and fourth sacral segments. Sympathetic innervation of the enteric plexus originates in the thoracic and lumbar segments (T2–L2) and forms synapses with postganglionic adrenergic fibers in the prevertebral ganglia of the celiac, superior mesenteric, inferior mesenteric, and pelvic plexuses. The esophagus is innervated by preganglionic fibers from spinal segments T2 to T7 and synapse with postganglionic fibers in the stellate ganglion and the sympathetic chain. The stomach and small intestine are supplied by preganglionic fibers from segments T6 to T9 and T6 to T11, respectively, and that follow the greater splanchnic nerves and form synapses with postganglionic fibers in the celiac ganglia. The large intestine is supplied by preganglionic fibers in segments T12 to L2.

## General Characteristics of Autonomic Nerve Fibers

Nerve fibers that serve a particular function normally have similar characteristics, including degree of myelination, diameter of axon, and type of nerve ending. Because of these similarities, generalizations can be made about the various components of the ANS.

### Diameter and Myelination

Most preganglionic fibers have myelinated axons of 1.5 to 4 $\mu$ diameter (group B fibers) with conduction velocities of 5 to 30 m/sec and all have cholinergic terminals. Postganglionic fibers are unmyelinated axons of approximately 0.1 to 1.5 $\mu$ diameter (group C fibers) with conduction velocities of only 0.5 to 2 m/sec, and they normally have either cholinergic or adrenergic nerve terminals. All postganglionic fibers from the craniosacral division have cholinergic terminals. Most of the postganglionic fibers in the thoracolumbar division have adrenergic terminals, but notable exceptions include fibers involved in active vasodilatation and those that innervate the sweat glands, which have cholinergic terminals.

### Density and Distribution of Innervation

Ganglia are a site of dispersal or distribution for peripherally bound nerve impulses. As a general rule, the closer the ganglion is to the CNS (i.e., pathways with shorter preganglionic fibers and longer postganglionic fibers), the larger is the region affected. Conversely, the closer the ganglion cells are to the target tissue, the smaller their region of influence.

### Terminations and Synapses

The terminal nerve endings of sympathetic postganglionic fibers normally exhibit branching, which form a plexus in the target tissue termed the *sympathetic ground plexus*. The plexuses are made up of numerous fine, interconnected axons that form a network over the surface of the smooth muscle cells and gland cells, which are their targets. The various branches of the plexus have, at regular intervals, spherical enlargements, where the neurotransmitters are synthesized and stored in small (~50-nm diameter) vesicles and from which neurotransmitter is released.[13] In some cases the distance between the surface of the plexus and the target tissue is only about 10 to 20 nm, and each smooth muscle cell may be served by a nerve terminal. In other cases the distance between the surface of the plexus and the target tissue is 100 nm or more and neurotransmitter released into the intracellular space affects more that one cell. Studies of the ultrastructure of the enertic plexus, for example, have revealed few synaptic structures; rather, the axons appear to merely run close to the smooth muscle cells. Because smooth muscle fibers are connected electrically by gap junctions (areas of electrical continuity between cells), excitation spreads from one smooth muscle fiber to others across the tissue in the absence of nerves. Parasympathetic nerve terminal endings look similar to the sympathetic endings, except that the vesicles of adrenergic terminals have a dense core whereas the vesicles in cholinergic terminals are clear.

## Physiologic Basis of Autonomic Function

The basis of nervous system function is a change in polarity of nerve cell membranes. Nerve cells have specialized membranes that actively maintain a relatively high electrical gradient (potential) across the membrane. Disruption of this electrical difference is the basis of initiating a nerve impulse in the sensory terminals, the propagation of impulses along axons, and transmission of the impulse across junctions, called *synapses,* between two nerve cells or between nerve cells and specialized tissue such as glands and striated or smooth muscle. This section of the chapter is about maintenance of the electrical difference across the membrane, initiation of impulses, and the characteristics of synaptic junctions in ANS pathways.

### *Nerves at Rest*

The membrane of the resting nerve cell is more permeable to some ions (potassium) than to others (sodium) and is altogether impermeable to some. This contributes to differences in intracellular and extracellular concentrations of ions and net elec-

trical charge. In addition, incorporated in the membrane is an active transport or pump mechanism (electrogenic pump) comprised of sodium ions, potassium ions, and adenosine triphosphatase (ATPase), which actively pumps sodium ions out of the cell and potassium ions into it. This pump is activated by sodium ions inside and by potassium ions outside the axon and actively moves them at a ratio of three sodium ions to two potassium ions.[14] Because the resting membrane is highly permeable to potassium, this pump is driven continuously by the presence of extracellular potassium. As a result of the pump, the concentration of potassium ions inside the axon is 30 to 70 times greater than outside the axon when the nerve is at rest. Conversely, the concentration of sodium and chloride ions is greater outside the axon than inside. These ion concentration gradients are responsible for the relatively high (about $-70$ mV to $-90$ mV) *electrical potential* (or *resting potential*) across the resting axon membrane and its polarized state at rest.

### *Conduction of Action Potential Along Axons (Figure 4-3)*

An action potential (nerve impulse) occurs when there is a sudden increase in membrane permeability to sodium, and the influx of sodium along its concentration gradient causes depolarization of the membrane. The impulse is propagated along unmyelinated axons via circuit currents that increase the sodium permeability of the axon but without loss of electrical strength, as the resting electrical potential is similar along the entire length of the axon. In myelinated fibers, permeability changes occur only at the nodes of Ranvier (see Figure 4-3), in which case circuit currents propagate impulses via jumps from one node to the next. Impulse propagation is faster in myelinated axons, where such jumps occur, than in unmyelinated axons. Repolarization occurs immediately after a depolarization, owing to reinstatement of a high potassium ion permeability and low sodium ion permeability,[15] and the action of the ATP-active transport pump in the membrane. Normally, a nerve is initiated at either a sensory terminal or a synaptic junction. In either case specialized molecules in the nerve cell membrane at these sites

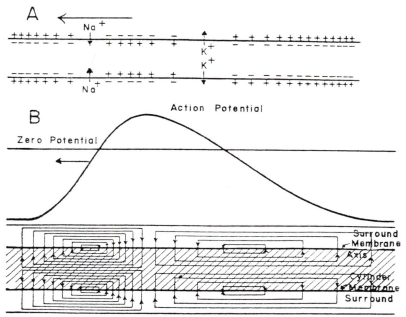

**Figure 4-3.** The movement of sodium and potassium across a nerve membrane during a nerve impulse traveling in the direction of the arrow. Upper curve indicates the potential difference along the nerve. Lower part of figure illustrates the flow of current inside and outside the nerve fiber. (From Schwartz IL, Siegel GJ. Excitation, conduction and transmission of the nerve impulse. In: Brobeck JR, ed. Best and Taylor's Physiological Basis of Medical Practice. Baltimore: Williams & Wilkins, 1975; 1–44, with permission.)

apparently increase sodium ion permeability in response to local stimuli (e.g., temperature, pressure, pain, pH, stretch) or to chemicals released by other nerve cells (neurotransmitter substances).

### Synaptic Transmission of Nerve Impulses (Figure 4-4)

#### Neurotransmitters

Loewi[16] was the first to demonstrate the existence of neurohumoral agents (chemicals involved in transmission of nerve impulses). His experiment used two isolated frog hearts, prepared for recording the contractions of each and arranged in series so they were perfused by the same fluid. Stimulation of the vagus of the first heart caused it to slow, and when the fluid that had perfused the first heart reached the second heart, its contraction rate also slowed. Similarly, stimulation of the sympa-

thetic nerve of the first heart not only accelerated its rate of contraction but also increased the heart rate of the second heart via a substance in the common perfusion fluid, thus demonstrating that synaptic transmission occurred by chemical rather than electrical means. Subsequent studies[17] found that the substances responsible for slowing and accelerating the second heart are, respectively, acetylcholine and norepinephrine. These substances (and others), synthesized in nerve terminals and stored in vesicles there, are responsible for transmission of nerve impulses from one neuron to the next and are therefore called *neurotransmitters.*

Until recently it was thought that only one neurotransmitter was associated with each nerve and that acetylcholine and norepinephrine were the only two neurotransmitters associated with peripheral autonomic fibers. Fibers with acetylcholine in their terminals are said to use *cholinergic transmission;* those with norepinephrine in their terminals use *adrenergic transmission.*[18] Now, how-

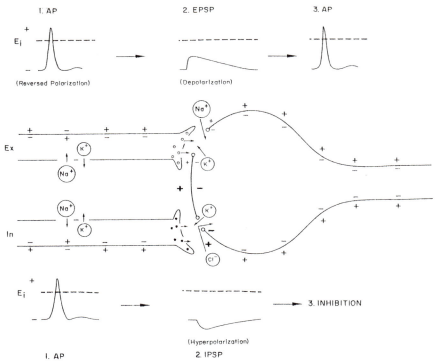

**Figure 4-4.** Steps involved in excitatory (Ex) and inhibitory (In) neurohumoral transmission.
1. The nerve action potential (AP), a self-propagated reversed polarization of the nerve membrane, reaching a nerve terminal causes the release of excitatory (o) or inhibitory (o) transmitter.
2. The excitatory transmitter's action on its postsynaptic receptor causes localized depolarization, the EPSP, by increasing ion permeability of the postsynaptic membrane. The inhibitory transmitter causes only a selective increase in permeability to small ions (potassium and chloride), which results in hyperpolarization of the membrane, the IPSP.
3. The EPSP can initiate an action potential in the postsynaptic nerve, but this can be inhibited by the hyperpolarization that accompanies IPSP. (From Koelle GB. Drugs acting at synaptic and neuroeffector junctional sites. In: Goodman LS, Gilman A, eds. The Pharmacological Basis of Therapeutics. New York: Macmillan, 1975; 414, with permission.)

ever, these substances are referred to as *classical transmitters* because other neurotransmitters have been identified. Furthermore, it has been shown that more than one neurotransmitter may be released from a single nerve terminal. Such *cotransmitters* are discussed further later.

The steps involved in the rupture of vesicles to release neurotransmitter, termed *exocytosis,* are still ill-understood, though it is known that calcium ions, thought to facilitate the joining of the vesicle membrane with the terminal membrane, are essential to exocytosis.

*Receptors*

When an action potential in the presynaptic fiber reaches the synaptic terminals, hundreds of quanta (the contents of one vesicle) of neurotransmitter are released into the synaptic cleft. The neurotransmitter diffuses across the 5- to 100-nm wide synaptic cleft and combines with a specific molecule (termed *receptor*) on the membrane of the postsynaptic cell. Several types of receptors (discussed in more detail later) have been identified for each of the well-known neurotransmitters involved in

ANS function. Thus, synaptic transmission is commonly classified not only in terms of the neurotransmitter involved but also in terms of the specific type of receptor affected on the target membrane, regardless of whether it is a nerve–nerve junction or a nerve–effector tissue junction.

Other substances that mimic neurotransmitter effects on receptors are called *agonists*. If they mimic acetylcholine, they may also be referred to as *parasympathomimetic*. If they mimic norepinephrine, they may be called *sympathomimetic*. Substances that block the receptor sites are called *antagonists* or *blocking agents* (or the term *blocker* is used with a prefix to identify the type of receptor being blocked). Still other substances that modulate either the release of the neurotransmitter at the presynaptic level or the effect of neurotransmitter on the postsynaptic membrane are called *neuromodulators*. Furthermore, there is evidence[19,20] that neurotransmitter release is regulated through *presynaptic autoreceptors* (e.g., receptors on the presynaptic terminal membrane that respond to the presence of neurotransmitter and affect the rate of further release of neurotransmitter substance).

In the resting condition small amounts of neurotransmitter are released continuously into the synaptic cleft. This amount of neurotransmitter is insufficient to stimulate an action potential in the target membrane, but it does cause small depolarizations (0.1 to 3.0 mV) called miniature end-plate potentials (MEPP) in the target membrane about once every second.[21] The continuous release of small, subthreshold amounts of neurotransmitter and associated neurochemicals from the resting presynaptic fibers is thought to play a role in maintaining the presynaptic and postsynaptic membrane in a state of readiness.[22,23] This has been particularly well-studied in relation to the neuromuscular junction and junctions at the effector tissue of the sympathetic nervous system.[24]

*Postsynaptic Impulse Generation and Propagation*

The combination of the neurotransmitter with its receptor creates increased ion permeability at the target membrane. There are two principal types of increased permeability to ions. If permeability to all ions is increased, depolarization of the target membrane occurs and an excitatory postsynaptic potential (EPSP) is created. The influx of sodium ions is of particular importance, as axons in the resting state are already permeable to potassium ions. If there is increased permeability to small ions only (potassium and chloride but not sodium), the membrane becomes hyperpolarized and causes an inhibitory postsynaptic potential (IPSP), which inhibits development of EPSPs in the target membrane. IPSPs and EPSPs acting on the same target membrane normally originate from different presynaptic fibers. They functionally oppose each other, so that the development of an action potential in the target membrane is determined by the algebraic sum of these IPSPs and EPSPs acting on that cell. Inhibition of synaptic junctions can also result from prolonged depolarization of the presynaptic membrane elicited by a neurotransmitter released by another nerve, but this can occur only if the appropriate receptors are present in that presynaptic membrane.

The effect of EPSP differs according to the tissue type. In postsynaptic neurons, cardiac, and skeletal muscle, EPSP results in an action potential being propagated along the target cell. In smooth muscle EPSP results in a localized contraction, which can affect neighboring cells via gap junctions (regions of electric continuity between cells). EPSPs in gland cells stimulates secretion.

Because neurotransmitter can be released at a rate of several hundred times a second, there has to be a mechanism for removing excess transmitter from the synaptic cleft if such repeated bursts of neurotransmitter are to result in repeated elicitation of EPSPs in the target tissue. For cholinergic transmission, the enzyme acetylcholinesterase acts rapidly to hydrolyze the transmitter. No such enzyme has been found at adrenergic synapses, and excess catecholamine transmitters are thought to be disposed of by rapid reuptake in the nerve terminals and diffusion in the tissue. Because of these differences, the effect of acetylcholine is localized and of short duration compared to the effect of norepinephrine.

***Autonomic Neurotransmission***

Knowledge about neurotransmitters, receptors, autoreceptors, blocking agents, and neuromodulators provides the basis of treatment with nonprescription and prescription drugs. Thus, understanding the pharmacology of the ANS is essential to development of pharmacologic treatments for autonomic dysfunction.

*Acetylcholine: Cholinergic Transmission*

Within the ANS, acetylcholine is responsible for synaptic transmission in all ganglia (i.e., between preganglionic and postganglionic fibers) and at the postganglionic nerve terminals in the craniosacral division (parasympathetic nerves). It is also the neurotransmitter responsible for active vasodilatation in the muscle and sweat gland function in the thoracolumbar division (sympathetic cholinergic fibers).

Acetylcholine is synthesized in the terminals of cholinergic fibers[25] and stored in vesicles.[26] These vesicles also contain cholinacetylase, an enzyme that promotes acetylcholine synthesis from choline and coenzyme A (Figure 4-5). It has been estimated that there are as many as 300,000 vesicles in a nerve terminal and that each vesicle contains 1000 to 50,000 acetylcholine molecules.

Identification of different types of receptors for a neurotransmitter—in this case acetylcholine—is based on observations of the different effects of cholinergic substances on different populations of cholinergic receptors. For example, two types of acetylcholine receptors were initially identified,

(1) cholinergic receptors in ganglia, which responded to nicotine in the same way they responded to acetylcholine (*nicotinic receptors*), and (2) cholinergic receptors in glands and smooth muscle, which did not respond to nicotine but did respond to muscarine in the same way they responded to acetylcholine (*muscarinic receptors*). The antagonist atropine blocks the muscarinic but not nicotinic effects of acetylcholine; thus, it is a muscarinic receptor blocker.

Muscarinic receptors have been further subdivided pharmacologically.[27,28] $M_1$ receptors are found in sympathetic ganglia, $M_2$ receptors in cardiac muscle, and $M_3$ receptors in glandular (salivary gland) and smooth muscle (ileum, bladder) tissue. There is some evidence that the $M_3$ receptors in glandular tissue differ from those in smooth muscle. Furthermore, the muscarinic receptors in vascular smooth muscle differ from cardiac ($M_2$) receptors, but their classification is still unresolved. Of particular interest is the observation, made from genetic cloning studies, that muscarinic receptors belong to the same family of receptors as adrenergic receptors.[29]

The pharmacologic evidence for these subtypes of muscarinic receptors is as follows: First, $M_1$ and $M_2$ receptors were differentiated on the basis of their affinity for pirenzepine: receptors in the sympathetic ganglia ($M_1$) having much higher affinity than receptors in the cardiac, ileum, bladder, or glandular tissue ($M_2$). Further differentiation of

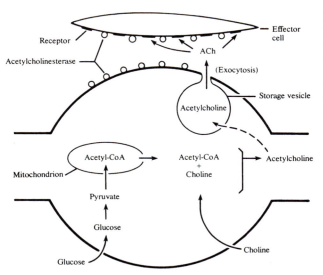

**Figure 4-5.** Schematic illustration of cholinergic nerve terminal varicosity and the process involved in the synthesis and storage of acetylcholine. Also illustrated is the release of acetylcholine (exocytosis) and its degradation by acetylcholinesterase. (From Craig CR, Stitzel RE. Modern Pharmacology. Boston: Little, Brown, 1986, with permission.)

the $M_2$ receptors into $M_2$ and $M_3$ receptors was based on their different affinity for the antagonists AF-DX 116 and 4-DAMP. Cardiac receptors ($M_2$) have a higher affinity for AF-DX 116 glandular receptors ($M_3$). Moreover, glandular and ileum receptors ($M_3$) have a higher affinity for 4-DMP than cardiac receptors ($M_2$). Evidence suggesting that $M_3$ receptors should be further differentiated into subtypes comes from the observation that glandular $M_3$ receptors have a 10-fold higher affinity for 4-DAMP than ileum $M_3$ receptors, but further supportive observations are needed. The muscarinic receptors in vascular tissue have not been conclusively identified, but investigations have measured affinity to the antagonists ipratropium and AF-DX 116. Cardiac receptors have 16- to 29-fold higher affinity for AF-DX 116 than do vascular receptors. Thus, it is concluded that vascular muscarinic receptors are not of the $M_2$ subtype found in the heart. Furthermore, vascular receptors involved in relaxation of vessels have a 10-fold higher affinity for ipratropium than do receptors involved in constriction of the same vessels. Thus, these physiologically different functions are probably mediated by different receptor types.

All nicotinic receptors can be blocked by *d*-tubocurarine (*d*-TC) but can be further subdivided pharmacologically into $N_1$ receptors, located in autonomic ganglia and capable of being blocked by decamethonium (C10) but not by hexamethonium (C6), and $N_2$ receptors located in striated muscle and blocked by C6 but not by C10.

Much of the acetylcholine released by the presynaptic nerve terminals is immediately hydrolyzed by acetylcholinesterase, which is abundant in the membrane of the postsynaptic fibers. The effect of acetylcholine is very localized because very little of it leaves the immediate vicinity of the presynaptic terminal. Several different cholinesterases are categorized either as true (specific) cholinesterase (acetylcholinesterase), which has only acetylcholine as a substrate, or as pseudo- (nonspecific) cholinesterase, which acts on a variety of substrates (acetylcholine, choline, noncholine esters) and is effective in hydrolyzing larger quantities of acetylcholine. The choline by-product of this hydrolysis is taken up by the presynaptic terminal for resynthesis of acetylcholine, as facilitated by cholinacetylase.

### Adrenergic Transmission

Norepinephrine is the commonly known neurotransmitter of the postganglionic adrenergic (i.e., sympathetic) fibers.[30–32] The principal events involved in the synthesis, storage, and release of norepinephrine into the synaptic cleft are illustrated in Figure 4-6. Norepinephrine and epinephrine are the end products of a class of compounds synthesized from tyrosine (hydroxyphenylalanine)

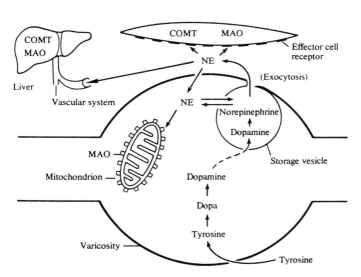

**Figure 4-6.** Schematic illustration of adrenergic nerve terminal varicosity and the processes involved in the synthesis and storage of norepinephrine. Also shown are its release (exocytosis) and multiple paths of degradation. Key: NE, norepinephrine; COMT, catechol-*o*-methyltransferase; MAO, monoamine oxidase. (From Craig CR, Stitzel RE. Modern Pharmacology. Boston: Little, Brown, 1986, with permission.)

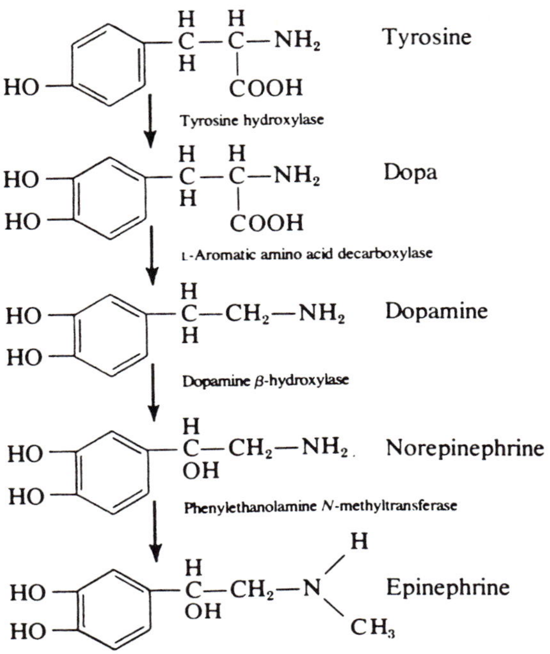

**Figure 4-7.** Steps in the enzymatic synthesis of dopamine, norepinephrine, and epinephrine. (From Craig CR, Stitzel RE. Modern Pharmacology. Boston: Little, Brown, 1986, with permission.)

(Figure 4-7).[33] The series of compounds includes L-epinephrine synthesized from L-norepinephrine (enzyme, phenylethanolamine), which is synthesized from dopamine (enzyme, dopamine β-hydroxylase), which is synthesized from L-dopa (enzyme, L-dopa decarboxylase), which is synthesized from L-tyrosine (enzyme, tyrosine hydroxylase).[33,34] The hydroxylation of tyrosine to dopa and the decarboxylation of dopa to dopamine (steps 2 and 3) occur in the axonal cytoplasm. Dopamine enters vesicles in the terminals, where the enzyme β-hydroxylase converts it to norepinephrine. Also present in the vesicles is ATP (its concentration is about 25% that of the catecholamines).

When a nerve impulse reaches the terminal end of the sympathetic adrenergic postganglionic fiber, the contents of some vesicles are expelled into the synaptic cleft. Some of the norepinephrine released from presynaptic terminals combines with receptors on the target membrane. Most of it is actively transported back into the presynaptic terminals and vesicles (termed *reuptake I*), and a smaller amount is taken up by chemical reactions in the surrounding tissue (termed *reuptake II*) or diffused into the circulation and is metabolically transformed by the enzymes monoamine oxidase (MAO; present in mitochondria, it deaminates norepinephrine) and catechol-*o*-methyltransferase (COMT; present in cytoplasm, it methylates norepinephrine).[35,36] Both enzymes are widely distributed in the body. The participation of nerve terminals in reuptake and storage of norepinephrine is supported by the observation that administered exogenously epinephrine or norepinephrine disappears more quickly in innervated than in denervated tissue.[37] At least two active transport mechanisms are involved in reuptake I, one at the axonal membrane and another at the vesicular membrane. The latter transport mechanism can establish a 200-fold concentration gradient and is blocked by reserpine. The axoplasmic transport mechanism is blocked by cocaine and tricyclic antidepressants.

The suggestion that different types of adrenergic receptors exist originates from the observation by Dale[38] that epinephrine causes some smooth muscles to contract and others to relax. Further investigation of the effects of different catecholamines on different tissues led Alquist[39] to classify them as two subtypes: α-*receptors* associated with vasoconstriction, intestinal relaxation, and dilatation of the pupil, and β-*receptors* associated with vasodilatation, intestinal and bronchiolar relaxation, and acceleration of the heart and cardiac inotropic responses. These subdivisions were confirmed pharmacologically by blocking agents. Phenoxybenzamine (an α antagonist), for example, blocks α-receptors but not β-receptors and propranolol (a β antagonist), for example, blocks β receptors but not α receptors. These groups of receptors have now been further subdivided on the basis of their location and pharmacologic evidence, with designations of $\alpha_1$- and $\alpha_2$-receptors, and $\beta_1$-, $\beta_2$-, and $\beta_3$-receptors. The $\alpha_1$-receptors are located predominantly on the postsynaptic membranes and are responsible for vasoconstriction, venoconstriction, uterine and splenic contraction, and glycogenolysis in the liver. The $\alpha_2$-receptors are found on presynaptic terminals, where they are involved in autoregulation of norepinephrine release, and perhaps on postsynaptic membranes.[40] The $\beta_1$-receptors are located principally in the heart and mediate sympathetic stimulation of heart rate acceleration, whereas $\beta_2$-receptors were originally identified in the bronchi[41,42] but have subsequently been found in vascular smooth muscle (vasodilatation), intestinal smooth muscle (relaxation), kidney (renin secretion), uterus (contraction during delivery), spleen (relaxation of capsule), liver (gluconeogenesis), and pancreas (increased secretion).

Very recently[43] another subtype of $\beta$-receptor, $\beta_3$-, was identified in adipocytes, liver muscle, and ileum that is functionally associated with control of metabolic rate, fat metabolism and thermogenesis, ileum relaxation, and glycogen synthesis in muscle and to which antidiabetic properties are attributed.

## Other Adrenergic Transmitters and Receptors

Other adrenergic transmitter substances include dopamine and epinephrine. Dopamine receptors have been identified in the peripheral autonomic nervous system and are classified as $DA_1$ receptors, which facilitate vascular smooth muscle relaxation, and $DA_2$ receptors, which act to inhibit norepinephrine release from postganglionic sympathetic fibers.[44,45]

Epinephrine is synthesized from norepinephrine in the adrenal medulla and, when released into the circulation during fight-or-flight responses, has widespread action. The adrenal medulla originates embryonically from cells that are precursors of sympathetic nerve cells, which migrate away from the neural tube and differentiate into sympathetic ganglia (in the sympathetic chain and prevertebral and terminal ganglia) and chromaffin cells located in the adrenal medulla. At birth, the adrenal medulla is composed primarily of sympathetic cells, which differentiate into chromaffin cells during the first 3 years of life. Synthesis of norepinephrine in the adrenal medulla occurs in the chromaffin cells in much the same way it does in adrenergic nerve terminals, but in chromaffin cells most of the norepinephrine leaves the vesicles and is methylated to form epinephrine in the cytoplasm (see Figure 4-10) and then is stored in a second type of vesicle. Epinephrine makes up about 80% to 90% of the total complement of catecholamine in the adrenal medulla.[46,47]

The adrenal medulla is innervated by sympathetic preganglionic cholinergic fibers via the lesser thoracic splanchnic nerve and celiac ganglion. Impulses along the preganglionic fibers release acetylcholine from the terminals, which acts on receptors in the chromaffin cell membranes and stimulates the release of catecholamines, principally epinephrine, into the circulation. Epinephrine has widespread effects on $\alpha$- and $\beta$-receptors throughout the body.

## Autonomic Ganglia

Some autonomic ganglia, primarily parasympathetic ones, have one preganglionic fiber to one postganglionic fiber synaptic relationships, but other autonomic ganglia, principally sympathetic ones, have very complicated or complex ganglionic synapses that involve interneurons within the ganglia, and a single ganglionic neuron may impact as many as 20 postganglionic fibers.

The principle neurotransmitter in the autonomic ganglia is acetylcholine, but other neurotransmitter substances, such as dopamine, epinephrine, or norepinephrine, are sometimes involved. Unlike the cholinergic junctions between postganglionic fibers

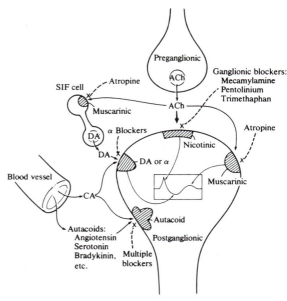

**Figure 4-8.** Schematic diagram of various types of autonomic ganglionic transmission. (From Craig CR, Stitzel RE. Modern Pharmacology. Boston: Little, Brown, 1986, with permission.)

and effector tissue or neuromuscular junctions, these ganglionic synapses have both nicotinic and muscarinic cholinergic receptors—and, on occasion, dopaminergic or adrenergic receptors.

In the more complicated ganglionic synapses (Figure 4-8) the release of acetylcholine by a preganglionic terminal results in a complex postsynaptic potential that has at least three components; (1) a fast EPSP, activated by the nicotinic receptors and responsible for the impulse generated in the postganglionic fiber, (2) a slow IPSP, activated by a muscarinic receptor that can be blocked by atropine or by dopamine receptor antagonist, and (3) a slow EPSP activated by another muscarinic receptor that can be blocked by atropine but not dopamine receptor antagonist. The slow IPSP is thought to be mediated through an intermediate cell (interneuron or small intensely fluorescent [SIF] cell), which releases dopamine neurotransmitter.

### Noncholinergic, Nonadrenergic Transmission

Some fibers in the gastrointestinal tract are neither cholinergic nor adrenergic.[48] Extensive investigation in the 1960s and 1970s resulted in the identification of ATP, 5-hydroxytryptamine, γ-aminobutyric acid, and dopamine as probable neurotransmitter substances, and they are now well-accepted as neurotransmitters.

### Putative Cotransmitters and Neuromodulators

### Neuropeptides

Several peptides (Table 4-1) have been identified that occur widely in nerve cells and nerve terminals and are referred to collectively as neuropeptides. Because more peptides are being identified all the time, Table 4-1 is a tentative list. These neuropeptides are found in sensory, motor, and autonomic fibers, which may contain just one peptide or a combination of peptides. Marti and coworkers[49] reported that an adultlike pattern of neuropeptide distribution coincides with adultlike maturity of afferent and efferent fibers and in humans occurs in late fetal life.

Although chemically distinct populations of

**Table 4-1.** Neuropeptides in the ANS

| Neuropeptide | Abbreviation |
| --- | --- |
| Calcitonin gene–related peptide | CGRP |
| Cystokinin | CCK |
| Dynorphin | DYN |
| Enkephalin | ENK |
| Galanin | GAL |
| Gastrin-releasing peptide | GRP |
| Neuropeptide Y | NPY |
| C-flanking peptide of NYP | CPON |
| Neurotensin | NT |
| Peptide HI | HI |
| Somatostatin | SOM |
| Substance P | SP |
| Neurokinin A, substance K | NA |
| Vasoactive intestinal peptide | VIP |

nerves can be identified, the correlation between the peptide content and the function of a nerve is still unclear.[48] For example, it has been shown that within a single vascular tree of large and small arteries and arterioles, neurons that innervate the consecutive vascular components contain unique complements of peptides,[50] but apparently functionally similar neurons in the same animal often have different complements of peptides.[50] Other studies of the ENS[51] have revealed correlations between peptide distribution and neurons that are anatomically and functionally distinct.

Several functions for neuropeptides have been proposed: (1) a role in determining the type of synaptic junction that develops or in maintaining a synapse in a functional state, and (2) that peptides act as primary neurotransmitters or cotransmitters[48] or as modulators of synaptic and nonsynaptic neural activity in central and peripheral nerves.[48,52] For example, it has been found that a peptide called *vasoactive intestinal peptide* (VIP) often occurs in cholinergic nerve terminals and may function as a modulator or cotransmitter to acetylcholine.[6] *Neuropeptide Y* (NPY) occurs in many adrenergic nerve terminals[53,54] but apparently only those serving vascular smooth muscle and not those innervating glands. There is substantial evidence that NPY acts as a neuromodulator at adrenergic synapses, and it has been suggested that it may act as a cotransmitter with norepinephrine.[55]

In summary, though it is clear that neuropeptides are present in autonomic (and sensory and motor) nerves fibers, and there are clear differences in the distribution of nerves with particular complements of peptides—and in electrophysiologic recordings from the neurons—the function of theses neuropeptides is ill-understood.

## Functions of the Autonomic Nervous System

The ANS affects the function of all cardiac and smooth muscle tissue and exocrine glands in the body. Most of these tissues and glands are innervated by both sympathetic and parasympathetic divisions, which apply opposing stimuli. For example, in the heart parasympathetic fibers are inhibitory and sympathetic fibers are facilitative, whereas in the digestive tract parasympathetic fibers are facilitative and sympathetic fibers inhibitory. Exceptions to the dual innervation trend include the sweat glands and cutaneous vasculature. Furthermore, the ANS does not provide the sole controlling stimuli for cardiac muscle and much of the visceral smooth muscle, as these tissues have intrinsic neural networks that can function independent of extrinsic input. In these tissues, function continues in the absence of extrinsic innervation or neurohumoral agents. In normal function, however, both intrinsic and ANS stimuli and extrinsic hormones contribute to the control of these tissues.

Although some of the ANS functions are of limited scope (i.e., degree of iris contraction), most are important in maintaining internal homeostasis. The latter is true of the autonomic effects on circulation (heart rate and contractile force, vascular resistance, blood pressure), digestion (motility of gut and secretion of digestive juices), kidney function, temperature regulation, and fluid balance (composition, distribution, volume), all of which contribute to maintaining a fairly stable internal environment favorable to the basic biochemical processes necessary for life.

### Pineal Gland (Table 4-2)

The pineal gland is involved in the synthesis and secretion of melatonin, a hormone that mediates our responses to photoperiod and exposure to the sun. The pineal gland is innervated by sympathetic adrenergic fibers, which are principally responsible for stimulating melatonin synthesis via the action of $\alpha_1$- and $\beta_1$-adrenoreceptors.[56,57] Photic signals originating in the retina travel via the retinohypothalamic tract, the suprachiasma, tuberal hypothalamus, medial forebrain bundle, reticular formation, and upper thoracic intermediolateral cell column to the superior cervical ganglion. From this ganglion the postganglionic sympathetic fibers pass via the tentorium cerebelli and conarian nerve to the pineal gland.[58] Additionally, the pineal gland has innervation directly from the brain[59] with several neuropeptides and amino acids such as γ-aminobutyric acid, glutamate, serotonin, acetylcholine, and dopamine, present and thought to be involved as transmitters or modulators in pineal gland control mechanisms.[57]

**Table 4-2.** Autonomic Innervation of Eye Structures and Pineal Gland

| Organs | ANS Division | Nucleus of Origin | Nerve(s) | Ganglion | Receptors | Response |
|---|---|---|---|---|---|---|
| Eye | | | | | | |
| Ciliary m. | Parasympathetic | Edinger-Westphal | Oculomotor | Ciliary | M | Focus of lens |
| Radial m. | Sympathetic | Intermediolateral | Ciliary | Superior cervical | $\alpha_1$ / M | Contraction of dilator / relaxation of dilator |
| Sphincter m. | Parasympathetic | Edinger-Westphal | Short ciliary | Ciliary | M | Contraction of constrictor |
| Lacrimal glands | Parasympathetic | Superior salivary | Facial | Pterygopalatine | M | Secretion |
| Pineal gland | Sympathetic | Intermediolateral | Conarian | Superior cervical | $\alpha_1$, $\beta_1$ | Melatonin synthesis/secretion |

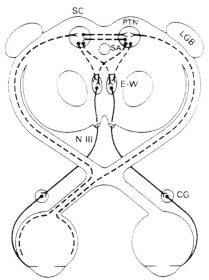

**Figure 4-9.** Schematic diagram of the pathways involved in pupillary dilatation. (From Smith SA. Pupillary function in autonomic failure. In: Bannister R, ed. Autonomic Failure. A Textbook of Clinical Disorders of the Autonomic Nervous System. Oxford: Oxford University Press, 1988; 393–412, with permission.)

### *Pupil diameter (Figures 4-9 and 4-10, Table 4-2)*

Pupil constriction in response to bright light and near vision occurs by contraction of the circular smooth muscle fibers of the sphincter pupillae in the iris. The pathways of the pupil's response to light are illustrated in Figure 4-9. Light transduced by the retina generates impulses that travel along the optic nerve tracts, pass through the optic chiasma where some of the fibers cross to the opposite hemisphere, and then proceed to form synapses in the *pretectal nuclei* in the midbrain. Fibers from both pretectal nuclei innervate the Edinger-Westphal nuclei in both hemispheres. The reflex for near vision descends from the cortex to the Edinger-Westphal nuclei without passing through the pretectal nuclei. From the Edinger-Westphal nuclei fibers proceed along the oculomotor nerve (cranial nerve III) and form synapses with postganglionic fibers in the ciliary ganglia. Postganglionic fibers release acetylcholine, which acts on muscarinic receptors in the sphincter pupillae smooth muscle fibers.[60,61]

Pupil dilatation occurs in response to both inhibition of Edinger-Westphal nuclei and sympathetic stimulation of the radial smooth muscle fibers in the dilator pupillae of the iris. The pathways involved in pupillary dilatation are illustrated in Figure 4-10. Postganglionic fibers release norepinephrine, which causes contraction of radial smooth muscle fibers in the dilator pupillae by acting on α-receptors.

There is evidence of muscarinic receptors on radial fibers, which may cause some relaxation to

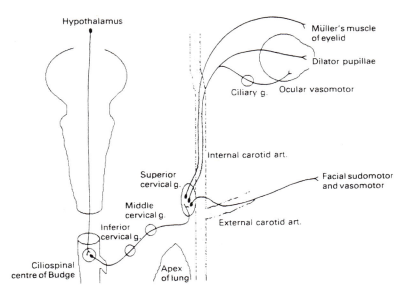

**Figure 4-10.** The pathway of the light reflex from the retina to the iris sphincter. Key: SC, superior colliculus; PTN, pretectal nucleus; LGB, lateral geniculate body; SA, sylvian aqueduct; E-W, Edinger-Westphal nucleus; N III, oculomotor (third cranial) nerve; CG, ciliary ganglion. (From Alexandridis E. The Pupil. Berlin: Springer-Verlag, 1985; 6–7, with permission.)

**Table 4-3.** Autonomic Innervation of the Respiratory Structures

| Organ | ANS Division | Nucleus of Origin | Nerve(s) | Ganglion | Receptors | Response |
|---|---|---|---|---|---|---|
| Nasopharynx | Parasympathetic | Superior salivary | Facial | Pterygopalatine | ? | Secretion |
| Lungs | | | | | | |
| Bronchial m. | Sympathetic | Intermediolateral T1–4 | Spinal | Chain | $\beta_2$ | Relaxation |
| | Parasympathetic | Dorsal vagal nucleus | Vagus (X) | Intramural bronchial | $M_2$ | Contraction |
| Bronchial glands | Parasympathetic | Dorsal vagal nucleus | Vagus (X) | Intramural bronchial | $M_2$ | Stimulation |
| Pulmonary vessels | Sympathetic | Intermediolateral T1–4 | Spinal | Chain | $\alpha_1$, $\beta_2$ | Constriction, dilatation |
| | Parasympathetic | Dorsal vagal nucleus | Vagus (X) | Intramural | M | Dilatation |

facilitate pupil contraction. Also, there is some evidence of β-receptors on the sphincter pupillae fibers, which may cause their relaxation during pupil dilatation.[61,62]

The integrity of pupil innervation is tested by (1) instillation of adrenaline, which has no effect on normally innervated pupils but causes dilatation in the presence of postganglionic denervation, (2) instillation of 4% cocaine, which causes dilation in normally innervated pupils but has no effect on pupils that lack sympathetic innervation, and (3) instillation of 2.5% methacholine, which has no effect on normally innervated pupils but constricts pupils that lack parasympathetic innervation.[63]

## Respiratory Tract Function (Table 4-3)

The respiratory vasculature and smooth muscle tissues in the larynx, trachea, bronchi, and lungs

are innervated by both sympathetic and parasympathetic fibers. Vasodilatation is under parasympathetic control, and vasoconstriction is mediated by sympathetic nerves and $\alpha_1$- and $\beta_2$-adrenoreceptors. Contraction of pulmonary smooth muscle is under parasympathetic control, and relaxation of smooth muscles is mediated by sympathetic fibers via $\beta_2$-adrenoreceptors. Secretion in nasopharyngeal and bronchial surfaces is under parasympathetic control.

## Digestion (Table 4-4)

The acts of eating and chewing are voluntary, but digestion of food is largely under involuntary control mediated by the autonomic sympathetic, parasympathetic, and enteric divisions of the nervous system. The processes involved in digestion include salivation, swallowing, passage of food to

**Table 4-4.** Autonomic Innervation of Digestive Tract Organs and Glands

| Organ | ANS Division | Nucleus of Origin | Nerve(s) | Ganglion | Receptors | Response |
|---|---|---|---|---|---|---|
| Salivary Glands | Sympathetic | Intermediolateral | | Superior cervical | $\alpha$, $\beta$ | Secretion of $K^+$, $H_2O$, amylase |
| | Parasympathetic | Inferior salivary | Glossopharyngeal | Submandibular, otic | M | Secretion of gland cells |
| Arterioles | Sympathetic | Intermediolateral | | Superior cervical | $\alpha$ | Constriction |
| | Parasympathetic | Inferior salivary | Glossopharyngeal | Submandibular, otic, pterygopalatine | $M_3$ | Dilatation |

**Table 4-4.** *Continued*

| Organ | ANS Division | Nucleus of Origin | Nerve(s) | Ganglion | Receptors | Response |
|---|---|---|---|---|---|---|
| Throat | Parasympathetic | Dorsal vagal nucleus | Vagus (X) | Submandibular, pterygopalatine | M ⎫ | Coordination of swallowing |
| Esophagus | Parasympathetic | Dorsal vagal nucleus | Vagus (X) | Myenteric, submucous | M ⎬ | |
| **Pancreas** | | | | | | |
| Acini | Sympathetic | Intermediolateral | Splanchnics | Celiac | $\alpha$ | Decreased secretion |
| | Parasympathetic | Dorsal vagal nucleus | Vagus (X) | Intramural pancreatic | $M_3$ | Secretion |
| Islets | Sympathetic | Intermediolateral | Splanchnics | Celiac | $\alpha$ | Increased secretion |
| | Sympathetic | Dorsal vagal nucleus | Vagus (X) | Intramural | $\beta_2$ | Decreased secretion |
| Gallbladder | Sympathetic | Intermediolateral | Splanchnics | Celiac | ? | Relaxation |
| | Parasympathetic | Dorsal vagal nucleus | Vagus (X) | Intramural | ? | Contraction |
| **Stomach** | | | | | | |
| Smooth muscle | Sympathetic | Intermediolateral | Splanchnics | Celiac | $\alpha_2$, $\beta_2$ | Decreased motility and tone |
| | Parasympathetic | Dorsal vagal nucleus | Vagus (X) | Myenteric plexus | $M_?$ | Increased motility and tone |
| Sphincters | Sympathetic | Intermediolateral | Splanchnics | Celiac | $\alpha$ | Contraction |
| | Parasympathetic | Dorsal vagal nucleus | Vagus (X) | Intramural | $M_?$ | Relaxation |
| Glands | Parasympathetic | Dorsal vagal nucleus | Vagus (X) | Submucous plexus | $M_3$ | Secretion |
| **Small Intestine** | | | | | | |
| Smooth muscle | Sympathetic | Intermediolateral | Splanchnics | Celiac | $\alpha_2$, $\beta_2$, $\beta_3$ | Decreased motility and tone |
| | Parasympathetic | Dorsal vagal nucleus | Vagus (X) | Intramural | $M_3$ | Increased motility and tone |
| Sphincters | Sympathetic | Intermediolateral | Splanchnics | Celiac | $\alpha$ | Contraction |
| | Parasympathetic | Dorsal vagal nucleus | Vagus (X) | Intramural | $M_?$ | Relaxation (usually) |
| Glands | Parasympathetic | Dorsal vagal nucleus | Vagus (X) | Submucous plexus | $M_3$ | Secretion |
| **Large Intestine** | | | | | | |
| Upper colon sm | Sympathetic | Intermediolateral | Splanchnics | Celiac | Adrenergic | Decreased motility |
| | Parasympathetic | Dorsal vagal nucleus | Vagus (X) | Intramural | M | Increased motility |
| Lower colon sm | Parasympathetic | Sacral | Pelvic | Intramural | M | Motility |
| | Sympathetic | Intermediolateral | Nervus erigens | Superior messenteric | Adrenergic | Motility |
| Vessels | Parasympathetic | Sacral | Pelvic | Intramural | $M_3$ | Blood flow to colon |
| Rectum (vessels) | Parasympathetic | Sacral | Pelvic | Inferior hypogastric plexus | M | Blood flow |
| sphincters | Parasympathetic | Sacral | Pelvic | Inferior hypogastric plexus | M | Contraction, relaxation |

the stomach, secretion of gastric and other digestive fluids, passage through the small and large intestines and colon, and defecation of unabsorbed material. The ANS regulates secretory processes and digestive tract blood flow and motility.

### Salivation

Saliva is the first digestive juice to contact food. Besides containing amylase to initiate digestion of food, it is essential to lubricate the food for swallowing. Saliva secretion in humans occurs principally from three pairs of salivary glands, the parotid (the largest), submaxillary, and sublingual glands, but many smaller mucous glands, including the lingual mucous glands, lingual serous glands, and mucous glands in the cheek, hard and soft palate, and surface of the pharynx, participate in the production of saliva. The salivary glands have both sympathetic and parasympathetic innervation. Parasympathetic stimulation provokes secretion by the gland cells (acinar cells) into collection ducts and dilatation of blood vessels in the glands. Sympathetic nerves mediate constriction of blood vessels, smooth muscle contraction, and secretion of potassium and amylase from the glands.

### Swallowing

Swallowing is a reflex under parasympathetic control via the hypoglossal, glossopharyngeal, and vagus nerves. The transducers that provoke the reflex are at the entrance to the oropharynx in the mucous membrane of the pillar of fauces, tonsils, soft palate, the base of the tongue, and the posterior wall of the pharyngeal region. Markwald[64] discovered a region at the base of the fourth ventricle that is essential to coordination of the various muscles involved in swallowing. This "swallowing center" is near (above and lateral) the respiratory center, but its complete independence is demonstrated by the observation that respiration is unaffected by destruction of the swallowing center, and vice versa. Efferent nerves that participate in the swallowing reflex include the hypoglossal and glossopharyngeal, which coordinate the initial stages in the mouth and pharynx, and the vagus, which mediates stimulation of both the striped muscle and smooth muscle components of the esophagus. The striped muscle is innervated directly, but the smooth muscle is innervated via an extensive local plexus similar to the myenteric plexus in other regions of the gastrointestinal tract.

### Stomach Gastric Glands

The gastric mucosa in innervated by both sympathetic and parasympathetic fibers.[65] The sympathetic fibers originate in the fifth through the tenth thoracic lateral horns in the spinal cord. Some of the preganglionic nerves form synapses in the paravertebral sympathetic chain, but most continue via the thoracic splanchnic nerves and form synapses in the celiac plexus ganglion. Postganglionic sympathetic fibers follow the arterial vascular supply to the stomach. The sympathetic nerves supply the mucosa and stimulate secretion by the pyloric glands.

Parasympathetic fibers originate in the dorsal vagal nucleus; preganglionic fibers traverse the left and right vagus nerves. The left vagus fibers supply the posterior surface of the stomach and the right vagus fibers, the anterior surface. Some fibers from both vagus nerves traverse the celiac plexus and travel with the sympathetic postganglionic fibers. The parasympathetic fibers form synapses with ganglionic cells in the myenteric plexus of Auerbach and the submucous plexus of Meissner in the smooth muscle layers of the stomach. These postganglionic fibers are very short. Parasympathetic fibers are responsible for gastric secretion (rich in pepsin) and for release of gastrin from the gastric antrum. Vagal fibers also control secretion of mucin by the surface epithelium of the gastric mucosa.[66]

Gastric emptying occurs as part of the stomach contents is pushed through the pyloric orifice during normal stomach movements. The rate of stomach emptying depends largely on the composition and volume of its contents.

### Pancreas

The structure of the pancreas is similar to that of the salivary glands. It is innervated by both the sympathetic and parasympathetic fibers. The sympathetic innervation travels via the splanchnic nerves to synapse in the celiac ganglion and associated ganglia. Postganglionic sympathetic fibers innervate pancreatic vasculature to affect blood flow.

Pancreas-bound parasympathetic fibers occur in both vagus nerves. They traverse the celiac plexus and travel along with the blood vessels supplying the pancreas (primarily the pancreaticoduodenal artery) to intramural ganglia cells in the pancreas tissue. The parasympathetic fibers are responsible for stimulating pancreatic secretion.

### Gallbladder

Gallbladder and Brunner's glands are innervated by sympathetic and parasympathetic fibers, but little is known of the role of each division in stimulating and inhibiting secretion of bile and digestive juices.

### Small Intestine

Foodstuffs leaving the stomach have been broken down into large molecules but are far from ready for absorption by the intestine. Further breakdown of the foodstuffs is helped by pancreatic juices that contain lipase to digest fats, and other enzymes for reducing protein to peptides and reducing starch and dextrose to maltose and glucose. Final preparation of food for absorption is accomplished by enzymes secreted from the mucosal lining and glands in the intestinal wall. Secretion by Brunner's glands located in the duodenum can be initiated by stimulation of the vagi but not by stimulation of sympathetics.[67] Secretion from the mucosa of the small intestine is stimulated principally by local mechanical and chemical stimuli[68] and, furthermore, the gut wall has an intrinsic ability to perform smooth muscle contractions. Although the gut wall is innervated by both sympathetic and parasympathetic nerves, their role and degree of participation in facilitating intestinal secretion and motility are ill-understood. Stimulation of parasympathetic tracts in the vagus nerves can increase secretion in the duodenum but not in the lower regions of the intestine. Stimulation of the sympathetic nerves does not increase secretion, but sectioning of these fibers results in significant increases in secretion, termed *paralytic secretion.* Paralytic secretion is increased by parasympathomimetic drugs and inhibited by atropine and sympathomimetic drugs. Thus, it is clearly a "cholinergic-mediated" response because of unopposed acetylcholine stimulation.

### Colon

The proximal part of the colon is innervated with parasympathetic fibers via the vagi. The distal portion is innervated via the sacral fibers and the nervus erigens. The simulation of parasympathetic fibers cause secretion in the colon,[69,70] but it should be remembered that the colon is principally a site of fluid absorption, so secretion is small. Sympathetic fibers do inhibit the secretion stimulated by parasympathetic fibers.

**Defecation.** Defecation is partly voluntary and partly involuntary reflex actions. The involuntary portion is stimulated by an increase in pressure in the rectum (equal to 20 to 25 cm $H_2O$) causing stretch-initiated impulses to pass to the sacral cord via lumbar colonic and hypogastric nerves. Reflex centers for defecation occur in the hypothalamus, the lower lumbar and upper sacral segments of the spinal cord, and the ganglionic plexus of the gut. The effector stimuli result in massive contractions of the colon, which propel its contents into the rectum, and finally in expulsion unless it is voluntarily inhibited. Defecation occurs, however, even in persons with complete spinal cord transection, as the intrinsic intestinal plexus and the sacral cord take over control of the reflexes involved.

**Micturition (Table 4-5, Figure 4-11).**[12,71] The urinary tract has sensory, somatic motor and autonomic innervation which works in an integrated fashion to maintain continence and effect micturition (urination). Mechanoreceptors in the bladder wall respond to bladder distension in a graded manner after a threshold tension of about 5 to 15 mm Hg is reached. Afferents important to micturition occur principally in the pelvic nerve but also are found in the hypogastric and inferior splanchnic nerves. There is somatic voluntary innervation of the striated muscle fibers in the urethra and periurethra. These fibers originate in Onuf's nucleus in the lateral ventral horn and travel via the pudendal nerve.

Parasympathetic fibers serving the detrusor muscle of the bladder originate in the intermediolateral column of segments S2 to S4 of the spinal

**Table 4-5.** Autonomic Innervation of Bladder and Urinary Tract Tissues

| Organ | ANS Division | Nucleus of Origin | Nerve(s) | Ganglion | Receptors | Response |
|---|---|---|---|---|---|---|
| Kidneys | Sympathetic | Intermediolateral TL | Splanchnics | Renal | $\beta_2$ | Renin secretion |
| | Parasympathetic | Intermediolateral S | Hypogastric | Intramural | $M_?$ | ? |
| Ureter | Sympathetic | Intermediolateral L | Hypogastric | Chain | $\alpha$ | Increased motility |
| Bladder detrusor sm. | Sympathetic | Intramediolateral L | Hypogastric | Chain | Adrenergic | Unknown ($\beta$ relaxation)? |
| | Parasympathetic | Intramediolateral S2–4 | Pelvic, pudendal | Pelvic plexus, intramural | M | Contraction |
| Urethra sm. | Sympathetic | Intermediolateral L | Hypogastric | Chain | $\alpha_1$ | Excitatory stimulus, contraction |
| | Parasympathetic | Intermediolateral S2–4 | Pelvic, pudendal | Intramural | Non-M | Inhibition of smooth muscle |
| Trigone, sphincter | Sympathetic | Intermediolateral L | Hypogastric | Chain | $\alpha_1$ | Excitatory stimulus, contraction |
| | Parasympathetic | Intramediolateral S2–4 | Pelvic, pudendal | Intramural | Non-M | Relaxation |

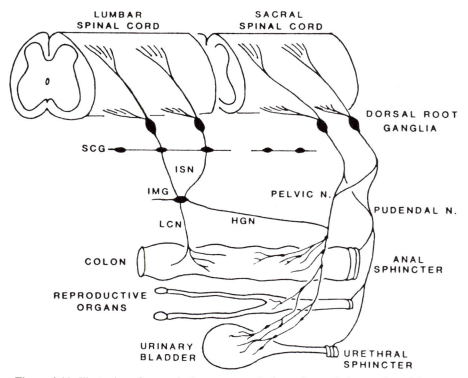

**Figure 4-11.** Illustration of sympathetic, parasympathetic, and somatic innervation of the colon, reproductive organs, and urinary tract of the cat. (From deGroat WC. Neuropeptides in pelvic afferent pathways. Experientia 1987; 43:801–813, with permission.)

cord and travel along the pelvic nerves to form synapses either in the pelvic plexus or with intramural ganglion cells in the bladder. These parasympathetic fibers effect bladder contraction by effecting release of acetylcholine from ganglion cells, which excites the smooth muscle fibers of the bladder. Cholinergic transmission is mediated by muscarinic receptors and can be blocked by atropine. Nonmuscarinic parasympathetic fibers inhibit smooth muscle of the urethra.[72]

Sympathetic fibers also innervate the detrusor smooth muscle, but its function is unclear. There is no evidence in the literature of sympathetic inhibitory action in humans, and in other mammals it is sometimes found to be inhibitory (cat and rhesus monkey) and sometimes not inhibitory (dog, rabbit). Similarly, the sympathetic nerves do not cause excitatory action in humans, but do result in excitatory contraction of the detrusor in ferrets, guinea pigs, and male goats. The $\alpha_1$-adrenergic fibers do provide excitatory innervation of the trigone and urethra.[73]

Stimulation of the pelvic nerves causes bladder contraction. Bilateral pelvic nerve section results in paralysis of the detrusor muscle, retention of urine, and incontinence due to overflow (see Chapter 19).

### Gonads (Table 4-6, Figure 4-11)

Both testes and ovaries have sympathetic (but no parasympathetic) innervation. The sympathetic supply to the ovaries occurs via the ovarian plexus and superior ovarian nerve.[74] A mechanism that facilitates either release or synthesis of progesterone is adrenergic. The opposing mechanism is non–$\alpha$-adrenergic.[75] Lumbar sympathectomy in guinea pigs, cats, and dogs results in depressed spermatogenesis in the week after section, but some recovery is apparent after 3 months.

The vas deferens, seminal vesicles, and prostate also have sympathetic, but no parasympathetic, innervation. Sympathetic nerves run via the hypogastric plexus and are mediated by $\alpha_1$-adrener-

**Table 4-6.** Autonomic Innervation of Reproductive Organs

| Organ | ANS Division | Nucleus of Origin | Nerve(s) | Ganglion | Receptors | Response |
|-------|-------------|-------------------|----------|----------|-----------|----------|
| Female Organs | | | | | | |
| Ovaries | Sympathetic | Intermediolateral | Ovarian plexus | Renal ganglion | $\alpha$ | Progesterone synthesis or release |
| Uterus | Sympathetic | Intermediolateral | Ovarian, hypogastric | Renal ganglion, intramural | $\beta_2$, $\alpha_1$ | Relaxation normally; contraction during pregnancy |
| | Parasympathetic | Intermediolateral | Pelvic splanchnic | Uterovaginal plexus | ? | Variable |
| External genitals | Sympathetic | Intermediolateral | Hypogastric | Uterovaginal plexus | ? | ? |
| | Parasympathetic | Intermediolateral | Pelvic | Uterovaginal plexus | ? | ? |
| Male Organs | | | | | | |
| Testes | Sympathetic | Intramediolateral | Testicular plexus | Renal ganglion | $\alpha_1$ | Ejaculation |
| Seminal vesicle, vas deferens, prostate | Sympathetic | Intermediolateral | Hypogastric | Pelvic plexus, intramural | $\alpha_1$ | Ejaculation |
| Erectile tissue | Sympathetic | Intermediolateral | Hypogastric | Inferior hypogastric plexus | $\alpha_1$ | Antierectile |
| | Sympathetic | Intermediolateral | Hypogastric | Inferior hypogastric plexus | ? (Not $\beta$) | Erectile |
| | Parasympathetic | Intermediolateral S2–3 | Pelvic | Prostate plexus | ? (Non-M) | Erection |

gic receptors. The smooth muscles in these tissues become activated during ejaculation, and electrical stimulation results in powerful synchronized contractions.

The erectile mechanism of the penis is mediated by both sympathetic and parasympathetic nerves. The parasympathetic fibers emerge from the spinal cord from S2 or S3 and enter the pelvic splanchnic plexus. They emerge and travel with the sympathetic erectile fibers coming from the thoracolumbar region along the prostate and urethra. Besides the sympathetic erectile fibers, there are sympathetic antierectile fibers, which are a $\alpha_1$ adrenergic. Both emerge from the spinal cord via thoracolumbar anterior nerve roots and travel via the hypogastric plexus. The exact route by which these fibers reach erectile tissues is not known. The receptors involved in sympathetic and parasympathetic erectile response also are not known, but it has been shown that the parasympathetic fibers are not muscarinic, since erection cannot be blocked with atropine, and that the sympathetic fibers are not β-adrenergic fibers.[76] Vasoactive intestinal peptide is considered a probable candidate as one transmitter, as it has been located in all the appropriate sites[77] and affects the appropriate smooth muscle response.[78]

*Circulation (Table 4-7, Figure 4-12)*

The cardiovascular system is responsible for delivering oxygen and other nutrients to various tissues of the body and for removing metabolic waste products, including heat. The three essential physiologic components of circulation are (1) cardiac output, the volume of blood pumped by the heart into the vascular network per unit time, (2) blood pressure, the force necessary to push that volume of blood through the vascular network at the appropriate velocity, and (3) vascular resistance, which functions to maintain the blood pressure and the appropriate amount of tissue perfusion and size of vascular space for the volume of blood in the system. Cardiac output, blood pressure, and peripheral vascular resistance are all largely regulated by the autonomic nervous system acting on the heart and the vascular network.

The heart has specialized cells in the sinus node intrinsically capable of providing the electrical stimulation for an organized heart contraction. Input from sympathetic and parasympathetic nerves affects both the frequency and the force of the heart contraction. Parasympathetic stimulation of the sinus and atrioventricular nodes via release of acetylcholine acts to slow heart rate, and sympathetic stimulation of the sinus node and ventricles acts to increase the heart rate and ventricular contractile force. In normal life, the ANS input to the heart contributes to the maintenance of proper tissue perfusion to vital organs. For example, to maintain blood pressure adequate for proper perfusion of the brain when a person assumes a standing posture there are adjustments in heart rate and contractility and peripheral vascular resistance. Without these cardiovascular adjustments there would be a loss of central blood pressure, insufficient blood and oxygen reaching the brain, and the person would "black out."

Arteries and arterioles are primarily innervated by sympathetic fibers that affect the degree of constriction. These sympathetic fibers are largely responsible for directing which tissues are perfused with blood at any given moment and which are not. They are essential to the maintenance of blood pressure by sustaining the proper degree of vascular resistance and the size of the vascular space. Loss of function in these nerves results in loss of vasoconstriction stimulus, a lack of control of the size of the vascular space and the direction of blood flow in the tissue, and increased difficulty in maintaining blood pressure. For a more detailed discussion of the cardiovascular system, see Chapter 5.

## Autonomic Assessment Based on Cardiovascular Responses to Standard Tests

Many of the tests directed at assessing the integrity of autonomic function in general or of specific pathways focus on cardiovascular responses, because these are most easily measured owing to accessibility and available techniques for monitoring them (as compared to other autonomic function such as gut motility or bladder contractility). Certain cardiovascular parameters are normally monitored. Blood pressure is measured intermittently using a sphygmomanometer or continuously using an arterial catheter attached to a pressure transducer. Heart rate is monitored continuously. Pe-

**Table 4-7.** Autonomic Innervation of Heart and Vasculature

| Organ | ANS Division | Nucleus of Origin | Nerve(s) | Ganglion | Receptors | Response |
|---|---|---|---|---|---|---|
| **Heart** | | | | | | |
| SA node | Sympathetic | Intermediolat-eral T1–4 | Middle & inferior cervical cardiacs | Middle cervical, stellate | $\beta_1$ | Increased heart rate |
| | Parasympathetic | Dorsal vagal nucleus | Cervical vagal cardiacs | Intramural cardiac | $M_2$ | Decreased heart rate |
| Atria | Sympathetic | Intermediolat-eral T1–4 | Middle & inferior cervical cardiacs | Middle cervical, stellate | $\beta_1$ | Increased contractility |
| | Parasympathetic | Dorsal vagal nucleus | Cervical vagal cardiacs | Intramural cardiac | $M_2$ | Decreased contractility |
| AV node | Sympathetic | Intermediolat-eral | Inferior cervical & thoracic | Stellate, chain | $\beta_1$ | Increased conduction velocity |
| | Parasympathetic | Dorsal vagal nucleus | Cervical vagal cardiacs | Intramural cardiac | $M_2$ | Decreased conduction velocity, AV block |
| His-Purkinje | Sympathetic | Intermediolat-eral | Inferior cervical & thoracic | Stellate, chain | $\beta_1$ | Increased conduction velocity |
| Ventricles | Sympathetic | Intermediolat-eral | Inferior cervical & thoracic | Stellate, chain | $\beta_1$ | Increased contractility, conduction, velocity, automaticity, idioventricular pacemakers |
| | Parasympathetic | Dorsal vagal nucleus | Cervical vagal cardiacs | Intramural cardiac | $M_2$ | Slightly decreased contractility |
| **Arterioles** | | | | | | |
| Cerebral | Sympathetic | Intermediolat-eral | Internal carotid n | Cervical chain | $\alpha$ | Constriction |
| Heart | Sympathetic | Intermediolat-eral | Inferior cervical & thoracic | Chain | $\alpha, \beta_2$ | Constriction, dilatation |
| Pulmonary | Sympathetic | Intermediolat-eral | Inferior cervical & thoracic | Chain | $\alpha_1, \beta_2$ | Constriction, dilatation |
| Abdominal vicera | Sympathetic | Intermediolat-eral | Thoracic splanchnics | Chain | $\alpha_1, \beta_2$ | Constriction, dilatation |
| Skin and epithelium | Sympathetic | Intermediolat-eral | Spinal | Chain | $\alpha$ | Constriction |
| Skeletal muscle | Sympathetic | Intermediolat-eral | Spinal | Chain | $\alpha_1, \beta_2$ | Constriction, dilatation |
| Veins | Sympathetic | Intermediolat-eral | Spinal | Chain | $\alpha_1, \beta_2$ | Constriction |

ripheral blood flow is measured intermittently using venous occlusion plethysmography or continuously by measuring superficial capillary perfusion using laser Doppler technique. Cardiac output is measured noninvasively with Doppler ultrasonography or resistance methods. Peripheral vascular resistance is calculated for peripheral blood flow measures and blood pressure.

Standard tests used to assess autonomic (cardiovascular) pathways are listed and discussed in

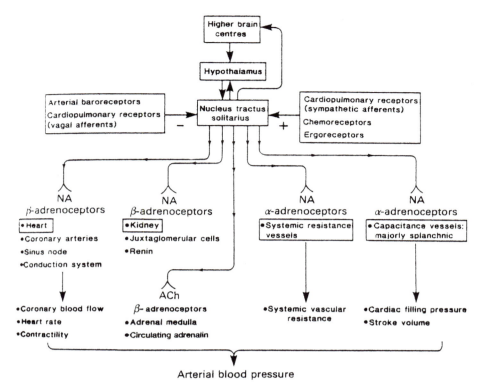

**Figure 4-12.** Diagram of reflex control in the cardiovascular system. The arterial baroreceptors and the cardiopulmonary receptors with vagal afferents tonically inhibit ( − ) the vasomotor centers in the nucleus tractus solitarius. The cardiopulmonary receptors with sympathetic afferents, the arterial chemoreceptors, and ergoreceptors in the skeletal muscles (when activated by their contraction) stimulate ( + ) the centers. As a consequence, sympathetic outflow is modified selectively to adjust appropriately the performance of the cardiovascular system. The norepinephrine (NA) released at the sympathetic terminals acts on β-adrenoceptors in the heart and the coronary vessels to accelerate heart rate and augment cardiac contractility and relax the main coronary arteries. Norepinephrine also acts on the β-adrenoceptors in the juxtaglomerular cells of the kidney to regulate the release of renin. The sympathetic outflow to the adrenal medulla regulates adrenaline release. The circulating adrenaline also activates the β-adrenoceptors. The noradrenaline released also activates α-adrenoceptors to cause constriction of the resistance vessels and a decrease in the capacitance of the splanchnic vascular bed. As a consequence, systemic vascular resistance and cardiac filling pressure (and, thus, stroke and cardiac output) are adjusted to maintain the arterial blood pressure at the appropriate level for perfusion of the organs and tissues of the body. (From Shepherd RFJ, Shepherd JT. Control of the blood pressure and the circulation in man. In: Bannister R, ed. Autonomic Failure. Oxford: Oxford University Press, 1988; 80–96, with permission.)

detail in the text *Autonomic Dysfunction*, edited by R. Bannister.[63]

## Temperature Regulation (Table 4-8)

The thermoregulatory mechanism is comprised of five functionally distinct types of elements: (1) temperature-sensitive structures (temperature sensors) in the skin[79] and inner body tissues,[80–87] (2) afferent pathways in trigeminal and spinal nerves that transmit information from the temperature transducers to the CNS, (3) a neural network within the spinal cord and brain that is largely responsible for the integration of afferent signals and stimulating appropriate effector responses, (4)

**Table 4-8.** Autonomic Innervation of Thermoregulatory Effector Tissues

| Organ | ANS Division | Nucleus of Origin | Nerve(s) | Ganglion | Receptors | Response |
|---|---|---|---|---|---|---|
| Adipose tissue | Sympathetic | Intermediolateral | Spinal | Chain | $\alpha_1$, $\beta_1$, $\beta_3$ | Lipolysis |
| Skin | | | | | | |
|   Sweat glands | Sympathetic | Intramediolateral | Spinal | Chain | $\alpha$?, $\beta$? | Secretion on palms, soles |
| | | | | | M | Thermoregulatory sweating over body surface |
|   Pilomotor muscles | Sympathetic | Intramediolateral | Spinal | Chain | $\alpha$ | Contraction, piloerection |
| Arterioles | | | | | | |
|   Skin, epithelium | Sympathetic | Intermediolateral | Spinal | Chain | $\alpha$, M | Constriction, dilatation |
| | | | | | M | Dilatation |
| Veins | Sympathetic | Intramediolateral | Spinal | Chain | $\alpha_1$, $\beta_2$ | Constriction, dilatation |

efferent sympathetic and motor pathways from the brain and the spinal cord to the effector tissues, and finally, (5) the effector tissues, the cutaneous vascular bed responsible for vasoconstriction to conserve heat and vasodilatation to transport heat to the skin surface, muscles for shivering thermogenesis, brown adipose tissue for nonshivering thermogenesis, and sweat glands for evaporative heat loss from the skin.

### Effector Mechanisms

Effector mechanisms include conservation of body heat by vasoconstriction followed by increased heat production by shivering and nonshivering thermogenesis in response to cold stress, and vasodilatation to increase heat flow to the skin followed by increased heat loss from the body surface via sweating.

Cutaneous vasoconstriction occurs principally at the arteriole level and is $\alpha$-adrenergic. Cutaneous venoconstriction, which occurs in response to cold stress or exercise,[88] is mediated by sympathetic adrenergic receptors and functions to shift blood volume from the skin to more central sites.[89,90] Shivering occurs in the striated muscle, which is served by motor neurons. It is an involuntary reaction to cold, but temporarily it can be consciously suppressed. Fully developed shivering is characterized by rhythmic grouped contractions. These are controlled by grouped discharges of the

motor neurons, though descending supraspinal pathways appear not to show rhythmic bursts of activity. Thus, the grouped discharges are assumed to evolve at the level of the spinal cord but are clearly under supraspinal influences, as shivering is a response to cold and can be induced by cooling the hypothalamus. Nonshivering thermogenesis is defined as an increase in metabolic heat production that is not attributable to increased motor activity.[91,92] It is controlled by the sympathetic nervous system acting principally on brown adipose tissue in newborns via $\alpha_1$-, $\beta_1$-, and $\beta_3$-receptors, but smooth muscle may also participate in the increased heat production.

Active cutaneous vasodilatation is known to occur principally in the proximal limbs and trunk regions, through sympathetic pathways by action on $\alpha_1$- and $\beta_2$-adrenergic receptors. Thermoregulatory sweating is mediated by sympathetic fibers acting on M receptors.

## References

1. Langley JN. The autonomic nervous system. Brain 1903; 26:1–26.
2. Langley JN. The Autonomic Nervous System. Cambridge: Heffer, 1921.
3. Cannon WB. Organization for physiological homeostasis. Physiol Rev 1929; 9:399–431.
4. Gaskell WH. The Involuntary Nervous System. London: Longmans, Green, 1916.

5. Reil JC.. In: Meyer I, ed. De Joahnnis Christiani Reilii in Physiologia Dignitate. Vratislaviae: 1857.

6. Uvnas B. Sympathetic dilator outflow. Physiol Rev 1954; 34:608–618.

7. Dale HH, Feldberg W, The chemical transmission of secretory impulses to the sweat glands of the cat. J Physiol (Lond) 1934; 82:121–128.

8. Langley JN. Unknown. 1989.

9. Furness JB, Costa M, Types of nerves in the enteric nervous system. Neuroscience 1980; 5:1–20.

10. Roze M. Neurohumerol control of gastrointestinal motility. Reprod Nutr Dev 1980; 20:1125–1141.

11. deGroat WC. Neuropeptides in pelvic afferent pathways. Experientia 1987; 43:801–813.

12. deGroat WC, Steers WD. Neural control of the urinary bladder and sexual organs: Experimental studies in animals. In: Bannister R, ed. Autonomic Failure. Oxford: Oxford University Press, 1988; 196–222.

13. Geffen LB, Livett GB, Synaptic vesicles in sympathetic neurons. Physiol Rev 1971; 51:98–157.

14. Armstrong CM. Ionic pores, gates and gating currents. Rev Biophysi 1974; 7:179–209.

15. Cole KS. Membranes, Ions and Impulses: A Chapter of Classical Biophysics. Berkeley: University of California, 1968.

16. Loewi O. Uber humorale Ubertragbarkeit der Herznervenwirkung. Pflugers Arch 1921; 189:239–243.

17. Feldberg W, Krayer O. Das Auftreten eines azetylcholinartigen Stoffes in Hervenenblut von Warmblutern bei Beizung der Nervi vagi. Arch Exp Pathol Pharmakol 1933; 172:170–193.

18. Dale HH. Nomenclature of fibers in the autonomic system and their effects. J Physiol London 1933; 80:10P–11P.

19. Starke K, Gothert M, Kilbinger H. Modulation of neurotransmitter release by presynaptic autoreceptors. Physiol Rev 1989; 69:864–989.

20. Starke K. Presynaptic autoregulation: Does it play a role? News Physiologic Sci 1989; 4:1–4.

21. Fatt P, Katz B. Spontaneous subthreshold activity at motor nerve endings. J Physiol Lond 1952; 117:109–128.

22. Hall ZW. Release of neurotransmitters and their interaction with receptors. Annu Rev Biochem 1972; 41:925–947.

23. Rang HP. Acetylcholine receptors. O Rev Biophys 1975; 7:283–397.

24. Miyamoto MD. The actions of cholinergic drugs on motor nerve terminals. Pharmacol Rev 1978; 29:226–247.

25. Ritchie AK, Goldberg AM. Vesicular and synaptoplasmic synthesis of acetylcholine. Science 1970; 173:489–490.

26. DeRobertis E, Bennett HS. Some features of the submicroscopic morphology of synapses in frog and earthworm. J Biophys Biochem 1955; 1:47–58.

27. Doods HN. Selective muscarinic antagonist for peripheral muscarinic receptor subtypes. In: Rand MJ, Raper C, eds. Pharmacology. Amsterdam: Excerpta Medica, 1987; 59–65.

28. Brown JH, Goldstein D, Masters SB. Biochemical evidence for muscarinic receptor subtypes. In: Rand MJ, Raper C, eds. Pharmacology. Amsterdam: Excerpta Medica, 1987; 55–58.

29. Dohlman HG, Caron MG, Lefkowitz RJ. A family of receptors coupled to guanine nucleotide regulatory proteins. Biochemistry 1987; 26:2657–2664.

30. Cannon WB, Bacq ZM. Studies on the conditions of activity in endocrine organs. Am J Physiol 1931; 96:392–412.

31. von Euler US. Identification of the sympathomimetic ergone in adrenergic nerves in cattle (sympathin N) with laevo-noradrenaline. Acta Physiol Scand 1948; 16:63–74.

32. von Euler US. Adrenergic neurotransmitter functions. Science 1971; 173:202–206.

33. Blaschko H. The specific action of L-dopa decarboxylase. J Physiol (Lond) 1939; 96:50P–51P.

34. Iversen LL. The catecholamines. Nature 1967; 214:8–14.

35. Axelrod J. Methylation reactions in the formation and metabolism of catecholamines and other biogenic amines: The enzymatic conversion of norepinephrine (NE) to epinephrine (E). Pharmacol Rev 1966; 18:95–113.

36. Kopin IJ. Metabolic degradation of catecholamines. The relative importance of different pathways under physiological conditions and after administration of drugs. In: Blaschko H, Muscholl E, eds. Catecholamines. Berlin: Springer-Verlag, 1972; 271–282.

37. Stromblad BC, Nickerson M. Accumulation of epinephrine and norepinephrine by some rat tissues. J Pharmacol Exp Ther 1961; 134:154–159.

38. Dale HH. On some physiological actions of ergot. J Physiol Lond 1906; 34:163–206.

39. Ahlquist RPA. A study of the adrenotropic receptors. Am J Physiol 1948; 153:586–600.

40. Langer SZ. Presynaptic regulation of catecholamine release. Biochem Pharmacol 1974; 23:1793–1800.

41. Lands AM, Arnold A, McAuliff JP, et al. Differentiation of receptor systems activated by sympathomimetic amines. Nature (Lond) 1967; 214:597–598.

42. Lands AM, Luduena FP, Buzzo HJ. Differentiation of receptors responsive to isoproterenol. Life Sci 1967; 6:2241–2249.

43. Emorine LJ, Marullo S, Briend-Sutren M-M, et al.

Molecular characterization of the human beta$_3$-adrenergic receptor. Science 1989; 245:1118–1121.

44. Goldberg LI, Kohli JD. Peripheral pre- and post-synaptic dopamine receptors: Are they different from dopamine receptors in the central nervous system. Commun Psychopharmacol 1979; 3:447–456.

45. Willems JL, Buylaert WA, Lefebvre RA, et al. Presynaptic, ganglionic and gastrointestinal dopamine receptors in the periphery. Pharmacol Rev 1985; 37:169–216.

46. Axelrod J. The formation, metabolism, uptake and release of noradrenaline and adrenaline. In: Varely H, Gowenluck AH, eds. The Clinical Chemistry of Monoamines. Amsterdam: Elsevier, 1963; 5–18.

47. von Euler US. Synthesis, uptake and storage of catecholamine in adrenergic nerves. The effects of drugs. In: Blaschko H, Muscholl E, eds. Catecholamines. Berlin: Springer-Verlag, 1972; 186–230.

48. Burnstock G. Autonomic neuromuscular junctions: Current developments and future directions. J Anat 1986; 146:1–30.

49. Marti E, Gibson SJ, Polack JM, et al. Ontogeny of peptide- and amine-containing neurons in motor, sensory, and autonomic regions of rat and human spinal cord, dorsal root ganglia, and rat skin. J Comp Neurol 1987; 266:332–359.

50. Gibbins IL. Morphological evidence for regional diversification of autonomic cotransmission in different parts of the cardiovascular system. Proc Int U Physiol Sci 1989; 17:28.

51. Llewellyn-Smith IJ. Neuropeptides and the microcircuitry of the enteric nervous system. Experientia 1987; 43:813–821.

52. Cuello AC. Peptides as neuromodulators in primary sensory neurons. Neuropharmacology 1987; 26:971–979.

53. Lundberg JM, Hokfelt T. Coexistence of peptides and classical neurotransmitters. Trends Neurosci 1983; 62:325–333.

54. Lundberg JM, Ternius L, Holkfelt T, et al. Neuropeptide Y (NPY)–like immunoreactivity in peripheral noradrenergic neurons and effects of NPY on sympathetic function. Acta Physiol Scand 1982; 116:479–480.

55. Lundberg JM, Pernow J, Lacroux JS. Neuropeptide Y: Synaptic cotransmitter and neuromodulator. News Physiol Sci 1989; 4:13–17.

56. Ebadi M, Govitrapong P. Neural pathways and neurotransmitters affecting melatonin synthesis. J Neural Trans Suppl 1986; 21:125–155.

57. Cardinali DP, Vacas MI. Cellular and molecular mechanisms controlling melatonin release by mammalian pineal glands. Cell Molec Neurobiol 1987; 7:323–337.

58. Kappers JP. Survey of the innervation of the epiphysis cerebri and the accessory pineal organs of the vertebrates. Prog Brain Res 1965; 10:87–153.

59. Korf HW, Moller M. The innervation of the mammalian pineal gland with special references to central pinealopetal projections. Pineal Res Rev 1984; 2:41–86.

60. Lowenstein O, Loewenfeld IE. The pupil. In: Davson H, ed. The Eye. New York: Academic Press, 1969; 3:255–337.

61. Smith SA. Pupillary function in autonomic failure. In: Bannister R, ed. Autonomic Failure. A Textbook of Clinical Disorders of the Autonomic Nervous System. Oxford: Oxford University Press, 1988; 393–412.

62. Lowenstein O, Loewenfeld IE. Mutual role of sympathetic and parasympathetic in shaping of the pupillary reflex to light. Pupillographic studies. Arch Neurol Psychiatry 1950; 64:341–377.

63. Bannister R, Mathias C. Testing autonomic reflexes. In: Bannister R, ed. Autonomic Failure. A Text Book of Clinical Disorders of the Autonomic Nervous System. Oxford: Oxford University Press, 1988; 289–307.

64. Markwald M. Uber die Ausbreitung der Erregung und Hemmung von Sckluckcentrum auf das Athemcentrum. Z Biol 1889; 7:1–54.

65. Grossman MI. Integration of neural and hormonal control of gastric secretion. Physiologist 1963; 6:349–357.

66. Vineberg AM. The activation of different elements of the gastric secretion by variation of vagal stimulation. Am J Physiol 1931; 96:363–371.

67. Florey HW, Harding HE. Further observations on secretion of Brunner's glands. J Pathol Bacteriol 1934; 39:255–276.

68. Florey HW, Harding HE. A hormonal control of the secretion of Brunner's glands. Proc R Soc London [Biol] 1935; 117:68–77.

69. Florey HW. The secretion of mucus by the colon. Br J Exp Pathol 1930; 11:348–361.

70. Wright RD, Florey HD, Jennings MA. The secretion of the colon of the cat. Q J Exp Physiol 1938; 28:207–229.

71. Lapides J. In: Campbell MF, Harrison JH, eds. Urology. Philadelphia: WB Saunders, 1970; 1343–1378.

72. Brindley GS. Autonomic control of the pelvic organs. In: Bannister R, ed. Autonomic Failure. Oxford: Oxford University Press, 1988; 223–237.

73. Awad SA, Downie JW, Lywood DW. Sympathetic activity in the proximal urethra in patients with urinary obstruction. J Urol 1976; 115:545–547.

74. Lawrence JE, Burden HW. The origin of the ex-

trinsic adrenergic innervation to the rat ovary. Anat Rec 1980; 196:51–59.

75. Weiss GK, Dail WG, Ratner A. Evidence for direct neural control of ovarian steroidogenesis in rats. J Reprod Fertil 1982; 65:507–511.

76. Brindley GS. Pilot experiments on the actions of drugs injected into the human corpus cavernosum penis. Br J Pharmacol 1986; 87:495–500.

77. Polak JM, Gu J, Mina S, et al. VIpergic nerves in the penis. Lancet 1981; ii:217–219.

78. Adaikan PG, Kottegoda SR, Ratnam SS. Is vasoactive intestinal polypeptide the principal transmitter involved in human penile erection? J Urol 1986; 135:638–640.

79. Hensel H, Andres KH, During M. Structure and function of cold receptors. Pflugers Arch 1974; 352:1–10.

80. Hammel HT, Hardy JD, Fusco MM. Thermoregulatory responses to hypothalamic cooling in unanesthetized dogs. Am J Physiol 1960; 198:481–486.

81. Simon E, Rautenberg W, Thauer R, et al. Die Ausvisung von Kaltezittern durch lokale Kuhlung im Wirbeikanal. Pflugers Arch 1964; 281:309–331.

82. Heath ME, Jessen C. Thermosensitivity of the goat's brain. J Physiol 1988; J Physiol (Lond) 1988; 400:61–74.

83. Rawson RO, Quick KP. Evidence of deep-body thermoreceptor response to intraabdominal heating of the ewe. J Appl Physiol 1970; 28:813–820.

84. Reidel W, Siaplauras G, Simon E. Intra-abdominal thermosensitivity in the rabbit as compared with spinal thermosensitivity. Pflugers Arch 1973; 340:59–70.

85. Riedel W. Warm receptors in the dorsal abdominal wall of the rabbit. Pflugers Arch 1976; 361:205–206.

86. Bligh J. Possible temperature-sensitive elements in or near the vena cava of sheep. J Physiol 1961; 159:85–86.

87. Blattis CM. Afferent initiation of shivering. Am J Physiol 1960; 199:697–700.

88. Shepherd JT, Vanhoutte PM. Veins and Their Control. Philadelphia: WB Saunders, 1989.

89. Rowell LB. Competition between skin and muscle for blood flow during exercise. In: Nadel ER, ed. Problems with Temperature Regulation During Exercise. Academic Press, 1989.

90. Rowell LB. Active neurogenic vasodilatation in man. In: Vanhoutte PM, Leusen I, eds. Vasodilatation. New York: Raven Press, 1981; 1–17.

91. Himms-Hagen J. Nonshivering thermogenesis. Brain Res Bull 1984; 12:151–160.

92. Rothwell NJ, Stock MJ. Nonshivering and diet-induced thermogenesis: The role of brown adipose tissue. In: Hales JRS, ed. Thermal Physiology. New York: Raven Press, 1985; 145–153.

93. Brain R. Clinical Neurology, ed 6. Oxford: Oxford University Press, 1985; 124–125.

94. Schwartz IL, Siegel GJ. Excitation, conduction and transmission of the nerve impulse. In: Brobeck JR, ed. Best and Taylor's Physiological Basis of Medical Practice. Baltimore: Williams & Wilkins, 1975; 1.44.

95. Koelle GB. Drugs acting at synaptic and neuroeffector junctional sites. In: Goodman LS, Gilman A, eds. The Pharmacological Basis of Therapeutics. New York: Macmillian, 1975; 414.

96. Craig CR, Stitzed RE. Modern Pharmacology. Boston: Little, Brown, 1986.

97. Alexandridis E. The Pupil. Berlin: Springer-Verlag, 1985; 6–7.

98. Shepherd RFJ, Shepherd JT. Control of the blood pressure and the circulation in man. In: Bannister R, ed. Autonomic Failure. Oxford: Oxford University Press, 1988; 80–96.

# Chapter 5

# Skeletal Muscle: Structure, Chemistry, and Function

JAMES S. LIEBERMAN
E. RALPH JOHNSON
DAVID D. KILMER

Most of the basic elements of skeletal muscle structure and function, and the mechanics of muscle contraction, have been known for many years. More definitive understanding of the anatomy, chemistry, and physiology of muscle contraction has come only with the development of modern investigative techniques such as election microscopy, x-ray diffraction studies, and magnetic resonance spectroscopy.

In this chapter we provide a concise overview of the development, anatomy, chemistry, physiology, and energetics of skeletal muscle and skeletal muscle contraction.

## Muscle Development

### Prenatal Development

Embryonic development of skeletal muscle is treated in standard textbooks,[1-3] most data being derived from nonhuman mammalian species. Skeletal muscles of the limbs and trunk are derived from mesodermal somites, whereas cervical and craniobulbar muscles originate in the branchial arches. By the 8th week of gestation the primordia of many individual muscles are identifiable as groups of primitive myotubes. These multinucleated syncytia contain the first traces of myofibrils in their cytoplasm. The myotubes are formed by fusion of mononucleate stem cells termed *myoblasts*.

Individual skeletal muscles are well-formed by the 10th week of gestation, and in the next 6 weeks myotubes proliferate by fusion with specific neighboring cells until the ultimate number of muscle fibers has been formed in a given muscle. Division by mitosis does not occur in striated muscle cells.[4] As myotubes mature, their myofibrils increase in number and size until they are densely packed, and the nuclei migrate to their familiar location beneath the sarcolemma, at which time they are termed *myofibers*. Maturation of the sarcotubular system and initiation of motor innervation occur concurrently. The first fetal movements at around 14 to 16 weeks' gestation probably reflect functionally active neuromuscular junctions. The second half of fetal life is associated with exponential growth of skeletal muscles, primarily by hypertrophy of individual muscle fibers.[5] Mean fiber diameter increases exponentially.[6]

Histochemical staining properties of fetal muscle are uniform until about the 5th month of gestation. At 20 weeks, a few type I fibers can be identified by staining characteristics, but they are sparse until 34 weeks, when they rapidly increase in number in a linear fashion to constitute 40% of total fibers at term.[6] Types IIA and IIB fibers gradually differentiate from fetal type II fibers, often called type IIC fibers. Maturity of the innervating motor neurons may be the determining factor in fiber type differentiation.[7]

### Postnatal Growth

Between birth and puberty, muscle mass increase is the result of both fiber hypertrophy and lengthening. Sarcomeres are added to the ends of the muscle fiber in series adjacent to the musculotendinous junction, resulting in increased fiber length.[8] The amount of muscle stretch seems to affect sarcomere growth. For example, immobilization of growing mouse muscle in a shortened position decreases the addition of sarcomeres, but the ability to fully recover is not affected by the period of immobilization or the stage of development.[9] Most of the increase in myofiber cross-sectional area is due to the increased number of myofibrils, though the number of nuclei per fiber also increases with age.[8]

## Muscle Structure

Muscles are divided into fascicles, each containing many muscle fibers. These vary in length up to 40 cm; diameter varies from 10 to 100 μ and generally runs the entire length of the fascicle without interruption. Owing to the pennate arrangement of most muscles, few fibers are longer than 10 cm and most are shorter than the overall length of the muscle.

### Connective Tissue

Muscle fibers are bound by collagenous connective tissue that has three separate components. The *epimysium* is the tough elastic envelope for the entire muscle merging at its end with the tendon. Connective tissue septa that divide fibers into fascicular bundles are termed the *perimysium*. The final connective tissue component, the *endomysium,* separates individual muscle fibers from each other.

Each individual muscle fiber is surrounded by a structural framework called the sarcolemma, a connective tissue scaffold made up of basal lamina and endomysial reticula. This is differentiated by anatomists from the plasmalemma, the cell membrane of each muscle syncitial fiber, but in practice these terms are often used interchangeably.

### Vascular Supply

The vascularization of skeletal muscle varies much. Generally, five main types of intramuscular arterial vascularization patterns are seen in muscles[10]: (1) Separate nutrient vessels enter the muscle throughout its length, forming an anastomotic chain (soleus and peroneus longus). (2) A single group of arteries form a longitudinal pattern, but they arise from a common stem and enter one end of the muscle (gastrocnemius). (3) A radiating pattern of collaterals is formed from a single vessel that enters the middle of the muscle (biceps brachii). (4) A series of anastomotic loops is present throughout the muscle length. The loops are formed from a succession of entering vessels (tibialis anterior, extensor hallucis longus, long leg flexors). (5) The final type is an open quadrilateral pattern with sparse anastomotic connections (extensor hallucis longus).

A significant capillary bed is present in muscle. At rest, few capillaries are open. With muscle contraction, however, a great number open.[10] As a general rule, in any particular muscle, blood flow at rest is proportional to the number of slow fibers, whereas during increasing muscle activity it is proportional to the number of fast fibers.[11]

### Nerve Supply

The nerve supply to a muscle enters near the endplate zone and may consist of one or several branches that contain both efferent and afferent fibers. In fact, only 50% to 60% of large myelinated fibers are typically efferent in a muscle branch[12] in the muscle itself. The major afferent fibers (types IA and IB) are from muscle spindles and Golgi tendon organs. Significant branching occurs at nodes of Ranvier, resulting in the presence of many intramuscular nerve bundles.[11] Efferent fibers are myelinated until the terminal portion of the nerve at the neuromuscular junction.[11]

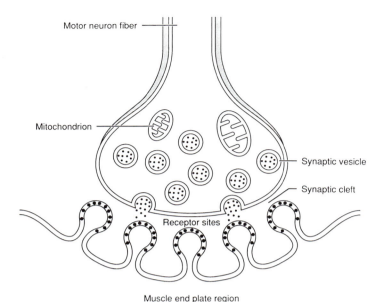

Motor neuron fiber

Mitochondrion

Synaptic vesicle

Synaptic cleft

Receptor sites

Muscle end plate region

**Figure 5-1.** Structure of the neuromuscular junction showing major structures and release of acetylcholine from synaptic vesicles.

## Neuromuscular Junction (Figure 5-1)

As a terminal axon of a muscle nerve nears its muscle fiber, it loses its myelin sheath and develops a slightly bulbous terminal. The terminal lies within a groove on the surface of the muscle fiber, and the presynaptic (neural) portion of the neuromuscular junction comes to within 50 nm of the postsynaptic (muscular) portion. This 50-nm gap is the synaptic cleft. One or more Schwann cells cover the nerve terminal and form the membrane of the postsynaptic portion of the muscle fiber.

The muscle membrane on the postsynaptic side is constructed with multiple folds that much increase its surface area. Within these junctional folds are acetylcholinesterase receptors and storage sites for acetylcholinesterase. The muscle sarcoplasm underlying the neuromuscular junction contains a large number of muscle nuclei and mitochondria.

On the presynaptic side, the nerve terminal contains a number of mitochondria as well as large numbers of 40- to 50-nm vesicles that contain the neurotransmitter acetylcholine. Although the vesicles are distributed diffusely within the terminal, they cluster at several thicker portions of the presynaptic membrane, the "active sites."[13]

## Muscle Fiber Histochemistry

With histochemical techniques it is possible to differentiate fiber types based on activity of key enzymes and constituents. This has important functional and metabolic consequences, as each individual muscle has a unique fiber makeup that generally supports its function in the body.

Originally, two major fiber types were identified, based on a difference in reactivity of myofibrillar adenosine triphosphatase (ATPase) at pH 9.4 and verified with histochemical activity of oxidative enzymes and phosphorylase. Type I fibers are characterized by high activity of oxidative enzymes and low relative activity of phosphorylase and myofibrillar ATPase at pH 9.4. They also have greater lipid and myoglobin concentrations as well as capillary density, but less glycogen storage. This suggests that type I fibers have greater capacity for oxidative metabolism.

Type II fibers have a contrasting profile with fibers specialized for anaerobic or glycolytic metabolism (Table 5-1). Type II fibers can be subgrouped into IIA, IIB (Figure 5-2), and IIC[14,15] by using the pH sensitivity of the myofibrillar ATPase reaction and acid preincubation. The IIA fibers seem to represent an intermediate class that

**Table 5-1.** Muscle Fiber Type Classification

|  | Type I | Type IIA | Type IIB | Type IIC |
|---|---|---|---|---|
| Color | Red | Red | White |  |
| Myoglobin content | High | High | Low |  |
| Glycogen content | Low | High | High |  |
| Capillary density | High | High | Low |  |
| Mitochondria | Many | Many | Few |  |
| Lipid content | High | Intermediate | Low |  |
| Muscle fiber type: contraction and metabolism | SO | FOG | FG |  |
| Physiologic motor unit type | S | FR | FF | F(int) |
| Contraction | Slow | Fast | Fast | Fast |
| Fatigue resistance | High | High | Low | Intermediate |
|  |  |  |  |  |
| Enzyme activity |  |  |  |  |
| ATPase (pH 9.4) | Low | High | High | High |
| ATPase (pH 4.6) | High | Low | Moderate | Moderate |
| ATPase (pH 4.3) | High | Low | Low | Low |
| Phosphorylase | Low | High | High |  |
| Oxidative enzymes | High | Intermediate | Low |  |

has both oxidative and glycolytic characteristics. Type IIC fibers may be intermediate as well, and they are often regarded as an immature fiber type.

An important finding is that muscle fibers that belong to a single motor unit are of a single histochemical type.[16,17] These fibers are not grouped together but are interspersed throughout a larger volume of muscle with many fibers from other motor units. Functionally, this spreads the contractile force generated by a single unit across a larger area of muscle.

Correlations between histochemical fiber type and physiologic properties demonstrate that type I fiber motor units contract slowly and are fatigue resistant.[16] Type IIB motor units tend to have the opposite characteristics (i.e., fast twitch and relative susceptibility to fatigue). As expected, type IIA units are intermediate, having both fast twitch and fatigue-resistant properties. In humans, predominantly tonic postural muscles such as the soleus contain primarily type I fibers, whereas phasic muscles such as the orbicularis oculi contain principally type II fibers.[18]

Although cross-innervation experiments demonstrate the ability to change the histochemical profile of a predominantly slow muscle,[19] until recently it was not considered possible to change fiber type proportions using specific training techniques or electrical stimulation, but there is now evidence to the contrary. Long-term low-frequency stimulation induces transformation of fast muscle fibers into slow ones in both rats and rabbits.[17,20] High-intensity interval training has been shown to increase the proportion of type I fibers in both rats[21] and humans[22] at the expense of type IIB. This suggests that the proportions of fiber types

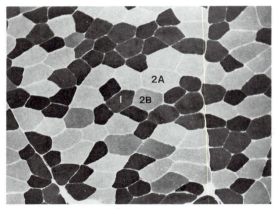

**Figure 5-2.** Photomicrograph of vastus lateralis from a 21-year-old man stained for ATPase at pH 4.6 showing type I, type IIA, and type IIB fibers (original magnification × 185). (Courtesy of Dr. William Ellis.)

may not be solely under genetic control and may respond to specific environmental influences.

## Structural Organization Within the Muscle

A skeletal muscle is composed of a number of discrete bundles of muscle fibers termed *fascicles,* each sheathed in connective tissue. Each muscle fiber, in turn, is composed of a number of myofibrils. The myofibrils are composed of myofilaments arranged in units called sarcomeres. There are two types of myofilaments, thin filaments containing actin, troponin, and tropomyosin, and thick filaments containing myosin. The arrangement of myofibrils into sarcomeres is responsible for the striated appearance of skeletal muscle under the light microscope; thus, the derivation of the term *striated muscle.*

## Ultrastructure

The sarcomere, the functional unit of the myofibril, can be seen with electron microscopy. One sarcomere is defined as extending from Z line to Z line (Figures 5-3, 5-4). The dark A band of the sarcomere is composed of thick myosin filaments and overlapping thin actin filaments, while the pale I band, transected at its midpoint by the Z line, is

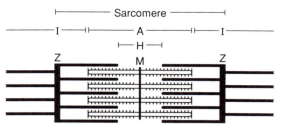

**Figure 5-4.** Diagram of the sarcomere shows thick filaments, thin filaments, cross-bridges, as well as subdivisions of the sarcomere, including Z lines, the M line, H zone, I band, and A band.

made up only of thin actin molecules. The H zone is the central area without filament overlap and is relatively lighter than the A band because it contains only myosin filaments. However, the H zone is darker than the I band, which contains only thin filaments. The dark central M line represents the point where myosin filaments are bound together with their neighbors, lending stability to the thick filaments during contraction.[23] The Z lines serve as the junction between sarcomeres and are the attachment point for thin filaments; thus, they appear to be the point of tension transmission between sarcomeres during muscle contraction.

Changes in the sarcomere during contraction were described by Huxley and Hanson, who noted that during stretch and contraction the size of the A band remained constant while the length of the I band and the H zone changed. From this they derived the sliding filament theory of muscle contraction.[24] That is, the thin filaments slide toward the center of the sarcomere (M line), while thick filaments remain stationary (Figure 5-5).

## Internal Noncontractile Structures

### Sarcoplasmic Reticulum[25]

The sarcoplasmic reticulum (SR) is a network of tubules and cisternae that surrounds the myofibrils. The SR maintains a specific relationship to the transverse tubular system (T system), which will be described presently. The SR consists mainly of tubules arranged longitudinally, parallel to the long axis of the myofibrils. At the junction of the A and I bands, where the SR is adjacent to the T

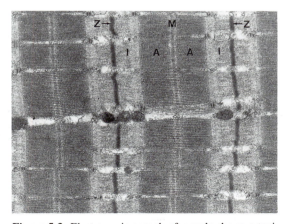

**Figure 5-3.** Electron micrograph of muscle shows a typical sarcomere. Major structures are labeled, including Z and M lines, and I and A bands (original magnification × 40,000.) (Courtesy of Dr. William Ellis.)

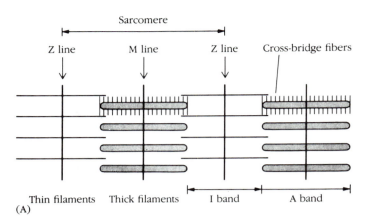

**Figure 5-5.** The sarcomere, showing the relationship between thick and thin filaments at A (rest) and B (during contraction), illustrating the sliding filament theory. (From Matthews GG. Cellular Physiology of Nerve and Muscle. Boston: Blackwell Scientific, 1986, with permission.)

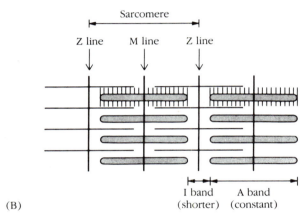

system, the SR tubules fuse to two terminal cisternae, one on either side of the T tubule.

The SR is the primary calcium storage and release site in muscle. Portions of the SR function as a calcium pump, and the terminal cisternae have the special ability to convert an electrical impulse from the T system into calcium release. In addition, the SR interior contains large amounts of calsequestrin, a protein that binds calcium.

### T System[25]

An extension of the plasma membrane, the T system, or tubule, penetrates the muscle fiber in the region of the terminal cisternae of the SR at the junction of the A and I bands. The T system assists in the propagation of electrical impulses from the surface to the interior of the muscle. The T system, with two transverse tubules per sarcomere, occu-

pies approximately 0.1% to 0.5% of the volume of the muscle fiber[26]; the SR occupies some >1.0% to >9.0% of muscle volume in some animal species.[27,28]

### Triads[25]

The combination of two SR terminal cisternae and one transverse tubule, known as a *triad* (Figure 5-6), is where the electrical impulse is converted into calcium release, which initiates muscle contraction.

At the triad there is a gap of 11 to 14 nm between the SR cisternae and the T tubule. Recently, periodic densities, called *feet*, have been described in this space.[29] It still is not clear whether these feet have a functional role in muscle contraction or only a structural one. Finally, a series of indentations in the terminal cisternae have

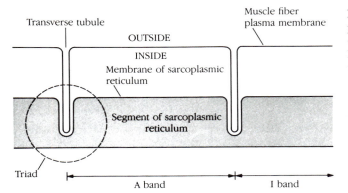

Figure 5-6. The transverse tubule and sarcoplasmic reticulum in the region of the triad. (From Matthews GG. Cellular Physiology of Nerve and Muscle. Boston: Blackwell Scientific, 1986, with permission.)

been described. At least one group of investigators[30] believe that these indentations mark sites of calcium release.

### Mitochondria

Muscle mitochondria are seen in two locations, between the myofibrils and beneath the plasmalemma. Most mitochondria between myofibrils are near the Z lines at the I-band level.

### Satellite Cells

Mature muscles include certain cells located in a characteristic position between the basal lamina and the plasma membrane of muscle fibers. These *satellite cells* retain their myogenic capabilities. They cannot be distinguished from normal muscle nuclei without special techniques. Their numbers increase and they show significant mitotic activity in growing, injured, or denervated muscle.[33]

## Skeletal Muscle Proteins

### Contractile Proteins

The force of skeletal muscle contraction is generated by thick filament myosin molecule projections (cross-bridges), which cyclically attach to adjacent actin thin filaments during contraction and relaxation.[34] Therefore, a review of muscle protein structure and chemistry is essential for understanding the mechanism of skeletal muscle contraction.

Each muscle fiber is composed of $10^2$ to $10^3$

myofibrils enveloped by SR and suspended in sarcoplasm containing potassium, magnesium, phosphate, and protein enzymes. Each myofibril is 1 to 3 $\mu$ in diameter. Mitochondria producing ATP are found between myofibrils.

Each myofibril has 1500 thick myosin filaments and 3000 thin actin filaments that interdigitate. The pattern of interdigitation in polarized light produces the sarcomere's typical appearance, with isotropic I light bands, which contain actin filaments, and anisotropic A dark bands, which contain myosin filaments and overlapping actin filaments (Figure 5-3). Actin filaments are attached to Z discs comprised of several filamentous proteins different from actin and myosin. These act as structural attachments for actin filaments. The length of the fully stretched sarcomere at rest is approximately 2.0 $\mu$.

### Thick Filaments

**Myosin.** The myosin filament is an essential functional component of the sarcomere. Each myosin filament contains some 200 to 300 myosin molecules of approximately 480 kd molecular weight, organized as six polypeptide chains, two heavy chains (weight 200 kd each) and four light chains (weight 20 kd each).[35,36]

Trypsin splits myosin into two components, light meromyosin (LMM), which forms the tail or rod portion of the molecule, and heavy meromyosin (HMM), primarily a globular protein termination of the molecule called a *head* (Figure 5-7). Papain splits HMM into an $S_1$ globular protein and a rodlike $S_2$ protein that is attached to LMM.

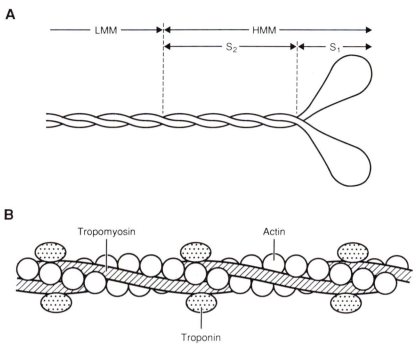

**Figure 5-7.** Structure of the contractile proteins. (*A*) The myosin molecule; (*B*) the thin filament showing actin, tropomyosin, and troponin.

The two myosin heavy chains are arranged in a double-stranded α-helix of 146 nm called the *tail* or *rod*. Each heavy chain terminates in an unstranded globular head of 17 to 20 nm. Each head contains two polypeptide light chains. One light chain can be phosphorylated and has a single site for binding bivalent cations, known as the P light chain. The second is the alkali or A light chain. Both light chains regulate actomyosin interaction.

The two heads of the myosin molecule are roughly pear shaped, 6 to 7 nm wide at the tip and 5.4 nm thick, and have a 3.5 to 4 nm, slightly curved neck.[37] Each head is mobile and rotates and angulates at the neck hinge or fulcrum, which is located at the junction of the $S_1$ and $S_2$ subfragments. A hinge in the myosin molecule at the junction of the $S_2$ and LMM provides additional flexibility, allowing a portion of the rod (rail) to act as a trunk or arm to move the head toward the actin filaments (Figure 5-8). The myosin head has ATPase activity, hydrolyzing ATP to release a high-energy phosphate bond.[38] The ATPase activity of myosin is located in the HMM or HMM-$S_1$

fragments and correlates with the shortening velocity of skeletal muscle contraction. The myosin head and neck form the cross-bridges (Figure 5-9).

*Thin Filaments*

**Actin, Tropomyosin, and Troponin.** The second essential component of the skeletal muscle sarcomere is the actin filament approximately 1 μ long and containing a double-stranded helix F actin, a polymer of 300 G-actin monomers of 42 kd molecular weight. Each G-actin monomer is attached to one molecule of adenosine diphosphate (ADP). Interaction between the actin and the myosin heads occurs at the ADP loci. These active sites are staggered every 2.7 nm. Each actin monomer interacts with three or four other actin monomers in the polymer as well as with tropomyosin and troponin.[37]

The thin filament is actually a complex of three proteins: actin, tropomyosin, and the troponin complex in a 7:1:1 ratio. Tropomyosin and the troponin complex are regulatory proteins that assist

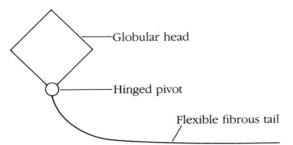

-----Globular head

-----Hinged pivot

-----Flexible fibrous tail

**Figure 5-8.** The myosin molecule, showing the flexible pivot area of the myosin head as well as the flexible portion of the fibrous tail. (From Matthews GG. Cellular Physiology of Nerve and Muscle. Boston: Blackwell Scientific, 1986, with permission.)

in the control of the actin-myosin interaction. These two regulatory proteins are a structural component of the thin filament (Figure 5-7).

Tropomyosin is an elongated polymer of approximately 70 kd molecular weight, 41 nm in length and 20 $\mu$ diameter, consisting of two $\alpha$-helix coiled chains located 180 degrees apart in two F-actin grooves.

Troponin is a complex of three separate proteins. Troponin T (TN-T, 30 kd molecular weight) binds the other two troponins to tropomyosin. Troponin-C (TN-C, 18 kd molecular weight) is a calcium receptor lying between TN-T and Troponin I (TN-I). Troponin I, (22 kd molecular weight) is involved with inhibition of the actin-myosin interaction during muscle relaxation. This inhibition

may be stereotactic. At concentrations of calcium less than $10^{-5}$ M TN-I participates in stereotactic blockage of the actin active site, which inhibits the attachment of myosin to actin.[39] One molecule of troponin complex containing one molecule of TN-I regulates the interaction of seven actin monomers with myosin.[40,41]

*Noncontractile Proteins*

**Thick Filaments.** C protein is a nonmyosin component of the thick filament, a monomer with a single polypeptide chain of 140 kd molecular weight. C protein binds to LMM and $S^2$ myosin fragments. Its function is not known. It has no ATPase activity.[42]

**Thin Filaments.** Alpha actinin is a protein localized to the Z line. Alpha actinin is believed to attach F actin to the Z line. Beta actinin is located at the free end of the actin filament and is believed to function as a polymerization terminator for actin.

*Sarcoplasmic Reticulum*

**Calsequestrin.** Calcium ions released from the SR are essential in initiating the actin-myosin interaction. Normal $Ca^{2+}$ concentration in myofibrillar cytosol is $10^{-7}$ M, too small to initiate the actin-myosin interaction. Maximal muscle contraction requires a calcium concentration of $10^{-5}$

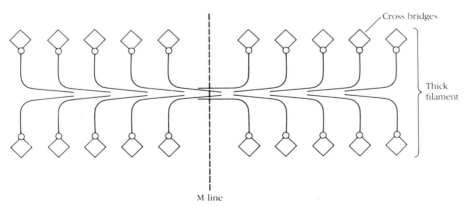

Cross bridges

Thick filament

M line

**Figure 5-9.** Structure of the thick filaments showing the formation of the cross-bridges by the myosin heads. (From Matthews GG. Cellular Physiology of Nerve and Muscle. Boston: Blackwell Scientific, 1986, with permission.)

M. There is an active calcium pump that concentrates $Ca^{2+}$ in the sarcoplasmic reticulum to $10^{-4}$ M. Calsequestrin is a sarcoplasmic reticulum protein that provides another 40-fold increase in calcium storage. Through these mechanisms the myofibrillar cytosol is essentially depleted of $Ca^{2+}$ during muscle relaxation. Excitation of the T tubules in the sarcoplasmic reticular system releases $Ca^{2+}$ to the myofibrillar fluid in concentrations as high as $2 \times 10^{-4}$ M. $Ca^{2+}$ release involves structurally complex proteins at loci that are dihydropyridine-sensitive receptors.[43] The receptor peptide has a molecular weight of 212 kd, binds dihydropyridine, is phosphorylated by ATP, and is similar to the large peptides of voltage-sensitive sodium channels.

**Parvalbumin.**   Parvalbumin[44] is an intracellular calcium-binding protein that may play a role in the diffusion of $Ca^{2+}$. Speed of relaxation is correlated with parvalbumin content in mammalian skeletal muscle. Fast skeletal muscle, which is rich in parvalbumin, relaxes much faster than slow fibers, which are almost devoid of it.

*Other Proteins*

**Myoglobin.**   Myoglobin functions as a store for oxygen and speeds its diffusion from the periphery into the muscle fiber.[45] Type I fibers are richer in myoglobin than type II fibers.

**Dystrophin.**   This is a recently described structural protein localized to the sarcolemma of the surface muscle membrane in the triad region. Its normal role is unknown. However, it is absent in Duchenne's muscular dystrophy and decreased in Becker's dystrophy.[46] It is believed to be the gene product of the Duchenne's dystrophy gene locus.

## Muscle Contraction

*Presynaptic Events*

Muscle contraction is initiated by the arrival at the synaptic terminal of a presynaptic nerve action potential. With the arrival of the action potential the synaptic terminal is depolarized, leading to the opening for calcium of voltage-sensitive membrane channels, which are closed when the terminal is in its resting state.

As the calcium concentration in the extracellular fluid is much greater than that inside the nerve terminal, calcium enters the terminal when the channels open. When the calcium concentration within the synaptic terminal reaches the appropriate level, acetylcholine is released from the presynaptic membrane.

The acetylcholine is packaged in the synaptic vesicles in multimolecule units termed *quanta,* each containing approximately 10,000 molecules of acetylcholine. In the resting state in a synaptic terminal, the release of single quanta of acetylcholine occurs regularly and spontaneously. This release can be recognized as the miniature end-plate potential (MEPP) when recording from the neuromuscular region with a microelectrode. Release of single quanta with their resultant MEPPs does not lead to propagation of a potential along the muscle fiber, so MEPPs do not stimulate muscle contraction.

A nerve action potential, however, leads to simultaneous release of 100 to 200 quanta of acetylcholine. The release of this amount of acetylcholine generates an end-plate potential (EPP) in the postsynaptic muscle fiber. The EPP is propagated along the muscle fiber, and muscle contraction follows.

*Postsynaptic Events*

The acetylcholine released from the nerve terminal enters the synaptic cleft and diffuses across the cleft to the postsynaptic muscle membrane. This membrane contains acetylcholine receptor sites, which act as gates controlling acetylcholine-sensitive sodium and potassium channels (Figure 5-10). These channels open when two acetylcholine molecules bind to them.

After acetylcholine binding has occurred the channel opens. This ion channel allows both sodium and potassium to cross the membrane in equal amounts. The equal permeability to sodium and potassium results in depolarization of the muscle membrane, as the relative concentrations of these two ions are changed in a direction that leads to depolarization of the muscle membrane. This depolarization is then propagated throughout the muscle, and contraction results. The contact of

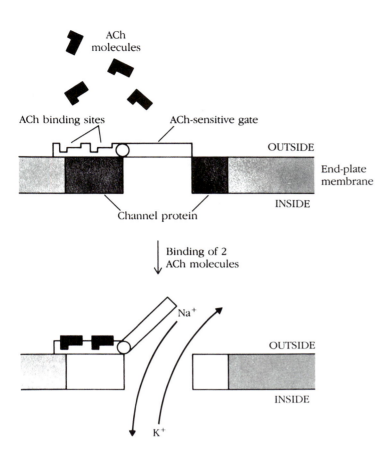

ACh
molecules

ACh binding sites

ACh-sensitive gate

OUTSIDE

End-plate
membrane

INSIDE

Channel protein

Binding of 2
ACh molecules

Na$^+$

OUTSIDE

INSIDE

K$^+$

**Figure 5-10.** The acetylcholine-sensitive channel in the end-plate membrane. (From Matthews GG. Cellular Physiology of Nerve and Muscle. Boston: Blackwell Scientific, 1986, with permission.)

acetylcholine with the receptor site lasts about 1 msec. At this time, acetylcholine is inactivated by acetylcholinesterase and is split into acetate and choline. The choline is taken up again by the nerve terminal and acetylcholine is resynthesized.

The calcium available for release from the sarcoplasmic reticulum accumulates because of a calcium pump in the SR membrane. The calcium pump causes the transport of calcium ions into the SR and utilizes ATP for energy. Following the release of calcium from the SR, actin-myosin interactions are triggered and actual contraction begins. The calcium pump also serves to terminate contraction by pumping calcium back into the SR after it has reacted with the protein troponin on the thin filament.

### Excitation-Contraction Coupling

Actual contraction of muscle with shortening of the sarcomere (see Figure 5-5), occurs because of

the interaction of the myosin head cross-bridges with myosin-binding sites on the actin filament. The myosin head contains an area that binds ATP, forming myosin ATP. A high-energy phosphate bond is then split off, yielding an "energized" myosin head (Figure 5-11) that is capable of binding to the myosin-binding site on the actin filament (Figure 5-12). After binding, energy is released and thin filament displacement occurs, as shown in the diagram.

The regulation of the actin-myosin interaction depends on the interrelationship between troponin, tropomyosin, and actin in the thin filament. Without regulation, as long as ATP was present every muscle would be constantly contracting because of continual actin-myosin head binding.

During the resting state, the myosin-binding sites on the thin filament are unavailable to the myosin head because they are blocked by tropomyosin held in position by troponin. The calcium released by the SR interacts with troponin to shift its position. As a result, the position of tropo-

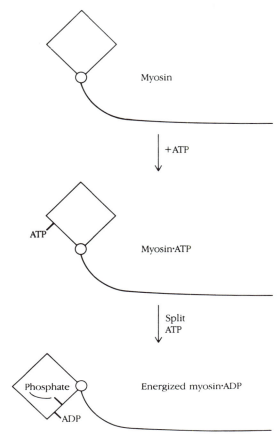

**Figure 5-11.** Binding of ATP by the myosin molecule, and the energized state of the myosin head with rotation of the head about the pivot point. (From Matthews GG. Cellular Physiology of Nerve and Muscle. Boston: Blackwell Scientific, 1986, with permission.)

myosin is also shifted and the myosin-binding sites become available to the myosin heads. These events are summarized in Figure 5-13.

Postsynaptic skeletal muscle plasma membrane depolarization is propagated when the resting membrane potential is raised from $-90$ mV to $-50$ mV and is conducted at a velocity of 4 m per second.[47] The electromotive force (EMF) changes during depolarization are rapidly spread to the sarcoplasmic T-tubule system at a radial propagation velocity of 0.064 m per second.[48–50] The wave of depolarization then travels via the T tubule from the surface to the interior of the muscle, where it causes release of calcium by the SR.

The exact molecular mechanism by which the electrical depolarization in the T tubule causes calcium release in the sarcoplasmic reticulum is unknown; however, both electrical and chemical mechanisms are possible, including calcium-induced calcium release. In this regard, it is interesting to note that T tubules contain $Ca^{2+}$-ATPase capable of concentrating and sequestering $Ca^{2+}$ in the tubule lumen.[51] Whatever the mechanism, the radially propagated EMF initiates a release of $Ca^{2+}$, raising the cytosol $Ca^{2+}$ concentration from $10^{-7}$ to $10^{-5}$ M.[52] This results in movement of tropomyosin and the uncovering of the myosin-binding site on the thin filament.

Myosin heads are then activated. The binding of a single calcium ion may activate both myosin heads. The hinged myosin rod and hinged myosin neck move to place the myosin heads at the active site[53] via the high myosin affinity for actin, thus producing an actomyosin complex.

The myosin heads then move or flip to a new position (Figure 5-14) initiating a more acute angle, with the myosin rod producing 5 to 7 nm of shortening or sliding of the myosin filament on the actin filament, which is stabilized at the Z line. ATP is hydrolyzed by the ATPase activity of myosin in the presence of actin to produce the energy required for contraction.[54,55] Myosin extracted from fast and from slow muscle fibers produces the same velocity of contraction.[56]

After the flip stroke of the cross-bridge actin-myosin interaction, sustained and continued contraction is produced by sequential attachment and angulation of myosin heads on adjacent actin-active sites. Muscle relaxation is initiated with rapid depletion of $Ca^{2+}$ by the pumping mechanism described previously. As the $Ca^{2+}$ concentration in the myofibrillar cytosol falls, the tropomyosin-troponin complex folds to cover the actin-active site and the contractile cycle ends.

## Energy Production

Energy for the various processes in muscle contraction and relaxation is derived from ATP. The ATP content of resting muscle is approximately $5 \times 10^{-6}$ mol/g. This "stored" energy can sustain maximal muscle contraction for only a few seconds; regeneration of ATP by phosphorylation of ADP is necessary for sustained contraction.

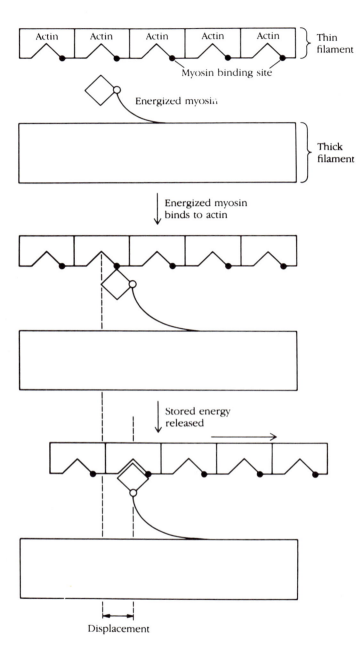

**Figure 5-12.** The interaction between energized myosin and actin according to the sliding filament hypothesis. (From Matthews GG. Cellular Physiology of Nerve and Muscle. Boston: Blackwell Scientific, 1986, with permission.)

Creatine phosphate provides a substrate for rapid resynthesis of ATP via the transfer of a phosphate bond to ADP in the presence of MM creatine kinase which is localized exclusively at the M line.[57] The energy bonds of creatine phosphate are present in four to six times the concentration of resting muscle ATP; however, the combined stored energy of ATP and creatine phosphate in muscle is adequate to maintain maximal contraction for only a few seconds more than resting ATP alone. Additional sources of ATP are required for sustained contraction.

Glycolytic breakdown of glucose via the Embden-Meyerhof pathway provides two ATP molecules per molecule of glucose degraded:

$$\text{Glucose} + 2\ \text{ADP} + 2\ \text{Pi} \longrightarrow 2\ \text{pyruvic acid} + 2\ \text{ATP}$$

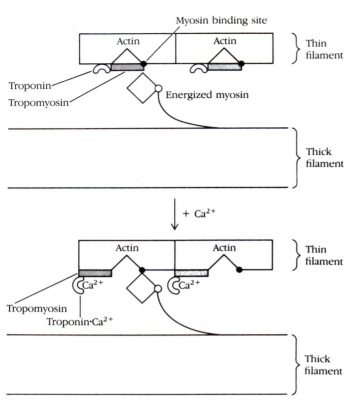

**Figure 5-13.** Regulation of the interaction between actin and myosin by calcium ions, troponin, and tropomyosin. (From Matthews GG. Cellular Physiology of Nerve and Muscle. Boston: Blackwell Scientific, 1986, with permission.)

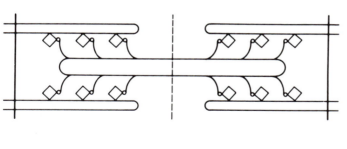

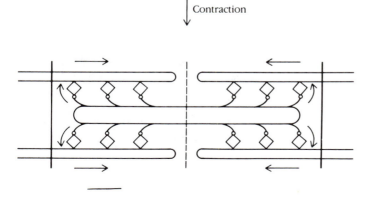

**Figure 5-14.** The mechanism of sarcomere shortening as well as the flip of the myosin heads during contraction. (From Matthews GG. Cellular Physiology of Nerve and Muscle. Boston: Blackwell Scientific, 1986, with permission.)

Glycolytic degradation of glucose produces new ATP two-and-one-half times as rapidly as oxidative mechanisms. However, glycolytic end products build rapidly to prevent maximal contraction beyond 1 minute.

Muscle glycogen provides a large source of the energy required for sustained muscle contraction. During 1 hour's heavy exercise muscle glycogen content falls to approximately zero, after which no further work can be done in the absence of regeneration or glycogen or oxidative mechanisms for ATP regeneration.[58] When glucose is infused to maintain a high serum concentration glycogen utilization is reduced only 25%, indicating that glycogen is the primary energy source for muscle contraction, even in the presence of a high serum glucose concentration.

Synthesis of mammalian skeletal muscle glycogen requires a cell permeable to the hexose molecule and an effective intracellular phosphorylating mechanism to produce glucose-6-phosphate. Insulin increases the permeability and transport of several hexoses and pentoses across the cell membrane. The pentose pathway is not utilized for mammalian muscle energy bond production. Skeletal muscle has high glucose phosphorylating capacity relative to glucose uptake, even at maximal insulin transport effect. Thus, there is no significant free intracellular glucose in resting muscle under normal conditions. Glucose is converted to glycogen by several mechanisms: (1) Phosphorylation of glucose to glucose-6-phosphate requires a high-energy phosphate bond:

Glucose + ATP — Glucose-6-phosphate + ADP

(2) Conversion of glucose-6-phosphate to glycogen occurs via several enzymes, including uridine triphosphorylases and glycogen synthase. Glucose-6-phosphate cannot be reconverted to free glucose in skeletal muscle, as it lacks glucose-6-phosphatase, which is present in liver, kidney, and small intestine.

Glycogen is a highly branched homopolymer of glucose that is stored predominantly in the I band sarcoplasm near the tubule system.[59] Fast twitch and slow twitch fibers have similar amounts of glycogen at rest. In 80% of both fiber types, glycogen content at rest is between 300 and 750 mmol/kg dry weight. At the end of 2 hours' work,

however, fast twitch fibers averaged 150 mmol/kg and slow twitch fibers 70 mmol/kg.[60]

Glycogenolysis of glycogen to glucose-6-phosphate requires several enzymes. Glucose-6-phosphate generated from glycogenolysis or glycolytic degradation of glucose is further metabolized to pyruvic acid, generating ATP via the citric acid–cytochrome oxidase aerobic pathway or lactic acid via the anaerobic pathway. Lactic acid is then converted to pyruvic acid when oxygen is available.

Complete oxidation of glucose to carbon dioxide and water yields 686,000 cal/mol or 38 ATP molecules per molecule of oxidized glucose. As 456,000 calories is available for production of ATP, 66% of the energy is converted to ATP while the remainder is released as heat. Complete degradation of a molecule of glycogen yields 39 ATP molecules per glucose unit. The one ATP difference occurs in the energy bond required to convert glucose to glucose-6-phosphate. Under anaerobic conditions glucose degradation stops at lactic acid and yields 56,000 cal/mol, an aerobic-anaerobic ratio of approximately 12:1.

## References

1. Carpenter S, Karpati G. General aspects of skeletal muscle biology. In: Pathology of Skeletal Muscle. New York: Churchill Livingstone, 1984;1–38.
2. Kukulas BA, Adams RD. Embryology and histology of skeletal muscle. In: Diseases of Muscle: Pathologic Foundation of Clinical Myology. Philadelphia: Harper and Row, 1985;3–60.
3. Landon DN. Skeletal muscle—normal morphology, development and innervation. In: Mastaglia FL, Walton J, eds. Skeletal Muscle Pathology. 1987; 1–87.
4. Kelly AM, Zacks SI. The histogenesis of rat intercostal muscle. J Cell Biol 1969; 42:135–153.
5. Stickland NC. Muscle development in the human fetus as exemplified by m. sartorius: A quantitative study. J Anat 1981; 132:557–579.
6. Schloon H, Schlottmann J, Lenard HG, et al. The development of skeletal muscles in premature infants. Eur J Pediatr 1979; 131:49–60.
7. Haltia M, Berlin O, Schucht H, et al. Postnatal differentiation and growth of skeletal muscle fibres in normal and undernourished rats. J Neurol Sci 1978; 36:25–39.

8. Williams PE, Goldspink G. Longitudinal growth of striated muscle fibres. J Cell Sci 1971; 9:751–767.

9. Williams PE, Goldspink G. The effect of immobilization on the longitudinal growth of striated muscle fibres. J Anat 1973; 116:45–55.

10. Jerusalem F. The microcirculation of muscle. In: Engel AG, Banker BQ, eds. Myology. New York: McGraw-Hill, 1986;343–356.

11. Slater CR, Harris JB. The anatomy and physiology of the motor unit. In: Walton J. eds. Disorders of Voluntary Muscle, ed 5. 1988;1–26.

12. Schmalbruch H. Motorneuron death after sciatic nerve section in newborn rats. J Comp Neurol 1984; 224:252–258.

13. Hubbard JI. Microphysiology of vertebrate neuromuscular transmission. Physiol Rev 1973; 53:674–723.

14. Brooke MH, Kaiser KK. Muscle fiber types: How many and what kind? Arch Neurol 1970; 23:369–379.

15. Gauthier F. Skeletal muscle fiber types. In: Engle AG, Banker BQ, eds. Myology. New York: McGraw-Hill, 1986;255–283.

16. Burke RE, Levine DN, Zajac FE III. Mammalian motor units: Physiological-histochemical correlation in three types in cat gastrocnemius. Science 1971; 174:709–712.

17. Kugelberg E, Edstrom L. Differential histochemical effects of muscle contractions on phosphorylase and glycogen in various types of fibres: Relation to fatigue. J Neurol Neurosurg Psychiatry 1968; 31:415–423.

18. Johnson MA, Polgar J, Weightman D, et al. Data on the distribution of fibre types in thirty-six human muscles: An autopsy study. J Neurol Sci 1973; 18:111–129.

19. Dubowitz V, Newman DL. Change in enzyme pattern after cross-innervation of fast and slow skeletal muscle. Nature (Lond) 1967; 214:840–841.

20. Pette D. Activity-induced fast to slow transitions in mammalian muscle. Med Sci Sports Exerc 1984; 16:517–528.

21. Luginbuhl AJ, Dudley GA, Staron RS. Fiber type changes in rat skeletal muscle after intense interval training. Histochemistry 1984; 81:55–58.

22. Simoneau JA, Lortie G, Boulay MR, et al. Human skeletal muscle fiber type alteration with high-intensity intermittent training. Eur J Appl Physiol 1985; 54:250–253.

23. Craig R. The structure of the contractile filaments. In: Engel AG, Banker BQ, eds. Myology. New York: McGraw-Hill, 1986;73–123.

24. Huxley H, Hanson J. Changes in the cross-striations of muscle during contraction and stretch and their structural interpretation. Nature 1954; 173:973–976.

25. Cullen MJ, Landon DN. The ultrastructure of the motor unit. In: Walton JN, ed. Disorders of Voluntary Muscle, ed 5. 1988; 27–73.

26. Eisenberg BR. Quantitative ultrastructure of mammalian skeletal muscle. In: Peachey LD, Adrian RH, eds. Handbook of Physiology, sect 10. Bethesda, Md: American Physiological Society, 1983;73–112.

27. Schmalbruch H. The membrane systems in different fiber types of the triceps surae muscle of cat. Cell Tissue Res 1979; 204:187–200.

28. Davey DF, Wong SYP. Morphometric analysis of rat extensor digitorum longus and soleus muscle. Aust J Exp Biol Med Sci 1980; 58:213–230.

29. Franzini-Armstrong C. Structure of sarcoplasmic reticulum. Fed Proc 1980; 39:2403–2409.

30. Dulhunty AF, Gage PW, Valoes AA. Indentations in the terminal cisternae of denervated rat extensor digitorum longus and soleus muscles. J Ultrastruct Res 1984; 88:30–34.

31. Mauro A. Satellite cells of skeletal muscle fibers. J Biophys Biochem Cytol 1961; 9:493–495.

32. Campion DR. The muscle satellite cell: A review. Int Rev Cytol 1984; 87:225–251.

33. Klein-Orgus C, Harris JB. Preliminary observations of satellite cells in undamaged fibres of the rat soleus muscle assaulted by a snake-venom toxin. Cell Tissue Res 1983; 230:617–676.

34. Huxley A. Prefactory chapter: Muscular contraction. Annu Rev Physiol 1988; 50:1–16.

35. Huxley HE. Electron microscope studies on the structure of natural and synthetic protein filaments from striated muscle. J Mol Biol 1963; 7:281–308.

36. Cooke R. The mechanism of muscle contraction. Crit Rev Biochem Mol Biol 1986; 21:53–118.

37. Elliott A, Offer G. Shape and flexibility of the myosin molecule. J Mol Biol 1978; 123:505–519.

38. Engelhardt WA, Ljubimowa MN. Myosine and adenosine triphosphatase. Nature 1939; 44:668–669.

39. Adelstein RS. Regulation and kinetics of the actin-myosin-ATP interaction. Annu Rev Biochem 1980; 49:921–956.

40. Perry SV, Cole HA, Head JF, et al. Localization and mode of action of the inhibitory protein component of the troponin complex. Cold Spring Harb Symp Quant Biol 1973; 37:251–262.

41. Perry SV. The regulation of contractile activity in muscle. Biochem Soc Trans 1979; 7:593–617.

42. Moos C, Mason CM, Besterman JM, et al. The binding of skeletal muscle C protein to F actin and

its relation to the interaction of actin with myosin subfragment 1. J Mol Biol 1978; 124:571–586.

43. Agnew WS. Proteins that bridge the gap. Nature 1988; 334:299–300.

44. Kretsinger RH. Calcium-binding proteins. Ann Rev Biochem 1976; 45:239–266.

45. Wittenberg JB. Myoglobin-facilitated oxygen diffusion: Role of myoglobin in oxygen entry into muscle. Physiol Rev 1970; 50:559–636.

46. Hoffman EP, Brown RH, Kunkel LM. Dystrophin: The protein gene product of the Duchenne muscular dystrophy locus. Cell 1987; 51:919–928.

47. Buchthal F, Guld C, Rosenfalck P. Propagation velocity in electrically activated muscle fibres in man. Acta Physiol Scand 1955; 34:75–89.

48. Huxley AF, Taylor RE. Local activation of striated muscle fibers. J Physiol (Lond) 1958; 144:426–441.

49. Costantin LL. The role of sodium current in the radial spread of contraction in frog muscles fibers. J Gen Physiol 1970; 55:703–715.

50. Nakajima S, Gilai A. Radial propagation of muscle action potential along the tubular system examined by potential-sensitive dyes. J Gen Physiol 1980; 76:751–762.

51. Brandt NR, Caswell AH, Brunschwig JP. ATP-energized Ca pump in isolated transverse tubules of skeletal muscle. J. Biol Chem 1980; 255:6290–6298.

52. Endo M. Calcium release from the sarcoplasmic reticulum. Physiol Rev 1977; 57:71–108.

53. Lehman W, Kendrick-Jones J, Szent-Gyorgi AG. Myosin-linked regulatory systems: Comparative studies. Cold Spring Harb Symp Quant Biol 1973; 37:319–330.

54. Goldman YE, Hibberd MG, Trentham DR. Relaxation of rabbit psoas muscle fibres from rigor by photochemical generation of adenosine-5-triphosphate. J Physiol 1984; 354:577–604.

55. Goldman YE, Hibberd MG, Trentham DR. Initiation of active contraction by photogeneration of adenosine-5-triphosphate in rabbit psoas muscle fibres. J Physiol 1984; 354:605–624.

56. Altringham JD, Yancey PH, Johnston IA. Limitations in the use of actomysin threads as model contractile systems. Nature 1980; 287:338–340.

57. Walliman T, Turner DC, Eppenberger HM. Localization of creatine kinase isoenzymes in myofibrils. J Cell Biol 1977; 75:297–317.

58. Bergstrom J, Hultman E. A study of the glycogen metabolism during exercise in man. Scand J Clin Lab Invest 1967; 19:218–228.

59. Wanson JC, Drochmans P. Rabbit skeletal muscle glycogen. A morphological and biochemical study of glycogen B particles isolated by the precipitation centrifugation method. J Cell Biol 1968; 38:130–150.

60. Essen B, Henriksson J. Glycogen content of individual muscle fibres in man. Acta Physiol Scand 1974; 90:645–647.

61. Matthews GG. Cellular Physiology of Nerve and Muscle. Boston: Blackwell, 1986.

# Chapter 6

# Receptors in Muscle and Their Role in Motor Control

JAMES GORDON

The idea that there is a "muscular sense," as Sherrington referred to it, was not definitively established until the end of the 19th century.[1] Before that time, the idea was a controversial one; indeed, the prevalent view was that our sense of movement derives not from peripheral receptors but rather from our estimate of the effort required to move. In the 19th century, however, detailed descriptions by Ruffini and Golgi of the receptors in muscles began to turn the tide.[2,3] The matter was definitively resolved in 1894, when Sherrington demonstrated that, when the ventral roots were cut a rich supply of afferent fibers to the muscles remained after the motor fibers degenerated.[4] The largest of these sensory fibers, as large as the motor fibers themselves, innervated two types of receptors, called *muscle spindles* and *Golgi tendon organs*. The muscle spindle, perhaps because of its intriguing combination of sensory and motor elements, became the focus of intensive study throughout this century.[5] Nevertheless, a full understanding of muscle spindle structure was slow to develop. It was not established until 1945 that its motor innervation is independent of the innervation of the skeletal muscles themselves, and many important details of its ultrastructure are still emerging today.

An explanation of the functional role of muscle receptors in motor control has been even more difficult to achieve. The early recognition that muscle spindles provide the stimulus for stretch reflexes, such as the well-known knee jerk, provided the impetus for intensive studies during the first half of this century of the properties of these reflexes. The principle that guided these studies was that simple reflexes such as stretch reflexes provide the nervous system with a set of building blocks from which to construct more complex behavioral acts, but the overly simplistic corollary—that voluntary movements can be reduced to simple reflexes chained together—fell gradually into disfavor, especially as evidence emerged that complex movements can be executed in the absence of sensory input. A more recent insight, which emerged along with the science of cybernetics at the end of World War II, was that muscle receptors and stretch reflexes could be profitably analyzed as components of feedback loops, capable of providing automatic compensation for errors in motor output. Nevertheless, while this type of analysis deepened our knowledge of the function of muscle receptors, it has gradually given way to the recognition that nature's round pegs do not so easily fit into the square holes of engineering theory.

The current attitude toward the functional role of muscle receptors has become more eclectic. The contemporary emphasis on motor control has brought with it the recognition that the properties of the musculoskeletal system are complex and change from moment to moment. Thus, in order to accurately plan motor commands, the brain requires information about the state of the musculoskeletal system, including the current length and tension of the muscles. This information derives in large part from muscle receptors and is undoubtedly used in myriad ways, depending on the external context and overall goal or intent.

In this chapter I present a basis for understanding the role of muscle receptors in motor control. No single theory is presented. Rather, the structure and functional properties of muscle receptors are discussed, their central connections are considered, and some of the current views of their role in motor control are reviewed. For more detailed information on these subjects, several excellent reviews are available.[2–4,6–12]

## Sensory Receptors in Muscle

The classic studies of Ruffini, Golgi, and Sherrington showed that skeletal muscles are richly supplied with a variety of receptors. Indeed, afferent axons outnumber efferent axons in most muscles.[2] The afferent fibers arising from muscle are classified according to a system introduced by Lloyd and Chang.[13] Because larger-diameter axons conduct impulses faster, these investigators were able indirectly to estimate the sizes of axons in peripheral nerves by measuring their conduction velocity. They found that the axons of myelinated fibers fall into three groups, according to their diameters (Table 6-1). Group I fibers are the largest and fastest-conducting afferent axons in the peripheral nervous system. Group II and group III fibers are smaller and conduct impulses more slowly. Unmyelinated axons are classified as group IV. Among the different receptors in muscles, two have been studied most thoroughly, the muscle spindles and the Golgi tendon organs. Muscle spindles are innervated by both group I and II axons. Tendon organs are innervated by group I axons. The group I axons from spindles are, on average, slightly larger than those from tendon organs and are referred to as group Ia axons, whereas those from tendon organs are referred to as group Ib axons.

### Muscle Spindles

The muscle spindle is a remarkable sensory receptor whose supporting structure has a complexity that is often compared to that of the eye. Each spindle consists of a set of specialized muscle fibers, called intrafusal fibers, embedded within

**Table 6-1.** Muscle Afferents and Efferents

| Afferent Axon Type | Receptor | Sensitive to: |
|---|---|---|
| Group Ia | Primary spindle ending | Muscle length and rate of change of length |
| Group Ib | Golgi tendon organ | Muscle tension |
| Group II | Secondary spindle ending | Muscle length (little rate sensitivity) |
| Group II | Nonspindle endings | Deep pressure |
| Groups III, IV | Free nerve endings | Pain, chemical stimuli, and temperature (important for physiologic response to exercise) |

| Efferent Axon Type | Innervation | Function |
|---|---|---|
| Alpha motor neurons (skeletomotor) | Extrafusal muscle fibers | Control tension of muscle |
| Beta fibers (skeletofusimotor) | Intrafusal muscle fibers (collaterals from alpha motor neurons) | Control sensitivity of spindles (no independent control of spindle sensitivity) |
| Gamma motor neurons (fusimotor) | Intrafusal muscle fibers | Control sensitivity of spindles (independently of alpha motor neuron activation) |

the normal, or extrafusal, muscle fibers. Each intrafusal fiber is innervated by one or more sensory receptors that are sensitive to stretch of the spindle. In addition, the spindle has motor innervation, which allows the central nervous system (CNS) to control the firing properties of the sensory endings. Thus, just as the brain can move the eyes and change the shape of the lens to focus on objects of interest, it can also control the degree of contraction of the muscle fibers on which the sensory endings terminate to adjust the sensitivity and dynamic range of the sensory output from the spindle.

This simple description of spindle structure and function disregards considerable complexity of both structure and function. Spindle endings transmit information about both dynamic and static aspects of muscle length, and the CNS can selectively control the sensitivity to these different aspects of length change. These physiologic properties of muscle spindles derive from the fine structure of the muscle spindle and, in particular, from differences in the physiologic properties of the different types of intrafusal fibers. Indeed, the most significant advances of the past 20 years of spindle research have been in working out the "internal operation" of the spindle.[11]

Muscle spindles are found in almost all skeletal muscles. In human muscles, counts of spindles have ranged from six in the small stylohyoideus muscle and 35 in the lumbrical muscles up to 500 in the triceps brachii and 1300 in the quadriceps femoris.[2,8] In general, they are more dense in the small muscles responsible for fine movement or postural control. The greatest density of spindles has been found in the small intervertebral muscles of the neck, whereas in large muscles such as the gluteus maximus, spindles are relatively less dense. There is no evidence for greater density of spindles in either extensor or flexor muscles.[2]

Spindles are encapsulated structures with a fusiform or spindle shape (Figure 6-1). They range in length from a few millimeters to 10 mm and usually lie deep within muscle bellies, close to the intramuscular nerve branches and blood vessels. Each spindle consists of a bundle of intrafusal muscle fibers (usually two to 12) arranged in parallel with each other and with the larger extrafusal fibers of the muscle within which they lie. The connective tissue capsule that surrounds the intrafusal fibers is thickest in the central region, giving the spindle its fusiform shape, and encloses within this region a gelatinous substance. Presumably this substance facilitates sliding of the intrafusal fibers on each other.

It was recognized as long ago as the 19th century that there were two morphologically distinct types of intrafusal fibers and that there were differences in the sensory and motor innervation of the two.[4] One type, referred to as a *nuclear bag fiber*, is distinguished by a concentration of many nuclei in the central region of the fiber, so that in cross-section three or four nuclei may be seen. The other type of fiber, referred to as a *nuclear chain fiber*, is shorter than the bag fiber and its nuclei are arranged in a row, so that only one is

visible at a time in cross-section. It is now understood that there are two distinct types of nuclear bag fibers that differ in structure, physiologic properties, and innervation. They are referred to as *dynamic* and *static* nuclear bag fibers. A typical mammalian muscle spindle contains two nuclear bag fibers, one of each type, and a variable number of chain fibers, usually about five. The different properties of these three intrafusal fiber types and their roles in how the spindle operates will be discussed presently.

The central region of each intrafusal fiber is noncontractile and is innervated by one or more sensory nerve endings that are sensitive to stretching of the central portion of the intrafusal fiber. In many cases the afferent terminals spiral around the intrafusal fiber in what is referred to as an annulospiral ending. The polar regions of the intrafusal fibers connect to the aponeuroses of the whole muscle, so that as the length of extrafusal fibers changes, the length of the intrafusal fibers changes in parallel. When the central region of an intrafusal fiber is lengthened, the rate of firing of the sensory endings accelerates; when it shortens, the rate of firing slows. Thus, the firing of the sensory endings of the muscle spindle encodes information about changes in length of the whole muscle.

There are two types of afferent terminals in muscle spindles, primary and secondary. A primary ending consists of multiple branches of a single group Ia axon that terminate on all the intrafusal fibers in the spindle, including dynamic bag, static bag, and chain fibers. There is usually just one primary ending on each spindle. A secondary ending consists of the terminations of a single group II afferent on one or more chain fibers or static bag fibers. There may be as many as five secondary endings in a muscle spindle. Both types of endings respond to stretch of the intrafusal fibers; however, the primary and secondary endings have different firing properties.

The polar regions of the intrafusal fibers are contractile and are innervated by small myelinated motor axons called *gamma motor neurons*. The motor axons that innervate extrafusal fibers are larger and are referred to as *alpha motor neurons*. Because the central region is noncontractile, contraction of the intrafusal fibers elongates the central region by pulling on it from both ends. Depending on the type of intrafusal fiber (see below) and the current state of the muscle, intrafusal contraction

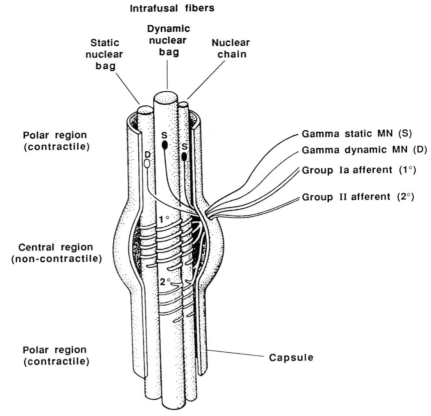

**Figure 6-1.** Simplified illustration of a muscle spindle. Capsule is cut away to show pattern of connections of afferent and efferent axons to different types of intrafusal fibers. Three intrafusal fibers are shown, one of each type; however, there are typically as many as five nuclear chain fibers in a spindle. Sensory endings wrap around the central regions of the intrafusal fibers; these are responsive to stretch of the intrafusal fibers. There are two types of sensory endings, each has different firing properties (see Figure 6-4). A primary (1°) ending consists of the terminations of a group IA afferent, usually on all three types of intrafusal fibers. A secondary (2°) ending consists of the terminations of a group II afferent, usually only on nuclear chain and static nuclear bag fibers. There are also two types of gamma motor neurons. Gamma dynamic motor neurons innervate only the dynamic nuclear bag fibers. Gamma static motor neurons innervate both static nuclear bag fibers and nuclear chain fibers. The gamma motor neurons regulate the sensitivity of the muscle spindle by causing contraction of the polar regions of the intrafusal fibers (see Figure 6-5). (From Hulliger M. The mammalian muscle spindle and its central control. Rev Physiol Biochem Pharmacol 1984; 101:1–110.)

may either increase the rate of firing of sensory endings or make them more sensitive to changes in length of the muscle. Thus, by controlling the firing rate of gamma motor neurons the central nervous system can modulate the sensitivity of the spindle.

## Golgi Tendon Organs

Golgi tendon organs are slender encapsulated structures about 1 mm long and 0.1 mm in diameter.[7] Like muscle spindles they are plentiful in almost all skeletal muscles. Though referred to as

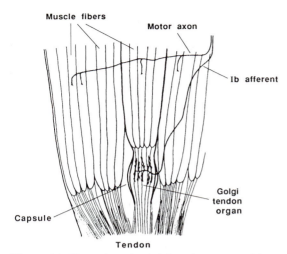

**Figure 6-2.** Illustration of a Golgi tendon organ and its relationship to muscle fibers. A capsule surrounds the collagen fibers that connect a set of muscle fibers to the common tendon. A group Ib afferent axon enters the capsule and splits into many fine, unmyelinated branches that intertwine among the collagen fibers. When the tendon is stretched, especially by a muscle contraction (see Figure 6-3B), these sensory endings are compressed and increase their firing rate. Note that each tendon organ is connected in series to a small number of muscle fibers (10 to 20), but because these are typically from different motor units, the firing rate of the afferent fiber is sensitive to the effects of recruitment. (From Houk JC, Crago PE, Rymer WZ. Functional properties of the Golgi tendon organs. In: Desmedt JE, ed. Spinal and Supraspinal Mechanisms of Voluntary Motor Control and Locomotion. Basel: S Karger, 1980; 33–43.)

*tendon organs,* they rarely are found within the tendon itself but more typically are located at the musculotendinous junction, where collagen fibers arising from the tendon attach to the muscle fibers (Figure 6-2). The tendon organs consist of bundles of such collagen fibers, which are in series with about 15 to 20 extrafusal muscle fibers.[8] Within the capsule of the tendon organ these collagen fibers have a braided appearance.

Each tendon organ is innervated by a single group Ib axon, which loses its myelination after it enters the capsule and branches into many fine endings, each of which intertwines among the fine collagen fibers. When the extrafusal muscle fibers contract, they cause the collagen fibers to straighten, compressing and stretching the nerve endings, which causes their firing rate to increase.

The braided arrangement of the collagen fibers gives them a significant mechanical advantage in deforming the nerve endings, making these axons sensitive to minute changes in muscle tension.[14] Moreover, because the muscle fibers in series with a given tendon organ are members of many different motor units, the firing rate of the tendon organ's afferent fiber is sensitive to the effects of recruitment.[15]

### Other Muscle Receptors

Relatively little is known about afferents that do not arise from spindles and tendon organs, even though they outnumber those that do. Most of these have smaller diameters and are classified as group III or IV. Most have free nerve endings and probably subserve nociceptive and thermoregulatory functions. It is presumed, but not proven, that some of these afferents play an important role in regulating the response of the body to exercise, including changes in blood pressure and breathing.[8] Some nonspindle afferents in the group II range respond to pressure, such as squeezing the muscle belly. There is indirect evidence that these afferents have significant influences on motor neurons and, so, may play some role in motor control.[16]

## Functional Properties of Spindles and Tendon Organs

### Complementary Information from Spindles and Tendon Organs

The functional differences between muscle spindles and Golgi tendon organs were first demonstrated by Matthews in 1933.[17] In the first direct recordings from muscle afferents, Matthews found that when he recorded from the afferent axon of a muscle spindle or a tendon organ and stretched the muscle, the spindle afferent increased its rate of discharge, whereas the tendon organ afferent showed only small and inconsistent increases in discharge rate. On the other hand, if the muscle was made to contract actively while still stretched (for example, by stimulating the motor neuron that innervates the muscle), the firing rate of the tendon

## A   Muscle stretch

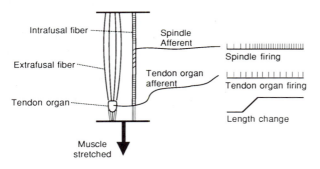

## B   Muscle contraction

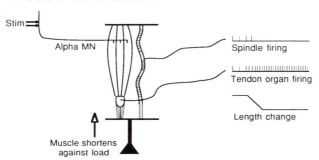

## C   Alpha-gamma coactivation

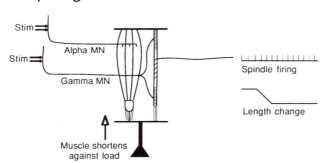

**Figure 6-3.** Functional properties of muscle spindles and Golgi tendon organs. The intrafusal muscle fibers of muscle spindles are arranged in parallel with extrafusal muscle fibers. Tendon organs are arranged in series with extrafusal fibers. Because of this difference in anatomic arrangement, the spindles sense changes in length of the muscle while the tendon organs sense changes in tension. (*A*) When the muscle is stretched, the spindle is also stretched, and its afferents increase their discharge rate. The tendon organ shows little response, because most of the stretch is taken up by the muscle tissue. (*B*) When the muscle contracts, the spindle shortens and its afferents decrease their firing rate and eventually fall silent as the intrafusal fiber becomes slack. The tendon organ is very sensitive to contraction because the tendon is pulled directly by the muscle fibers. (*C*) The nervous system can prevent the muscle spindle from slackening during muscle contraction by activating the gamma motor neurons. The resulting contraction of the polar regions of the intrafusal fibers maintains the central region taut and allows the spindle to continue to sense small changes in length during muscle shortening.

organ increased markedly, but the firing rate of the spindle decreased or it ceased altogether to fire.

The main reason for this difference in response lies in the different anatomic relationships of the two types of receptor to extrafusal muscle fibers. The muscle spindles are arranged in parallel with the extrafusal fibers, whereas the Golgi tendon organs are arranged in series (Figure 6-3). Passive stretching of the muscle elongates and distorts the spindle receptors, leading to an increased firing rate. The tendon organ is relatively less responsive to stretch than the muscle spindle, since the collagen fibers emanating from the tendon are stiffer than muscle fibers. Therefore, most of the stretch is taken up by the more compliant muscle fibers and little direct stretching of the tendon organ takes place. When the muscle contracts, however, the muscle fibers pull directly on the collagen fibers and thus transmit more effective stretch to the tendon organ. As a result, tendon organs always respond more robustly to muscle contraction than to passive stretch of the muscle. The arrangement in series of tendon organs therefore makes them most responsive to the tension of muscles. Spindles, on the other hand, decrease their firing rate when the muscle contracts, because, as the extrafusal fibers shorten with active contraction the parallel intrafusal fibers also shorten. The resultant unloading of the intrafusal fibers causes them to slacken, often to the point of "kinking," leading to a decrease in or cessation of firing. Thus, the muscle spindles, because of their parallel relationship to extrafusal fibers, are sensitive to changes in length of the muscles. Because the length of a muscle is directly related to the angle of the joint or joints it crosses, muscle spindles indirectly provide the central nervous system with information about the positions of the limbs in space.

Therefore, although muscle spindles and tendon organs are both sensitive to stretch, because of their different anatomic arrangements within muscles they provide the CNS with complementary information about the state of the muscle. The muscle spindles inform the nervous system about changes in length of the muscle; the tendon organs signal changes in tension exerted by the muscle. The complementary information coming from spindles and tendon organs is thought to be important in allowing the CNS to distinguish between changes in internal state of the muscle (e.g., fatigue) and changes in external loads acting on the muscle.[8]

### Primary and Secondary Endings of Muscle Spindles

When a muscle is stretched or released from a stretch we can distinguish two phases of the change in length: a dynamic phase, the period during which length is changing, and a static phase, after a new steady-state length is achieved (Figure 6-4). The primary and secondary endings of muscle spindles respond quite differently during the dynamic phase of a change in length.[18] While both receptors discharge similarly when the muscle is held at a constant or static length, the primary ending shows a distinct high-frequency burst during the dynamic phase of a stretch, whereas the secondary ending does not.

Thus, the firing rates of both primary and secondary endings always reflect the final static or steady-state length. When a muscle is stretched to a longer length, both endings respond by increasing their firing rates to a higher steady-state level. When a muscle shortens, both endings decrease their firing rates to a lower rate, reflecting the shorter final length. The primary endings of the muscle spindle are additionally sensitive to the rate of change in length, a property sometimes referred to as *velocity sensitivity*. During the dynamic phase of stretch of the muscle the primary ending shows a distinct burst in firing, achieving much higher rates than during the later steady-state phase. The firing rate of the secondary ending increases more gradually, and the firing rate is not much higher during the dynamic phase than during the steady-state phase. The instantaneous rates of firing in the primary ending that occur during a change in muscle length reflect the rate of length change; higher rates occur during faster stretches. A similar velocity sensitivity is also present for shortening of muscle; the primary ending often shows a pause in firing during a fast shortening before achieving a new steady-state firing rate. Because primary endings are so sensitive to phasic length changes, they typically fire in bursts in response to stimuli such as vibration or quick taps of the muscle. As these stimuli do not change the steady-state length of the muscle, the secondary endings are relatively unaffected by them.

The high degree of rate sensitivity of primary endings implies that the firing rates of spindles can encode both the length of a muscle and the velocity of length change, thus allowing the CNS to compute the speed of movements as well as the static positions of joints. The strength of this interpretation must be tempered, however, by several additional properties of primary endings.[3,8] First, and most important, primary endings are most sensitive to very small changes in length (less than 0.1 mm). For large changes the dynamic sensitivity of the primary endings decreases dramatically. This high degree of sensitivity of primary endings to very small stretches is often reflected by a transient increase in firing rate at the very beginning of a stretch (Figure 6-4). Second, the primary ending has the ability to reset its responsiveness to small stretches after it comes to a new length. Consequently, it is able to sense small changes in length at whatever new length it comes to. Third, these first two properties indicate that the actual rela-

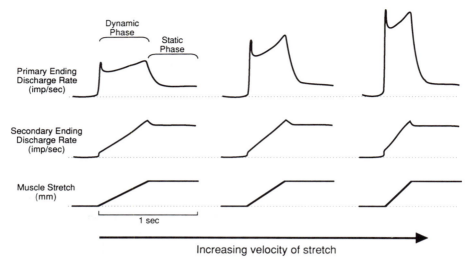

**Figure 6-4.** Differences in the firing properties of primary and secondary endings of muscle spindles. The traces show the time-varying changes in discharge rate of the afferent axons during muscle stretches of different velocities. During the static phase, when the muscle has stabilized at a new, longer length, the firing rate of both types of endings is faster than before the stretch. The firing rate during this phase is roughly proportional to the length of the muscle. During the dynamic phase, when the muscle is stretching, the firing rate of the primary ending increases. The magnitude of this transient increase in discharge rate reflects the velocity of the length change. Thus, the primary ending has the additional capacity for signaling the velocity of length change. Note also the brief increase in firing of the primary ending at the beginning of muscle stretch. This occurs because the primary ending is most sensitive to very small changes in length.

tionships of muscle length and rate of length change to rate of spindle firing are highly nonlinear, that is, they depend in complex ways on multiple factors, such as the initial length and the recent history of spindle firing. This has confounded physiologists attempting to "decode" signals from muscle spindles: it means that there are no simple formulas by which the nervous system can compute muscle length and velocity of length change from spindle firing. It thus appears that primary endings are most useful for detecting small movements or unexpected changes in rate of length change, rather than for direct velocity transduction.

### Dynamic and Static Gamma Motor Neurons

Although it was known since Ruffini's descriptions of the spindle in the 19th century that intrafusal fibers had motor innervation, an understanding of the source and function of this innervation awaited a series of classic studies in the period between 1945 and 1955. Until this time it was believed that the motor innervation of the spindle derived from the same motor axons that innervated the extrafusal muscle fibers, as had been demonstrated in amphibian muscle spindles. However, in 1945 Leksell used pressure to block conduction in the large alpha motor axons in ventral roots so that stimulation of the ventral roots excited only smaller motor axons, classified as gamma motor neurons.[19] He discovered that while such excitation of the gamma fibers produced no significant increase in muscle tension, multiunit recordings of spindle afferents showed a greater discharge rate. These findings were soon refined and confirmed by Hunt and Kuffler, who developed a method for stimulating single gamma efferents and simultaneously recording from single spindle afferents.[20] Their experiments established that the motor innervation of the spindle derived from a separate

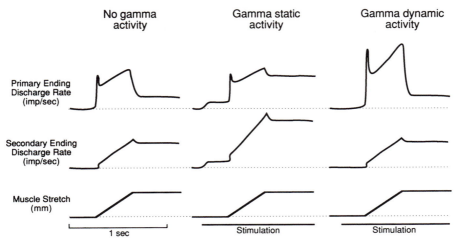

**Figure 6-5.** The effects of activating different types of gamma motor neurons on the firing properties of primary and secondary endings of muscle spindles. Here, as in Figure 6-4, each trace shows the discharge rate of spindle afferents during muscle stretch. In the middle column, the effect of stimulating a gamma static motor neuron is shown. Both types of ending show increases in discharge rate during the static phase. Note that because the firing rate during the static phase increases without any change in the firing rate during the dynamic phase, the primary ending shows relatively less dynamic responsiveness. In the column on the right, the effect of stimulating a gamma static motor neuron is shown. This increases the sensitivity of primary endings during the dynamic phase of length change but has little effect on the secondary ending. Thus, the nervous system can, by selective activation of these two types of gamma motor neurons, adjust the input from the spindles so that it predominantly reflects either steady-state length or rate of length change.

system of smaller gamma efferents and that excitation of these efferents led to higher rates of discharge of spindle afferents. The separate system of efferents to spindles is often referred to as the *fusimotor system;* the alpha motor neurons that innervate extrafusal muscle fibers are referred to as the *skeletomotor system.*

The gamma efferents do more than simply change afferent discharge, however. The changes in contractile state of intrafusal fibers that result from modulation of gamma discharge alter the sensitivity of spindle endings to changes in length. Moreover, there are two types of gamma motor neurons, *static* and *dynamic,* which selectively alter the dynamic and static responsiveness of spindle afferents (Figure 6-5). This was demonstrated in an experiment carried out by Crowe and Matthews in 1964.[21] They recorded from isolated Ia afferent fibers while stretching the muscle at a controlled rate. The primary ending typically showed a high rate of discharge during the dynamic phase of the stretch and a higher steady

state rate during the static phase. They then repeated the procedure many times, while at the same time stimulating different gamma motor neurons. Activation of some gamma motor neurons produced marked enhancement of the steady-state discharge from the primary afferent during the static phase with little effect on the dynamic responsiveness of the afferent. These efferents are thus classified as gamma static motor neurons. Activation of gamma static motor neurons has a similar effect on the output of secondary endings, increasing their firing rate at a given length. Activation of other neurons produced marked enhancement of the high-frequency burst during the dynamic phase with only slight enhancement of the static responsiveness. These efferents are classified as gamma dynamic motor neurons.

Because activation of gamma static motor neurons increases the static discharge rate of spindle afferents relative to their dynamic response, it diminishes the relative intensity of the dynamic response (the dynamic response is that over and above the final steady-state firing level; see Figure 6-5). Thus, selective activation of gamma static motor neurons has the overall effect of making the ensemble spindle input to the CNS more related to current length of the muscle, while selective activation of gamma dynamic motor neurons makes the overall spindle input more phasic (that is, related to small and quick changes in muscle length).[11] The central nervous system therefore has the capacity to modify the predominant quality of the information it is receiving.

### Relationships Between Structure and Function

The reason for the different actions of the two types of gamma motor neuron, as well as the different firing properties of primary and secondary afferents, is not that the neurons themselves have intrinsically different properties, but rather that they innervate different types of intrafusal fiber (see Table 6-2).[2,8] Primary spindle endings terminate on all the intrafusal fibers within a spindle, including dynamic bag fibers, static bag fibers, and nuclear chain fibers. Therefore, the firing pattern of primary endings derives from the combined influence of all three types of fiber. Secondary endings, on the other hand, innervate principally chain fibers but some static bag fibers. Their firing patterns, therefore, reflect only the properties of these intrafusal fibers. Gamma dynamic motor neurons innervate only the dynamic nuclear bag fibers. Gamma static motor neurons innervate nuclear chain fibers as well as static nuclear bag fibers.

**Table 6-2.** Different Types of Intrafusal Muscle Fibers

| Type | Sensory Innervation | Motor Innervation |
|---|---|---|
| Dynamic nuclear bag | Primary ending (Ia) | Gamma dynamic |
| Static nuclear bag | Primary ending (Ia) | Gamma static |
| | Secondary ending (II) | |
| Nuclear chain | Primary ending (Ia) | Gamma static |
| | Secondary ending (II) | |

The dynamic sensitivity of primary afferent fibers derives from the mechanical behavior of the dynamic nuclear bag fibers, referred to as *intrafusal creep*.[22] This type of intrafusal fiber has non-uniform characteristics along its length. The central region acts much like a spring, whereas the polar regions exhibit a kind of viscous friction. Thus, when the intrafusal fiber is stretched, the central region lengthens immediately and the polar regions only gradually stretch out to the new length. As the polar regions slowly stretch, the initially lengthened central region "creeps" back to a slightly shorter length. Because the sensory endings are located in the central region, they respond to the stretch with a burst of firing, which then adapts to a lower level as the central region shortens. Furthermore, the contraction of these fibers is not propagated throughout its length, as in normal muscle fibers. Activation of these fibers by gamma dynamic motor neurons leads not to shortening of the intrafusal fiber but rather to stiffening of the polar regions, with a concomitant increase in the viscous friction. This has the effect of enhancing the intrafusal creep and, in turn, the dynamic sensitivity of the primary ending, without much effect on the steady-state discharge rate.

Nuclear chain fibers, on the other hand, have properties much more like those of ordinary skeletal muscle. They exhibit a fast, propagated contraction when stimulated, leading to shortening of the intrafusal fiber. Thus, stimulation of these fibers by gamma static efferents brings about an increase in steady-state discharge rate of both primary and secondary endings. The static nuclear bag fibers seem to have intermediate properties, but at present the view is that they behave more like nuclear chain fibers.

### Role of the Gamma System

An important role of gamma motor neurons was first suggested by Hunt and Kuffler in the early 1950s.[20,23] They reasoned that during large muscle contractions the spindle becomes slackened and therefore is unable to signal further changes in muscle length. They suggested that one role of the fusimotor system is to maintain tension in the muscle spindle during and after active contraction, in order to maintain its responsiveness at different lengths. Experiments carried out by Hunt and Kuffler demonstrated the feasibility of this hypothesis.[24] If the discharge rate of spindle afferents is recorded while alpha motor neurons are stimulated, the firing of the afferent shows a characteristic pause during the contraction, because the muscle is shortening, and therefore unloading (slackening) the spindle (see Figure 6-3B). If, however, a gamma motor neuron is activated at the same time as the alpha motor neuron, the pause becomes filled in because contraction of the intrafusal fibers keeps their central regions loaded, or under tension (see Figure 6-3C).

Thus, an essential role of fusimotor innervation is to prevent the spindle from falling silent when the muscle shortens as a result of active contraction, thus enabling it to signal length changes over the full range of muscle lengths. This mechanism maintains the spindle firing rate within an optimal range for signalling length changes, whatever the actual length of the muscle. If alpha motor neurons were activated more or less in parallel with gamma motor neurons, a pattern referred to as *alpha-gamma coactivation*,[25] automatic maintenance of sensitivity, would result.

It is now known that, in addition to gamma efferents there are collaterals from alpha motor neurons that innervate intrafusal fibers.[9, 11] These are referred to as *skeletofusimotor* or beta efferents. A significant, though still unquantified, amount of skeletofusimotor innervation has been found in both cat and human spindles. These efferents provide the equivalent of alpha-gamma coactivation; when skeletofusimotor neurons are activated, unloading of the spindle by contraction of extrafusal fibers is at least partially compensated by loading due to intrafusal contraction. Nevertheless, the existence of a skeletofusimotor system, with its forced linkage of extrafusal and intrafusal contraction, serves to highlight the importance of the independent fusimotor system, the gamma motor neurons. Apparently, mammals have evolved a mechanism that allows for uncoupling the control of muscle spindles from the control of their parent muscles. On logical grounds, this would give the organism greater flexibility in controlling the spindle output in different functional contexts; however, the degree to which such independent control is achieved remains a matter of controversy and will be taken up again later in this chapter.

## Role of Muscle Spindles in Perception of Limb Position and Movement

One of the most venerable controversies in neurophysiology is whether muscle receptors, particularly spindles, are responsible for our conscious perception of limb position and movement. This controversy has raged for at least 100 years, since Helmholtz attributed our ability to perceive limb position and movement to a "sense of effort" (that is, we know where our limbs are by monitoring the neural output that has gotten them to where they are).[1] Sherrington, on the other hand, proposed that there is a "muscular sense" that accounts for position and movement sense, and he used the term *proprioception* to refer to the general sense of where limbs are in relation to each other. The notion that muscles are insentient and that our sense of position derives purely from monitoring neural effort became less attractive as the rich sensory innervation of muscles was detailed by different investigators. Thus, for a time, Sherrington's view that muscle receptors are the source of proprioception became the accepted account.

More recently, however, the controversy was revived. Many investigators argued that, rather than muscle receptors, receptors in the joints themselves were the chief source of information about the positions of the limbs. These receptors respond to tension in the joint capsule and often show a preferential joint angle at which they fire; usually at the extremes of range. In 1956, Skoglund[26] showed that some slowly adapting joint receptors discharged at intermediate joint angles and argued that these could be used to detect joint position. This idea held sway for about a decade, until Burgess and Clark[27,28] in extremely detailed studies, showed that the overwhelming majority of joint receptors fire at the extremes of range. The few receptors found that fired at intermediate angles could not possibly account for our sense of position. Thus, the notion that joint receptors account for position sense became less tenable.

At the same time, a number of psychophysical experiments lent weight to Sherrington's original idea that it was the muscle spindles that account for position sense. Perhaps the most dramatic of these was performed by Goodwin and colleagues.[29–31] They showed that vibration of a muscle, known to be a powerful stimulus to primary endings of spindles, induced large errors in sense of position. If, for example, a vibration was applied to the biceps muscle of a subject, the subject perceived the elbow as being more extended than it actually was. Often these errors could be as great as 40 degrees. Thus, the error in perception was consistent with a stimulus to the spindle, since if the spindle was active, the CNS would interpret this as a stretching of the biceps muscle, leading to a perception that the elbow was extended.

The current consensus, therefore, is that muscle spindles play a primary role in our sense of position and movement.[1] It is believed that joint receptors and cutaneous receptors also play a role in position sense, but the relative importance of their contributions is still unclear.[32]

## Reflex Connections of Spindles and Tendon Organs

Until now, we have been discussing spindles and tendon organs as sensory receptors, transducers of muscle length and tension, but the intrinsic role of these receptors in motor control cannot be fully appreciated without discussing their participation in stretch reflexes. Stretch reflexes are automatic contractions of muscle in response to passive lengthening of the muscle. Though once thought to result from intrinsic properties of muscles themselves, Sherrington's demonstration at the turn of the century that stretch reflexes could be abolished by cutting either the dorsal or the ventral roots established that they require sensory input from the muscle to the spinal cord and a return path to the muscles.[11]

Sherrington carried out an extensive series of investigations of the properties of stretch reflex.[33] For these experiments, he used decerebrate cats, that is, cats whose brain stem had been surgically transected at the level of the midbrain, between the superior and inferior colliculi. Decerebrate animals have simplified and usually heightened spinal reflexes, making it is easier to examine the factors controlling their expression. Sherrington found that the stretch reflex has two components: a brisk but short-lived phasic component, which is triggered by the change in muscle length, and a weaker but longer-lasting tonic component, which is determined by the static stretching of the mus-

cles at the new longer length. The phasic component can be seen in isolation in intact animals by briskly tapping a muscle or its tendon, a response referred to as a tendon jerk. Tonic stretch reflexes are more subtle and less obvious in intact animals. Typically they are not seen unless the muscle is already contracting. A critical finding of Sherrington's was that stretching one muscle often produced effects in other muscles. Synergist muscles, that is muscles with a similar mechanical action, also contracted. Most interestingly, when a muscle was stretched its antagonist muscles tended to relax. Sherrington referred to this as reciprocal innervation.

Though Sherrington believed that the receptor responsible for the stretch reflex was the muscle spindle, it remained for other investigators to definitively identify the afferent fibers responsible and to work out the spinal circuitry. Investigators such as Lloyd[13,34,35] and Eccles[36,37] using increasingly refined techniques, have given us a fairly complete picture of the central connections of Ia fibers, and it is now known that these afferents are largely responsible for the phasic component of the stretch reflex.

### Spinal Connections of Group Ia Afferents

Ia fibers from muscle spindles enter the spinal cord through the dorsal roots and immediately diverge into numerous collateral fibers (Figure 6-6). Some collaterals pass to the ventral horn of the gray matter, where they make direct (monosynaptic) excitatory connections with alpha motor neurons that innervate the same muscles (homonymous motor neurons). The distribution of Ia fibers to alpha motor neurons supplying homonymous muscles is quite extensive. A single Ia afferent makes monosynaptic connections with virtually all of the motor neurons innervating the same muscle from which the Ia afferent arises. Thus, Ia afferent fibers provide a strong excitatory drive to the muscle in which they originate, a phenomenon referred to as *autogenic excitation*. Other Ia collaterals make monosynaptic excitatory connections with alpha motor neurons innervating synergist muscles. These connections, though widespread, are not quite as strong as the connections to homonymous motor neurons. The strength of these connections

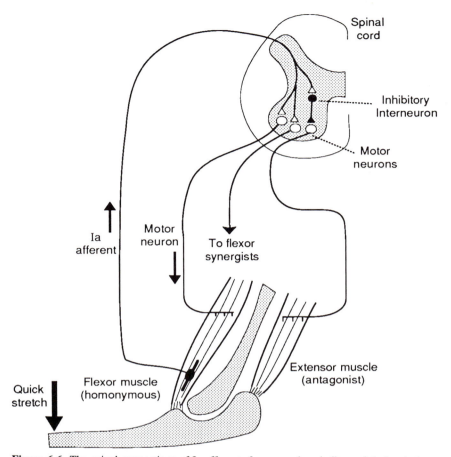

**Figure 6-6.** The spinal connections of Ia afferents from muscle spindles and their role in the stretch reflex. IA afferents make excitatory connections (*unfilled triangles*) to motor neurons that innervate the same muscle and synergist muscles. They make inhibitory connections (*filled triangles*) through an interneuron to motor neurons that innervate antagonist muscles. The primary endings of muscle spindles respond to a quick stretch with an increase in firing rate of the Ia afferent. This increase in firing rate causes the motor neurons to fire and the muscle contracts briskly. At the same time, the antagonist muscle is inhibited. The stretch reflex thus enhances the intrinsic stiffness of the muscle because it acts to oppose stretch of the muscle.

varies from muscle to muscle in a complex way, according to the similarity of the mechanical actions of the synergists.

Ia collaterals also make excitatory connections with a special class of inhibitory interneurons that project to alpha motor neurons supplying muscles that are antagonistic to the muscles from which the Ia fibers originate. Thus, Ia afferents inhibit antagonist motor neurons disynaptically (that is, through an interposed inhibitory neuron). This connection accounts for the reciprocal innervation

observed by Sherrington. As motor neurons supplying homonymous and synergist muscles are excited, motor neurons to antagonist muscles are reciprocally inhibited.

Many Ia collaterals make connections with propriospinal and other interneurons, whose targets and functions are not well understood. Besides the monosynaptic stretch reflex, Ia afferents also participate in other, more complex reflex pathways. Finally, some Ia collaterals ascend in the dorsal columns to the brain stem, where they make connections to sensory tracts that ultimately reach the cerebral cortex and other higher centers.

### The Monosynaptic Stretch Reflex

How does this spinal circuitry account for the stretch reflex? Brisk passive extension of the limb lengthens the flexor muscles (see Figure 6-6), causing an increase in the discharge rate of Ia fibers arising in these muscles. The Ia fiber discharge excites both homonymous and synergist muscles monosynaptically, causing a contraction that tends to oppose the passive lengthening. By virtue of the Ia afferent's connection to inhibitory interneurons, antagonist motor neurons are inhibited, and the antagonist muscles tend to relax, an action that indirectly assists the reflex resistance to the imposed stretch.

Thus, it would appear that the stretch reflex acts to resist changes in joint position. It certainly functions in this way in decerebrate cats, whose standing position is maintained by virtue of tonic stretch reflexes in the extensor muscles. In intact animals tonic stretch reflexes are not nearly strong enough to prevent changes in joint position, and the monosynaptic stretch reflex produced by Ia afferents is primarily phasic. Because Ia afferents terminate in primary endings, which are highly sensitive to the dynamic phase of a length change, it is usually necessary to quickly stretch the muscle to elicit an observable reflex. A sharp tap on a tendon, for example, produces brief but effective stretching of most or all of the spindles in a muscle. The ensuing volley of Ia afferent discharge reaches the homonymous and synergist motor neurons synchronously, and, owing to the widespread divergence and convergence patterns of Ia afferents, the result is both temporal and spatial summation of excitatory potentials in the motor neurons. This leads to a brisk phasic contraction in the stretched muscles, sometimes referred to as a *tendon jerk* or a *deep tendon reflex*. Despite the widespread clinical use of this terminology, it must be emphasized that the receptors responsible are in the muscle and not the tendon. In fact, it is now believed that tapping a tendon with a reflex hammer causes a wave of vibration to pass through the whole muscle, which gives a powerful stimulus to many if not most of the primary endings within the muscle.[38]

### Spinal Connections of Group II Spindle Afferents

The central connections of group II afferents from the secondary spindle endings have proved more difficult to trace, primarily because there are other afferent fibers in the group II diameter range that arise from nonspindle receptors and free nerve endings. Group II spindle afferents from the secondary endings do participate in the monosynaptic stretch reflexes, though this connection is thought to be relatively weak.[39,40] Early findings by Eccles and Lundberg[41] suggested that group II afferents were excitatory to motor neurons innervating flexor muscles and inhibitory to those innervating extensor muscles and that these connections were polysynaptic, as the latencies of these effects were relatively long. It is clear now that at least some of the afferents producing these effects arise from free nerve endings and are not directly involved in sensing muscle length.[16] These connections are now seen as part of a widespread system of reflex pathways, referred to as *flexion reflex afferent* (FRA) pathways. Lundberg recently suggested that the spinal reflex pathways in which group II afferents participate can be switched on and off by higher centers.[42–44] He further proposes that these pathways are important for organizing whole limb movements, as for locomotion, and that the afferent input serves to reinforce muscle contraction and modulate its timing.

### Spinal Connections of Group Ib Afferents from Golgi Tendon Organs

Group Ib afferents from Golgi tendon organs also show widespread divergence in the spinal cord. Stimulation of tendon organ afferents produces disynaptic or trisynaptic inhibition of homonymous motor neurons, called autogenic inhibition, and excitation of antagonist motor neurons. Because stimulation of Golgi tendon organs produces an effect that seems opposite to that of stimulating the spindle afferents, this is often referred to as an inverse myotatic reflex.

The action of Ib afferents is a good deal more complex than this, however, primarily because the interneurons that mediate these effects receive convergent input from many different types of receptors as well as descending pathways. Moreover,

Ib afferents make more diffuse connections than Ia afferents, with significant effects on motor neurons innervating remote muscles. Therefore, the central connections of tendon organ afferents, like those of group II afferents, are thought to be part of spinal reflex networks responsible for regulating whole limb movements.[45]

Golgi tendon organs were originally thought to have a protective function, preventing damage to muscle, since it was assumed that they fired only when high tensions were achieved. In 1966, however, Houk and Henneman[46] demonstrated that they signal minute changes in muscle tension, thus providing the nervous system with precise information about the state of contraction of the muscle. Lundberg[45] has proposed that the convergence of afferent input from tendon organs, cutaneous receptors, and joint receptors onto interneurons that inhibit motor neurons allows for precise spinal control of muscle tension in activities such as active touch. Combined input from these receptors would inhibit muscle contraction when the limb contacts an object.

## The Stretch Reflex in Motor Control

Historically, the analysis of stretch reflexes has served as a useful "model system" in which to examine the processes by which neurons communicate with each other and by which neural signals are integrated. Indeed, well before modern techniques for intracellular recording were developed, Sherrington and his contemporaries, by careful measurement of muscle responses to stretch and other stimuli, were able to infer the basic rules governing synaptic transmission, including excitation and inhibition, as well as spatial and temporal summation.[25,47] Modern neurobiology continues to exploit simple reflexes as model systems for analyzing the elementary mechanisms of neural processing.

Because of the relative simplicity of the neural circuits responsible for the monosynaptic stretch reflex, testing the strength of phasic stretch reflexes is also an extremely useful tool in clinical diagnosis. Absence or weakness of phasic stretch reflexes often indicates a disruption of one or more of the peripheral components of the reflex arc—peripheral motor or sensory axons, the cell bodies of motor neurons, or the muscle itself. However,

because the excitability of motor neurons is dependent on both excitatory and inhibitory descending influences, hypoactive (decreased relative to normal) stretch reflexes can also result from lesions of the central nervous system. This is especially evident after transection of the spinal cord, which produces a phenomenon referred to as spinal shock, in which all spinal reflexes are depressed. The spinal shock is usually transient, lasting several days to weeks, and reflex excitability usually increases gradually, with the result that stretch reflexes ultimately become hyperactive (increased relative to normal). Hyperactive stretch reflexes always result from central lesions that disrupt the normal balance of excitatory and inhibitory influences on the motor neurons. Hyperactive stretch reflexes are often associated with spasticity, a condition in which muscles show abnormally high resistance to passive stretch, especially rapid muscle stretches. The association of hyperactive stretch reflexes with weakness or paralysis and spasticity is often referred to clinically as upper motor neuron disease, as it is presumed that, either directly or indirectly, the lesion disrupts the descending motor pathways that converge on the alpha (lower) motor neurons.

Despite the experimental and clinical significance of the stretch reflex, its role in normal motor control has not been easily defined. Nevertheless, the spinal stretch reflex is the only known monosynaptic reflex in the mammalian nervous system, and its afferent and efferent neurons are among the fastest-conducting of the nervous system. Thus, it provides a relatively fast system for influencing motor neuron excitability. Furthermore, the sheer magnitude of spindle input to the spinal cord, with widespread convergence and divergence patterns, implies that these reflex pathways play an important role in motor control. Some possible explanations of the functional role of stretch reflexes are therefore considered.

### *Reflex Generation of Posture and Movement*

During the first half of this century it was generally believed that stretch reflexes were directly responsible for triggering many simple motor acts, especially in relatively automatic behaviors. For example, postural adjustments in standing were thought to result from simple stretch reflexes.

Thus, if the body swayed forward, posterior muscles of the legs would be stretched, initiating reflex contractions that would resist the sway. Rhythmic behaviors, such as locomotion, that require alternation between flexion and extension, were believed to be generated by alternating reflex contractions. In this scheme, flexion movements of the legs would trigger stretch reflexes in the extensor muscles that would initiate the next phase of the cycle, and so on.

More recent research, however, indicates that even automatic behaviors such as postural adjustments and locomotion are controlled by central neural circuits that generate relatively complex sequences of muscle contractions. Postural adjustments, for example, typically occur in advance of a disturbance, if that disturbance can be anticipated, and they involve synergic contractions of groups of muscles.[48,49] Furthermore, the alternating patterns of muscle contraction seen in locomotion persist even when all afferent information from the limbs is blocked.[50,51] Nevertheless, even though stretch reflexes may not be directly responsible for generating these motor actions, they still play an important role in modulating and refining the motor output. Under certain conditions stretch reflexes may reinforce certain motor patterns; in other situations they may assist in correcting for unanticipated disturbances.

### The Stretch Reflex as a Feedback Loop

An important class of functional hypotheses about stretch reflex function depends on the idea that the stretch reflex can function not only as a discrete reflex but also as a closed feedback loop (Figure 6-7). For example, stretch of a muscle produces an increase in spindle discharge, leading to muscle contraction and consequent shortening of the muscle. But this muscle shortening leads to a decrease in spindle discharge, a reduction of muscle contraction, and a lengthening of the muscle. Thus, the stretch reflex loop, in theory, can act continuously, tending to keep muscle length close to a constant value. This is referred to as *feedback* because the output of the system (a change in muscle length) is "fed back" and becomes the input. The stretch reflex is a *negative* feedback system because it tends to counteract or reduce deviations from a reference value of the regulated variable, that is, it tends to keep muscle length

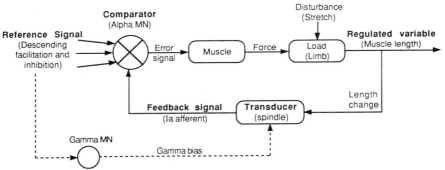

**Figure 6-7.** The stretch reflex as a feedback loop. The spindle acts as a transducer, sensing changes in the regulated variable, muscle length. If the actual length is different from the intended or reference length, the motor neuron either increases or decreases its firing rate, producing the appropriate change in muscle force to bring the muscle back to the intended length. Such a system can in principle act to maintain an intended posture at the joint, but in normal situations the stretch reflex is not strong enough to overcome a large disturbance. It is more probable that it acts to correct for small perturbations. The dotted lines show the hypothetical effect of activating gamma motor neurons. This gamma bias could produce indirect activation of muscles by inducing the spindles to signal a change in length (see text). In effect, the gamma bias would signal the intended length of the muscle. This hypothesis that the stretch reflex acts as a servomechanism for initiating movement has not been validated, but it did stimulate intensive interest in the stretch reflex as a feedback loop.

constant. The reference value is set by descending signals that act on the alpha motor neurons. Because the regulated variable is length, the spindle feedback loop enhances the springlike properties of muscle, tending to resist changes in length.

How might such a feedback loop function in motor control? In 1952, Merton[52,53] put forward an ingenious hypothesis that, although it was ultimately proven erroneous, drew attention to the possible roles of feedback in motor control. Merton suggested that the higher centers might activate muscles indirectly, by way of gamma motor neurons, rather than directly, through the alpha motor neurons (see Figure 6-7). Activation of gamma motor neurons would cause contraction of the intrafusal fibers, thereby activating Ia afferent neurons. The Ia afferent neurons would then activate alpha motor neurons, causing the muscles to contract. The advantage of indirect activation through this gamma loop would be that the amount of gamma activity (referred to as gamma bias) would in effect signal the intended length of the muscle. The automatic stretch reflex would continue to produce contraction of the muscle until it shortened to the point where the spindle was unloaded, at which point stable equilibrium would be achieved. According to Merton's hypothesis, the stretch reflex serves as a servomechanism, that is, a feedback loop in which the output variable (actual muscle length) automatically follows a reference value (intended muscle length). This mechanism would therefore bring the muscle to the intended length, regardless of the actual load being moved. Thus, the nervous system could produce a movement of a given distance without having to know in advance the actual load or weight to be moved.

Merton's hypothesis was attractive because it postulated a mechanism for simplifying movement control. Unfortunately, such compelling and explicit hypotheses often turn out to be oversimplifications, and such was the case here. A central prediction of Merton's hypothesis is that a voluntary movement is initiated in a specific sequence of events in peripheral axons: (1) activation of gamma motor neurons, (2) activation of Ia afferent neurons, (3) activation of alpha motor neurons. In the early 1970s, Swedish investigators developed a technique known as microneurography for recording from the larger afferent neurons in peripheral nerves, and this method allowed direct testing of Merton's hypothesis. In 1972, Vallbo[54] recorded from Ia afferent neurons while at the same time recording the electromyographic (EMG) activity in muscles (EMG activity is an indirect measure of the activation of alpha motor neurons). Vallbo's experiments demonstrated conclusively that Ia afferent activity always followed EMG activity, so the initial activation of the muscle could not be through the gamma loop.

Nevertheless, the fact that Ia fibers increase their rate of discharge during the movement in Vallbo's recordings indicates that gamma motor neurons must have been activated, not before, but rather in synchrony with the alpha motor neurons. If there were no gamma activation, spindle discharge should decrease or pause during a contraction, because of unloading of the spindle. This finding led Vallbo and others[4,55,56] to suggest a revision of the Merton hypothesis, referred to as *servo-assistance*. They argued that the afferent discharge from the spindle is insufficient to bring about large changes in muscle length, especially when significant loads are to be moved. Further, muscle spindles are most sensitive to very small changes in length. Therefore, according to this view, alpha and gamma motor neurons are normally coactivated during shortening contractions. The stretch reflex feedback loop then serves to compensate for small disturbances, allowing automatic correction of small errors in the movement trajectory.

### Alpha-Gamma Coactivation versus Independent Modulation

While alpha-gamma coactivation may often be employed, especially in the slow, precise movements that Vallbo studied, it is by no means the only possible mode of interaction of the fusimotor and skeletomotor systems. Though it is inherently difficult to record simultaneously from alpha and gamma motor neurons during natural movements, indirect evidence strongly suggests that the nervous system adjusts fusimotor activation in different ways, according to the specific task. For example, Loeb and Hoffer[57] recorded from Ia afferents in hind limb muscles during locomotion in cats and showed that they behaved differently depending on whether the muscle they originated from was lengthening or shortening. During certain phases of locomotion, muscles contract while shortening; during these phases, gamma motor neurons appear to be activated, presumably to maintain sensitivity of the spindle. During other phases, however, some muscles contract while lengthening; during these phases, there appears to be relatively little gamma activation. Loeb points out that gamma activation is not necessary for maintaining sensitivity of the spindle during lengthening contractions, and it might even be counterproductive, since spindle firing would saturate, that is, reach its highest level and become unresponsive to further increases in muscle length. Thus, Loeb emphasizes the importance of different patterns of gamma activation for maintaining optimal sensitivity of the spindle as a transducer.[10]

A particularly elegant series of experiments aimed at discovering natural patterns of gamma activation was carried out by Prochazka and colleagues[12,58–60] These investigators recorded, during natural movements of cats, the activity of Ia afferents and the movements of the associated joints. They then electrically stimulated gamma motor neurons in anesthetized cats while at the same time reproducing the exact joint movements with a computer-controlled motor and recording from Ia afferents with similar characteristics to those they had recorded in awake animals. By using a computer to adjust the fusimotor stimulation until the patterns of Ia discharge exactly matched the records in natural movements, they were able to "reconstruct" the specific type of gamma activation that had been employed.

The overall results of these experiments indicate that, rather than a strict linkage of alpha and gamma activation, the amount and type of gamma activation (static or dynamic) is preset at a certain tonic level, depending on the specific task or context. Prochazka and coworkers[59] referred to this as *fusimotor set*. A summary of some of their findings is illustrated in Table 6-3. Gamma static activation predominates when the animal is carrying out slow and predictable movements. On the other hand, high levels of gamma dynamic activation appear to be preset when the animal is moving fast or attempting a difficult or unpredictable task, such as beam walking. Thus, it would

**Table 6-3.** Relative Activity of Gamma Static and Gamma Dynamic Motor Neurons in Cats During Different Motor Activities

| Motor Activity | Gamma Static Firing | Gamma Dynamic Firing |
|---|---|---|
| Resting | 0 | 0 |
| Sitting | + | 0 |
| Standing | + | 0 |
| Slow walking | + + | 0 |
| Fast walking | + + + | + |
| Imposed movements | + | + + + |
| Paw shaking | + | + + + |
| Beam walking | + + + | + + + |

Adapted from Prochazka A, Hulliger M, Trend P, et al. Dynamic and static fusimotor set in various behavioural contexts. In: Hrik P, Soukop T, Vejsada R, et al., eds. Mechanoreceptors. New York: Plenum, 1988; 417–430.

appear that the nervous system is capable of tuning the spindles so that they provide information most appropriate for the specific task conditions.

### Adaptive Control of Muscle Tone

Stretch reflexes play an important role in the neural regulation of muscle tone (that is, the force with which a muscle resists being lengthened). One component of muscle tone derives from the intrinsic elasticity, or stiffness, of the muscles themselves. Muscles have both series and parallel elastic elements, which resist lengthening; thus, a muscle behaves like a spring. In addition to this intrinsic stiffness, however, there is a neural contribution to muscle tone; the stretch reflex also acts to resist lengthening of the muscle. Thus, stretch reflexes enhance the springlike quality of muscles.

Normal muscle tone serves several important functions. First, the tone of muscles helps maintain posture. As we sway back and forth while standing, the muscles resist being stretched, preventing the amount of sway from becoming too large. Second, muscles, like springs, can store energy and release it later. This is particularly important in walking and running. As weight is accepted on a limb, the muscles stretch and store mechanical energy. When the leg pushes off, some of this energy is released and assists the active contraction of muscles. Thus, the elasticity of muscles makes locomotion more efficient: less active contraction of muscles is required to propel the body forward. Finally, the springlike qualities of muscles help to smooth movements. If muscles acted simply like the motors that control a robot's limbs, movements would be jerky, with sudden starts and stops. The elasticity of muscles smooths out these jerks, because the muscle achieves an equilibrium length more gradually, like a spring.

The neural circuits responsible for stretch reflexes provide the higher centers of the nervous system with a mechanism for adjusting muscle tone under different circumstances. For example, during walking, the strength of monosynaptic stretch reflexes is continuously modulated to provide greater stiffness during the period when weight is being accepted on the limb and reduced stiffness when the limb is swinging.[61] Descending pathways regulate stretch reflex sensitivity, both directly, through synaptic connections with alpha and gamma motor neurons, and indirectly, through interneurons.

Because stretch reflexes are controlled by higher brain centers, disorders of muscle tone are frequently associated with lesions of the motor systems, especially those that interfere with descending motor pathways. These may involve both abnormal increases (hypertonus) and abnormal decreases (hypotonus) in tone. The most common form of hypertonus is spasticity, which is characterized by hyperactive tendon jerks and an increase in velocity-dependent resistance to muscle stretch.[62] In a patient with spasticity, slowly applied stretch of a muscle may elicit little resistance, but as the speed of the stretch is progressively increased, resistance to the stretch progressively increases in magnitude (see Figure 6-8). Thus, spasticity is principally a phasic phenomenon. An active reflex contraction occurs only during a rapid stretch; when the muscle is held in a lengthened position, the reflex contraction subsides. In some patients, however, there is also a tonic component to the hypertonus; that is, the reflex contraction continues even after the muscle is no longer being lengthened.[62]

The pathophysiology of spasticity is still unclear. It was long thought that the increased gain of stretch reflexes in spasticity resulted from hyperactivity of the gamma motor neurons. Recent experiments, however, have cast doubt on this

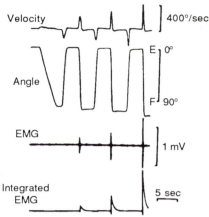

**Figure 6-8.** EMG responses in the quadriceps muscle of a spastic patient to stretches of different velocities. The downward changes in knee angle stretch the quadriceps muscle, causing a phasic reflex contraction of the muscle. Each successive stretch is faster, as indicated by the progressively higher-velocity peaks in the top trace. A normal subject would show little or no EMG activity under these conditions. Note that there is no EMG activity except during the stretches, even when the muscle is fully lengthened. Thus, spasticity is a phasic phenomenon, reflecting an abnormal increase in the velocity-dependent stretch reflex. (From Burke D. Spasticity as an adaptation to pyramidal tract injury. In: Waxman SG, ed. Functional Recovery in Neurological Disease. New York: Raven Press, 1988; 401–423.)

explanation.[63] While gamma overactivity may be present in some cases, it is probable that changes in the direct input to alpha motor neurons and interneurons play a more important role. Thus, the presence of spasticity is clear evidence of disordered descending input to motor neurons.

It would logically seem that spasticity in certain muscles should interfere with rapid movements in which the antagonist muscles are spastic. This assumption has led to attempts to reduce spasticity with drugs, biofeedback, nerve blocks, and physical therapy techniques. Often, however, little functional improvement has been associated with reduction in spasticity.[64,65] The inability of spastic patients to make rapid movements is more likely due to direct impairments of motor unit control than indirect resistance by overactive stretch reflexes,[66,67] though in some patients overactive stretch reflexes may indeed interfere with fast movement.[68] It is therefore important to keep in mind Landau's caution that spasticity is a positive symptom and cannot necessarily explain negative symptoms also associated with upper motor neuron syndromes.[69]

### Long-Loop Stretch Reflexes

It should be emphasized that the monosynaptic reflexes are not the only means for providing active resistance to stretch. When a muscle that is already contracting is stretched, it typically contracts after a short latency (about 20 to 30 msec in arm muscles), a response that can be attributed to monosynaptic spinal circuits. This contraction is associated with a brief burst in the EMG signal from the muscle. Usually, however, the muscle shows later EMG bursts (about 40 to 60 msec); these are often larger than the short-latency burst and provide greater resistance to stretch than the monosynaptic component. Voluntary responses to stretch, that is, those that can be consciously controlled and modulated, take at least 100 to 120 msec to appear in the EMG record. The neural circuits responsible for the medium-latency responses, often referred to as *long-loop* stretch reflexes, have not been definitively identified. Some have argued for a transcortical loop[70]; others contend that polysynaptic spinal circuits can account for these responses.[71]

Whatever their mechanism, long-loop stretch reflexes are functionally important. As Hughlings Jackson argued more than a century ago, there is a continuum between reflex and voluntary control.[72] Short-latency stretch reflexes provide the quickest response to stretch, and they help to compensate for intrinsic irregularities in the initial passive response of a muscle tissue to stretch.[73] The long-loop stretch reflexes fall somewhere in the middle of the continuum. They are under greater adaptive control than monosynaptic stretch reflexes. In contrast to monosynaptic stretch reflexes, which are most automatic and stereotyped, long-loop responses can vary considerably, according to prior expectations and intentions of subjects.[74] Voluntary responses to stretch provide the greatest degree of intentional control. Rather than viewing each of these as a discrete entity, we should perhaps view the entire response to stretch, from monosynaptic to voluntary, as providing a smooth stiffness with progressively greater adaptive control over its strength as the response unfolds.[75]

### Conclusion

Since the end of last century the study of muscle receptors, especially spindles, and their central connections has attracted the attention of succeeding generations of motor physiologists. Though much has been learned, especially about their structure and basic physiology, there is still no clear picture of the roles they play in motor control. Nevertheless, there can be no doubt that proprioceptive input from the limbs is crucial for motor control. Several groups have recently examined motor control in patients with generalized sensory neuropathies that primarily affect the large afferent fibers that transmit proprioceptive input from the muscles and joints. Though there is no disorder in the motor axons of these patients, they have severe impairments in both feedback control and programming of movement.[76–78] Moreover, their movements are poorly coordinated, their balance is poor, and, because they must rely on vision to substitute for absent proprioception, they move slowly and awkwardly. Patients with lesions of the somatosensory areas of the cerebral cortex, where proprioceptive information is processed, have similar problems.[79]

Though the lack of consensus concerning the role of muscle receptors in motor control initially may be discouraging to beginning students, an appreciation for the elegance of their structure and operation, and for their usefulness in clinical diagnosis, should more than compensate. Moreover, we should expect that continuing interest in muscle receptors will soon resolve at least some of the questions about how the brain uses them to control movement.

### References

1. Matthews PBC. Where does Sherrington's "muscular sense" originate? Muscles, joints, corollary discharges? Ann Rev Neurosci. 1982; 5:189–218.
2. Boyd IA, Smith RS. The muscle spindle. In: Dyck PJ, et al., eds. Peripheral Neuropathy, ed 2. Philadelphia: WB Saunders, 1989; 171–202.

3. Matthews PBC. Muscle spindles: Their mesages and their fusimotor supply. In: Brooks VB, ed. Handbook of Physiology, sec. 1, The Nervous System, vol. 2. Motor Control, part 1. Bethesda, Md: American Physiological Society, 1981; 189–228.

4. Matthews PBC. Mammalian Muscle Receptors and Their Central Actions. London: Arnold, 1972.

5. Granit R. Comments on history of motor control. In: Brooks VB, ed. Handbook of Physiology, sec. 1, The Nervous System, vol. 2, Motor Control, part 1. Bethesda, Md: American Physiological Society, 1981; 1–16.

6. Baldissera F, Hultborn H, Illert M. Integration in spinal neuronal systems. In: Brooks VB, ed. Handbook of Physiology, sec. 1, The Nervous System, vol. 2, Motor Control, part 1. Bethesda, Md: American Physiological Society, 1981; 509–595.

7. Crago PE. Golgi tendon organs. In: Dyck PJ, et al., eds. Peripheral Neuropathy, ed 2. Philadelphia: WB Saunders, 1989; 203–209.

8. Hasan Z, Stuart DG. Mammalian muscle receptors. In: Davidoff RA, ed. Handbook of the Spinal Cord, vol. 2&3: Anatomy and physiology. New York: Marcel Dekker, 1984; 559–607.

9. Hulliger M. The mammalian muscle spindle and its central control. Rev Physiol Biochem Pharmacol. 1984; 101:1–110.

10. Loeb GE. The control and responses of mammalian muscle spindles during normally executed motor tasks. Exer Sports Sci Rev 1984; 12:157–204.

11. Matthews PBC. Evolving views on the internal operation and functional role of the muscle spindle. J Physiol (Lond) 1981; 320:1–30.

12. Prochazka A, Hulliger M. Muscle afferent function and its significance for motor control mechansims during voluntary movements in cat, monkey, and man. In: Desmedt JE, ed. Motor Control Mechanisms in Health and Disease. New York: Raven Press, 1983; 93–132.

13. Lloyd DPC, Chang H-T. Afferent fibers in muscle nerves. J Neurophysiol 1948; 11:199–207.

14. Swett JE, Schoultz TW. Mechanical transduction in the Golgi tendon organ: A hypothesis. Arch Ital Biol 1975; 113:374–382.

15. Houk JC, Crago PE, Rymer WZ. Functional properties of the Golgi tendon organs. In: Desmedt JE, ed. Spinal and Supraspinal Mechanisms of Voluntary Motor Control and Locomotion. Basel: S Karger, 1980; 33–43.

16. Rymer WZ, Houk JC, Crago PE. Mechanisms of the clasp-knife reflex studied in an animal model. Exp Brain Res 1979; 37:93–113.

17. Matthews BHC. Nerve endings in mammalian muscle. J Physiol (Lond) 1933; 78:1–53.

18. Cooper S. The responses of primary and secondary endings of muscle spindles with intact motor innervation during applied stretch. Q J Exp Physiol 1961; 46:389–398.

19. Leksell L. The action potential and excitatory effects of the small ventral root fibres to skeletal muscle. Acta Physiol Scand Suppl 1945; 10:1–84.

20. Hunt CC, Kuffler SW. Stretch receptor discharges during muscle contraction. J Physiol (Lond) 1951; 113:298–315.

21. Crowe A, Matthews PBC. The effects of stimulation of static and dynamic fusimotor fibres on the response to stretching of the primary endings of muscle spindles. J Physiol (Lond) 1964; 174:109–131.

22. Boyd IA, Ward J. Motor control of nuclear bag and nuclear chain intrafusal fibres in isolated living muscle spindles from the cat. J Physiol (Lond) 1975; 244:83–112.

23. Kuffler SW, Hunt CC, Quilliam JP. Function of medullated small-nerve fibers in mammalian ventral roots: Efferent muscle spindle innervation. J Neurophysiol 1951; 14:29–54.

24. Kuffler SW, Hunt CC. The mammalian small-nerve fibers: A system for efferent nervous regulation of muscle spindle discharge. Res Publ Assoc Res Nerv Ment Dis 1952; 30:24–47.

25. Granit R. The Basis of Motor Control. London: Academic Press, 1970.

26. Skoglund S. Anatomical and physiological studies of knee joint innervation in the cat. Acta Physiol Scand 1956; 124:1–99.

27. Burgess PR, Clark FJ. Characteristics of knee joint receptors in the cat. J Physiol (Lond) 1969; 203:317–335.

28. Clark FJ, Burgess PR. Slowly adapting receptors in cat knee joint: Can they signal joint angle? J Neurophysiol 1975; 38:1448–1463.

29. Goodwin GM, McCloskey DI, Matthews PBC. The contribution of muscle afferents to kinaesthesia shown by vibration induced illusions of movement and by the effects of paralysing joint afferents. Brain 1972; 95:705–748.

30. Eklund G. Position sense and the state of contraction: The effects of vibration. J Neurol, Neurosurg, Psychiatry 1972; 35:606–611.

31. Roll JP, Vedel JP. Kinaesthetic role of muscle afferents in man, studied by tendon vibration and microneurography. Exp Brain Res 1982; 47:177–190.

32. Ferrell WR, Gandevia SC, McCloskey DI. The role of joint receptors in human kinaesthesia when intramuscular receptors cannot contribute. J Physiol (Lond) 1987; 386:63–71.

33. Liddell EGT, Sherrington CS. Reflexes in response to stretch (myotatic reflexes). Proc R Soc Lond [Biol] 1924; 96:212–242.

34. Lloyd DPC. Conduction and synaptic transmission of the reflex response to stretch in spinal cats. J Neurophysiol 1943; 6:317–326.

35. Lloyd DPC. Integrative pattern of excitation and inhibition in two-neuron reflex arcs. J Neurophysiol 1946; 9:439–444.

36. Eccles JC, Fatt P, Koketsku K. Cholinergic and inhibitory synapses in a pathway from motor-axon collaterals to motoneurones. J Physiol (Lond) 1954; 126:524–562.

37. Eccles JC. The Physiology of Synapses. Berlin: Springer-Verlag, 1964.

38. Lance JW, McLeod JG. A Physiological Approach to Clinical Neurology. London: Butterworths, 1981.

39. Matthews PBC. Evidence that the secondary as well as the primary endings of the muscle spindles may be responsible for the tonic stretch reflex of the decerebrate cat. J Physiol (Lond) 1969; 204:365–393.

40. Kirkwood PA, Sears TA. Monosynaptic excitation of motoneurones from secondary endings of muscle spindles. Nature 1974; 252:243–244.

41. Eccles JC, Lundberg A. Synaptic actions in motoneurones by afferents which may evoke the flexion reflex. Arch Ital Biol 1959; 97:199–221.

42. Lundberg A, Malmgren K. Schomburg ED. Reflex pathways from group II muscle afferents. 1. Distribution and linkage of reflex actions to α-motoneurones. Exp Brain Res 1987; 65:271–281.

43. Lundberg A, Malmgren K, Schomburg ED. Reflex pathways from group II muscle afferents. 2. Functional characteristics of reflex pathways to α-motoneurones. Exp Brain Res 1987; 65:282–293.

44. Lundberg A, Malmgren K, Schomburg ED. Reflex pathways from group II muscle afferents. 3. Secondary spindle afferents and the FRA: A new hypothesis. Exp Brain Res 1987; 65:282–293.

45. Lundberg A, Malmgren K, Schomburg ED. Convergence from Ib, cutaneous and joint afferents in reflex pathways to motoneurones. Brain Res 1975; 87:81–84.

46. Houk JC, Henneman E. Responses of Golgi tendon organs to active contractions of the soleus muscle of the cat. J Neurophysiol 1967; 30:466–481.

47. Sherrington CS. The Integrative Action of the Nervous System. New Haven, Conn: Yale University Press, 1947.

48. Marsden CD, Merton PA, Morton HB. Human postural responses. Brain 1981; 104:513–534.

49. Cordo PJ, Nashner LM. Properties of postural adjustments associated with rapid arm movements. J Neurophysiol 1982; 47:287–302.

50. Forssberg H. Spinal locomotor functions and descending control. In: Sjolund B, Bjorklund A, eds. Brain Stem Control of Spinal Mechanisms. New York: Elsevier, 1982; 253–271.

51. Grillner S, Wallen P. Central pattern generators for movement, with special reference to vertebrates. Ann Rev Neurosci 1985; 8:233–261.

52. Merton PA. Speculations on the servo-control of movement. In: Wolstenholme GEW, ed. The Spinal Cord. London: Churchill Livingstone, 1953; 247–255.

53. Merton PA. How we control the contraction of our muscles. Sci Am 1972; 226:30–37.

54. Vallbo ÅB. Discharge patterns in human muscle spindle afferents during isometric voluntary contractions. Acta Physiol Scand 1970; 80:552–566.

55. Granit R. The functional role of muscle spindles–facts and hypotheses. Brain 1975; 98:531–556.

56. Stein RB. The peripheral control of movement. Physiol Rev 1975; 54:215–243.

57. Loeb GE, Hoffer JA. Muscle spindle function during normal and perturbed locomotion in cats. In: Taylor A, Prochazka A, eds. Muscle Receptors and Movement. London: MacMillan, 1981; 219–228.

58. Prochazka A, Wand P. Independence of fusimotor and skeletomotor systems during voluntary movement. In: Taylor A, Prochazka A, eds. Muscle Receptors and Movement. London: MacMillan, 1981; 229–243.

59. Prochazka A, Hulliger M, Zangger P, et al. 'Fusimotor set': New evidence for α-independent control of γ-motoneurones during movement in the awake cat. Brain Res 1985; 339:136–140.

60. Prochazka A, Hulliger M, Trend P, et al. Dynamic and static fusimotor set in various behavioural contexts. In: Hnik P, Soukop T, Vejsada R, et al., eds. Mechanoreceptors. New York: Plenum, 1988; 417–430.

61. Stein RB, Capaday C. The modulation of human reflexes during functional motor tasks. Trends Neurosci 1988; 11:328–332.

62. Burke D. Spasticity as an adaptation to pyramidal tract injury. In: Waxman SG, ed. Functional Recovery in Neurological Disease. New York: Raven Press, 1988; 401–423.

63. Burke D. A reassessment of the muscle spindle contribution to muscle tone in normal and spastic man. In: Feldman RG, Young RR, Koella WP, eds. Spasticity: Disordered Motor Control. Miami, Fla: Symposia Specialists, 1980; 261–278.

64. McLellan DM. Co-contraction and stretch reflexes in spasticity during treatment with baclofen. J Neurol, Neurosurg, Psychiatry 1977; 50:30–38.

65. Neilson PD, McCaughey J. Self-regulation of spasm and spasticity in cerebral palsy. J Neurol, Neurosurg, Psychiatry 1982; 45:320–330.

66. Sahrmann SA, Norton BJ. The relationship of voluntary movement to spasticity in the upper motor neuron syndrome. Ann Neurol 1977; 2:460–465.

67. Tang A, Rymer WZ. Abnormal force-EMG relations in paretic limbs of hemiparetic human subjects. J Neurol, Neurosurg, Psychiatry 1981; 44:690–698.

68. Corcos DM, Gottlieb GL, Penn RD, et al. Movement deficits caused by hyperexcitable stretch reflexes in spastic humans. Brain 1986; 109:1043–1058.

69. Landau WM. Spasticity: The fable of a neurological demon and the emperor's new therapy. Arch Neurol 1974; 31:217–219.

70. Marsden CD, Merton PA, Morton HB. Stretch reflexes and servo actions in a variety of human muscles. J Physiol (Lond) 1976; 259:531–560.

71. Ghez C, Shinoda Y. Spinal mechanisms of the functional stretch reflex. Brain Res 1978; 32:55–68.

72. Walshe FMR. Contributions of John Hughlings Jackson to neurology: A brief introduction to his teachings. Arch Neurol 1961; 5:119–131.

73. Nichols TR, Houk JC. Improvement in linearity and regulation of stiffness that results from actions of stretch reflex. J Neurophysiol 1976; 39:119–142.

74. Houk JC. Participation of reflex mechanisms and reaction-time processes in the compensatory adjustments to mechanical disturbances. In: Desmedt JE, ed. Cerebral Motor Control in Man: Long Loop Mechanisms. Basel: S Karger, 1978; 193–215.

75. Brooks VB. The Neural Basis of Motor Control. New York: Oxford University Press; 1986.

76. Rothwell JL, Traub MM, Day BL, et al. Manual motor performance in a deafferented man. Brain 1982; 105:515–542.

77. Sanes JN, Mauritz K-H, Dalakas, MC, et al. Motor control in humans with large-fiber sensory neuropathy. Hum Neurobiol 1985; 4:101–114.

78. Ghez C, Gordon J, Ghilardi MF, et al. Roles of proprioceptive input in the programming of arm trajectories. Cold Spring Harbor, Symp Quant Biol 1990; 55:837–847.

79. Jeannerod M. The Neural and Behavioral Organization of Goal-Directed Movements. Oxford: Clarendon Press, 1988.

# Chapter 7

# Cardiopulmonary Physiology

JONATHAN R. MOLDOVER
JOEL STEIN

Efficient and coordinated functioning of the cardiopulmonary system is essential for supplying oxygen to the tissues of the body and removing carbon dioxide. The central organs (heart and lungs) and the distribution system (blood vessels) must quickly respond to the varying metabolic demands of each of the body's tissues. In this chapter we review the structure and function of each of the system's components and describe the system's regulation at rest and during exercise, and its adaptation to training.

## Heart

### Anatomy

The human heart consists of four chambers, two atria and two ventricles, connected in series. Blood is circulated from the left ventricle through the systemic circulation, arterial to venous, then to the right atrium and ventricle and through the pulmonary circulation to return to the left atrium and then the left ventricle, completing its circuit. Unidirectional flow of blood from and to the heart is made possible through a system of valves. Atrial contraction increases the diastolic filling of the ventricles, thus increasing ventricular stroke volume, contributing 15% to 20% of the cardiac output.[1] The atrial contribution varies with heart rate, being greater at higher heart rates. The atrial contribution also increases in disease states when there is decreased diastolic compliance of the ventricle.

The heart's special metabolic and functional requirements have led to the development of specialized muscular and electrical conduction apparatuses. Cardiac muscle fibers are histologically and functionally distinct from both the skeletal muscle and smooth muscle fibers found elsewhere in the body. Their branched connections allow for propagation of electrical depolarizations, and cardiac muscle fibers are uniquely able to sustain, lifelong, the required frequent contractions of the heart.

The electrical system of the heart is comprised of specially adapted muscle cells that provide careful coordination of the heart's muscle activity. Electrical impulses normally originate in the sinoatrial (SA) node, located in the right atrium. The cells comprising the SA node have the shortest period between spontaneous depolarizations and act as the heart's natural pacemaker. The electrical impulse generated in the SA node travels through three atrial bundles (internodal pathways) to the atrioventricular (AV) node, located in the lower part of the intraatrial septum. The electrical impulse is then transmitted to the bundle of His, which extends into the ventricular septum where it divides into two main branches, the right and left bundles. The left bundle further divides into an anterior and a posterior fascicle. Small branches of these major divisions carry the impulses to the myocytes.

A close-fitting fibrous sac, the pericardium, surrounds the heart. It provides some physical protection for the heart and contains a small amount of fluid that provides lubrication for the constantly moving heart. Its resistance to distention prevents rapid changes in cardiac chamber size, though it gradually enlarges to accommodate cardiac dilatation or large pericardial effusions. Surgical removal or congenital absence of the pericardium generally is tolerated well.

### Coronary Circulation

The coronary vasculature is of paramount importance; disease of the coronary arteries remains the leading cause of death in the United States. The major epicardial arteries originate in the cusps of Valsalva, at the root of the aorta. The two vessels are the left main coronary artery, and the right coronary artery. The left main artery promptly bifurcates into the left circumflex artery and the left anterior descending artery. The right coronary artery typically supplies the majority of the right ventricular wall as well as the inferior left ventricular wall. The left circumflex artery supplies the lateral wall of the left ventricle. The left anterior descending artery supplies the anterior wall and apex of the left ventricle, as well as most of the interventricular septum. In approximately 60% of persons the right coronary artery gives off the posterior descending artery, which supplies a portion of the interventricular septum. Such persons are said to have *right-dominant* coronary circulation. In 30%, the posterior descending artery is supplied equally by the right and left circumflex arteries, and in the remaining 10%, the posterior descending artery is given off by the left circumflex artery *left-dominant* circulation; (Figure 7-1).

The venous drainage of the heart consists primarily of the coronary sinus, which runs in the atrioventricular groove. The coronary sinus, a continuation of the great cardiac vein, empties into the right atrium, near the inferior vena cava.

The microcirculation of the heart has been receiving increasing attention, particularly as a cause of the syndrome of microvascular angina.[2] Persons with microvascular angina have objective evidence of ischemia in the absence of angiographically determined stenosis of the epicardial blood ves-

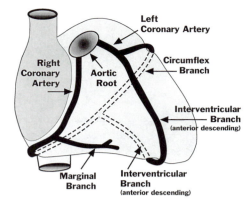

**Figure 7-1.** The coronary arteries of the heart.

sels. Impaired vasodilator reserve of both the coronary and systemic arterial beds has been found in these persons.[3]

### Myocardial Metabolism

The heart is one of the most metabolically active organs in the body. Oxygen extraction (measured by comparing aortic oxygen content with coronary sinus oxygen content) is approximately 65% to 70%, as compared with 36% for the brain, and an average of 26% for the entire body.[4] The heart is versatile in its use of substrates for energy metabolism, and uses glucose, lactate, ketones, or fatty acids, as available. Normally, carbohydrates contribute approximately 35% to 40% and the remainder is primarily fatty acids.[5] When adequate oxygen is available cardiac energy is produced through oxidative metabolism; it shifts to anaerobic metabolism when necessary.

The high oxygen extraction in the resting heart precludes significant increases in extraction with increasing metabolic demand. Therefore, increases in metabolic demand must be met by increased coronary artery flow. Regulation of the coronary circulation is locally controlled. Many substances produce dilatation, including acetylcholine, substance P, serotonin, thrombin, histamine, bradykinin, prostaglandins, and adenosine compounds.[6] Prostacyclin, with a half-life of approximately 3 minutes, exerts a relaxing effect on vascular smooth muscle in addition to inhibiting aggregation of platelets.[7] An important common pathway for vasodilatation of both peripheral and cardiac blood vessels is mediated by the endothelium-derived relaxing factor (which has been shown to be nitric oxide[6,8,9]) which is produced from an L-arginine precursor and has a half-life of about 3 to 6 seconds. Its effects are mediated intracellularly by cyclic guanosine 3′,5′-monophosphate. In addition to the chemical agents that induce its release, flow-induced shear stresses within the vessels stimulate release of endothelium-derived relaxing factor. A potent endothelium-derived vasoconstricting factor is postulated, possibly endothelin, a peptide produced by endothelial cells.[6,10]

Coronary perfusion takes place primarily during diastole, as during systole the increased intramural tension within the myocardial wall prevents, and may even transiently reverse, forward blood flow in the coronary vessels.[11] During early diastole, myocardial wall tension is as its lowest while the perfusion pressure within the aortic root remains high, owing to the elasticity of the aorta, permitting coronary perfusion (Figure 7-2).

### The Frank-Starling Mechanism

Cardiac output increases in response to increased venous return; this relationship is called the *Frank-Starling mechanism*. It derives from the relationship between myocardial fiber length and the force generated with each contraction. At rest there is

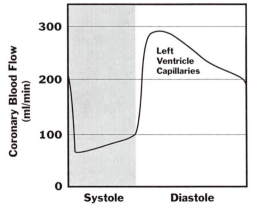

**Figure 7-2.** The relationship of coronary blood flow to the contraction of the left ventricle. (Adapted from Guyton AC. Textbook of Medical Physiology, ed 7. Philadelphia: WB Saunders, 1986.)

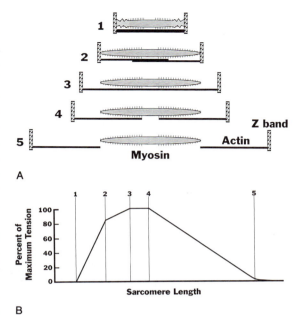

**Figure 7-3.** (*A*) The relationship between the myosin and actin filaments during stretching of myocardial fibers, demonstrating that the number of available cross-bridges increases to a point but then decreases if the fiber is stretched too far. (*B*) The relationship between fiber length and contractile force.

overlap between the thin actin fibers of the myocardium, reducing the area available for forming cross-bridges with thick myosin fibers. As the sarcomere is stretched, the overlap between the thin fibers is eliminated, and a larger area is available for interaction with the myosin fibers; this allows increased contractile force to be generated. As the sarcomeres are stretched farther, the 'a' band of each actin fiber is no longer available to form cross-bridges with the myosin fibers, and the force generated declines (Figure 7-3A). The relationship between fiber length and contractile force is represented graphically in Figure 7-3B.

The relationship between end-diastolic volume and ventricular stroke volume is analogous to (and physiologically based upon) the relationship between myocardial fiber length and contractile force. Accordingly, increasing end-diastolic volume causes an increase in ventricular stroke work. The relationship between end-diastolic volume and stroke output may be modified by a decrease in the contractile function of the heart, as in a dilated cardiomyopathy (Figure 7-4).

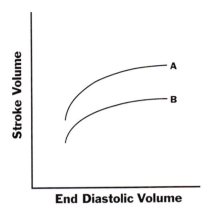

**Figure 7-4.** The relationship between end-diastolic volume and stroke volume in (A) a normal heart and (B) dilated cardiomyopathy.

The Frank-Starling mechanism is an important homeostatic mechanism, as it provides a means of compensating for temporary imbalances in the circulation. For example, if the right ventricle receives increased venous return, it increases its output without a change in heart rate, owing to the increased stroke volume ejected. When the left side of the heart is presented with this same fluid challenge, it too experiences greater diastolic filling, and owing to the Frank-Starling mechanism, a greater stroke volume is ejected.

### Cardiac Response to Exercise

#### Oxygen Consumption

In reviewing the cardiac response to exercise it is necessary first to understand the concepts of oxygen consumption ($V_{O_2}$) and maximal oxygen consumption ($V_{O_2}$max), as the intensity of exercise is usually expressed in these terms. $V_{O_2}$ is calculated by measuring from the expired air at the mouth, thus representing whole body oxygen consumption. During exercise there is increased consumption, primarily owing to metabolism of the working skeletal muscle. For any given constant submaximal workload the $V_{O_2}$ increases over the first 3 to 6 minutes and then reaches a steady-state level. With increasing work intensity the steady-state level increases until a point is reached where increasing the work further does not produce any increase in $V_{O_2}$. If the various steady-state levels are plotted against the workloads, the result is a straight line with a short horizontal plateau at the top, representing the $V_{O_2}$max (Figure 7-5). The slope of this line represents the mechanical efficiency of the exercise being performed. Activities that require muscle contraction to stabilize the trunk (e.g., upper extremity ergometry) or activities performed by persons with spastic cocontraction have steeper slopes for the linear increase in oxygen consumption with increasing workload, representing a reduction in mechanical efficiency.[12,13] When plotting various cardiac and pulmonary parameters against increasing work intensity the independent variable is usually expressed as the percentage of the subject's $V_{O_2}$max, though the absolute $V_{O_2}$ (e.g., liters of oxygen per minute or milliliters per kilogram body weight per minute) or a mechanical measure of work intensity (e.g., watts or kiloponds) is sometimes used.

#### Cardiac Output

The cardiac output (expressed in liters of blood per minute) is a function of the heart rate and the stroke volume. The relationship between the cardiac output and $V_{O_2}$ is linear, at least for nonathletes (Figure 7-6).[14] As we get older the line shifts downward, but there is no significant change in linearity or slope. The relationship of cardiac output to $V_{O_2}$ during submaximal work performed in the upright position is parallel to but below the line of work performed when the subject lies supine. Maximum cardiac output in the supine position is less than during upright exercise, as is the $V_{O_2}$max.[15] The increasing cardiac output with increasing $V_{O_2}$ in the supine position is produced by an increase in heart rate while the stroke volume remains constant. During "upright exercise" both heart rate and stroke volume increase. In the pres-

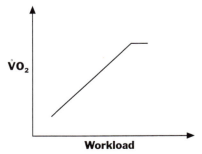

**Figure 7-5.** The relationship between steady-state oxygen consumption and workload.

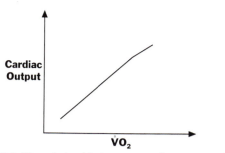

**Figure 7-6.** The relationship between cardiac output and oxygen consumption.

ence of a fixed (paced) heart rate the cardiac output increases by means of increasing stroke volume.[16]

*Heart Rate*

The relationship between heart rate and $V_{O_2}$ is also linear (Figure 7-7). Maximal heart rate is a function of age, whereas the slope of the line is determined by the level of physical conditioning. The increase in heart rate with increasing $V_{O_2}$ is regulated through the autonomic nervous system (vagal tone versus sympathetic beta-adrenergic tone) and by circulating catecholamines.[16–18]

*Stroke Volume*

There is greater variability in the stroke volume response to exercise than in the response of cardiac output or heart rate. For example, during increasing work in the supine position the stroke volume may increase, decrease, or stay the same. If there

is a change from the resting level, the stroke volume levels out when the $V_{O_2}$ reaches 40% of $V_{O_2}$max. Resting stroke volume in the upright position is approximately 60% of that while supine, and with increasing work the stroke volume increases by 50%, but never to the supine value (Figure 7-8). Older persons demonstrate a smaller increase in stroke volume with exercise in either position.[15,19]

*Myocardial Oxygen Consumption*

Though the preceding cardiac parameters form the foundation of most discussions of the cardiac response to exercise, it is myocardial $V_{O_2}$ that has the greatest implications for clinical decision making in rehabilitation medicine. Patients with atherosclerotic coronary artery disease develop problems (angina pectoris, arrhythmias, myocardial infarction, sudden death) when the myocardial $V_{O_2}$ required by an activity exceeds the maximum oxygen supply the coronary circulation can deliver. The clinician needs to understand the factors that influence myocardial $V_{O_2}$, in order to perform appropriate patient evaluation and program modification.

*Indirect Measurement of Myocardial Oxygen Consumption*

It is not practicable to measure myocardial $V_{O_2}$ directly in most clinical settings, so we must utilize more easily measurable parameters that correlate with it—heart rate, blood pressure, ventricular wall tension, rate of fiber shortening, venous return, and systemic arterial pressure the heart must pump against (afterload). It has been shown empirically that only the heart rate and systolic blood

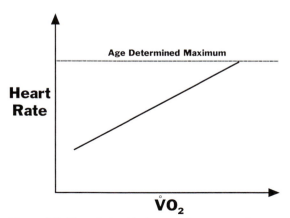

**Figure 7-7.** The relationship between heart rate and oxygen consumption.

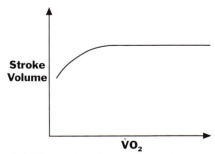

**Figure 7-8.** The relationship between stroke volume and oxygen consumption.

pressure need be measured to obtain a reasonable assessment of myocardial $Vo_2$.[20] The rate-pressure product (RPP) is calculated by multiplying the heart rate by the systolic blood pressure and dividing by 100; this correlates well ($r = .85-.90$) with the directly measured myocardial $Vo_2$ under a variety of clinical situations.[20-22] The RPP increases in a linear fashion with $Vo_2$ until the anginal threshold is reached (Figure 7-9). The anginal threshold is the point where there is evidence of an imbalance between myocardial $Vo_2$ and the available oxygen supply, as manifested by anginal pain or electrocardiographic abnormality.

### The Effect of Isometric Muscle Contraction

The cardiovascular response to isometric exercise has been well-described by Donald.[23] Contractions as small as 10% of the maximal voluntary con-

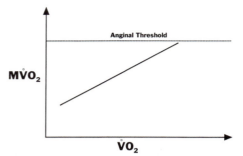

**Figure 7-9.** The relationship between myocardial oxygen consumption and total body oxygen consumption.

traction produce an increase in heart rate that leads to an increase in systolic blood pressure, thus increasing the myocardial $Vo_2$ out of proportion to the physical work being performed (Figure 7-10). During sustained contractions that are less than 15% of maximum, a steady-state cardiac response is reached, whereas with stronger contractions the

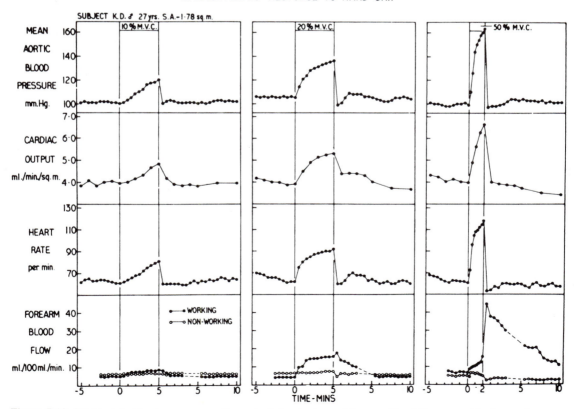

**Figure 7-10.** Increases in blood pressure, cardiac output, heart rate, and forearm blood flow caused by isometric contractions are proportional to the relative intensity of the contraction.

RPP continues to rise until fatigue limits the duration of the contraction. This response is proportional to the maximal voluntary contraction for the muscle in use, regardless of the mass of that muscle, and is thought to be a cardioaccelerating reflex initiated by potassium ion flux in the contracting muscle. Stroke volume and total peripheral resistance do not change. It is important to note that the increase in myocardial $V_{O_2}$ caused by the isometric contraction is superimposed on the metabolic response to any isotonic work being performed at the same time (Figure 7-11). Thus, a strong hand grip on a cane or walker may create a myocardial oxygen demand out of proportion to the metabolic demands of the slow ambulation of a rehabilitation patient.

*The Effect of Upper Extremity Exercise*

Both the heart rate and the systolic blood pressure are higher for any given submaximal $V_{O_2}$ if the work is performed with the upper extremities instead of the lower ones (Figure 7-12).[24,12] The difference between upper and lower extremity work becomes more significant as the workload increases.[12] The values during combined upper and lower extremity exercise are the same as for lower extremity work alone at each submaximal $V_{O_2}$.[24]

*The Effect of Posture*

The effect of upright versus supine posture on the myocardial oxygen consumption (as reflected by the RPP) depends on the relative workload. With lower-intensity exercise the RPP is higher for supine than for upright exercise at the same $V_{O_2}$.[12,25] At higher intensities the situation is reversed: then upright exercise produces the higher RPP (Figure 7-13).[24] This distinction is important in rehabilitation when prescribing supine mat exercises for patients who have coexisting coronary artery dis-

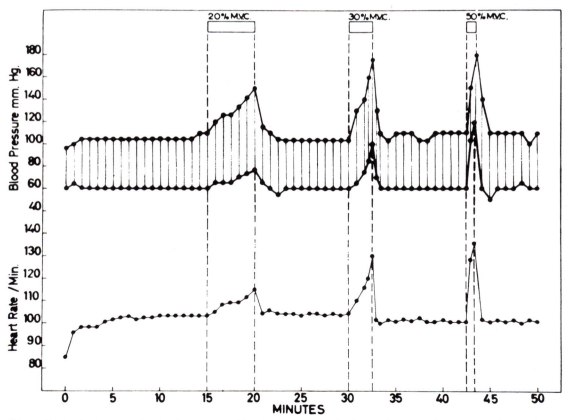

**Figure 7-11.** The increases in blood pressure and heart rate generated by isometric contractions are superimposed on the increases from aerobic work.

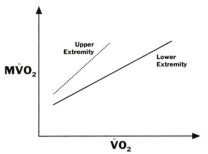

**Figure 7-12.** A comparison of the relationship between myocardial oxygen demand and total body oxygen consumption for upper and lower extremity work.

ease. Such supine exercises may create higher myocardial oxygen demand than ambulation or other upright activities, especially if the exercise contains an isometric component (e.g., bridging).

*The Effect of Bed Rest*

Though short periods of bed rest are commonly prescribed for acutely ill and convalescent patients, prolonged bed rest has a deleterious effect on the cardiac response to exercise. Saltin subjected five volunteers to 20 days' strict bed rest and measured various metabolic parameters as well as the cardiopulmonary response to exercise.[26] He found that the average $VO_2max$ decreased 27%; the maximum heart rate remained constant, whereas the maximum stroke volume and cardiac output decreased. At a submaximal workload the cardiac output and stroke volume were lower, and the heart rate higher, after the period of bed rest. There was no significant change in mean arterial pressure at rest or during submaximal exercise following bed rest.

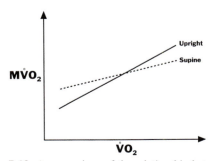

**Figure 7-13.** A comparison of the relationship between myocardial oxygen demand and total body oxygen consumption for upright and supine work.

*The Effect of Training*

Aerobic training programs modify the cardiac response to exercise. Such programs involve exercising three times a week for approximately 30 minutes utilizing large muscle groups in a repetitive fashion, as by running, jogging, swimming, cycling, "aerobic" calisthenics, rowing, or circuit training with exercise intense enough to produce a heart rate of 60% to 70% of the maximum heart rate. The changes in the cardiac response to exercise described in the following sections should be evident within 4 to 6 weeks after the onset of training.

The change in the cardiac response to exercise is most evident when the muscles undergoing training are the same muscles used to generate the cardiac response in testing before and after the training. Thus, if the subject trains with a walking or running program, the cardiac response measured on a treadmill will change significantly, whereas the cardiac response to armcrank ergometry will change little, if at all.

Another key concept for studying the changes in the cardiac response to exercise is that the changes may be different during rest, submaximal exercise, and maximal exercise. Differences during submaximal work are the ones most relevant to rehabilitation.

*The Effect of Training on Oxygen Consumption*

With aerobic training $VO_2max$ is increased but the $VO_2$ at rest and during any given submaximal load remains unchanged (Figure 7-14). Although most people, especially those in rehabilitation programs, never exercise to their $VO_2max$, the increase is still relevant, because each submaximal activity represents a smaller percentage of the $VO_2max$ after training, thus generating a smaller increase in the heart rate, systolic blood pressure, and myocardial $VO_2$.

*The Effect of Training on Cardiac Output*

The maximal cardiac output increases with training, but there is no change in the cardiac output at rest or at any submaximal workload (Figure 7-15). There is a difference, however, in how the

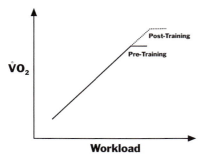

Figure 7-14. The effect of training on the relationship between oxygen consumption and workload.

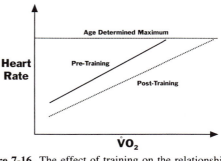

Figure 7-16. The effect of training on the relationship between heart rate and oxygen consumption.

submaximal cardiac output is generated and distributed. (The changes in the heart rate and stroke volume that determine the cardiac output will be described presently.) The distribution of the peripheral blood flow is different in trained subjects. For example, less blood is shunted to the working muscles because they are able to extract and use oxygen more efficiently. This change in distribution produces less of an increase in the total peripheral resistance, and thus less afterload for the heart and a lower systolic blood pressure response to exercise.

### The Effect of Training on Heart Rate

Training causes the heart rate to be lower at rest and during any submaximal workload, but the maximal heart rate does not change (Figure 7-16). This bradycardia of training is the most noticeable and clinically important change that occurs with aerobic conditioning and it is primarily due to an increase in vagal tone combined with a decrease in sympathetic tone and lower levels of circulating catecholamines.[27,28] As noted previously, the change in heart rate with exercise is seen only during exercise with the trained muscles. The muscle changes of endurance training are discussed in Chapter 15.

### The Effect of Training on Stroke Volume

After an aerobic training program the stroke volume is usually greater at rest during submaximal and maximal exercise (Figure 7-17). The increase in stroke volume is reciprocal to the decrease in heart rate, maintaining a stable submaximal cardiac output, and is due to both a longer diastolic filling period resulting from the slower heart rate and increased venous return caused by the exercise-induced increase in blood volume.

### The Effect of Training on Myocardial Oxygen Consumption

The myocardial $VO_2$ is lower at rest and during submaximal exercise following an effective training program, but the angina threshold is unchanged (Figure 7-18). The decrease in myocardial

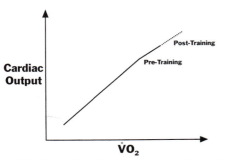

Figure 7-15. The effect of training on the relationship between cardiac output and oxygen consumption.

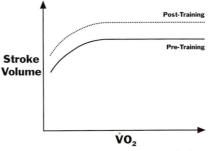

Figure 7-17. The effect of training on the relationship between stroke volume and oxygen consumption.

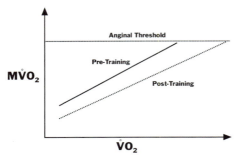

**Figure 7-18.** The effect of training on the relationship between myocardial oxygen demand and total body oxygen consumption.

$V_{O_2}$ is due primarily to the lower heart rate. The systolic blood pressure response to exercise may also be lower, owing to a decrease in peripheral vascular resistance created by less shunting of blood from visceral capillary beds to supply working muscle. The reduced myocardial $V_{O_2}$ at submaximal loads explains the effectiveness of properly designed cardiac rehabilitation programs in increasing the work capacity of persons with coronary artery disease even though exercise does not raise the angina threshold. The fact that the angina threshold does not change suggests that aerobic training does not increase perfusion through the diseased coronary bed. This finding is consistent with the lack of convincing evidence that collateral circulation develops in the coronary beds of humans who follow an exercise program.

## The Peripheral Circulation

### Anatomy

The blood vessels constitute the "plumbing" of the body, carrying blood to and from all organ systems. Arteries by definition carry blood from the heart to the target organ system, and veins carry blood back to the heart. Arteries contain blood rich with oxygen (with the prominent exception of the pulmonary arteries). Veins carry blood that contains less oxygen and more carbon dioxide, though again the exception is the pulmonary veins. There are several *portal* systems in the body, in which a portion of the blood supply to an organ derives from venous blood collected from a capillary bed, including the portal systems supplying the liver and the anterior pituitary gland.

Arteries are muscular, thick-walled vessels that are exposed to high pressure. The arteries originate from the aorta and form a branching, and to some degree anastamosing, network. Distally the smaller arteries branch farther to form arterioles, which give rise to metaarterioles or directly to capillaries. Gas, nutrient, and waste exchange with the tissues occurs through the capillary walls. The effluent from the capillaries goes to the venules, which in turn give rise to the smaller veins, later to join to form the large veins, and then the superior and inferior vena cava.

The wall of the aorta contains a large amount of elastic tissue and a relatively small amount of muscle tissue. Farther down the arterial system this ratio is reversed: there, arterioles contain a high concentration of smooth muscle cells and a small amount of elastic tissue. The elastic aorta serves to buffer and damp the pulsatile pressure of the cardiac output. During systole the aorta expands to accommodate rapid ejection of blood. During diastole, when cardiac output has ceased, the aorta maintains perfusion pressure by contracting by elastic recoil (Figure 7-19). If the arterial system were completely inelastic the diastolic blood pressure would fall to zero, and, conversely, if the aorta were infinitely distensible blood pressure would remain at a constant level.

The veins have thinner walls than the arteries, though they are still muscular, and they contain valves to assist in the unidirectional flow of blood. The veins freely form anastomoses and serve as a capacitance reservoir for the circulation. They can contract or expand the volume of blood contained within them to adjust for volume loss or overload. The veins constitute the primary reservoir of blood for the body, normally containing 67% of the intravascular volume*; the arteries contain only 11% and the capillaries 5%. The remaining 17% is contained in the heart (5%) and the pulmonary circulation (12%).

The valves in the veins allow skeletal muscle to function as an auxiliary pump, particularly in the lower extremities. The contraction of the calf muscles causes compression of the veins in the lower leg, forcing the blood toward the heart. The

---

*Values are extrapolated from animal studies.[30]

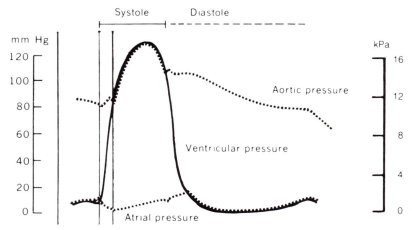

**Figure 7-19.** The maintenance of aortic pressure during diastole is the result of the elasticity of the aortic wall (From Åstrand P-O, Rodahl K. Textbook of Work Physiology, ed 3. New York: McGraw-Hill, 1986, with permission.)

veins then passively fill during relaxation of the muscles, completing the cycle and preventing the large increases in hydrostatic pressure that would otherwise occur in the legs.[29]

The cross-sectional area of the circulation increases gradually from the aorta to the arterioles, with a large increase at the level of the capillaries. The capillaries, owing to their immense number, have a cross-sectional area on the order of 60 times that of the arterioles, and 1000 times that of the aorta.[4] Autoregulation of the microcirculation limits the effective cross-sectional area of the small blood vessels at any given time, but the effective cross-sectional area remains quite large in comparison with that of the larger blood vessels. Given an essentially closed system in which total capillary blood flow must equal the aortic blood flow, it follows that the velocity of the blood in the capillaries is much slower than in the aorta, allowing more time for exchange of gases and nutrients in the capillary beds.

The arterioles contain a circular band of smooth muscle that enables them to vary the resistance to blood flow within their lumens. The arterioles contribute the bulk of the resistance to blood flow and also function to damp the pulsatile pressure of arterial blood flow, providing the capillaries with a more continuous supply. The ability of the arterioles to vary the resistance they provide allows for regulation of blood flow and redistribution of

blood flow to reflect changing metabolic needs (e.g., exercise).

Laplaces's law, which describes how an acceptable blood vessel wall stress is maintained throughout the circulation, states that wall tension is proportional to the transluminal pressure and to the radius of the vessel. Calculation of wall stress takes into account wall thickness, with stress being inversely proportional to the thickness of the wall. The full equation can be stated thus:

$$S = Pr/v$$

where S is wall stress, P is transluminal pressure, r is radius, and v is vessel thickness. As vessels become smaller the wall tension falls in proportion to the vessel radius. This permits a decrease in vessel wall thickness in smaller vessels without causing an increase in wall stress.

Poiseuille's law describes the laminar flow of an idealized fluid in a smooth round tube:

$$Q = \frac{\pi(P_1 - P_2)r_4}{8v1}$$

where Q is the rate of flow, r is the radius of the tube, $v$ is the viscosity of the fluid, $P_1$ and $P_2$ are the pressures at the ends of the tube, and 1 is the length of the tube. This equation can be used to approximate blood flow through a vessel. From the preceding equation it is apparent that blood flow varies with the fourth power of the radius of the blood vessel. Thus, even small decreases in the radius of a vessel from atherosclerosis have a significant effect on its maximal flow. Resistance is defined as the ratio of the change in pressure to flow, and is proportional both to the length of the vessel and to the inverse of the radius to the fourth power.

Turbulence, another important consideration, can be predicted by Reynold's number:

$$N_r = \frac{pDv}{v}$$

where $N_r$ is Reynold's number, p is density, D is diameter, v is mean velocity, and $v$ is viscosity. Turbulence becomes more likely as $N_r$ increases. $N_r$ varies proportionally with the diameter of a vessel, and inversely with the viscosity of the blood. Atherosclerosis has been shown to have a predilection for areas of high turbulence such as ostia and bifurcations.[31]

The lymphatics are small, thin-walled vessels that carry lymphatic fluid from the periphery to the central circulation. They provide drainage for the interstitial and extravascular spaces. Lymphatics also contain valves to ensure unidirectional flow, and they operate at very low pressures. The lymphatics contain some smooth muscle and also utilize transient increases in local tissue pressure (as during muscle contraction) to pump lymphatic fluid. Lymph passes through one or more lymph nodes before being collected in the larger lymphatics and returning to the circulation via the thoracic duct or the right lymphatic duct.

## The Circulation at Rest

### Tissue Perfusion

The hydrostatic forces present in the capillaries derive from the mean arterial blood pressure, attenuated by the arterioles, which function as the main resistive component of the circulation. The resulting hydrostatic pressure within the capillary ranges from 32 mm Hg at the arteriolar end of the capillary to 15 mm Hg at the venular end. This varies with tissue location: dependent tissues have higher hydrostatic pressure. The counterpressure exerted by the tissue interstitial fluid is small (close to, or perhaps even slightly less than, zero).

Filtration of plasma across the capillary membranes that would result from hydrostatic pressure would cause unacceptable amounts of fluid transudation were it not for the counterpressure or pull exerted by osmotically active substances in the blood. Osmotically active substances are molecules too large to be filtered across the capillary wall (molecular weight approximately 60 kd), the most important being albumin. The osmotic pressure exerted by albumin is greater than would be expected from its concentration and size. This discrepancy can be accounted for by albumin's negative charge, which essentially keeps cations (primarily sodium) in the intravascular compartment, thus increasing the osmotic force generated.

The relationship between the hydrostatic forces and the opposing osmotic forces can be expressed in relation to fluid movement across the capillary walls. Starling's hypothesis can be stated as follows:

$$F = k[Pc + Oi - (Pi + Op)]$$

where F is fluid movement, K the filtration constant of the capillary membrane, Pc the capillary hydrostatic pressure, Oi the osmotic pressure, and Op the osmotic pressure of the capillary fluid.[32] Fluid moves from the capillary to the interstitium when F is positive and from the interstitium to the capillary when F is negative. Only a small fraction (0.02%) of the fluid that passes through the capillaries is filtered. Of this amount, 85% is reabsorbed by the capillaries and venules and the remainder forms the lymphatic fluid.[5]

### Control of The Circulation

Blood flow to different organ systems is based both on the size of the organ and its metabolic requirements (Table 7-1); the flow to each organ is regulated by the size of its supplying arteries and by neural, humoral, and local mechanisms. The blood vessels are supplied by autonomic adrenergic—and in some cases cholinergic—fibers. This innervation allows for centrally directed rapid response to changing conditions, such as autonomic sympathetic response seen when a person is confronting danger. Sympathetic adrenergic fibers release norepinephrine at the resistive vessels (arterioles), exerting influence over blood pressure at that site. Sympathetic fibers also provide stimulation to the capacitance vessels (primarily but

**Table 7-1.** Distribution of Blood Flow to Organs at Rest

| Organ | Percentage | Volume (ml/min) | Volume (ml/min/100 g) |
|---|---|---|---|
| Brain | 14 | 700 | 50 |
| Heart | 4 | 200 | 70 |
| Bronchi | 2 | 100 | 25 |
| Kidneys | 22 | 1100 | 300 |
| Muscle (inactive) | 15 | 750 | 4 |
| Liver | 27 | 1350 | 95 |
| Bone | 5 | 250 | 3 |
| Skin (cool weather) | 6 | 300 | 3 |
| Thyroid gland | 1 | 50 | 160 |
| Adrenal glands | 0.5 | 25 | 300 |
| Other tissues | 3.5 | 175 | 18 |
| Total | 100 | 5000 | |

From Guyton AC. Textbook of Medical Physiology. ed 7. Philadelphia: WB Saunders, 1986, with permission.

not exclusively venules) to increase venous return as needed. The β-adrenergic receptors are also present at the arteriolar level; they mediate a vasodilating response to catecholamines and increase blood flow to selected structures such as skeletal muscles.[33]

A secondary means of controlling vascular tone via the sympathetic nervous system involves the sympathetic cholinergic fibers. These fibers cause vasodilatation in the resistance vessels in skeletal muscle, at least in the extremities. Their functional importance in humans remains unclear, but they may play a part in the fight-or-flight response by increasing muscle readiness for action.

The release of catecholamines (epinephrine and norepinephrine) from the adrenal medulla provides a humoral means to influence the peripheral circulation. In small amounts epinephrine produces a vasodilating response, owing to the selective stimulation of the β-adrenergic receptors in the arterioles. In larger amounts, epinephrine's α-adrenergic stimulation predominates, causing a pressor response. Norepinephrine, which is much more selective for the alpha receptors, produces vasoconstriction at all doses. During normal physiologic functioning, however, the physiologic significance of circulating catecholamines released from the adrenal medulla is small relative to that released from the sympathetic nerve fibers innervating the vessels.[5]

Reactive hyperemia provides a useful model of local responses of the vasculature to stress. When the blood supply to an extremity is transiently interrupted and then allowed to resume, the tissue increases its blood flow by relaxing the arteriolar sphincters. The degree of reactive hyperemia is related to the length of the occlusion: longer occlusion causes greater hyperemia. Reactive hyperemia is not neurally mediated, as it is not eliminated by complete denervation or sympathectomy.[34] The mediators of reactive hyperemia are many of the substances that normally mediate local control of vascular tone.

Local control of vascular tone is exerted through several mechanisms. The relative contributions of each mechanism remain somewhat uncertain, and vary in different tissues. Among the mediators of this mechanism are prostaglandins, adenosine phosphates, endothelium-derived relaxing factor (nitric oxide) and endothelium-derived contracting factors.

### Blood Pressure

Normal blood pressure ranges from 100 to 120 mm Hg systolic and 60 to 80 mm Hg diastolic. It is influenced by cardiac output and the peripheral resistance at the level of the arterioles. The mean arterial pressure is approximately equal to the diastolic pressure plus one third the difference between the systolic and diastolic pressures, based on the (generally accurate) assumption that systole lasts one third of the cardiac cycle. The mean arterial pressure depends on cardiac output and on peripheral resistance. The pulse pressure, defined as the difference between diastolic and systolic blood pressure, is a function of the stroke volume and of arterial capacitance.

The overall control of blood pressure is complex and involves several components. The fluid component of blood volume is controlled largely through the renin-angiotensin-aldosterone axis. The juxtaglomerular apparatus in the kidney, located adjacent to the afferent arteriole and the glomerulus, is responsible for the secretion of renin into the circulation. Renin converts renin substrate, an α-globulin produced in the liver, to angiotensin I. Angiotensin I is converted in the pulmonary capillary beds to angiotensin II. Angiotensin I is an apparently inactive substance, but angiotensin II is a potent vasoconstrictor and also stimulates secretion of aldosterone by the adrenal cortex. Aldosterone, in turn, is responsible for sodium and water reabsorption in the renal tubules. The increased plasma volume and increased blood pressure resulting from this cascade cause inhibition of the juxtaglomerular apparatus, and complete the feedback loop (Figure 7-20).

Atriopeptin, or atrial natriuretic factor, is a recently characterized polypeptide released from atrial cells in response to stretch. It promotes loss of sodium and water by increasing the glomerular filtration rate and by decreasing renin secretion. Its role in the maintenance of normal blood pressure and in hypertension remain under investigation.[35]

The neural control of blood pressure is mediated through the autonomic nervous system and the adrenal medullary catecholamines. The baroreceptors are located in the carotid body and along the arch of the aorta, responding to changing hemodynamic needs. Stimulation of these baroreceptors, as with increased blood pressure, causes a decrease in sympathetic tone and an increase in vagal tone to the heart, to produce bradycardia and a decrease in peripheral resistance. A fall in blood pressure, as on rising from a supine position, causes a decrease in the tonic firing of the baroreceptors, with an increase in sympathetic vasomotor tone and tachycardia. The baroreceptors accommodate to persistent changes in blood pressure, effectively changing their "set point." Thus, baroreceptors provide effective moment-to-moment control of blood pressure but have little effect overall on blood pressure, which is controlled primarily through the renal mechanisms already discussed.

### Circulatory Response to Exercise

The circulation responds to exercise by shunting blood away from the gut, kidneys, and skin toward the skeletal muscles involved in the exercise. The vasoconstriction in the viscera and skin is accomplished through the sympathetic nervous system. The vasodilatation of the active muscle groups is largely locally mediated, through several factors, including increases in potassium ion concentration, increases in osmolarity, changes in adenosine nucleotide concentrations, and falling pH. An increase in muscle blood flow up to 15 to 20 times the baseline value may accompany the arteriolar dilatation associated with vigorous exercise,[36] and oxygen extraction increases severalfold as well.[37]

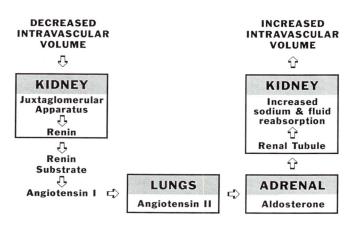

**Figure 7-20.** The role of the renin-angiotensin system in responding to decreased intravascular volume.

The arteriolar dilatation in active muscle groups during vigorous exercise more than offsets the increased resistance in the viscera and skin circulation, and during vigorous exercise causes total peripheral resistance to fall perhaps to 50% of the resting value. The cardiac output increases even more, primarily through increases in heart rate, which causes an increase in blood pressure despite the decreased total peripheral resistance. The increase in blood pressure is both systolic and diastolic, though the systolic increase is greater.

## The Lungs

### Anatomy

The lungs consist of two spongelike organs separated by the mediastinal structures. The functional unit of the lung is the alveolus. There are approximately 300 million alveoli in an adult lung, and they provide a surface area on the order of 85 m$^2$ for gas exchange with the capillaries.[38] The multibranched structure of the bronchial tree makes possible this large surface area in a compact volume. Each alveolus is constructed of thin-walled alveolar cells that are heavily invested with capillaries, allowing for diffusion of gases.

The muscles of respiration consist of the diaphragm, the intercostal muscles, sternocleidomastoids, scalene muscles, and the abdominal muscles. The diaphragm is a dome-shaped muscle with a tendinous central portion that separates the thoracic and the abdominal cavity. It performs most of the work of quiet breathing. The other muscles of respiration become more active during forceful inspiration and expiration, as discussed below. The crural part of the diaphragm has no attachments to the rib cage, and causes abdominal displacement only while inflating the lungs.[39] Because of this different action, as well as its separate embryonic origin and segmental innervation, it may be thought of as a muscle distinct from the rest of the diaphragm.[40]

The surface of the lung is enveloped by the pleura, which is reflected to cover the parietal surface as well. The area between the two pleural surfaces is known as the *pleural space,* though in fact it is primarily a potential space in normal healthy persons, containing only a small amount of lubricating fluid.

The lungs have a dual blood supply. The pulmonary arteries carry blood with low oxygen tension. A low-pressure system, with normal systolic pressures in the vicinity of 22 mm Hg, it allows gas exchange in the alveoli. The bronchial arteries constitute the secondary blood supply. They originate directly from the aorta and contain blood with a high oxygen tension and at systemic pressures, providing nutrition to the pulmonary tissues.

The lungs are divided into five lobes. The right lung consists of the right upper, right lower, and right middle lobe. The left lung contains only an upper and a lower lobe. The lingula is considered the left lung's anatomic correlate of the right middle lobe. Each lobe is further divided into segments, a total of nineteen for the two lungs.

The diaphragm is innervated by the phrenic nerves. Each intercostal muscle is supplied by the corresponding intercostal nerve, which runs in the neurovascular bundle. The parietal pleura, unlike the visceral pleura, is capable of providing sensory information, such as pain or touch, to the brain. It is supplied in part by the intercostal nerves and in part by the phrenic nerves.

The nerve supply to the lungs includes both sympathetic fibers from the sympathetic chain and parasympathetic fibers from the vagus nerve.

### Lung Volumes

The normal volume of air exchanged during quiet respiration is termed the *tidal volume* (TV). After a normal expiration, the volume of air that remains in the lung is known as the *functional residual capacity* (FRC). Upon completion of a maximal expiration, the volume remaining in the lungs is called the *residual volume* (RV). The *vital capacity* (VC) is the amount of air exhaled after a maximal inspiration and subsequent maximal expiration. *Total lung capacity* (TLC) consists of the *vital capacity* VC plus RV (Figure 7-21). Approximately 150 ml of air remains in the nasopharynx, trachea, and bronchial tree during respiration and is thus unavailable for gas exchange in the alveoli. This volume is the *anatomic dead space*. The volume of air that ventilates alveoli that are not fully perfused by blood is the *physiologic dead space*.

In addition to these static volumes, a number of dynamic volumes are useful in evaluating patients with pulmonary or neuromuscular problems.

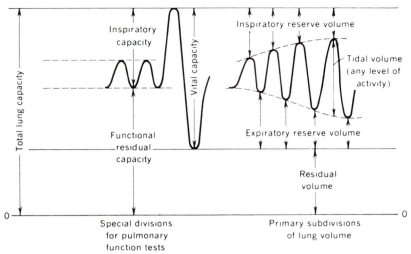

**Figure 7-21.** The relationship of the various lung volumes to the total lung volume. (From Åstrand P-O, Rodahl K. Textbook of Work Physiology, ed 3. New York: McGraw-Hill, 1986, with permission.)

*Forced expiratory volume* (FEV) is the volume of air that can be exhaled with maximal effort during a specified unit of time, usually expressed as a percentage of the VC. The time, in seconds, is denoted by a subscript (e.g., $FEV_1$ is the volume of air exhaled during the first second of a forced expiration). The FEV is particularly useful for evaluating patients with obstructive pulmonary disease. *Maximal voluntary ventilation* (MVV) is the volume of air exhaled during a period of time as the patient is told to breathe as rapidly and deeply as possible. Data are usually collected for a short time (15 seconds) and the results are extrapolated to the volume per minute. MVV is influenced by the mechanical and neuromuscular status of the chest wall and lungs.

### Mechanics of Respiration

Before inspiration, the intrapleural pressure is approximately $-5$ cm $H_2O$. This negative pressure is generated by the elastic recoil of the lungs, and the pressure in the alveoli immediately prior to inspiration is zero relative to the environment. With inspiration, negative pressure is generated in the pleural space by diaphragmatic contraction. This negative pressure (approximately 8 to 10 mm Hg) results in a negative pressure in the airways,

causing the movement of air into the lungs. Quiet expiration is a passive process, driven by the elastic recoil of the lungs and of the chest wall.

Deeper inspiration is accomplished by the additional use of the external intercostal muscles, which contract and cause the ribs to move upward and forward, increasing both the anteroposterior dimension and side-to-side dimensions of the thoracic cage (Figure 7-22). Maximal inspiratory efforts make use of the sternocleidomastoid and the scalene muscles, which raise the sternum and first two ribs, respectively.

Forced expiration uses the internal intercostal muscles to move the ribs downward and backward, an action opposite to that effected by the external

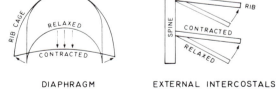

DIAPHRAGM          EXTERNAL INTERCOSTALS

**Figure 7-22.** The effect of the mechanical action of the diaphragm and external intercostal muscles on chest wall dimensions. (From Haas A, Pineda H, Haas F, et al. Pulmonary Therapy and Rehabilitation: Principles and Practice. Baltimore: Williams & Wilkins, 1979, with permission.)

intercostal muscles. This leads to a decrease in both anteroposterior and side-to-side dimensions of the thorax. The abdominal musculature (rectus abdominis, internal and external obliques, and the transversus abdominis) also contribute to forced expiration by increasing intraabdominal pressure, pushing the diaphragm upward.[41] Expiratory muscles are able to exert the greatest force when the lung volume approaches TLC, by virtue of a favorable length-tension relationship. Conversely, the inspiratory muscles can exert the greatest force at lung volumes approaching RV. Maximal expiratory force averages 230 cm $H_2O$ for males aged 20 to 55 years and 150 cm $H_2O$ for females of the same age. Maximal inspiratory force averages 125 cm $H_2O$ for men aged 20 to 55, and 90 cm $H_2O$ for women in this age group.[42]

During quiet respiration, the resistance to air flow derives primarily from the medium-sized bronchi. The terminal bronchioles contribute less than one fifth of the resistance.

The energy requirement, or cost of respiration, is due to the resistance to flow of air and the elasticity of the lungs and chest wall. The relative contributions of these two vary individually and according to breathing pattern. Breathing deeply increases the elastic work of breathing disproportionately, while breathing at faster rates increases the proportion of work due to airway resistance. The work performed on the lung can be graphically represented by plotting pleural pressure versus lung volume (Figure 7-23).

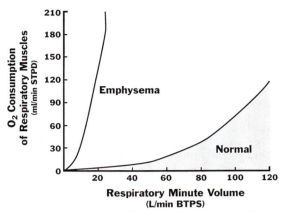

**Figure 7-24.** The work of breathing in a normal individual compared with a patient with emphysema. (Adapted from Mountcastle VB: Medical Physiology. St. Louis: CV Mosby, 1974.)

The normal energy requirements of quiet breathing through the nose is approximately 1 Calorie per minute. This may increase to 20 to 25 Cal per minute with a minute ventilation of 70 L.[43] The oxygen consumption of the respiratory muscles is 0.5 to 1.0 ml per liter of ventilation at rest, representing approximately 1% to 2% of the body's total oxygen consumption.[31] This rises rapidly with increased ventilation (Figure 7-24), reaching 5 ml per liter of ventilation when minute ventilation reaches 180 L.[44] Endurance training can increase maximal oxygen consumption of the respiratory muscles as much as 67%.[44]

Expiration is normally a passive process for a person at rest, but with increased ventilatory demands becomes active and consumes a considerable portion of the energy required by the respiratory muscles. During forced expiration by a normal individual, 80% of the lung volume is exhaled in the first second. Similarly, early inspiration contains the bulk of the inspired volume. These facts allow for considerable increases in respiratory rate without impairing the ability to exchange full tidal volumes with each breath.

*Alveolar ventilation* is the volume of air that each minute reaches the alveoli for gas exchange and is calculated by subtracting anatomic dead space from tidal volume and multiplying the result by the respiratory rate. Rapid shallow breathing thus provides less effective ventilation for a given volume of air breathed.

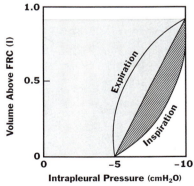

**Figure 7-23.** The pressure-volume curve of the lung demonstrating the work of inspiration overcoming elastic (*shaded area*) and viscous (*cross-hatched area*) forces. (Adapted from West JB. Respiratory Physiology—The Essentials, ed 3. Baltimore: Williams & Wilkins, 1989.)

The fundamental purpose of the lung is gas exchange. For this to be effective a mechanism for transporting oxygen from the air in the alveoli to the blood, and carbon dioxide in the reverse direction, is needed. Transport of carbon dioxide is facilitated by its higher solubility in blood (20 times greater than oxygen), by formation of bicarbonate in the red blood cells through carbonic anhydrase, and through the formation of carbamino compounds through the nonenzymatic combination of carbon dioxide with the terminal amine groups on proteins, primarily hemoglobin.

The amount of oxygen that can dissolve in blood is quite small, approximately 0.3 ml per 100 ml of arterial blood at a partial pressure of oxygen ($P_{O_2}$) of 100 mm Hg. Hemoglobin is responsible for the remainder of oxygen transport and can bind 20.8 ml of oxygen per 100 ml of blood.[45] The affinity of hemoglobin for oxygen varies with the $P_{O_2}$, a relationship described by the hemoglobin-oxygen dissociation curve (Figure 7-25A). The advantages of this curve include allowing for a relatively small drop in oxygen content per decrement in $P_{O_2}$ in the upper, flatter part of the curve, and a large release of oxygen during the steep midportion of the curve. Thus, oxygen content of the blood is minimally affected by small changes in ambient $P_{O_2}$ or mild alveolar hypoventilation, and a large amount of oxygen can be delivered to the body tissues as the blood $P_{O_2}$ falls during passage through the periphery.

The hemoglobin-oxygen dissociation curve may be shifted by a number of factors. Acidosis, elevated temperature, and increased $P_{CO_2}$ all cause the curve to shift to the right, in association with a decrease in the affinity of hemoglobin for oxygen (Figure 7-25B). Hypoxia causes an increase in red blood cell 2,3-diphosphoglycerate, which also causes a shift to the right. These adaptations allow for delivery of more oxygen to the peripheral tissues, especially during times of stress, when tissue oxygen demand may be increased.

Movement of oxygen and carbon dioxide across the alveolar wall takes place through diffusion. The rate of diffusion (Vgas) is described by Fick's law and is proportional to the difference in the

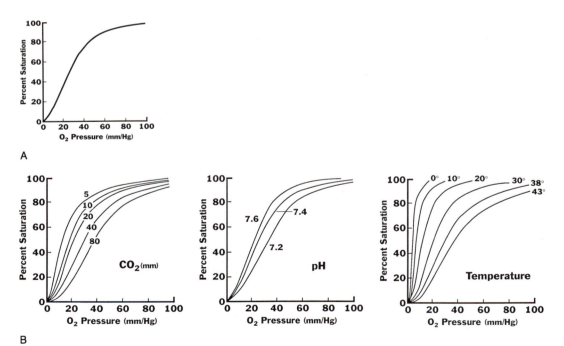

**Figure 7-25.** (*A*) The oxyhemoglobin dissociation curve. (*B*) The effect of carbon dioxide, pH, and temperature on the oxyhemoglobin dissociation curve. (From Åstrand P-O, Rodahl K: Textbook of Work Physiology, ed 3. New York: McGraw-Hill, 1986, with permission.)

partial pressures of the gas $(P_1 - P_2)$, the surface area available for diffusion, and a diffusion constant. It is inversely proportional to the thickness of the barrier. The diffusion constant is determined by the solubility and molecular weight of the gas. Thus:

$$\text{Vgas} \propto \frac{\text{Area}}{\text{Thickness}} \times \text{Diffusion constant} \times (P_1 - P_2)$$

### Regulation of Respiration

#### Neural Factors

The control of the basic respiratory pattern appears to be centered in clusters of neurons in the medulla, which form a central pattern generator.[46,47] This center receives inhibitory impulses from the rostral pons as well as from the pulmonary stretch receptors, which send feedback via vagal afferents. The inhibition from the stretch receptors is known as the *Hering-Breuer reflex*. This basic mechanism is influenced by many other factors, including cortical, extrapyramidal, and peripheral neural input, as well as chemical factors. The situation is further complicated by the individual's inability to exert a significant amount of voluntary control on the process and by the effects of emotional expression.

#### Central Chemoreceptors

The central chemoreceptors are located on the surface of the medulla. These receptors respond to changes in the pH of the cerebrospinal fluid, which in turn is influenced by the $P_{CO_2}$ of arterial blood. Activation of these receptors results in an increased rate of firing of the pattern generator as well as an increased threshold for neurons that respond to inhibitory influences, thus increasing the depth of respiration. The minute ventilation is thus increased by a combination of increased ventilatory rate and increased tidal volume in response to an increase in the $P_{CO_2}$.

Salicylates increase the depth and rate of respiration by directly stimulating the medulla, increasing the sensitivity of the central chemoreceptors to carbon dioxide.[48] This greater increased sensitivity interacts with increased carbon dioxide production caused by the uncoupling of oxidative phosphorylation in the skeletal muscles.

#### Peripheral Chemoreceptors

The peripheral chemoreceptors are located in the carotid and aortic bodies. These clusters of epithelioid cells have a very high metabolic rate and are very sensitive to decreases in $P_{O_2}$. The hypoxic drive may be generalized due to hypoxemia or local due to decreased blood flow. Decreased blood flow at the receptors may be due to either generalized hypotension or a local decrease in blood flow caused by sympathetic activation or circulating catecholamines. It is important to remember that it is the local $P_{O_2}$ at the receptor sites, not the arterial $P_{O_2}$ or the oxygen saturation, that determines the activation of these receptors. At least part of the hyperventilation caused by salicylates appears to be related to stimulation of these peripheral chemoreceptors,[49] a phenomenon that is independent of the inhibition of prostaglandin synthesis.[50]

### The Respiratory Response to Exercise

The stimulation and regulation of respiration during exercise remain controversial; the relative importance of neural and chemical factors are undetermined.[51] The minute ventilation increases in a linear fashion with increasing work intensity *up to a point,* and then the response becomes much steeper (Figure 7-26). During most of this increase there is no measurable change in $P_{CO_2}$, $P_{O_2}$ or pH. With greater loads there is a decrease in the pH

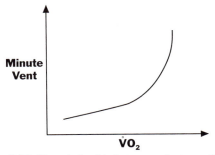

**Figure 7-26.** The relationship between minute ventilation and oxygen consumption.

that is not proportional to the ventilatory response, and with very high loads $P_{O_2}$ may fall.

Both factors are involved, though the precise mechanisms of control still are not clear. There is a rapid ventilatory response to exercise; this is mediated by neural mechanisms, through somatosensory feedback from working muscles and moving joints stimulating the medullary centers. As exercise continues, additional control is exerted by the effect of acidosis on the medullary chemoreceptors and hypoxia on the peripheral chemoreceptors. The hypoxic effect is exaggerated by the activation of the sympathetic nervous system and circulating catecholamines, depending on the relative stress of the exercise (i.e., the fitness of the individual).

The typical ventilatory response to exercise described above refers to dynamic exercise. The response to isometric exercise is exaggerated in the same way that the cardiac response is exaggerated when an isometric component is superimposed on dynamic exercise.[52] The rapid onset and offset of the increased ventilation, out of proportion to the metabolic demands, suggests a neural reflex. The stimulus for this reflex is not clear.

Physical training has less of an effect on the ventilatory response to exercise than the cardiac response. In general, the rate of respiration is somewhat slower and the depth greater at any given submaximal load, but the minute ventilation remains essentially unchanged.

# References

1. Ruskin J, McHale PA, Harley A, et al. Pressure-flow studies in man: Effects of atrial systole on left ventricular function. J Clin Invest 1970; 49:472.
2. Brush JE Jr, Cannon RO 3rd, Schenke WH, et al. Angina due to coronary microvascular disease in hypertensive patients without left ventricular hypertrophy. N Engl J Med 1988; 319:1302–1307.
3. Sax FL, Cannon RO 3d, Hanson C, et al. Impaired forearm vasodilator reserve in patients with microvascular angina, evidence of a generalized disorder of vascular function? N Engl J Med 1987; 317:1366–1370.
4. Guyton AC. Textbook of Medical Physiology, ed 7. Philadelphia: WB Saunders, 1986.
5. Berne RB, Levy MN. Cardiovascular Physiology. St. Louis: CV Mosby, 1986.
6. Furchgott RF, Vanhoutte PM. Endothelium-derived relaxing and contracting factors. FASEB J 1989; 3:2007–2018.
7. Gryglewski RJ, Botting RM, Vane JR. Mediators produced by the endothelial cell. Hypertension 1988; 12:530–548.
8. Ignarro LJ. Endothelium-derived nitric oxide: Actions and properties. FASEB J 1989; 3:31–36.
9. Moncada S, Palmer RM, Higgs EA. The discovery of nitric oxide as the endogenous nitrovasodilator. Hypertension 1988; 12:365–372.
10. Vanhoutte PM, Auch-Schwelk W, Boulanger C, et al. Does endothelin-1 mediate endothelium-dependent contractions during anoxia? J Cardiovasc Pharmacol 1989; 13(suppl 5):S124–128.
11. Klocke FJ, Mates KE, Canty JM Jr, et al. Coronary pressure-flow relationships: Continued issues and probable implications. Circ Res 1985; 56:310–323.
12. Moldover JR, Downey JA: Cardiac response to exercise: Comparison of 3 ergometers. Arch Phys Med Rehabil 1983; 64:155–159.
13. Lundberg A. Oxygen consumption in relation to work load in students with cerebral palsy. J App Physiol 1976; 40:873–875.
14. Faulkner JA, Heigenhauser GF, Schork MA. The cardiac output–oxygen uptake relationship of men during graded bicycle ergometry. Med Sci Sports 1977; 9:148–154.
15. Ekelund LG, Holmgren A. Central hemodynamics during exercise. Circ Res 1967; 20(suppl 1):I33–I43.
16. Braunwald E, Sonnenblick EH, Ross J, et al. An analysis of the cardiac response to exercise. Circ Res 1967; 20(suppl 1):I44–I58.
17. Kotchen TA, Hartley LH, Rice TW, et al. Renin, norepinephrine, and epinephrine responses to graded exercise. J Appl Physiol 1971; 31:178–184.
18. von Euler US. Sympatho-adrenal activity in physical exercise. Med Sci Sports 1974; 6:165–173.
19. Bevegård S, Holmgren A, Jonsson B. The effect of body position on the circulation at rest and during exercise, with special reference to the influence on the stroke volume. Acta Physiol Scand 1960; 49:279–298.
20. Kitamura K, Jorgensen CR, Gobel FL, et al. Hemodynamic correlates of myocardial oxygen consumption during upright exercise. J Appl Physiol 1972; 32:516–522.
21. Jorgensen CR, Wang K, Wang Y, et al. Effect of propranolol on myocardial oxygen consumption and its hemodynamic correlates during upright exercise. Circulation 1973; 48:1173–1182.
22. Nelson RR, Gobel FL, Jorgensen CR, et al. Hemodynamic predictors of myocardial oxygen consumption during static and dynamic exercise. Circulation 1974; 50:1179–1189.

23. Donald KW, Lind AR, McNicol GW, et al. Cardiovascular responses to sustained (static) contractions. Circulation Res 1967; 20(suppl 1):I15–I30.

24. Stenberg J, Åstrand P-O, Ekblom B, et al. Hemodynamic response to work with different muscle groups, sitting and supine. J Appl Physiol 1967; 22(1):61–70.

25. Lecerof H. Influence of body position on exercise tolerance, heart rate, blood pressure, and respiration rate in coronary insufficiency. Br Heart J 1971; 33:78–83.

26. Saltin B, Blomqvist G, Mitchell JH, et al. Response to exercise after bed rest and after training. Circulation 1968; 38(suppl 7):1–50.

27. Ekblom B, Lundberg A. Effect of physical training on adolescents with severe motor handicaps. Acta Paediatr Scand 1968; 57:17–23.

28. Winder WW, Hagberg JM, Hickson RC, et al. Time course of sympathoadrenal adaptation to endurance exercise training in man. J Appl Physiol 1978; 45:370–374.

29. Guyton AC. The venous system and its role in the circulation. Mod Concepts Cardiovasc Dis 1958; 27:483.

30. Milnor WR. Hemodynamics. Baltimore: Williams and Wilkins, 1982.

31. Otis AB. The work of breathing. In: Fenn WO, Rhan H, eds. Handbook of Physiology, vol 1, Sec 3, Respiration. Washington: American Physiological Society, 1964; 463–476.

32. Starling EH. On the absorption of fluids from the connective tissue spaces. J Physiol 1986; 19:312.

33. Weiner N, Tatlor P. Neurohumoral transmission: The autonomic and somatic motor nervous systems. In: Gilman AG, Goodman LS, Rall TW, et al., eds. The Pharmacological Basis of Therapeutics, ed 7. New York: Macmillan, 1985; 72–73.

34. Duff F, Shepard JT. The circulation in the chronically denervated forearm. Clin Sci 1953; 12:407–416.

35. Genest J, Larochelle P, Cusson RJ, et al. The atrial natriuretic factor in hypertension. Am J Med Sci 1988; 295:299–304.

36. Shephard RJ. Physiology and Biochemistry of Exercise. New York: Praeger, 1982; 232.

37. Berger RA. Applied Exercise Physiology. Philadelphia: Lea & Febiger, 1982.

38. West JB. Respiratory Physiology—The Essentials, ed 3. Baltimore: Williams & Wilkins, 1985.

39. De Troyer A, Sampson M, Sigrist S, et al. The diaphragm: Two muscles. Science 1981; 213:237–238.

40. Roussos C, Macklem PT. The respiratory muscles. N Engl J Med 1982; 307:786–797.

41. Taylor AE, Rehder K, Hyatt RE, et al. Clinical Respiratory Physiology. Philadelphia: WB Saunders, 1989.

42. Black LF, Hyatt RE. Maximal respiratory pressures: Normal values and relationship to age and sex. Am Rev Respir Dis 1969; 99:646–702.

43. Roussos C, Campbell EJM. Respiratory muscle energetics. In: Fishman AP, ed. Handbook of Physiology. sec 3. Bethesda, Md: American Physiological Association, 1986; 500.

44. Bradley M, Leith D. Ventilatory muscle training and the oxygen cost of sustained hypernea. J Appl Physiol 1978; 45:885–892.

45. West JB. In: Best and Taylor's Physiological Basis of Medical Practice, ed 12. Baltimore: Williams & Wilkins, 1991; 564.

46. von Euler C. On the central pattern generator for the basic breathing rhythmicity. J Appl Physiol 1983; 55:1647.

47. Åstrand P-O, Rodahl K. Textbook of Work Physiology, ed 3. New York: McGraw-Hill, 1986.

48. Cameron IR, Semple SJ. The central respiratory stimulant action of salicylates. Clin Sci 1968; 35:391–401.

49. McQueen DS, Ritchie IM, Birrell GJ. Arterial chemoreceptor involvement in salicylate-induced hyperventilation in rats. Br J Pharmacol 1989; 98:413–424.

50. Kuna ST, Levine S. Relationship between cyclooxygenase activity (COA) inhibition and stimulation of ventilation by salicylates. J Pharmacol Exp Ther 1981; 219:723–730.

51. Cunningham DJC. Regulation of breathing in exercise. Circ Res 1967; 20(suppl 1):I122–I131.

52. Wiley RL, Lind AR. Respiratory responses to simultaneous static and rhythmic exercises in humans. Clin Sci Mol Med 1975; 49:427–432.

# Chapter 8

# Physiology of Synovial Joints and Articular Cartilage

JERALD R. ZIMMERMAN
VAN C. MOW

Joints are formed as a connection between any two bones. The type created during embryogenesis depends on the function to be performed. Three types of joints are found in the human body; they vary by the amount of relative motion they allow.[1] Diarthrodial or synovial joints, such as the hip and knee, are capable of large amounts of motion. Synarthroses or fibrous joints, such as the coronal sutures, allow no relative motion. Amphiarthroses or cartilaginous joints, such as the intervertebral disc and symphysis pubis, provide little or no relative motion.

Of these three types of joints, diarthrodial joints have come under the greatest scrutiny. One of their primary functions is to facilitate the movement of body segments and locomotion. All body movements involve diarthrodial joints. Under normal conditions, these joints provide efficient bearing systems with excellent friction, lubrication, and wear properties, that undergo little deterioration throughout an individual's life.[2,3] They must be able to withstand loads up to six times body weight on a repetitive basis, for up to a million cycles per year, depending on the specific joint and function. Wear-and-tear breakdown of diarthrodial joints leads to degenerative joint disease and arthritis, resulting in severe limitations in joint function and body movement.[4–7]

Although individual anatomic forms and material properties vary, two components are common to all diarthrodial joints: synovial fluid and soft connective tissues. Structures formed by connective tissue include articular cartilage, capsule, meniscus, and ligaments.[1] Abnormalities in any of these structures of the joint can lead to significant pain and loss of function.[4–7]

Articular cartilage covers the ends of the bones and serves the primary load-bearing functions in the joint, doing so with excellent frictional characteristics[2,3] It also provides a highly wear-resistant surface that allows one end of the joint to move efficiently over the other with little or no attrition.[8] Most arthritic changes begin with focal lesions on the cartilage surface, eventually leading to complete wearing away of the tissue and to arthritis. Because this tissue plays a unique role in the function of the diarthrodial joint, researchers have made great efforts to understand its biology, molecular structure, biochemistry, and biomaterial properties (see, for example, references 2 through 13).

Disease and dysfunction of diarthrodial joints, such as osteoarthritis and rheumatoid arthritis, are due to the destruction of articular cartilage and to bony changes such as osteophyte formation.[4,5] Osteoarthritis is a universal problem involving metabolic, biochemical, enzymatic, and biomechanical abnormalities.[2–12] Knowledge of the biochemical and mechanical properties of joint cartilage is essential to understanding the normal working and pathophysiology of diarthrodial joints. In this chapter we discuss the gross anatomy and ultrastructure of these joints, followed by a more detailed discussion of the mechanical properties of normal articular cartilage. Finally, the biochemical and biomechanical response of cartilage in several well-known clinical settings, immobilization and aging, are presented, and we conclude with some thoughts on the pathogenesis of osteoarthritis. This information helps to provide a valid rationale for rehabilitation of joints affected by degenerative joint disease.

## Joint Structures and Anatomy

### Synovium

The synovial membrane lines the inside of the entire joint except the articular cartilage.[1] It is composed of loose connective tissue on which the densely packed surface cells are arranged in epithelium-like fashion. This synovial lining secretes synovial fluid and nutrients and absorbs the metabolic waste products produced by the chondrocytes in cartilage and by other avascular soft tissues inside the joint.

### Synovial Fluid

Synovial fluid is clear and colorless or slightly yellow,[15,16] and its volume is very small compared to the volume of the joint. In most joints it is just 0.2 ml, but a large joint such as the knee may contain up to 5 ml. Biochemically, synovial fluid is an exudate of blood plasma that contains a hyaluronic acid protein complex with a molecular weight of approximately $2 \times 10^6$.[15,16] The presence of this macromolecule produces the non-Newtonian flow properties of synovial fluid (e.g., viscosity or resistance to shearing of the fluid decreases as the rate of shearing increases).[15–19] These flow behaviors play important roles in joint lubrication[2,3] and protect the cartilage from wear.[14] Synovial fluid samples obtained from osteoarthritic joints show that many of these flow properties are diminished.

Synovial fluid also provides necessary nutrients for the articular cartilage. Low–molecular weight solutes, such as glucose, appear to be transported by passive diffusion. The transport mechanism of the larger molecules, such as serum albumin, is less clear. One theory suggests that it may be due to a mechanical pumping effect induced by movement of the joint.[8,20,21] The compression of cartilage causes interstitial fluid flow, which then carries the dissolved substances by convection.

### Cartilage

The thickness of the layer of articular cartilage in any given joint depends on the species, the particular joint, and the location in the joint.[22,23] It is usually in the range of 0.5 to 1.5 mm thick, though on the patella it may be as thick as 7.5 mm. The cartilage is comprised of both a solid phase, consisting of chondrocytes, collagen, and proteoglycans (PG), and a fluid phase composed of water. The chondrocytes account for less than 1% of the wet weight of the articular cartilage.[24] These cells, which are of mesenchymal origin, manufacture, secrets, and maintain the organic components of the extracellular matrix (ECM). The ECM consists of two networks: a permanent network of collagen fibrils and a network of PGs that exhibits rapid turnover. These two networks are enmeshed within each other, forming a strong, cohesive, fiber-reinforced solid matrix that is porous and permeable.

The collagen fibrils of the ECM are mainly type II collagen and are produced by the tissue chondrocytes.[10,25,26] They comprise 20% of the wet weight of normal tissue and 65% of the dry weight of the ECM. The collagen fibrils have an average diameter of 25 to 40 nm. Covalent cross-links exist between the tropocollagen molecules, allowing the formation of fibrillar networks within the matrix.[25,26]

### Proteoglycans

PGs contribute an additional 5% to the wet weight of the articular cartilage and approximately 25% to the dry weight of the solid matrix. They are charged protein-polysaccharide molecules that exist in the ECM generally as aggregates linked to a hyaluronate filament.[10,11] A PG monomer consists of a long protein core to which approximately 150 sulfated glycosaminoglycan (GAG) chains are attached. The two sulfated GAGs found in articular cartilage, keratan sulfate and chondroitin sulfate, are composed of repeating disaccharide units.[10,11] There is a heterogeneous distribution of the GAGs along the protein core, consisting of a region rich in keratan sulfate and a region rich in chondroitin sulfate. This structural arrangement gives a "bottle brush" appearance to the PG monomer (Figure 8-1A). Each PG monomer is not structurally identical, however, and they can vary in length, weight, and composition. A link protein is required to stabilize the non-covalent bond between a PG monomer and the hyaluronate filament.[10,11] This link protein also provides structural rigidity to the aggregate, thus imparting strength to the ECM of cartilage.[27] Loss of this link protein owing

to aging or an arthritic condition weakens the ECM, increasing the propensity of cartilage to develop further mechanical damage.[9,10,27–29]

The hyaluronate to which PG monomers are attached is a nonsulfated disaccharide chain that can be as long as 4 μ. The molecular weight of this molecule is approximately $10^6$. Figure 8-1B provides a schematic representation of a PG aggregate. Figure 8-1C shows an electron micrograph of a cartilage-PG aggregate in solution, confirming the organization of the molecule.

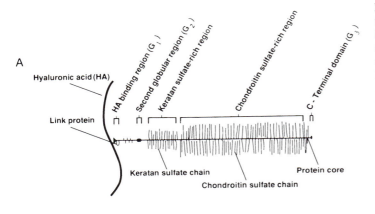

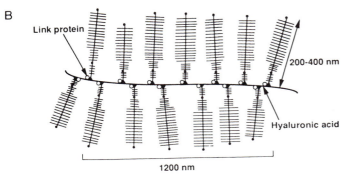

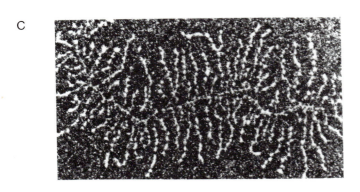

**Figure 8-1.** (*A*) Schematic depiction of the molecular structural arrangement of a PG monomer, giving it a "bottle brush" appearance. (*B*) The PG aggregate with many PG monomers attached to a hyaluronate chain whose molecular weight is approximately 400 kd. The aggregate is stabilized by the link protein. (*C*) An electron micrograph of a cartilage proteoglycan aggregate confirming the organization of the molecule.[28] (From Buckwalter JA, Rosenberg LC. Structural changes during development in bovine fetal epiphyseal cartilage. *Collagen Rel Res* 1983; 3:489–504.)

*Water*

Water, the most abundant component of articular cartilage, accounts for the remaining 70% to 75% of the total wet weight. The distribution of water in cartilage decreases with depth in a nearly linear fashion, from approximately 80% near the joint surface to 65% at the subchondral bone.[35–37] Approximately 70% of the total volume of water is found in the intermolecular space between the PGs and the collagen. Most of the remaining water is located in the intrafibrillar spaces of the collagen, and a small percentage is intracellular. The water serves several important functions in the maintenance of the cartilage: (1) It maintains the PGs in solution. (2) It modulates, together with the PGs, the diameter of the collagen fibrils. (3) Its movement from the ECM controls the compressibility of the cartilage under loading conditions and contributes to the lubrication of the joint. (4) It permits transport of nutrients and waste products between the chondrocytes in the cartilage and the surrounding synovial fluid.

## Ultrastructure of Articular Cartilage

In addition to the molecular structures of collagen and proteoglycans, articular cartilage also has an elaborate microscopic organization.[10,13,38,39] The most salient organizational feature of cartilage is the layering of its major components (collagen, PGs, and chondrocytes) throughout its depth.[37–39] This has often been depicted simply as a three-layer model (Figure 8-2) in which the superficial tangential zone accounts for 10% to 20% of the total tissue thickness. It contains sheets of densely packed collagen fibers that are randomly woven in planes roughly parallel to the articular surface (Figure 8-2B). In the middle zone, which accounts for 40% to 60% of the total thickness, the distance between the collagen fibers is greater. These fibers are more evenly distributed throughout the middle zone. Finally, in the deep zone, the fibers form anastomoses to make larger, radially oriented bundles that cross the tidemark and insert into the calcified cartilage,[40] forming a system that anchors the cartilage to the subchondral bone. Figure 8-3

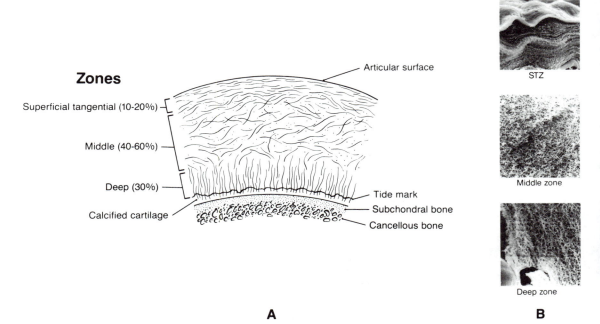

**Figure 8-2.** (*A*) Schematic model of joint cartilage collagen ultrastructure depicts the four zones of the tissue: the superficial tangential zone, the middle zone, the deep zone, and the calcified cartilage.

also depicts the chondrocyte arrangement through-out the tissue. The morphology and arrangement of these cells closely resemble the collagen ultra-structure.

If the surface of the cartilage is punctured with an awl, *split line patterns* are produced that are believed to demonstrate the orientation of the col-lagen fibers in the superficial tangential zone (Fig-ure 8-4).[41,42] The split line patterns can be impor-tant when evaluating the effect of the orientation of the collagen fibers on the mechanical properties of the cartilage. Though the total amount of col-lagen is similar in each zone, the PG content in-creases with depth from the surface and reaches a maximum in the middle zone. This nonhomoge-neous distribution of PG serves an important func-tion by providing an osmotic pressure gradient against rapid fluid efflux from the tissue.[35]

Visually, the surface of articular cartilage ap-pears smooth. Microscopically, however, the smooth appearance disappears; the relatively rough surface has four distinct orders of contours: (1) primary anatomic contours; (2) secondary irregu-larities less than 0.5 mm in diameter; (3) tertiary hollows 20 to 45 μ in diameter and 0.5 to 2.0 μ deep; and (4) quarternary ridges 1 to 4 μ in di-ameter and 0.1 to 0.3 μ deep.[43] The quarternary

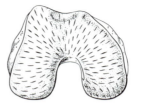

**Human Femoral Condyles**

**Figure 8-4.** Pattern of "split lines" is produced when small, round holes are punctured into the joint surface. This pattern is believed to reflect the orientation of the collagen fibers in the superficial tangential zone.[41,42]

ridges first appear in the second decade of life and become more common with age. Knowledge of the surface topology is important in determining the mechanisms involved in joint lubrication. Scanning electron micrographs of normal and os-teoarthritic cartilage show a wide range of varia-tions in surface topology (Figure 8-5). Osteoar-thritic changes dramatically alter normal surface texture (see Figure 8-5B, C) and can adversely affect the efficacy of the natural lubrication mech-anisms in synovial joints, accelerating the destruc-tive processes.

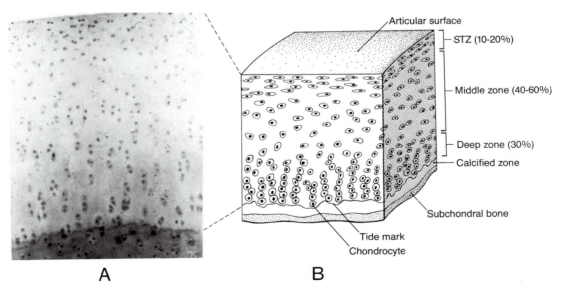

A                                    B

**Figure 8-3.** Arrangement of chondrocytes throughout the articular cartilage shows the three zones in the uncalcified tissue.

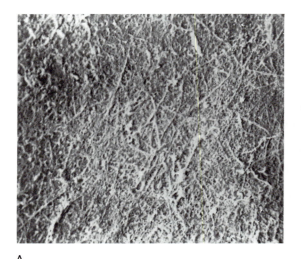

A

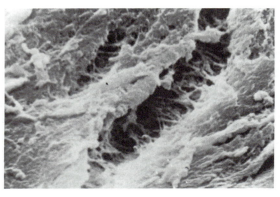

C

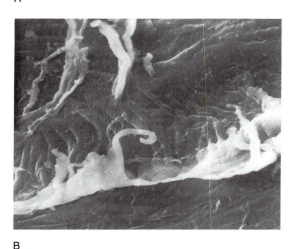

B

**Figure 8-5.** (*A*) Scanning electron micrographs of normal human articular cartilage show smooth texture, without preferred fiber directions.[3] (*B*) An example of human osteoarthritic cartilage shows peeling of the superficial collagen sheets.[3] (*C*) An example of human osteoarthritic cartilage shows a surface crack spanned by many collagen fibers in the deeper zones. (Mow VC, Mak AF. Lubrication of diadiarthrodial joints. In: Shalak R, Chein S, eds. Handbook of Bioengineering. New York: McGraw-Hill, 1986; 5.1–5.34.)

## Mechanical Behavior of Articular Cartilage

Because direct experimental measurements of stresses and strains in cartilage, meniscus, ligaments, and other tissues of diarthrodial joints are limited and very difficult to obtain,[44–47] theoretical models are often used to predict these quantities. The accuracy of these model-based predictions depends on the accuracy of the measured material properties and on the ability of theories to describe the experiment. In general, the material properties are controlled not only by the components of the tissue (e.g., collagen and PG) but by their reciprocal interactions. In this section, a theoretical model describing cartilage is presented to illustrate those processes, along with a review of the properties of normal articular cartilage.[8,9]

## Basic Concepts in Material Testing

Some knowledge of engineering concepts is necessary to understand (1) the basics of deformation, (2) the relationships between stresses and strains, and (3) the types of experiments required to measure the material properties.

### Stress and Strain

When a material body is subjected to an external force, the resulting deformation depends on the intrinsic mechanical properties of the object and on its geometric shape. There are two types of stresses (which is defined as force per area): normal stress and shear stress (Figure 8-6). Normal

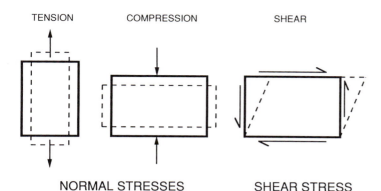

TENSION          COMPRESSION          SHEAR

NORMAL STRESSES          SHEAR STRESS

**Figure 8-6.** Normal stress acting on a material may be tension or compression. Shear stress tends to change angles between two non-colinear material elements.

stresses may be in tension or compression. They tend to elongate or shorten the material in the direction of the applied load. Shear stresses tend to change the angle between two non-colinear material elements (see Figure 8-6). When a material is stretched, the force necessary to produce a certain deformation is proportional to the original cross-sectional area whereas the change in length is proportional to the original length. In order to remove these geometric influences on the force-deformation behavior of the material, stress and strain are used to determine its properties. Stress ($\sigma$) is defined as the force (F) per unit of original area (A):

$$\sigma = F/A$$

and strain ($\epsilon$) is defined as the change in length ($\Delta l$) per unit of the original length ($l_o$:

$$\epsilon = \Delta l/l_o.$$

Defined in this manner, the stress-strain relationship of any material is independent of its geometric form and its stiffness is determined solely by its intrinsic mechanical properties. An example is steel versus wood. The intrinsic stiffness of a material is defined by a constant known as a modulus.

### Modulus, Stiffness, and Strength

When an object is subject to an arbitrary loading condition, the stresses and strains inside the object may be quite complex. The objective of a carefully designed material test is to simplify the loading condition so that the resulting stresses and strains may be easily analyzed. For these material tests, it is necessary to have specimens with known cross-sectional areas and lengths. It is also necessary to apply a specified stress or strain (tensile, compressive, or shear) precisely and predictably onto the specimen. If a constant strain rate is applied then the resulting stress-strain graph is obtained. Figure 8-7A shows a typical tensile stress-strain relationship for a linear material such as

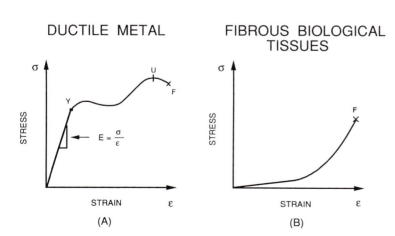

DUCTILE METAL          FIBROUS BIOLOGICAL TISSUES

$E = \dfrac{\sigma}{\epsilon}$

(A)          (B)

**Figure 8-7.** (A) A typical tensile stress-strain relationship for an elastic ductile material such as steel (B) A typical tensile stress-strain behavior for a soft, fibrous biologic material.

steel. The slope of the stress-strain graph (below the yield point Y) defines Young's modulus ($E = \sigma/\epsilon$). The ultimate stress (U) is the largest stress that develops in the material (i.e., strength of material); the failure stress (F) is the stress at which the sample fractures. Figure 8-7B shows typical tensile stress-strain behavior for a soft biologic material. For such materials, the values of U and F often coincide (Figure 8-7B). It can be seen that these two types of tensile behaviors are very different, representing the macroscopic manifestations of their intrinsic differences in composition and microscopic organization. For steel, Young's modulus E is 200 GPa, for bone, 3 GPa, for ligaments, 200 MPa, and for cartilage, 10 MPa. For cartilage in compression, Young's modulus is 0.6 MPa. If a test specimen is sheared and its response is linear, then the shear modulus (G) is defined as the ratio between the shear stress ($\tau$) and the shear strain ($\gamma$): $G = \tau/\gamma$. The shear modulus is also known as the modulus of rigidity. For normal articular cartilage, the shear modulus is 0.3 MPa.

## Theoretical Models of Material Behavior

### Linear Elasticity

A material is linearly elastic if (1) the strain is reversible when the stress is removed, (2) the material response is rate insensitive, and (3) the stress and strain are linearly related, as seen in Figure 8-7A. These materials follow Hooke's law (1678), which states that deformations produced by forces are linearly proportional to each other. When the deformation is expressed in terms of strain and force is expressed in terms of stress, the constant of proportionality is known as Young's modulus (1807) for tension and compression and the shear modulus, as described above. Isotropic linearly elastic materials have elastic properties that are independent of orientation. Therefore, the two moduli completely define their stress-strain behavior. For anisotropic linearly elastic materials, which have different mechanical properties in different directions, more elastic constants are required. Examples of anisotropic materials are wood and bone. Wood is orthotropic, requiring nine elastic constants, and bone is transversely

isotropic, requiring five elastic constants to define their respective stress-strain behaviors. The complete set of elastic constants for these materials is very difficult to obtain, and at present no complete set of these constants exists for either wood or bone. Within certain limits, many engineering materials obey this law of linearly elastic behavior. This theory, however, does not explain the time-dependent stress-strain responses of plastics and most soft biologic materials. These time-dependent properties are attributable to viscoelastic effects.

### Linear Viscoelasticity

For many materials, including polymers and biologic materials, the requirements of the linear elasticity law cannot be met. For these materials, the proportionality between stress and strain is not constant but varies with time. Viscoelastic materials exhibit time-dependent behaviors known as *creep* and *stress relaxation,* and their stress-strain responses are strongly sensitive to strain rate. These viscoelastic characteristics result from a combination of the elastic and viscous elements within the material. *Elasticity* is a term that applies to solids and their time-independent behavior, whereas *viscosity* is generally used to describe fluids and their time-dependent behavior. Solids are modeled by springs, which are linearly elastic, and fluids are modeled by dashpots, which are linearly viscous (Figure 8-8A). A viscous fluid or viscous dashpot is one in which the shear stress is linearly proportional to the rate of shear (Figure 8-8B). The constant of proportionality is called the *coefficient of viscosity.* Thus, a linear viscoelastic material is modeled by linear springs linked together by linear viscous dashpots. Figures 8-8C and 8-8D depict two very simple linear viscoelastic materials, one with the spring and dashpot linked in parallel (Figure 8-8C) and the other with them linked in series (Figure 8-8D). The parallel arrangement is known as a *Kelvin-Voigt material* (1855) and the series arrangement is known as a *Maxwell material* (1870).

A creep test consists of applying and maintaining a constant load on a viscoelastic material, and measuring the resulting deformation as a function of time. A stress-relaxation test consists of imposing and maintaining a constant strain and measur-

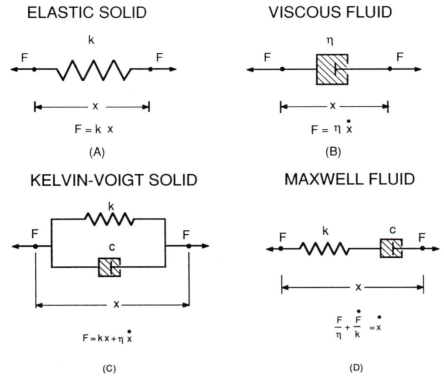

ELASTIC SOLID

$$F = k\,x$$

(A)

VISCOUS FLUID

$$F = \eta\,\dot{x}$$

(B)

KELVIN-VOIGT SOLID

$$F = k\,x + \eta\,\dot{x}$$

(C)

MAXWELL FLUID

$$\frac{F}{\eta} + \frac{\dot{F}}{k} = \dot{x}$$

(D)

**Figure 8-8.** (A) A linear elastic solid is often represented by a spring (Hooke's law), where the force (F) in the spring (k) is directly related to the stretch (x), given by the relationship $F = kx$. (B) A viscous fluid or viscous dashpot is described by Newton's law, where the force (F) is directly proportional to the rate of shear (x) given by the equation $F = \nu x$. The dot symbol (·) refers to a time derivative. (C) The Kelvin-Voigt solid is a model of a viscoelastic solid where a spring (k) and a dashpot ($\nu$) are linked in parallel series. This material exhibits both creep and stress relaxation. The relationship between the force (F) and the displacement is given by $F = kx + \nu x$. (D) The Maxwell material is a model of a viscoelastic fluid where a spring and a dashpot are linked in series. This material exhibits both creep and stress relaxation. The relationship between the force (F) and displacement (x) is given by $(F/\nu) + (F/k) = x$.

ing the force required to do so as a function of time. An elastic solid exibits neither creep nor stress relaxation. Figure 8-9 shows the creep behaviors of the Kelvin and Maxwell materials. These two materials show distinctly different responses because of the way the springs and dashpots are arranged—in parallel or in series. The specifics of their creep behaviors (i.e., the initial response, the rate of creep, and the equilibrium response) are governed by the manner in which the spring and the dashpot are connected and by the set of constants (K,$\nu$) that characterize the elements comprising the material (Figure 8-9). The Kelvin-Voigt material does not creep indefinitely,

because the spring is in parallel with the dashpot, limiting the creep. It is characteristic of a solid. Therefore, the Kelvin-Voigt material is a viscoelastic solid. The Maxwell material creeps indefinitely, as long as the load is maintained, because of the behavior of the dashpot. It is characteristic of a fluid. Thus, a Maxwell material is a viscoelastic fluid. Figure 8-10 shows the stress-relaxation results for both the Maxwell fluid and the Kelvin-Voigt solid. More complex behavior of real materials may be described by simply connecting a number of springs and dashpots in series or parallel.[48] The most commonly used model for a viscoelastic solid is one in which the spring is

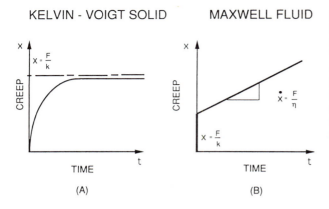

**Figure 8-9.** Graph shows the creep behavior of a Kelvin-Voigt solid under an applied load $F$. The equilibrium creep displacement is given by $x = F/k$. The rate of creep is given by the retardation time constant ($\lambda = \mu/k$). ($B$) The creep behavior of a Maxwell fluid under an applied load $F$. Because of the dashpot, this viscoelastic material will creep indefinitely. The rate of creep is determined by the viscous resistance of the dashpot and the applied force.

connected to a Kelvin-Voigt model. This is known as the standard or three-element viscoelastic material.[49]

A theoretical model is successful in describing a material if the general trends of the creep and stress-relaxation responses are similar to those measured from material tests. The material coefficients ($K, \nu$) are determined by matching the actual experimental data with a theoretical creep or stress-relaxation curve. Several investigators have proposed such a viscoelastic model to describe the compressive and shear behaviors of cartilage.[48,50] An even more comprehensive theory, the quasi-linear viscoelastic theory, was developed by Fung to describe the viscoelasticity in tension of biologic soft tissues such as ligaments and tendons.[49,51] However, these viscoelastic models are not always consistent with known information about the structure and composition of biologic tissue. To understand how the high degree of hydration in biologic tissues influences their mechanical behaviors is particularly important.

## The Biphasic Theory

Both the elastic and viscoelastic models for cartilage treat it as a single-phase material, ignoring the large component of fluid in the tissue. Studies have long suggested that water is an essential component to the proper functioning of articular cartilage.[52–54] More recently, a biphasic model was developed by Mow and coworkers to account for the influence of interstitial fluid on the mechanical properties of cartilage.[8,9,55] In this model two phases exist: (1) the collagen-PG solid matrix, which is assumed to be linearly elastic and incompressible, and (2) an interstitial fluid, which is assumed to be incompressible. In this model, the stresses and strains in each phase are combined to explain time-dependent phenomena such as creep and stress relaxation. Mow and his colleagues theorized that the time-dependent behavior of biphasic materials came from the frictional drag associated with interstitial fluid flow. These interactive forces act between the interstitial fluid and

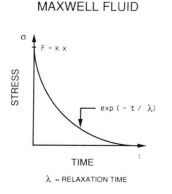

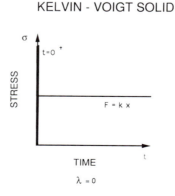

**Figure 8-10.** ($A$) Graph shows the stress-relaxation behavior of a Maxwell fluid. The rate of stress relaxation is given by the relaxation time constant $\lambda = (\nu/k)$. ($B$) The stress-relaxation behavior of a Kelvin-Voigt solid under a given stretch ($x$). The equilibrium value of the force is given by $F = kx$. This viscoelastic material has an indefinitely fast relaxation rate.

the solid pore walls as the former flows through the latter, dissipating energy and retarding the response of the elastic porous-permeable solid matrix. The biphasic theory shows that the frictional drag coefficient is inversely proportional to the permeability coefficient, which may be measured experimentally, as shown below. The biphasic model has provided consistent and excellent correlations between its theoretical predictions and experimental data.[8,9,55]

## Mechanical Properties of Normal Cartilage

### Compression Tests

A number of experiments have been performed to determine the intrinsic compressive modulus of the porous-permeable solid matrix and the permeability of articular cartilage. The most commonly used experiment is the confined compression test, in which the specimen is restricted to moving in only one direction.[8,9,55] Both creep and stress-relaxation measurements may be taken. Figure 8-11 depicts the biphasic creep phenomenon in this experiment. Here, the surface of the specimen is loaded by a rigid porous-permeable plate that allows free fluid exudation to occur at the surface. The rate of fluid exudation is the rate of volume loss from the tissue, thus the permeability governs the rate of compressive creep. At equilibrium, fluid movement stops, and the internal flow-induced friction vanishes. Load supported by the cartilage is then borne entirely by the elastic collagen-PG solid matrix. In this manner, the intrinsic elastic modulus of the solid matrix is deter-

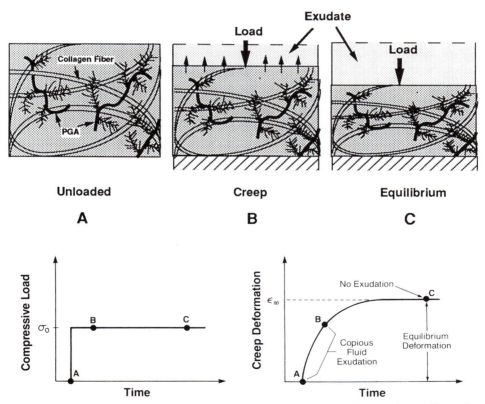

**Figure 8-11.** Illustration of the biphasic creep in the confined compression experiment. The surface of the specimen is loaded by a rigid porous-permeable plate, allowing free fluid exudation. The rate of fluid exudation is the rate of volume loss from the tissue. At equilibrium, fluid movement stops, no internal flow friction exists, and load support is borne entirely by the elastic solid matrix.

mined.[8,9,55] Note that the frictional drag associated with fluid flow produces falsely high values of the compressive modulus if measurements are taken before equilibration occurs (i.e., the "2-second modulus" proposed by Kempson and coworkers.[56]). These moduli are not to be confused with the intrinsic modulus of the solid matrix. For a 2.0-mm thick normal cartilage, it takes 20,000 seconds to reach equilibrium. Figure 8-12 provides the equilibrium or flow-independent compressive modulus of the porous-permeable solid matrix as functions of its water and proteoglycan contents.

Cartilage permeability has been calculated using the rate of creep data from the tests mentioned above.[8,9,55] It has been shown that cartilage permeability increases with water content and decreases with PG content. However, the correlations between the permeability coefficient and these cartilage components have been less significant than for the equilibrium compressive modulus.[8,9] This is because cartilage permeability is not constant but decreases as the tissue is compressed.[8,55,57] Compression decreases both the pore size of cartilage and the water content while increasing PG density; thus, tissue permeability would decrease with increased compression. These effects introduce additional confounding variables that make the simple calculation for the permeability coefficient from the compression creep data more difficult to interpret. Holmes and coworkers (1985) have developed advanced theories to account for these nonlinear changes. Reference 58 provides a detailed explanation of this theory.

### Uniaxial Tension Tests

The compression test described above assumes that cartilage is homogeneous and isotropic throughout its depth. Though these assumptions are satisfactory for the compression behavior of cartilage, they do not provide a good description of its tensile behaviors. Indeed, the tensile response of all connective tissue is strongly dependent on its collagen content and organization.[51,56,59,60] To demonstrate the inhomogeneous and anisotropic tensile response of articular cartilage, thin (about 200 μ) test strips of the tissue are "microtomed" from various layers of cartilage[51,56,59,60] in directions parallel or perpendicular to the split lines.[41,42] These tests can be performed at either a constant strain rate or as creep or stress-relaxation experiments. A slow strain rate is required to defeat the biphasic flow-dependent viscoelastic effect, so that the intrinsic tensile behavior of the collagen-PG solid matrix can be determined. The intrinsic modulus can also be determined from the equilibrium measurements of the stress-relaxation experiments.

The tensile stress-strain behavior due to a constant strain rate exhibits an initial "toe region" which is not linear, followed by a linear stress-strain response. This is the force response that develops from the straightening of the initially "crimped' or ''wavy'' collagen fibrillar organization in the specimen, and the linear response provides a measure of the true tensile stiffness of the collagen fibrils. Thus, strictly speaking, Hooke's law is not valid for this material, and Young's modulus cannot be used. For simplicity, however, many investigators have used the proportionality between the linear stress and strain response in the latter portion of the curve as a measure of cartilage stiffness,[51,56,59] referring to it as Young's modulus.

The equilibrium tensile stress-strain relationship (i.e., the flow-independent property) was found to be linear for strains up to 15%.[60,61] In general, these equilibrium modulus values are much lower than those obtained from the constant–strain rate tension tests. This difference is due to fluid pressurization in the collagen-PG solid matrix caused by the constant–strain rate test.[62] Figure 8-13 provides data on the equilibrium tensile modulus of human knee joint cartilage. Here, *HWA* and *LWA* denote cartilage specimens harvested from regions of high- and low-weight bearing.[60] All specimens were tested in the direction parallel to the predominant collagen fibers. The results show that in tension HWA cartilage is less stiff than LWA cartilage. This finding corresponds to a lower collagen-PG ratio in the HWA cartilage than in the LWA cartilage. The results also show that there is significant tissue inhomogeneity; for both

**Figure 8-12.** (A) Variation of the equilibrium or flow-independent compressive modulus of the solid matrix as functions of its water content. (B) Variation of the equilibrium or flow-independent compressive modulus of the solid matrix as a function of its PG content.

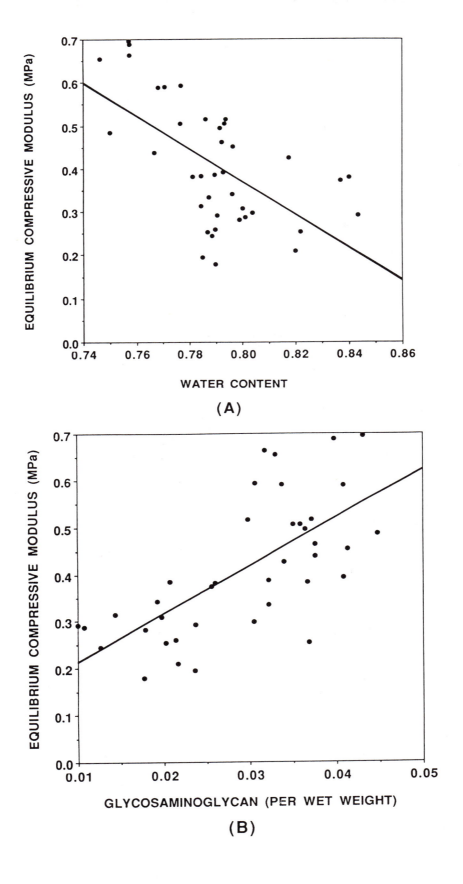

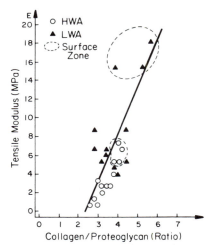

**Figure 8-13.** Variation of the equilibrium tensile modulus of human knee joint cartilage: HWA and LWA denote high and low weight-bearing areas. All specimens were tested in the direction parallel to the split line direction. (From Akizuki S, Mow VC, Muller F, et al. Tensile properties of knee joint cartilage: I. Influence of ionic conditions, weight bearing, and fibrillation on the tensile modulus. J Orthop Res 1986; 4:379–392.)

the HWA and LWA cartilage specimens the surface specimens are stiffer than those from the deeper regions. This trend is not always observed true. For immature bovine cartilage, as evidenced by the presence of a growth plate, tissues from deeper zones are as stiff as those from the surface zones.[59]

### Swelling Behavior of Cartilage

In solution, the PGs that are embedded in the collagen are both highly hydrophylic and compressible. In the extracellular matrix, the negatively charged PGs are confined to approximately 20% of their free solution volume.[10,54] The high density of negatively charged sulfate and carboxyl groups of the PGs packed into the collagen meshwork cause tissue expansion through charge-to-charge electrostatic repulsion (see Figure 8-1).[8,63,64] The high concentration of fixed charges also attracts a high molar concentration of small, freely mobile counter ions (e.g., $Na^+$) in the interstitial fluid, which, in turn, produces a large Donnan (ionic) osmotic pressure effect.[21,35,64,65] These physicochemical and electromechanical forces are the cause of water gain or loss in the tissue in response

to change in either the external ion solution or mechanical loading. The swelling pressure created by the PGs trapped in the collagen network is resisted by tension that develops in the collagen.[64,65] This balance of internal forces within the extracellular matrix dictates the equilibrium water content of the tissue, which in turn controls the cartilage's mechanical properties.

The equilibrium water content of the cartilage matrix is important: an increase in water content has long been known to be one of the earliest signs of cartilage damage due to osteoarthritis.[8–10,65–69] Such changes are detrimental to joint function, as they adversely affect the material properties of cartilage and its ability to carry load. Biochemical and biomechanical experimental evidence from studies of normal and degenerate tissue suggest that the mechanisms for increased tissue hydration are: loss of PGs, damage of collagen network, or both.

The equilibrium swelling behavior due to the change in water content and osmotic pressure associated with changes in the pH or ion concentration of the external bathing solution have been studied extensively.[20,21,35,65–69] In contrast, the kinetics of swelling has only recently been investigated.[61,63,64,70,71] The fundamental mechanism that controls cartilage swelling is the modulation of the PG domain by the concentration of counterions (e.g., $Na^+$) in solution surrounding the molecules.[10,63,64,71] Therefore, the rate of $Na^+$ diffusion into the tissue would dictate the rate of change of solution domain occupied by PG molecules. As PGs are entirely and firmly enmeshed in the collagen network[10,73] the rate of tissue swelling would be determined by the rate of $Na^+$ diffusion into the tissue.[61–64,70,74] The rate of $Na^+$ diffusion has been studied by investigators performing isometric tests in tension or compression, where the tissue sample size was maintained constant.[61,63,64,70,74] By studying the rate of change of force required to maintain the same size (isometric) with a sudden change of $Na^+$ concentration, the diffusion coefficient of the tissue may be calculated.[61,63,70,74] Figure 8-14 shows an actual stress-relaxation curve for a thin strip of canine cartilage. This cartilage was taken parallel to the local split line direction and held in isometric tension after a sudden increase of $Na^+$ concentration in the external bathing solution. The diffusion

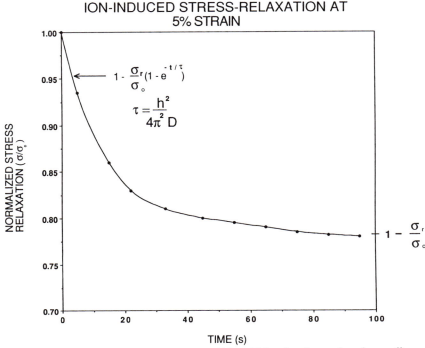

ION-INDUCED STRESS-RELAXATION AT
5% STRAIN

$$1 - \frac{\sigma_r}{\sigma_o}(1 - e^{-t/\tau})$$

$$\tau = \frac{h^2}{4\pi^2 D}$$

$$1 - \frac{\sigma_r}{\sigma_o}$$

**Figure 8-14.** A stress-relaxation curve for a 200-μ thick strip of normal canine cartilage taken parallel to the split line direction. The specimen is stretched and held in isometric tension. After a sudden increase of $Na^+$ concentration, stress relaxation occurs. This provides a method of calculating $Na^+$ diffusion coefficient in cartilage.

coefficient calculated this way for strips of tissue is very similar to those determined from radioassay studies for whole chunks of tissue.[21,36,61,63,70,74] The isometric test data demonstrate zonal variation that exists for the diffusion coefficient for cartilage.[61,70] The results of these calculations show that surface zone cartilage has the lowest diffusion coefficient ($D = 0.6 \times 10^{-9}$ $m^2$/sec). For the middle zone it is $D = 0.9 \times 10^{-9}$ $m^2$/sec and for the deep zone $D = 1.2 \times 10^{-9}$ $m^2$/sec. These variations correspond well with the variability of cartilage permeability.[8,20,21,35]

In summary, articular cartilage is a complex hydrated material that acts mechanically as a porous-permeable, fiber-reinforced composite. The cohesiveness of the solid matrix is maintained by the interactions between the collagen fibrils and PGs. The viscoelastic properties of cartilage are determined by: (1) the intrinsic viscoelastic properties of the collagen-PG solid matrix and (2) the permeability of the porous-solid matrix. The intrinsic elastic properties of the solid matrix depend on: (1) the tensile stiffness and strength of the collagen network; (2) the resistance of the PGs to compression; and (3) the swelling pressures generated by the PGs. The intrinsic properties of the solid matrix also depend on the ultrastructural arrangement of the type II collagen and various PG populations throughout the tissue. The physical and chemical interactions between these structural molecules dictate the inhomogeneities and anisotropies of its mechanical responses to loading. As a whole, this exquisite arrangement endows articular cartilage with its unique mechanical behavior, providing a load-bearing capacity that lasts throughout life. The friction-, lubrication-, and wear-related functions of the articular bearing surfaces depend on these structure-function relations.

## Lubrication of Synovial Joints

The major weight-bearing joints of the body, the hips, knees and ankles, are exposed to large ranges of relative motion in multiple directions as well as to loads that are often as great as six times body-weight during a normal gait cycle.[2,3,75] Under normal conditions, these loads must be sustained for seven or eight decades by the diarthrodial joints. These joints must have low friction and wear, as well as effective lubrication characteristics that allow them to function effectively in a physically isolated environment. In this section we deal with these biotribologic aspects of joint function. (*tribology* is the study of physics and chemistry of two interacting moving surfaces. The major components of tribology are friction, lubrication and wear. Biotribology is the study of two interacting biologic moving surfaces.)

### Friction

Friction develops when there is a relative sliding motion between two contracting surfaces. It is caused by energy-dissipating mechanisms that come from two sources, (1) interfacial shear stresses due to the adhesion of one surface to the other or viscous dissipation in the lubricant separating the two moving surfaces, and (2) internal dissipation of energy caused by viscoelasticity within the contacting bodies.[2,3] Adhesion is produced most frequently between metal surfaces, at contact points at the tips of the microirregularities of the surfaces. Internal dissipation is caused by the deformations within the bodies in contact. This is called *plowing friction*. The coefficient of friction ($\mu$) is a measure commonly used to quantify frictional resistance. It is the ratio of the magnitude of the tangential frictional force (T) that resists the motion, to the magnitude of the normal force (N) that presses the surfaces together ($\mu = T/N$).

### Lubrication

Two modes of lubrication exist between contacting surfaces, (1) boundary lubrication and (2) fluid film lubrication.[2,3] Boundary lubrication depends on the chemical adsorption of a monolayer of lubricant molecules to the contacting surfaces. During relative motion, the surfaces are protected by the lubricant molecules sliding over each other, preventing adhesion and abrasion of the naturally occurring asperities of the surface (Figure 8-15).

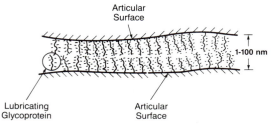

**Figure 8-15.** Boundary lubrication depends on the chemical adsorption of a monolayer of lubricant molecules to the contacting surfaces. This molecule has been isolated and is called the lubricating glycoprotein (LGP) fraction of synovial fluid.

The molecule thought to be responsible for boundary lubrication in synovial joints has been isolated and is called the *lubricating GP* (LGP) *fraction* of synovial fluid.[76,77] It consists of a single polypeptide chain containing only oligosaccharides, with a molecular weight of approximately 250 kd.

For fluid film lubrication a much thicker layer of lubricant, as compared to the molecular size of LPG, is necessary, which causes relatively wide separation of the two surfaces. The load on the bearing surface is supported by pressure generated in this fluid film. This pressure is generated in four different ways (Figure 8-16). If the noncongruent articulating surfaces are moving tangentially to each other, a converging wedge of fluid is formed (see Figure 8-16A). The viscosity of the fluid causes it to be dragged into the gap between the surfaces, generating a lifting pressure. This is known as hydrodynamic lubrication. If the surfaces are moving perpendicularly toward each other, the fluid must be squeezed out from the gap between the two surfaces, (see Figure 8-16B). The load-carrying capacity afforded by the pressure generated in the fluid film by this mechanism is known as *squeeze-film lubrication*. If the bearing material is relatively soft, like articular cartilage, then the pressure in the fluid film may cause substantial deformation of the articulating surfaces. These deformations may beneficially alter the film and surface geometry, leading to greater restriction to fluid escape, a longer-lasting fluid film, and an increase in its load-carrying capacity. This is known as elastohydrodynamic lubrication.

Alternatives to synovial fluid as a source of the lubricant have been postulated. Lubricant fluid film may be generated between the surfaces by the natural compression of the cartilage during joint

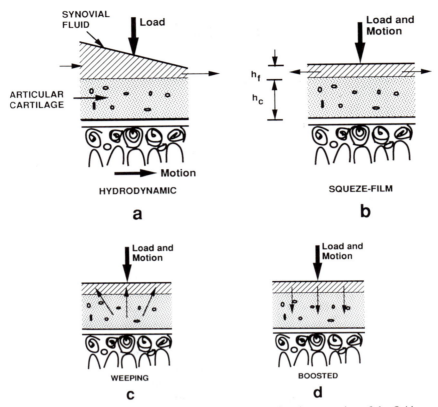

**Figure 8-16.** (*A*) Hydrodynamic lubrication is caused by the viscous action of the fluid being dragged into the gap between the two articulating surfaces. The flow of the viscous lubricant into the narrowing gap requires a hydrodynamic pressure, which in turn generates a lifting force, separating the two sliding surfaces. (*B*) The load-carrying capacity during squeeze film is generated by the hydrodynamic pressure required to force the lubricant from the gap. (*C*) The hypothesis for weeping lubrication requires cartilage to yield its interstitial fluid into the gap.[79] (From McCutchen CW. The frictional properties of animal joints. Wear 1962; 5:1.) This is an alternative source for the lubricant fluid film. (*D*) High pressure in the lubricant film causes the filtrate of synovial fluid to flow into articular cartilage.[80,81] (From Walker PS, Dowson D, Longfield MD, et al. Boosted lubrication in synovial joints by fluid entrapment and enrichment. Ann Rheum Dis 1968; 27:512–520. Walker PS, Unsworth A, Dowson D, et al. Mode of aggregation of hyaluronic acid protein complex on the surface of articular cartilage. Ann Rheum Dis 1970; 29:591–602.) This filtration process leaves a concentrated layer of hyaluronate gel in the gap, protecting the articular surfaces. This mechanism is dominant during prolonged standing.[82] (From Hou JS, Holmes MH, Lai WM, et al. Effects of changing cartilage stiffness, poisson ratio and permeability on squeeze film lubrication. Bioeng Trans ASME 1989; 103–105.)

use, exuding a fluid over the articulating surface into the joint cavity (see Figure 8-16C). This has been called *weeping lubrication*.[2,3,78,79] Since articular cartilage is porous and permeable, however, the high pressure in the fluid film also causes the synovial fluid, without the hyaluronate, to flow into the tissue, leaving a concentrated gel in the gap protecting the articulating surfaces (Figure 8-

16D). This is called *boosted lubrication*.[2,3,80,81] Recent theoretical calculations show that boosted lubrication (Figure 8-16D) is more likely to occur in the joint than weeping lubrication (Figure 8-16C).[82] As articular cartilage is not smooth, it may be that the thickness of the fluid film is of the same order of roughness as the bearing surfaces, and contact between the surface irregularities may occur (Figure 8-17). A mixed lubrication mechanism may develop, with the load being carried by both the pressure in the partial fluid film and boundary lubricated contacts.

The mode of lubrication depends on the way the load is applied as well as the relative velocities of the surfaces. Boundary lubrication is important when microsurface asperities of the surfaces come into contact or when, under prolonged severe loading conditions, the fluid film is depleted. At high speeds and low loads, fluid-film lubrication is likely to be in the form of either the hydrodynamic or elastohydrodynamic models. Loads applied suddenly may be supported for a time by a squeeze film mechanism.[2,3] Evidence about the likely mode of lubrication in diarthrodial joints can be obtained from experimental measurements of the coefficient of friction.

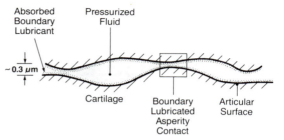

**Figure 8-17.** The surface roughness of normal articular cartilage (less than 50μ) is similar to the thickness of the lubricant film in the gap. Contact between the surface irregularities may occur, causing a mixed mode of lubrication—boundary and fluid film.

### Measurements of Coefficient of Friction

As stated above, friction has two components: (1) shear stresses on the two surfaces sliding over each other and (2) plowing (deformation) of the two surfaces. In boundary lubrication, the shear stresses are independent of the relative velocity of the two surfaces. If a fluid film exists, changes will be observed in the coefficient of friction, resulting from changes in either the relative velocity or the applied load. Investigators have employed these basic characteristics to determine modes of lubrication at the articular surfaces.[2,3] However, if a mixed lubrication mechanism is in place, as is most likely in articular cartilage, gross friction measurements alone will not be sufficient to determine the mode of lubrication.

The coefficient of friction in intact synovial joints is extremely low (Table 8-1). The original experiments used a pendulum machine; the joint acts as the fulcrum.[2,83,84] Investigators soon learned, however, that such measurements were not sensitive enough to enable them to differentiate between mechanisms of lubrication. Their results suggested the existence of a fluid film at loads up to body weight.[83,84] They also noted that in an unlubricated joint, the coefficient of friction rapidly returned to normal as load was applied (Figure 8-18). This implies that at physiologic loads either the fluid film is being generated by the cartilage itself or boundary lubrication is occurring.

Another experimental design used for friction testing is one[79,85] that slides small pieces of cartilage over another surface (Figure 8-19). In these experiments the entire surface is loaded, eliminating the plowing effect.[85] In this study, Malcom found that synovial fluid caused less friction than a buffer lubricant and that there was a much greater

**Table 8-1.** Coefficient of Friction in Synovial Joints Lubricated with Synovial Fluid

| Investigator (year) | Coefficient of Friction | Joint |
|---|---|---|
| Barnett and Cobbold (1962) | 0.015–0.03 | Canine ankle |
| Charnley (1960) | 0.005–0.02 | Human knee |
| Clark et al. (1975) | 0.01 –0.03 | Human hip |
| Linn (1968) | 0.005–0.01 | Canine ankle |
| Radin and Paul (1971) | 0.009–0.03 | Bovine ankle |
| Swanson (1973) | 0.003–0.01 | Human hip |
| Unsworth et al. (1975) | 0.01 –0.04 | Human hip |

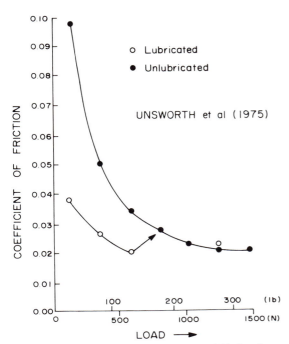

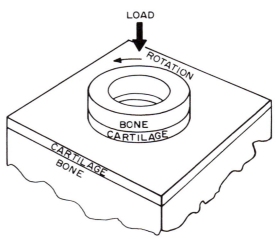

**Figure 8-18.** Comparison of coefficients of friction for an unlubricated hip and a lubricated hip at various load levels.[84] (Unsworth A, Dowson D, Wright V. The frictional behavior of human synovial joints: I. Natural joints. J Lubr Tech ASME 1975; 97:360–376.) At physiologic load levels, the coefficient of friction of the unlubricated hip approaches that of the lubricated hip.

**Figure 8-19.** Another experimental design used for measuring the surface friction of cartilage.[85] (Malcom LL. An Experimental Investigation of the Frictional and Deformational Responses of Articular Cartilage Interfaces to Static and Dynamic Loading, PhD Thesis, University of California, San Diego, 1976.) In this experiment the entire surface of one specimen is sliding over the other, thus eliminating friction due to plowing.

reduction in friction if the vertical loads were oscillated rather than held static (Figure 8-20). This second effect was thought to be due to the expression of interstitial fluid from the cartilage; thus, the lubrication mechanism is changed from boundary to fluid film.

In summary, synovial joints are able to function under a wide range of loading and moving conditions, such as (1) lightly loaded high-speed motions, (e.g., the swing phase of gait); (2) loads of large magnitude and short duration (e.g., jumping); and (3) fixed steady loads (e.g., standing for long periods). These joints enjoy remarkable lubricating mechanisms in place, allowing them to function with almost negligible resistance in practically any situation. It is unlikely that such varied demands can be satisfied by a single mode of lubrication. Elastohydrodynamic fluid films of both the sliding and squeeze type probably play a vital role in the lubrication of the joint. The source

of the fluid film appears to come from both synovial fluid and interstitial fluid of the extracellular matrix. As the loading conditions become more severe, the rate of fluid movement slowly deceases. The joint, though, can remain protected through an adsorbed layer of boundary lubricant. It is impossible, however, to state under which conditions a particular lubrication mechanism may be in effect. It is possible that a combination of mechanisms may be operating at any one time. It must be remembered, however, that currently no comprehensive theory exists to describe diarthrodial joint function.

## Response of Cartilage to Immobilization

Immobilization of a joint results in removal of the normal physiologic loading conditions of the joint and cartilage. Clinically, this may involve a loss of motion (e.g., plaster immobilization for fracture healing), loss of normal joint loading (e.g., prolonged bed rest), paralysis of a limb, or a combination of these situations. The lack of clinical specimens has generally precluded studies of human material.[86,87] The few that have been done

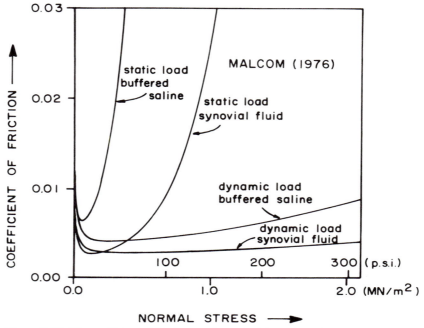

**Figure 8-20.** The coefficient of friction, as determined from the Malcom experiment.

have shown significant changes in the morphology and biochemistry of the cartilage. Therefore, a number of animal models have been developed to examine the effects of immobilization on articular cartilage.[88–92]

Palmoski and coworkers and others found that after 8 weeks' immobilization the gross appearance of the cartilage was normal—white and smooth.[93,94] There were no synovial effusions, and the x-ray appearance was normal except for slight bone demineralization. In spite of the grossly normal appearance, progressive loss of staining by safranin O indicated a reduction in the content of PG in the cartilage. This was accompanied by a reduction in PG synthesis and gradual but complete loss of PG aggregation. This aggregation defect appeared to be in the hyaluronate-binding region of the core protein. There was also atrophy of the cartilage, with a 30% to 50% decrease in its thickness and a reduction in the number of cells per unit area. After 3 weeks' immobilization, the water content had already increased by 20%. Other investigators have found the surface characteristics of the cartilage to be disturbed after as little as 1 week of immobilization.[31,90]

It has been observed that all of these changes are completely reversible after ad lib remobilization. Palmoski found that cartilage appeared to recover within 2 weeks, becoming indistinguishable from control specimens.[33] With remobilization, the chondrocytes are stimulated to increase production of the PG monomers and link proteins.[33,34] With the hyaluronate present, these molecules are assembled into PG aggregates again, restoring cartilage to its original form. Laboratory results have shown recovery of cartilage after immobilization, although motion of the joint without loading is insufficient for recovery.[33,88] Excessive mechanical loading, such as running after removal of a cast, also inhibits reversal of atrophic changes in knee cartilage.[93] In some cases it may take 8 to 12 weeks for cartilage to recover and revert to normal.[34,91,95] Recovery is stimulated by joint function and loading. Sometimes, despite the increased synthesis of PGs by the chondrocytes, PG synthesis is insufficient to maintain normal homeostasis. The newly synthesized PGs are lost, either because they cannot aggregate appropriately with the hyaluronate in the tissue or because the collagen network is damaged or weakened.

A few investigators have directly addressed the effects of immobilization on the intrinsic tensile properties of the collagen network of articular cartilage. Setton and associates used an isometric tension test to determine the flow-independent tensile modulus and diffusion coefficient of cartilage from canine knees that were subjected to 4 weeks' immobilization.[96] Specimens were taken from the lateral femoral condyle (LFC) and the patellofemoral groove (PFG). The equilibrium tensile modulus of the LFC cartilage of the immobilized joints was significantly lower than the controls', and this reduction in tensile stiffness was associated with a significant reduction in the ratio of hexuronate to hydroxyproline. For cartilage specimens from the PFG, where there is ongoing contact loading despite immobilization, the tensile modulus remained unchanged. Jurvelin and coworkers found similar results performing indentation tests on immobilized canine cartilage, with the compressive modulus decreasing between 17% and 25%.[31] They also noted the smallest reductions in the compressive stiffness in the patellofemoral groove. Recent findings by Pita and coworkers support the hypothesis that immobilization results in PG disaggregation and loss of PG monomers from the tissue, with hyaluronate remaining in the collagen network.[32] Recovery from immobilization-induced atrophic changes requires that newly synthesized PG monomers aggregate with the hyaluronate. If the collagen is damaged, as evidenced by the tensile studies of Setton and coworkers, the hyaluronate will also be lost, in which case recovery is not possible.

In summary, local mechanical factors, in the form of both joint loading and joint motion, appear to play important physiologic roles in the maintenance of normal articular cartilage. The changes described in these models of immobilization bear a striking resemblance to those seen in the experimental models of osteoarthritis described in the next section, though changes due to immobilization appear to be reversible under certain conditions whereas osteoarthritic changes are progressive with time. Thus, immobilization alone may not be a good osteoarthritis model. Immobilization, in combination with strenuous exercise, may prove to be a more accurate model of osteoarthritis, though this model has not been studied extensively.

## Response of Cartilage to Aging and Osteoarthritis

It has been shown that articular cartilage is a remarkable structure that can withstand large cyclic loads of many times body weight over decades of use without significant deterioration in function. However, loss of joint stability due to permanent strains around the joint (e.g., collateral and cruciate ligaments around the knee), loading that is excessive in light of past injuries, or loss of range of motion, may lead to cartilage damage, and eventually to osteoarthritis.[4–7] Osteoarthritis is a disabling disease affecting one joint or many. The morbidity and economic costs resulting from osteoarthritis are staggering when measured in terms of loss of function, medical costs, and lost wages. At present, it is estimated that more than 35 million Americans suffer this disabling disease.

How does osteoarthritis develop when there is no obvious antecedent injury to either the joint or the cartilage? This question has been studied extensively but no clear answers have been found. In this section the changes that occur in articular cartilage during this degenerative process are presented, followed by some thoughts on the etiology of osteoarthritis.

### Histologic and Morphologic Changes

Macroscopic evidence of osteoarthritis can be observed on gross examination of the cartilage surface. The earliest findings in osteoarthritis include flaking and pitting of the surface.[4–7,97] As the degenerative process continues, deep fissuring occurs, giving the cartilage a frayed appearance known as *cartilage fibrillation*. The final stage of this process is a completely denuded surface exposing the underlying eburnated bone (Figure 8-21).

Attempts have been made to quantify the amount of surface damage. Emery and Meachim described a technique in which the cartilage surface is stained with India ink and then rinsed off lightly with Ringer's solution.[97] Ink particles lodge in any surface irregularities, causing a dark stain. The degree of staining can then be graded as minimal, moderate, or severe, providing a macroscopic view of articular surface damage. Micro-

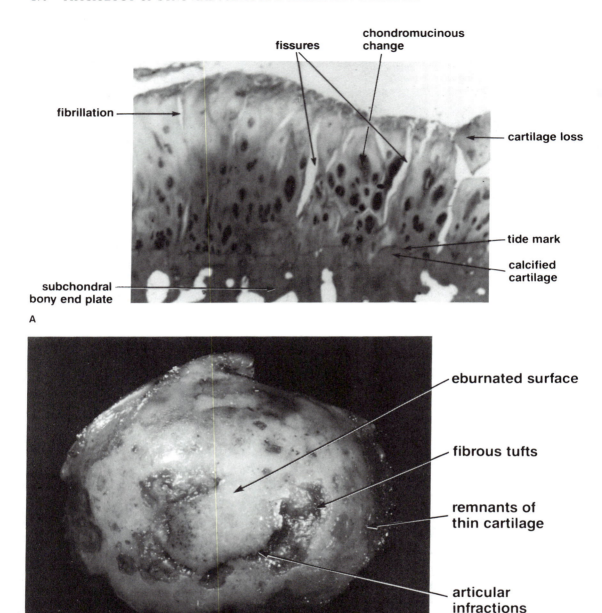

**Figure 8-21.** (*A*) Typical histologic appearance of advanced stages of osteoarthritic cartilage showing surface disruptions, deep fissures, chondrocyte cloning, and loss of metachromasia. (*B*) Photograph shows the sclerotic and eburnated bony surface on the humeral head, where all the articular cartilage has been worn off. Fibrous tufts are often evident on such bony surfaces.

scopically, cellular injury may be evident, showing only the ghost outlines of the chondrocytes remaining. The structural integrity may change microscopically, with clefts and fissures that traverse the ECM. There also may be loss of PGs, as noted on safranin O staining. Finally, there is loss of tidemark integrity as blood vessels cross the tidemark to affect a reparative response. Mankin and coworkers developed a semiquantitative grading scheme to evaluate the histologic and histochemical changes in the cartilage (see Table 8-2). These scores are generally accepted as providing a semiquantitative measure of cartilage degeneration during osteoarthritis.[4,5,98]

Microscopic evidence also exists that demonstrates the presence of reparative cartilage in osteoarthritis. This reparative cartilage comes from two sources: (1) the damaged cartilage itself, in the form of cell proliferation and new matrix synthesis, and (2) tissue outside the joint, located on the periphery of the joint, the subchondral bone, or both.[5–7] Cartilage from the joint margin may be seen as a cellular layer of cartilage extending over, or dissecting into, existing cartilage. From denuded bone, small nodules of fibrocartilage develop (see Figure 8-21B).[99,100] Microscopically, fibrocartilage is a fibrous-appearing tissue in which the cells are spindlelike, with a higher density within the tissue. The collagen formed is much more likely type I than type II.[101] In some joints these nodules of fibrocartilage may form an apparently continuous layer of tissue over the denuded surface (see the fibrous tufts in Figure 8-21B).

Osteoarthritis is a disease that begins in the articular cartilage but eventually involves the surrounding tissues, bone, and synovium. When the cartilage is absent from the articular surface, the underlying bone is subject to greater local stresses. By Wolff's law of bone remodeling, new bone formation at these areas is expected, resulting in the bony sclerosis that is often seen on radiographs of arthritic joints.[102] Subarticular bone cysts are also commonly seen on x-rays. They exist only in the absence of overlying cartilage. Bone cysts are a result of the transmission of intraarticular pressure into the narrow spaces of the subchondral bone. The cysts increase in size until the pressure in them is equal to the intraarticular pressure. If the joint becomes covered with reparative cartilage, the cysts may regress.[103] Finally, because of the breakdown of both cartilage and bone,[4,5] a chronic inflammatory response is produced in the synovium of the joint.

It should be remembered that joint function depends on the anatomy of the entire joint. The reparative changes that are observed are directed towards restoration of joint anatomy, presumably to increase joint stability. Remodeling of the bone occurs at the joint margins through the formation of osteophytes. Osteophytes form as a result of enchondral ossification of both the existing cartilage and reparative cartilage from the joint margin. Remodeling of the joint can be considerable. The presence of osteophytes in clinically asymptomatic joints confirms that this reparative process can be effective in increasing joint stability.[4]

**Table 8-2.** Histologic Grading System of Mankin and Coworkers[99]

|  | Grade |
|---|---|
| I. Structure | |
| a. Normal | 0 |
| b. Surface irregularities | 1 |
| c. Pannus and surface irregularities | 2 |
| d. Clefts to transitional zone | 3 |
| e. Clefts to radial zone | 4 |
| f. Clefts to calcified zone | 5 |
| g. Complete disorganization | 6 |
| II. Cells | |
| a. Normal | 0 |
| b. Diffuse hypercellularity | 1 |
| c. Cloning | 2 |
| d. Hypocellularity | 3 |
| III. Safranin O staining | |
| a. Normal | 0 |
| b. Slight reduction | 1 |
| c. Moderate reduction | 2 |
| d. Severe reduction | 3 |
| e. No stain noted | 4 |
| IV. Tidemark integrity | |
| a. Intact | 0 |
| b. Crossed by blood vessels | 1 |

From Bennett GA, Bauer W, Maddock SJ. A A study of the repair of articular cartilage and the reaction of normal joints of adult dogs to surgically created defects of articular cartilage, "joint mice" and patellar displacement. Am J Pathol 1932; 8:499–524.

### Biochemical Aspects of Osteoarthritis

The earliest changes in the development of osteoarthritis in humans have not been elucidated because specimens cannot be obtained early in the process. Only when the disease has advanced so far that surgery is being contemplated are the remnants of cartilage available for testing. Therefore, experimental animal models have been designed to mimic the development of human osteoarthritis.[104–111] These models allow examination of early osteoarthritic changes in cartilage, and afford access to control tissue from the same animal. A large variety of animal models have been developed. All produce alterations in the normal mechanics of the joint, usually the knee, by sectioning of ligaments, removal of a meniscus and other tissues, or repetitive, impulsive loading and impact, to create osteoarthritic lesions in the cartilage. One of the most commonly used animal models is described by Pond and Nuki: the anterior cruciate ligament is surgically resected, resulting in joint instability.[105] The progressive changes in cartilage histology and biochemistry are very similar to those seen in early human osteoarthritis.[106] This model has been demonstrated to be both reliable and reproducible.

The earliest changes seen in this model are an increase in tissue water content and enhanced extractability of the PGs. This response is followed by progressive loss of the PGs from the extracellular matrix and altered biomechanical properties. These biochemical and biomechanical changes are seen throughout the cartilage and precede any gross degenerative changes.[107,111–113] Subsequently, it has been suggested that the chondrocytes revert to a metabolically immature stage.[5–7] As in the immobilization model, the chondrocytes in this cartilage, despite an elevated metabolic level, are unable to stop the loss of PGs, possibly owing to the disruption of the collagen network. The effects of early osteoarthritis on the collagen network have also been studied morphologically.[114] Collagenase was noted to be present in cartilage 2 weeks after surgery, and total collagenolytic activity was significantly more pronounced in the diseased cartilage. As a correlation, electron microscopy demonstrates disruption of the collagen in the midzone cartilage as early as 2 weeks postoperatively.

The progression of all these changes simulates the changes in human osteoarthritis. Metabolic studies on human cartilage in which osteoarthritis is present have shown increases in both anabolism and catabolism when compared to normal cartilage. Though the rate of synthesis of PG in osteoarthritic cartilage is elevated, the half-life of these new PGs is reduced compared to controls.[115] Investigators have described several agents that may interrupt the normal metabolic equilibrium. These include the cytokines interleukin 1 and tumor necrosis factor. In culture both substances increase the rate of PG loss and inhibit biosynthesis.[116] Low levels of interleukin 1 are normally found in the synovial fluid of osteoarthritic joints. The cytokine response may be activated by the inflammatory response that develops in the synovium, perpetuating the cartilage damage.

## Effects of Osteoarthritis on Biomechanical Properties of Cartilage

The mechanical properties of normal articular cartilage have been studied in depth and were reviewed earlier in this chapter. The potential loss of the ability to withstand daily stresses remains a central issue. It is vital to know how the mechanical properties of the cartilage change with age and degeneration and how they correlate with the biochemical composition of the tissue.

### Effects of Age

Roth and Mow examined the variation of the intrinsic tensile modulus of normal bovine articular cartilage with age, as determined by an open or closed joint physis.[59] They found significant differences in the failure stress of the open and closed physis groups. For cartilage from the open physis group, the failure stress of the surface was 12 MPa and that of the deep zone was 24.5 MPa. For cartilage from the closed physis group, these values were 12 MPa for the surface and 3 MPa for the deep zone. No statistical differences were found for the tensile strength of the superficial zone. These findings indicate that, with aging, the subsurface levels of the cartilage may become mechanically inferior compared to the surface layer. Armstrong and Mow examined the intrinsic compressive properties of human articular cartilage over a wide spectrum of age and disease.[9] They found that the equilibrium compressive modulus decreased with increasing age. However, Sokoloff did not find changes in either the compressive modulus or the water content with aging.[117] Thus, it may be concluded that the decrease of compressive modulus observed by Armstrong and Mow is due to a pathologic increase in water content, as seen in osteoarthritis.

### Effects of Degeneration

Many changes take place in the mechanical responses of cartilage during the degenerative process. Armstrong and Mow showed significant negative associations between the compressive mechanical properties of cartilage and its water content. As shown above, the modulus, as well as the frictional resistance, decreased significantly with increasing water content, but there was no correlation between increased water content and any of the light microscopic histologic grades (Table 8-3).

Akizuki and coworkers performed isometric tension tests on normal, fibrillated, and osteoarthritic specimens of human knee cartilage to determine the swelling- and flow-independent tensile properties of the collagen-PG solid matrix.[60,70] Though there was no significant decrease in the flow-independent tensile modulus between normal and mildly fibrillated cartilage, there was a trend in this direction. Dramatic decreases were observed from the cartilage adjacent to frank osteoar-

thritis lesions.[60] The swelling parameters are defined as the stress peak ($\sigma_p$) and stress relaxation ($\sigma_r$) for these human knee cartilage specimens.[70] The magnitude of $\sigma_p$ is a measure of PG movement in the collagen-PG solid matrix, and $\sigma_r$ is a measure of the stiffness of the collagen network. In fibrillated cartilage there was a general increase in $\sigma_p$ and a decrease in $\sigma_r$. Thus, the results of these swelling studies confirm the notion that PG are more mobile in osteoarthritic cartilage and the collagen network is less stiff and strong.

### Biochemical and Biomechanical Correlations

Correlations have been made between the intrinsic tensile modulus and a number of biochemical parameters.[60] As discussed earlier, for normal knee joint cartilage there are strong correlations, either positive or negative, between the tensile modulus and some major biochemical parameters (e.g., collagen content, hexosamine content, and collagen-proteoglycan ratio). In abnormal tissue these correlations disappear, except with the collagen-PG ratio for fibrillated specimens. These data show that the highest tensile modulus, and the highest collagen-PG ratio, occurs in the surface zone, where the PG is least concentrated.

The statistical correlations between the swelling parameters and the biomechanical parameters also change considerably when abnormal tissue is

**Table 8-3.** Summary of Statistically Significant Positive ( + ) and Negative ( − ) Correlations Between Age, Histologic Grade, India-Ink Staining, Water Content, Thickness, Permeability, and Compressive Modulus[9]

|  | Age | Permeability | Modulus | Thickness |
|---|---|---|---|---|
| Age |  |  | − |  |
| Thickness |  | + + + |  |  |
| Histologic grade |  |  |  |  |
| I | + + + |  | − |  |
| II |  |  |  |  |
| III | + + |  |  |  |
| IV | + |  |  |  |
| Total | + + + |  |  |  |
| India-ink staining | + + + |  |  |  |
| Water content | + + | + + + | − − − | + + |

tested.[60,70] These data support the hypotheses that (1) collagen is important for the tensile properties of articular cartilage; (2) PG is important for the compressive and fluid flow properties of the tissue; and (3) the collagen-PG ratio is important for the shear properties and the cohesiveness of the ECM.

## Factors in the Etiology of Osteoarthritis

Articular cartilage, despite its ability to stand up to decades of use, has some limited capacity to repair itself. This allows the joint to function in a normal capacity when injured or involved by osteoarthritis. At present there is no clear, concise theory to explain the development of osteoarthritis. How the earliest changes in osteoarthritis take place—increased water content and weakening of the ECM of the cartilage—remains a mystery. The surface layer of the cartilage appears to play an important role in maintaining the structural integrity of the cartilage as a whole. When the surface layer is disrupted, the remaining zones of the cartilage, as well as the subchondral bone, may be subjected to much higher stresses than normal, leading to further cartilage destruction. Mechanical and chemical changes during osteoarthritis appear to act in concert, making it impossible, at present, to determine a single causative factor for osteoarthritis. Ongoing research into the etiology of osteoarthritis continues in the various animal models and with the microscopic, biochemical, and biomechanical studies described in this chapter. Our understanding of joint pathology has increased immensely over the past two decades. Scientists do not yet have complete answers, but there is hope that the cause and cure for osteoarthritis can be found. Readers are advised to study some of the literature cited in this chapter to share the excitement of scientific discoveries now occurring in this field of biomedical research.

## References

1. Goss CM. Gray's Anatomy of the Human Body. Philadelphia: Lea & Febiger, 1972
2. Dowson D. Basic tribology. In: Dowson D, Wright V, eds. Introduction to the Biomechanics of Joints and Joint Replacement. London: Mechanical Engineering Publications, 1981; 49–60.
3. Mow VC, Mak AF. Lubrication of diarthrodial joints. In: Skalak R, Chein S, eds. Handbook of Bioengineering. New York: McGraw-Hill, 1986; 5.1–5.34.
4. Howell DS. Etiopathogenesis of osteoarthritis. In: Moskowitz RW, Howell DS, Goldberg VM, et al. eds. Osteoarthritis: Diagnosis and Management. Philadelphia: WB Saunders, 1984; 129–146.
5. Buckwalter JA, Rosenberg LC, Hunziker EB. Articular cartilage: Composition structure, response to injury and methods of facilitating repair. In: Ewing JW, ed. Articular Cartilage and Knee Joint Function: Basic Science and Arthroscopy. New York: Raven Press, 1990; 19–56.
6. Mankin HJ. The reaction of articular cartilage to injury and osteoarthritis: Part I. N Engl J Med 1974; 291:1285–1292.
7. Mankin HJ. The reaction of articular cartilage to injury and osteoarthritis: Part II. N Engl J Med 1974; 291:1335–1340.
8. Mow VC, Holmes MH, Lai WM. Fluid transport and mechanical properties of articular cartilage. J Biomech 1984; 17:377–394.
9. Armstrong CG, Mow VC. Variations in the intrinsic mechanical properties of human articular cartilage with age, degeneration, and water content. J Bone Joint Surg 1982; 64A:88–94.
10. Muir H. Proteoglycans as organizers of the extracellular matrix. Biochem Soc Trans 1983; 11:613–622.
11. Hardingham TE. Proteoglycans: Their structure, interactions and molecular organization in cartilage. Biochem Soc Trans 1981; 9:489–497.
12. Poole AR, Pidoux I, Reiner A, et al. Immuno-electron microscope study of the organization of proteoglycan monomer, link protein and collagen in the matrix of articular cartilage. J Cell Biol 1982; 93:921–937.
13. Buckwalter JA, Hunziker EB, Rosenberg LC, et al. Articular cartilage: Composition and structure. In: Woo SL, Buckwalter JA, eds. Injury and Repair of the Musculoskeletal Soft Tissues. Park Ridge, Ill: American Academy of Orthopaedic Surgeons, 1988; 405–425.
14. Lipshitz H, Glimcher MJ. In-vitro studies of the wear of articular cartilage. II. Characteristics of the wear of articular cartilage when worn against stainless steel plates having characterized surfaces. Wear 1979; 52:297–339.
15. Balazs EA, Watson C, Duff IF, et al. Hyaluronic acid in synovial fluid: I. Molecular parameters of hyaluronic acid in normal and arthritic human fluids. Arthritis Rheum 1967; 10:357–376.

16. Sundblad L. In: Balazs EA, Jeanloz RW, eds. The Amino Sugars, Glycosaminoglycans and Glycoproteins in Synovial Fluid. New York: Academic Press, 1965; 229–250.

17. Bloch B, Dintenfass L. Rheological study of human synovial fluid. Aust NZ J Surg 1963; 33:108–113.

18. Lai WM, Kuei SC, Mow VC. Rheological equations for synovial fluids. J Biomech, ASME 1978; 100:169–186.

19. Schurz J, Ribitsch V. Rheology of synovial fluid. Biorheology 1989; 24:385–399.

20. Maroudas A, Bullough P, Swanson SAV, et al. The permeability of articular cartilage, J Bone Joint Surg 1968; 50B:166–177.

21. Maroudas A. Biophysical chemistry of cartilaginous tissues with special reference to solute and fluid transport. Biorheology 1975; 12:233–248.

22. Simon WH. Scale effects in animal joints. I. Articular cartilage thickness and compressive stress. Arthritis Rheum 1970; 13:244–256.

23. Soslowsky LJ, Ateshian GA, Pollock RG, et al. An in-situ method to determine diarthrodial joint contact areas using stereophoto-grammetry. Adv Bioeng ASME 1989; 129–130.

24. Stockwell RA. The cell density of human articular and costal cartilage. J Anat 1967; 101:753–763.

25. Eyre DR. Collagen: Molecular diversity in the body's protein scaffold. Science 1980; 207:1315–1322.

26. Nimni ME, Harkness RD. Molecular structure and functions of collagen. In: Nimni ME, ed. Collagen. Boca Raton, Fla: CRC Press, 1988; I:1–78.

27. Mow VC, Zhu W, Lai WM, et al. Link protein effects on proteoglycan viscometric flow properties. Biochem Biophys Acta 1989; 112:201–208.

28. Buckwalter JA, Rosenberg LC. Structural changes during development in bovine fetal epiphyseal cartilage. Collagen Rel Res 1983; 3:489–504.

29. Buckwalter JA, Kuettner KE, Thonar EJM. Age-related changes in articular cartilage proteoglycans: Electron microscopic studies. J Orthop Res 1985; 3:251-257.

30. Kiviranta I, Jurvelin J, Tammi M, et al. Weight-bearing controls glycosaminoglycan concentration and articular cartilage thickness in the knee joints of young beagle dogs. Arthritis Rheum 1987; 30:801–809.

31. Jurvelin J, Kiviranta I, Tammi M, et al. Softening of canine articular cartilage after immobilization of the knee joint. Clin Orthop Res; 207:246–252.

32. Pita JC, Manicourt DH, Muller FJ. Centrifugal and biochemical comparison of two populations of proteoglycan aggregates from articular cartilage of immobilized dog joints. Trans Orthop Res Soc 1990; 15,17.

33. Palmoski M, Perricone E, Brandt KD. Development and reversal of a proteoglycan aggregation defect in normal canine knee cartilage after immobilization. Arthritis Rheum 1979; 22:508–517.

34. Tammi M, Paukkonen K, Kiviranta I, et al. Joint loading–induced alterations in articular cartilage. In: Helminen HJ, et al., eds. Joint Loading. Bristol: Wright, 1987; 64–88.

35. Maroudas A. Physicochemical properties of articular cartilage. In: Freeman MAR, ed. Articular Cartilage. Tunbridge Wells, England: Pitman Medical, 1979; 215–290.

36. Torzilli PA, Rose DE, Dethmers DA. Equilibrium water partition in articular cartilage. Biorheology 1982; 19:519–537.

37. Lipshitz H, Etheredge R, Glimcher MJ. Changes in the hexosamine content and swelling ratio of articular cartilage as functions of depth from the surface. J Bone Joint Surg 1976; 58A:1149–1153.

38. Clark IC. Articular cartilage: A review and scanning electron microscope study—1. The interterritorial fibrillar architecture. J Bone Joint Surg 1971; 53B:732–750.

39. Lane JM, Weiss C. Review of articular cartilage collagen research. Arthritis Rheum 1975; 18:553–562.

40. Redler I, Zimny ML, Mansell J, et al. The ultrastructure and biomechanical significance of the tidemark of articular cartilage. Clin Orthop 1975; 112:357–362.

41. Hultkrantz W. Ueber die Spaltrichtungen der Gelenkknorpel. Ver Anat Gesellschaft 1898; 12:248–256.

42. Benninghoff A. Form und Bau der Gelenkknorpel in ihren Beziehungen zur Funktion: Zweiter Teil. Der Aufbau des Gelenkknorpels in seinen Beziehungen zur Funktion. Z Zellforsch Mikrosk Anat 1925; 2:783–862.

43. Gardner DL, MacGillivray DC. Living articular cartilage is not smooth. Ann Rheum Dis 1971; 30:3–9.

44. Brown TD, Shaw DT. In-vitro contact stress distributions in the natural hip. J Biomech 1983; 16:373–384.

45. Brown T, Shaw DT. In-vitro contact stress distribution on the femoral condyles. J Orthop Res 1984; 2:190–199.

46. Ahmed AM, Burke DL. In-vitro measurement of static pressure distribution in synovial joints—Part I: Tibial surface of the knee. J Biomech Eng 1983; 105:216–225.

47. Ahmed AM, Burke DL. In-vitro measurement of static pressure distribution in synovial joints—Part

II: Retropatellar surface. J Biomech Eng 1983; 105:226–236.

48. Hayes WC, Mockros LF. Viscoelastic properties of human articular cartilage. J Appl Physiol 1971; 31:562-568.

49. Fung YC. Biomechanics: Mechanical Properties of Living Tissues. New York: Springer-Verlag, 1981.

50. Sprit AA, Mak AF, Wassell RP. Nonlinear viscoelastic properties of articular cartilage in shear. J Orthop Res 1988; 7:43–49.

51. Woo SL-Y, Mow VC, Lai WM. Biomechanical properties of articular cartilage. In: Skalak R, Chein S, eds. Handbook of Bioengineering. New York: McGraw-Hill, 1987; 4.1–4.44.

52. Fessler JH. A structural function of mucopolysaccharide in connective tissue. Biochem J 1960; 76:124–132.

53. Linn FC, Sokoloff L. Movement and composition of interstitial fluid of cartilage. Arthritis Rheum 1965; 8:481–494.

54. Edwards J. Physical characteristic of articular cartilage. Proc Inst Mech Eng (Lond) 1967; 181:16–24.

55. Mow VC, Kuei SC, Lai WM, et al. Biphasic creep and stress relaxation of articular cartilage in compression: Theory and experiments. J Biomech Eng 1980; 102:73–84.

56. Kempson GE Mechanical properties of articular cartilage. In: Freeman MAR, ed. Adult Articular Cartilage, ed. 2. Tunbridge Wells, England: Pitman, 1979; 333–414.

57. Mansour JM, Mow VC. The permeability of articular cartilage under compressive strain and at high pressures. J Bone Joint Surg 1976; 58A:509–516.

58. Holmes MH, Lai MW, Mow VC. Singular perturbation analysis of the nonlinear, flow-dependent, compressive stress-relaxation behavior of articular cartilage. J Biomech Eng 1985; 107:206–218.

59. Roth V, Mow VC. The intrinsic tensile behavior of the matrix of bovine articular cartilage and its variation with age. J Bone Joint Surg 1980; 62A:1102–1117.

60. Akizuki S, Mow VC, Muller F, et al. Tensile properties of knee joint cartilage: I. Influence of ionic conditions, weight bearing, and fibrillation on the tensile modulus. J Orthop Res 1986; 4:379–392.

61. Myers ER, Lai WM, Mow VC. A continuum theory and an experiment for the ion-induced swelling behavior of articular cartilage. J Biomech Eng 1984; 106:151–158.

62. Li JT, Armstrong CG, Mow VC. The effect of strain rate on mechanical properties of articular cartilage in tension. Symp Biomech ASME 1983; AMD56:9–12.

63. Eisenberg SR, Grodzinsky AJ. Swelling of articular cartilage and other connective tissues: Electromechanochemical forces. J Orthop Res 1985; 3:148–159.

64. Lai WM, Hou JS, Mow VC. A triphasic theory for articular cartilage swelling. Proc Biomech Symp ASME 1989; AMD98:33–36.

65. Maroudas A. Balance between swelling pressure and collagen tension in normal and degenerate cartilage. Nature 1976; 260:808–809.

66. Bollett AJ, Nance JL. Biochemical findings in normal and osteoarthritic articular cartilage. 2. Chondroitin sulfate concentration and chain length, water and ash content. J Clin Invest 1966; 45:1170–1177.

67. Maroudas A, Venn M. Chemical composition and swelling of normal and osteoarthritic femoral head cartilage. II: Swelling. Ann Rheum Dis 1977; 36:399–406.

68. Jaffe FF, Mankin HJ, Weiss C, et al. Water binding in the articular cartilage of rabbits. J Bone Joint Surg 1974; 56A:1031–1039.

69. Mankin HJ. The water of articular cartilage. In: Simon WH, ed. The Human Joint in Health and Disease. Philadelphia: University of Pennsylvania Press, 1978; 37–42.

70. Akizuki S, Mow VC, Muller F, et al. The tensile properties of human knee joint cartilage II: The influence of weight bearing, and tissue pathology on the kinetics of swelling. J Orthop Res 1987; 5:173–186.

71. Myers ER, Armstrong CG, Mow VC. Swelling pressure and collagen tension. In: Hukins DWL, ed. Connective Tissue Matrix. London: MacMillian Press, 1984; 161–168.

72. Pasternack SG, Veis A, Breen M. Solvent-dependent changes in proteoglycan subunit conformation in aqueous guanidine hydrochloride solutions. J Biol Chem 1974; 239:2206–2211.

73. Pottenger LA, Lyon NB, Hecht JD, et al. Influence of cartilage particle size and proteoglycan aggregation on immobilization of proteoglycans. J Biol Chem 1982; 257:11479–11485.

74. Grodzinsky AJ, Roth V, Myers ER, et al. The significance of electromechanical and osmotic forces in the non-equilibrium swelling behavior of articular cartilage in tension. J Biomech Eng 1981; 103:221–231.

75. Paul JP. Joint kinetics. In: Sokoloff L, ed. The Joints and Synovial Fluid, vol II. New York: Academic Press, 1978; 146–176.

76. Radin EL, Swann DA, Weisser PA. Separation of

a hyaluronate-free lubricating fraction from synovial fluid. Nature 1970; 228:377–378.

77. Swann DA, Silver FH, Slayter HS, et al. The molecular structure and lubricating activity of lubricin from bovine and human synovial fluids. Biochem J 1985; 225:195–201.

78. Lewis PR, McCutchen CW. Lubrication of mammalian joints. Nature 1960; 185:920–921.

79. McCutchen CW. The frictional properties of animal joints. Wear 1962; 5:1.

80. Walker PS, Dowson D, Longfield MD, et al. Boosted lubrication in synovial joints by fluid entrapment and enrichment. Ann Rheum Dis 1968; 27:512–520.

81. Walker PS, Unsworth A, Dowson D, et al. Mode of aggregation of hyaluronic acid protein complex on the surface of articular cartilage. Ann Rheum Dis 1970; 29:591–602.

82. Hou JS, Holmes MH, Lai WM, et al. Effects of changing cartilage stiffness, Poisson ratio and permeability on squeeze film lubrication. Adv Bioeng Trans ASME 1989; 15:103–105.

83. Unsworth A, Dowson D, Wright V. The frictional behavior of human synovial joints: I. Natural joints. J Lubr Tech ASME 1975; 97:360–376.

84. Unsworth A, Dowson D, Wright V. Some new evidence on human joint lubrication. Ann Rheum Dis 1975; 34:277.

85. Malcom LL. An Experimental Investigation of the Frictional and Deformational Responses of Articular Cartilage Interfaces to Static and Dynamic Loading. Thesis, University of California, San Diego, 1976.

86. Enneking WF and Horowitz M. The intra-articular effects of immobilization on the human knee. J Bone Joint Surg 1972; 54A:973–985.

87. Perricone E, Palmoski M, Brandt K. The effect of disuse of the joint on proteoglycan (PG) aggregation in articular cartilage. Clin Res 1977; 25:616.

88. Palmoski M, Colyer R, Brandt K. Joint motion in the absence of normal loading does not maintain normal articular cartilage. Arthritis Rheum 1980; 23:325–334.

89. Eronen I, Videman T, Friman C. et al. Glycosaminoglycan metabolism in experimental osteoarthrosis caused by immobilization. Acta Orthop Scand 1978; 49:329–334.

90. Finsterbush A, Friedman B. Early changes in immobilized rabbit knee joints: A light and electron microscope study. Clin Orthop 1973; 92:305–319.

91. Jurvelin J. Kiviranta I, Saamanen AM, et al. Partial restoration of immobilization-induced softening of canine articular cartilage after remobiliza-

tion of the knee joint. J Orthop Res 1989; 7:352–358.

92. Caterson B, Lowther DA. Changes in the metabolism of the proteoglycans from sheep articular cartilage in response to mechanical stress. Biochim Biophys Acta 1978; 540:412–422.

93. Palmoski M, Brandt K. Running inhibits the reversal of atrophic changes in knee cartilage after removal of a leg cast. Arthritis Rheum 1981; 24:1329–1337.

94. Palmoski M, Perricone E, Brandt K. Development and reversal of a proteoglycan aggregation defect in normal canine knee cartilage after immobilization. Arthritis Rheum 1979; 22:508–517.

95. Sood SC. A study of the effects of experimental immobilization on rabbit articular cartilage. J Anat 1981; 108:497–507.

96. Setton LA, Zimmerman JR, Mow VC, et al. Effects of disuse on the tensile properties and composition of canine knee joint cartilage. Trans Orthop Res Soc 1990; 15:155.

97. Emery IH, Meachim G. Surface morphology and topography of patellofemoral cartilage fibrillation in Liverpool necropsies. J Anat 1973; 116:103–120.

98. Mankin HJ, Dorfman H. Lippiello L, et al. Biochemical and metabolic abnormalities in articular cartilage from osteoarthritic human hips. II. Correlation of morphology with biochemical and metabolic data. J Bone Joint Surg 1971; 53A:523–537.

99. Bennett GA, Bauer W, Maddock SJ. A study of the repair of articular cartilage and the reaction of normal joints of adult dogs to surgically created defects of articular cartilage, "joint mice" and patellar displacement. AM J Pathol 1932; 8:499–524.

100. Meachim G, Roberts C. Repair of the joint surface from subarticular tissue in the rabbit knee. J Anat 1971; 109:317–327.

101. Furukawa T, Eyre DR, Koide S, et al. Biochemical studies on repair cartilage resurfacing experimental defects in the rabbit knee. J Bone Joint Surg 1980; 62A:79–89.

102. Wolff J. The Law of Bone Remodeling, 1892, translated to English by Maquet P, Furlong R. Berlin: Springer-Verlag, 1986.

103. Telhas H, Lindberg L. A method for inducing osteoarthritic changes in rabbits' knees. Clin Orthop 1972; 86:214–223.

104. Macys JR, Bullough PG, Wilson PD. Coxarthrosis: A study of the natural history based on a correlation of clinical, radiographic and pathologic findings. Semin Arthritis Rheum 1980; 10:66–80.

105. Pond MJ, Nuki G. Experimentally induced os-

teoarthritis in the dog. Ann Rheum Dis 1973; 32:387–388.

106. Moskowitz RW, Howell DS, Goldberg VM, et al. Cartilage proteoglycan alterations in an experimentally induced model of rabbit osteoarthritis. Arthritis Rheum 1979; 22:155–162.

107. McDevitt C, Gilbertson E, Muir H. An experimental model of osteoarthritis; early morphologic changes and biochemical changes. J Bone Joint Surg 1977; 59B:24–35.

108. Radin EL, Martin RB, Burr DB, et al. Effects of mechanical loading on the tissue of rabbit knee. J Orthop Res 1984; 2:221–234.

109. Donohue JM, Buss D, Oegema TR Jr, et al. The effects of indirect blunt trauma on adult canine articular cartilage. J Bone Joint Surg 1983; 65A:948–957.

110. Armstrong CG, Mow VC, Wirth CR, Biomechanics of impact-induced microdamage to articular cartilage: A possible genesis for chondromalacia patella. In: Finerman G, ed. Symposium on Sports Medicine: The Knee. St. Louis: CV Mosby, 1985; 70–84.

111. Altman RD, Tenenbaum J, Latta L, et al. Biomechanical and biochemical properties of dog cartilage in experimentally induced osteoarthritis. Ann Rheum Dis 1984; 43:83–90.

112. Myers ER, Hardingham TE, Billingham MEJ, et al. Changes in the tensile and compressive properties of articular cartilage in a canine model of osteoarthritis. Trans Orthop Res Soc 1986; 11:231.

113. Hock DH, Grodzinsky AJ, Kobb TJ, et al. Early changes in material properties of rabbit articular cartilage after meniscectomy. J Ortho Res 1983; 1:4–12.

114. Pelletier JP, Martel-Pelletier J, Altman RD, et al. Collagenolytic activity and collagen matrix breakdown of the articular cartilage in the Pond-Nuki dog model of osteoarthritis. Arthritis Rheum 1983; 26:866–874.

115. Teshima R, Treadwell BV, Trahan CA, et al. Comparative rates of proteoglycan synthesis and size of proteoglycans in normal and osteoarthtic chondrocytes. Arthritis Rheum 1983; 26:1225–1230.

116. Ratcliffe A, Tyler JA, Hardingham TE. Articular cartilage cultured with interleukin 1: Increase release of link protein, hyaluronate-binding region, and other proteoglycan fragments. Biochem J 1986; 238:571–580.

117. Sokoloff L. Elasticity of aging cartilage. Proc Fed Am Socs Exp Biol 1966; 25:1089–1095.

# Chapter 9

# Physiology of the Skin

JANET H. PRYSTOWSKY
LEONARD C. HARBER

## Embryonic Development[1]

The skin, the body's largest organ, contains the most extensive vascular supply. It maintains body temperature by regulating heat loss, prevents external organisms such as bacteria, fungi, and viruses from entering the body, protects it against environmental insults such as ultraviolet radiation, and relays diverse information to the central nervous system. This information is mediated by sensory receptors to heat, cold, pain, pressure, and touch.

The skin has three distinct anatomic compartments: epidermis, dermis, and subcutaneous tissue (Figure 9-1). The epidermis has an outer inert keratin layer above a 5- to 10-cell thickness of keratinocytes (Figure 9-2). The epidermal compartment is highly cellular, and approximately as thick as a sheet of paper. The acellular non-metabolizing stratum corneum is 10 to 20 $\mu$, the cellular epidermis 40 to 150 $\mu$, and the epidermis ranges 40 to 150 $\mu$ (see Figure 9-1). The cutis is relatively acellular, 10 to 20 times thicker, and primarily composed of connective tissue fibers. The subcutaneous tissue consists mainly of fat-laden cells divided into lobules by connective tissue septa. It varies considerably in thickness (see Figure 9-1).

The embryonic skin becomes distinct as early as the third week of fetal life, when a single layer of cells, the periderm, constitutes the outer layer. Within days, a second layer, the germinative cell layer, develops. This cell layer is the ancestor of all the appendageal glands as well as the stratified squamous epithelium cells of the epidermis (Figure 9-3). During the second month, connective elements of mesodermal origin are visible; these are noted in a vascular background. The third compartment, the subcutaneous tissue, is not rigidly demarcated, but during the third month of fetal life it contains clearly recognizable lipid-laden cells.

## Cellular and Glandular Components

### Epidermis

#### Epidermal Cells

The epidermis consists of multiple layers of ectodermal cells, called *keratinocytes* because of their abundant production of the tonofilament keratin. In addition to keratinocytes, made from progenitor cells in the skin, the epidermis normally has immigrant cells, called Langerhans' cells (LCs), that are derived from the bone marrow and have a macrophage lineage. During pathologic events, erythrocytes and leukocytes may also be seen in the epidermis. Finally, melanocytes, which are responsible for the formation of melanin pigment, are derived from neuroectodermal elements in neural crest. They, too, migrate to the skin and then locally replicate in the skin.

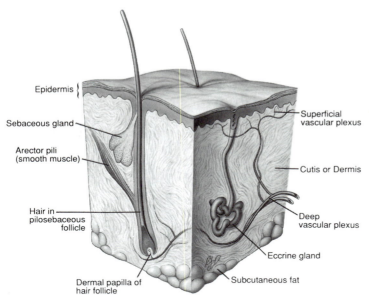

**Figure 9-1.** Constituents and structures of skin: epidermis, cutis, subcutaneous tissue, pilosebaceous units, and appendiceal glands.

**Differentiation.** Keratinocytes undergo many changes, known as *differentiation,* during their life cycle. The epidermis has three compartments (Figure 9-2). The first consists of the basal layer of cells and part of the overlying suprabasal layer. It is also called the *stratum germinativum,* because the cells in the basal and suprabasal layers are mitotically active germinative cells responsible for producing new keratinocytes to replace those shed externally by the epidermis. The second compartment, the *stratum spinosum,* consists of metabolically active cells that have entered into a differentiation process that leads finally to formation of cornified cells in the outermost and third compartment, the stratum corneum.

The first compartment (germinative cells) and second compartment (differentiating cells) constitute the viable portion of the epidermis. A transitional zone, the *stratum granulosum,* contains elongated, flattened cells. The third compartment is the outer layer (stratum corneum), consisting of nonviable cellular components that protect the skin from the environment. Shedding of the stratum corneum completes the cellular turnover process of the epidermis (i.e., differentiating cells must constantly replace the shedding stratum corneum to maintain this layer and its protective function). Thus, normally, a germinative cell in the basal or suprabasal compartment gives rise to a differentiating cell, which has lost its proliferative capacity

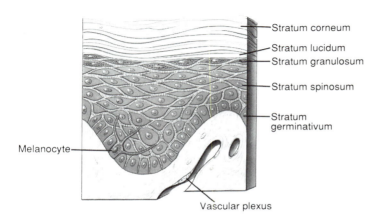

**Figure 9-2.** Epidermal cell layers.

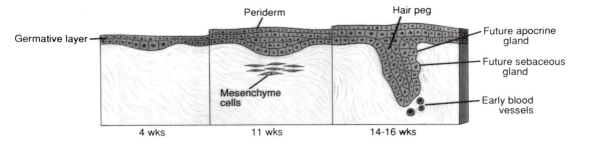

**Fetal Skin**

**Figure 9-3.** Embryonic development of the epidermis and adenexal glands.

and terminally differentiates into a cornified non-viable component of the stratum corneum.

The precise mechanisms and controls over epidermal proliferation and differentiation remain unclear; however, studies in vivo and in vitro have revealed numerous details of the process. Studies in vitro have shown that proliferation and differentiation are inversely regulated: when proliferation is promoted, differentiation is suppressed, whereas when keratinocytes differentiate they lose the ability to proliferate. The proliferative process has both irreversible and reversible growth arrest states, depending on the composition of the tissue culture medium (e.g., growth factors, amino acid composition).[2]

Furthermore, the concentration of calcium in the medium is a critical regulator of differentiation. Cells in medium containing 0.1 mM of calcium remain undifferentiated, proliferate rapidly, and do not stratify, whereas addition of 1.2 to 2.0 mM of calcium is associated with induction of differentiation.[2,3] Differentiation of keratinocytes is demonstrated by colony formation, stratification, and expression of highly organized elements such as specific antigens, involucrin, and keratin tonofilaments. When keratinocytes enter the differentiating process the synthesis of DNA decreases and is totally inhibited within 24 hours.[3] Other mediators such as retinoids have a marked effect on keratinocyte differentiation, particularly with respect to keratin gene expression.

Keratins are a group of at least 19 proteins referred to as intermediate filaments because they function as structural components of the cytoskeleton.[4] They range in molecular weight from approximately 40 to 70kd. The keratins synthesized in squamous "keratinizing" epithelium are higher in molecular weight than the keratins found in nonsquamous nonkeratinizing epithelial (mucosal) surfaces.

Differentiation in cultured human epidermal cells is dependent on the absence or presence of retinoids in the medium and on whether the cultures are submerged in medium or grown on a collagen support to allow keratinocyte maturation at an air-water interface.[5] When keratinocytes are grown submerged in medium containing retinoids the keratins synthesized reflect those found in mucosal surfaces (lower–molecular weight keratins) and the cells do not cornify. The higher–molecular weight keratins associated with terminal differentiation are not made in the presence of retinoic acid. In contrast, cultures grown submerged in retinoid-deficient medium show high–molecular weight keratin production that reflects what is typically found in vivo in epidermis. Similarly, keratinocytes cultured at an air-water interface with retinoids in the medium below also follow a keratinization process that reflects the situation in vivo by production of the high–moleculor weight keratins seen in terminal differentiation.[5] Thus, under conditions in vivo, the delivery of retinoids from plasma to the outer layers of the epidermis may be quite limited; terminal differentiation and cornification processes may occur as the keratinocytes progressively become more retinoid deficient in the outer layers of the epidermis.

The advances in culturing human keratinocytes in vitro have now made it possible to propagate autologous keratinocytes for grafting onto full-thickness wounds for massive burned areas.[6] Similarly, patients with the inherited disorder epidermolysis bullosa have large areas of denuded skin, owing to defective or absent structural components for the epidermis to adhere to the dermis. These patients can benefit from grafts of autologous epidermis to denuded dermis.

**Cell Kinetics.** Evidence suggests that at any given time, only a fraction of the cells in the germinative compartment are actually cycling, or undergoing mitotic division. The remainder are in a "resting" phase, called $G_0$. Cells in $G_0$ (Figure 9-4) enter the actively cycling pool, $G_1$, in response to proliferative stimuli.[7] The population of actively dividing cells also appears to be heterogeneous, some cells being more likely than others to undergo cell division.[8,9]

Once cells have entered into the differentiation compartment they are no longer mitotically active. A steady state exists when the production of cells from the germinative compartment is equal to the cell loss through desquamation from the stratum corneum. The time a cell takes to move from the basal layer to a scale sloughed or shed from the stratum corneum is referred to as the transit or epidermal turnover time. This period has two phases. The first is the time required for a basal cell to reach the stratum corneum; the second is the time required for the cellular material that becomes a component of the stratum corneum to be sloughed (Table 9-1).

The thickness of the epidermis depends on the number of keratinocytes between the basal layer and the stratum corneum; it may be altered by changes in the production rate of keratinocytes from the basal layer, epidermal turnover time, or the cell cycle time. Chronic inflammatory states such as psoriasis may cause significant increases in the epidermal thickness (hyperplasia).

The cell cycle time is the period required for a basal cell in $G_1$ (Figure 9-5) to undergo mitosis. As mentioned, at any given time only a fraction of the germinative cells are cycling; many cells remain in the $G_0$ or resting phase.

Cell cycle time cannot be measured directly; mathematical formulae (reviewed by Bauer[10]) are needed to determine these kinetic data. Historically, cell cycle time has been calculated from autoradiographic studies following incorporation of radioactive DNA precursors into actively cycling cells. More recently, flow cytometry of epi-

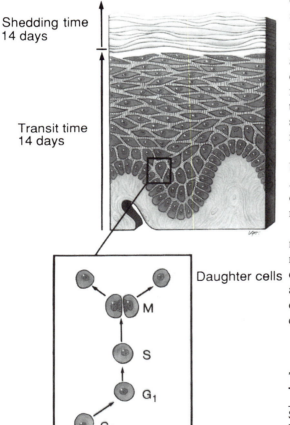

Shedding time
14 days

Transit time
14 days

Daughter cells

**Figure 9-4.** Epidermal cell kinetics. The stages of cell cycling are composed of the following steps: $G_0$, resting stage; $G_1$, cell has entered into cycling process; S, active DNA-synthesizing phase; M, mitotic cell division giving rise to daughter cells.

**Table 9-1.** Cellular Kinetics in Normal Skin*

| Cell Cycle | Time | Reference |
|---|---|---|
| S phase | 10 hr | 10 |
| Entire cell cycle ($G_1$–M) | 37 hr | 10 |
| Transit time (of basal epidermal cell to stratum corneum) | 14–18 d | 10 |
| Turnover time (of stratum corneum) | 14 d | 11 |

*Estimated.

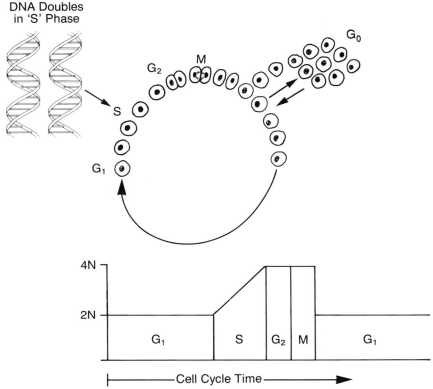

DNA Doubles in 'S' Phase

**Figure 9-5.** Epidermal cell cycle. $G_1$, cell is in cycling process; S, active DNA synthesis stage; $G_2$, cell prior to division containing a diploid quantity of DNA; M, mitotic phase; $G_0$, cell in resting phase, not undergoing cycling process.

dermal cell suspensions has been utilized to distinguish between diploid (2N DNA content) cells in $G_1$, $G_0$, and differentiated cells (no longer cycling), and cells in S, $G_2$, and M states that contain greater quantities of DNA (between diploid and tetraploid in S and tetraploid in $G_2$ and M). This is a possible because the DNA-specific fluorochrome utilized emits a signal proportional to the cells' content of DNA. The cell cycle time and duration of the S phase in normal skin is presented in Table 9-1.

Cell cycle times, as reported in the literature, show tremendous variability.[10] Probably the largest single responsible factor is the difficulty of accurately assessing the proportion of cells in $G_0$ (i.e., those not actively cycling). Figure 9-5 illustrates the multiple points at which significant alterations may occur in epidermal cell kinetics in normal cutaneous responses (e.g., irritation, pharmacologically induced changes, and disease states, such as psoriasis).

Cellular kinetic data are useful for understanding skin disease processes and suggesting therapeutic approaches. In psoriasis, for example, the rated cellular turnover of the epidermis is about four to six times faster than normal.[10,11] It is not surprising that this results in a hyperplastic epidermis that may be two to five times thicker than normal skin (Figure 9-6). Additionally, the production rate is increased, suggesting that the number of cells cycling is approximately 20 times greater than in normal skin. Thus, cells that would normally be in the resting ($G_0$) state have been influenced to enter $G_1$. Predictably, many of the most widely used therapeutic modalities for psoriasis interfere with DNA synthesis (e.g., metho-

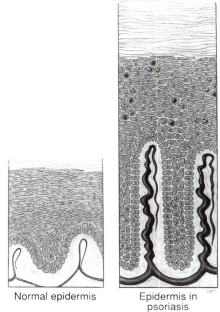

Normal epidermis          Epidermis in
                          psoriasis

**Figure 9-6.** Hyperplastic epidermis, a characteristic feature of psoriasis. The psoriatic skin has a hyperplastic epidermis with marked tortuosity of superficial vasculature within the dermis. Leukocytes are interspersed between epidermal cells in psoriasis.

trextate, PUVA, anthralin, tar,) or with recruitment of cells from $G_0$ into $G_1$ (corticosteroids).[10]

*Melanocytes*

Melanocytes are normally found interspersed amongst the basal cells of the epidermis. They are specialized ectodermal cells that embryonically are of a neural crest origin (Figure 9-7A); their biologic function is the production of the melanosome, a granular structure shaped like a cucumber. Within this protein structure, a light-opaque high-molecular weight tyrosine polymer, melanin, is synthesized. The epidermal cell melanin content is primarily responsible for skin color. All races have essentially similar numbers of melanocytes; tyrosine activation is the rate-limiting factor in melanin synthesis. Albinos, whose tyrosinase activity is genetically shut down, synthesize virtually no melanin, whereas the blackest Africans, skin type VI, have approximately 1 g of melanin. The melanocyte's sole function appears to be to manufacture melanin. This dense, opaque polymer is insoluble in aqueous solutions and in most organic solvents and has been demonstrated to have widespread survival value throughout the animal world. The squid's protective behaviors provide a good example. This creature has a contractile sac that ejects melanin in its ink to lay down a "smokescreen" and permit it to escape from a predator. Many animals such as frogs and chameleons use melanin to blend in with their environments. Under neurohormonal control melanin is rapidly synthesized and moved to various locations. Flounders have an extremely well-developed camouflage pattern that employs melanin to mimic a changing sandy background. This is also accomplished by a highly developed ability to rapidly disperse melanin granules.

In humans the major function of melanin is to protect the skin against solar radiation, and the epidermal cells in particular against ultraviolet radiation.[12] Through an adaptive mechanism, the melanocytes, located primarily in the basal cell layer, have developed long dendritic processes that have contact with as many as 30 to 40 adjacent epidermal cells, often referred to as the *epidermal melanocyte unit* (see Figure 9-7B). Through incompletely understood mechanisms, they "inject" their pigment granules, melanosomes, into the epidermal cells. These melanosomes, now within epidermal cells, tend to congregate in a supranuclear pattern that, by absorbing and blocking photons of ultraviolet light, affords protection for DNA. Humans exposed to excessive solar radiation show a direct correlation between the amount of melanin and the incidence of basal and squamous cell skin cancer. Severe episodes of acute sunburn in fair-skinned persons are associated with a high incidence of melanoma. The biochemical mechanism of melanin formation in humans is well-known, but the hormonal influence on this process needs clarification. A pituitary hormone, melanocyte-stimulating hormone (MSH), has been isolated and synthesized. When injected into humans, diffuse pigmentation (except in albinos) is noted within 2 or 3 days. Adrenocorticotropic hormone (ACTH), a pituitary hormone biochemically similar to MSH, has a similar but less pronounced effect. It is of interest that estrogen, whether administered systemically or applied topically, can cause darkening (melanization) of the

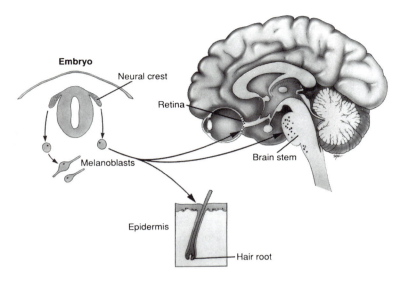

**Figure 9-7.** (*A*) Embryonic development and migratory pattern of melanocytes. (*B*) Epidermal melanocyte. The dendritic processes of a single melanocyte may inject melanosomes into 30 to 40 epidermal cells. This affords a protective mechanism against UV radiation.

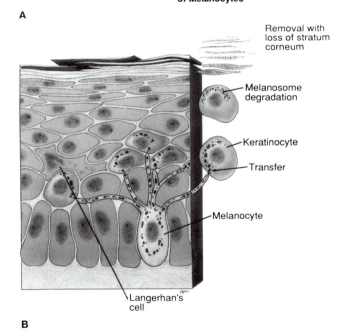

nipple and areolar area of the breast. The skin of patients after hypophysectomy or large doses of radiation to the pituitary often becomes lighter in appearance. It is well-documented that inflammation of the skin associated with heat, trauma, x-ray, and particularly ultraviolet light stimulates melanocytes to synthesize more melanin. Whether or not melanin formation following injury involves a common mechanism is controversial. Although direct neural pathways with melanocytes are present in other species, none have been demonstrated in humans.

*Langerhans' Cells*

Paul Langerhans, as a medical student in 1868, first described the morphology of the unique epidermal dendritic cell that today bears his name.

Until recently the LCs embryonic origin, uniqueness of structural components, and biologic function were controversial.[13]

Paul Langerhans identified LCs by their staining properties with a gold chloride solution that showed their cell structure contained an extensive network of darkly staining dendritic processes. Because it resembled a melanocyte this feature led to the speculation that the LC was also of neuroectodermal origin and that it had simply lost the capacity to synthesize melanin and thus could be considered an "effete melanocyte." The fact that LCs, in this vestigial role, constituted close to 4% of all epidermal cells was dismissed as just another anatomic curiosity; however, the LC is now well-established as a crucial component of the immune system and is known to be of mesodermal origin, originating from stem cells residing in the bone marrow.

The anatomic observation that led to our present morphologic identification of LC cells was made by Birbeck in 1968 (Figure 9-8). He identified a characteristic cytoplasmic organelle of rod-shaped lamellar appearance with a terminal protuberance that suggested a tennis racket. This ultrastructural unit, Birbeck's granule, was soon found in other sites such as lymph nodes, thymus, tonsils, and histiocytic cells. LCs are also characterized by an irregularly shaped, highly convoluted nucleus and the absence of tonofilaments and melanosomes in the cytoplasm and of desmosomes on the cell membrane. Other properties include intense staining with adenosine triphosphatase (ATPase). A characteristic cell membrane marker known as the *Ia antigen* can also be detected by fluorescent antibody labeling. This is helpful in distinguishing LCs from normal epidermal cells and melanocytes. Like other members of the mesodermal macrophage series, LC membranes contain receptors for the Fc portion of immunoglobulin G (IgG) and the C3b component of complement.[14]

The origin of these IA-bearing cells within the epidermis was unclear until 1979, when Katz and coworkers isolated Ia-bearing cells from the bone marrow of donor mice.[15] This was accomplished through the use of isotropically labeled marrow cells injected into the bone marrow of syngeneic recipient animals that had been rendered immunodeficient by lethal doses of x-irradiation. They were therefore devoid of epidermal LCs. The skin of these recipient animals was then shown to contain the labeled "Ia-positive" cells within 48 hours, indicating that these cells had migrated from the bone marrow compartment and were derived from residual bone marrow cells.[16,17]

Silberberg and Baer[18] made the initial suggestion that LCs have an immune function. In 1973 they offered a startlingly innovative concept based

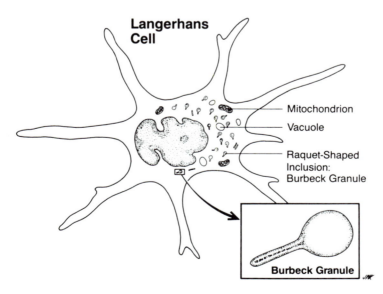

**Langerhans Cell**

Mitochondrion

Vacuole

Raquet-Shaped Inclusion: Burbeck Granule

**Burbeck Granule**

**Figure 9-8.** Langerhans' cell. These dendritic cells are characterized by a convoluted nucleus and cytoplasmic structures (Burbeck's granules) shaped like a tennis racket. The Langerhans' cell, after migrating from the bone marrow, resides in the epidermis and appears crucial for processing antigens.

on studies conducted to compare the cutaneous response to primary irritants and contact allergens in humans previously sensitized to contact allergens.[19] Silberberg and coworkers observed by ultrastructural analysis that in specimens obtained from immunized subjects Langerhans' cells and T lymphocytes were closely apposed. In contrast, this type of response was not observed in a primary irritant response. On the basis of these observations, Silberberg and Baer postulated that in allergic contact dermatitis a specific interaction occurs between LCs and lymphocytes that is crucial for eliciting the immune response.[18] Further studies showed that LCs could be identified in draining lymph nodes, suggesting that these cells play an important role in the presentation of contact allergens to the immune system.[19] Later studies showed that LCs also had phagocytic properties and could take up ferritin, suggesting the ability to ingest and process antigens.

Bergstresser (1980) provided additional evidence of the crucial role of LCs in allergic contact dermatitis. In an ingenious experiment based on the observation of regional differences in the density of LCs in the dorsal skin and tail of rats,[20] Bergstresser demonstrated that the degree or ability to induce allergic sensitization varied dramatically in these two sites. Indeed, the high degree of sensitization following the application of a hapten to the back correlated directly with the large number of LCs there, as compared to markedly less sensitization when the tail site, which contained relatively few LCs, was used. Attempts to induce sensitization in tail skin resulted in the induction of immune suppression or tolerance.

Thus LCs have been shown to be crucial for the induction of allergic contact sensitization in the skin: conversely, when LCs are reduced or absent, skin exposure to a contact sensitizer tends to result in tolerogenic or suppressor responses rather than sensitization.

Studies by Kripke in 1974 indicate that the LC may be one of the major regulators in tumor surveillance.[21] Thus, the LC, a previously obscure resident of the epidermis, is now considered vital to the development of an immune response to inert and viable environmental agents. LCs also appear to play a crucial role in tumor immunity. Studies of this cell's role in wound healing time and prevention of cutaneous infection should have the highest priority.

### Epidermal Appendages and Structures

#### Sebaceous Glands

Three types of cutaneous adnexal glands derive from epidermal tissue, the sebaceous, apocrine, and eccrine glands. Sebaceous glands (Figures 9-1 and 9-9) vary regionally in density, size, and shape: the face has the most per unit area and the largest gland size.[22] Although their role is still debated, the final destination of the sebaceous gland cells (sebocytes) is the skin surface, where they form an amorphous lipid-rich material called *sebum*. This terminal differentiation or disintegration obliterates all traces of earlier cellular identity. Because of the complete *(whole)* disappearance of the cells, they are often referred to as *holocrine glands*. Sebaceous glands show no neural pattern of innervation; but they are very responsive to hormonal stimuli.

The embryonic development of sebaceous glands, like that of other adnexal structures, is

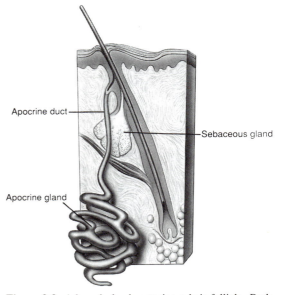

**Figure 9-9.** Adnexal glands entering a hair follicle. Both apocrine and sebaceous glands enter the pilosebaceous duct, which delivers their contents to the skin surface.

ectodermal in origin (Figure 9-3). As their origin is identical with that of the epidermal cells producing stratum corneum, they retain this function and serve as important components of the wound-healing process. The development of a sebaceous gland can be noted in the epithelium of the hair follicle by the 14th week of gestation (see Figure 9-3).[23] It appears as a spherical bud that grows laterally from the hair follicle and develops into a multilobulated gland (see Figure 9-9). In adult life this glandular tissue surrounds more than 50% of the circumference of each hair follicle. The gland's products enter the hair follicle through a short pilosebaceous duct rather than traveling directly to the skin surface.

By the 6th month of gestation a basement membrane surrounds the basal cell layer of sebocytes. As cells are viewed inwardly from the peripheral portion of the gland they become larger and paler and form fat droplets, which increase in size as cellular identity fades. This mechanism is fully operative before term.

Humans have more sebaceous glands than any other mammal. The density ranges from 400 to 900 glands per square centimeter of skin surface and is greatest on the forehead. Other high-density sites are the scalp, face, and genitalia. The upper chest and back show intermediate sebaceous gland density and concentrations of 10% or less of the forehead level are found on the wrists and ankles. Sebaceous glands do not occur on the palms and soles. The density distribution of sebaceous glands coincides with the sites at which acne vulgaris lesions most frequently are noted. All sebaceous glands, regardless of size or location, empty into the follicular duct of the hair follicle (see Figure 9-9). This may be related ontologically to their vital importance in protecting aquatic birds' feathers by forming a lipid coating. Their absence is associated with loss of luster and brittleness that affects flight. In mammals the sebum may similarly help protect hair and fur from environmental insults. The proliferation of sebocytes, most pronounced at puberty and accompanied by a massive increase in sebaceous lobule size and accumulation of lipids, is recognized as a growth process initiated, and probably regulated, by direct hormone stimulation.

Increased sebaceous gland proliferation coincides with other signs of puberty such as the emergence of a beard and deep voice in males and of mammary tissue and body contour in females. Microscopic examination of the basal cell sebocytes shows a marked increase in mitotic activity during puberty.[24] The historical clinical data that identified hormonal control of sebocyte proliferation was the observation that sebaceous hyperplasia and acne did not occur in prepubertal castrates and eunuchs, though following testosterone injections hyperplasia and acne developed.[25,26] Additional studies in humans have demonstrated that large doses of estrogen have an inhibitory effect on sebaceous gland hyperplasia. Females who develop acne probably do so from androgenic hormones elaborated by the adrenal cortex such as dehydroepiandrosterone. In general, males have higher excretory levels of sebum than females and older males have lower levels than those of middle age.[27,28] Sebum production correlates with age-related testosterone levels.[29,30]

Though no specific role for sebum on the skin surface of humans is demonstrable at present, many feel that dry skin and winter itch can be minimized by preventing excessive transepidermal water loss. The role of the sebaceous excretory products may be to form a lipid layer on the skin surface that inhibits insensible water loss.[31] Others feel the epidermal cell lipids of the skin are sufficient for this purpose.[32–34] Another possible function of sebum is the production of 7-dehydrocholesterol (provitamin D). The action of ultraviolet B radiation converts this compound to vitamin D, which is important in preventing rickets and osteomalacia in persons whose diet is deficient in vitamin D.

In summary, sebaceous gland activity may aid in maintaining a skin surface lipid level that protects against water loss. Under abnormal hormonal effects, disorders ranging from mild acne to disabling folliculitis may occur.

*Apocrine Glands*

Apocrine glands (see Figure 9-9) secrete chemical substances related to scent called *pheromones*. Though in many species pheromones elaborate odors that act as sexual attractants or delineate territorial domains, there is no evidence of this in humans. Indeed, apocrine glands may well be vestigial sweat glands rather than a scent unit.

The highest concentration of apocrine glands is found in the axillary and genital regions; smaller concentrations are found in the umbilical and perianal zones and the areolar area of the nipples. A modified form of an apocrine gland, the gland of Moll, is found in the eyelids. From an embryonic basis, the glandular tissue of the breast per se can be regarded as an apocrine structure.[35] The embryonic development of the apocrine gland is similar to that of the sebaceous gland and is intimately involved with the hair follicle (see Figure 9-3). Apocrine glands are minute structures that have a ductal connection with hair follicles (see Figure 9-9). The glands can be considered principally as adrenergic response organs, and secretion is stimulated by emotional episodes or by systemic or local injection of epinephrine.[36]

Uncontaminated apocrine sweat is difficult to obtain because of cannulation problems. In pure form it is a viscous, milky white fluid that is odorless until it is acted upon by residual bacteria in the pilosebaceous apparatus and skin surface. Following decomposition by bacterial enzymes a pungent odor, often termed *BO* (body odor), emerges.

The apocrine glands are nonsecretory until puberty; their growth and development is apparently under hormonal control. After development of their glandular structure, apocrine glands can be readily distinguished from eccrine glands. Specifically, the secretory portion of this coiled gland consists of a single layer of palely staining cells with a convex border projecting into a lumen. The base of the secretory cells is surrounded by contractile myoepithelial cells. These contractile cells rhythmically contract, producing a pulsatile secretion.

As noted, the highest concentration of apocrine glands are in the axillary, perianal, genital, and umbilical areas. Inflammation of the adnexal glands at these sites may be associated with a chronic infection known as hidradenitis suppurativa.[37,38] From the viewpoint of the practitioner of rehabilitation medicine, apocrine glands serve principally as elaborators of unpleasant odors that can be controlled by appropriate antiperspirant and hygienic procedures.[39,40]

In summary, apocrine glands appear to be vestigial appendiceal glands in humans. Their hormonal development and adrenergic responsiveness are well-documented.

*Eccrine Glands*

Eccrine glands are appendiceal glands that empty directly onto the skin surface (Figure 9-10). They markedly influence body temperature through regulation of water loss.[41,42]

During routine activities, noneccrine gland mechanisms of water loss include invisible secretion of sweat and respiratory water vapor loss through exhaling. These two physiologic processes, often referred to as *insensible water loss,* are continuous and normally play a limited role in temperature control and water regulation. In contrast, eccrine gland activity is crucial for heat reg-

**Eccrine Gland**

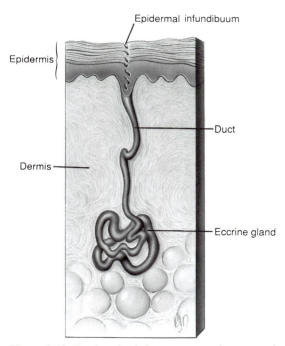

**Figure 9-10.** Eccrine gland. In contrast to sebaceous and apocrine glands, the eccrine gland extends deep into the dermis and has an independent duct that carries its secretions directly to the skin surface.

ulation. At normal internal and external temperatures, the radiation and convection of the insensible water loss maintains homeostasis.

Under conditions of extreme heat, however, the evaporation of the eccrine gland secretion provides the major cooling effect. This cooling process is augmented by peripheral vasodilatation and hyperpnea. In very hot environments and in response to extreme physical stress all these cooling mechanisms may prove insufficient and hyperthermia and death may occur.

The average adult human has more than 2 million eccrine glands (see Figure 9-10). They are found in highest concentration on the palms and soles, where they may number more than 300 glands per square centimeter. About half this number are found on the forehead, dorsum of the hands, chest, and abdomen. Concentrations are lowest on the buttocks, thighs, medial aspect of the legs, and nape of neck. The actual size of the sweat glands, as measured in biopsy specimens, averages $5 \times 10^{-3}$ per cubic millimeter (variation 50%). The rate of sweat secretion appears to correlate with gland size.[43] Sweat delivered to the skin surface is a colorless hypotonic solution with a pH of approximately 5.0.

**Embryology.**    Eccrine gland cells can be identified in the fourth week of fetal life (see Figure 9-3) as the lower cellular layer (germinative) beneath the periderm. These cells are completely distinct from embryo sebaceous and apocrine gland cells. The germinate cells multiply into small buds and migrate downward, but they always maintain direct contact with their original connection to the epidermis. The descent of the glandular cells is completed when they approach the lower portion of the dermis. During this downward migration, which is virtually complete by the fifth to sixth fetal month, the eccrine glands acquire a ductal portion, which communicates directly with the skin surface, as well as vasculature and a nerve supply derived from dermal elements (see Figure 9-17). By the eighth month of fetal life the coiled eccrine gland has a double cell layer with a clearly discernible lumen. The ectodermal cells lining the eccrine duct unit retain the ability to regenerate a functional epidermis similar to the pilosebaceous units and are very important in wound healing.

**Regulation of Thermal Sweating.**    The major afferent message controlling internal heat is probably the result of warmed blood reaching the hypothalamic center of the brain. Under extreme febrile stress sweat volume may exceed 2 L per hour. Local heating of any portion of the body from a sufficiently hot external stimulus can also cause sweating by a reflex mechanism.[45,46]

A modified thermal response occurs in the eccrine glands of the palms, soles, and forehead. Emotional stimuli—anxiety, fear, pain—trigger their maximal response. These same glands are significantly less responsive to thermal stimuli. The glands of the upper lip release acetylcholine in response to "sharp" and spicy foods. This third type of response is often referred to as *localized gustatory sweating.*

Diseases of the central nervous system have long been recognized to influence eccrine activity. Damage to the cortex of parietal brain tissue is associated with hyperhidrosis of the contralateral side, where motor paralysis may be observed. Transection of the spinal cord also can be associated with distal hyperhidrosis. This and the parietal lesions suggest a role for an undefined inhibitory substance in eccrine secretion. In contrast, destructive lesions of peripheral nerves (Hansen's disease) are frequently associated with hypohidrosis or anhidrosis.

**Pharmacologic (Hormonal) Responses of the Eccrine Gland and Duct.**    Fibers of the automatic nervous system that innervate the eccrine gland are sympathetic in anatomic structure, but acetylcholine rather than norepinephrine is released at their nerve endings, with resultant stimulation of eccrine secretion. These postganglionic anatomically adrenergic fibers to the eccrine glands are thus called sympathetic cholinergic fibers because of their physiologic role. In addition, deinnervated eccrine sweat glands still secrete when acetylcholine is applied directly. The minimal secretions from the direct glandular effects of norepinephrine are considered secondary to norepinephrine acting on the myoepithelial cells surrounding the gland.[47] Atropine and probanthine, by blocking the receptor site, decrease the response to acetylcholine. Physostigmine blocks acetylcholinesterase and, in so doing, intensifies sweating.[48,49]

The reabsorption of sodium from the eccrine sweat duct is strongly influenced by the adrenal cortical hormone aldosterone. Indeed, the initial secretory product from the gland is hypertonic compared to the plasma; that leaving the duct at the skin surface is hypotonic. Thus, the reabsorption of sodium is an active tubular process. The final eccrine product appears to have lower concentrations of sodium and chloride than serum, whereas sweat has higher concentrations of lactate, potassium, and urea. The increased urea may be a ductal metabolic product rather than a selective secretion effect. Though there are similarities to the renal tubular reabsorption process, this is probably an oversimplification.[50,51]

In summary, thermal regulation, a crucial requirement for human survival, is the major function of this cutaneous appendiceal gland. However, in debilitated febrile patients this process increases maceration, particularly in the inframammary and genital areas. If maceration is not adequately controlled, patients may suffer fungal and bacterial infections.

*Hair Follicles and Hair*

**Embryology of Hair Follicle and Hair.** Hair follicle cells are derived from ectodermal basal cells (see Figure 9-3).[52] These embryonal basal cells form the hair germ cells, which are bilateral and symmetrically distributed throughout the skin. They descend in a slanted caudal direction and become merged with a mesodermal component that becomes the dermal papilla and the fibrous root sheath (Figure 9-11). This is accomplished by mesodermal cells of the hair germ surrounding the ectodermal follicle cells. A cuplike invagination of epithelial cells that they abut forms the dermal papilla. Active hair growth is associated with the union of the matrix cells with an abundant vascular supply.

Hair represents the end product of highly active hair matrix cells located at the base of the follicle, a site characterized by a high rate of keratin synthesis. Keratin, biochemically a highly insoluble protein, is the basic constituent of hair. Only drastic environmental measures, such as a "permanent wave," alter its structure.

Hair, a terminal protein of epidermal cells, is similar biochemically to nail and is found in all

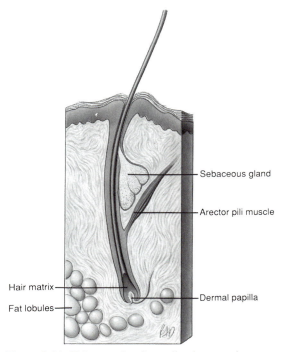

**Figure 9-11.** Hair emerging from pilosebaceous duct. The abundant vasculature of the dermal papilla supplies the rapidly dividing ectodermal cells of the hair matrix with sufficient nutrients to produce the keratin product, hair.

Labels in figure: Sebaceous gland; Arector pili muscle; Dermal papilla; Hair matrix; Fat lobules

mammals. Hair has several roles in human survival—heat conservation, tactile probing, and physical protection of the skin surface. For humans, hair may serve only a minor sensory tactile function, but it is of considerable aesthetic and cosmetic import in terms of location, quantity, and quality.

Hairs are best conceived of as nonmetabolizing keratin fibers produced from the hair matrix and discharged from hair follicles. The hair follicle is an epidermal appendage that embryonically descended into the dermis. The hair follicle is characterized by sebaceous glands that proliferate and excrete sebum into its common duct. The two structures are commonly known as *pilosebaceous unit* (Figure 9-11). They are found universally throughout the body, except on the palms and soles. The emerging hair, compact α-keratin, is divided into two groups, terminal and vellus. the terminal hairs comprise more than 95% of the hair on the scalp, trunk, and extremities of males. The vellus hairs are much shorter, grow slower, and are more numerous in women.

Hairs do not grow continuously; the matrix cells cycle through anagen and telogen phases, periods of growth with high metabolic activity and periods of rest. Hairs are shed during the telogen phase (Figure 9-12). A shed scalp hair may be 3 years old and have achieved a length of more than 2 feet. Average growth rates depend on metabolic activity of the matrix cells and vary with season; they are greatest in the summer, when scalp hair can grow an inch in 8 weeks. Approximately 90% of terminal hairs on a normal scalp are in the anagen phase. Acute febrile episodes, typhoid fever, or hormonal changes such as occur after pregnancy may abruptly terminate the anagen phase. The resulting transient hair loss is called *telogen effluvium*.

The growth of hairs from a given follicle is determined by androgenic hormones, and the responsiveness of a follicle to hormones is genetically determined. Hair follicles from the lateral portion of the scalp produce hairs when transplanted to the bald midportion if hormone levels remain constant. Loss of scalp hair (alopecia) is strongly under hereditary control and is referred to as *male pattern baldness* or *androgenetic alopecia*.

When hairs are visualized in cross-section they are usually oval and consist of multiple sections. The major ones are a central medulla and a compact cortex. Interspersed in the cortex is melanin, which adds color to the otherwise translucent hair.

## Nails[53]

The nail, a rigid keratin plate (Figure 9-13), is continuously being produced by rapidly dividing epidermal cells called the *nail matrix*.[54] This relatively small site, proximal to visible nail, under normal conditions is the only site of nail plate synthesis (Figure 9-14). Fingernails grow at the rate of 0.1 mm a day, in unlikely situations where no trauma or friction intervened they have grown to 12 inches or more. Under normal physiologic conditions fingernails have a constant thickness of approximately 0.6 mm. Toenails grow significantly more slowly than fingernails but are about 1.2 mm thick.

The embryonic origin of the nail can be detected during the 10th week of fetal life. It consists of a wedge of basal cell–like epithelial cells at the future site of the terminal interphalangeal joint. By the 12th week, a definite matrix group of proliferating basal cells has produced nail. The distal portion of these keratin-synthesizing cells is the distal portion of the pale lunula of the nail (see Figure 9-13). The nail rests on a nail bed of epidermal cells. After the 20th week, no granular layer is noted in the nail bed. The lateral margins of the nail plate are encased by lateral nail folds. The nail bed overlies a rich vasculature; however, no subcutaneous tissue develops and underlying bone intimately approximates the nail bed.[55,56]

The hyponychium, the region between the distal portion of the nail bed and the distal nail

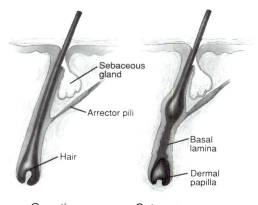
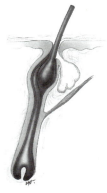

Anagen Growth Phase    Catagen    Telegen Shedding

**Figure 9-12.** Three stages of hair growth. Under normal conditions more than 90% of scalp hairs are in the actively growing (anagen) stage. A negligible number are in the catagen phase. Fewer than 10% are normally found to be falling out (telogen phase).

Sebaceous gland

Arrector pili

Hair

Basal lamina

Dermal papilla

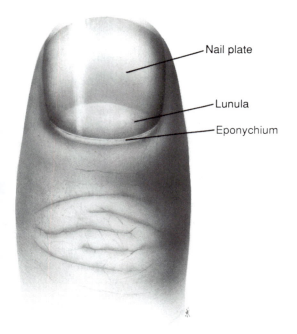

**Figure 9-13.** External appearance of nail. The distal portion of all 10 digits contains a hard nail plate of keratin produced from matrix cells proximal to the lunula.

Nail plate

Lunula

Eponychium

groove, is another portion of the nail unit. Clinically, the hyponychium appears as a hard, keratinous growth that prevents debris from entering beneath the distal portion of the nail. Though the nail can be considered a relatively vestigial organ, it can be affected by numerous external and systemic agents. Because it is produced by rapidly dividing cells it is particularly influenced by acute disease states.

*Dermis*

*Basement Membrane*

The cutaneous basement membrane refers to the extracellular structures organized at the interface between the epidermis and dermis. Recent research has led to a much better understanding of the details of composition, organization, and function in this region.[57]

Congenital defects in the basement membrane may result from either a lack of production of basement membrane constituents or synthesis of defective components. These abnormalities result in poor cohesion between the epidermis and dermis. Clinically, this shows as vesicles, blisters, and bullae following the application of minimal frictional forces.

Fortunately, inherited mechanobullous disorders are uncommon. Commonly encountered processes such as blistering inflammatory dermatoses, autoimmune blistering disorders, friction blisters, and coma bullae are caused by damage to the basement membrane at the dermoepidermal junction.

The epidermal basement membrane lies between the epidermis and the dermis and is responsible for the bonding of these two layers of the skin (Figure 9-15). The epidermal basement membrane begins at its attachment to the plasma membrane of the basal epidermal cells. These basal cells are predominantly keratinocytes, but Merkel cells and melanocytes are also found in this cell layer. Electron microscopy shows three morpho-

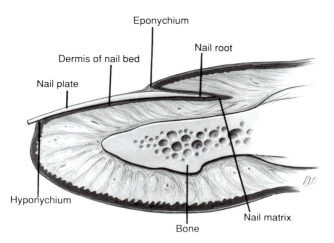

Eponychium

Nail root

Dermis of nail bed

Nail plate

Hyponychium

Bone

Nail matrix

**Figure 9-14.** Longitudinal section of nail unit. The nail, a nonviable, rigid keratin structure, covers the nail bed and protects the dermal vasculature and bone.

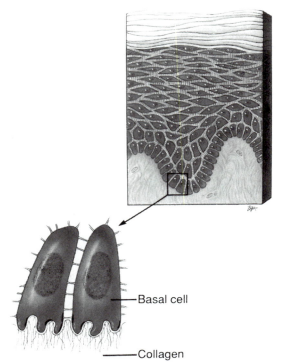

Figure 9-15. Basement membrane uniting epidermis and cutis (macro). The epidermis and cutis are firmly joined by a basement membrane.

logically distinct layers of epidermal basement membrane: (1) the lamina lucida, (2) the lamina densa, and (3) the sub–lamina densa fibrillar zone (reticular zone; Figure 9-16).

The lamina lucida is located subjacent to the plasma membrane of basal epidermal cells and is 20 to 40 nm thick. As its name implies, this layer is relatively electron lucent; it contains anchoring filaments, laminin, and fibronectin. The anchoring filaments connect the epidermal cell plasma membranes to deeper structures by traversing this region. The lamina lucida also contains the bullous pemphigoid antigen, a glycoprotein identified by antibodies in the sera of patients with this disorder. Other less well-characterized antigens have been localized to this region by antibodies in the sera of patients with other blistering disorders such as herpes gestationis and scarring pemphigoid.[58]

The lamina densa is an electron-dense band immediately below the lamina ludica that runs parallel to the epidermal cell lower border. It is approximately 30 to 60 nm thick. The major component of this region is type IV collagen; other components include heparin sulfate and proteoglycan, but the strength of the basement membrane is in large part attributable to type IV collagen. Laminin and type IV collagen bind to each other. A noncollagenous antigen, KF-1, has been identified in the lamina densa by a skin-specific monoclonal antibody.[58]

The sub–lamina densa fibrillar zone lies between the lamina densa above and dermal stroma below. This layer is principally composed of anchoring fibrils and to a lesser extent finer fibrils called *elastic microfibrils* (oxytalan fibers) and interstitial collagen fibrils composed of type III collagen. Two antigens, AF-1 and AF-2, are localized to the sub–lamina densa as well as the antigens associated with epidermolysis bullosa acquisita.[58]

The anchoring fibrils are cross-banded structures extending from the lamina densa into the dermis. They occasionally form loops linking one portion of the lamina densa to another while anchoring around dermal collagen bundles. The finer fibrils move deeply into the dermis and sometimes are associated with elastic fibers.

The epidermal cells are attached to the basement membrane by hemidesmosomes. The anchoring filaments in the lamina lucida are attached to the basal epidermal cell hemidesmosomes, which are situated along the dermal surface of the basal keratinocytes.

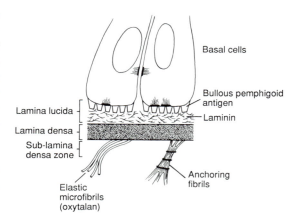

Figure 9-16. Basement membrane uniting epidermis and cutis (micro). Cohesion between the epidermis and cutis is well-served by a discrete multilayered structure, the basement membrane, which is composed of the lamina lucida, lamina densa, and sub–lamina densa.

**Relationships to Disease.** Defects in the structure of the basement membrane are thought to be responsible for the inherited blistering disorder epidermolysis bullosa. For example, in junctional epidermolysis bullosa the blistering arises within the lamina lucida and is associated morphologically with rudimentary and sparse hemidesmosomes.[57] In dystrophic epidermolysis bullosa blistering occurs beneath the lamina densa and morphologically is associated with abnormal anchoring fibrils.[57]

In autoimmune disorders such as bullosa pemphigoid, bullous systemic lupus erythematosus, and dermatitis herpetiformis, deposition of antibodies within the basement membrane zone has been visualized by immunofluorescence- and immunoelectron microscopy. Presumably, the presence of the antibodies alters the structural function of the antigenic component of the basement membrane, thus causing dyshesion. Alternatively, or additionally, antigen-antibody complexes may stimulate inflammatory destructive processes (e.g., activation of complement).

The mechanism by which mechanical or frictional bullae develop has not been well characterized, but it appears to involve stress-induced injury to the structional components of the basement membrane. In bullae associated with coma, anoxia of the skin occurs from prolonged periods of pressure caused by the patient's weight while he or she remains in one position.[59] The anoxia presumably results in destruction of the structional integrity of the basement membrane and leads to formation of blisters. In extreme cases, when this occurs over bony prominences decubitus ulcers form.

*Vasculature*[60]

Compared to other organs the dermis of the skin has a disproportionately large blood supply. This extensive network of vessels is functionally involved in heat transfer and in serving the metabolic needs of the large numbers of eccrine and sebaceous glands in the cutis. Embryonically, all three elements of the vasculature—arteries, veins, and lymphatics—are mesodermal in origin and accordingly can regenerate with relative ease.

Anatomically, the dermis' major vascular network consists of two parallel systems of blood vessels traversing it in a pattern horizontal to the epidermis (Figure 9-17). These two units are connected vertically by communicating vessels oriented perpendicular to the epidermis. The anatomic origin of the cutaneous vasculature can be traced to perforating vessels emerging from muscular arteries that in turn penetrate through the

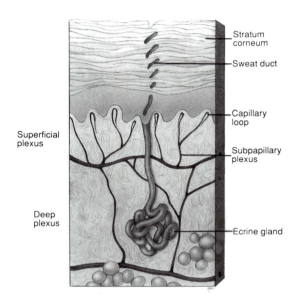

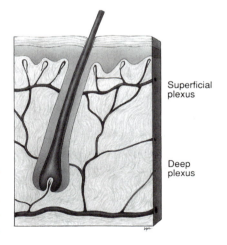

**Figure 9-17.** (*A*) Vasculature of the cutis. The cutaneous blood supply is characterized by two parallel branches of vessels connected by communicating branches perpendicular to the skin surface. (*B*) Vascular plexus of the cutis. The superficial and deep plexus of vessels provide the blood supply for the cutis.

subcutaneous fascia and then traverse in a direction perpendicular to the skin surface. The vessels that pass directly through the subcutaneous tissue bypass the subcutaneous fat by traversing within the fibrous septa, which separate fat lobules.

The deepest vascular plexus, the transverse one, supplies principally the adnexal glands (sebaceous and eccrine), whereas the more superficial ones form the papillary plexus. This plexus, which is rich in capillaries, is localized in the dermal papillae abutting the epidermis (see Figure 9-17B). The superficial and the deep vascular plexus have numerous anastomoses and form an exceedingly abundant blood supply. Blood returns through an almost identical venous pattern of vessels located in close apposition to the arteries. Under most circumstances the arterial venous communications are mediated by a rich capillary network, though the capillary beds may be bypassed by direct shunts between arteries and venules known as *glomus bodies* (Figure 9-18). These are particularly effective in regulating heat loss in these acral areas.

The vascular blood flow is controlled principally by the resistance of arterioles. They constrict following adrenergic stimulation of unmyelinated sympathetic fibers. Hormonal effects on the smooth muscles of arterioles of the skin include a vasopressor action from angiotensin and adrenalin. Histamine, alcohol, prostaglandins, and heat are associated with vasodilatation.

*Mast Cells*

Mast cells are derived from the bone marrow and distributed via the bloodstream to all tissues and organs of the body except solid bone and cartilage. Mast cells contain myriad mediators that are preformed and stored within granules or produced following mast cell activation. The group that are preformed can be further divided into those that are soluble following mast cell degranulation and those that are insoluble and remain associated with the extruded granules.[61] Table 9-2 lists representative mast cell mediators. Mast cells in humans form two groups, based on their proteinase content. One group contains tryptase; the other, a tryptase and a chymotryptase. In any given anatomic site more than one subpopulation of mast

**Table 9-2.** Mast Cell Mediators[61]

| Released in Soluble Form | Stored in Granules Released Within Granules (Insoluble) | Synthesized Upon Mast Cell Activation |
| --- | --- | --- |
| Histamine | Proteoglycans | Platelet-activating factors |
| Serotonin | Proteases | Leukotrienes |
| Proteases | Inflammatory factors | Prostaglandins |
| Exoglycosidases | Peroxidase | Adenosine |
| Chemotactic Factors | Superoxide dismutase | |

cells may be present, and differences are observable in their mediators.

Although the IgE receptor and the IgE antibody-antigen induction processes have been studied extensively in relation to the activation of the mast cell, a vast array of other mediators and stimuli have also been found to initiate mast cell activation. For example, selected neuropeptides, endogenous opioids, hormones, T-cell factors, complement (C3a, C5a), and interleukin 1 have been found to stimulate histamine secretion. The major rationale for the wide use of antihistamines is to block histamine receptors on target cells and so prevent allergic responses resulting from mast cell histamine release. Corticosteroids inhibit secretion of mast cell mediators and are widely used, systemically and topically, for allergic reactions and for other mast cell disorders such as urticaria pigmentosa.[62]

The mast cell, with its diverse array of mediators, is involved in many biologic activities, but the precise role of the mast cell and its mediators in such activities is under investigation and has been reviewed.[61,63,64] Broadly, the mast cell participates in inflammatory responses (both immediate and delayed hypersensitivity), angiogenesis, immunoregulation, and fibrosis. Thus, the skin mast cells are found to accumulate or be activated in the following disorders: (1) normal wound healing, (2) keloids, (3) neurofibromas, (4) mastocytosis, (5) eosinophilic fasciitis, and (6) scleroderma.

*Collagen*

Collagen, a protein widely distributed throughout all organs and tissues, comprises 70% to 80% of the dry weight of human skin.[65] Collagen functions principally in a structural role, maintaining form and limiting deformation. It also participates in blood clotting, inflammation, and tissue repair.

Fifteen distinct types of collagen exist; each has a characteristic tissue distribution. All collagens are composed of three polypeptide chains, referred to as $\alpha$ chains, which consist of repeating tripeptides gly-X-Y. One third of the X and Y residues are proline or 4-hydroxyproline. Alpha chains are of 18 different types that combine to form the 15 different types of collagen.[66] Variation between collagen types also depends on the extent of glycosylation of hydroxylysine residues and the hydroxylation of proline.

Type I collagen is the most abundant form and the only collagen type in bone and tendon. The predominant form in adult human skin, Type I collagen is composed of two distinct $\alpha$ polypeptide chains (two $\alpha_1$, and one $\alpha_2$ chain to form the triple helix). Type II, composed of three identical $\alpha$ chains, is found in cartilaginous tissues. Type III collagen consists of three identical $\alpha$ chains and is distributed widely throughout the body, including the skin. Type IV collagen is a major component of the basement membrane. Type V collagen is present in small amounts throughout the body and can be detected in the dermis. Type VII collagen is present in the skin as part of the anchoring fibril complex.

Granulation tissue contains increased amounts of types I, III, and V collagens. Collagen types I, II, and III form broad, banded, extracellular fibers and are called *interstitial collagens*. Collagen types IV to X are minor collagens that do not form banded fibers.

Collagen has a low rate of cell turnover; the half-life of collagen is estimated to be 2 1/2 years. The continuous remodeling and degradation of collagen makes it a valuable material to study for changes associated with aging. Studies in vitro of the rate of cutaneous collagen synthesis show increases up to age 30 to 40 years, after which synthesis remains approximately constant.[66]

Collagen is synthesized by fibroblasts in the dermis. Each $\alpha$ chain has a distinct gene and corresponding mRNA. A triple helix structure is formed as the collagen chains are released from polysomes. Procollagen is secreted from the cells and is converted to collagen in the extracellular space by the action of neutral endoproteases that remove propeptides (Figure 9-18).

The largest fibrils of type I collagen are 50 to 300 nm in diameter. Electron microscopy shows a 67-nm repeating banding pattern caused by the staggered alignment of individual collagen molecules. Aggregates of these collagen molecules form fibrils. Cross-linking between collagen molecules occurs through post-translational modification of lysine and hydroxylysine residues. Four enzymes are important in these modifications: (1) prolyl-4-hydroxylase, (2) lysyl hydroxylase, (3) galactosyl transferase, and (4) glucosyl transferase. The activity of all these enzymes decreases in human skin with aging. The activity of prolyl hydroxylase depends on oxygen and vitamin C intake. Thus, malnutrition or poor circulation would be expected to compromise tissue viability and collagen repair processes.

As collagen matures and stabilizes in the extracellular matrix it becomes progressively less soluble. Collagen in skin is more susceptible to pepsin digestion than intestinal collagen. Pepsin digestin is inversely related to the extent of cross-linking. The greater solubility of skin collagen may therefore be related to greater turnover of skin collagen. Weight changes alter the need for more skin, and damage resulting from external environmental changes may affect skin collagen and enhance turnover. Many of the factors important in regulating collagen synthesis are only partially understood; however, hydrocortisone and fluorinated corticosteroids applied topically or delivered intradermally inhibit collagen synthesis. This may in part explain the dermal atrophy observed with continued use of these agents.[67]

With increasing age, collagen throughout the body shows physical changes that are due to progressive cross-linking or chemical stabilization. These changes may be responsible for the loss of skin elasticity with age. Collagen is associated with glycosaminoglycans in the dermis. These polymers are lost with aging, and this results in decreased water-binding capacity, or hydration of the skin, leading to a dry, wrinkled appearance.[65]

*Elastic Tissue*

Elastic tissue, a connective tissue component of the dermis, constitutes about 0.6% to 2% of its

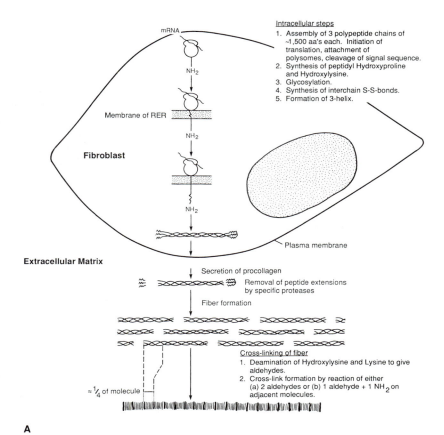

Intracellular steps
1. Assembly of 3 polypeptide chains of
   ~1,500 aa's each. Initiation of
   translation, attachment of
   polysomes, cleavage of signal sequence.
2. Synthesis of peptidyl Hydroxyproline
   and Hydroxylysine.
3. Glycosylation.
4. Synthesis of interchain S-S-bonds.
5. Formation of 3-helix.

mRNA

NH$_2$

Membrane of RER

NH$_2$

Fibroblast

NH$_2$

Plasma membrane

Extracellular Matrix

Secretion of procollagen

Removal of peptide extensions
by specific proteases

Fiber formation

Cross-linking of fiber
1. Deamination of Hydroxylysine and Lysine to give
   aldehydes.
2. Cross-link formation by reaction of either
   (a) 2 aldehydes or (b) 1 aldehyde + 1 NH$_2$ on
   adjacent molecules.

≈ $\frac{1}{4}$ of molecule

A

**Figure 9-18.** (A) Collagen synthesis and assembly. Procollagen is synthesized and secreted into the extracellular matrix by fibroblasts. Collagen fibers are formed in the extracellular compartment by a specific enzymatic cross-linking process.

total dry weight. All elastic tissue components derive from a mesodermal stem cell; the mature fibroblast is the parent of both collagen and elastic fibers. The formation of elastic fibers appears to result from active secretion of a protein-rich microfibril that polymerizes along the cell surface of the fibroblast.[68] This glycoprotein forms tubular bundles that encase an amorphous protein, elastin.

In a mature elastic fiber the elastin component accounts for more than 90% of the total weight. Elastin is an amorphous insoluble protein that when fully mature, is arranged in sheets. The relative insolubility of elastin is due principally to covalent linkages of elastin polypeptides by desmosine and isodesmosine, which are unique to elastic fibers. Conclusive data demonstrate that human fibroblasts also synthesize elastin, and, in-

deed, the presence of a gene controlling elastin synthesis has been demonstrated in fibroblasts by Davidson.[68] Elastin messenger RNA has also been identified. An enzyme, lysyl oxidase, which is a crucial initial step in the cross-linking of elastin by deaminating lysyl residues, has recently been purified. Lysyl oxidase requires copper for biologic activity.[69]

Skin turgor or tone (the ability of skin that has been extended by a force to return rapidly to its original position) is the primary function of elastic tissues.[70] Defects in or damage to elastic fibers can alter this property and contribute to old-looking skin.[71-73]

**Dermal Matrix.**    The dermal matrix or ground substance represents the third component of the

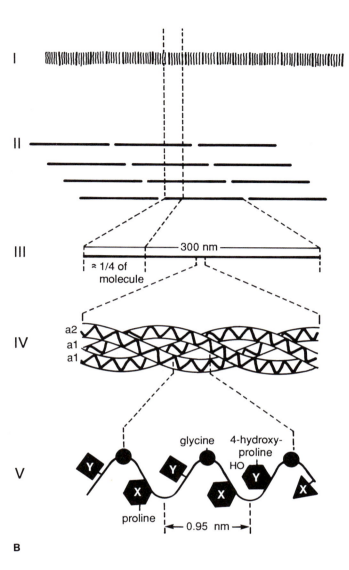

**B**

**Figure 9-18.** (*continued*) (*B*) Collagen structure: I, The banding pattern of collagen seen by electron microscopy; II, the alignment of collagen fibers that accounts for the banding pattern seen in I; III, the 300-nm banding pattern repeats that consist of overlapping collagen fibers; IV, a collagen fiber consists of three collagen chains that are helically arranged; V, the repeating primary amino acid structure of collagen. (*B* from Uitto J, et al. Collagen: Its structure, function, and pathology. In: Progress in Diseases of the Skin, vol 1. New York: Grune and Stratton, 1981; 103.)

dermis. It consists primarily of protoglycan and glycosaminoglycans (GAGs). Its gross appearance is mucoid and it contains a high percentage of mucopolysaccharides. Quantitatively, ground substance represents less than 1% of the dry weight of the dermis. It is not a primary source of major cutaneous diseases.

*Innervation*

More than 1 million afferent nerve fibers located within the skin monitor the external environ-ment—heat, cold, touch, and pain. The terminal endings of these fibers are located principally at the dermoepidermal junction, adnexal structures, or deep cutis (Figure 9-19). They consist of two types of nerve endings: *corpuscular*, which are in direct contact with cutaneous structures, and *free* nerve endings, which traverse the cutis. The latter envelop the majority of hair follicles (see Figure 9-19).[74] Specific sensory functions of both the free nerve endings and encapsulated receptors remain controversial. It appears that significant overlap exists in the reception of external stimuli (energies) that are cortically perceived in terms of temperature, touch, and pain (see Figure 9-19).

*Corpuscular nerve units* were originally (but are no longer) considered as specific for heat, pain, touch, and cold. The types of units may be generally defined as follows: *Pacinian corpuscles* are ovoid structures that on cross-section are laminar, like an onion (see Figure 9-18). They are found extensively on the soles and, therefore, may subserve pressure. *Meissner corpuscles* are found in the papillary dermis of glabrous skin. They may be related to tactile sensations. They are found primarily on fingertips, palms, and soles. These lobulated nerve endings are found in all mammals.[75] *Merkel cells* may resemble LCs and frequently are located in the epidermal rete ridges. They communicate with nerve fibrils and may be important as specialized cells adapted to touch reception. *Ruffini structures* are present in heavy concentration in the digits and are connected to myelinated afferent fibers and appear to be related to fine perception.

**Somatic Sensory Innervation of the Skin.**

FREE NERVE ENDINGS. Within the papillary dermis an extensive network of ectodermally derived unmyelinated nerve fibers course in a horizontal path. Their external sheath is composed of Schwann cells in direct contact with the cells of the dermoepidermal junction or enveloping the adnexal glands (see Figure 9-19). A particular group of these fibers, called *thick myelinated Aβ fibers,* appear most receptive to touch and vibration, whereas the thinner Aγ are most sensitive to light touch and pressure. The thinnest, known as Aδ, transmit pain, temperature, and "causal" or physiologic itching. A poorly localized sensation of pruritus, often a feature of various chronic dermatologic conditions, appears to be carried by still other nerve fibers that are anatomically deeper and unrelated to pain perception.[76]

Receiving information on the external environment is a prerequisite to human survival and is probably related to the evolutionary development and present overlap of a complex cutaneous sensory network of receptor fibers.

Pruritus (itching) has often been described as a stimulus transmitted to the cortex that elicits a desire to scratch.[77] Although no hard evidence exists, itching may have had survival value in protecting against parasites, fleas, and other insects that were vectors for systemic disease. The mediation of the itch sensation remains controversial. Relatively strong clinical data indicate that pain and itching are separable sensations; it ap-

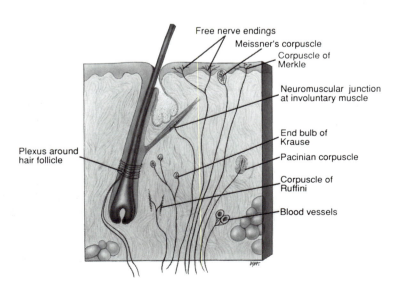

**Figure 9-19.** Corpuscular structure and free nerve endings innervating the skin. Temperature, pressure, touch, and pain are received as afferent stimuli by diverse corpuscular structures and free nerve endings.

pears that the papillary dermis has an extensive network of superficial unmyelinated nerve fiber endings, C fibers, that as receptors transmit impulses for both mild cutaneous pain and itching. Indeed, patients with central cord lesions of syringomyelia lose pain sensation but not touch, suggesting that C fibers are polymodal, with varying thresholds of responsiveness.

In chronic, extremely pruritic, widespread skin conditions, the unmyelinated fibers appear to be mediating pruritus solely when minimally excited. In contrast, the sensory fibers of the δ type mediate the mild localized casual itching as well as cutaneous pain in the same fiber. Again, an arbitrary distinction between structure and function in the superficial dermal fibers is difficult if not impossible to make. It is noteworthy that when areas of skin are denuded and devoid of epidermis and dermal papillae itching is not elicited; rather, severe pain is felt. This reinforces the concept that superficial and deep sensory nerve receptors may not be function specific.

What chemical stimuli discharge nerve receptors is also unclear. Current evidence indicates that proteases brought by an inflammatory white blood cell response to an eczematous process provide the stimuli. In other cases, mast cell degranulation liberates several diverse-acting pruritic agents. Recent studies document that epidermal cells may secrete proteases that they themselves have manufactured. These chemicals or their substrates may be the true initiators of pruritus.

The list of mediators involved in pruritic sensation is constantly expanding. The majority have the chemical structure of peptides. It is probable that each agent has a preferential role in selective sites or situations. Currently under study, in addition to the classical pruritic agent histamine, are serotonin, slow-reacting substance, bradykinins, endorphins, and endopeptidases.[78,79]

### Subcutaneous Tissue

Beneath the dermis is the hypodermis or subcutaneous tissue layer (see Figure 9-1). Its origin in midfetal life derives from mesenchymal cells that give rise to lipocytes and fibrocytes.[80] These in turn give rise to a fully mature fibrous tissue and a lobulated adipocyte layer that is in direct apposition to the dermis above and the fascia below (see Figure 9-1). Within the fibrous septa surrounding the lipocytes course nerve fibers, blood vessels, and lymphatics. Under normal conditions the unstained lipocytes have a characteristic clear cytoplasm, the nucleus being compressed and displaced against the cell membrane. The largest biochemical constituent of lipocytes is triglycerides. Subcutaneous tissue stores energy in the form of fat, provides insulation against heat loss, and cushions internal structures against environmental trauma or pressure.[81]

## Selected Functions

### Vitamin D Synthesis

Vitamin D is photosynthesized in keratinocytes following irradiation with ultraviolet B (UVB, 290 to 320 nm; Figure 9-20). The synthetic pathway begins with 7-dehydrocholesterol being converted to pre–vitamin $D_3$ (cholecalciferol) by UVB. Pre–vitamin $D_3$ undergoes thermal conversion to vitamin $D_3$. Vitamin $D_3$ is released into the bloodstream bound to vitamin D–binding protein (DBP) and is transported to the liver for hydroxylation to form 25-hydroxycholecalciferol and then to the kidney to finally form 1,25-dihydroxy vitamin $D_3$, the most metabolically active form of vitamin D.[82]

Following exposure to intense UVB, not all of the 7-dehydrocholesterol is converted to pre–vitamin D, because alternative pathways exist for the formation of less active metabolites. These alternative routes of metabolism may be an important mechanism whereby excessive ultraviolet exposure does not lead to hypervitaminosis D.

Vitamin D deficiency results in rickets in children and osteomalacia in adults. It may occur in instances of low dietary intake or inadequate exposure to UV radiation. Sunscreen lotions have been shown to block cutaneous synthesis of vitamin D following UV exposure, presumably by blocking transmission of the 295-nm wavelength necessary for the photochemical synthesis of vitamin D. Because elderly persons are cautious about aging changes and skin cancer as hazards of excessive sun exposure, their vitamin D status is

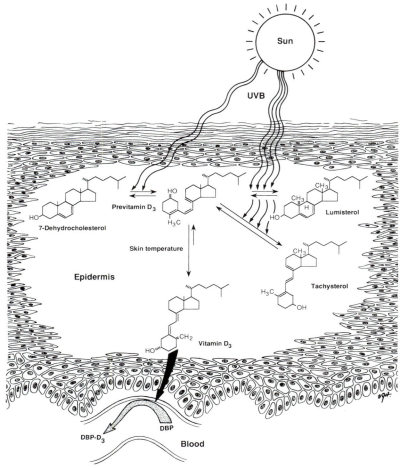

**Figure 9-20.** Synthesis and metabolism of vitamin D in the skin. Pre–vitamin D is formed following the UVB irradiation of 7-dehydrocholesterol. Thermal catalysis converts pre–vitamin $D_3$ to vitamin $D_3$. Excessive ultraviolet radiation causes pre–vitamin $D_3$ to form the less active metabolites, lumisterol and tachysterol. Vitamin D–binding protein (DBP) binds and transports the vitamin $D_3$ to the liver for hydroxylation.

a concern. Their dietary intake of vitamin D is poor, and they often avoid the sun or wear sunscreen.[83]

Vitamin D and its active metabolites form an endocrine system important in the absorption of calcium from the diet, conservation of calcium by the kidney, mineralization of bones, and maintenance of normal plasma levels of calcium (important for normal neuromuscular conduction). These processes were comprehensively reviewed by DeLuca.[101]

The cellular effects of 1,25-dihydroxy vitamin $D_3$ are mediated through interaction with a nuclear receptor protein of 55,000 kd that belongs to a superfamily of receptors that bind steroid hormones, retinoic acid, and thyroid hormone.[84] The 1,25-dihydroxy vitamin $D_3$ receptor protein is expressed in practically all tissues, including keratinocytes and fibroblasts from the skin.[84] Autoradiography of frozen tissue sections using labeled 1,25-dihydroxy vitamin $D_3$ has suggested the presence of the nuclear receptor in tissues that were not previously considered to be target tissues for vitamin D, such as the parathyroid gland, pancreatic islets, some bone marrow cells, and cutaneous keratinocytes. Another finding is that approximately 60% of all cancer cell lines have large amounts of the receptor.

A number of genes have been recognized to be regulated by 1,25-dihydroxy vitamin $D_3$: calcium metabolism–related proteins (e.g., preproparathyroid hormone, calcitonin, calbindin), oncogenes (c-*myc*, c-*fos*, and c-*fes*), the 1,25-dihydroxy vitamin $D_3$ receptor, and several others, among them type I collagen, fibronectin, prolactin, interleukin, and I L 2. For each of these genes, levels of mRNA accumulation have been shown to be either increased or decreased by 1,25-dihydroxy vitamin $D_3$.[84]

During the past decade researchers have identified actions of 1,25-dihydroxy vitamin $D_3$ in addition to its role in mineral metabolism. These actions include influences on differentiation and proliferation of the hematopoietic cells, cancer cells, and epidermal cells (keratinocytes)[84] and thus may be responsible in part for the clinical findings associated with rickets (i.e., increased infections, impaired neutrophil phagocytosis, anemia, decreased cellularity of the marrow, extramedullary hematopoiesis.

Receptors for 1,25-dihydroxy vitamin $D_3$ are present in a variety of cancer cell lines, including melanoma.[84] Large doses of 1,25-dihydroxy vitamin $D_3$ have inhibited melanoma xenografts in mice. Also, 1,25-dihydroxy vitamin $D_3$ stimulates fibronectin production by human cancer cell lines, and it has been suggested that this may mediate an antimetastatic effect for vitamin D. Future studies will evaluate the potential therapeutic use of vitamin D and its analogues for chemoprevention or therapy of human malignancies.

In cultured skin cells 1,25-dihydroxy vitamin $D_3$ induces antiproliferative changes such as decreased DNA synthesis and promotes terminal differentiation toward nonadherent cornified squamous cells. Synthesis of 1,25-dihydroxy vitamin $D_3$ occurs in neonatal, but not adult, skin. The possibility exists that 1,25-dihydroxy vitamin $D_3$ produced in the skin may exert local effects on keratinocyte proliferation and differentiation. Preliminary studies of orally or topically administered 1,25-dihydroxy vitamin $D_3$ to patients with psoriasis have shown that the skin lesions improve. Psoriasis, a benign skin disorder characterized by hyperproliferation of keratinocytes resulting in the formation of thickened plaques, remains a therapeutic problem. Flattening of lesions following therapy with 1,25-dihydroxy vitamin $D_3$ has been reported and is consistent with the antiproliferative effects of 1,25-dihydroxy vitamin $D_3$ observed in cultured epidermal skin cells. The role of vitamin D and its analogues in the treatment of psoriasis and other cutaneous disorders requires further study to evaluate its efficacy.

### Percutaneous Absorption

A major function of the skin is as a barrier or interface between the rest of the body and the external environment. This barrier is selective, allowing some molecules that come in contact with the skin to penetrate to various levels within the epidermis and dermis and others, most notably moisture, to escape from the epidermis to the ambient environment.

The penetration of compounds through the skin has been intensively studied by researchers evaluating chemicals used in cosmetics and for topical therapy and those encountered in occupational settings. Determination of the rate and degree of penetration of chemicals into the skin is complex and is dependent upon (1) concentration, (2) type of vehicle, (3) skin region, (4) skin condition, and (5) extent of occlusion.[85]

Chemicals have very different skin penetration rates; the differences may exceed four orders of magnitude.[85] When injury or disease alters the structure of the skin, making it thinner, thicker, or discontinuous, the rate of absorption may be affected significantly. The stratum corneum, or horny layer, normally varies in thickness from less than 0.01 mm in eyelid skin to 1 mm in palmar or plantar skin. Nevertheless the ease with which certain agents penetrate the skin of the palms or soles may be great despite the thickness of the stratum corneum in these areas. The stratum corneum is still considered the rate-limiting barrier in cutaneous absorption, unless it is absent owing to skin disease or injury. Once the agent or drug has penetrated the stratum corneum it may diffuse transcellularly or through intercellular spaces to reach the basement membrane and dermis. From the dermis, agents or their cutaneous metabolites are taken up into systemic circulation.

The chemical structure, size, polarity, and degree of hydration are important factors in determining the diffusivity of the compound. Small lipophilic compounds lacking polar groups or ionic charges diffuse most readily. When a lipophilic compound is applied to the skin dispersed in a hydrophilic vehicle, it diffuses into the stratum corneum more effectively than when it is applied in a lipophilic vehicle. In addition to penetration of the epidermis, compounds may also enter the skin via the pores associated with skin appendages (i.e., sweat ducts, hair follicles, sebaceous glands; Figure 9-21).

The hazards from percutaneous absorption of noxious chemicals include (1) direct toxic effects on the skin (e.g., caustic agents); (2) systemic toxicity from absorption through the skin; and (3) induction of contact dermatitis, either the allergic or primary irritant type. Tables of compounds that are particularly hazardous for skin exposure have been made in many countries. These lists may be used to establish guidelines for protective skin covering requirements to prevent toxic exposure, especially in the workplace.

In addition to the general process of percutaneous absorption there is a phenomenon referred to as the *reservoir effect*. This is best exemplified in the absorption of topical glucocorticosteroids. Topical steroids accumulate in the stratum corneum following initial application. When, long after the last application of the topical steroid, the skin is covered with plastic wrap, the hydration of the stratum corneum and the remainder of the epidermis increases. This results in increased systemic absorption of the topical steroid because more drug can penetrate the epidermis to reach the circulation.

Percutaneous absorption requires special caution in premature and full-term infants. First, the ratio of the surface area to total body weight is much greater in a newborn than in an adult. Thus, in a newborn a percutaneous dose systemically absorbed is estimated to be about 2.7 times greater per kilogram of body weight than the same topical dose per unit area in an adult. The skin of a term infant is considered to be an intact barrier, though, because the stratum corneum may be thinner than an adult's the neonate may absorb more drug. The skin of the premature infant is considered to be an immature barrier that allows greater percutaneous drug absorption and skin water loss. The epidermis matures from weeks 23 to 33 of gestation.[86] Premature babies born during this period have an

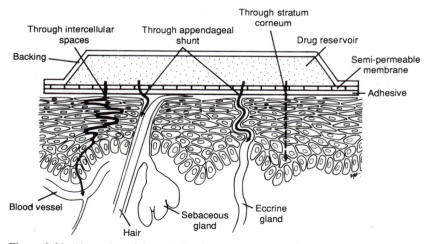

**Figure 9-21.** Absorption of drugs delivered transcutaneously from transdermal patches applied to the skin. This drug delivery system has the following potential routes for transcutaneous absorption of the drug to the blood vessels: (1) intercellular spaces, (2) appendiceal shunts such as the hair follicle or sweat duct, and (3) across cells without partitioning significantly between cells.

incomplete epidermal barrier and characteristically suffer increased transepidermal water loss and increased drug absorption per unit of surface area.[86] Following birth, the premature infant's skin quickly matures, and by postnatal week 2 or 3 its epidermal barrier approximates that of term infants, children, and adults.[86]

Inadvertent drug toxicity has been reported in newborns; often the toxicant is a disinfectant used in nurseries or laundry detergent.[87] Newborn infants have developed cutaneously derived toxic reactions, most commonly from diaper agents, topical antiseptics, and skin preparations. Premature infants are at greatest risk owing to their incomplete epidermal barrier and the greater likelihood of intensive care that requires invasive procedures. In this regard the following observations are offered:

1. Routine skin or umbilical care does not require an antiseptic.
2. Isopropyl alcohol swabs or aqueous chlorhexidine used sparingly is adequate to prepare the skin for invasive procedures.
3. Alcohol solutions, iodine, hexachlorophene, and neomycin-containing sprays are particularly hazardous and should not be used.

Several commonly used dermatologic preparations have associated risks and complications, particularly for newborns (Table 9-3).

**Table 9-3.** Dermatologic Preparations with High Risk Potential for Infants

| Topical Agent | Toxicity |
| --- | --- |
| Steroids | Adrenal suppression, particularly when the epidermal barrier is disrupted |
| Boric acid | Gastrointestonal, neurologic, dermatologic complications |
| Lindane | Well documented in animals and may similarly affect infants. |
| Epinephrine | Applied to bleeding sites, (e.g., after circumcision) can cause tachycardia and heart failure |
| Urea cream (10%) | When applied for ichthyosis BUN can get very high despite normal creatinine value |
| Estrogens | May produce feminization in males and pseudoprecocious puberty in females |

### Percutaneous Drug Absorption as Therapy

A number of drugs can be delivered effectively and safely transdermally. The drug, dissolved in a suitable vehicle, penetrates a microporous membrane to deliver drug, which is then absorbed through the skin. Nitroglycerine, scopolamine, clonidine, estrogen, and testosterone are among the drugs delivered this way (Figure 9-21).

The advantages of transdermal drug delivery include (1) avoidance of irregularities in gastrointestinal absorption of drug, avoidance of first-pass metabolism by the liver, and continuous drug delivery. The effective use of transdermal drug delivery is limited to drugs that are active systemically in small quantities, are not irritating or sensitizing to skin, and are absorbed well across the stratum corneum and into the bloodstream.

## Wound Healing

Wound healing is a dynamic process influenced by multiple factors: (1) local structural repair elements of the dermis and epidermis, (2) host defenses against external pathogens that gain entry into the wound, (3) inflammatory mediators and growth factors produced locally at the site of injury or delivered via the bloodstream, (4) immigrant cells derived from the bone marrow and the quality of the regional circulation to a wound, as well as the amount of pressure, tension, and movement at the wound surface. An abnormality in any of these factors impairs the ability of host mechanisms to promote wound healing (Figure 9-22).

### Epithelial Repair

Epithelial cells actively divide at the wound edge and roll over each other to reepithelialize the wound surface. At the same time, the basement membrane to which the epithelial cells become attached is laid down beneath them. Bullous pemphigoid antigen is synthesized first, followed by laminin, and finally type IV collagen. Type IV collagen is synthesized when the entire wound is reepithelialized (e.g., 4 to 6 days after wounding).

Epithelial cells migrate only over viable tissue, because they are dependent upon underlying tis-

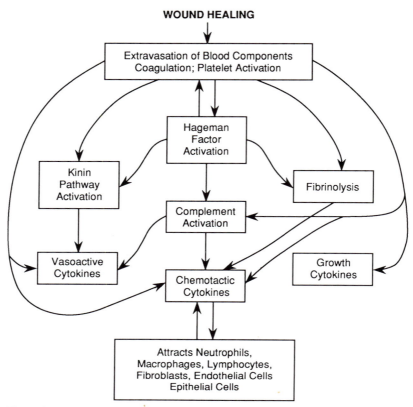

**WOUND HEALING**

**Figure 9-22.** Wound healing involves a complex process whereby many mediators and cytokines interplay to orchestrate an inflammatory response, removal of debris, and growth of new tissue.

sues for nutrients. Migration has been demonstrated to occur more readily over a moist wound bed. Crusts or eschars impede epithelial migration. It occurs more gradually as the new epithelium fights its way beneath the eschar.

Thus, epithelialization occurs during wound healing by the migration of keratinocytes to the wound site and by their subsequent proliferation. Recent studies have demonstrated that several mediators (extracellular matrix molecules and soluble peptide factors) modulate cultured keratinocyte motility and proliferation and may be important in vivo (Table 9-4).[88]

*Dermal Repair*

Following tissue injury, perivascular fibroblasts become activated and proliferate. Fibroblasts are responsible for the synthesis of collagen, elastin, glycosaminoglycans, and proteoglycans; all are components of the extracellular matrix.[89] During the early phase of wound repair, fibroblasts synthesize embryonic type III collagen, which as the wound matures is eventually replaced by adult type I collagen. New collagen is present in the wound within the first day after injury. In partial-thickness wounds, collagen synthesis peaks on the second or third day after injury, whereas in full-thickness wounds the rate of collagen synthesis peaks between the fifth and seventh days after injury. Collagen synthesis is accelerated as long as a year after injury, but is accompanied by simultaneous degradation by collagenases as the wound is remodeled. In addition to collagen, the elastin, proteoglycans, and glycosaminoglycans are restored to the connective tissue structure of the dermis. Angiogenesis, the development of new blood vessels, is an important component of wound healing, as it restores nutrient delivery. For example, angiogenesis is needed to bridge the vasculature from

**Table 9-4.** Effects of Wound Healing Factors on Keratinocytes[88]

| Agent | Keratinocyte Migration | Proliferation |
|---|---|---|
| Fibronectin | + + | |
| Thrombospondin | + | |
| Laminin | − | |
| High calcium | − | |
| growth factor = β* | + | |
| Epidermal growth factor* | + | + |
| Somatomedin C[†] | | + |
| Interferon-γ | − | − |
| Radiation | | − |

* May stimulate migration by induction of fibronectin production.
[†] Stimulates thrombospondin production.

grafts to the underlying blood supply, to rejoin vessels across a wound, or to provide new vasculature to a tissue defect. Lymphatics also regenerate, but permanent damage may result in an edematous wound that is susceptible to infection.

*Wound Contraction*

Following full-thickness excision of rodent skin, the defect closes itself by a process referred to as wound contraction. The edges of the wound are brought together by a centripetal action attributed to contraction of myofibroblasts at the wound edge. In some areas of human skin (e.g., perineum), this process occurs more readily and is more complete than in other areas. Epithelialization is necessary to achieve complete wound closure. Wound contractures across joints can limit mobility.

*Abnormal Wound Repair*

When the modeling of scars is defective, excessive scar tissue may accumulate over time. Some patients form keloids, abnormal tissue growths at the site of tissue injury. They are hypercellular, containing a more concentrated population of fibroblasts and an increased number of mast cells compared to normal dermal tissue. Hypertrophic scars consist of excessive scar tissue but are less prominent than keloids. Both hypertrophic scars and keloids are more likely to occur in areas of increased skin tension.

Poor healing can also complicate wound repair. It is associated with many local factors as well as multiple systemic conditions, as noted in Table 9-5.

*Malnutrition and Wound Healing*

Malnutrition causes delayed wound healing and is associated with patients who suffer from malabsorption, inability to receive enteral nutrition, or hypermetabolic or catabolic states. The inability to synthesize wound repair components adequately may result from deficiencies of a vitamin, mineral, protein, carbohydrate, or lipid. Infection may be a major problem secondary to immunodeficiency caused by malnutrition. Finally, edema from hypoalbuminemia poses physical stress on wound edges and can interfere with healing.[90]

Patients with significant wounds should be assessed for nutritional status and requirements. Intervention, as needed, must be a part of the overall approach to the patient with a healing wound.[91]

*Vascular Supply and Wound Healing*

Oxygen delivery to wounds is often a problem in patients with significant peripheral vascular disease. Determination of transcutaneous oxygen partial pressures has helped identify optimal sites of limb amputation for ischemic arterial disease. Unfortunately, the use of these measurements to predict venous ulcer healing does not distinguish which ulcers will heal. Clearly, many additional factors are involved in wound healing. Though oxygen tension is an important factor, venous ul-

**Table 9-5.** Factors That Promote Poor Wound Healing

| Local | Systemic |
|---|---|
| Suboptimal surgical technique | Chronic illness |
| Drugs (e.g., steroids, antineoplastics, aspirin) | Malnutrition |
| | Diabetes |
| Ischemia (arteriosclerosis, pressure occlusion) | Cushing's syndrome |
| Infection | Old age |
| Trauma | Vasculitis |
| Skin disease (e.g., psoriasis) | |
| Foreign body | |
| Neuropathy | |

cers with relatively poor oxygen tension have been shown to be capable of healing.[92]

## Wound Dressings

It is now widely accepted that wounds kept moist and free from infections epithelialize faster. Thus, occlusive and semiocclusive dressings are preferred over the formation of a thick eschar that occurs when wounds are kept open to the air. Eschar formation appears to impede keratinocyte migration; however, despite enhanced reepithelialization, return of the cutaneous barrier functions, as measured by transepidermal water loss, does not return more quickly when these dressings are utilized (see Figure 9-23).[93]

## New Approaches to Wound Healing

To aid in the healing of deep wounds and to diminish wound contraction, animal models have been developed that demonstrate the feasibility of using synthetic extracellular matrices for regeneration of skin. Extracellular matrices have been synthesized from cross-linked collagen-glycosaminoglycan polymers. Feeding these matrices with fibroblasts and keratinocytes has decreased wound contraction as skin regenerates.[94] To be optimally effective these matrices must be highly porous and show partial resistance to collagenase digestion.

The foregoing approach to wound healing has been extended to incorporate specific growth factors into the collagen matrix, to enhance angiogenesis and epidermal proliferation. For example, heparin-binding growth factor 2 and epidermal growth factor have been covalently bound to biotinylated collagen. This growth factor–enhanced matrix has been shown to sustain accelerated growth rates of human epidermal keratinocytes.[95] Future studies of this modified collagen in synthetic extracellular matrices could potentially enhance our ability to heal deep wounds.

Growth factors are also being applied directly to wounds to stimulate wound healing. Epidermal growth factor (10 μg/ml) in silver sulfadiazine cream, applied to skin graft donor sites, has been found to accelerate wound healing when compared with control sites treated with silver sulfadiazine cream only.[96]

## Retinoids

Pretreatment of patients for 2 weeks with topical all-*trans*-retinoic acid has been shown to decrease the time required for epithelialization following dermabrasion. Animal studies have further demonstrated that treatment of pig skin with retinoic acid prior to partial-thickness wounding resulted in enhanced epithelialization.[97] Continuation of the retinoic acid treatment after wounding, however, retarded epithelialization. Priming skin sites with external agents prior to surgical wounding may increase the capacity of tissues to heal.

Systemic 13-*cis*-retinoic acid has been helpful in healing, and eventually inducing remission, of severe nodulocystic acne. Approximately 5% of acne patients develop exuberant granulation tissue in acne lesions while receiving 13-*cis*-retinoic acid therapy. The mechanism for this retinoid effect is not well-characterized. As shown in a guinea pig model, animals treated with large doses (10 mg/kg) of 13-*cis*-retinoic acid exhibited delayed wound contraction.[98] When the retinoid therapy was discontinued, wound healing proceeded. As

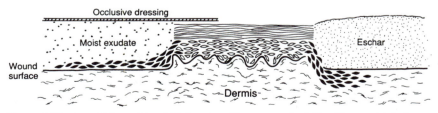

**Figure 9-23.** A multichannel hand FNS system ("neuroprosthesis") with completely implantable motor and sensory electrodes, lead wires and receiver/stimulator, powered and controlled by radio frequency and an external portable computer. (Keith MW, Peckham PH, Thrope GB, Buckett JR, Stroh KC, Menger V: Functional neuromuscular stimulation neuroprosthesis for the tetraplegic hand. Clin. Orthop. Rel. Research 1988, 233:25-33, by permission)

more patients may be treated with systemic retinoids for acne, psoriasis, and other cutaneous disorders, their management at the time of injury or surgery will require careful assessment, and possibly interruption of retinoid therapy to optimize tissue repair.

*Lasers*

Recently it was demonstrated that treatment of skin wounds with low-power laser irradiation enhanced healing.[99]

In summary, advances in wound healing are proceeding at a rapid pace. Improved treatment modalities involving molecular approaches are at present seen at the bedside, as exemplified by the use of recombinant epidermal growth factor in topical wound care.[96]

*Decubitus Ulcer*

The term *decubitus ulcer* is often used synonymously with the more frequently encountered expressions *bed sores* and *pressure ulcers*. All describe end-stage damage or death of the skin and subcutaneous tissues after ischemia over a bony prominence.[91,100] They vary in severity through a pattern of broad-spectrum tissue destruction that may be arbitrarily divided into the three stages (Figure 9-24).

The first stage is simply sharply demarcated, reversible erythema. In chronic cases there may be diapedesis of red blood cells leading to deposition of hemosiderin. At the end of this stage the central area may be cyanotic, with a periphery of erythema overlying the bony prominence. The affected area is often warm and painful.

When a break in the skin ensues, stage II is operative. It is characterized by a minor abrasion of the epidermis with more extensive damage to connective tissue. Experimental studies[101] indicate that, following pressure, subcutaneous tissue and muscle are more susceptible to necrosis than the epidermis. This contributes to the undermining frequently noted (see Figure 9-24). Small vesicles enlarging to form bullae may be noted in early decubitus ulcers. Secondary bacterial invasion frequently follows. With appropriate therapy and absence of pressure, the ulcer of stage II heals within a few weeks.

When the subcutaneous tissue is involved the

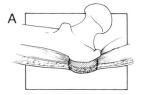
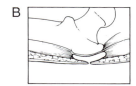
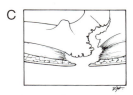

**Figure 9-24.** Decubitis ulcer formation. (*A*) Pressure over the greater trochanter results in anoxia of overlying skin and tissue friability. (*B*) Continued anoxia results in tissue breakdown and undermining of the ucler edges, causing wound extension. (*C*) Long-standing tissue necrosis permits entry of pathogens into the joint capsule, with attendant osteomyelitis and bone destruction.

ulcer is rapidly associated with fat necrosis and development of a thick, rigid, black eschar. Continued pressure leads to necrosis of fascia, muscles, and ligaments, and involvement of periosteal coverings. Bacterial infection is invariably present. Under most conditions, healing usually will not occur, even after several months, without extensive surgical intervention.

In the absence of therapy, stage III rapidly develops. It is characterized by bone necrosis, osteomyelitis, and fistula formation. The mortality rate for hospital patients with such advanced lesions exceeds 25%.

Decubitus ulcers occur most frequently where external pressure is exerted over bony prominences covered by minimal subcutaneous (adipose) tissue. In order of decreasing frequency these sites are the sacral bone, greater trochanter, ischial tuberosity, and lateral malleolus. As one might anticipate, the incidence of decubitus ulcers is highest in elderly, bedridden patients[100] and next highest among persons with spinal cord injuries that are complicated by urinary and fecal incontinence. Shearing forces such as those incurred when a patient slides in a wheelchair or is pulled across a bed sheet are other major contributing factors. Additional factors that are difficult to rank but that may place patients at increased risk include heavy smoking, hypoalbuminemia, xerotic (dry) skin, and anemia (hemoglobin less than 12 g/100 ml). Several factors found in the National Health Survey[91] to be unrelated include obesity, hypertension, and readily palpable femoral and dorsal pedis pulses.[101,102]

Decubitus ulcers can be diagnosed readily by their location and appearance. In selected cases the differential diagnosis includes pyoderma gangrenosum, stasis ulcer, ulceration secondary to ionizing radiation, and vasculitis.

No unique biochemical factors are found in decubitus ulcers, but during the earliest or initial phase of ulcer formation[103] lower pH, decreased $PO_2$, and increased $PCO_2$ can be demonstrated. Ferguson-Pell and Hagisawa believe that an increase in the eccrine sweat lactate concentration, demonstrated by pilocarpine administration, may be of some diagnostic aid.[103]

The role of fibrinolysin remains controversial and is based on the following circumstantial evidence: in numerous reports of the histopathologic findings at ulcer margins, fibrin is present in relative abundance. It is particularly noticeable within and without the microvascular system. Fibrin thrombi within dilated capillaries are in turn encircled by a perivascular mononuclear cell infiltrate embedded in a fibrin network. Larger vessels have also been found to contain intra-arteriolar fibrin thrombi. Cherry and Ryan[104] felt that a lack of, or defect in, fibrinolytic activity might contribute to the genesis of the decubitus ulcer. Larsson and Risberg[105] have demonstrated experimentally that, following prolonged ischemia that had no effect on fibrinolysis, there was marked deposition of fibrin when blood flow was reestablished.

During this period decreased fibrinolytic activity could be demonstrated. It was speculated[104] that pressure ischemia resulted in damage to epidermal cells, which then released an inhibitor of fibrinolysis.[105] The role of fibrin in the pathogenesis would thus be twofold: first as vascular thrombi increasing anoxia, and second as accumulations of perivascular fibrin in amounts large enough to inhibit vascular regrowth and healing of the ulcer, as is routinely observed in classical wounds.

Though this chapter omits consideration of therapy, all therapeutic regimens for decubitus ulcers must include measures to facilitate restitution of the vascular bed and control of the bacterial infection that inevitably ensues. These measures, plus active debridement and good nursing, facilitate ultimate closure of the ulcer site.[106,107]

# References

1. Holbrook KA, Wolff K. The structure and development of skin. In: Fitzpatrick TB, et al., eds. Dermatology in General Medicine. New York: McGraw-Hill, 1987.
2. Wilke MS, Hsu BM, Wille JJ Jr, et al. Biologic mechanisms for the regulation of normal human keratinocyte proliferation and differentiation. Am J Pathol 1988; 131:171–182.
3. Hennings H, Michael D, Cheng C, et al. Calcium regulation of growth and differentiation of mouse epidermal cells in culture. Cell 1980; 19:245–254.
4. Benz EW. Intermediate filament proteins: A molecular basis for tumor diagnostics. Biotechniques 1985; 3:412–421.
5. Kopan R, Traska G, Fuchs E. Retinoids as important regulators of terminal differentiation: Examining keratin expression in individual epidermal cells at various stages of keratinization. J Cell Biol 1987; 105:427–400.
6. Pittelkow MR, Scott RE. New techniques for the in vitro culture of human skin keratinocytes and perspectives on their use for grafting of patients with extensive burns. Mayo Clin Proc 1986; 61:771–777.
7. Gelfant S. On the existence of non-cycling germinative cells in human epidermis in vivo and cell cycle aspects of psoriasis. Cell Tissue Kinetics 1982; 14:393–397.
8. Lavker RM, Sun TT. Epidermal stem cells. J Invest Dermatol 1983; 81(Suppl):121–127.
9. Potten CS. Kinetic organization in squamous epithelium. In: Wright NA, Camplejohn RS, eds. Psoriasis: Cell Proliferation. Edinburgh: Churchill Livingstone, 1983.
10. Bauer FW. Cell kinetics. In: Mier PD, van de Kerkhof PCM, eds. Textbook of Psoriasis. Edinburgh: Churchill Livingstone, 1986.
11. Rothberg S, Crounse RG, Lee JL. Glycine-$^{14}$C incorporation into the proteins of normal stratum

corneum and the abnormal stratum corneum of psoriasis. J Invest Dermatol 1961; 37:497–505.

12. Bickers D, Harber L, Kopf A. Nonmelanoma skin cancer and melanoma. In: Harber L, Bickers D, eds. Photosensitivity Diseases. Toronto: BC Decker, 1989.

13. Ebling FJG. Homage to Paul Langerhans. J Invest Dermatol 1980; 75:3.

14. Green I, Stingl G, Shevach EM, et al. Antigen presentation and allogeneic stimulation by Langerhans cells. J Invest Dermatol 1980; 75:44.

15. Katz S, et al. Epidermal Langerhans cells are derived from cells originating in the bone marrow. Nature 1979; 282:324.

16. Stingl G, Katz SI, Green I, et al. The functional role of Langerhans cells. J Invest Dermatol 1980; 74:315.

17. Silberberg I. Apposition of mononuclear cells to Langerhans cells in contact allergic reactions. An ultrastructural study. Acta Dermatol Venereol 1973; 53:1–12.

18. Silberberg I, Baer RL, Rosenthal SA. The role of Langerhans cells in allergic contact hypersensitivity. A review of findings in man and guinea pigs. J Invest Dermatol 1976; 66:210.

19. Thorbecke GJ, Silberberg-Sinakin I, Flotte TJ. Langerhans cells as macrophages in skin and lymphoid organs. J Invest Dermatol 1980; 75:32.

20. Toews GB, Bergstresser PR, Streilein JW. Langerhans cells: Sentinels of skin associated lymphoid tissue. J Invest Dermatol 1980; 75:78.

21. Bickers D, Harber LC, Kripke M. Photo-Immunology. In: Harber L, Bickers D, eds. Photosensitivity Diseases. Toronto: BC Decker, 1989.

22. Ellis RA, Henrickson RC. The ultrastructure of the sebaceous glands in man. In: Montagna WB, ed. Advances in Biology of Skin, vol 4. New York: Pergamon Press, 1963.

23. Serri F, Huber WM. The development of sebaceous glands in man. In: Montagna WB, ed. Advances in Biology of Skin, vol 4. New York: Pergamon Press, 1963.

24. Pochi PE, et al. Age-related changes in sebaceous gland activity. J Invest Dermatol 1979; 73:108.

25. Pochi PE, et al. Skin surface lipid composition, acne, pubertal development, and urinary excretion of testosterone and 17-ketosteroids in children. J Invest Dermatol 1977; 69:485.

26. Pochi PE, Strauss JS. Sebaceous gland response in man to the administration of testosterone, delta[4]-androstenedione, and dehydroepiandrosterone. J Invest Dermatol 1969; 52:32.

27. Pochi PE, Strauss JS. Sebaceous gland suppression with ethinyl estradiol and diethylstilbesterol. Arch Dermatol 1973; 108:210.

28. Ebling FJ. Hormonal control and methods of measuring sebaceous gland activity. J Invest Dermatol 1974; 62:161.

29. Shuster S, Thody AJ. The control and measurement of sebum secretion. J Invest Dermatol 1974; 62:172.

30. Pochi PE, Strauss JS. Endocrinologic control of the development and activity of the human sebaceous gland. J Invest Dermatol 1974; 62:191.

31. Downing DT, Strauss JS. On the mechanism of sebaceous secretion. Arch Dermatol Res 1982; 272:343.

32. Jakubovic HR, Ackerman AB. Development, morphology and physiology. In: Moschella SL, Hurley HJ, eds. Dermatology, ed 2. vol I. Philadelphia: WB Saunders, 1985.

33. Pochi PE. Sebum: Its nature and physiopathologic responses. In: Moschella SL, Hurley HJ, eds. Dermatology, ed 2. vol 1. Philadelphia: WB Saunders, 1985.

34. Downey D, Stewart M, Strauss J. Biology of sebaceous glands. In: Fitzpatrick, et al., eds. Dermatology in General Medicine. New York: McGraw-Hill, 1987.

35. Montagna W. The Structure and Function of Skin. New York: Academic Press, 1962.

36. Bell M. Proceedings: The ultrastructure of human axillary apocrine glands after epinephrine injection. J Invest Dermatol 1974; 63:147–159.

37. Robertshaw D. Apocrine sweat glands. In: Goldsmith LA, ed. Biochemistry and Physiology of the Skin, vol 1. Oxford: Oxford University Press, 1983.

38. Shelley WB. Apocrine sweat. J Invest Dermatol 1951; 17:255.

39. Tani M, Yamamoto K, Mishima Y. Apocrine acrosyringeal complex in human skin. J Invest Dermatol 1980; 75:431–435.

40. Robertshaw D. Biology of apocrine sweat glands. In: Fitzpatrick, et al., eds. Dermatology in General Medicine. New York: McGraw-Hill, 1987.

41. Gisolfi CV, Wenger CB. Temperature regulation during exercise: Old concepts, new ideas. Exerc Sport Sci Rev 1984; 12:339–372.

42. Itoh S. Physiological responses to heat. In: Yoshimura, et al., eds. Essential Problems in Climatic Physiology. Kyoto: Nankado, 1960.

43. Sato K. Biology of eccrine sweat glands. In: Fitzpatrick, ed. Dermatology and General Medicine, vol II. publ. 1986.

44. Gagge AP, Nishi Y. Heat exchange between human skin surface and thermal environment. In: Handbook of physiology: Reactions to environmental agents. Bethesda: American Physiological Society, 1977.

45. Conn JW. The mechanism of acclimatization to heat. Adv Inter Med 1949; 3:373–393.

46. Clark G, Magoun HW, Ranson SW. Hypothalmic regulation of body temperature. J Neurophysiol 1939; 2:61–80.
47. Hyndman OR, Wolkin J. The pilocarpine sweating test. I. A valid indicator in differentiation of preganglionic and postganglionic sympathectomy. Arch Neurol Psychiatry 1941; 45:992–1006.
48. Keller A. Descending nerve fibers subserving heat maintenance functions coursing with cerebrospinal tracts through the pons. Am J Physiol 1948; 154:82–86.
49. Myerson A, Loman J, Rinkel M. Human autonomic pharmacology: General and local sweating produced by acetyl-beta-methyl-choline chloride (mecholyl). Am J Med Sc 1937; 194:75–79.
50. Bijman J. Transport processes in the eccrine sweat gland. Int Kidney 1987; 32:S109–S112.
51. Sato K. Biology of eccrine sweat glands. Fitzpatrick et al., eds. Dermatology in General Medicine. New York: McGraw-Hill, 1987.
52. Ebling FJ. Biology of hair follicles. In: Fitzpatrick et al., eds. Dermatology in General Medicine. New York: McGraw-Hill, 1989.
53. Baden H, Zaias N. Biology of nails. In: Fitzpatrick et al., eds. Dermatology in General Medicine. New York: McGraw-Hill, 1987.
54. Baden HP. The physical properties of nail. J Invest Dermatol 1970; 55:115–122.
55. Hashimoto K. Ultrastructure of the human toenail. II. Keratinization and formation of the marginal band. J Ultrastruct Res 1971; 36:391–410.
56. Hashimoto K, Gross BG, et al. The ultrastructure of the skin of human embryos. III. The formation of the nail in 16- to 18-weeks-old embryos. J Invest Dermatol 1966; 47:205–217.
57. Eady RAJ. The basement membrane. Interface between the epithelium and the dermis: Structional features. Arch Dermatol 1988; 124:709–712.
58. Katz SI. The epidermal basement membrane zone-structure, ontogeny, and role in disease. J Am Acad Dermatol 1984; 11:1025-1037.
59. Woodley DT. Importance of the dermal-epidermal junction and recent advances. Dermatologica 1987; 174:1-10.
60. Tan O, Stafford, TJ. Cutaneous circulation In:Fitzpatrick et al., eds. Dermatol Gen Med. New York: McGraw Hill, 1987; 357–367.
61. Befus D, Fujimaki H, Lee TDG, et al. Mast cell polymorphisms. Present concepts, future directions. Dig Dis Sci 1988; 33:16S–24S.
62. Barton J, Lavker RM, Schechter NM, et al. Treatment of urticaria pigmentosa with corticosteroids. Arch Dermatol 1985; 121:1516–1523.
63. Schwartz LB. Mediators of human mast cells and human mast cell subsets. Ann Allergy 1987; 58:226–235.
64. Peters SP, Schleimer RP, Naclerio RM, et al. Am Rev Repir Dis 1987; 135:1196–1200.
65. Kohn RR, Schnider SL. Collagen changes in aging skin. (p121 -139) In: Balin AK, Kligman AM, eds. Aging and the Skin. New York: Raven Press, 1989.
66. Uitto J. Connective tissue biochemistry of the aging dermis. Clin Geriatr Med 1989; 5:127-147.
67. Uitto J, Eisen A. Collagen. In: Fitzpatrick, et al., eds. Dermatology in General Medicine. New York: McGraw-Hill, 1987; 259–287.
68. Davidson JM, et al. Elastin production in human skin fibroblasts: Reduced levels in the cells of a patient with atrophoderma. Clin Res 1984; 32:147A.
69. Pinnell SR, Martin GR. The cross-linking of collagen and elastin: Enzymatic conversion of lysine in peptide linkage to alpha-aminoadipic-delta-semialdehyde (allysine) by an extract from bone. Proc Natl Acad Sci USA 1968; 61:708–716.
70. Sandberg LB. Elastin structure, biosynthesis and its relation to disease states. N Engl J Med 1981; 304:566–579.
71. Davidson JM, et al. Regulation of elastin synthesis in developing sheep nuchal ligament by elastin mRNA levels. J Biol Chem 1981; 257:747–754.
72. Foster JA. Elastin structure and biosynthesis: An overview. Methods Enzymol 1982; 82A:559–570.
73. Uitto J. Biochemistry of the elastic fibers in normal connective tissues and its alterations in diseases. J Invest Dermatol 1979; 72:1–10.
74. Montagna W. Morphology of cutaneous sensory receptors. J Invest Dermatol 1977; 69:4.
75. Hashimoto K. Fine structure of the Meissner corpuscle of human palmar skin. J Invest Dermatol 1973; 60:20.
76. Soden C, Pierson DL, Rodman OG. A classification of cutaneous receptors. J Assoc Milit Dermatol 1981; 7:5.
77. Herndon JH. Itching: The pathophysiology of pruritus. Int J Dermatol 1975; 14:465–484.
78. Hagermark O, Hokfelt T, Pernow B. Flare and itch induced by substance P in human skin. J Invest Dermatol 1978; 71:233–235.
79. Bernstein JE, Hamill JR. Substance P in the skin. J Invest Dermatol 1981; 77:250.
80. Jakubovic H, Ackerman AB. Development, morphology and physiology. In: Moschella S, Hurley, eds. Dermatology. Philadelphia: WB Saunders, 1985; 45–46.
81. Braverman IM, Yen AK. Ultrastructure of the human dermal microcirculation III. The vessel in the mid and lower dermis and subcutaneous fat. J Invest Dermatol 1981; 77:297.
82. DeLuca HF. The vitamin D story: A collaborative

effort of basic science and clinical medicine. FASEB J 1988; 2:224-236.

83. Prystowsky JH. Photoprotection and the vitamin D: Status of the elderly. Arch Dermatol 1988; 124:1844–1848.

84. Reichel H, Koeffler HP, Norman AW. The role of the vitamin D endocrine system in health and disease. N Engl J Med 1989; 320:980–991.

85. Grandjean P, Berlin A, Gilbert M, et al. Preventing percutaneous absorption of industrial chemicals: The "skin" denotation. Am J Ind Med 1988; 14:97–107.

86. Rutter N. Percutaneous drug absorption in the newborn: Hazards and uses. Clin Perinatol 1987; 14:911–930.

87. Besunder JB, Reed MD, Blumer JL. Principles of drug biodisposition in the neonate. A critical evaluation of the pharmacokinetic-pharmacodynamic interface, (part I). Clin Pharmacokinet 1988; 14:189–216.

88. Nickoloff BJ, Mitra RS, Riser BL, et al. Modulation of keratinocyte motility. Am J Pathol 1988; 132:543–551.

89. Alvarez OM, Goslen JB, Eaglstein WH, et al. Wound healing. In: Fitzpatrick, et al., eds. Dermatology in General Medicine. 1987; 321–336.

90. Young ME. Malnutrition and wound healing. Heart and Lung 1988; 17:60–67.

91. Guralnik JM, Harris TB, White LR, et al. Occurrence and predictors of pressure sores in the National Health and Nutrition Examination Survey follow-up. J Am Geratr Soc 1988; 36:807–812.

92. Nemeth AJ, Eaglstein WH, Talanga V. Clinical parameters and transcutaneous oxygen measurements for the prognosis of venous ulcers. J Am Acad Dermatol 1989; 20:186–190.

93. Silverman RA, Lender J, Elmets CA. Effects of occlusive and semiocclusive dressings on the return of barrier function to transepidermal water loss in standardized human wounds. J Am Acad Dermatol 1989; 20:755-760.

94. Yannas IV, Lee E. Orgill DP, et al. Synthesis and characterization of a model extracellular matrix that induces partial regeneration of adult mammalian skin. Proc Natl Acad Sci USA 1989; 86:933–937.

95. Stompro BE, Hansbrough JF, Boyce ST. Attachment of peptide growth factors to implantable collagen. J Surg Res 1989; 46:413–421.

96. Brown GL, Nanney LP, Griffen J, et al. Enhancement of wound healing by topical treatment with epidermal growth factor. N Engl J Med 1989: 321:76–79.

97. Hung VC, Lee JY, Zitelli JA, et al. Topical tretinoin and epithelial wound healing. Arch Dermatol 1989; 125:65–69.

98. Arboleda B, Cruz NI. The effect of systemic isotretinoin on wound contraction in guinea pigs. Plast Reconstr Surg 1989; 83:118–121.

99. Rochkind S, Rousso M, Nissare M, et al. Systemic effects of low-power laser irradiation on the peripheral and central nervous system, cutaneous wounds, and burns. Lasers Surg Med 1989; 9:174–182.

100. Allman RM. Pressure ulcers among the elderly. N Engl J Med 1989; 850–853.

101. Daniel RK, Priest DL, Wheatly DC. Etiologic factors in pressure sores: An experimental model. Arch Phys Med Rehabil 1981; 62:492–498.

102. Andersen KE, Jensen O, Kvorning SA, et al. Prevention of pressure sores by identifying patients at risk. Br Med J 1982; 284:1370.

103. Ferguson-Pell M, Hagisawa S. Biochemical changes in sweat following prolonged ischemia. J Rehabil Res Dev 1988; 25:57–62.

104. Cherry GW, Ryan TJ. The effects of ischemia and reperfusion on tissue survival. Major Prob Dermatol 1976; 7:93–115.

105. Larsson J, Risberg B. Ischemia-induced changes in tissue fibrinolysis in human legs. Bibl Anat 1977; 15:556–558.

106. Petersen NC, Bittman S. The epidemiology of pressure sores. Scand J Plast Reconstr Surg 1971; 5:62.

107. Seiler WO, Stahelin HB. Recent findings on decubitus ulcer pathology: Implications for care. Geriatrics 1986; 41:47–57.

## Bibliography

Domonkos AN, Arnold HL, Odom RB. Andrews' Diseases of the Skin: Clinical Dermatology, ed 7. Philadelphia: WB Saunders, 1982.

Jarrett A. The Physiology and Pathophysiology of the Skin, vol II. New York: Academic Press, 1973.

Goldsmith LA, ed. Biochemistry and Physiology of the Skin, vol II. New York: Oxford University Press, 1983.

Montagna W, Parakkal PF. The Structure and Function of the Skin. New York: Academic Press, 1974.

Moschella SL, Hurley HJ. *Dermatology,* ed 2, vol I. Philadelphia: WB Saunders, 1985.

Parrish JA. Dermatology and Skin Care. New York: McGraw-Hill, 1975.

Pillsbury DM. A Manual of Dermatology. Philadelphia: WB Saunders, 1971.

Rothman S. Physiology and Biochemistry of the Skin. Chicago: University of Chicago Press, 1954.

# Chapter 10

# Nerve Conduction and Neuromuscular Transmission

ROBERT E. LOVELACE
STANLEY J. MYERS

Nerve conduction and neuromuscular transmission, together with electromyography (EMG, see Chapter 11), are the basis of electrodiagnosis of neuromuscular disease. Because nerve and muscle have specific anatomic and chemical compositions that relate to their preeminent electrical activity, inferences can be made about dysfunction.[1,2] Conduction velocity is related to diameter, and in nerve to the thickness, efficiency, symmetry, and presence of the myelin sheath. The motor unit potential, representing the individual muscle fiber potentials in the anatomic motor unit, enables the examiner to assess the number of active units and any breakup in the final common motor path.[3]

The nerve fiber is a rodlike structure surrounded by a membrane composed of lipid-protein dipoles with an internal medium containing predominantly $K^+$ cations and an external medium comprising principally $Na^+$ cations. Divalent cations ($Ca^{++}$ and $Mg^{++}$) are also present in the external medium, but in much smaller concentrations. The anions are principally $Cl^-$ and $HCO3^-$ externally; internally there are mainly complex organic anions of protein type and a very low concentration of $Cl^-$. By means of these differences in concentration, and because of the biologic activity of the membrane, with its variable permeability and ion extrusion pump, a negative charge is maintained on the inside of the membrane relative to the outside, giving rise to the *membrane potential*. This axon membrane, which is between 5 and 10 nm thick, occupies only 0.15 of the total volume of the neuron but is of predominant importance in

conduction. The membrane of both the axon and the muscle fiber has various anatomic ion channels.[4] Each ion channel has its own specific mechanism for generating charge and is governed by electrical charges. The ion channels have also been found to have specific genetic representations, and subunits of postjunctional receptors are similarly encoded.[5]

During excitation, the resting equilibrium is disturbed by depolarization of the membrane, during which the internal negativity is reduced toward zero. When this depolarization reaches a critical level (i.e., a threshold), an action potential is produced in the nerve and the internal potential overshoots, past zero to a positive value. Upon repolarization, the internal potential returns to its negative value. Unless conductivity is blocked the axonal potential is self-propagating in either direction along the nerve and is followed by an electrical and chemical recovery phase. This electrical manifestation of the action potential can be explained by postulating potential-dependent changes (condensor-battery system) in a selectively permeable membrane (pore or aperture theory) along with extrusion pumps.[6] An alternative explanation considers the resting and active states of the membrane in terms of variation of its cation exchange properties.[7] Certainly, the axonal protoplasm is completely unnecessary for conduction.[8] Removal of the divalent cations from the external medium leads to loss of excitability, whereas, under proper conditions, complete elimination of univalent cations may not result in total loss of excitability,[8] though the amplitude of the action potential is markedly diminished.[9] In the normal state, a depolarizing stimulus coursing outward through the membrane drives the internal univalent ($K^+$) ions by electrophoresis into the inner layers of the membrane and finally into the outer layer, displacing the divalent cations (i.e., $Ca^{++}$).[7] Abrupt depolarization occurs at a critical level, as is shown by a sudden change in the relationship of univalent membrane cation concentration to membrane conductance.

Our knowledge of these various aspects of nerve conduction derives either from voltage clamp experiments, in which the internal potential is kept at constant voltage, or from perfusion experiments, in which internal and external electrolyte concentrations are varied. Turbidity, birefringence of nerves, and intensity of fluorescence of stained nerves also vary during excitation, and these changes have been explained by postulating alterations in orientation of the membrane macromolecules during the active state.[10]

Intracellular potentials are measured with glass micropipettes filled with hypertonic electrolytic solution (KC1 3M) (Figure 10-1).[11] With a balanced bridge, the same setup can be used for stimulation and for recording events.[12] In most animal muscle and nerve tissue, the resting potential value is about −90 mV, and it varies slightly, according to whether the readings are made in vitro on excised tissue,[13] in situ with an open-pool method,[14] or in situ with a closed (percutaneous) method.[15] In the percutaneous technique, as yet applied only to muscle, a microelectrode is passed through a hollow insertional electrode placed in a muscle belly.[16–18] Recordings from single nerve fibers are achieved easily only in crustaceans and some other invertebrates. Particular success is possible using the giant axon of the squid, but studies by Eliasson[19] with a voltage clamp applied to a mammalian single fiber have confirmed the presence of an electron leak at the node of Ranvier, the physiology of which is discussed later. A more "physiologic" recording from a single muscle or nerve, or even the end-plate region by a very local breach of the membrane at the electrode tip, is called the *patch clamp method*.[20,21] If the single-fiber action potential is recorded intracellularly with an internal or crushed-end reference recording, the curve is usually monophasic, rising from a negative membrane potential.

More often, recording is made from surface electrodes on single fibers or whole nerves, with biphasic potentials being recorded (Figure 10-2A). If crushed-end reference recording is used, on the other hand, the potentials are monophasic (Figure 10-2B). In clinical practice, the recording electrodes usually pick up potentials from many fibers and at a variably greater distance from these active fibers in the nerve, giving rise to compound nerve

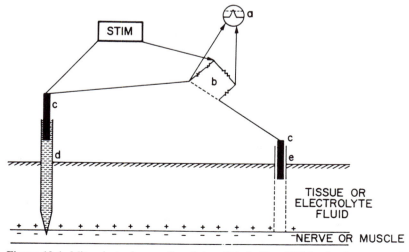

**Figure 10-1.** Microelectrode recording (intracellular). Key: STIM, stimulator; a, oscilloscope recording; b, balanced Wheatstone bridge; c, anodized silver electrodes; d, recording electrode: glass micropipette (3 M KCl filled); e, indifferent or reference electrode.

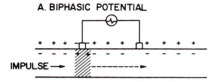
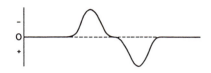

A. BIPHASIC POTENTIAL

IMPULSE →

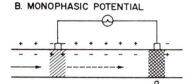
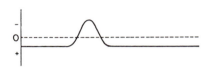

B. MONOPHASIC POTENTIAL

a

**Figure 10-2.** Surface recording (extracellular). (*A*) The derivation of a biphasic potential with surface-active and reference electrodes is shown. Second phase is produced by impulse travelling to and activating reference electrode. (*B*) Demonstration of a monophasic potential using an injury or crushed-end reference (a) electrode that cannot be activated by the transmitted impulse.

action potentials. These are at least biphasic and may be irregular in form, owing to summation of temporally dispersed responses.[22] Such waveforms, as seen on direct measurement, can be computed from the addition of individual fiber responses. In recording at a distance in this fashion, from either a single fiber or a bundle of fibers (as in a peripheral nerve), the initial phase is usually negative, which in EMG is generally recorded by upward deflection of the beam on the cathode ray oscilloscope. Nerve action potentials so recorded usually are biphasic or triphasic.[23]

At this stage it is useful to summarize some of the properties and characteristics of neurons[24,25]:

1. The *all-or-none response* is the ability of nerve fibers to respond completely and with a propagated impulse when the stimulus reaches threshold.

2. The *refractory period* is the length of time following an effective stimulus during which the nerve fiber will not respond to a further stimulus.

3. *Two-way conduction* is the property of a neuron whereby a propagated action potential is transmitted in both directions from the site of the stimulus.

4. *Subthreshold stimuli* may sometimes summate to give a threshold stimulus, with a resulting response.

5. *Accommodation* occurs in nerves and is mani-

fested by a decrease of excitability with prolonged subthreshold stimulation.

6. *Depolarization* block may be produced by subthreshold stimuli, by excessive external potassium, by anoxia, or by injury. This block is counteracted by hyperpolarization.

7. Impulses are duplicated at the branching points of nerves (which always correspond to nodes of Ranvier), so that the undiminished impulse is propagated down each branch.

8. Interaction between adjacent fibers in a neuron by *volume conduction* may give rise to a change in threshold of up to 10% in apparently inactive neurons. Occasionally, current flow generated by active fibers can stimulate a previously inactive adjacent fiber to above-threshold levels. This phenomenon is called *ephaptic stimulation*.

## Volume Conduction

The problem of volume conduction recurs frequently in recording biologic electrical potentials. Although basically it constitutes the application of Ohm's law to the electrolytic conduction around the axon, this phenomenon of volume conduction is complicated in vivo by the nonuniformity of the excitable tissues and the inhomogeneity of the conducting medium: $I_l = KV/r$ where $I_l$ is longitudinal current, V is axoplasmic potential, r is axoplasmic resistance, and K is a constant, related to the units employed. The equation is Ohm's law applied to a neuron.

## Conduction Velocity

Conduction velocity varies directly with the diameter of a nerve fiber, and is much increased in the presence of a myelin sheath. An impulse can pass along an unmyelinated nerve fiber at the relatively slow rate of 0.4 to 1 m/per second, and its speed is directly proportional to the square root of the diameter of the fiber. The more rapid transmission of the impulse along the myelinated fiber results from the insulation of the nerve segments by a myelin sheath. These insulated segments are separated by the myelin-free areas (1 μ) at the nodes of Ranvier. At the node of Ranvier there is an electron leak and easy depolarization relative to the greater stability of the internode. Excitation, therefore, appears to jump from node to node, as the electrical field from one node becomes sufficient to activate the next. This phenomenon is called *saltatory conduction* (Figure 10-3). There is some longitudinal current traveling at a finite rate in the internode, so it is not strictly correct to state that in saltatory conduction the nerve impulse jumps from node to node without some latency being referable to the internode.[26] Alternatively, this more rapid conduction may be related to the low membrane capacity in the internode of the medullated fiber.[27] Thus, two thirds of the membrane's charge is at the tiny nodal region.

A safety factor is present in myelinated fibers,

so that in nerve conduction the impulse can sometimes pass across one or even two nodes that have been narcotized (see Figure 10-3).[28] This is relevant only to experimental situations. Using multiple recording points, in demonstrating passage of impulses on a computer model of charge buildup at the node of Ranvier, Bostock and Sears[29] indicate how the impulse passes to the next internode or is pathologically blocked. The chemical correlates of this have been worked out well by Waxman and Ritchie,[30] who currently describe as many as seven physiologically active molecules or channels in the membrane of the myelinated fiber. At least four of these—the voltage-sensitive sodium channels, the fast and slow potassium channels, and the sodium-potassium–adenosine triphosphatase (ATPase) system are found in the nodal or paranodal areas and modulate or maintain saltatory conduction. As noted, in myelinated fibers conduction velocity is directly proportional to diameter, and it can vary from as fast as 120 m per second in some motor and sensory fibers[31] (e.g., cat) to as slow as 4 m per second in some slow myelinated fibers (A or delta). The velocity of nerve transmission also varies with the internodal distance, as there is a direct relationship between the separation of the nodes of Ranvier and the time required for the electrical field to produce appropriate depolarization in saltatory conduction.

Returning to the compound nerve action potential, if this is recorded at progressively greater distances from the stimulation point, the various spikes of the dispersed potentials become separated into distinct velocity groups (Figure 10-4).[32] This method provides one of the electrical methods of classifying nerve fibers. Three components, al-

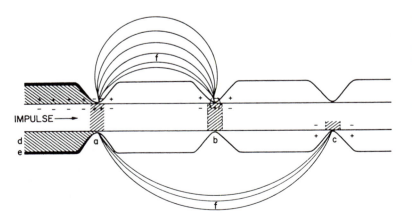

**Figure 10-3.** Saltatory conduction in a myelinated fiber. Key: a, depolarized membrane at node of Ranvier; b, partially depolarized membrane at node of Ranvier (near threshold); c, beginning depolarization of membrane at node of Ranvier; d, myelin sheath; e, Schwann cell; f, electrical field.

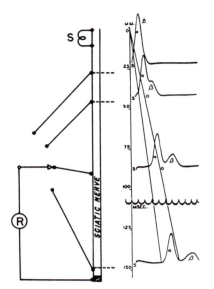

**Figure 10-4.** Compound action potential of frog sciatic nerve recorded at different distances from site of stimulation. (*Left*) Diagram of recording apparatus. Key: S, stimulus; R, recorder. (*Right*) Only the first two elevations, α and β, are shown. As conduction increases, α and β became clearly separated in time (temporal dispersion) because they reflect activity of fibers' conduction at different rates. Diagonal straight lines are drawn through onsets of α and β deflections; slopes of these lines give conduction rates of most rapidly conducting α and β fibers. (From Ruch TC, Patton HD. Physiology and Biophysics. Philadelphia: WB Saunders, 1965.)

1. Muscular nerves
   a. Myelinated
      Motor and proprioceptive afferent
      Group I, 12 to 21 μ ⎱
      Group II, 6 to 12    ⎰ alpha ⎱ A fibers
      Group III, 1 to 6 μ } delta ⎰
   b. Unmyelinated
      Group IV, 0.4 to 1.2 μ — C fibers
2. Cutaneous nerves
   a. Myelinated
      6 to 17 μ   alpha ⎱ A fibers
      1 to 6 μ    delta ⎰
   b. Unmyelinated
      0.4 to 1.2 — C fibers

Conduction velocity is affected by physical factors such as temperature and metabolic rate; a decrease of either factor reduces velocity. In disease, slow conduction velocities occur in regenerating fibers of small diameter and in the presence of primary or segmental demyelination of nerves.

## Applied Aspects

Basic anatomic and physiologic knowledge of nerve conduction can be applied in health and disease by recording the effects of nerve and muscle stimulation.[33] The equipment consists of an amplified cathode ray oscilloscope (CRO) system, on which potentials may be recorded and demonstrated on the screen. Preamplification is needed to adequately visualize potentials in the microvolt to millivolt range. Differential amplification enables the appropriate frequency range to be chosen, which in EMG and nerve conduction is between 20 and 8000 Hz (cycles per second). The signal-to-noise ratio can be increased by the appropriate use of an input transformer. Records are usually taken from surface electrodes placed over appropriate nerves or muscles, but they may also be made from needle electrodes placed in the muscle or adjacent to nerves. The CRO is connected to a loudspeaker and also to a stimulator, which usually drives the sweep of the oscilloscope. The stimulator, isolated from ground, is capable of delivering a short-duration pulse (between 0.05 and 2 msec) with a maximum voltage of 300 V. Further refinements include the use of a stimulator capable of delivering trains and multiple stimuli at given separations. A permanent recording of the tracing can be made using 35-mm film, polaroid film, fiberoptic recording systems, magnetic tape, laser

pha, beta, and delta, can be distinguished by the velocity of each group. Another electrical distinction is shown by differences in threshold for stimulation: the threshold is lower in the faster fibers and higher in the fibers with slow conduction velocity. Mixed nerves contain components of all three velocity or threshold groups, but cutaneous nerves usually contain only alpha (faster) and delta (slower) fibers.

Nerves can also be classified functionally into groups. Group A fibers are myelinated somatic, being both afferent and efferent. Group B fibers are also myelinated, but are efferent and preganglionic in the autonomic system. Group C fibers are unmyelinated and are of two subgroups: sympathetic (sC), the efferent, postganglionic, sympathetic axons, and dorsal root sensory (drC), the small, unmyelinated afferent axons found in peripheral nerves and dorsal roots (Table 10-1).

Finally, fiber diameter may be used as a basis for classification.

**Table 10-1.** Properties of Mammalian Nerve Fibers

|  | A | B | sC | drC |
|---|---|---|---|---|
| Fiber diameter (μ) | 1–22 | ≤3 | 0.3–1.3 | 0.4–1.2 |
| Conduction speed (m/sec) | 5–120 | 3–15 | 0.7–2.3 | 0.6–2.0 |
| Spike duration (msec) | 0.4–0.5 | 1.2 | 2.0 | 2.0 |
| Absolute refractory period (msec) | 0.4–1.0 | 1.2 | 2.0 | 2.0 |
| Negative afterpotential amplitude (% of spike) | 3–5 | None | 3–5 | None |
| Duration (msec) | 12–20 | . . . . | 50–80 | . . . . |
| Positive afterpotential amplitude (% of spike) | 0.2 | 1.5–4.0 | 1.5 | * |
| Duration (msec) | 40–60 | 100–300 | 300–1000 | * |
| Order of susceptibility to asphyxia | 2 | 1 | 3 | 3 |
| Velocity-diamater ratio | 6 | ? | ? | 1.73 average |

* Postspike positivity 10–30% of spike amplitude and decaying to half size in 50 msec is recorded from drC fibers. This afterpositivity differs from the positive afterpotential of other fibers.

From Ruch TC, Patton HD: Physiology and Biophysics. Philadelphia: WB Saunders, 1965.

printout, or computer floppy disk. A storage oscilloscope is used to study the form of motor unit potentials in electromyography and the variation of potentials following repetitive stimulation in nerve stimulation studies. Averaging devices are used to demonstrate low-amplitude nerve action potentials, which would otherwise be buried in the baseline noise level. For single-fiber EMG, a delay line and triggering device for superimposing or averaging potentials is added,[34] and memory and digitalization enable data to be recalled and numerical reports to be generated. For the final analysis, complex diagnostic expert systems are programmed for sequential tests to be performed to solve specific problems.

Galvanic and faradic stimulation at the motor point of a muscle are now of historical interest only, and even the more elegant demonstration of the effects of direct stimulation of muscle by constructing a strength-duration curve is rarely employed. Minimal excitability[35] offers a simpler method for assessing prognosis early in cases of facial or Bell's palsy.

### *Motor Nerve Conduction*

The velocity of motor nerve conduction is measured by stimulating a nerve at two points along its course and in each instance recording the muscle action potential of a peripheral muscle this nerve supplies. To ensure that all nerve fibers are appropriately excited, the intensity of stimulus should be supramaximal (i.e., 50% above that sufficient to produce a maximum muscle response). For example (Figure 10-5), the median nerve is stimulated at the elbow and at the wrist, and the evoked potentials from the thenar muscles are recorded. The time it takes the impulse to reach the muscle (the latency) is usually measured on a CRO

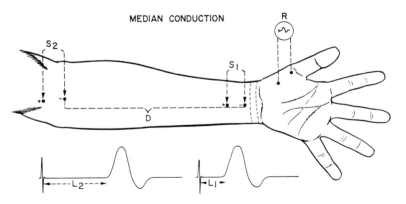

MEDIAN CONDUCTION

**Figure 10-5.** Procedure for motor conduction measurement in median nerve. Key: $S_1$, stimulus distally (wrist); $S_2$, stimulus proximally (elbow); R, recording electrode over thenar muscle; $L_1$, distal latency (wrist to muscle); $L_2$, proximal latency (elbow to muscle); D, distance between stimulating electrodes $S_1$ and $S_2$.

Conduction velocity =
$$D/(L_2 - L_1)$$

from the stimulus artifact to the onset of the evoked potential. The shorter distal latency from the wrist stimulation is subtracted from the longer proximal latency of the stimulation at the elbow, to give the conduction time between the two points. The conduction velocity of the nerve from elbow to wrist is then calculated by dividing the difference between the latencies into the distance between stimulation points.[36] Each latency represents the time required for the impulse to pass from the distal point of stimulation to the instant that the electrical reaction begins in the muscle. This, of course, also includes the time in the arborized axon and the time for neuromuscular transmission, which is eliminated in the calculation (above) of conduction velocity. Other important parameters of the evoked muscle potential from nerve stimulation are amplitude, duration, and complexity. The voltage and duration of the stimulus required at various points are also of value, and in a few cases the latency from threshold, and supramaximal stimulation, should be recorded. Absolute and relative refractory periods were used by the late Gilliatt and colleagues.[37]

### Sensory Nerve Conduction

Sensory nerve conduction can be measured orthodromically by stimulating digits with ring electrodes and recording at one or more points proximally utilizing surface or deeper needle electrodes, with or without averaging. It is important to measure the inflexional latency rather than the peak latency, to obtain true conduction velocity. This is even more accurate if more than one proximal recording or stimulation point is used.[38] Alternatively, the nerve can be stimulated more proximally and recording made by the digital electrodes in the antidromic method. The sensory potential can be obscured or misinterpreted owing to interference by the evoked motor response. If the nerves are stimulated directly at the wrist or ankle, and the recording is made over more proximal parts of the nerve, a mixed motor and sensory compound potential will be obtained unless sensory evoked potentials are recorded over the spinal cord or brain. The latter way, the method for recording somatosensory evoked potential (SSEPs), is discussed in more detail in Chapter 12. Although it incidentally assesses the peripheral pathways,

this method is much more useful for assessing central conduction, particularly in demyelinating diseases.

In peripheral nerves the special techniques of Buchthal and Rosenfalck,[38] with isolation transformers and near-nerve stimulating and recording electrodes,[39] have enabled us to demonstrate slower fiber groups in the compound nerve action potential. This is seen well in the illustration taken from Trojaborg (Figure 10-6),[40] which shows how the radial sensory fibers can be fully evaluated by wrist stimulation and axillary recording and how this can be enhanced by the multiple averaging techniques that are also used for SSEPs. Averaging of sensory nerve action potentials is now common practice, particularly those under 5 μV, as the noise level of most equipment varies between 2 and 5 μV.[41] Stegeman and DeWeerd[42] have shown that the amplitude and area of the sensory nerve

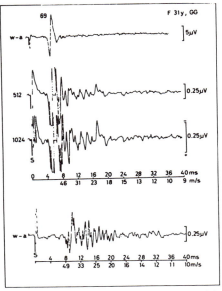

**Figure 10-6.** Recordings of sensory action potentials over the radial nerve at axilla (*a*) evoked by stimulation of the nerve at wrist (*w*). The first three traces are from a 31-year-old normal subject, and the fourth trace is from a 46-year-old woman with a pressure palsy. Electronic averaging of 512 stimuli (*second trace*) and of 1024 stimuli (*third and fourth traces*) was carried out to determine minimum conduction velocity. The last component was conducted at 18 m per second in the normal subject, and at 12 m per second in the patient. The figure above the first trace indicates the velocity of the fastest conducting fibers from *w* to *a*.

action potential are important. Because they correlate well with a number of fibers of different diameter within a nerve, their calculated nerve action potential should indicate the number and type of fibers that remain active in a damaged nerve. Other ways of recording this slow-fiber component are by measuring (1) the latency between the first and second impulses with the collision methods of Thomas and coworkers[43] or (2) the span between the slow and fast fibers, as described by Hopf.[44] In addition to the five nerves most commonly used for sensory studies, (ulnar, median, radial, sural, superficial peroneal), other nerves that can be investigated include the saphenous and lateral femoral cutaneous in the leg and the musculocutaneous (lateral cutaneous) of the forearm and ulnar dorsal cutaneous[45] nerves in the arm. Velocity in sensory nerves is in the same general range as that of motor nerves but about 5 m per second faster. Cold skin and limbs drastically reduce velocity (5% for every 1°C in a nonlinear fashion), so due care should be taken to maintain limb temperature.[46] Temperature can be monitored with skin and intramuscular thermometers or thermistors, as Trojaborg and coworkers have demonstrated for the sural nerve.[47]

### Clinical Measurements and Application

Normal values of nerve conduction velocity are usually in the range of 50 to 60 m per second in upper limb nerves of the distal segments (below the elbow) and between 60 and 80 m per second between shoulder and elbow. In the legs, normal values are usually between 40 and 50 m per second (Table 10-2). Standards from the EMG Laboratory of the Neurological Institute of New York[48–50] and others[4,51] give full details on different normal values and techniques. Trojaborg[52] just published a reference of normal values in many different sensory nerves. He used near-nerve techniques, and emphasized the importance of age and maturity in assessing velocity.

Nerve conduction velocity in human infants at birth is about 40% of the adult value, owing to the small size of the fiber and to the fact that at this age a portion of the nerve fibers are incompletely myelinated.[53] Maturation occurs mainly over the first year, and by the end of the second year[54] most myelinated peripheral nerves are conducting at rates in the normal range. The median nerve is an exception; in it full velocity may not be achieved until age 5 to 7 years.[55] Other studies do not confirm this finding.[56–59] In premature infants there is a correlation, which is important for gauging prematurity, between the postconceptional age and nerve conduction velocity in median, ulnar, peroneal, and tibial nerves.[60] Studies on twins, triplets, quadruplets, and quintuplets confirm these findings (Figure 10-7).[60]

Conduction velocity can be measured directly from a nerve or fascicle of a nerve that has been atraumatically removed during open surgical biopsy, if care is taken to avoid ischemia and to place the nerve immediately into an oxygenated medium (Figure 10-8). This is done both in human

**Table 10-2.** Normal Values for Motor and Sensory Nerve Conduction*

| Nerve | Motor Conduction Velocity (m/sec) | | | |
|---|---|---|---|---|
| | Mean | SD | Lower Limit | Patients (N) |
| Median | 57.2 | 4.2 | 48.8 | 25 |
| Ulnar | 60.0 | 5.8 | 48.4 | 188 |
| Peroneal | 51.0 | 3.26 | 44.5 | 69 |
| Post. tibial | 48.7 | 3.5 | 41.7 | 12 |

| | Sensory Distal Latency (m/sec) | | | |
|---|---|---|---|---|
| | Mean | SD | Upper Limit | Patients (N) |
| Median | 2.8 | .30 | 3.4 | 70 |
| Ulnar | 2.3 | .29 | 2.9 | 28 |

* SD (standard deviation) of measurement. Lower limit is regarded as mean value −2 SD measurement.
From Lovelace RE, Horwitz SJ. Peripheral neuropathy in long-term diphenylhydantoin therapy. Arch Neurol 1968; 18:69–77.

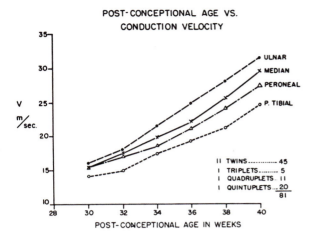

POST-CONCEPTIONAL AGE VS. CONDUCTION VELOCITY

```
ULNAR
MEDIAN
PERONEAL
P. TIBIAL

II TWINS.............. 45
I  TRIPLETS......... 5
I  QUADRUPLETS.. 11
I  QUINTUPLETS... 20
                   81
```

POST-CONCEPTIONAL AGE IN WEEKS

**Figure 10-7.** Postconceptional age versus conduction velocity. V, velocity; m/sec, meters per second. Number of studies on multiple births is indicated. (From Koenigsberger MR, Curtin J, Lovelace RE. Motor conduction velocities as a measure of gestational age in premature infants. A study of multiple births. Neurology 1970;20:381.)

tissue[61] and in rat nerve, using the Lorente-de-No chamber.[62,63] The velocity obtained correlates well with the composition of the fiber population with respect to diameters. This makes it possible to record C fibers. The faster components of the nerve (usually sural) are evaluated at one oscilloscope speed and the C-fiber potentials at a slower sweep speed. This technique has been used for a number of neuropathic situations, particularly by Lambert, Dyck, and colleagues.[64–67] Low amplitude and delayed primary potentials (representing slow conduction) are seen in the hypertrophic neuropathies of the Charcot-Marie-Tooth type (hereditary motor and sensory neuropathy [HMSN]), where the C-fiber potential is well-retained. The

C-fiber potential is also retained in Friedreich's ataxia, where the primary potential is of low amplitude but relatively normal velocity with respect to the degree of retention of the fast fibers. In the amyloid neuropathies, with the involvement of autonomic and slow sensory fibers, the C-fiber potential is absent, and this is also seen in hereditary sensory neuropathy type I. We have noted the absence of C-fiber potentials in the Shy-Drager type of autonomic neuropathy, and its presence in milder neuropathies[68] associated with myotonic dystrophy. It is possible to correlate demyelination and the absence of small fibers with histologic analysis using nerve fiber–teasing techniques. It is also possible to compare diabetic autonomic neu-

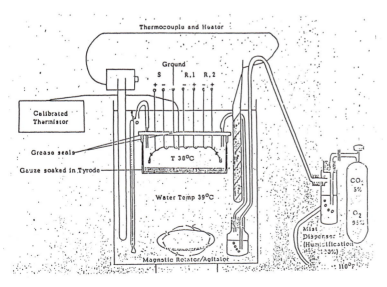

**Figure 10-8.** Nerve constant temperature apparatus.

ropathy with absence of C-fiber potentials with other axonal neuropathies such as those related to the paraproteinemias, where the C-fiber potentials may be retained.

### Varieties of Nerve Lesions

The three main parts of the nerve are the axon, the myelin sheath, and the cell of Schwann. Both the first and the last have endoplasm and a membrane as well as oxidative and phosphorylation mechanisms, and the nerve axon has a complicated nutrient system of axon flow. It is rare for one structure to be affected in isolation, and different structures may be affected at different times in the development of neuropathy.

**Axonal Disorders.** Axonal lesions are usually vascular, toxic, or traumatic; however, nerve trauma can affect all aspects of the nerve structures, and it does do differentially.

Axonal lesions may be localized, and when they are due to vascular insufficiency or destructive nerve trauma, conduction is interrupted at that level and is followed by progressive failure of nerve conduction in a distal direction. In a complete nerve lesion we can expect conduction velocity to fall suddenly by as much as 30% as the recorded muscle action potential (MAP) falls, perhaps as the large fast-conducting fibers cease functioning first. Then, depending on the length of the distal segment, conduction fails completely in 1 to 6 days,[69] a process that may be related to interruption of the axonal flow. Unusual and partial distributions of nerve territory lesions can result from specific involvement of the vascular supply of individual fascicles in large nerves, such as the sciatic.[70,71] Reinnervation from sprouting usually reaches recordable levels as muscle contact is made.

If the nerve lesions are proximal to the dorsal root ganglion[72] sensory nerve action potentials (SNAPs) may be retained and can be recorded distally.

Multiple axonal lesions may occur in mononeuritis multiplex[73] and many generalized toxic neuropathies can produce focal lesions with axonal atrophy and atresia. This results first in a differential fall in amplitude of MAPs and SNAPs, and especially if partial, it can produce dispersed ac-

tion potentials without true block. Like local lesions, they are usually associated with denervation and can be seen in renal and diabetic neuropathy. Sarcoid neuropathy is an important differential consideration here and it can be definitely diagnosed only by biopsy.[74] Near-nerve recording, as practiced by Buchthal[38,75] and Trojaborg[40,52,76–80] and their colleagues, has permitted more detailed evaluation of the nerve action potential form, so that not only variable involvement of slow, intermediate, and fast fiber groups can be assessed, but variable slowing, or even nerve blocks, in different segments of the nerve can be evaluated. We can, therefore, utilize clinical neurophysiologic methods to give comparable and complementary information to that obtained by serial sections of nerve.

Neuropraxia is a temporary disturbance of nerve conduction not associated with an obvious histologic change. It is a true nerve block, usually temporary, but rare cases (particularly associated with multifocal conduction block (CB) neuropathologies) last more than the traditional limit of 3 to 4 months.[81–83] A clear illustration of neuropraxia[84] with a proximal block in the ulnar nerve at the elbow is shown in Figure 10-9, where it is possible to see the lesion classically defined: no or very reduced conduction when stimulating from above (or proximal to) the level of the lesion and recording distally, and a normal MAP and conduction velocity with stimulation below the level of the lesion. The site can sometimes be exactly defined by inching distalward when a polarity-reversed (usually positive) deflection[85] precedes the MAP as the level is reached, but latency of the MAP onset remains constant until the normally functioning nerve is reached and stimulated. This is due to volume conduction. According to the definition of pure conduction block, no prolonged duration low-amplitude potential should be elicited by stimulation proximal to the lesion, which could be due to differential slowing across the lesion with phase cancellation within the dispersed part of the MAP or SNAP.[86] If the physiologic block is partial, the low-amplitude responses from proximal stimulation should resemble in form the large ones from distal stimulation. Such blocks can last a few days to several weeks, but rarely longer than a few months, though exceptional examples of prolonged CB of neuropraxic type occur. In varying degrees, if further recovery does not take place, demyelination and slow conduction across

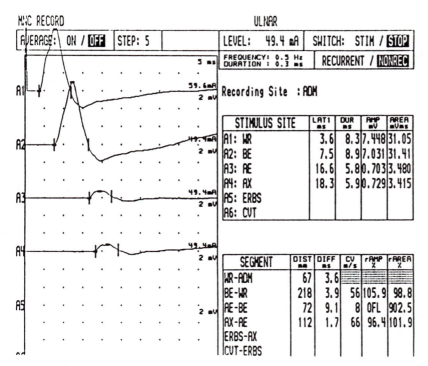

**Figure 10-9.** Ulnar nerve conduction; raster, showing 90% block around eblow with normal velocity above (axilla to above elbow) and below (below elbow to wrist), concordant amplitude and area changes and insignificant change in duration.

the site may develop with additional MAP or SNAP dispersion. Alternatively, axonal lesions may develop when all the amplitudes produced from every stimulation site fall to about the same level. This may also occur in the presence of proximal dispersion due to large-fiber involvement. In evaluation of motor neuron disease and multifocal CB simulating motor neuron disease[87] a distinction is made among (1) pure CB, in which amplitude and area are decreased but duration is normal, (2) mixed CB with temporal dispersion, where the duration is increased, and finally, (3) pure temporal dispersion mimicking CB, in which the increased duration compensates for the amplitude drop to give a normal area. These varieties of CB can occur in association with predisposing conditions such as renal and endocrine disease, which can produce neuropathy, in various toxic neuropathies (particularly those due to alcohol), in malnutrition, in bony compression, such as rheumatoid and other arthropathy, and in some familial neuritides such as predisposition to pressure palsies and familial brachial neuritis. Classical acute CB is seen in the acute phase of the inflammatory neuropathy of the Guillain-Barré syndrome. Sudden exacerbations of chronic progressive and relapsing neuropathy can temporarily cause neuro-

pratic lesions, which can also be seen in patients with unusual occupations, such as window dressers and choreographers, with particular involvement of the peroneal nerve; jackhammer operators and shock–weight lifters with involvement of the deep ulnar nerve in the palm, and in similar other entrapment situations. These entrapment lesions are postulated to be of mixed etiology, the result of both chronic pressure leading to demyelination and vasa nervorum occlusion leading to ischemia and axon pathology. CB usually is not seen in the Charcot-Marie-Tooth group of familial neuropathies.

Diffuse axonal lesions usually produce distal manifestations and give rise to marked lowering of the MAP or SNAP amplitudes with relatively normal velocity. When there is axon atresia and atrophy, as in diabetes and some chronic toxic neuropathies, conduction velocity can be lowered by 40% to 50%.[88] This correlates with the much smaller diameter of fibers in these conditions because of either loss of large fibers or the presence of small diameter regenerating fibers. Alcoholic neuropathy is a prototype of such a disorder, and varying degrees of denervation in the muscle are present, depending on the acuteness of the situation.[89] The amplitude of the SNAPs may be so low as to require averaging techniques or near-nerve recording. The pathologic lesion is usually diffuse multifocal wallerian degeneration with distal emphasis or crescendo. As well as toxic neuropathies most of the neuropathies associated with vasculopathy as well as those with diabetes and with the infections of Lyme disease are of this axonal type. In a number of instances the toxic neuropathies appear to have an element of familial and genetic susceptibility.[90]

### Myelin Sheath Disorders

Disorders of the myelin sheath can be divided into the more unusual genetic neuropathies with dysmyelination and hypomyelination, the commoner genetic neuropathies with diffuse demyelination, onion bulb formation in peripheral nerve and hypertrophic nerves, and the acquired demyelinating disorders. The last group is illustrated by some varieties of diabetic neuropathy, other endocrine neuropathies, the dysimmune neuropathies (Guillain-Barré syndrome and chronic relapsing demyelinating neuropathy), and rare toxic neuropathies such as that due to perihexiline maleate.[91] The significant distinction to be made here is that the demyelination, often called *segmental demyelination,* is diffuse, and concordantly so in the genetic neuropathies, but more discordant between individual nerves and with distal emphasis in these acquired neuropathies.[92] The emphasis is usually distal in these dysimmune acquired neuropathies, but it is not uncommon for proximal slowing of conduction (also representing demyelination) to occur with evolution of the disorder. This is seen in some examples of the early recovering phase of the Guillain-Barré syndrome, where absent F waves may develop into very prolonged-latency ones.[4,93] In the acquired neuropathies, remyelination can take some 6 to 12 weeks, as Kaeser and Lambert[94] described in their experimental studies. Here supramaximal stimulation is very important, as patients with demyelinating neuropathies may have much increased stimulation thresholds.

Demyelination can of course be found in the entrapment neuropathies, and the experimental work of Ochoa and coworkers[95] has indicated how axonostenotic lesions can produce invagination of the nerve at the edges of pressure with disturbance of the symmetric myelin patterns and a loss of

nodes of Ranvier. Distal latency, however, may be prolonged owing to small, regenerating axons or to entrapment and distal demyelination. Thus, in the Guillain-Barré syndrome, prolonged distal latencies can be seen in both the acute and the chronic phase.

### Additional Stimulation Techniques

To investigate proximal conduction, McLean[96] described nerve root stimulation with distal small hand muscle or foot muscle recording. By this method conduction velocities can be measured distally from the nerve root. By using spinal and more proximal evoked potentials, velocity can also be recorded proximally from the root entry to the spinal cord. As described by Mills and Murray,[97] and others,[98] spinal root stimulation can also be performed from the surface of the skin using a high-voltage hand-held stimulator. The potentials evoked by this method compare well with those produced by proximal and distal limb stimulation. Inouye and Buchthal[99] described similar placement of needle electrodes in cervical nerve root locations using radiographic control and then digital and near-nerve wrist stimulation with proximal root recording. Finally, the methods of magnetic stimulation[100] can be applied to proximal conduction. This includes both cortical and spinal cord stimulation with recording distally.

Microneurography, originally devised by Hagbarth[101] is a technique for recording from proprioceptive and nocioceptive myelinated fibers using small tungsten microelectrodes inserted into peripheral nerves. This method has been developed clinically by Valbo and associates[102] in Europe and Ochoa and associates[103] in the United States and has proved valuable for the assessment of mechanoreceptor function and also in C fiber and Aδ fiber function. In Australia, Berke and colleagues[104] have extended its use, particularly in unmyelinated fibers.

Finally, it should be noted that stimulation does not always activate the fibers one expects from individual nerves, and when unusual discrepancies are observed it is important to stimulate nearby nerves and record from other distal sites. Four-point stimulation with the ulnar and median nerves in the arm enables the different anomalous innervations of the Martin Gruber[105] anastamosis to be evaluated, and similarly in the foot, when ankle stimulation produces a much smaller MAP than knee stimulation in the peroneal nerve recording from extensor digitorum brevis. This latter anomalous lateral peroneal distal motor branch can be discovered[106] by moving the ankle-stimulating electrode laterally over the lateral malleolous.

## Late Responses

Two late responses are frequently used to assess proximal conduction, the H reflex and the F wave.[107]

### H Reflex

The H reflex is that produced by low-threshold stimulation of a muscle nerve so that the large, myelinated sensory fibers from the muscle spindles are activated but the stimulus to the direct motor fibers is subthreshold. The response in the muscle occurs, therefore, via a reflex pathway through the spinal cord. This is thought to represent the time of a single-synapse reflex arc. The spindle afferent conduction velocity may thus be estimated by the H-reflex measurement. As an example, the H reflex may be produced in the gastrocnemius muscle at a latency of approximately 30 msec by stimulating the posterior tibial nerve behind the knee when the stimulating cathode is directed proximally. In a normal adult this is practically the only convenient site for H-reflex recording, but in the first few years of life H reflexes can be recorded from other nerves, including the ulnar.[108] In adults, abnormal H reflexes can be recorded in the presence of spinal cord disease at the appropriate level.[109] Though H reflexes have been reported from other muscle nerve systems,[110] especially when single-fiber recording techniques are used,[111] its main clinical use is for the evaluation of function in the S-1 root.[112] Unilateral absence provides supportive evidence for S-1 root disease, but the other side must always be tested because bilateral absence is not necessarily abnormal.

### F Waves

Though they can be found in most muscle nerve systems, F waves, so called because they were originally recorded in the small foot muscles,[113] have much more variable latency and form and probably involve only the motor axon[114] and no synapse. The impulse passing proximally (antidromically) with supramaximal stimulation, unlike the threshold stimulation required for H reflex, alters the excitability of the anterior horn cell or the surrounding central area, so that a variable number of anterior horn cells fire, giving rise to this late response, the F wave. It is not obliterated when the M response appears. This is the most helpful of the late responses. F-wave latency determinations are useful in measuring abnormal neurodisorders of the nerve root zone, as in the early stage[115,116] of acute polyradiculoneuritis or the Guillain-Barré syndrome (now also called acute *inflammatory demyelinating polyneuropathy* [AIDP]). This is of particular value at a time of severe limb paralysis, when the motor conduction of the fastest fibers is normal distally and the F wave is absent, indicating a proximal neuropractic block or an immature developing axonal lesion.[117]

When prolonged distal latencies are reported in the late stage of Guillain-Barré syndrome, low-amplitude F waves may be present concurrently and also have prolonged latency[118] In other demyelinating neuropathies such as chronic inflammatory demyelinating polyneuropathy (CIDP) F-wave latencies[119] may be very markedly prolonged, but in diabetic neuropathy the prolongation is more modest. In the genetic demyelinating neuropathies (e.g., Charcot-Marie-Tooth disease[120] of the demyelinating type [HMSN I], the neuropathy of Refsum's disease, and the neuropathy of familial amyloidosis), F-wave latencies are also prolonged but are quite comparable and concordant with the slowing of distal conduction of these conditions. Abnormal manifestations of the F wave in root or proximal plexus disorders, such as those due to chronic pressure or trauma, are less consistent[121] and can include absence or chronic dispersion or delayed latency responses.[122]

Other late responses include the so-called C response,[123] axon reflexes,[124] long-loop reflexes,[125] and the sympathetic skin response,[126] and can vary from modest latencies of 20 msec to very prolonged latencies greater than 100 msec. The long-loop reflexes and C responses appear to be multisegmental and occur at various epochs, depending on the length of the pathway. They are useful in analysis of central EMG, especially for evaluating spasticity and movement disorders. The axon reflex is short, with a latency between the M and F responses, and it can be recognized by its constant appearance, latency, and fixed relationship to the M response. The axon reflex occurs with neurogenic muscle atrophy followed by reinnervation, as may be seen in genetic neuropathies, plexopathies, and entrapments. It represents sprouting, usually distal to the nerve lesion. Thus, the impulse passes proximally or antidromically to the sprouting branch and then orthodromically down the branch to give the second muscle evoked response. Investigators assessing nerve function and spinal cord disorders need to correlate these late responses with the results of spinal and cerebral evoked potentials (discussed in other chapters). The sympathetic skin response is nonspecifically evoked by a variety of stimuli, has very prolonged latency (1.3 to 1.6 seconds), and is assessed by its absence rather than amplitude or latency change. It is useful for evaluating for autonomic neuropathies, particularly those of diabetes mellitus.

The blink reflex[4] is used for assessing peripheral and central facial function by stimulating the trigeminal nerve via the supraorbital branch and recording from the orbicularis oculi and upper facial muscles.[127] The ipsilateral early response (between 8 and 12 msec) is probably a simple (or oligosynaptic) reflex, whereas, ipsilateral and contralateral late reflexes (between 28 and 42 msec) are polysynaptic. They are, respectively, called $R_1$ for the early, and $R_2$ for the late response.[128,129] Naturally, both the $R_1$ and $R_2$ responses are absent or delayed on the side of a lower motor neuron facial palsy or Bell's palsy, without reference to the side of the afferent or trigeminal stimulation. $R_1$ may be abnormal in conditions where the reflex arc is interrupted such as trigeminal sensory disorders or demyelination from multiple sclerosis. $R_2$ alterations, either prolongation or absence, occur more frequently in lesions in the lateral medulla, such as Wallenberg's syndrome, when the interruption is of the afferent type. Reduced levels of consciousness (e.g., coma) as well as impaired appreciation of pain may reduce the $R_2$ component. In severe demyelinating neuropathy such as Charcot-Marie-Tooth disorder (HMSN I) there may be so much dispersion of the responses that

the distinction between $R_1$ and $R_2$ may be obliterated.

Finally, the facial condition of hemispasm can be investigated by recording ephaptic conduction responses at just less than twice the normal facial distal latency, as Kamp-Nielsen[130] has done, proving that the responses are ephaptic by using collision studies. This is of some importance, as a proportion of patients with facial hemispasm have an aberrant artery compressing the facial nerve, a condition that is surgically treatable.[131]

## Clinical Correlations

Neuropraxia and axonal degeneration or axonal injury with so-called axonotmesis has already been discussed, but when the primary damage is to the Schwann cell—whether by toxins, antibodies (including cell damage), compression, or anoxia—primary demyelination or Gombault's[132] degeneration takes place. If the axon nevertheless remains intact, conduction is possible, but at a much slower rate. With remyelination there may be a great variation in the internodal distance, which also causes slow conduction velocity.[133] Fibrosis around a peripheral nerve, which may be associated with this segmental demyelination, increases the threshold of stimulus needed to activate the nerve and reduces conduction velocity, relative to the degree of demyelination.

From these considerations the clinical significance of retarded conduction velocity may be appreciated, and it correlates well with demyelination in peripheral nerves.[134,135] This may be generalized, as in the metabolic neuropathies. Diabetic neuropathy was originally cited as a good example, but it is now thought to be mainly secondary demyelination following axon disease. Hypothyroidism and hepatic neuropathies are other examples of metabolic neuropathy. Other demyelinating neuropathies include allergic or autoimmune disorders (AIDP and CIDP), the familial neuropathies of Charcot-Marie-Tooth disorder,[136,137] and sulphatide storage disorders in metachromatic leukodystrophy.[138] Infections also produce demyelinating neuropathy—leprosy, diphtheria, and some of the rarer forms of Lyme disease. Focal slowing is seen in chronic nerve compression syndromes such as tardy ulnar palsy, peroneal palsy, and carpal or tarsal tunnel syndrome.

The other electrical parameters of importance in studying peripheral nerves are threshold amperage and the amperage necessary for maximal stimulation, both of which rise in the acute neuropathies such as the Guillain-Barré syndrome and Bell's palsy, and particularly in the chronic neuropathies of CIDP, Charcot-Marie-Tooth disorder, and diabetes.

Anterior horn cell and muscle disorders do not usually show nerve conduction changes, though occasionally low-amplitude muscle evoked potentials may represent spared fascicles of slower-conducting fibers so that in anterior horn cell disease some slower velocities than normal may occur.[139] Another condition that simulates anterior horn cell disease is the multifocal conduction block syndrome.[140] Another reason for slowing of motor nerve conduction is the effect of local cold on the nerve trunk, which reduces conduction velocity by about 5% for every 1°C drop in temperature.[144]

Primary axonal neuropathies, as in acute intermittent porphyria, most drug and industrial toxic neuropathies, some alcoholic neuropathies, early acute renal neuropathy, and lead neuropathy, may not show reduction of conduction velocity, but nerve action potentials and muscle evoked potentials are often significantly reduced. Overall, the velocity distinctions between axonal and demyelinating neuropathies have been made by observations on single teased nerve fibers stained for myelin, and, as suggested by Gilliatt, it is better to think of neuropathies as showing scanty or extensive demyelination[69] rather than as being exclusively axonal or demyelinating.

On this basis, the toxic neuropathies are those with scanty or no demyelination, and they have been classified as *axonal*. Examples include chemical poisoning, as by organophosphates, or the neuropathies resulting from drugs, such as thalidomide or vincristine.[90] It is generally thought that the primary nerve disorder in diabetes is an axonal neuropathy that merely develops secondary demyelinating features with a variable degree of slowing of conduction velocity. In porphyria, though some demyelination is seen, the major involvement is axonal. The neuropathy of the neuronal form of Charcot-Marie-Tooth disorder (Charcot-Marie-Tooth type II or HMSN II) is also

of axonal type, and similarly the severe sensory involvement of Friedreich's ataxia[142] would be classified as mainly an axonal neuropathy.

The most important examples of the demyelinating neuropathies with slow conduction are those associated with autoimmune diseases—specifically, the chronic inflammatory demyelinating[143] and acute inflammatory demyelinating neuropathies.[144] They have been discussed, but their slow conduction is related, as shown in earlier work by McLeod and associates,[145] to the presence of moderate or marked demyelination, particularly segmental demyelination. Although demyelination clearly is found in the hypertrophic form of Charcot-Marie-Tooth disorder, it appears to be most extensive in the familial hypertrophic polyneuritis called *Dejerine-Sottas disorder* and now classified as CMT type III or HMSN III.[146] Again, the most important distinction between the genetic and the acquired neuropathies is the presence of concordance in the first group. In these there may be concordance not only of the degree of slowing of conduction velocity, and therefore of demyelination both from one side of the body to the other in individual nerves, but also concordance of slowing of conduction velocity between the distal and proximal portions of each nerve. Even with the axonal genetic neuropathies, this same concordance in the degree of denervation or of reduction of nerve action potential is noted. Many of the demyelinating neuropathies may also have central demyelination; this is well-described in the neuropathies of abetalipoproteinemia (the Bassen-Kornzweig syndrome)[147] and Tangier disease[148] (serum-lipoprotein deficiency). Similar involvement, both proximally in the central nervous system and distally in the peripheral neuraxis, is noted in the neuropathies of metachromatic leukodystrophy, in children and sometimes in adults, and of the adult-onset leukodystrophies.[149]

In patients with myopathy and myositis conduction velocity is generally normal.

Sensory conduction may be lost in any lesion of the sensory pathway distal to the dorsal root ganglion, and testing of sensory conduction velocity is valuable for distinguishing a brachial plexus disorder from involvement of the anterior horn cell. Normal sensory nerve action potentials may be recorded from or at the wrist by digital stimulation when anesthesia or analgesia is present if sensory pathways are only involved proximal to the dorsal root ganglion as in a spinal cord lesion like syringomyelia. Thus, the distal ganglion-axon sensory system remains intact and can sustain impulse transmission. Distal latencies may be increased or sensory nerve action potentials may be lost in a variety of conditions associated with neuropathies, a good example being Friedreich's ataxia,[150–152] a hereditary neuropathy of Charcot-Marie-Tooth type with prominent areflexia. In the rare neurogenic thoracic outlet syndrome associated with entrapment of the lower trunk of the brachial plexus over an aberrant cervical rib or band, the sensory potentials recorded in the hand, particularly from the ulnar nerve, are lost or of low amplitude.[153] The distal sensory velocities from wrist to elbow would be normal in this situation, and such examples of cervical rib or band entrapment must be diagnosed with extreme care.[154] When a spinal cord lesion or root avulsion causes appropriate segmental sensory loss, the sensory nerve action potentials in these areas are typically retained[72] as the lesions are proximal to the neuronal sensory cells in the dorsal root ganglion. In subliminal nerve lesions associated with subclinical neuropathy, threshold conduction velocity may be valuable, as shown in the past by Preswick in carpal tunnel syndrome[155] Provocative ischemia may give rise to nerve conduction failure or slowing earlier than would normally be expected for such lesions.[156] Subclinical diabetic and uremic neuropathies may also be demonstrated by nerve conduction studies,[157] and these studies of subclinical involvement of nerves have proved valuable in epidemiologic studies of nerve toxicity.[158]

## A Technique of Nerve Conduction Development

Here, we list possible steps in the evaluation of nerve conduction studies:

1. Choose relevant nerves for clinical assessment, which would vary from those most appropriate for early disease presentation to those only moderately affected clinically (and therefore, still recordable from) in severe disorders.
2. Age and temperature control evaluations are important.

3. Noninvasive surface methods of stimulation and recording should be tried first.
4. Pickup active electrodes moved around the end-plate region (motor point) to give a sharp negative takeoff of MAP and larger negative spikes. If MAP has an abnormal shape, check that correct filters are in place.
5. For sensory conduction place active electrodes directly over the nerve and reference electrodes 2 cm to the side and proximal.
6. Beware of motor spike if antidromic sensory stimulation is used.
7. Always build up voltage at shortest duration unless there are overriding reasons for single-shock studies (e.g., in children).
8. Use loudspeaker at low level to detect very slow conduction MAPs not on the oscilloscope screen sweep.
9. Stop at supramaximal level or volume conduction to nearby nerves may occur.
10. Beware of interpretation as to site or nerve supply of low-amplitude potentials.
11. If MAP from distal stimulation is greater than that from proximal stimulation, consider nerve block.
12. If MAP from distal stimulation is smaller than that from proximal stimulation, consider cross-over or anomolous innervation.
13. Always record late potentials: Distinguish (1) late components of dispersed MAP, (2) axon reflexes (can block only over a significant distance), (3) ephaptic transmission (useful in facial hemispasm), (4) F waves (useful in proximal neuropathies, less so in root disorders), (5) H reflex (if it appears on building up potentials, consider associated pyramidal disorder).
14. Double stimulation studies to elucidate slow components of MAP/SNAP.
15. Near-nerve stimulation and recording.
16. Averaging techniques (also useful for the full compound nerve action potential).
17. Root or cord stimulation for plexus lesions (using needle or surface electrodes with high-voltage stimulation).
18. Segmental and sensory nerve stimulation evoked potentials for root and plexus lesions.
19. Root stimulation evoked potentials.
20. Microneurography.

Such a philosophy might be called *The Compleat Nerve Conductioner.*

## Neuromuscular Transmission

### Motor End-Plate Anatomy, Immunochemistry, and Physiology

*Neuromuscular transmission* describes the passage of the nerve impulse in motor nerve fibers across the neuromuscular junction to the muscle fiber. This results in a propagated muscle fiber action potential and the contraction of the muscle fiber (twitch). It is achieved by a complex mechanism of acetylcholine generation and release at the nerve terminal via specific ion channels and acetylcholine's conjugation with receptors on the end-plate region of the muscle fiber, which process generates electrical potentials. Both the ion channels on the nerve terminal and the receptors on the muscle are liable to immune-mediated and chemical disorders that disturb neuromuscular transmission.[159–161]

The size and shape of end-plates vary with species, but generally end-plates are circular or oval and usually of a diameter smaller than 70 μ. There is usually one motor end-plate for each muscle fiber, situated entrally and supplied by one terminal twig from a neuron.[162] Histologically, the end-plate consists of three portions: (1) the terminal apparatus of the nerve, (2) the specialized region of muscle fiber surface in contact with this terminal apparatus, and (3) the area of teloglia surrounding it.

The area of teloglia contains the "sole nuclei" and appears to be continuous with the Schwann cell envelope of the myelinated fiber. The end-plate of the muscle is separated from the terminal apparatus of the nerve by a space of less than 1 μ called the *synaptic cleft*. Electron microscopic studies (see Figure 10-10) indicate that in mammalian (including human) tissue, the end-bulb of the nerve has a curved surface that is cupped into a partially concave footplate on the muscle, forming a primary cleft. The footplate of the muscle is further subdivided into numerous secondary clefts. In disease, the primary cleft may become distorted and the secondary clefts abnormal in shape and number. Developing end-plates of the fetus are similar to the abnormal end-plates in diseases of neuromuscular transmission.[163] Organization of the end-plate with maturity involves the development of the primary and secondary clefts.

The function of the end-plate region has been studied by chemical and electrical means. Following the response of repeated stimulation on the nerve, the muscle contracts in forms that vary from single twitches to completely fused tetanus. End-plates can transmit frequencies up to 40 per second continuously without fatigue and, when considering relatively limited periods of activity, fatigue in the normal system does not begin until the frequency exceeds 50 per second. The basic electrical potential produced in the muscle end-plate is the miniature end-plate potential (or MEPP).[164] The first step is mobilization of the stores (or reserves) of acetylcholine in order to provide readily available acetylcholine, which can then be incorporated into the vesicles that pass to the end-bulb of the neuron.[165] The discharge of these vesicles is com-

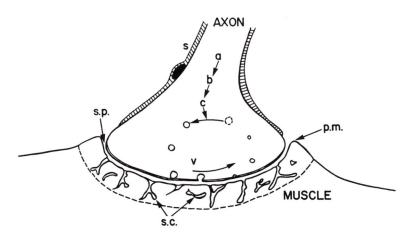

**Figure 10-10.** Motor end-plate (diagram). Key: s, Schwann cell; S.P., synaptic space: primary cleft; s.c., secondary clefts; p.m., postjunctional membrane; a, synthesis of acetylcholine; b, store (reserve) of acetylcholine; c, readily available acetylcholine; v, discharge and recharge cycle of synaptic vesicles.

plicated and is governed by the calcium receptor protein at the calcium ion channels.[161]

When discharged, the packet of acetylcholine is subject to the destructive effect of the cholinesterase in the primary cleft or synaptic space,[166] but sufficient acetylcholine reaches the receptor protein sites around the "mouths" of the secondary clefts, which in the normal state appear to be nicely juxtaposed to the release sites.[160] It is believed that the vesicles containing the acetylcholine in the end-bulb of the nerve are recycled and recharged with acetylcholine.[167]

The transmission across the small gap of the primary cleft is thought to be chemical, with fairly equal-sized multimolecular packets (quanta) of acetylcholine, each containing about 5,000 to 10,000 molecules. The safety factor across the tiny distance of 15 nm (300 to 500 Angstroms) is excellent.[168] At the muscle end-plate the combination of the acetylcholine with its receptor produces the small depolarization of about 1 mV (as measured by microelectrodes), the MEPP. If the system is driven by a propagated nerve action potential producing acetylcholine quanta, usually numbering about 100, then sufficient MEPPs are produced to summate and create depolarization of the postjunctional membrane in excess of the threshold of this membrane. This produces a muscle action potential, which is propagated.[169] The action potential triggers the mechanical contraction of the muscle by an excitation-contraction-coupling reaction.[162] To account for the speed of this change, there is a mechanism for rapid transmission of information from the surface to the center of the fiber that involves the transverse tubular system of the sarcoplasmic reticulum (see Chapter 9). Calcium has an important role: there is an influx of calcium ions when the nerve action potential reaches the nerve terminal, and the release of acetylcholine is calcium dependent.[170] Thus, increasing the concentration of extracellular magnesium eventually increases the ratio of magnesium to calcium ions near the prejunctional membrane of the end-bulb, reducing the number of quanta released and so reducing the end-plate potential to a subthreshold level and blocking transmission.

The end-plate mechanism appears to be acutely dependent on the concentrations of divalent cations. If we consider an end-plate potential to be produced as a result of the discharge of 100 to 200

quanta (each equivalent to an MEPP) of acetylcholine from the nerve terminals, the magnitude of the action potential depends on the ability of the terminal ending of the nerve to produce an adequate quantity of acetylcholine.[168] Sufficient acetylcholine is usually produced only when the action potential arriving at the terminal nerve ending increases the quantal release of acetylcholine and when the depolarization produced by the nerve impulse is large enough.

Reducing the concentrations of external calcium and raising that of external magnesium may reduce the number of quanta produced per impulse; thus, the action of calcium appears to be to increase the release of these quanta caused by the action potential in the nerve terminal.[169] This corresponds to raising the frequency of the miniature end-plate potentials. Further studies with curarized mammalian preparations have indicated that, at the start of repetitive stimulation using "low calcium–high magnesium–treated" preparations, a potentiation under normal physiologic conditions is masked. Such masking could be attributed to reduced available store of acetylcholine in the nerve terminal, and that would certainly fit in with the fall of end-plate amplitude on repetitive stimulation in a curarized preparation. Following a train of nerve impulses to a normal physiologic endplate, potentiation of neuromuscular transmission occurs.[170] Studies with preparations blocked by magnesium and d-tubocurarine have indicated that this posttetanic potentiation results from an increase in the store of available acetylcholine and that it reaches a peak in about 100 msec. Secondary potentiation, reaching a peak in 4 to 7 seconds, may result from increased mobilization of the acetylcholine, building up the available store.[171]

### Clinical Applications and Immunology: Genetics

Of historical interest is the Jolly[172] reaction—clinical muscle fatigue in response to repeated stimulation of the appropriate nerve. One of the simplest methods of demonstrating the efficiency of the neuromuscular junction is to observe single-firing motor unit potentials.[84] The motor unit potential is composed of the many single-fiber potentials that make up one motor unit (a group of muscle fibers and its single neuron). If every muscle fiber in the motor unit fires consistently with each neuronal impulse, the shape of the motor unit potential recorded from the same position on each occasion should be exactly comparable. In practice, there is a small variation (up to 5%) in amplitude and duration. When, however, individual end-plates with their muscle fibers show excessive fatigue, the motor unit potential becomes lower in amplitude or fragmented as individual muscle fiber potentials disappear. Thus, a significant variation in amplitude of a single motor unit potential, repetitively firing, appears with defects of neuromuscular transmission such as myasthenia gravis. This may take the form of a simple progressive decrement of the motor unit potential as more fibers become fatigued, or it may present with variations in amplitude of one motor unit potential.

In a similar fashion, the amplitude and numbers of potentials firing in a maximal interference pattern of motor unit potentials produced by a strong contraction decrease in the presence of a defect of neuromuscular transmission. When such a fall-off in the interference pattern is observed during needle EMG of a patient with myasthenia gravis, intramuscular or intravenous administration of an anticholinesterase drug preserves acetylcholine in the synaptic cleft and corrects the defect of neuromuscular transmission for as long as the drug acts.[24]

An extension of this is single-fiber EMG using semi-microphysiologic techniques with electrode tips of 25 μ, so that the second safety level of the neuromuscular mechanism at the motor unit level can be investigated. Here, individual spikes can be recorded instead of the enigmatic profile of the motor unit potential ("the blanket effect") described so well by Payan.[173] This is usually the utmost miniaturization we can reach in the clinical neurophysiology laboratory,[174] and, in fact, it measures the variability of the interval between two closely recorded spikes from adjacent muscle fibers of one motor unit.[34] This variability, called *jitter*,[175] is contributed to by conduction over three areas in the neuromuscular mechanism, neuromuscular transmission, terminal nerve fiber conduction, and muscle fiber conduction.[176] It is excessive in disorders of neuromuscular transmission such as myasthenia gravis,[177,178] Lambert-Eaton syndrome,[179] and botulism, and an appropriate

measurement can be made. A factor called the mean consecutive difference (MCD) can be derived, and the number of times the second potential blocks (or as it is called *blocking*) can be recorded. It is said that the increased diagnostic sensitivity of electrophysiologic tests in myasthenia gravis using single-fiber EMG may double, to 80%[180] and Stalberg and Trontelj[181] claim 92% abnormal results. The most frequently used muscles are the extensor digitorum communis and the frontalis. The latter may be helpful in cranial or purely ocular myasthenia gravis.

MEPPs can be recorded from excised muscle in a suitable constant-temperature nutrient bath medium. In excised muscle, microelectrode studies[182,183] have consistently shown that in myasthenia gravis the MEPPs are reduced in amplitude but not significantly in frequency. When small macroelectrodes are inserted at the motor point into mammalian[184] and human muscle, MEPPs can also be recorded extracellularly with amplitudes of 30 to 60 μV, and these are also abnormal in myasthenia gravis.[185] This is because myasthenia gravis produces a morphologic change at the end-plate due to immune-mediated destruction of the postjunctional membrane receptor sites.

Elmquist and Lambert[186] in a series of beautiful studies in vitro on small strips of excised intercostal muscle, have shown the low-amplitude MEPPs described above and have elucidated the microphysiologic features of the Lambert-Eaton syndrome[187] (normal amplitude MEPPs in reduced numbers) and of botulism and the animal model of experimental autoimmune myasthenia gravis. This in vitro method, certainly the most accurate method of defining the defect, has been used in five or six new defects of congenital myasthenias described by Engel and Lambert[188]: end-plate esterase deficiency and small nerve terminals, abnormalities of the acetylcholine-induced ion channels, and defects of acetylcholine resynthesis and mobilization.[189] The last one is not unlike the blocking effect of hemicholinium in normal muscles.

Today, newly discovered defects of neuromuscular transmission are usually analyzed by this excised muscle technique, and the effects of different antibodies on both the end-bulb and the footplate are described. It is quite likely that at least two antibody mechanisms are associated with both the Lambert-Eaton syndrome and myasthenia gravis.[190]

The standard laboratory test for myasthenia gravis uses repetitive stimulation and supramaximal stimulation levels[191,192] and investigates the third level of the safety factor or the whole muscle. If the evoked potential from muscle produced by supramaximal stimulation is recorded with surface electrodes in such a fashion that consistent results can be produced using this technique, the effects can be interpreted to describe the function of the neuromuscular junction. At stimulation rates between one and five per second in normal muscle there is no significant variation in the amplitude of the supramaximally evoked potential. At more rapid rates, in normal patients posttetanic potentiation results in a rise in amplitude of some 5% to 20%. This becomes more apparent at stimulation rates up to 40 per second, and usually repetitive stimulation up to 50 per second is not associated with any significant decrement. In disorders of neuromuscular transmission, decrement usually appears at the slow rates of stimulation best seen at two and five per second; with prolonged stimulation further decrement usually occurs.

The commonest disorder that exhibits this type of decrement is myasthenia gravis, and decrements greater than 20% are often noted when testing a weak muscle. Anticholinesterase therapy tends to correct this decrement and may invalidate results of tests on a patient who is receiving continuous therapy. At high rates of stimulation in patients with myasthenia gravis, potentiating effects may be noted following an initial decrement,[193] but prolonged stimulation usually produces further decrement. Thus, posttetanic facilitation usually is not lost in disorders of neuromuscular transmission such as myasthenia gravis, but in fact is very easily recognized. With repetitive stimulation, lesser, somewhat irregular, decrements are also noticed in neuronal muscle wasting diseases such as amyotrophic lateral sclerosis, syringomyelia, and carcinomatous neuromyopathy. Some patients with myotonic muscular dystrophy may also show unusual decrements.[194] In patients with myasthenia gravis who have only mild defects the decrement can be potentiated with prolonged exercise for up to 1 minute,[195] and ischemia of the system may be needed to bring out a decrement using repetitive stimulation.[196] Different laboratories use different stimulation rates for basic slow stimulation, some

use two per second, others three. When the median-thenar system is used, decrements, to be abnormal, should be between 8% and 10%, and they are usually most evident by the fourth or fifth potential. Desmedt has shown that a decrement as small as 5% or 6%[197] may be obtained in a well-stabilized ulnar hypothenar system. Similarly, he concurs that the greatest decrement is usually present by the fifth potential, after which partial recovery occurs. Thus, part of the testing procedure would be brief exercise, about 10 seconds, which would be sufficient to bring out posttetanic potentiation, and vigorous exercise for 1 minute, which would be sufficient to show increased decrement in a patient with myasthenia gravis.[50] Other sites of stimulation include proximal regions such as the accessory-trapezius, axillary-deltoid, and facial systems.[198,199]

Occasionally, a paradoxical myasthenic reaction is seen principally in patients, with small-cell carcinoma of the bronchus. This has been called the *myasthenic syndrome*[200] or *Lambert-Eaton syndrome* and has been investigated extensively by Newsom-Davis,[190] who found antibodies located on the end-bulb or nerve side of the neuromuscular junction (prejunctional). Patients have a fatiguing type of muscle weakness and may have frank neuropathy, but they do not have the specific exercise fatigue so characteristic of myasthenia gravis. Clinicians sometimes feel they can identify the disorder by noting slow clinical onset to the hand grip. The characteristic findings are seen on electrical stimulation using supramaximal stimuli after the muscle is well relaxed. Occasionally, even at very low rates, there can be quite marked potentiation. The initial amplitude of the supramaximally evoked potential is in most instances markedly reduced from normal, but stimulation rates even as slow as one per second[200] can produce increments of about 200%, and with faster rates of two to 50 per second, increments as great as 500% to 700% can be seen. Repetitive stimulation at higher rates produces increasing potentiation, and the greatest potentiation typically is seen at 50 per second, but since this is somewhat uncomfortable, vigorous exercise is now used in its place after the muscle-nerve system has been fully relaxed and without any stimuli for at least 2 minutes.[49] The other feature in both myasthenia gravis and the Lambert-Eaton syndrome is EMG variation in the amplitude of single–motor unit potentials, and both, of course, show excessive jitter and blocking on single-fiber EMG. Coexistence of myasthenia gravis and the Lambert-Eaton syndrome has been reported,[201–203] both being immune-mediated diseases, as has intercurrent multiple sclerosis and myasthenia gravis.[204] Intracellular investigations in the Lambert-Eaton syndrome have already been discussed. In this disorder there are many subthreshold end-plate potentials, which are rapidly advanced to threshold level by mobilization of stores and released with repetitive stimulation. Immunohistochemical methods are available, and, indeed, are preferable, for treatment of both this and myasthenia gravis, but in the Lambert-Eaton syndrome administration of guanidine improves the condition and increases the amplitude of the end-plate potentials, perhaps by increasing the number of quanta of acetylcholine.[205] Use of this drug has since been discontinued, owing to its many toxic side effects. Eventually it may be replaced by diaminopyridine. In some ways the defect of neuromuscular transmission in the myasthenic syndrome is similar to that produced experimentally by excess circulating magnesium ($Mg^{++}$).[205]

Abnormal neuromuscular transmission can be accentuated by the administration of curare. Patients with myasthenia gravis are markedly sensitive to curare, and this is the rationale underlying a curare test. A dose one tenth the ''curarizing'' dose is given intravenously divided in eight aliquots under anesthesiology surveillance.[206]. A number of studies have shown that patients with myasthenia gravis become weak after the first two or three aliquots of curare.[206] This is because part of the defect of the disorder is related to the acetylcholine concentration in the vesicles. Thus blocking the primary receptor sites for acetylcholine with the curare can reduce the safety factor in the myasthenia gravis end-plate mechanism and give rise to the excessive paralysis easily produced by small doses of curare. A shorter version of this test is the regional or localized curare test,[207] in which curare is introduced intravenously distal to an arterial occlusive cuff, allowing it to diffuse back into the muscle. In some hands, and if the procedure is performed carefully, it appears to be without significant risk. Horowitz has described the use of single-fiber EMG with the regional curare test to increase the percentage yield for detecting myasthenia gravis.[208]

Finally, various chemicals and toxins may act on the end-plate. In particular, the mycin antibiotics, such as neomycin and kanamycin, can produce disorders of neuromuscular transmission resembling myasthenia gravis and may seriously exacerbate symptoms in patients with this diagnosis. Other substances that can affect the end-plate mechanism include quinine and quinidine.

Botulinum toxin probably produces its effects by presynaptic action or by disturbance in the synthesis or storage of acetylcholine.[209] It may also produce a rather profound distal axonopathy.[210] Clearly, electrophysiologic testing of adults poisoned with the toxin from anaerobic bacteria in improperly canned or bottled foods is important. In botulism there is a blockade of synchronized transmitter release, as shown in Stanley and Drachman's studies[211] and the role of antidromic backfiring induced by a stimulus may explain a rapid decrement, with a maximum at the second response, followed by recovery.[212] This is called the *DI* (decrement-increment) *phenomenon,* and in this case true posttetanic fascilitation does not occur. There is also a childhood or infantile botulism syndrome in which these bacteria produce the toxin in constipated intestines. Findings of repetitive stimulation of infants are subject to the same less stringent normal values as nerve conduction, owing to immaturity.[213] It should be mentioned that carefully administered minute doses of botulinum toxin have been shown to give significant relief of disabling movement disorders such as torticollis, blepharospasm, hemifacial spasm, and spasmodic or dystonic dysphonia,[214] presumably because it interrupts the aberrantly firing pathways by denervation (followed later by reinnervation).[215]

# References

1. Katz B. Nerve, Muscle and Synapse. New York: McGraw-Hill, 1966.
2. Tasaki I. Conduction of the nerve impulse. In: Handbook of Physiology. Washington, DC: American Physiological Society, 1959;75–121.
3. Lovelace RE. Clinical neurophysiology of neuromuscular disease. In: JP Mohr, ed. Manual of Clinical Problems in Neurology. Boston: Little, Brown, 1989.
4. Kimura J. Electrodiagnosis in Disease of Nerve

and Muscle: Principles of Practice, ed. 2. Philadelphia: FA Davis, 1988.

5. Beeson D, Jeremiah S, West LF, et al. Assignment of the human nicotinic acetylcholine receptor genes: The and subunit genes to chromosome 2 and the subunit gene to chromosome 12. Ann Hum Genet 1990; 54:199–208.

6. Hodgkin AL, Keynes RO. Active transport of cations in giant axons Sepia and Loligo. J Physiol (Lond) 1955; 128:28–60.

7. Tasaki I. Nerve Excitation. Springfield, Ill.: Charles C Thomas, 1953.

8. Cole KS. Membranes, Ions and Impulses. Los Angeles: University of California Press, 1968.

9. Tasaki I, Barry W, Carnay L. Optical and electrophysiological evidence for confirmational changes in membrane macromolecules during nerve excitation. In: Physical Principles of Biological Membranes. Coral Gables Conference, Gordon and Breach, 1968;17–34.

10. Tasaki I, Carnay L, Watanabe A. Transient changes in extrinsic fluorescence of nerve produced by electrical stimulation. Proc Nat Acad Sci USA 1969; 64:1362–1368.

11. Ling G, Gerard RW. The normal membrane potential of frog sartorius fibers. J Cell Comp Physiol 1949; 34:383–396.

12. Tasaki I, Mizuguchi K. The changes in electrical impedance during activity and the effect of alkaloids and polarization on the biological processes in the myelinated nerve fiber. Acta Biochem Biophys 1949; 3:484–493.

13. Elmquist D, Hofmann WE, Kugelberg J, et al. An electrophysiological investigation of neuromuscular transmission in myasthenia gravis. J Physiol (Lond) 1964; 174:417–434.

14. Johns RJ. Microelectrode studies of muscle membrane potentials in man. Res Publ Assoc Nerv Ment Dis 1958; 38:704–713.

15. McComas A, Johns RT. Potential changes in the normal and diseased muscle cell. In: Walton J, ed. Disorders of Voluntary Muscle. Boston, Little, Brown, 1969;877–907.

16. Beranek R. Intracellular stimulation myography in man. Electroencephalogr Clin Neurophysiol 1964; 16:301–304.

17. Goodgold J, Eberstein AF. Transmembrane potentials of human muscle cells in vivo. Exp Neurol 1966; 15:338–346.

18. Riecker C, Bolte HD. Membran Potentiale einzelner Skeletmuskelzellen bei hypokaliamischer periodischer Muskel-paralyse. Klin Wschr 1966; 44:804–807.

19. Eliasson SG. Properties of isolated nerve cells from alloxanized rats. J Neurol Neurosurg Psychiatry. 1969; 32:525–529.

20. Maselli RA, Soliven BC. Analysis of the organophosphate-induced electromyographic response to repetitive stimulation: Paradoxical response to edrophonium and D-turocurarine. Muscle Nerve 1991; 14:1182–1188.

21. Akaike N, Tokutomi N, Kijima H. Kinetic analysis of acetylcholine-induced current in isolated frog sympathetic ganglion cells. J Neurophysiol 1988; 61:283–290.

22. Gasser HS, Grundfest M. Axon diameters in relation to spike dimensions and conduction velocity in mammalian fibers. Am J Physiol 1939; 127:393–414.

23. Lenman JAR, Ritchie AE. Clinical Electromyography. Philadelphia: JB Lippincott, 1970.

24. Lovelace RE, Myers SJ. Nerve conduction and synaptic transmission. In: Darling RC, Downey JA, eds. Physiological Basis of Rehabilitation Medicine. Philadelphia: WB Saunders, 1971; 85–106.

25. McComas A. Neuromuscular function and disorders. Butterworths, 1977.

26. Stampfli R. Saltatory conduction in nerve. Physiol Rev. 1954; 34:101–112.

27. Rasminsky M, Sears TA. Saltatory conduction in demyelinated nerve fibers. In: Desmedt JE, ed. New Developments in Electromyography and Clinical Neurophysiology, vol 2. Basel: S Karger, 1973;158–165.

28. Tasaki I. Nervous transmissions. Springfield, Ill.: Charles C Thomas, 1968.

29. Bostock H, Sears TA. The internodal axon membrane: Electrical excitability and continuous conduction in segmental demyelination. J Physiol (Lond) 1978; 280:273–301.

30. Waxman SG, Ritchie JM. Molecular dissection of the myelinated axon. Ann Neurol 1993; 33:121–136.

31. McDonald WI. Nerve conduction in muscle afferent fibers during experimental demyelination in cat nerve. Acta Neuropathol 1962; 1:425–432.

32. Gasser HS, Erlanger J. Electrical Signs of Nervous Action. Philadelphia: University of Pennsylvania Press, 1937.

33. Sumner AJ, ed. The Physiology of Peripheral Nerve Disease. Philadelphia: WB Saunders, 1980.

34. Ekstedt J, Stalberg E. A method of recording extracellular action potentials of simple muscle fibers and measuring their propagation velocity in voluntary activated human muscle. Bull Am Assoc Electromyogr Electrodiagn 1963; 10:16.

35. Devi S, Challenor Y, Duarte N, et al. Prognostic value of minimal excitability of facial nerve in Bell's palsy. J Neurol Neurosurg Psychiatry 1978; 41:649–652.

36. Hodes R, Larrabee MG, German W. The human electromyogram in response to nerve stimulation and the conduction velocity of the motor axons. Arch Neurol Psychiatry 1948; 60:340–365.

37. Gilliatt RW, Meer J. The refractory period of transmission in patients with a carpal tunnel syndrome. Muscle Nerve 1990; 13:445–450.

38. Buchthal F, Rosenfalck A. Evoked action potentials and conduction velocity in human sensory nerves. Brain Res, 1966; 3:1–122.

39. Rosenfalck A. Early recognition of nerve disorders by near-nerve recording of sensory nerve action potentials. Muscle Nerve 1978; 1:360–367.

40. Trojaborg W. Early electrophysiological changes in conduction block. Muscle Nerve 1978; 1:400–403.

41. Lovelace RE, Myers SJ, Zablow L. Sensory conduction in peroneal and posterior tibial nerves using averaging techniques. J Neurol Neurosurg Psychiatry 1973; 36:942–950.

42. Stegeman DF, DeWeerd JPC. Modelling compound action potentials of peripheral nerves in situ. I. Model description, evidence for a nonlinear relation between fiber diameters and velocity. Electroencephalogr Clin Neurophysiol 1982; 54:436–448.

43. Thomas PK, Sears TA, Gilliatt RW. The range of conduction velocity in normal motor nerve fibers to the small muscles of the hand and foot. J Neurol Neurosurg Psychiatry 1959; 22:175–181.

44. Hopf HC. Electromyographic study on so-called mononeuritis. Arch Neurol 1963; 9:307–312.

45. Jabre J. Ulnar nerve lesions at the wrist: New technique for recording from the sensory dorsal branch of the ulnar nerve. Neurology 1980; 30:873–876.

46. Stegeman DF, DeWeerd JPC. Modelling compound action potentials of peripheral nerves in situ. II. A study of the influence of temperature. Electroencephalogr Clin Neurophysiol 1982; 54:516–529.

47. Trojaborg W, Moon A, Andersen DB, et al. Sural nerve conduction parameters in normal subjects related to age, gender, temperature and height: A reappraisal. Muscle Nerve 1992; 15:.

48. Lovelace RE, Horowitz SJ. Peripheral neuropathy and long term diphenylhydantoin therapy. Arch Neurol 1968; 18:69–77.

49. Rosenberg RN, Lovelace RE. Mononeuritis multiplex in lepromatous leprosy. Arch Neurol 1968; 19:310–314.

50. Lange DJ. Electrodiagnostic studies of neuromuscular disease: A primer for clinicians. In: Rowland LP, ed. Merritt's Textbook of Neurology update 6, Philadelphia: Lea & Febiger, 1991;3–18.

51. Oh SJ. Clinical Electromyography: Nerve Conduction Studies. Baltimore: University Park Press, 1984.

52. Trojaborg W. Sensory nerve conduction: Near-nerve recording. Methods Clin Neurophysiol. 1992; 3:17–40.

53. Marinacci AA. In: Applied Electromyography. Philadelphia: Lea & Febiger, 1968;1–22.

54. Thomas JE, Lambert E. Ulnar nerve conduction velocity and H reflex in infants and children. J Appl Physiol 1960; 15:1–9.

55. Gamstorp I. Normal conduction velocity of ulnar, median and peroneal nerves in infancy, childhood and adolescence. Acta Paediatr Scand 1963; 146 (Suppl):68–76.

56. Wagner AL, Buchthal F. Motor and sensory conduction in infancy and childhood: A reappraisal. Dev Med Child Neurol 1972; 14:189–216.

57. Koenigsberger MR. Electrodiagnostic studies in infants and children. In: Kelley VC, ed. Practice of Pediatrics. Philadelphia: Harper and Row, 1981;1–7.

58. Parano E, Uncini A, DeVivo DC, et al. Electrophysiologic correlates of peripheral nervous system maturation in infancy and childhood. J Child Neurol 1993;8:336–338.

59. Rathke HW. Motor conduction in normal infants and children. Helv Paediatr Acta 1964; 24:390.

60. Koenigsberger MR, Curtin J, Lovelace RE. Motor nerve conduction velocities as a measure of gestational age in premature infants. A study of multiple births, twins, triplets and quadruplets. Neurology 1970; 20:381.

61. Dyck PJ, Lambert EH. Numbers and diameters of nerve fibers and compound nerve action potentials of sural nerves: Controls and hereditary neuromuscular disorders. Trans Am Neurol Assoc 1966; 91:214–217.

62. Chiu DTW, Lovelace RE, Yu LT, et al. Comparative electrophysiologic evaluation of nerve grafts and autogenous vein grafts as nerve conduits: An experimental study. J Reconstr Microsurg 1988; 4:304–310.

63. Lovelace RE. Experimental diabetic neuropathy: Pathophysiology and reversal. Muscle Nerve *Special Lambert Symposium* 1982; 5:S161–S162.

64. Lambert EH, Dyck PJ. Compound action potentials of sural nerve biopsies. Electroencephalogr Clin Neurophysiol 1968; 25:399–400.

65. Dyck PJ, Lambert EH. Dissociated sensation in amyloidosis: Compound action potential, quantitative, histologic and teased fiber and electron microscopic studies of sural nerve biopsies. Arch Neurol 1969; 20:480–507.

66. Dyck PJ, Lambert EH, Sanders K, et al. Severe hypomyelination and marked abnormality of conduction in Dejerine-Sottas hypertrophic neuropa-

thy: Myelin thickness in compound action potentials of sural nerve in vitro. Mayo Clin Proc 1971; 46:432–436.

67. Dyck PJ, Lambert EH, Nichols PC. Quantitative measurement of sensation related to compound action potentials and number and sizes of myelinated and unmyelinated fibers of sural nerve in health, Friedreich's ataxia, hereditary sensory neuropathy and tabes dorsalis. In: Cobb WA, ed. Handbook of Electroencephalography and Clinical Neurophysiology. Amsterdam: Elsevier, 1971; 9:83–118.

68. Roohi F, List T, Lovelace RE. Slow motor conduction in myotonic dystrophy. J Electromyogr Clin Neurophysiol 1981; 21:91–106.

69. Gilliatt RW. Recent advances in the pathophysiology of nerve conduction. In: Desmedt JE, ed. New Developments in Electromyography and Clinical Neurophysiology, vol 2. Basel: S Karger, 1973;2–18.

70. Parry GJG. Mononeuritis multiplex (AAEE case report). Muscle Nerve. 1985; 8:493–498.

71. Korthals JK, Korthals MA, Wisniewski HM. Progression of regenerations after nerve infarction. Brain Res 1991; 552:41–46.

72. Bonney G, Gilliatt RW. Sensory nerve conduction after traction lesions of the brachial plexus. Proc R Soc Med 1958; 51:365–367.

73. Lovelace RE. Mononeuritis multiplex in polyarteritis nodosa. Neurology 1964,14:434–442.

74. Oh SJ. Sarcoid polyneuropathy: A histologically proved case. Ann Neurol 1980,7:178.

75. Buchthal F. Sensory and motor conduction in polyneuropathies. In: Desmedt JE, ed. New Developments in Electromyography and Clinical Neurophysiology, vol 2. Basel: S Karger, 1973; 259–271.

76. Trojaborg W, Sindrup EH. Motor and sensory conduction in different segments of the radial nerve in normal subjects. J Neurol Neurosurg Psychiatry 1969; 32:354–359.

77. Buchthal F, Rosenfalck A. Trojaborg W. Electrophysiological findings in entrapment of the median nerve at wrist and elbow. J Neurol Neurosurg Psychiatry 1974; 37:340–360.

78. Trojaborg W. Motor and sensory nerve conduction along the musculocutaneous nerve. J Neurol Neurosurg Psychiatry 1976; 39:840–899.

79. Trojaborg W. Prolonged conduction block of axonal degeneration. J Neurol Neurosurg Psychiatry 1977; 40:50–57.

80. Trojaborg W. Electrophysiological findings in pressure palsy of the brachial plexus. J Neurol Neurosurg Psychiatry 1977; 40:1160–1167.

81. Gilliatt RW. Nerve conduction in human and experimental neuropathies. Proc R Soc Med 1966; 59:989–993.

82. Smith T, Trojaborg W. Clinical and electrophysiological recovery from peroneal palsy. Acta Neurol Scand 1986; 74:328–335.

83. Lange DJ, Blake DM, Hirano M, et al. Multifocal conduction block neuropathy: Diagnostic value of stimulating cervical roots. Neurology 1990; 40:182.

84. Lambert EH. Electromyography and electric stimulation. In: Clinical Examinations in Neurology, ed 4. Philadelphia: WB Saunders, 1976.

85. McDonald WI. The effects of experimental demyelination on conduction in peripheral nerve. A histological and physiological study. II Electrophysiological observations. Brain 1963; 86:501–524.

86. Trojaborg W, Lange DJ, Latov N, et al. Conduction block and other abnormalities in motor neuron disease: A review of 110 patients. Neurology 1990; 40:182.

87. Lange DJ, Trojaborg W, Latov N, et al. Multifocal motor neuropathy with conduction block: Is it a distinct entity? Neurology 1992; 42:497–505.

88. Buchthal F, Behse F. Polyneuropathy. Fact and fancies. In: Cobb WA, Van Duijn H, eds. Contemporary Clinical Neurophysiology EEG, suppl 34. Amsterdam: Elsevier, 1978;373–383.

89. Behse F. Buchthal F. Alcoholic neuropathy. Clinical electrophysiological and biopsy findings. Ann Neurol 1977; 2:95–110.

90. Kremer M. Clinical aspects of toxic neuropathies. In: Biochemical Aspects of Neurological Disorders. ser 2, Oxford: Blackwell, 1965;89–100.

91. Bouche P, Bousser MG, Peytour MA, et al. Perhexiline maleate and peripheral neuropathy. Neurology 1979; 29:739–745.

92. Lewis RA, Sumner AJ. The electrodiagnostic distinctions between chronic, familial and acquired demyelinative neuropathies. Neurology 1982; 32:592–596.

93. Shahani BT, Potts F, Domingue J. F response studies in peripheral neuropathies. Neurology 1980; 30:409.

94. Kaeser HE, Lambert EH. Nerve function studies in experimental polyneuritis. Electroencephalogr Clin Neurophysiol 1962; 22 (suppl):29–35.

95. Ochoa J, Fowler TJ, Gilliatt RW. Changes produced by a pneumatic tourniquet. In: Desmedt JE, ed. New Developments in Electromyography and Clincial Neurophysiology, vol 2. Basel: S Karger, 1973;174–180.

96. McLean IC. Nerve root stimulation to evaluate conduction across the lumbosacral plexus. Acta Neurol Scand 1979; 73 (suppl):270.

97. Mills KR, Murray NMF. Electric stimulation over the human vertebral column: Which neural elements are excited? Electroencephalogr Clin Neurophysiol 1986; 63:582–589.

98. Plasman BL, Gondevia SC. High voltage stimulation over the human spinal cord: Sources of latency variation. J Neurol Neurosurg Psychiatry 1989; 52:213–217.

99. Inouye Y, Buchthal F. Segmental sensory innervation determined by potentials recorded from cervical spinal nerves. Brain 1977;100:731–748.

100. Berardelli A. Electrical magnetic spinal and cortical stimulation in man. Curr Opin Neurol Neurosurg 1991; 4:770–776.

101. Hagbarth KE. Microneurography: In vivo exploration of impulse traffic in human peripheral nerves. In: Shahani BT, ed. Electromyography in CNS Disorders: Central EMG. Boston: Butterworths, 1984;19–28.

102. Vallbo AB, Hagbarth HE, Wallin BG. Somatosensory, proprioceptive and sympathetic activity in human peripheral nerves. Physiol Rev 1979; 59:919–957.

103. Ochoa J, Torebjork HE, Culp WJ, et al. Abnormal spontaneous activity in single sensory nerve fibers in humans. Muscle Nerve 1982; 5:S74–S77.

104. Burke D, Sundhof G, Wallin BG. Postural effects on muscle nerve sympathetic activity in man. J Physiol (Lond) 1977; 272:399–415.

105. Uncini A, Lange DJ, Lovelace RE. Anomalous intrinsic hand muscle innervation in median and ulnar nerve lesions: An electrophysiological study. Ital J Neurol Sci 1988; 9:497–503.

106. Lambert EH. The accessory deep peroneal nerve. Neurology 1969; 19:1169–1176.

107. Fisher MA. H reflexes and F waves: Physiology and clinical indications. Muscle Nerve 1992; 15:1223–1233.

108. Magladery JW, Porter WE, Park AM, et al. Electrophysiological studies of nerve and reflex activity in normal man. Bull Johns Hopkins Hosp 1951; 88:499–519.

109. Magladery JW, Teasdall RD, Park AM, et al. Electrophysiological studies of reflex activity in patients with lesions in the central nervous system. Bull Johns Hopkins Hosp 1952; 91:219–275.

110. Jabre JF. Surface recording of the H reflex of the flexor carpi radialis. Muscle Nerve 1981; 4:435–438.

111. Trontelj JV. A study of the H reflex by single-fiber EMG. J Neurol Neurosurg Psychiatry 1973; 36:951–959.

112. Braddom RI, Johnson EW. Standardization of the H reflex and diagnostic use in S1 radiculopathy. Arch Phys Med Rehabil 1974; 55:161–166.

113. Magladery JW, McDougal DB. Electrophysiological studies of nerve and reflex in normal man. 1. Identification of certain reflexes in the eletromyogram and the conduction velocity of the peripheal nerve fibers. Bull Johns Hopkins Hosp 1950; 86:265–290.

114. McLeod JG, Wray SH. An experimental study of F wave in the baboon. J Neurol Neurosurg Psychiatry 1966; 29:196–200.

115. Graham J. Studies on the F wave and the Guillain-Barré syndrome. Thesis, Cardiff University, Wales, 1970.

116. King D, Ashley F. Conduction velocity in the proximal segments of a motor nerve in the Guillain-Barré syndrome. J Neurol Neurosurg Psychiatry 1976; 39:538–544.

117. Kimura J, Butzer JF. F wave conduction velocity in the Guillain-Barré syndrome. Assessment of nerve segments between axilla and spinal cord. Arch Neurol 1975; 32:524–529.

118. Walsh JC, Yiannikas C, McLeod JG. Abnormalities of proximal conduction in acute idiopathic polyneuritis. Comparison of short latency evoked potentials and F waves. J Neurol Neurosurg Psychiatry 1984; 47:197–200.

119. Lovelace RE. Chronic inflammatory demyelinating polyneuropathy. Riv Pediatr Sicil 1991; 46:577–587.

120. Kimura J. F wave velocity in the central segment of the median ulnar serves. A study in normal subjects and patients with the Charcot-Marie-Tooth disease. Neurology 1974; 24:539–546.

121. Wulff CH, Gilliatt RW. F waves in patients with hand wasting caused by cervical rib and band. Muscle Nerve 1979; 2:452–457.

122. Panayiotopoulos CP. F chronodispersion: A new electrophysiological method. Muscle Nerve 1979; 2:68–72.

123. Struppler A. A control of isometric contractions in patients suffering from various lesions of the sensorimotor system. In: Shahani BT, ed. Electromyography in CNS Disorders: Central EMG. Boston: Butterworths, 1984;129–142.

124. Fullerton PM, Gilliatt RW. Axon reflexes in human motor nerves. J Neurol Neurosurg Psychiatry 1965; 28:1–14.

125. Marsden DC, Rothwell JC, Ray BL. The stretch reflex: Human spinal and long loop reflexes. In: Shahani BT, ed. Electromyography in CNS Disorders: Central EMG. Boston: Butterworths, 1984;45–75.

126. Uncini A, Pullman SL, Lovelace RE, et al. The sympathetic skin response: Normal values, elucidation of afferent components and application limits. J Neurol Sci 1988; 87:299–306.

127. Kimura J. The blink reflex as a test for brain stem and higher nervous (central) system function. In: Desmedt GE, ed. New Developments in Electromyography and Clinical Neurophysiology, vol 3. Basel: S Karger, 1973;681–691.

128. Soliven B, Meer J, Uncini A, et al. Physiologic and anatomic basis for contralateral R1 in blink reflex. Muscle Nerve 1988; 11:848–851.

129. Kimura J. Clincal uses of the electrically elicited blink reflex. In: Desmedt JE, ed. Brain and Spinal Mechanisms of Movement Control on Man: New Developments in Clinical Applications. New York: Raven Press, 1982.

130. Nielsen VK. Electrophysiology of the facial nerve in hemifacial spasm: Ectopic/ephaptic excitation. Muscle Nerve 1985; 8:545–555.

131. Janetta, PJ, Abbasy M, Maroon NJ, et al. Etiology and definitive microsurgical treatment of hemifacial spasm. J Neurol Neurosurg 1977; 47:321–328.

132. Gombault A. Contribution of l'etude anatomique de le neurite parenchymateuse subaigue et chronique neurite segmentaire peri-axile. Arch Neurol Paris 1880; 1:11–38.

133. Rasminsky M, Sears TA. Internodal conduction in undissected demyelinated nerve fibers. J Physiol (Lond) 1972; 227:323–350.

134. Gilliatt RW. Electrophysiology of peripheral neuropathies—an overview. Muscle Nerve 1982; 5:S108–S116.

135. Donofrio PD, Albers JW. Polyneuropathy: Classification by nerve conduction studies and electromyography. Muscle Nerve 1990; 13:889–903.

136. Brust JCM, Lovelace RE, Devi A. Clinical and electrodiagnostic features of the Charcot-Marie-Tooth syndrome. Uncomplicated and complicated cases. Acta Neurol Scand 1978; 58 (Suppl 68):1–150.

137. Lovelace RE, Brust JCM, Devi S. Clinical and electrodiagnostic features of typical Charcot-Marie-Tooth disease. In: Serratrice G, Roux H, eds. Peroneal Atrophies and Related Disorders. New York: Masson, 1979;23–38.

138. Fullerton PM. Peripheral nerve conduction in metachromatic leukodystrophy (sulphatide lipidosis). J Neurol Neurosurg Psychiatry 1964; 27:100–105.

139. Lambert EH. Diagnostic value of electrical stimulation of motor nerves. Electroencephalogr Clin Neurophysiol 1962; 22 (Suppl):29–35.

140. Parry GJ, Clarke S. Multifocal acquired demyelinating neuropathy masquerading as motor neuron disease. Muscle Nerve 1988; 11:103–107.

141. Petajan JH, Daube JR. Effects of cooling the arm and hand (on neuromuscular function). J Appli Physiol 1965; 20:1271–1274.

142. Harding AE. Friedreich's ataxia: A clinical and genetic study of 90 families with an analysis of early diagnostic criteria and intrafamilial clusters of clinical features. Brain 1981; 104:589–620.

143. Szmidt-Salkowska E, Saines N, Lovelace RE. Relapsing neuropathy: A clinical neurophysiology study (abstr). Electroencephalogr Clin Neurophysiol 1983; 56:180.

144. McLeod JG. Electrophysiological studies in Guillain-Barré syndrome. Ann Neurol 1981; 9(Suppl):20–27.

145. McLeod JG, Prineas JW, Walsh JC. The relationship of conduction velocity to pathology in peripheral nerves: A study of the sural nerve in 90 patients. In: Desmidt JE, ed. New Developments in Electromyography and Clinical Neurophysiology. Basel: S Karger, 1973; 248–258.

146. Ouvrier RA, McLeod JG. Hereditary motor and sensory neuropathy: Type III. In: Lovelace RE, Shapiro HK, eds. Charcot-Marie-Tooth Disorders: Pathophysiology, Molecular Genetics and Therapy. New York: Wiley-Liss, 1990;27–48.

147. Brin MF, Pedley Ta, Lovelace RE, et al. Electrophysiological features of abetalipoproteinemia: Functional consequences of vitamin E deficiency. Neurology 1986; 36:669–673.

148. Pollock M, Nukada H, Frith RW, et al. Peripheral neuropathy in Tangier disease. Brain 1983; 106:911–928.

149. Vercruyssen A, Martin JJ, Marcellis R. Neurophysiological studies in adrenomyeloneuropathy: A report on five cases. J Neurol Sci 1982; 56:327–336.

150. Brust JCM, Lovelace, Devi S. Clinical electrodiagnostic features of Charcot-Marie-Tooth disease plus additional neurological featues. In: Serratrice G, Roux H, eds. Peroneal Atrophies and Related Disorders. New York: Masson, 1979;39–47.

151. Preswick G. The peripheral neuropathy of Friedreich's ataxia. Presented at the 2nd International Congress of Electromyography, Glasgow, Scotland, 1967.

152. McLeod JG. An electrophysiological and pathological study of the peripheral nerves in Friedreich's ataxia. J Neurol Sci 1971; 12:333.

153. Gilliatt RW. Wasting of the hand associated with a cervical rib or band. J Neurol Neurosurg Psychiatry 1970; 32:615–624.

154. Lovelace RE. Brachial and lumbar plexopathies. Cur Opin Orthop 1991; 2:246–251.

155. Preswick G. The effect of stimulation intensity in the carpal tunnel syndrome. J Neurol Neurosurg Psychiatry 1963; 26:398–401.

156. Fullerton PM. The effect of ischemia on nerve conduction in the carpal tunnel syndrome. J Neurol Neurosurg Psychiatry 1963; 26:385–397.

157. Mulder DW, Lambert EH, Bastron JA, et al. The

neuropathies associated with diabetes mellitus: A clinical and electromyographic study of 103 unselected diabetic patients. Neurology (Minneap) 1961; 11:275–284.

158. Feldman RE. Peripheral neuropathy in arsenic smelter workers. Neurology 1979; 29:939–944.

159. Penn AS. Myasthenia gravis. In: Rosenberg RN, ed. Comprehensive Neurology. New York: Raven Press, 1991;623–638.

160. Albuquerque EX, Rash JE, Mayer RF, et al. An electrophysiological and morphological study of the neuromuscular junction in patients with myasthenia gravis. Exp Neurol 1976; 51:536–563.

161. Newsom-Davis J. Myasthenia gravis and myasthenic syndromes: Autoimmune disease of the neuromuscular junction. Curr Opin Neurol Neurosurg 1991; 4:683–688.

162. Fatt P. Skeletal neuromuscular transmission. In: Handbook of Physiology, vol 1. Washington, DC: American Physiological Society, 1959; 199–213.

163. Engel AG. Myasthenia gravis and myasthenic syndromes. Ann Neurol 1981; 16:519–534.

164. Fatt P, Katz B. Spontaneous subthreshold activity at motor nerve endings. J Physiol 1952; 117:109–128.

165. Barnett RJ. Ultrastructural histochemistry of normal neuromuscular junction. Ann NY Acad Sci 1966; 135:27–34.

166. Barnes JM, Duff JI. The role of cholinesterase at the neuromuscular junction. Br J Pharmacol 1953; 8:334–339.

167. Hubbard JL. Mechanism of transmitter release from the nerve terminal. Ann NY Acad Sci 1971; 183:131–146.

168. Nastuk WL. Fundamental aspects of neuromuscular transmission. Ann NY Acad Sci 1966; 135:110–135.

169. Liley AW. The effects of presynaptic polarization on the spontaneous activity of the mammalian neuromuscular junction. J Physiol 1956; 134:427–443.

170. Otsuka M, Endo M, Nonomura Y. Presynaptic nature of neuromuscular depression. Jpn J Physiol 1962; 12:573–584.

171. Hubbard J. Repetitive stimulation at the mammalian neuromuscular junction and emobilization of transmitter. J Physiol 1963; 169:641–652.

172. Jolly F. Uber Myasthenia gravis pseudoparalytica. Klin Wschr 1895; 33:4.

173. Payan J. The blanket principle: A technical note. Muscle Nerve 1978; 1:423–426.

174. Lovelace RE, Zablow L, Hoefer PFA. Single fiber stimulation in intact human muscle. Bull Am Assoc Electromyogr Electrodiagn 1965; 12:12.

175. Ekstedt J, Nilsson G, Stalberg E. Calculation of the electromyographic jitter. J Neurol Neurosurg Psychiatry 1974; 37:526–539.

176. Ekstedt J, Stalberg E. Single fiber electromyography for the study of the microphysiology of the human muscle. In: Desmedt JE, ed. New Developments in Electromyography and Clinical Neurophysiology. Basel: S Karger, 1973;84–112.

177. Stalberg E, Ekstedt J. Single fiber EMG and microphysiology of the motor unit in normal and diseased muscle. In: Desmedt JE, ed. New Developments in Electromyography and Clinical Neurophysiology. Basel: S Karger, 1973;113–129.

178. Stalbert E, Ekstedt J, Broman A. Neuromuscular transmission in myasthenia gravis studied with single fiber electromyography. J Neurol Neurosurg Psychiatry 1974; 37:540–547.

179. Schwartz MS, Stalberg E. Myasthenic syndrome studied with single fiber electromyography. Arch Neurol 1975; 32:815–817.

180. Sanders DB, Howard JF. Single fiber electromyography in myasthenia gravis. Muscle Nerve 1986; 9:809–819.

181. Stalberg E, Trontelj JV. Single Fiber Electromyography. Old Woking, IK: Miravalle Press, 1979; 1–244.

182. Elmquist D, Hofman WW, Kugelberg J et al. An electrophysiological investigation of neuromuscular transmission in myasthenia gravis. J Physiol (Lond) 1964; 174:417–434.

183. Thesleff S. Acetylcholine utilization in myasthenia gravis. Ann NY Acad Sci 1966,135:195–206.

184. Weiderholt WL. End plate noise. Neurology 1970; 20:214–224.

185. Lovelace RE, Stone R, Zablow L. A new test for myasthenia gravis: Recording a miniature endplate potential in situ. Neurology 1970; 20:385.

186. Elmquist D. Neuromuscular transmission defects. In: Desmedt JE, ed. New Developments in Electromyography and Clinical Neurophysiology. Basel: S Karger, 1973; 1:229–240.

187. Lambert EH, Elmquist D. Quantal component of the end-plate potentials in the myasthenic syndrome. Amer NY Acad Sci 1971; 183:183–199.

188. Engle AG, Lambert EH, et al. Recently recognized congenital myasthenia syndromes. Ann NY Acad Sci 1981; 377:614–637.

189. Engel AG, Lambert EH, et al. A new myasthenic syndrome with end-plate acetylcholinesterase deficiency, small nerve terminals and reduced acetylcholine release. Ann Neurol 1977; 1:315–330.

190. Newsom-Davis J. Myasthenia gravis and myasthenic syndromes: Autoimmune disease at the neuromuscular junction. Curr Opin Neurol Neurosurg 1991; 4:683–688.

191. Harvey AM, Masland RL. A method for the study of neuromuscular transmission in human subjects. Bull Johns Hopkins Hosp 1941; 44:161–166.

192. Lambert EH. Neurophysiological techniques use-

ful in the study of neuromuscular disorders. Res Publ Assoc Nerve Ment Dis 1960; 38:247–273.

193. Ozdemir C, Young RR. Electrical testing in myasthenia gravis. Am NY Acad Sci 1971; 183:287–302.

194. Desmedt JE. Observatia sur la reaction myotonique en stimulo-detection. Rev Neurol 1964; 110:324–336.

195. Kelly JJ, Daube JR, Lennon VA, et al. The laboratory diagnosis of mild myasthenia gravis. Ann Neurol 1982; 12:238–242.

196. Desmedt JE, Borenstein S. Double-step nerve stimulation for myasthenic block; sensitization of postactivation exhaustion by ischemia. Ann Neurol 1977; 1:55–64.

197. Desmedt JE. The neuromuscular disorder in myasthenia gravis. In: Desmedt JE, ed. New Developments in Electromyography and Clinical Neurophysiology, Basel: S Karger, 1973;241–302, 305–342.

198. Sanders DB. Electrophysiological study of disorders of neuromuscular transmission. In: Aminoff M, ed. Electrodiagnosis in Clinical Neurology, ed 2. Edinburgh: Churchill Livingstone, 1986;307–332.

199. Oh SJ, Eslami N, Nishirera T, et al. Electrophysiological and clinical correlations in myasthenia gravis. Ann Neurol 1982; 12:348–354.

200. Lambert EH, et al. Myasthenic syndrome associated with bronchial neoplasia. In: Viets HR, ed. Myasthenia Gravis, 2nd International Symposium. Springfield, Ill: Charles C Thomas, 1961;352–410.

201. Fetell MR, Shin HS, Penn AS, et al. Combined Eaton-Lambert syndrome and myasthenia gravis. Neurology 1978; 28:398.

202. Gieron, MA, Korthals JK, Lewis J. Lambert-Eaton syndrome in association with hypothyroidism and featuers of myasthenia gravis. J Florida Med Assoc 1987; 74:336–338.

203. Newsome-Davis J, Leys K. Vincent A, et al. Immunological evidence for the co-existence of the Lambert-Eaton syndrome and myasthenia gravis in two patients. J Neurol Neurosurg Psychiatry 1991; 54:442–453.

204. Patten MB, Hart A, Lovelace RE. Multiple sclerosis associated with defects in neuromuscular transmission. J Neurol Neurosurg Psychiatry 1972; 35:385–396.

205. Elmquist D, Lambert EH. Detailed analysis of neuromuscular transmission in a patient with the myasthenic syndrome sometimes associated with bronchogenic cancer. Mayo Clin Proc 1968; 43:89–113.

206. Rowland LP, Aranow HJ, Hoefer PFA. Observations on the curare tests in the diagnosis of myasthenia gravis. In: Viets HR, ed. Myasthenia gravis. Springfield, Ill: Charles C Thomas, 1961;411–434.

207. Foldes FF, et al. A new curare test for the diagnosis of myasthenia gravis. JAMA 1968; 203:649–653.

208. Horowitz SH, Jenkins G, Kornfeld P, et al. Electrophysiological diagnosis of myasthenia gravis in the regional curare test. Neurology 1976; 26:410–417.

209. Cherington M. Botulism: Electrophysiological and therapeutic observations. In: Desmedt JE, ed. New Developments in Electromyography and Clinical Neurophysiology. Basel: S Karger, 1973;375–379.

210. Gutmann L, Pratt L. Pathophysiological aspects of human botulism. Arch Neurol 1976; 33:175–179.

211. Stanley EF, Drachman DB. Botulinum toxin blocks quantal but not non-quantal release of ACH at the neuromuscular junctions. Brain Res 1983; 261:172–175.

212. Besser R, Vogt T, Gutmann L, et al. Impaired neuromuscular transmission during partial inhibition of acetylcholinesterase: The role of stimulus-induced backfiring in the generation of the decrement-increment phenomenon. Muscle Nerve 1992; 15:1072–1080.

213. Koenigsberger MR, Patten B, Lovelace RE. Studies of neuromuscular function in the new born: 1. Comparison of myoneural function in the full term in the premature infant. Neuropediatrie 1973; 4:350–361.

214. Brin MF, Blitzer A, Fahn S, et al. Adductor laryngeal dystonia (spastic dysphonia): Treatment with local injections of botulinum toxin (BOTOX). Movement Dis 1989; 4:287–296.

214. Lovelace RE, Blitzer A, Ludlow CL. Clinical laryngeal electromyography. In: Blitzer A, Brin MF, Sesaki CT, et al., eds. Neurological Disorders of the Larynx. New York: Thieme, 1991; 66–81.

# Chapter 11

# The Motor Unit and Muscle Action Potentials

STANLEY J. MYERS
ROBERT E. LOVELACE

In the broadest sense, electromyography (EMG) is electrophysiologic recording and study of nerve conduction and of the electrical activity of muscle. It can be more narrowly defined as recording and study of insertional, spontaneous, and voluntary electric activity of muscle.[1] Contemporary practice favors the latter definition; today, the broader description falls under the general heading of *clinical neurophysiology.*

EMG plays a significant role in diagnosis and prognosis and in physiologic and kinesiologic research. Redi postulated in 1666 that electricity was generated from muscle, a fact not demonstrated until 1838, by Matteucci, using an improved galvanometer. DuBois-Reymond confirmed this work and, in 1851, performed the first human EMG study, using jars of liquid as electrodes and recording action currents in a subject's contracting arm. The development of more sophisticated apparatus, especially Einthoven's string galvanometer, made possible further investigations of muscle action potentials and allowed correlation of laboratory findings with normal human muscle potentials. The first extensive clinical EMG study was done in Germany by Piper, who published the first book on electromyography in 1912. In 1929, Adrian and Bronk introduced the coaxial (concentric) needle electrode, which made it possible to record potentials from a single muscle fiber. They also amplified the muscle action potentials through a loudspeaker, as an additional aid in interpreting results. The introduction of the cathode ray oscilloscope (CRO) by Erlanger and Gasser (1937) freed workers from the limitations of mechanical galvanometers. Later developments in instrumentation, including the use of analog-digital converters, computers and expanded memory, extended the use of existing recording devices and permitted the development of even more sophisticated systems for data recording, storage, and analysis.

In this chapter we will review current understanding of the physiology of the motor unit and how it is affected by internal and external changes resulting from what might be called *normal conditions* such as aging and temperature, as well as by disease processes.

## Motor Unit

### Definition

The motor unit was defined as the anatomic unit of muscle function by Liddell and Sherrington in 1925. A motor unit consists of a single anterior horn cell (motor neuron), its axon cylinder (including the terminal and subterminal branching within the muscle body), the motor end-plates (neuromuscular junction), and all the muscle fibers innervated by that neuron (Figure 11-1).

### Anatomic and Physiologic Makeup

The motor axon branches many times to provide end-plates for its multiple muscle fibers. Most of

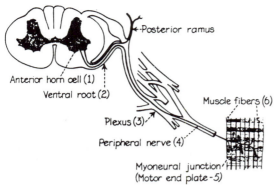

**Figure 11-1.** The motor unit. Terminal and subterminal branching of the nerve fiber occurs between points 4 and 5. (From Rodriquez, Oester. Fundamentals of electromyography. In: Licht S, ed. Electrodiagnosis and Electromyography. New Haven, E. Licht, 1971;321.)

the divisions occur within the terminal intramuscular nerve bundles at the points of branching of the nerve bundles proper at a node of Ranvier.[2] Normally, the divisions form two groups of fibers of approximately equal caliber containing 10 to 50 nerve fibers each, which, after emerging from the bundle as subterminal nerve fibers, run in isolation across the muscle fibers to terminate in the endplates. In humans, only 1.5% to 10% of nerve fibers branch after they leave as subterminal nerve fibers.

*Motor Unit Counting*

The number of muscle fibers in each motor unit can be estimated in humans by counting the total number of fibers in a muscle and dividing by the total number of motor nerve fibers.[3,4] The innervation ratio is the ratio of the total number of extrafusal muscle fibers to the number of motor axons supplying a specific muscle, which provides a measure of the average size of the motor unit. Muscles responsible for finer function tend to have a lower ratio than those for coarser movements. Some representative values of the number of muscle fibers per motor unit are these: opponens pollicis, 13; superior rectus, 23; platysma, 25; biceps brachii, 163; sartorius, 300; rectus femoris, 305; first dorsal interosseus, 340; gracilis, 527; anterior tibial, 610; gastrocnemius, 2037. These estimates assume that 60% of the nerve fibers in muscle are

motor fibers, as determined from measurements on the nerves to the anterior tibial and gastrocnemius muscles in cats. No correction is made for motor nerve fibers supplying intrafusal muscle fibers. Furthermore, it is unlikely that the proportion of motor nerve fibers is the same in functionally different muscles. Thus, the estimate of the number of muscle fibers per motor unit is imprecise and is likely to be on the low side. In 1971, McComas and coworkers[5] described a non-invasive method for counting the number of motor units in a muscle. By delivering small, graded electrical stimuli to the deep peroneal nerve, they were able to induce an incremental response in the evoked action potential of the extensor digitorum brevis, assuming that each increment of voltage was a result of the excitation of a single motor unit. By taking the average of approximately 10 motor units and using this to divide into the maximum compound potential amplitude evoked in a muscle by a supramaximal motor nerve stimulus, it was possible to obtain an estimate of the number of motor units in that muscle. This technique has a number of difficulties: lower threshold units are preferentially evaluated, the number of motor units sampled is relatively small, and it is not possible to distinguish between two or more motor units that have the same threshold. Over the years, this technique has been modified in a number of ways.[6,7] These methods are best applied to distal muscles. More recently, Brown and colleagues[8] presented a new method for estimating the number of motor units in human subjects. It can be used with proximal muscles, and it eliminates the error from overlap between thresholds of different motor units. This method combines isometric contraction, intramuscular needle electrode recordings, and spike-triggered averaging techniques to measure the sizes of motor unit potentials as recorded in the innervation zone with surface electrodes. The number of motor units is then estimated by dividing the maximum (M) potential evoked by supermaximal stimulation of the motor nerve recorded with the same surface electrodes by the mean of at least 10 surface-recorded motor unit potentials. This method obviates graded stimulation of motor nerves and can be applied to proximal muscle groups as well as distal ones. The authors used the method to study the biceps brachii, which showed a mean motor unit estimate of $911 \pm 254$ (ISD) for subjects younger than 60 years. This spike-triggered averaging-based technique has been further refined by using intramuscular potentials recorded with a macroelectrode. Slawnych and colleagues reviewed the techniques employed to estimate the number of motor units in a muscle.[9]

*Motor Unit Territory*

Individual muscle fibers extend throughout the length of most muscles and are arranged in parallel, except in the gracilis and sartorius, where they are arranged in series. Most researchers agree that there is intermingling and wide scattering of fibers from different motor units.

If single ventral root fibers innervating the rat anterior tibial muscle are isolated and stimulated repeatedly, the glycogen in the muscle fibers that respond to the stimulation of the single axon is exhausted. Immediately after stimulation, the whole muscle is excised and frozen. Cross-sections are cut and stained by periodic acid–Schiff (PAS) technique for glycogen, so that the muscle fibers of the stimulated motor unit can be identified. Such preparations show moderate variation in the total number of muscle fibers and motor unit territory and diffuse scattering of the muscle fibers throughout the territory of that motor unit.[10] The vast majority of fibers—approximately 70% of the motor unit—have no contact with other fibers of the same unit. A motor unit occasionally contains groups of muscle fibers, each group consisting usually of two fibers, and rarely more than three.

In humans, Buchthal and coworkers have developed indirect methods of analysis using a multilead electrode. They constructed different multielectrode setups of up to 14 leads, to study volume conduction of the spike of motor potentials, total muscle cross-section, and the territory of the motor unit.[11,12] The spatial spread of action potentials from a given motor unit so obtained indicates the territory occupied by the fibers of a motor unit. With two multielectrodes perpendicular to each other and transverse to the fiber direction and another situated at periphery of the motor unit field, it is found that the territory of a motor unit is roughly circular (ovoid in some muscles) with an average diameter of 5 mm (range, 2 to 22 mm).

Within the same muscle, the territory of different motor units varies by a factor of 4. The area of territory of a single motor unit may encompass fibers of as many as 30 motor units. For example, in the biceps brachii, with an average territory of 4 to 6 mm, theoretically there is space for the fibers of 10 overlapping motor units. In fact, as many as six different motor units were identified in the same lead, owing to different rates of discharge.[12] These findings agree with the histologic evidence of overlap between fibers of different motor units.

The concept of a subunit arrangement of fibers, with groups of up to 30 muscle fibers from the same unit being adjacent to each other, has been shown to be erroneous. Researchers thought that the clean, smooth spikes of motor unit potentials resulted from contraction of up to 30 perfectly synchronized, tightly packed fibers. This, however, can result from a single fiber.

The spatial distribution of muscle fibers within the territory of a motor unit was studied in the soleus and tibialis anterior of adult cats.[13] Results indicate that a motor unit is distributed over only a portion of the muscle cross-section and that this varies for different muscles and for different parts of an individual muscle, being 25% to 75% of the muscle cross-section for the soleus and 12% to 26% for the tibialis anterior. Although motor unit fibers were more localized in the tibialis anterior, the absolute areas of the territories were similar in the two muscles. The density of fibers appears to be relatively constant across units, with the size of the motor unit territory varying as a function of the number of motor unit fibers. This study indicates that the spatial distribution of fibers belonging to a motor unit is not randomly scattered or homogeneously dispersed. There is much variation in fiber densities in a single motor unit territory. The high-density areas usually were not located in the center of the territory. There appears to be some subgrouping (not subunits) of fibers within the motor unit territory, together with areas apparently void of motor unit fibers also within the territory. The closely associated motor unit fibers may be a consequence of the branching pattern of a motor axon. These clusters are separated by distances generally shorter than 500 μ and contain many more than 30 fibers. The distribution of fibers within each of the subgroups appears to be random, as determined by adjacency, nearest neighbor, and interfiber distance analysis.

*Multiple Innervation*

It is not known definitely whether multiple innervation of muscle fibers occurs. There is evidence that it may be present in cats, dogs, and frogs,[14–16] but there is no reliable evidence that it plays any significant role in humans. In the case of the animals mentioned above, the evidence was obtained mostly indirectly, from the measurement of tensions produced by stimulation of single motor nerve fibers and comparison with the tension produced by stimulation of two or more fibers together. Most muscle fibers do not seem to have more than two motor end-plates, and it has not been determined if these doubly innervated fibers receive their nerve from branches of the same neuron, from separate axons, or from nerve fibers supplied by different cord segments.

Double and multiple innervation has been reported in human gracilis and soleus muscles; the findings are based on histochemical staining of muscle fibers for motor end-plates. Other studies that used the muscles of stillborn infants do not support these conclusions.[3] In most muscles, motor end-plates are found in the middle of the muscle fibers. The gracilis and sartorius are exceptions: in the gracilis, two end-plate bands are noted; in the sartorius the end-plates are disseminated. In the sartorius, the end-plates correspond to the numerous short muscle bundles seen in serial longitudinal sections and are developed from a chain of myoblasts in series, each supplied with only one end-plate. In adult muscles, these longitudinal fiber chains fuse together and create the impression that one is dealing with multiple innervation and multiple end-plates in a single muscle fiber.

The location of the end-plates in the middle portion of the muscle belly affords the fastest activation of all its contractile material, and multiple nerve endings may increase the rate at which tension is developed by the muscle fiber. If nerve impulses reach terminations synchronously at several points along the muscle fiber, impulses are initiated and spread over the length of the muscle fiber in less time than if activity begins at one locus only.

The biceps brachii and opponens pollicis muscles of humans have been demonstrated to have 1.3 to 1.5 motor end-plates per muscle fiber,[3] and this, too, has been interpreted as indicating multiple innervation of some fibers. The end-plate zone in these muscles is centrally located, as in most other muscles. Therefore, if present, the two end-plates are only a short distance from each other, and multiple innervation can play only a limited role in reducing the activation time.

*Excitation and Depolarization*

In many ways, muscle fibers and nerve fibers resemble one another in the response of the surface membranes to excitatory stimuli. The physiology of the membrane potential is summarized here and is dealt with in more detail in other chapters.

The differences in potential between the inside and outside of single muscle cells have been measured by microelectrodes. The resulting potential difference between the interior of the muscle cell and the extracellular space is approximately 100 mV in mice and somewhat lower (60 to 80 mV) in humans.[17] The resting membrane has a high impedance (10 MΩ) and low permeability for most ions. The extracellular concentration of sodium ions is high and of potassium ions low; the opposite is the case inside the cells. Potassium ions are 32 to 50 times more permeative than sodium ions. However, the continuous flux of sodium ions across the membrane by virtue of a metabolic sodium pump in the cell membrane keeps the ion distribution constant. Because of the higher intracellular concentration, potassium ions diffuse through and accumulate at the outer surface of the membrane, to be held there by the negatively charged impermeable anions at the inner surface. This equilibrium is responsible for the positive polarization of the membrane; its magnitude can be predicted correctly from theoretical laws (Nernst's equation).

Initiation of the excitatory state occurs at the myoneural junction. Small disturbances are rapidly attenuated, but when a stimulus of critical current density is applied to a susceptible membrane area, a propagating electrical potential results. This ''action potential'' follows an all-or-none law: it travels the length of the muscle fiber with constant velocity and undiminished amplitude. The action potential is due to a specific increase in the permeability of the membrane to sodium ions (the reverse of the resting situation), as shown by the fact that (1) the absence of sodium in the surrounding fluid renders the muscle nonexcitable and (2) the action potential can be made smaller or larger by altering the extracellular sodium concentration.[18] At the height of excitation, there are more sodium ions (cations) entering than there are potassium ions leaving, so the membrane potential changes from the potassium equilibrium potential ($-100$ mV inside) through zero when the membrane is depolarized, to an overshoot, the sodium equilibrium potential ($+30$ mV). Repolarization occurs with the passive outward flux of potassium ions and the restoration of sodium ions by active pumping. The action potential of the muscle fiber differs from that of the nerve fiber, in that the repolarization curve for muscle fiber takes longer because of events in the submembrane tubular structure.

Qualitatively, muscle action potentials are similar to nerve action potentials, as is their mechanism of excitation. Along the membrane, conduction velocity for mammalian skeletal muscle is about 3 to 5 m per second. A refractory period (about 2 msec) allows for repolarization before the fiber can be reexcited. Because of shunting of most of the potential difference by nonactive tissue and surrounding fluids, the recorded action potential from muscles is only a fraction of the resting membrane potential. (This is so whether it is from a single fiber, a motor unit, or a group of fibers.) Because, as noted previously, most fibers in the muscle are arranged in parallel, the voltage from a muscle containing many thousands of fibers cannot be greater than the full, unshunted voltage of a single fiber. The muscle action potential initiates the resultant mechanical twitch response.

## Recording of Muscle Action Potentials

Muscle is a source of electrical activity and is surrounded by a low-resistance conducting medium (the interstitial fluid, blood, and other tissue) usually referred to as a *volume conductor*. This,

in turn, is surrounded by skin, the surface of which consists of a layer of horny, dead and dying cells that have a high electrical resistance. EMG is the recording of electrical changes in muscle by electrodes that are either in contact with the skin over the muscle area or inserted into the muscle.

### Surface Electrodes

Surface electrodes consist of paired metal (often silver or platinum) plates or pads placed on skin that has been cleaned and prepared with alcohol or lightly abraded to reduce impedance. The electrodes are usually round, but they can be square, rectangular, in strip form, or expandable (e.g., a ring electrode to fit around a digit). Electrode paste or another electrically conductive substance can be used to facilitate recording and minimize artifact. One electrode is usually placed over the motor end-plate area of the muscle to be studied and the other over the electrically inactive tendon or some distance away on the same muscle. A ground electrode must also be used. Though summated electrical potentials are recorded, rapid, low-amplitude potentials are attenuated and fine detail of individual motor units cannot be routinely obtained because of alterations in electrode position, varying degrees of skin and subcutaneous tissue thickness, and the large areas encompassed. Surface electrodes have been used to give a broad survey of action potentials from a whole group of fibers and can be of value in studying kinesiologic patterns such as time relationships and correlation with muscle tension. Clinical applications include muscle reeducation and biofeedback.

### Needle Electrodes

The two principal types of clinical recording needle electrodes—monopolar (unipolar) and concentric (coaxial)—are now available in disposable and reusable forms. Single-fiber needle electrodes and multilead electrodes are being used with increasing frequency, clinically and for research (Figure 11-2).

The concentric (coaxial) needle electrode, introduced by Adrian and Bronk in 1929 and still in use today, consists of a steel hypodermic injection–type needle with a centrally mounted insu-

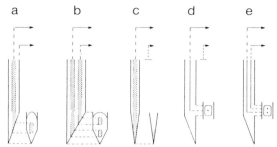

**Figure 11-2.** Schematic illustration of (*a*) concentric or coaxial, (*b*) bipolar, (*c*) monopolar, and (*d, e*) single-fiber needles. Dimensions vary, but the diameters of the outside cannulas shown resemble 26-gauge hypodermic needles (460 μ) for *a, d* and *e,* a 23-gauge needle (640 μ) for *b,* and a 28-gauge needle (360 μ) for *c.* The exposed tip areas measure 150 by 600 μ for *a,* 150 by 300 μ with spacing between wires of 200 μ center to center for *b,* 0.14 mm² for *c,* and 25 μ in diameter for *d* and *e.* A flat-skin electrode completes the circuit with unipolar electrodes shown in *c* and *d.* (From Kimura J. Electrodiagnosis in Diseases of Nerve and Muscle. Philadelphia, FA Davis, 1989;39.)

lated wire of stainless steel, silver, or platinum. The tip of the central exploring electrode is exposed flush with the bevel of the cannula. Voltage differences are measured between the center core, whose recording area usually ranges from 0.02 mm² to 0.07 mm², and the outer cannula, whose diameter ranges from 0.3 mm to 0.64 mm. The usual lengths of these needles are from 12 mm to 75 mm. As with other needle electrodes to be discussed, it should be noted that the recording area can vary, depending on the particular manufacturer, whether the needle is reusable or disposable, and on intentional (custom) variations in a particular needle type. The concentric needle selectively records potentials in the direction determined by the bevel, which is about a 15-degree angle (Figure 11-3).

The monopolar (unipolar) needle electrode was introduced by Jasper and Ballem in 1949. As used today, it consists of a thin wire, usually stainless steel, insulated with Teflon, except at its tip. The outer diameter is normally 0.35 to 0.46 mm, and the bare tip has a recording area of 0.15 to 0.30 mm². Voltage differences are recorded between the needle tip acting as the exploring electrode in the muscle and a more distant reference electrode, usually a metal plate on the skin surface.

The bipolar needle electrode, now less commonly used on a routine basis, may still have some application. This needle electrode consists of two insulated central cores, often of copper or platinum, cemented side by side in a grounded steel cannula. The tips of the electrodes are flush with the bevel of the cannula and can be parallel in the bevel or in tandem. This needle is also known as a *dual concentric needle.* The recording area of the core electrodes is usually between 0.015 and 0.03 mm²; the needle diameter ranges from 0.5 mm to 0.65 mm. As with the concentric needle electrode, the angle of the bevel determines the recording surface of the core as well as ease of muscle penetration.

### Recording Characteristics

Lundervold,[19] using a single needle that could be used for monopolar, concentric or bipolar recording observed that the amplitude of motor unit or fibrillation potentials as recorded by the monopolar lead, was only slightly larger than that with the concentric but usually considerably larger than that measured with the bipolar electrode. The duration of the negative spike of the action potential was shortest with bipolar and longest with monopolar leads and concentric needle recordings. The electrode records a mean value of the potential, which is spread over the sampling area.[20] The smaller the sampling area, the less the amplitude variation and the higher the amplitude. The amplitude of the potential is also a function of the distance between the recording surface of the electrode and the current source.

With monopolar electrodes the shape and duration of the motor unit action potential (MUAP) is determined by the fact that the muscle acts as a volume conductor, picking up more distant fibers and units, though there is a limit to the recording range and the absolute duration is still probably representative of a relatively small number of muscle fibers not too distant from the recording electrode. With bipolar electrodes the duration of the potential is considerably shorter because of the short distance between the recording cores. There is partial canceling of the initial and terminal portions of the potentials recorded by each of the inner cores. The advantage of bipolar needle electrodes is that, with maximal interference patterns, it may

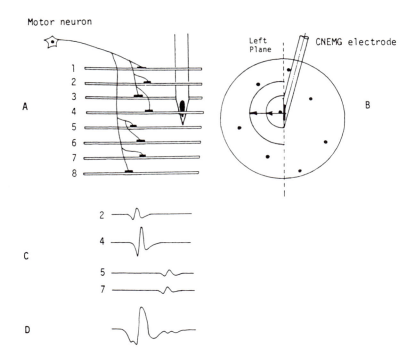

Motor neuron

**Figure 11-3.** Schematic of an MUAP recording with a concentric needle (CN) EMG electrode. (*A*) Longitudinal and (*B*) cross-sectional views of the MU with recording electrode are shown. Only the action potentials of fibers in the left plane (fibers 2, 4, 5, and 7) are recorded by the active electrode (*C*). The MUAP (*D*) is produced when the potential recorded by the cannula (not shown) is subtracted from the sum of action potentials in *C*. (From Nandedkar SD, Sanders DB, Stålberg EV, et al. Simulation of concentric needle EMG motor unit action potentials. Muscle Nerve 1988;11:152.)

be possible to analyze individual muscle action potentials. The recording range, however, is too limited for routine clinical EMG. The overall diameter of the bipolar electrode tends to be greater than in monopolar or concentric needle electrodes; this produces more discomfort and trauma for the patient.

Using an automatic method for decomposing complex EMG interference patterns into their constituent motor unit action potentials, Howard and coworkers[21] compared the configurational and firing properties of more than 7000 MUAPs recorded with either concentric or monopolar needle electrodes from the brachial biceps and anterior tibial muscles of 10 healthy young adults. In both muscles, mean MUAP amplitude, rise rate, and number of turns were significantly greater when recorded with monopolar needle electrodes at three tested levels of isometric contractile force. There was no significant difference between electrode types on measurement of mean MUAP duration or firing rate. Using both concentric and monopolar needle electrodes, Pease and Bowyer[22] examined the extensor digitorum communis muscle of 15 healthy volunteers. They found no significant difference in amplitude or duration of the MUAPs. Though they note that amplitude measurements

have been as much as twice as large when taken from monopolar needle electrodes as from concentric needle electrodes, they point out that the technique of manipulating the needle electrode may play a role. Rather than randomly inserting the needle electrode into the muscle, the EMG needle was manipulated so that a maximum peak-to-peak amplitude for the potential was obtained.

Nandedkar and Sanders[23] compared the recording characteristics of concentric needle (reusable) and monopolar needle (disposable) electrodes. They positioned the electrodes within the muscles so that a sharp MUAP was recorded. The MUAPs recorded by the monopolar needle electrode had higher amplitudes and larger areas and were more frequently complex than those seen with the concentric needle electrode. The MUAP's duration and area-amplitude ratio were similar for both electrode types. Each monopolar needle electrode was used once, and there was no wearing down of the Teflon coating. The monopolar needle electrode was thought to be more selective: the amplitude of a single muscle fiber action potential fell more rapidly as the distance from the muscle fiber increased than when recorded by the concentric needle electrode. Nandedkar and Sanders postulate that because the spike component of the

MUAP is produced predominantly by the muscle fibers close to the active recording surface of the electrode and because the monopolar needle electrode has a circular recording territory, it registers action potentials from more fibers than the concentric needle electrode, providing for greater MUAP amplitude and area (Figure 11-4). There is also less temporal coincidence, owing to the differences in the action potential propagation velocity and distances between the electrode and the muscle fiber end-plates resulting in complex MUAPs. Durations are similar, as there is a greater decline of action potentials with the monopolar electrodes, resulting in distant fibers falling out and not being recorded, counteracting the smaller semicircular recording territory obtained from the beveled concentric needle electrode. Because the monopolar needle electrode has a large recording surface, researchers might, theoretically, expect that the amplitude of the MUAP would be smaller than that recorded with the concentric needle electrode, where the muscle fiber surface would occupy a proportionately larger surface on the recording electrode. However, Nandedkar and Sanders reason that in a monopolar needle electrode, the current density is likely nonuniform, being greater near the electrode tip, and, therefore, the monopolar electrode behaves as though it had a much smaller recording surface than it actually does.

Thus, most studies do indicate that monopolar needle electrodes tend to record larger-amplitude MUAPs than concentric needle electrodes. No significant differences in duration are noted.

Factors to consider in recording characteristics include directionality of beveled needle tips; the wearing down and peeling of insulative coating on monopolar needle electrodes resulting in an enlarged tip area (lower MUAP amplitude); and the distance between the monopolar needle recording electrode and the indifferent recording electrode (reference electrode), which is usually placed over a tendon or other electrically inactive site to minimize interference from surface recording. Variation in electrode impedance, depending on the manufacturer and needle type, is another consideration, though most modern high-input impedance amplifiers can minimize the significance of

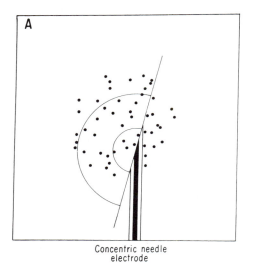

Concentric needle
electrode

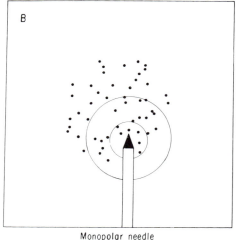

Monopolar needle
electrode

**Figure 11-4.** The distribution of muscle fibers in a motor unit. (*A*) The CN electrode has a semicircular recording territory but records action potentials from distant fibers. (*B*) The MN electrode does not record action potentials of distant muscle fibers but has a circular recording territory. The semicircular (*A*) and circular (*B*) boundaries enclose fibers that contribute to the spike component (small radius) and the duration of MUAPs (large radius). The larger boundary encloses similar numbers of muscle fibers for both electrodes; however, the smaller boundary contains more fibers for the MN electrode. (From Nandedkar SV, Sanders DB. Recording characteristics of monopolar EMG electrodes. Muscle Nerve 1991;14:111.)

this. The filter setting is also important. Filtering out low-frequency components results in shorter potential duration and enhanced reproducibility.

Recording and physical characteristics of disposable concentric needle EMG electrodes and reusable ones were compared.[24] Motor unit action potentials recorded by the reusable electrodes had greater amplitude and area values. The results obtained might be explained by the fact that it is more difficult to optimize the position of the disposable electrode so that the recording tip is positioned close to the muscle fiber of the motor unit under study. A strong correlation was found between the difference in MUAP amplitudes measured by the two electrode types and the difference in resistance of the needle tips measured in saline, but there was no difference between the duration of the MUAPs. In all, the research confirms that for routine clinical EMG studies, disposable electrodes are quite satisfactory.

### *Special Purpose Needle Electrodes*

The single fiber electrode is usually a variant of the concentric needle electrode, which has a very small area of recording surface (approximately $25\mu$ diameter) exposed several millimeters from the tip of the needle. This electrode has very limited pick-up area and is obviously directional, enabling single muscle fiber action potentials to be recorded when proper technique is used. Other variations of this electrode use several recording surfaces. When there is only one recording electrode surface on the single fiber EMG needle, the indifferent recording electrode is usually a skin surface one. The macro EMG electrode is a modified single fiber EMG electrode; it will be discussed later in the section on macro EMG.

Multilead electrodes can contain three or more insulated wires, usually with an exposed surface on the side of the cannula that is considerably larger (1 mm$^2$) than that seen in the multilead single fiber needle electrode. As many as 14 recording surfaces may be present. One of the wires is the indifferent electrode, and the cannula serves as the ground. Characteristics vary, depending on the distance between the recording electrodes. This type of electrode is used predominantly to measure motor unit territory.

Fine wire electrodes are most often used for kinesiologic recording. An electrode consisting of two fine, insulated wires, usually platinum and about 0.07 mm in diameter, is introduced into the muscle by an injection needle that is subsequently withdrawn.[25] These fine wires cause little discomfort, but their position can be altered only by withdrawing them through the insertion channel created by the needle.

## Muscle Action Potentials—EMG Findings

The electrode registers the average potential over its leading-off area, the recording surface of which is in direct contact with about eight muscle fibers, only one or two of which belong to the same motor unit. The sharp spike of the recorded potential is primarily the result of the excitation of a single muscle fiber.[26] This reflects the potential of the motor unit of which it is a part, but it is not the whole motor unit potential.

The amplitude of the action potential depends on several variables, particularly the distance between the recording electrode and the contracting muscle fibers. There is some correlation between the number of muscle fibers per unit and the amplitude of the potential, because summated spikes of contracting fibers near the electrode contribute to the spike component. Buchthal and coworkers[11] have demonstrated the relationship between the leading-off surface area of the electrode and the amplitude recorded. They estimated that eight muscle fibers can be in contact with the surface of a 0.1 by 0.4 mm concentric needle electrode, but at most three of the eight fibers belong to the same unit and contribute to the potential, which totals approximately 4.0 mV. With smaller-surface electrodes, such as a multilead electrode, the higher proportion of contracting fiber to surface area produces a larger potential (e.g., 10 mV). Also, muscles that have larger-diameter fibers produce potentials of greater amplitude.

The duration of a muscle action potential depends on, but is not proportional to, the mean size of the motor unit.[27] For example, eye muscles, which have small units, produce potentials with a duration of only 1.6 to 1.8 msec, whereas the potential of the platysma, with larger units (25 fibers), has an average duration of 4.9 msec. Potentials from the medial head of the gastrocnemius (1600 to 2000 fibers per unit) have a duration of 9.6 msec.

Nerve impulses have been demonstrated to arrive synchronously at all the end-plates of the motor unit under normal circumstances; transmission of the muscle action potentials from different fibers at varying distances from the recording electrode lead to a broadening of the resultant potential curve. Variation in synaptic delay also plays a role in modifying the duration of the action potential. For the human biceps brachii, there is little difference in conduction velocity for the individual muscle fibers of one motor unit (4 to 5.5 m per second at 36.5°C).[26] This constant velocity has been explained in part by the low external resistance of the extracellular fluid around the muscle fibers, which facilitates mutual interaction between fibers of different diameters.

The shape of the muscle action potential is influenced by factors similar to those that affect amplitude and duration (i.e., the number, distance, and distribution of fibers of the same unit in relation to the recording electrode). A slight temporal dispersion of the component spikes can cause potentials with several phases or humps. The muscle acts as a volume conductor, so the gradual onset and tail of the muscle action potential may be distorted by potentials picked up from more distant motor units.

Thus, it can be seen that the amplitude, duration, and shape of the recorded muscle action potential can vary with the size and type of the electrode and the actual positioning of the electrode within the muscle, amplitude being most dependent on proximity of the electrode to the firing muscle fibers. The rise time—the time lag from the initial baseline level or positive peak to the negative peak—provides a guideline to this distance. (By convention, in EMG recording the negative deflection is upward.) The needle electrode should be positioned so that the fastest rise time can be recorded, to obtain most consistent results. A unit accepted for quantitative measurement should have a shorter rise time than 500 μsec, preferably 100 to 200 μsec.[28]

With monopolar or concentric needle electrodes, bi- and triphasic potentials comprise about 80% of all potentials recorded in normal adult subjects (Figure 11-5); a phase is the portion of a wave between the departure from baseline and the

return to it.[29] In a complex or serrated action potential, the waveform shows several changes in direction, or turns, that do not cross the baseline.[1] These have a voltage range of 100 to 3000 μV and a duration from 2 to 10 msec. The duration of the sharp negative spike is approximately 2 msec. Action potential parameters vary from one muscle to another, as the innervation ratio is not the same. Mono- and polyphasic potentials are seen in 1% to 12% of all potentials recorded. Polyphasic potentials, by definition,[1] contain five or more phases and occur with increased frequency in neuropathic and myopathic disorders, though they comprise 1% to 3% of normal potentials (Figure 11-5).

### Spontaneous Activity

Spontaneous activity is recorded from a muscle at rest after insertional activity has subsided and in the absence of a voluntary contraction or external stimuli. The major types of spontaneous activity are fibrillation potentials, end-plate activity, positive sharp waves, fasciculation potentials and repetitive discharges, such as myokymic discharges, complex repetitive discharges, and variations of continuous muscle activity. These last few are not always spontaneous but can be a form of involuntary activity triggered by a stimulus such as needle insertion or voluntary muscle contraction.

### The Fibrillation Potential

Fibrillation potentials are muscle action potentials of short duration that result from firing of single muscle fibers, spontaneously or from mechanical irritation such as needle insertion. They are not visible at the skin surface but may be seen in an exposed muscle or on the tongue. Fibrillation potentials most characteristically have been noted with denervation. When a nerve to a muscle is sectioned there is a period of wallerian degeneration. Fibrillation potentials are usually observed in human denervated muscle after approximately 1 to 3 weeks. They are not exclusively indicative of lower motor neuron disease. Some 10% to 15% of apparently normal subjects have demonstrated a single region of fibrillation potentials.[30] These should not be confused with end-plate potentials

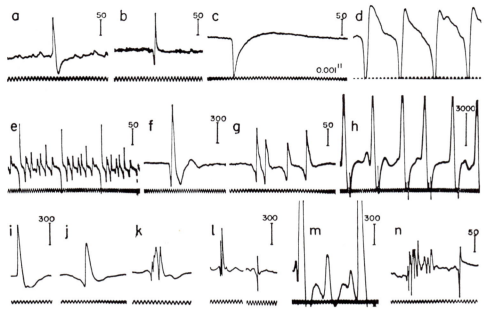

**Figure 11-5.** Muscle action potentials (MAPs) in electromyography. (*a*) end plate potential; (*b*) fibrillation potential, and (*c*) positive wave from denervated muscle; (*d*) myotonic discharge; (*e*) bizarre high frequency discharge; (*f*) fasciculation potential, single discharge; (*g*) fasciculation potential, repetitive or grouped discharge; (*h*) synchronized repetitive discharge in muscle cramp; (*i*) diphasic, (*j*) triphasic, and (*k*) polyphasic MAPs from normal muscle; (*l*) short-duration MAPs in progressive muscular dystrophy; (*m*) large potentials in anterior horn cell disease; (*n*) reinnervation "nascent" units. Calibration scales are in microvolts; time scales are in milliseconds. An upward deflection indicates a change of potential in the negative direction at the needle electrode. (From Mayo Clinic: Clinical Examinations in Neurology. Ed 3. Philadelphia, WB Saunders, 1971;276.)

(see below). According to Stöhr,[31] the rhythm of these normal or "benign" fibrillation potentials is almost always irregular. Fibrillation potentials are also noted in some 15% to 100% of primary myopathic diseases (if carefully sought) such as Duchenne's muscular dystrophy and polymyositis.[32]

Fibrillation potentials recorded with standard monopolar or concentric needle electrodes are most commonly diphasic discharges with an initial positive deflection (Figure 11-5). The usual amplitude is 50 to 150 μV, but potentials up to 3 mV have been recorded. Kraft recorded that the amplitude of fibrillation potentials was largest during the first several months following onset in patients with nerve injury, but a sharp drop in amplitude occurred during the first 6 months.[33] The amplitude decay then slowed considerably and was very gradual over the remaining years, but no fibrillation potentials larger than 100 μV were noted after the first year. Fibrillation potentials can persist as

long as 10 years following nerve injury, though it is unlikely that the fibrillating muscle fiber is the same. The usual duration of fibrillation potentials is 0.5 to 2.0 msec. Because of reinnervation or muscle fiber necrosis, with time the overall firing frequency of fibrillation potentials is reduced. Fibrillation potentials most commonly fire in a regular rhythmic pattern with a frequency of 1 to 30 impulses per second. Arrhythmic firing may indicate potentials from more than one muscle fiber, though arrhythmic firing from a single muscle fiber, in the range of 0.1 to 25Hz, may also be noted.[34] Studies employing intracellular microelectrode techniques on living white mice have shown that the resting potential remains near the normal level of 100 mV following denervation, until the muscle begins to fibrillate, at which time the potential falls rapidly, ultimately reaching 77 mV.[35] It is postulated that denervation causes absolute or relative alteration of the sodium pump mechanism, wherein the increased extrusion of sodium caused by the active fibrillatory process results in lowering of the membrane resting potential. Recordings from denervated muscles in vivo showed that spontaneous action potentials in denervated muscles were initiated by biphasic membrane oscillations of increasing amplitude. There is a correlation between membrane potential and the critical level for action potential generation; this relationship is most marked in denervated muscle at levels around the resting membrane potential (−60 to −79 mV).[36] Irregularly firing fibrillation potentials are thought to be triggered by spontaneous oscillations in the decreased resting membrane potential of the denervated muscle.[36] The irregularly discharging fibrillation potentials result from random discrete spontaneous depolarizations of nearly constant amplitude.[34] Hypoxia or cooling decreases the frequency of fibrillation potentials, and ischemia can abolish them. Neostigmine (cholinesterase inhibitors) increases the frequency, as does reduction in extracellular calcium concentration. Kraft,[37] in studies performed on guinea pigs, found that fibrillation potential amplitude is more closely related than any other physical measure of atrophic muscle fibers to the surface area or diameter of type I fibers. Other evidence from studies of rats suggests that fibrillation potentials may not originate in type I fibers.[38]

If the end-plate is excised from actively fibrillating muscle, the fibrillation continues in the strip bearing the end-plate but ceases in the other sections as soon they are cut off.[39] The membrane at the denervated end-plate zone seems to have properties that are different from the rest of the muscle fiber membrane. Cathodal currents applied to the denervated end-plate area increased fibrillatory frequency, whereas anodal currents decreased the frequency. Currents of a similar magnitude did not change fibrillation frequency when applied to other areas of the muscle fiber. In certain concentrations, acetylcholine and norepinephrine also increase the frequency of fibrillations when applied to the muscle at the denervated end-plate zone, and larger doses of acetylcholine depress fibrillation frequency. In spite of the fact that these two agents induce membrane potential changes (depolarization) wherever they are applied, fibrillation frequency is affected only when these agents act on the end-plate area. Thus, the denervated end-plate

region acts as a pacemaker site for fibrillation potentials and has chemical and electrical properties different from the rest of the denervated muscle fiber membrane.[40] In light of this information, further studies are necessary to reproduce these findings or to reevaluate the idea that in patients with myopathies fibrillation potentials can arise from fiber splitting (which may not occur unless there is also incomplete terminal reinnervation of these split-off fibers). Because fibrillation potentials are abolished after ischemia, a circulating substance appears to be involved. Administration of curare does not abolish fibrillation potentials, which suggests that acetylcholine hypersensitivity alone is not responsible. Sensitivity to circulating catecholamine may have a more important role than increased susceptibility to acetylcholine in the production of fibrillation potentials.

Muscle studies in premature infants (prior to innervation) and in patients with meningomyelocele (where complete innervation is prevented) showed fibrillation potentials.[41] Muscle fibers of a fetus apparently fibrillate until innervated. This preinnervation activity differs from denervation fibrillations only in its low amplitude (usually less than 15 μv) and slow frequency (fewer than 10 per second). Fibrillatory activity decreases as the time of normal gestation approaches and innervation is accomplished.

Fibrillation potentials and positive sharp waves may appear in muscles following needling for various procedures, but this is felt to be secondary to local trauma to the muscle membrane.

Spontaneous activity also can be seen within weeks of the onset of an upper motor neuron lesion such as hemiplegia. Though they are not always present, these spontaneous discharges can be noted even in the absence of associated lower motor neuron involvement. The mechanism for this has not been clearly defined; transsynaptic neuronal degeneration remains a possibility. (See the section on upper motor neuron lesions later in this chapter.)

### End-Plate Activity

Fibrillation potentials are to be distinguished from potentials recorded in the area of the neuromuscular junction (Figures 11-6 and 11-7).[42,43] These potentials are of two types. *Monophasic potentials*

## END-PLATE ACTIVITY

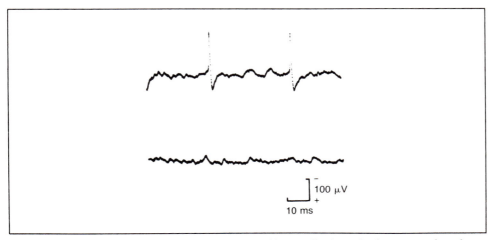

**Figure 11-6.** Spontaneous electrical activity recorded with a needle electrode close to muscle end-plates may be of two forms: (1) *Monophasic* (both traces): Low-amplitude (10- to 20-μV), short-duration (0.5 to 1 msec), monophasic (negative) potentials occur in a dense, steady pattern and are restricted to a localized area of the muscle. Because of the multitude of different potentials, the exact frequency, though it appears to be high, cannot be defined. These nonpropagated potentials are probably miniature end plate potentials recorded extracellularly. This form of end-plate activity has been referred to as *end-plate noise* or *seashell sound* (seashell noise or roar). (2) *Biphasic* (upper trace): Moderate-amplitude (100- to 300-μV), short-duration (2 to 4 msec), biphasic (negative-positive) spike potentials occur irregularly in short bursts with a high frequency (50 to 100 Hz) restricted to a localized area within the muscle. These propagated potentials are generated by muscle fibers excited by activity in nerve terminals. They have been called *biphasic spike potentials, end-plate spikes,* and, incorrectly, *nerve potentials*. (From AAEE Glossary of terms in clinical electromyography. Muscle Nerve 1987;10:G40.)

are spontaneous, localized, nonpropagated potentials of less than 100 μV (usually 10 to 20 μV), short duration (0.5 to 1 msec), and relatively high frequency (up to 1000 Hz). These are thought to be miniature end-plate potentials recorded extracellularly and have also been described as end-plate *noise* or *seashell sound*. These potentials are negative discharges. *Biphasic potentials* are spontaneous spikes of low amplitude (usually between 100 and 300 μV), usually diphasic with a sharp initial negative deflection, that fire irregularly with a frequency of approximately 50 to 100 Hz. These propagated potentials are thought to be due to firing of single muscle fibers in the end-plate area. They resemble fibrillation potentials, except that the initial deflection is negative rather than positive. These potentials have previously been mislabeled *nerve potentials*. If the needle recording electrode is somewhat distant from the end-plate, the initial deflection may be positive, giving the erroneous impression of a fibrillation potential.

*Positive Sharp Waves*

Positive sharp waves are spontaneous potentials often seen in association with fibrillation potentials (usually after denervation) that can appear days or weeks before the onset of fibrillation potentials. They may also be associated with myopathy. They are initiated by needle insertion but also fire spontaneously (Figure 11-7). The rhythm is usually regular; frequency ranges from 1 to 50 Hz. Positive sharp waves have an initial rapid positive (downward) deflection that is followed by an exponential negative charge that can continue into a prolonged low-voltage negative phase. The duration of the positive component is usually less than 5 msec and the amplitude up to 1 mV; the negative

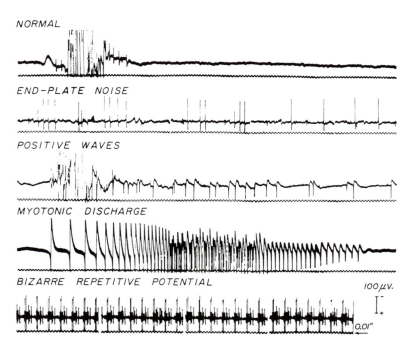

**Figure 11-7.** Insertion potentials evoked by insertion of a needle electrode into muscle. Normally, this consists of a brief discharge of electrical activity lasting little longer than the movement of the needle. (From Mayo Clinic. Clinical Examinations in Neurology, ed 3. Philadelphia, WB Saunders, 1971;279.)

phase can have a duration of 10 to 100 msec and lower amplitude (Figure 11-5). It is thought that positive sharp waves, like fibrillation potentials, arise from single muscle fibers and are due to the placement of the recording electrode adjacent to a blocked or damaged (depolarized) region of the muscle fiber (Figure 11-8).

*Fasciculation Potentials*

Fasciculations are involuntary muscle twitches that can often be seen on the surface of the skin or on the tongue. The electrically recorded fasciculation potentials result from spontaneous discharges of a whole or a portion of a motor unit. They are irregular in rhythm (firing frequency less than 5 Hz), form, voltage, and duration (see Figure 11-5). Fasciculation potentials are noted in many conditions, including benign myokymia, nerve root compression, ischemia, various forms of muscle cramps, and anterior horn cell disease. Though they are characteristically associated with the last condition, in themselves fasciculation potentials are not pathognomonic.

There is some controversy as to the site of origin of fasciculation potentials, but both distal

and more proximal sites are likely. Using a collision method, the origin of at least 80% of fasciculations in various lower motor neuron lesions was determined to be the distal extremity of the axon, regardless of the type of lesion, its duration, or the severity of the denervation.[44] Section of the motor nerve in cases of advanced disease of anterior horn cells (ALS) is followed by the same degree of fasciculation for several days before wallerian degeneration begins,[45] and spontaneous muscle fasciculations may not be affected by spinal anesthesia or peripheral nerve block. Neostigmine produces or increases fasciculations, even during spinal anesthesia. Curare abolishes spontaneous fasciculations and prevents induction of fasciculations by neostigmine in normal subjects. The impulse is presumed to start in the area of the end-plate and to spread antidromically to involve other axon branches, thus accounting for the frequently observed polyphasic nature and prolonged duration of the potentials.[46] Conradi and colleagues[47] studied fasciculation potentials in 10 patients with amyotrophic lateral sclerosis (ALS). EMG recordings of single MUAPs from the extensor digitorum brevis muscle on maximal voluntary effort and on supramaximal electrical stim-

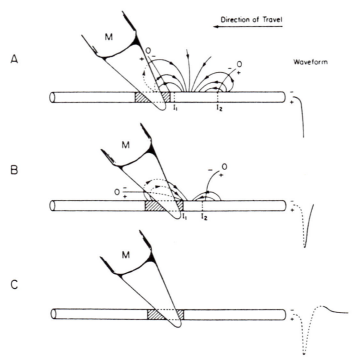

**Figure 11-8.** The generation of a positive sharp wave employing volume conduction theory. (*A*) A fibrillation potential approaches a monopolar electrode (M) placed next to a denervated muscle fiber. A positive source current is initially detected and the cathode ray tube records a positive deflection. (*B*) As the negative sink approaches the region of the membrane deformed by the needle electrode (hashed region), it cannot invade this portion of the membrane. As sodium inactivation and potassium efflux continue, the spatial extent of the negative sink ($I_1$ and $I_2$) diminishes. The current distribution and density are subsequently altered. This may be reflected as a decreasing positive or slightly negative potential. If the nonconducting portion of the membrane extends beyond the immediate vicinity of the electrode, a negative phase may not be observed and only a monophasic positive potential is recorded. (*C*) With failure of conduction to or beyond the electrode and absence of the negative sink, the CRT trace returns to baseline. (From Dumitru D. Volume conduction: Theory and application. In: Dumitru D, ed. Physical Medicine and Rehabilitation: State of the Art Reviews, vol 3, no 4. Philadelphia: Hanley & Belfus, 1989; 678.)

ulation of the peroneal nerve were evaluated. In a series of fasciculations, the shapes of the EMG potentials varied, whereas in a series of voluntary twitch activations of electrical nerve stimulations, EMG potentials were, on the whole, constant. Fasciculations were followed by antidromic impulses in the test unit axon, as judged from collision tests, and they persisted after lidocaine blockade of the nerve to the muscle. These findings are compatible with distal multifocal triggering of fasciculations. Wettstein[48] used collision technique to determine the origin of fasciculations in motor units from patients with ALS and other diseases involving motor neurons. In this study, some 60% of subjects

had only fasciculations of proximal origin, approximately 10% only of distal origin, and the rest had mixed-origin fasciculations.

Fasciculation potentials may be caused by a central mechanism, as well as a peripheral one.[49] Giant, bizarre, spontaneous potentials are seen in ALS and related diseases, and, unlike other fasciculations, these may be eliminated by nerve block. The anatomic basis for these abnormal potentials may in part be intramuscular axon budding or collateral regeneration from normal to denervated elements. EMG studies of motor unit territory in patients with ALS indicate that the motor units are expanded beyond what can be accounted for by intramuscular sprouting. In some instances, several neural elements at the same spinal level interact to produce synchronous fasciculations in different muscles, which seem to originate from a spinal locus of hyperexcitability. Intraspinal axonal sprouting occurs in ALS patients; it is uncertain whether this sprouting is analogous to the intramuscular collateral regeneration of partially denervated muscle.

After nerve section, fasciculation potentials disappear with the development of wallerian degeneration. Immature terminal and collateral sprouts of motor neurons were found in biopsies from fasciculating muscle regions in patients with ALS.[27] These immature neuromuscular junctions may be more sensitive to humoral agents, and thus fasciculation twitches may be initiated by normal levels of neurohumoral transmitters (such as acetylcholine). Fine, beaded nerve fibers are seen in the intramuscular nerve bundles of patients with motor neuron diseases. These fibers are unmyelinated, and many do not have Schwann cell cover. It is possible that ephaptic transmission across these fibers could produce fasciculatory movements.

Idiopathic "benign" fasciculations and muscle cramps often occur in the calf muscles; they can be associated with salt depletion and often are facilitated by ischemia. The twitches are irregular and variably polyphasic; they can be stopped by voluntary activity. Their polyphasic form seems to indicate that they arise in the terminal branches of the lower motor neuron and have a changing focus of origin. Single or grouped fasciculation potentials can also be present in other normal muscles. The frequency of firing of potentials recorded from normal muscle may be greater (average interval 0.8 seconds, compared with 3.5 seconds in patients with motor neuron disease).[50]

The fasciculation potentials that occur after root compression are often of simple diphasic form and are usually associated with signs of denervation, such as positive sharp waves and fibrillation potentials.

## Myokymic Discharges

Motor unit action potentials may discharge repeatedly. This is visible on the surface of the skin as a quivering or undulating movement known as *myokymia* (Table 11-1). The firing units have a uniform appearance, and discharge may be brief, repetitive firing of single units for a short period (doublets, triplets, or "multiplets" up to a few seconds) at a uniform rate of 2 to 60 Hz, followed by 2 or 3 seconds of silence then repetition of the same sequence for a particular potential. Less commonly, the potential recurs continuously at a fairly uniform firing rate of 1 to 5 Hz.[1] Myokymia is more common in facial than in extremity muscles. Myokymic discharges can be present in patients with brain stem tumors, multiple sclerosis, Guillain-Barré syndrome, or radiation plexopathy. Myokymic discharges arise spontaneously at some portion of the motor axon where the axon membrane is hyperexcitable.[51] Hyperventilation (hypocalcemia) enhances the discharges where the hyperexcitable area of the nerve is extramedullary (peripherally), as in Guillain-Barré syndrome.[52]

## Complex Repetitive Discharges

These are repetitive discharges of serrated (complex) or polyphasic potentials, which are relatively uniform in appearance, firing at a regular rate, though the frequency of discharge for each particular burst can vary from 5 to 100 Hz (see Figure 11-8). Amplitude ranges from 400 μV to 1 mV. The discharges characteristically start and stop relatively abruptly. They can begin spontaneously or be induced by needle insertion. These discharges have also been called *bizarre high-frequency potentials* or *pseudomyotonia*, but use of these terms is not encouraged. A single fiber in the complex apparently acts as a pacemaker, which then stimulates other fibers ephaptically, continuing the cycle until blocking occurs.[53] These discharges are seen in a number of disorders, including Duchenne's muscular dystrophy, polymyositis, radiculopathies, motor neuron disease, and chronic polyneuropathy.

## Neuromyotonic Discharges

Neuromyotonic discharges are bursts of motor unit action potentials originating in the motor axons and firing at high rates (150 to 300 Hz) for a few seconds. They often start and stop abruptly. The amplitude of the response typically wanes. Discharges can occur spontaneously or be initiated by needle insertion, voluntary effort, or ischemia.[1]

**Table 11-1.** Electromyographic Characteristics of Repetitive Discharges

| | Induction | Rate of Discharge (Hz) | MUAP Forms | Run |
|---|---|---|---|---|
| Myokymia | Spontaneous | a. 2–60<br>b. 1–5 | Uniform appearance | a. Up to several sec followed by 2–3 sec silence<br>b. Continuous |
| Complex repetitive discharges | Spontaneous or insertional | 5–100 | Complex and/or polyphasic | Regular rate for each burst |
| Neuromyotonic discharges | Spontaneous, insertional, or voluntary contraction | 150–300 | MUAPs | Few seconds, often starts and stops abruptly; amplitude usually wanes |
| Cramp discharges | Spontaneous muscle contraction | Usually high-frequency, up to 150 | MUAPs | Discharge frequency and number of MUAPs increase gradually and then subside gradually |
| Myotonic discharges | Spontaneous, insertional, or voluntary contraction | 20–80 | a. Bursts of positive waves 5 to 20 msecs<br>b. Biphasic positive-negative spike potentials usually less than 5 msec | Amplitude and frequency of potentials increase or decrease in a waxing and waning and can last several seconds |

Clinically, continuous muscle fiber activity is manifested as muscle rippling and stiffness.

### Cramp Discharges

A cramp discharge consists of involuntary repetitive firing of motor unit action potentials of high-frequency (up to 150 Hz) in a large area of muscles, usually associated with painful muscle contraction. Both discharge frequency and the number of motor unit action potentials that are firing increase gradually during development, and both subside gradually with cessation.[1]

Myokymic discharges, complex repetitive discharges, neuromyotonic discharges, and cramp discharges are differentiated one from the other by frequency and firing pattern rather than by appearance of individual potentials, which are often similar.

### Insertional Activity

When the needle is inserted briskly into the muscle, a burst of potentials can be recorded. These potentials are thought to arise from single muscle fibers whose membranes have been injured mechanically by the needle. Obviously, even under normal circumstances, the duration of this insertional activity depends on the speed and duration of the insertion itself. This measurement, therefore, is only semiquantitative. Examiners should attempt to standardize their insertion movements, making them relatively brisk. Under most circumstances, the duration of the burst of normal insertional activity is 50 to 100 msec. In the presence of reduced muscle bulk, as with fibrosis or necrosis, insertional activity is reduced. An increase in insertional activity can be seen when the muscle cell membranes are hyperirritable, as in acute denervation, inflammatory diseases of muscle, and myotonia. The potentials observed after cessation of the needle movement are even more significant from a clinical point of view, as needle insertion can provoke more prolonged runs of fibrillation potentials, positive sharp waves, complex repetitive discharges, and myotonic discharges. Normally, insertional activity lasts only a few milliseconds after needle movement ceases. Since recorded insertional activity is thought to be due to induced injury to the muscle membrane, several positive waves may be recorded, even in normal subjects immediately after needle insertion. Thus, this alone should not be attributed to a clinically pathologic condition. Increased insertional activity, manifested as brief runs of positive sharp waves or more rarely fibrillation potentials, may appear early in denervation, before the regular spontaneous activity.

*Myotonic Discharges*

Myotonic discharges occur spontaneously but can also be produced by needle insertion, voluntary muscle contraction, nerve stimulation, or mechanical stimulation such as muscle percussion. The discharges occur at a rate of approximately 20 to 80 Hz, and characteristically the amplitude and frequency of the potentials wax and wane. (see Figure 11-8). The characteristic audio manifestation is a "dive bomber" sound. The myotonic discharges recorded are of two types. (The total duration of the run can be as long as several seconds for both types.) One type consists of bursts of positive waves of 5 to 20 msecs' duration; the other is biphasic positive-negative spike potentials in which the negative component may predominate, though these potentials can resemble fibrillation potentials and last less than 5 msecs. The exact form of the potential recorded is thought to be related to the position of the recording electrode surface relative to the firing muscle fibers.

Myotonic discharges persist after procaine block of the nerve or after curarization, which suggests they originate in muscle. During intracellular recording of human myotonic muscle, Norris[54] found spontaneous slow depolarization of the muscle membrane leading to repetitive spikes or an abortive spike followed by further slow depolarization.

Though myotonic discharges are due to abnormalities of the muscle fiber membrane, apparently different mechanisms are involved, depending on the underlying disorder (see page 278). There is also a relation between myotonic discharges and increased serum potassium level.

*Myoclonus*

Myoclonus is one of the involuntary movements characterized by sudden, jerky, irregular contractions of a muscle or group of muscles not associated with loss of consciousness. There are various causes for this condition, as there are sites of involvement, rhythmicity, and provoking factors. It is thought that most myoclonic disorders are due to central nervous system (in particular cortical) involvement. Further discussion, therefore, is not warranted in the context of this section.

**Interference Patterns and Recruitment**

Needle EMG examination of a normal skeletal muscle at rest reveals an isoelectric baseline (i.e., electrical silence). Recruitment is successive activation of the same and additional motor units with increasing strength of voluntary muscle contraction. With minimal voluntary contraction one or several motor units are activated, usually low-amplitude ones (500 µV). As tension increases, the firing frequency of the individual potential increases. If the amplitude increases at the same time, it is assumed that the number of muscle fibers activated in the motor unit has increased, presumably because all the end-plates of a unit are not in an identical state of physicochemical readiness. Other evidence comes from studies with protected microelectrodes of the human rectus femoris and gastrocnemius muscles in which it was noted that motor unit potentials tended to increase in amplitude with heightened tension during isometric contraction.[55] This increase is attributed to an increase in the number of active muscle fibers involved in successive discharges of a single motor unit.

With increase in tension, additional motor units are recruited, some of higher amplitude. Buchthal and coworkers[20] found the amplitude of the second and third recruited units to be larger than that of the first and attributed this to decreasing distance between the recording electrode and the active unit as the strength of contraction increased. With further increases in tension, even more units are recruited, and temporal and spatial summation of potentials from multiple motor units produces a characteristic interference pattern, so that with monopolar and concentric needle electrodes, muscle action potentials from individual units no longer can be clearly distinguished.

There is an order of recruitment of motor units. At low strength of contraction, only a few motor units are active, and these have a slow rate of discharge and relatively low amplitude. These low-threshold, early-activated units produce relatively small forces used for fine motor control and postural adjustment, and the muscle fibers making up these units are of the S type (slow-fatigue, type I). Increasing tension increases the frequency of discharge by the active motor unit and recruitment of previously inactive units. The higher-threshold units have larger force contributions, and muscle fibers are of the FF (fast-fatigue) or FR (fatigue-resistant) types.[56] Motor neuron soma diameter, axon diameter, and conduction velocity are highly correlated.[56] The *size principle* holds that motor units are recruited in order of size, from small to large. This is most easily demonstrated for slowly developing muscle contraction.[57] In the presence of a normal, smooth, clinically sustained contraction of a muscle, motor units fire at a rate, and in relation to each other, so that fusion of muscle contraction results in a smooth, continuous, nonjerky contraction. In various states of tremor, fatigue, and denervation this relationship breaks down.[56] In the human biceps brachii, the slower-firing, low-threshold units tend to be located deep in the muscle, whereas the rapid-firing, higher-threshold units are more superficial.[58]

The recruitment interval is the interdischarge interval between two consecutive discharges of an MUAP at the point where a second motor unit potential is recruited with gradually increasing strength of voluntary muscle contraction (Figure 11-9). The recruitment frequency, or firing rate, is the firing rate of a motor unit action potential when a different MUAP first appears with gradually increasing strength of voluntary muscle contraction, and it is the reciprocal of the recruitment interval. These are quantitative measures and are most ac-

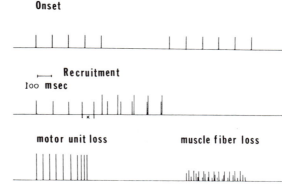

**Figure 11-9.** Essential features of motor unit recruitment are shown in the diagram. Onset level of firing is near threshold for activation, and lapses in firing may occur. Recruitment rate is the rate just before recruitment of a second motor unit during slowly increasing muscle force (innervation). Loss of motor units to disease results in the appearance of individual, easily distinguished single MUAPs firing at a high rate. Loss of muscle fibers results in recruitment of many different motor units at minimal effort. (From Petajan JH. Motor unit recruitment. Muscle Nerve 1991;14:494.)

curately evaluated when a fixed, low-level percentage of maximal voluntary contraction (MVC) of a particular muscle (25% to 30%) is maintained, rather than a fixed weight, which can represent a different MVC for different subjects. In neuropathic disease the recruitment interval is shortened because fewer motor units are available. The first unit is usually firing more rapidly at the moment when the second is recruited, shortening the recruitment interval and increasing the recruitment frequency. The converse takes place early in myopathic diseases, as the first unit is firing more slowly at the moment when the second unit is recruited because the first-recruited, slower-firing motor unit is not completely knocked out, and each motor unit has fewer functioning muscle fibers and is weaker.[59] Another useful value is the ratio of the average firing rate to the number of active units. In normal subjects it is less than 5:1 (e.g., three units firing fewer than 15 impulses per second). If two units are firing more than 20 impulses per second, the ratio exceeds 10:1, indicating loss of motor units.[60]

As noted, when individual motor unit potentials are analyzed during needle EMG examination in normal subjects, those potentials most readily isolated and clearly distinguished are the low-threshold, type I, low-frequency firing units. This is not necessarily the case in various disease states, e.g., in steroid myopathy with loss of type I fibers, the first-recruited fibers fire more frequently. Under normal circumstances, the principal mechanism for increasing force output is to add more motor units (i.e., spatial recruitment).[56] In different pathologic conditions, further recruitment may not be possible, so motor units fire at much greater than normal rates. This is also seen in very rapid force generation. It appears that recruitment has a more important role in grading of activity than does changing the frequency, except at very low and very high contraction strengths. Frequencies of firing of individual MUAPs above 50 per second are rarely observed. Under most conditions (25% to 75% MVC), the fastest units respond at frequencies between 25 and 35 Hz. Over the tension range of 5% to 60% MVC, the firing starts and stops abruptly and the frequency increases, but not in proportion to strength. For example, in one unit observed, the firing commenced at 20 Hz when the tension was 15% of maximum and increased with the tension rise, but only to 30 Hz.[61] Units that are active at tensions below 5% MVC usually have a lower starting frequency (5 to 7 Hz) and a greater frequency range and irregular discharge rates, even during constant contraction.

### Synchronization

In anterior horn cell diseases such as poliomyelitis, ALS, or syringomyelia, "synchronization" is demonstrated when action potentials are obtained simultaneously from two or more widely separated recording electrodes. The cause of this phenomenon is not clear. One speculation is that there is an intraspinal mechanism for synchronization of discharge rhythm in a number of different motor units supplied by the same spinal segment.[48] Another possibility is that in a given muscle single units of very large area (as noted with reinnervated muscle in anterior horn cell disorders) are responsible.

The occurrence of occasional true synchronization of motor units in a number of muscles in human subjects and animals has not received valid confirmation. An electronic model and statistical analysis of EMG records made under a variety of conditions seem to demonstrate the absence of true synchronization of motor neuron activity and voluntary contractions,[62] though grouping of discharges may be seen in the single action potential of the tendon jerk, and partial synchronization and grouping in clonus and various tremors.[63]

### Effect of Age

The normal mean duration of the muscle action potential increases with age, so that at age 70 to 80 years the average duration is as much as 75% longer than in children younger than 4 years.[20] This is explained as a decrease in the propagation velocity of the impulse over the muscle fiber. Peterson and Kugelberg[64] noted that in young persons normal values are obtained from the first-recruited low-threshold muscle action potentials, whereas aging may selectively destroy muscle fibers with the largest calibers and lowest thresholds.

Brown,[65] using the McComas method for counting number of motor units, studied median innervated thenar muscles and showed a drop in the number of motor units, especially in subjects older than 60 years. The mean motor unit count of subjects aged 70 years and older was less than half that of the subjects 39 years and younger. There was no evidence of denervation in the form of fibrillation potentials, nor any evidence for reduction in the size of individual motor units. It was postulated that the reduced motor unit count could be the result of asymptomatic injury to the median nerve, but distal latencies were essentially normal. Using a different method, combining isometric contraction, intramuscular needle electrode recordings, and spike-triggered averaging techniques to measure the sizes of motor unit potentials as recorded in the innervation zone with surface electrodes, the number of motor units in the biceps brachialis muscles of healthy subjects was estimated.[8] Here, too, estimates in subjects older than 60 years were half those of subjects in the third decade of life. None of the subjects reported symptoms or had physical findings suggestive of cervical radiculopathy, and EMG did not indicate denervation or reinnervation in the biceps or brachialis muscles. Slawnych and coworkers[9] reviewed a number of studies estimating the number of motor units in elderly subjects and in younger ones; these showed general agreement for reduced motor unit estimates in the extensor digitorum brevis of elderly subjects, though the extensor digitorum brevis and thenar muscles were more severely affected than the hypothenar muscles. Stalberg and Thiele[66] performed a single-fiber EMG study on the extensor digitorum communis muscle in subjects aged 10 to 89 years and noted that fiber density increases slowly throughout life and progresses faster after age 70 years. There was an indication that impairment of nerve or neuromuscular impulse transmission increases at the same time, suggesting that degenerative loss of motor neurons with aging was compensated for by reinnervation. Motor unit density in the tibialis anterior muscle decreased with age, as measured by macro EMG,[67,68] which could indicate loss of motor units with increasing age. Distal muscles show more extensive changes than proximal ones, and not all muscles are uniformly affected.

Few studies of humans have actually looked at age-related changes in motor neuron numbers in the spinal cord. In one such study[69] spinal cords of 47 subjects aged 13 to 95 years who died suddenly were examined. There was no evidence for loss of motor neurons up to age 60, but beyond that age, though individual counts varied considerably, there was evidence for a diminishing motor neuron population. After age 60 years, several cases showed counts only 50% those of younger subjects. Cell loss appeared to be uniform throughout all segments and was not accompanied by any other striking morphologic change. There was no history of preexisting weakness beyond what was "reasonable for age." (It is generally accepted, however, that clinical weakness usually is not noted until 40%–60% of muscle fibers have been lost.) Unfortunately, peripheral nerve and muscle were not examined. In another study[70] of the L-3 to L-5 spinal cord segments of 18 cases, progressive loss of large motor neurons was noted for all ages examined.

Although the total number of muscle fibers of the rat soleus muscle decreases with age, no difference was found in the number of alpha motor nerve fibers to the muscle.[71] It is possible that there is little or no loss of motor nerve cells in the spinal cord until aging is more advanced (after age 60 to 70 years in humans) and that peripheral loss

of muscle fibers is out of proportion to these findings. Evidence to substantiate this supposition is provided by the random degeneration of the endplates and some terminal end-plate regeneration. These factors may explain the longer duration of action potentials and the greater number of polyphasic potentials associated with aging in the absence of signs of acute denervation.

### Effect of Temperature

As the intramuscular temperature drops, the mean duration of the muscle action potential increases by 10% to 30% and the mean amplitude decreases by 2% to 5% for every 1°C reduction. The number of polyphasic potentials can increase as much as 10-fold with a 10°C fall in temperature.[20] This prolongation of duration is due to the temperature coefficient of the propagation velocity. The slower propagation velocity of the impulse over the muscle fiber and the terminal nerve fibers can cause temporal dispersion of fibers within the motor unit.

### Fatigue

Neuromuscluar fatigue can be defined as any reduction in the force-generating capacity of the total neuromuscular system, regardless of the force required in any given situation.[72] In the absence of fatigue, the sum of electrical activity, recorded by surface electrodes of a muscle, bears a simple linear relation to the force developed.[73] The increase in force is due to the activation of more motor units and, to a lesser degree, to their greater frequency of discharge. In fatiguing muscle, the relative force developed, and the sum of electrical activity, also remain linearly related until the level of mechanical activity cannot be maintained. In the fatigued muscle, however, each increment of physical force requires a larger volume of electrical activity, presumably because of a deficiency in the contractile process rather than changes in electrical propagation. Transmission across the neuromuscular junction may also be modified (especially with high-frequency stimulation), but it probably plays no significant role in normal subjects. The EMG recorded with surface electrodes reveals increased amplitude of the summated potentials and a decrease in their frequency with fatigue,[74] as a result of grouping of firing units.

This disrupts the normal smooth muscle contraction, resulting in a jerky firing pattern. Needle EMG study confirms that discharges of fibers from different motor units tend to group during fatiguing muscle work; there is also an increase in the total number of active motor units. The individual MUAPs are decreased in amplitude, but duration of the potentials is little changed. The number of polyphasic potentials is increased with fatigue,[73] presumably owing to incomplete synchronization between fibers of different motor units[20] or to endplate alterations with more irregular firing of individual fibers of the motor unit occurring in the vicinity of the needle electrode tip. Using tungsten microelectrodes, uncontaminated, single-unit potentials from the adductor pollicis of normal human subjects were recorded during maximal voluntary contractions.[75] Their amplitude, duration, and shape showed them to be action potentials from single muscle fibers. In brief, nonfatiguing, maximal contractions, the average firing rate of more than 200 units recorded from five subjects was $29.8 \pm 6.4$ Hz. During prolonged maximal effort, both force and firing rate always declined. Between 30 to 60 seconds and 60 to 90 seconds after the onset of the contractions, the rates were $18.8 \pm 4.6$ Hz and $14.3 \pm 4.4$ Hz, respectively. The percentage of decline in mean motor neuron firing rate paralleled, and appeared to account for, that of the surface EMG recorded simultaneously. These results are direct evidence for a reduction of motor neuron firing rates during this type of fatigue.

After a fatiguing muscle contraction, fewer motor unit spikes per second are needed to maintain a certain low level of force than before the contraction.[76] A significant reduction in spikes per second was found to occur in multiple regions of the biceps muscle examined and in other arm flexors. In addition, surface-rectified, integrated EMG, which measures electrical activity in a larger area of the muscle than the needle electrode, declined in parallel with the decrease in spike counts, indicating that other areas of muscle did not appear to be compensating for a more fatigued portion. These results imply that force can be maintained with a lower level of excitation after fatigue than before. It is thought that fatigue decreases the contraction-relaxation rate of muscle fibers, which lowers the funsion frequency. Thus, lower rates of motor unit activation can result in the maintenance of constant force. A feedback system from muscle to the central nervous system likely senses this slowing and leads to the spike count reduction.

### Effect of Disuse

In muscles with disuse atrophy, polyphasic potentials of more than four phases accounted for 25% of all action potentials, compared with 1 to 3% in normal muscle.[77] A reduction or increase in duration of the MUAPs occasionally is noted, which may be due to alteration in fiber conduction velocity. Spontaneous activity has not been reported as being present in disuse atrophy in the absence of superimposed denervation or primary muscle trauma. No significant changes of muscle fiber membrane characteristics have been demonstrated in animals up to a month after disuse was induced by section of the spinal cord at a higher level than the muscle supply and after sectioning of the dorsal roots.[78] In these animals, in which total flaccid paraplegia without lower motor neuron denervation was produced, a reversible fall of 10 mV in the resting membrane potential was noted in the first week only.

## Analysis of the Electromyogram and Special EMG

### Single-Fiber Electromyography

Standard EMG records compound action potentials from many muscle fibers making up the motor unit and from multiple motor units. The single-fiber needle electrode permits recording of individual muscle fibers belonging to a single motor unit. Because this technique looks at very restricted areas of the motor unit, it is prudent also to use information obtained from routine EMG examination, to allow for valid extrapolation of the functioning of the motor unit and the muscle as a whole. As previously noted, the single-fiber needle electrode, by having a small lead-off surface of approximately 25 $\mu$ diameter, can selectively record from single muscle fibers close to it. The recording surface is 3 to 4 mm along the shaft from the cutting point of the needle tip (Figure

11-2). There can be a separate indifferent recording electrode, or selectivity can be enhanced by a second electrode on the shaft a short distance (200 μ) from the first. The pickup area is approximately a hemisphere of 150 to 300 μ. These electrodes have a very high impedance, so the amplifier input impedance must also be quite high (100 mΩ) in order to have a high signal-to-noise ratio and an adequate common mode rejection ratio.[79] Baseline noise and low-frequency discharges from distant potentials must be filtered out, so a low-frequency filter of 500 Hz is used. The amplitude of the single-fiber potential can vary considerably, from 0.2 mV to 100 times that, but a range of 1 to 7 mV is most common. A triggering device usually set to trigger on the fastest slope of the deflection is necessary, together with a delay line, so that the initial portion of the potential can be recorded. Clinical single-fiber EMG records from voluntary contractions of individual muscle fibers while the patient attempts to maintain minimal contraction with a stable firing rate. The potential is biphasic with an initial positive deflection, and the rise time from positive to negative peak should be less than 300 μsec, and the peak-to-peak amplitude should exceed 200 μV. The shape should be constant with repetitive firing.

*Jitter*

Ekstedt[26] showed that the difference in arrival time at the electrode of two muscle fiber action potentials from the same motor unit was not constant from discharge to discharge. This *jitter phenomenon* was on the order of 10 to 30 μsec in the mutual time interval between the spike components of the composite potentials. This phenomenon can be seen with repetitive nerve stimulation and with voluntary contraction of muscle and can be due to variability in conduction along the terminal nerve fibers, neuromuscular junctions, and muscle fibers. Variability in transmission time at the neuromuscular junction plays the greatest role in normal subjects. Jitter, therefore, is the variability with consecutive discharges of the interpotential interval between two muscle fiber action potentials belonging to the same motor unit (Figure 11-10).[1] It is usually expressed quantitatively as the mean of the differences between the inter-

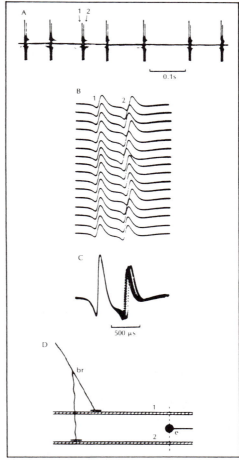

**Figure 11-10.** Single-fiber EMG recordings. (*A*) At a slow oscilloscope sweep speed, repetitive firing of one pair of potentials can be seen. (*B*) At a faster sweep speed, with the sweep triggered by the rising phase of potential 1, the same potential pairs are delayed and displayed rastered. (*C*) Ten sweeps are superimposed, demonstrating the variable interpotentials intervals (i.e., the neuromuscular jitter). (*D*) The recording position of the SFEMG electrode (e). (From Sanders DB, Phillips LH. Single Fiber Electromyography. AAEE Workshop, 1984;2. Courtesy of E. Stålberg.)

potential intervals of successive discharges (the mean consecutive difference, MCD). Newer digital equipment automatically analyzes jitter. Under certain conditions, jitter is expressed as the mean value of the difference between interpotential intervals arranged in order of decreasing interdischarge intervals (the mean sorted difference, MSD).[1] Jitter varies, depending on technique (fast sweep speeds are necessary for good resolution), age, and specific muscles tested. The extensor digitorum communis is the muscle most frequently used for single-fiber EMG recording, because it is superficial and easily accessible, does not normally show age-related abnormalities, and can easily be activated, controlled, and supported in a good position. Before the use of computer analysis, 50 potential pairs (10 groups of five or five groups of 10 potentials) were recorded and the MCD calculated. Values are abnormal if 10% or more of fiber pairs have jitter that exceeds the upper limit of normal for fiber pairs (55 μsec for extensor digitorum communis) or the mean jitter of all fiber pairs exceeds the upper limit of mean jitter for that muscle (34 μsec for extensor digitorum communis). Blocking—failure to fire of the second potential because of failure of end-plate depolarization—is also abnormal when observed (Figure 11-11). In normal muscles, jitter increases with drops in temperature or during ischemia. (Not to be confused with reduced decrement in amplitude of evoked potentials noted with repetitive nerve stimulation.) Abnormally increased jitter values and blocking are found in patients with myasthenia gravis who have only ocular manifestations and show relative sparing of extremity muscles. More

diffuse abnormalities can be present, depending on the severity of the generalized myasthenia gravis. Jitter is abnormal in any condition of impaired neuromuscular transmission, so abnormally increased jitter values and blocking can be found in patients with motor neuron disease, peripheral neuropathy, or myopathy. (Some patients with myopathy, such as Duchenne's muscular dystrophy, may have jitter values less than the normal range, possibly resulting from recording of potentials from split muscle fibers with the same innervation.[80]) Abnormal jitter values alone should not be used as a criterion for differentiating neurogenic and myopathic diseases. In patients with myasthenia gravis, edrophonium can decrease abnormal jitter and reduce the incidence of blocking. Increased jitter in patients with myopathy could be a result of prolonged propagation time of the muscle fibers or fragmentation of damaged muscle fibers with collateral reinnervation.

*Fiber Density*

As previously noted, the single-fiber electrode can record from a hemisphere area of approximately 200 to 300 μ. Random single-fiber EMG electrode insertion in a slightly contracting normal muscle usually records one single-fiber action potential; in about 20% of random insertions two muscle fibers of a single motor unit found are recorded. In fiber density measurement, the electrode is randomly inserted in 20 sites. The amplitude of the triggering potential is maximized, and the number of action potentials that are time locked and meet the criteria for single-fiber potentials (amplitude greater than 200 μV, rise time less than 300 μsec) are counted (Figure 11-12). The fiber density, therefore, provides a measure of the number of muscle fibers from a single motor unit presented as the mean value of the number of spikes recorded at 20 sites. Loss of muscle fiber normally is not detected, since the lowest possible value is 1.0. Normal fiber density varies, depending on the muscle examined, and also increases with age, being most marked after age 70 years. Fiber density is increased in conditions in which collateral sprouting and fiber grouping occur. Therefore, as would be expected, fiber density measurements are a sensitive indicator of chronic motor neuron disease, though in-

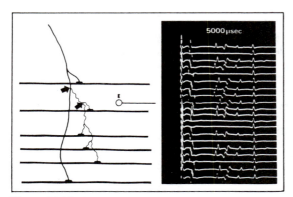

**Figure 11-11.** Concomitant blocking. A recording from six muscle fibers from the same motor unit. The middle four spike components intermittently block together. They also have a large common jitter in relation to the remaining two components. The block is most likely situated in the nerve twig common to the four blocking muscle fibers (i.e., between the arrows in the schematic drawing). (From Stålberg EV. In: AAEE International Symposium on Peripheral Nerve Regeneration, 1989;40.)

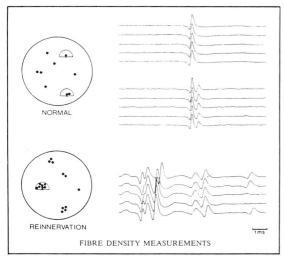

**Figure 11-12.** Method for measuring fiber density (FD). In normal muscle, usually one or two single–muscle fiber action potentials from the same motor unit are seen. After reinnervation, the chance to record from many fibers in one motor unit is increased, owing to grouping. (From Stålberg EV. In: AAEE International Symposium on Peripheral Nerve Regeneration. 1989;37.)

creased density is are also found in peripheral neuropathies, disorders of neuromuscular transmission, and myopathies.

## Macro EMG

Macro EMG provides information about the entire motor unit. The macro EMG needle electrode uses a 15-mm section of the length of the cannula from the tip as the principal recording surface for territorial pickup. Since the territory of most motor units is 5 to 10 mm, the 15-mm insertion length is both mechanically practical from an insertional point of view and long enough to encompass the area of the motor unit. One channel records the signal between the electrode shaft and a reference electrode (surface or subcutaneous needle electrode); the second channel is a modified single-fiber EMG electrode approximately halfway (7.5 mm) from the tip of the exposed electrode shaft that records a single-fiber EMG signal between the exposed 25-μm diameter platinum wire and the shaft of the same electrode. The sweep is triggered

by the single-fiber EMG recording, so that synchronously firing muscle fibers from the same motor unit are time-locked to the single-fiber EMG trigger. The signal is averaged until a smooth baseline occurs and the signal parameters do not change (Figure 11-13).[81] An attempt is made to obtain 20 different macro MUPs recorded at different depths in the muscle, using two to five different skin insertion points. Usually, a voluntary contraction of less than 30% of maximum is used, so that recordings are, therefore, obtained from relatively low-threshold motor units. Technical factors, such as filter settings, proper gain, sweep speed, and triggering, are all important. The presence of jitter and tremor also affects the results; the former causes a more prolonged signal with reduced amplitude and the latter an increase in am-

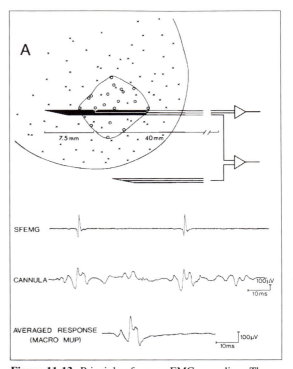

**Figure 11-13.** Principle of macro EMG recording. The small surface in the macro EMG electrode is positioned to record action potentials from one muscle fiber. This is used to trigger the averager to which the activity recorded with the cannula is fed. (From Stålberg EV. Methods in Clinical Neurophysiology: Macro EMG. Dantec, 1990;2.)

plitude as a result of synchronicity between different motor units. The characteristics of the potential are affected by the depth of penetration, as there may be different sizes of superficial and deep motor units, and also by the relationship between the electrode and the center of the motor unit (maximum amplitude being reduced when the electrode is at the periphery of the unit). The distance from the end-plate zone also affects the amplitude, with a diminution in amplitude and area being associated with the temporal dispersion. Because the higher-threshold motor units are larger than first-recruited units, this is also reflected in the mean amplitude of the macro EMG potential. Scanning EMG recordings, whereby a concentric needle electrode is pulled in steps of 50 μm through the motor unit, suggests that the peaks seen in macro EMG correspond to fractions of the motor unit, each of which seems to represent muscle fibers innervated by one nerve branch in the nerve tree of the motor unit.[82] Simulation studies show a positive correlation between macro MUP amplitude and area and the number and size of muscle fibers. The macro MUP represents the spatial and temporal summation of individual single-fiber action potentials. Muscle fiber atrophy decreases the macro MUP amplitude, however,

shrinkage or shortening of distances between individual fibers causes a packing effect and tends to increase the amplitude of the macro MUP. Both atrophy and shrinkage can occur together, and the net effect, therefore, can vary, depending on the balance between the two. Reinnervation with fiber type grouping can increase amplitude if the total number of fibers is increased (Figure 11-14). The amplitude of macro EMG MUAPs increases with age, especially after age 60.[68] In primary myopathies, the macro EMG amplitude is normal or slightly reduced. In the presence of reinnervation, the macro MUAP usually increases. In many pathologic conditions this situation is dynamic and not stable, and findings can change with time. Information obtained from single-fiber EMG (jitter and fiber density), macro EMG, and conventional EMG provides a better understanding of the anatomic and pathophysiologic changes that occur.

### Quantitative EMG and Automatic Analysis

Automatic analysis provides for rapid online readouts, replaces qualitative information with more precise quantitation, and reduces laborious manual computations and sources of human error in inter-

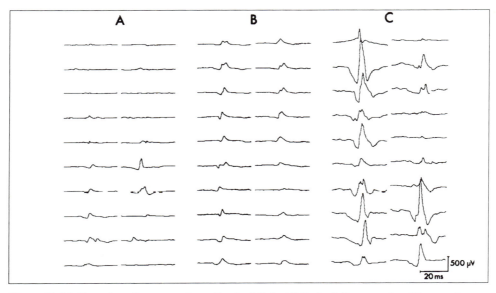

**Figure 11-14.** Examples of macro motor unit potentials in (A) limb girdle myopathy, (B) normal muscle, and (C) ALS. (From Stålberg EV. Methods in Clinical Neurophysiology: Macro EMG. Dantec, 1990;10.)

pretation. Quantitative studies of motor unit potential parameters are most often made by manually isolating 20 different motor units in each muscle. Computer analysis then helps plot out histograms of the number of phases, amplitude, duration, and other parameters. A computer can be used to identify and select stable units near the needle tip.

Dorfman and McGill reviewed automatic quantitative EMG,[83] breaking down those properties of interference patterns and motor unit action potentials that lend themselves to measurement (Figure 11-15). The EMG is a dynamically changing signal that is affected by many internal and external factors, including force of contraction, time, position of the recording electrode, and presence of pathology.

As defined by Dorfman and McGill,[83] the lowest-level computer-aided approach is to automate only measurement of MUAP properties once the operator has identified the MUAPs. More sophisticated techniques require automatic identification of the MUAP as well as measurements of parameters. Predetermined criteria must be set up for selection of presumed MUAPs on the basis of waveforms and recurrences.

Most methods of automatic motor unit potential analysis rely on template recognition with matching and sorting. The EMG signal from a particular epoch is stored, and recognized potentials are compared and matched with those from subsequent periods. There are differences in techniques, and results can be displayed as histograms, averaged potentials, or individual motor unit potentials, or as a comparison between normal, neuropathic, and myopathic units.[84–87] The various programs have different degrees of sensitivity and selectivity. Stalberg and colleagues[88] have reviewed and compared several different methods and proposed standardized terminology and criteria for measurement, which would have practical value.

The ANOPS computer method bridges the gap between analysis of individual motor unit potentials and the breakdown of more complex interference patterns into component potentials. This technique does not need the signal-processing complexities required for identification and classification, and total recognition may not relate to

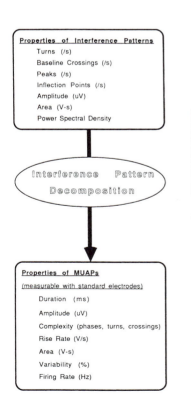

**Figure 11-15.** Properties of interference patterns (IPs) and motor unit action potentials (MUAPs). (From Dorfman LJ, McGill KC. AAEE Minimonograph No29: Automatic quantitative electromyography. Muscle Nerve 1988;11:805.)

single motor unit potentials if there is superimposition and noise bursts. MUAPs with faster firing rates are counted more often, so this is called a *frequency-weighted automatic analysis*. This technique traditionally averages 64 potentials at each of 16 sites (1024 single potentials). Results can be displayed in histograms of amplitude, duration, and phases of potentials. The method is rapid and less precise, but findings have been consistent compared with conventional manual quantitative analysis.[89,90]

*Interference Pattern Analysis*

Motor unit potential analysis usually requires signals derived from near-threshold muscle contractions to visualize individual motor unit potentials.

As force of the muscle contraction increases, the EMG signal becomes more complex, with superimposition of motor unit potentials from different units and ultimate obliteration of the baseline, so that individual motor unit potentials cannot be distinguished. With a submaximal contraction, the interference pattern is less full, but it can be difficult to visually distinguish individual motor unit potentials under normal circumstances, though this can be done with a contraction of relatively low force, such as 5 percent of MVC.[83] The units seen in such a low-force contraction are the lowest-threshold type I units, unless a lesion is present. Ideally, a system of analysis that is capable of breaking down a complex interference pattern into individual motor unit potentials during forceful contraction can also look at the status of higher-threshold units.

One of the earliest methods of interference pattern analysis to be described was that of Willison,[91] which attempted to systematize the change in phase of motor unit potentials with reference to a given integer of amplitude and the frequencies arising out of this. Baseline crossings, peaks, and inflection points are related to each other, and one parameter, calibrated amplitude steps (turns), can adequately describe them. During a preselected fixed contraction, the number of notches of the waveform "spikes" or "turns" (i.e., shifts from positive to negative phase or vice versa) is automatically counted. Using turns of 100 $\mu$V, the turns counts per second and the mean amplitude are compared with results from normal controls. This can show whether the recruited potentials are of high amplitude with only a few turns or of low amplitude with numerous turns. A problem with this method is that is does not adequately measure the important parameter of duration of MUAPs, which is useful in defining myopathy, though in primary muscle disease a marked elevation of the turns count was usually noted, as compared to a mean amplitude of more than 2 standard deviations from normal used as the criterion for denervation. Newer computer programs are able to refine this technique. Stalberg and coworkers[92] described the scatter plot or "clouds," in which mean amplitude per turn is plotted against turns per second, thus eliminating the need to maintain a constant contractile force. In myopathy, excessive turns of low amplitude occur; in neurogenic disease, increased amplitude with a reduced turn count. This comparison technique has been further augmented, providing for automatic measurements of the amplitude of the EMG envelope. When the force of contraction is increased, the interference potential signal contains more MUAP discharges and, therefore, the numerical value of activity increases. The EMG envelope (ENAMP) increases with the force of contraction and reflects the recruitment of motor units with large-amplitude MUAPs. Thus, plotting of ENAMP against activity enables one to study the number and size of MUAPs when the force of contraction is increased. When the numerical value of activity is greater than 500 msec, the interference pattern (IP) signal appears "full" on visual inspection. Examination of normal clouds show that if the activity values are greater than 500 msec (i.e., if the IP is full) and ENAMP is less than 2 mV, the data point is likely to be outside and below the normal area. This indicates a myopathy. Similarly, when the activity values are less than 500 msec (i.e., reduced IP) and ENAMP values are greater than 6 mV, the data are outside and above the normal cloud, indicating a neurogenic abnormality (Figure 11-16). The shape of the normal turns-amplitude is affected by the maximum effort at which recordings are made,[93] so care should be taken to avoid the false interpretation of a neurogenic abnormality when subjects exert near maximum force, though, in most clinical settings the

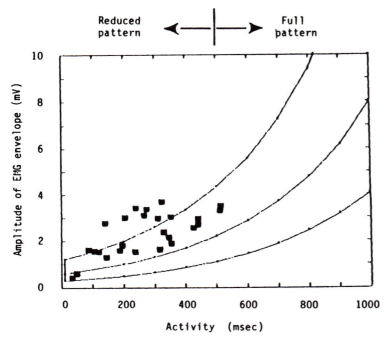

**Figure 11-16.** Analysis of IP in a patient with neuropathy. All but two epochs had activity values less than 500 msec, indicating reduced IP. The ENAMP values are on the upper side of the normal cloud, indicating a neurogenic abnormality. (From Nandedkar SD, Sanders DB. Measurement of the amplitude of the EMG envelope. Muscle Nerve 1990;13:937.)

clouds described should be adequate and sensitive for EMG analysis.

A number of methods are available for extracting MUAPs from partial interference patterns; however, many of these techniques require complicated computer equipment and are not capable of on-line measurements.[94,95] Automatic decomposition EMG (ADEMG, Figure 11-17)[96] is specifically oriented toward clinical application and can analyze contractile forces corresponding to up to 30% MVC using standard EMG electrodes. The signal is decomposed into constituent MUAPs in relatively short order, less than 1 minute. Only steady isometric contractions are decomposed, so that MUAP wave shapes and firing rates can be estimated even with incomplete identification. As many as 15 simultaneously active MUAPs can be identified at a single site.

A number of expert systems are now in use. Some of these have been developed by and are in use in small laboratories, others are available as part of the equipment package supplied by commercial manufacturers of electrodiagnostic instruments. Though these expert systems have the potential for providing enhanced accuracy of investigation, recording, and reporting, clinicians

should be cautious when evaluating results, since standardization and comparisons between systems are not yet readily available.

Power spectrum analysis of the interference pattern, using fast Fourier transformation, can break down an EMG signal for a particular period of time into frequency components. There is a shift from high to low frequency with increasing force. The percentage of low-frequency components also increases as fatigue occurs. For a given percentage of maximum force, the frequency spectrum is shifted toward the higher frequencies in patients with myopathy and toward the lower frequencies in those with neuropathy. When used with other methods of motor unit analysis, such as the turns amplitude analysis and manual measurement of MUP duration, power spectrum analysis supplemented these methods, increasing diagnostic yield.[97]

## Clinical Applications

This section is not intended to be a clinical manual, and though specific disease entities may produce characteristic EMG findings, these are not discussed in detail except to illustrate pathophysio-

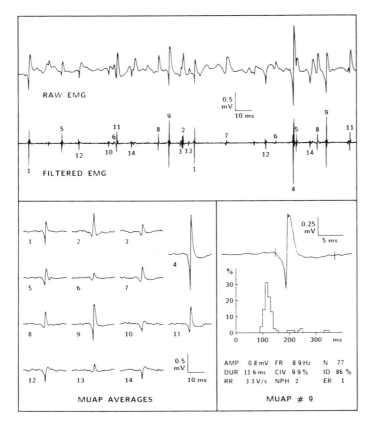

**Figure 11-17.** Decomposition of an IP using ADEMG. In the top portion of the figure, the uppermost trace shows a segment of raw IP signal and just below it the corresponding signals after application of a digital prefilter. The filtered spikes are numbered according to the order in which they were recognized by the ADEMG program. The left lower portion of the figure shows the waveforms of the 14 different MUAPs identified in the full 10-second EMG record, a segment of which is illustrated above. In the lower right, MUAP 9 is shown magnified, as an example, together with its histogram of interspike intervals (firing rate) and its set of descriptive statistical estimates. (From Dorfman LJ, McGill KC. AAEE Minimonograph No29: Automatic quantitative electromyography. Muscle Nerve, 1988;11:813, with permission.)

logic changes that apply to a group of disorders as a whole. The general electrodiagnostic texts more than adequately cover the clinical areas,[27,98] and there is also a recent specific review.[99]

Diseases that affect the motor unit pathway at any point from the anterior horn cell to the muscle fiber itself can produce an abnormal pattern in the EMG. In addition, the higher nervous centers influence the motor neuron apparatus, so that upper motor neuron lesions may alter EMG findings.

Monopolar or concentric needle electrodes are used for routine clinical EMG. The electrical activity produced by the insertion of the needle, any spontaneous activity in the relaxed, resting muscle, the character of the individual motor unit action potentials during weak or submaximal contraction, and the interference pattern in full forceful contraction against resistance are all recorded. More sophisticated quantitative motor unit analysis, SFEMG and other techniques that can provide additional supplemental information to help establish a diagnosis may be used. A muscle

is examined in several locations, and it is often helpful to amplify the sound equivalent of the potentials, as the ear is quite sensitive to variations.

### Lower Motor Neuron Disease

The electromyogram in lower motor neuron disease has certain general characteristics. These can include increased insertional activity, fibrillation potentials and positive sharp waves, fasciculation potentials, increased amplitude and average duration of MUAPs together with increased incidence of polyphasic potentials, and decreased number of MUAPs observed during full effort (Figure 11-18). Some of these changes also occur in myopathy, so a single criterion is insufficient to characterize the level of involvement along the motor unit pathway.

Brief comment should be made on collateral and terminal regeneration (Figure 11-19). Collat-

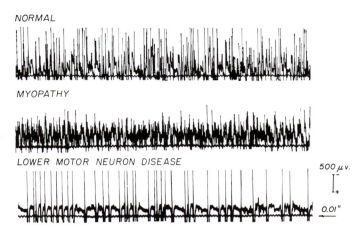

NORMAL

MYOPATHY

LOWER MOTOR NEURON DISEASE

500 μv.

0.01"

**Figure 11-18.** MUAPs during maximal voluntary contraction (biceps brachii). (From Mayo Clinic. Clinical Examinations in Neurology, ed 3. Philadelphia, WB Saunders, 1971;286.)

eral regeneration consists of the ingrowth of branches from intact nerve fibers to adjacent denervated muscle fibers. This axonal sprouting has been demonstrated in humans for both sensory and motor nerve fibers. The reinnervated muscle fibers take on the type characteristics of the intact axon. Terminal regeneration occurs in interrupted nerve fibers, whereby new end-plate connections are established by the peripherally regenerating terminal axon branches within the muscle fibers. A normal mean terminal innervation ratio (TIR) of $1.11 \pm 0.05$ was found for the biceps, palmaris longus, flexor carpi radialis, vastus medialis, and tibialis anterior muscles, with no significant difference in mean TIR between these muscles and no variation with age.[100] TIR was increased in 97% of patients with denervation and weakness and 74% of clinically normal muscles in patients with chronic polyneuropathy. TIR was normal in 82% of patients with muscular dystrophies (100% of patients with Duchenne's muscular dystrophy). TIR was increased in patients with myotonic dystrophy and was normal in those with myasthenia gravis.[101]

*Anterior Horn Cell Disorders*

The anterior horn cell is involved in disorders such as poliomyelitis, ALS, the progressive spinal muscular atrophies (e.g., Werdnig-Hoffman disease), and in hereditary degenerative conditions such as Charcot-Marie-Tooth disease. The characteristic features and clinical course vary according to the

particular entity, but in general, fibrillation potentials are common and fasciculation potentials may be seen. The degree of spontaneous activity diminishes with chronicity and reinnervation. There is a decrease in total number of motor units but an increase in the number of fibers that make up each individual unit, provided, of course, that the destruction is not so severe that further regeneration cannot occur. Most MUAPs have prolonged duration and increased amplitude that are more pronounced than those associated with impairment of peripheral nerves or roots (Figure 11-20). Early studies showed that motor unit territory may be increased by 80% to 140%, and the maximum voltage can be five to eight times the normal value in severely involved muscles.[102] As noted, though more recent data confirm that the size of the motor unit is increased (increased fiber density and increased amplitude of macro EMG signal), the overall territory of the motor unit seems to be less enlarged than was previously thought to be the case, and the more dense motor units remain mainly in their original territories.[103]

Findings depend on the rate of progression. In cases that progress very rapidly, single-fiber EMG shows increased jitter with a high degree of blocking while fiber density is only moderately increased, but in more chronic conditions, the fiber density increases, as does the total size of the motor unit, with less jitter and blocking. There is extensive collateral regeneration, since the degenerated nerve fibers are scattered over wide areas, and intact and degenerated nerve fibers often lie close together, giving rise to tremendous collateral

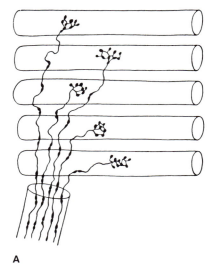

**A**

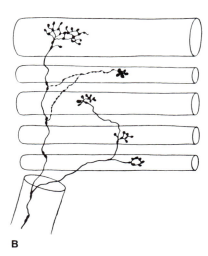

**B**

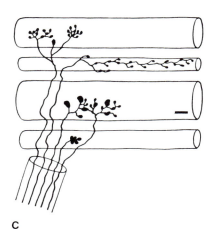

**C**

branching from the surviving fibers. In ALS, polyphasic fasciculations of increased duration may be observed in atrophic muscles and also in muscles that show no weakness or wasting. EMG findings suggest that this is caused by the firing of a single motor unit rather than the synchronous firing of two or more units, and the fact that the twitching muscle region is larger than that that normally corresponds to a single unit may be explained by the collateral branching that results in a pathologically enlarged motor unit. The action potentials are often polyphasic and of increased duration, again because of temporal dispersion of the enlarged unit together with variable distal conduction in the involved terminal nerve and muscle fibers.

Satellite potentials are small late components of the main motor unit action potential separated by an isoelectric interval and firing in a time-locked relation to the main action potential.[1] These potentials, also called *parasite potentials* or *linked potentials,* usually follow the main action potential (but can precede it) and are due to slow conduction from a sprouting immature twig. Satellite potentials are found in conditions in which there is chronic reinnervation, such as ALS and other motor neuron diseases. The time-locked relation to the main action potential should prevent confusion with separate low-amplitude units usually associated with myopathies.

*Nerve Root and Plexus Lesions*

A nerve root or plexus lesion causes denervation in the involved segments, manifested by fibrillation potentials and possibly occasional fascicula-

**Figure 11-19.** (*A*) Normal arrangement of terminal innervation. Note 1:1:1 relationship (one nerve fiber, one end plate, one muscle fiber). (*B*) Collateral sprouting and reinnervation. Degeneration has taken place in all but one nerve fiber. A sprout has arisen from the intact axon at a node of Ranvier and invaded the Schwann column of a degenerated fiber. One nerve fiber now innervates five muscle fibers, and there is variation in the form of the end-plates. (*C*) Probable mechanism of development of changes in terminal innervation in distal neuropathies and also in cases with primary degeneration of muscle fibers. Note tendency for nerve fibers to form several end-plates (more than one on most muscle fibers). (From Coërs, Woolf. The Innervation of Muscle. Springfield, Ill: Charles C Thomas, 1959.)

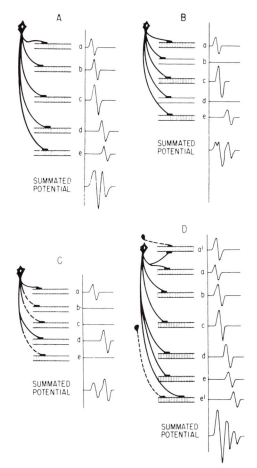

**Figure 11-20.** Simple diagrams to illustrate possible mechanisms for normal and abnormal motor unit potentials. (A) Normal situation with muscle fiber (**c**) closest to the electrode. The summated potential differs from any component action potential. (B) Myopathy with loss of fibers (**b, d**) causes bizarre alteration of summated potential. (C) Early terminal regeneration after a nerve lesion. The regenerated axon branches (**a, d**) excite muscle fibers (**a, d**) after increased latency; regeneration is incomplete in the other axon branches (*dashed*), and the corresponding muscle fibers are not activated. (D) Motor neuron degeneration with collateral growth from healthy axon branches to innervate muscle fibers (**a′, e′**). This summated potential is a giant potential. (From Norris. The EMG. New York: Grune and Stratton, 1963.)

tions, reduced numbers of MUAPs under voluntary control, and complex polyphasic units, often of increased duration. In the acute phase there may be electrical silence with fibrillation potentials and positive sharp waves appearing only as wallerian degeneration occurs. The peripheral nerve supply to individual muscles is composed of fibers from several spinal cord segments; as a result, normal and diseased motor units may be observed together. When atrophic changes occur in the muscle fibers, spontaneous activity can disappear or the firing and amplitude of fibrillation potentials may be reduced, and evidence of chronic denervation with reinnervation is noted in the muscles supplied by the affected cord segments. Plexus lesions can be differentiated from nerve root lesions by examination of the paraspinal muscles, which are supplied by the posterior primary division of the ventral nerve root proximal to the plexus. In root lesions the paraspinal muscles innervated in part by the involved root manifest signs of denervation. On the other hand, the paraspinal muscles are normal in the more distal plexus lesions.

*Peripheral Nerve Disorders*

A peripheral nerve damaged by disease or trauma may exhibit temporary loss of conductivity or varying degrees of degeneration.

In physiologic block (neuropraxia), continuity of the nerve sheath is maintained without wallerian degeneration, and the condition is characterized by electrical silence at rest. There is no voluntary action potential if the block is complete and a reduced number of normal potentials if the block is partial.

Immediately after the nerve trunk is severed, no voluntary muscle action potentials are seen. The axon cylinder begins to fragment about the third day, and at this time nerve conduction velocity distal to the site of injury rapidly decreases. The motor end-plate retains its excitability for another 5 to 10 days. Not until the end-plate is reduced to the same degree of excitability as the muscle fiber do fibrillation potentials begin to appear. Fibrillation potentials and positive sharp waves (see Figure 11-5) are noted approximately 10 days after the injury and occur in all areas of the muscle receiving their supply distal to the site of injury. Fibrillation potentials last until the regenerating axon arrives at the surface of the muscle fiber and penetrates the end-plate or until the muscle fibers atrophy. Fibrillation potentials have been observed for as long as 18 years,[104] but it can be questioned whether it is the same muscle fibers that are fibrillating or if other fibers break down and show fibrillation potentials or new denervation is occurring. As previously noted, the size of the fibrillation potentials and the rate of firing can be helpful to clinicians seeking to evaluate the chronicity of lesions.

The voluntary motor unit potentials first seen with return of function are of low amplitude, of long duration, and polyphasic. These potentials are called *nascent* units, but the term is not recommended, because the potential configuration is not, in itself, diagnostic. They are due to early terminal reinnervation of a reduced unit as well as to varying rates of distal conduction. As reinnervation progresses, the motor unit increases in area and number of fibers, so that by 3 months after injury the motor unit territory can be within normal limits and the maximum voltage ranges from normal to 1.8 times normal. Eight months or longer after nerve injury the maximum voltage is 2.5 to 3.5 times normal, and the motor unit territory is increased by an average of 15% to 40%.[102] Single-fiber EMG shows increased fiber density, and macro EMG also reveals that the total number of fibers in the motor unit is increased. The changes in motor unit territory and maximum voltage do not correlate with the degree of paresis as measured by muscle testing. Normal-looking action potentials are usually indicative of the return of near-synchronous discharge of fibers in the unit. Giant or large spike potentials—up to 15 mV—may be seen 3 to 5 years after regeneration.[105] Owing to the presence of blocking (increased jitter) in early lesions, the motor unit potential may be unstable, but with reinnervation that is relatively complete, more stable large-amplitude motor unit potentials with no variation in shape or duration are present.

In peripheral neuropathy both axonal degeneration and demyelination can occur. With denervation, fibrillation potentials and positive sharp waves proportional to the severity and extent of the lesion are seen at rest. If progressive degeneration occurs distally before the onset of (or in the absence of) nerve regeneration, there is gradual loss of muscle fibers in the unit, which causes a decrease in amplitude and fragmentation of the action potentials. As the degeneration spreads, there is a reduction of low-voltage initial and terminal deflections of the action potential. This relatively rare EMG picture of distal neuronitis is indistinguishable from that seen with the myopathies. In peripheral neuropathies, with primary axonal degeneration, spontaneous recovery is possible if there is anatomic continuity of the myelin sheaths. The recovery time depends on removal of the pathologic agent, the site of the lesion, and the distance through which regeneration must take place (Figure 11-21).

Recovery occurs by collateral and terminal regeneration. During and following reinnervation, the potentials are complex and of long duration because of temporal dispersion of the motor unit and alterations of conduction velocity along the regenerating distal nerve branches and across the immature end-plates. With time, in stable patients, MUAPs can develop a normal appearance.

*Motor End-Plate Disturbances*

A defect in transmission across the neuromuscular junction, as in myasthenia gravis, is characterized by a decrease in amplitude of the successively evoked potentials on repeated low-frequency stimulation. Amplitude of single motor units with voluntary contraction varies[106] until, because of fatigue, the unit may fail to respond. A normal pattern may be restored by an injection of neostigmine or edrophonium chloride (cholinesterase inhibitors). The change in amplitude is explained by blocking of excitation at the end-plate to a variable number of muscle fibers supplied by the neuron with fibers recovering at different rates. This may also account for the "myopathic picture" that is sometimes seen of complex polyphasic potentials of normal to decreased amplitude and normal to decreased duration. Myasthenia gravis is thought to be an autoimmune disease in which the defect is at the postsynaptic junction. Defects in neuromuscular transmission have been noted in other conditions, such as ALS and disseminated carcinomatosis.

**Myasthenic Syndrome (Lambert-Eaton Myasthenic Syndrome).** In patients with neoplasms, most commonly malignant intrathoracic tumors (and, at times, in patients who have no malignancy),

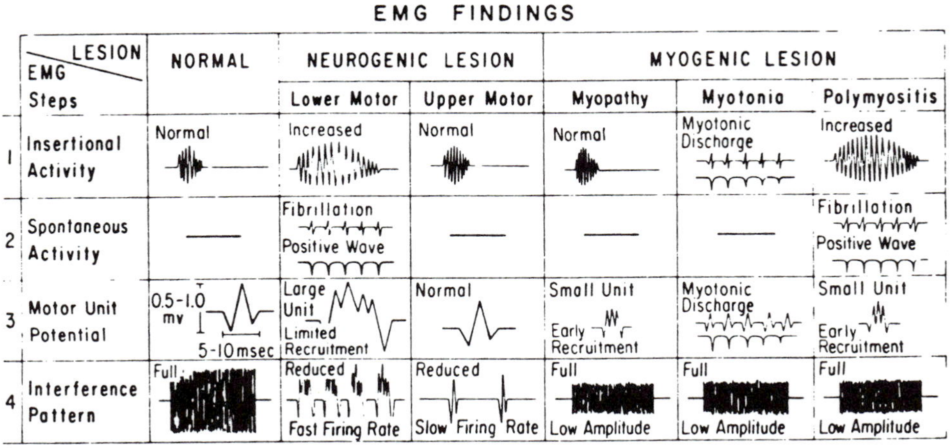

## EMG FINDINGS

| LESION / EMG Steps | NORMAL | NEUROGENIC LESION | | MYOGENIC LESION | | |
|---|---|---|---|---|---|---|
| | | Lower Motor | Upper Motor | Myopathy | Myotonia | Polymyositis |
| 1. Insertional Activity | Normal | Increased | Normal | Normal | Myotonic Discharge | Increased |
| 2. Spontaneous Activity | — | Fibrillation / Positive Wave | — | — | — | Fibrillation / Positive Wave |
| 3. Motor Unit Potential | 0.5-1.0 mv / 5-10 msec | Large Unit / Limited Recruitment | Normal | Small Unit / Early Recruitment | Myotonic Discharge | Small Unit / Early Recruitment |
| 4. Interference Pattern | Full | Reduced / Fast Firing Rate | Reduced / Slow Firing Rate | Full / Low Amplitude | Full / Low Amplitude | Full / Low Amplitude |

**Figure 11-21.** Typical findings in lower and upper motor neuron disorders and myogenic lesions. (From Kimura J. Electrodiagnosis in Diseases of Nerve and Muscle. Philadelphia, FA Davis, 1989;252.)

signs suggestive of a neuromuscular transmission defect have been noted. Clinically, the weak, resting patient becomes weaker with continuing muscle contraction or stimulation after an initial period of enhanced strength. Unlike with myasthenia gravis, the initial response to a supramaximal nerve stimulus is only a fraction of normal amplitude, and as contraction continues a period of facilitation occurs that is characterized by increasing responses, but these are often short of normal expected amplitude. The defect in the myasthenic syndrome is in the presynaptic region, as is that associated with botulinum toxin.

### Myopathy

Myopathy can be difficult to diagnosis on electrodiagnostic examination. Many of the findings observed are nonspecific, and the EMG may vary, depending on the stage of the disease. Fibrillation potentials have been noted in many myopathies. The mechanism for these abnormal spontaneous muscle potentials is not completely clear. In progressive muscular dystrophy and hyperkalemic periodic paralysis these spontaneous discharges may be related to the increase in excitability resulting from low levels of intracellular potassium.[30] It is also possible that in the dystrophies the degenerating muscle fibers may lose their terminal innervation. In the myositides Coers and Woolf[2] have demonstrated inflammatory involvement of the

subterminal intramuscular nerve endings and endplate areas. Segmental fiber necrosis and longitudinal fiber splitting may also result in fibrillation potentials. Complex repetitive discharges are often noted in myositis. These are high-frequency runs of similar-looking potentials, usually polyphasic, that start and stop abruptly.

In the myopathies, most of the EMG changes in the MUAPs are due to a reduction in the number of muscle fibers of the individual unit, changes in diameter of muscle fibers affecting conduction, and replacement with fibrous connective tissue. Unless the disease is very advanced, the total number of motor unit potentials remains unchanged, so while muscle force and summated voltage are decreased, the number of potentials is maintained with increased frequency of discharge (Figure 11-18).[107] More electrical activity of action potential spikes is necessary to achieve the amount of force that was attained prior to the illness. Because of the random degeneration of muscle fibers and of blocking, the smooth summated effect of the normal muscle action potential is lost and complex potentials of low amplitude are noted. The fibers farthest from the recording electrode are likewise decreased, so the duration of the recorded potentials is shortened. Fiber density is increased and macro MUP amplitudes are normal or only slightly reduced. Occasionally, long duration, larger amplitude units can be seen together with an increase in macro MUPs, possibly caused by fiber hypertrophy, splitting, and some collateral reinnervation.[99] This picture is most likely to be observed in patients with polymyositis after several years.[108]

*Myotonia*

Myotonia is an abnormally sustained contraction and difficulty in relaxation. The EMG shows runs of repetitive high-frequency, waxing and waning discharges, usually of positive waves or biphasic potentials whose initial deflection is positive (Figure 11-7).

In humans, myotonic discharges may be seen in patients with a dominantly inherited form of muscular dystrophy (myotonia dystrophica), myotonia congenita, associated with periodic paralysis (principally the hyperkalemic type) or with Pompe's disease (glycogenosis accompanied by acid maltase deficiency of muscle), or paramyotonia congenita. Clinical myotonia, a sustained contraction of muscle following voluntary effort or electrical or mechanical stimulation, can be present in the absence of myotonic discharges, but the reverse is also true. Procainamide and diphenylhydantoin are often used to reduce the intensity of clinical myotonia in patients with myotonic muscular dystrophy, and as these drugs are thought to reduce membrane permeability to ions, their stabilizing effect on the myotonic membrane may indicate a membrane permeability disorder. The slow depolarization of the membrane leading to repetitive spikes and the lower resting membrane potential are also found in denervated striated muscle. With voluntary contraction, the EMG may show short-duration, polyphasic, low-amplitude MUAPs as well as normal-looking potentials. High-voltage polyphasic potentials of prolonged duration have also been observed,[109] suggesting denervation with reinnervation. The subterminal nerve fibers have been noted to grow and ramify to form large multiple end-plates. They also can extend parallel to the muscle fibers, giving off short collateral sprouts that terminate in diminutive expansions on the muscle fiber. This, together with the central position of the nuclei in the extrafusal fibers in myotonic dystrophy, suggests conversion of normal extrafusal muscle fiber innervation into the multiple motor innervation characteristic of the intrafusal muscle fibers at the spindles. Thus, the conversion of the innervation of the muscle fibers

from an extrafusal to an intrafusal form can lead to hyperexcitable "pseudo–muscle spindles" that are spread throughout the involved muscles and are accompanied by resultant depolarization and membrane changes. The exact mechanism for the membrane disturbances responsible for the myotonia may not be the same for the different disorders—for example myotonia congenita, decreased number of calcium channels; myotonia dystrophica, abnormal sodium channel function; paramyotonia congenita, abnormal temperature dependence of the sodium channel kinetics.[110]

### *Upper Motor Neuron Lesions*

Hoefer and Putnam's[111] classic 1940 study of action potentials in spastic conditions noted that voluntary contraction produced a pattern of decreased frequency and amplitude, but these parameters were proportional to the strength of the contraction. The results of examination of individual discharges were essentially normal. In spastic muscles studied during clonus, there was a strong tendency to synchronization with alternating activity between protagonist and antagonist groups.

Physiologically, the higher nervous centers influence the lower motor neuron in normal motor activity. There has been some doubt that disease of the upper motor neurons affects the motor unit proper, but EMG findings of positive sharp waves and fibrillation potentials have been reported in some muscles of patients with upper motor neuron lesions who have not shown abnormal nerve conduction studies or findings suggestive of lower motor neuron pathology. One study of hemiplegic patients has shown a 57% prevalence of fibrillation potentials and a 70% prevalence of positive sharp waves.[112] Another study recorded a 73.5% prevalence of spontaneous activity in involved hemiplegic limbs, but a 9% prevalence of fibrillation potentials was also observed on the unaffected side.[113] In patients with high-level spinal cord lesions, fibrillation potentials have been observed in muscles innervated by nerve root segments quite distal to the level of injury. Nepomuceno and colleagues[114] also observed positive sharp waves and fibrillation potentials in patients with upper motor neuron lesions without conditions that involved the lower motor neuron. They studied these potentials to ascertain if there were differences in characteristics between those found in upper motor neuron and lower motor neuron lesions. They found interlesion differences in the mean frequency of occurrence ratio of positive sharp waves to fibrillation potentials: a ratio of 5:1 positive sharp waves to fibrillation potentials in those patients with upper motor neuron lesions and a ratio of 3:1 in those with lower motor neuron lesions. The positive sharp waves associated with lower motor neuron lesions had a longer duration than those seen in patients with upper motor neuron lesions ($P<.015$). The explanation for these differences is not clear at this time.

A number of theories have been proposed to explain the association of fibrillation potentials and positive sharp waves with upper motor neuron lesions. These include transsynaptic neuronal degeneration,[112] membrane instability,[115] and antifibrillation factor.[116]

## References

1. AAEE. Glossary of terms in clinical electromyography. Muscle Nerve 1987; 10 (8S):G1–G60.
2. Coërs C, Woolf AL. The Innervation of Muscle. Oxford: Blackwell, 1959.
3. Christensen E. Topography of terminal motor innervation in striated muscles from stillborn infants. Am J Phys Med 1959; 38:65–77.
4. Feinstein B, Lindegard B, Nyman E, et al. Morphologic studies of motor units in normal human muscles. Acta Anat 1955; 23:127–142.
5. McComas AJ, Fawcett PRW, Campbell MJ, et al. Electrophysiological estimation of the number of motor units within a human muscle. J Neurol Neurosurg Psychiatry 1971; 34:121–131.
6. Ballantyne JP, Hansen S. A new method for the estimation of the number of motor units in a muscle. 1. Control subjects and patients with myasthenia gravis. J Neurol Neurosurg Psychiatry 1974; 37:907–915.
7. Milner-Brown HS, Brown WF. New methods of estimating the number of motor units in a muscle. J Neurol Neurosurg Psychiatry 1976; 39:258–265.
8. Brown WF, Strong MJ, Snow R. Methods for estimating numbers of motor units in biceps-brachialis muscles and losses of motor units with aging. Muscle Nerve 1988; 11:423–432.
9. Slawnych MP, Laszlo CA, Hershler C. A review of techniques employed to estimate the number of motor units in a muscle. Muscle Nerve 1990; 13:1050–1064.
10. Brandstater ME, Lambert EH. A histological study of the spatial arrangement of muscle fibers in single motor units within rat tibialis anterior muscle. Bull Am Assoc Electromyogr Electrodiagn 1969; August 15–16:82.
11. Buchthal F, Guld C, Rosenfalck P. Volume conduction of the spike of the motor unit potential investigated with a new type of multielectrode. Acta Physiol Scand 1957; 38:331–354.
12. Buchthal F, Guld C, Rosenfalck P. Multielectrode study of the territory of a motor unit. Acta Physiol Scand 1957; 39:83–105.
13. Bodine-Fowler S, Garfinkel A, Roy RR, et al. Spatial distribution of muscle fibers within the territory of a motor unit. Muscle Nerve 1990; 13:1133–1145.
14. Brown MC, Matthews PBC. An investigation into the possible existence of polyneuronal innervation of individual skeletal muscle fibers in certain hind limb muscles of the cat. J Physiol 1960; 151:436–457.
15. Hunt CC, Kuffler SW. Motor innervation of skeletal muscle: Multiple innervation of individual muscle fibers and motor unit function. J Physiol 1954; 126:293–303.
16. Walker LB Jr. Multiple motor innervation of individual muscle fibers in the m. tibialis anterior of the dog. Anat Rec 1961; 139:1–11.
17. Brooks JE, Hongdalarom T. Intracellular electromyography. Resting and action potentials in normal human muscle. Arch Neurol 1968; 18:291–300.
18. Nastuk WL, Hodgkin AL. The electrical activity of single muscle fibers. J Cell Compar Physiol 1950; 35:39–73.
19. Lundervold A, Li C. Motor units and fibrillation potentials as recorded with different kinds of needle electrodes. Acta Psych Neurol Scand 1953; 28:201–212.
20. Buchthal F, Pinelli P, Rosenfalck P. Action potential parameters in normal human muscle and their physiological determinants. Acta Physiol Scand 1954; 32:219–229.
21. Howard JE, McGill KC, Dorfman LJ. Properties of motor unit action potentials recorded with concentric and monopolar needle electrodes: ADEMG analysis. Muscle Nerve 1988; 11:1050–1055.
22. Pease WS, Bowyer BL. Motor unit analysis: Comparison between concentric and monopolar needle electrodes. Am J Phys Med 1988; 67:2–6.
23. Nandedkar SD, Sanders DB. Recording characteristics of monopolar EMG electrodes. Muscle Nerve 1991; 14:108–112.

24. Nandedkar SD, Tedman B, Sanders DB. Recording and physical characteristics of disposable concentric needle EMG electrodes. Muscle Nerve 1990; 13:909–914.

25. Basmajian JV. Muscles Alive, ed 2. Baltimore: Williams & Wilkins, 1967.

26. Ekstedt J. Human single muscle fibre action potentials. Acta Physiol Scand 1964; 51 (suppl 226):1–96.

27. Wohlfart G. Clinical considerations on innervation of skeletal muscle. Am J Phys Med 1959; 38:223–230.

28. Kimura J. Electrodiagnosis in Diseases of Nerve and Muscle: Principles and Practice ed 2. Philadelphia: FA Davis, 1989.

29. Buchthal F, Guld C, Rosenfalck P. Action potential parameters in normal human muscle and their dependence on physical variables. Acta Physiol Scand 1954; 32:200–218.

30. Buchthal F. Spontaneous and voluntary electrical activity in neuromuscular disorders. Bull NY Acad Med 1966; 42:521–550.

31. Stöhr M. Benign fibrillation potentials in normal muscle and their correlation with end-plate and denervation potentials. J Neurol Neurosurg Psychiatry 1977; 40:765–768.

32. Wilbourn AJ. The EMG examination with myopathies. AAEE Course A: Myopathies, Floppy Infant and Electrodiagnostic Studies in Children 1987; 7–20.

33. Kraft GH. Fibrillation potential amplitude and muscle atrophy following peripheral nerve injury. AAEE International Symposium on Peripheral Nerve Regeneration 1989; 45–50.

34. Buchthal F. Fibrillations: Clinical electrophysiology. In: Culp WJ, Ochoa J, eds. Abnormal Nerves and Muscles as Impulse Generators. Oxford: Oxford University Press, 1982; 632–662.

35. Ware F Jr, Bennett AL, McIntyre AR. Membrane resting potential of denervated skeletal muscle measured in vivo. Am J Physiol 1954; 177:115–118.

36. Thesleff S, Ward MR. Studies on the mechanism of fibrillation potentials in denervated muscle. J Physiol 1975; 244:313–323.

37. Kraft GH. Fibrillation potential amplitude and muscle atrophy following peripheral nerve injury. Muscle Nerve 1990; 13:814–821.

38. Tsubahara A, Chino N, Mineo K. Fibrillation potentials and muscle fiber types. Muscle Nerve 1990; 13:983.

39. Hayes GJ, Woolsey CN. The unit of fibrillary activity and the site of origin of fibrillary contractions in denervated striated muscle. Fed Proc 1942; 1:38.

40. Belmar J, Eyzaguirre C. Pacemaker site of fibrillation potentials in denervated mammalian muscle. J Neurophysiol 1966; 29:425–441.

41. Marinacci AA. Applied Electromyography. Philadelphia: Lea & Febiger, 1968.

42. Goodgold J, Eberstein A. The physiological significance of fibrillation action potentials. Bull NY Acad Med 1967; 43:811–818.

43. Wiederholt WC. End-plate noise in electromyography. Neurology 1970; 20:214–224.

44. Roth G. The origin of fasciculations. Ann Neurol 1982; 12:542–547.

45. Forster FM, Alpers BJ. The site of origin of fasciculations in voluntary muscle. Arch Neurol Psychiatry 1944; 51:264–267.

46. Richardson AT. Muscle fasciculation. Arch Phys Med Rehabil 1954; 35:281–285.

47. Conradi S, Grimby L, Lundemo G. Pathophysiology of fasciculations in ALS as studied by electromyography of single motor units. Muscle Nerve 1982; 5:202–208.

48. Wettstein A. The origin of fasciculations in motoneuron disease. Ann Neurol 1979; 5:295–300.

49. Norris FH Jr. Synchronous fasciculation in motor neuron disease. Arch Neurol 1965; 13:495–500.

50. Trojaborg W, Buchthal F. Malignant and benign fasciculations. Acta Neurol Scand 1965; 41(suppl 13):251–254.

51. Gutmann L. Facial and limb myokymia. Muscle Nerve 1991; 14:1043–1049.

52. Brick JF, Gutmann L, McComas CF. Calcium effect on generation and amplification of myokymic discharges. Neurology 1982; 32:618–622.

53. Trontelj J, Stålberg E. Bizarre repetitive discharges recorded with single fiber EMG. J Neurol Neurosurg Psychiatry 1983; 46:310–316.

54. Norris FH Jr. Unstable membrane potential in human myotonic muscle. Electroencephalogr Clin Neurophysiol 1962; 14:197–201.

55. Norris FH Jr, Gasteiger EL. Action potentials of single motor units in normal muscle. Electroencephalogr Clin Neurophysiol 1955; 7:115–126.

56. Petajan JH. Motor unit recruitment. Muscle Nerve 1991; 14:489–502.

57. Henneman E. The size principle of motoneuron recruitment. In: Desmedt JE, ed. Motor Unit Types, Recruitment and Plasticity in Health and Disease: Progress in Clinical Neurophysiology. Basel: S Karger, 1981;26–60.

58. Clamann HP. Activity of single motor units during isometric tension. Neurology 1970; 20:254–260.

59. Johnson EW. The EMG examination. In: Johnson EW, ed. Practical Electromyography ed 2. Baltimore: Williams & Wilkins, 1988;1–21.

60. Daube JR. Needle examination in clinical electromyography. Muscle Nerve 1991; 14:685–700.
61. Bigland B, Lippold OCJ. Motor unit activity in the voluntary contraction of human muscle. J Physiol 1954; 125:322–335.
62. Taylor A. The significance of grouping of motor unit activity. J Physiol 1962; 162:259–269.
63. Denny-Brown D. Interpretation of the electromyogram. Arch Neurol Psychiatry 1949; 61:99–128.
64. Petersen I, Kugelberg E. Duration and form of action potential in the normal human muscle. J Neurol Neurosurg Psychiatry 1949; 12:124–128.
65. Brown WF. A method for estimating the number of motor units in thenar muscles and the changes in motor unit count with aging. J Neurol Neurosurg Psychiatry 1972; 35:845–852.
66. Stålberg E, Thiele B. Motor unit fiber density in the extensor digitorum communis muscle: Single fiber electromyographic study in normal subjects at different ages. J Neurol Neurosurg Psychiatry 1975; 38:874–880.
67. DeKoning P, Wieneke GH, Van Der Most Van Spyke D, et al. Estimation of the number of motor units based on macro EMG. J Neurol Neurosurg Psychiatry 1988; 51:403–411.
68. Stålberg E, Fawcett PRW. Macro EMG in healthy subjects of different ages. J Neurol Neurosurg Psychiatry 1982; 45:870–878.
69. Tomlinson BE, Irving D. The number of limb motor neurons in the human lumbosacral cord throughout life. J Neurol Sci 1977; 34:213–219.
70. Kawamura Y, O'Brien P, Okazaki H, et al. Lumbar motoneurons of man. J Neuropathol Exp Neurol 1977; 36:861–870.
71. Gutmann E, Hanzliková V. Motor unit in old age. Nature 1966; 209:921–922.
72. Bigland-Ritchie B. Changes in EMG and neural control during human muscle fatigue. Am Assoc Electromyogr Electrodiagn Didactic, program 1983:21–26.
73. Scherrer J, Bourguignon A. Changes in the electromyogram produced by fatigue in man. Am J Phys Med Rehabil 1959; 38:148–158.
74. Myers SJ, Sullivan WP. Effect of circulatory occlusion on time to muscular fatigue. J Appl Physiol 1968; 24:54–59.
75. Bigland-Ritchie B, Johansson R, Lippold OCJ, et al. Changes in motoneuron firing rate during sustained maximal voluntary contractions. J Physiol 1983; 340:335–346.
76. Gooch JL, Newton BY, Petajan JH. Motor unit spike counts before and after maximal voluntary contraction. Muscle Nerve 1990; 13:1146–1151.
77. Pinelli P, Buchthal F. Muscle action potentials in myopathies with special regard to progressive muscular dystrophy. Neurology 1953; 3:347–359.
78. Brooks JE. Disuse atrophy of muscle. Arch Neurol 1970; 22:27–30.
79. Stålberg E, Trontelj J. Single Fibre Electromyography. Surrey: Miraville Press, 1979.
80. Hilton-Brown P, Stålberg E, Trontelj J, et al. Causes of the increased fiber density in muscular dystrophies studied with single fiber EMG during electrical stimulation. Muscle Nerve 1985; 8:383–388.
81. Stålberg E. Macro EMG. Methods Clin Neurophysiol 1990 (Dantec); 1:1–14.
82. Stålberg E, Antoni L. Electrophysiological cross section of the motor unit. J Neurol Neurosurg Psychiatry 1980; 43:469–474.
83. Dorfman LJ, McGill KC. Automatic quantitative electromyography. Muscle Nerve 1988; 11:804–818.
84. Bergmans J. Computer-assisted on-line measurement of motor unit potential parameters in human electromyography. Electromyography 1971; 11:161–181.
85. Leifer LJ, Pinelli P. Analysis of motor units by computer aided electromyography. 3rd International Congress of Electrophysiology and Kinesiology, Pavia, Italy. 1976;1–14.
86. Stålberg E, Antoni L. Computer-aided EMG analysis. In: Desmedt JE, ed Computer-aided Electromyography. Basel: S Karger, 1983;186–234.
87. Coatrieux JL. Interference electromyogram processing. Electromyogr Clin Neurophysiol 1983; 23:229–242.
88. Stålberg E, Andreassen S, Falck B, et al. Quantitative analysis of individual motor unit potentials: A proposition for standardized terminology and criteria for measurement. J Clin Neurophysiol 1986; 3:313–348.
89. Hausmanowa-Petrusewicz I, Kopec J. Quantitative EMG and its automation. In: Desmedt, JE, ed. Computer-Aided Electromyography. Basel: S Karger, 1983;164–185.
90. Kopec J, Hausmanowa-Petrusewicz I. Diagnostic yield of an automated method of quantitative electromyography. Electromyogr Clin Neurophysiol 1985; 25:567–577.
91. Willison RG. Analysis of electrical activity in healthy and dystrophic muscles in man. J Neurol Neurosurg Psychiatry 1964; 27:386–394.
92. Stålberg E, Chu J, Bril V, et al. Automatic analysis of the EMG interference pattern. EEG Clin Neurophysiol 1983; 56:672–681.
93. Nandedkar SD, Sanders DB, Stålberg EV. On the shape of the normal turns-amplitude cloud. Muscle Nerve 1991; 14:8–13.

94. LeFever RS, DeLuca CJ. A procedure for decomposing the myoelectric signal into its constituent action potentials. Technique, theory and implementation. IIEE Trans Biomed Eng BME 1982; 29:149–157.

95. Guiheneuc P, Calamel J, Doncarli C, et al. Automatic detection and pattern recognition of single motor unit potentials in needle EMG. In: Desmedt JE, ed. Computer-Aided Electromyography. Basel: S Karger, 1983; 73–127.

96. McGill KC, Dorfman LJ. Automatic decomposition electromyography (ADEMG): Validation and normative data in brachial biceps. EEG Clin Neurophysiol 1985; 61:453–461.

97. Fuglsang-Frederiksen A. Power spectrum of the needle EMG in normal and diseased muscles. Methods Clin Neurophysiol 1990 (Dantec) 2:1–8.

98. Johnson EW, ed. Practical Electromyography, ed 2. Baltimore: Williams & Wilkins, 1988.

99. Stålberg E. Invited review: Electrodiagnostic assessment and monitoring of motor unit changes in disease. Muscle Nerve 1991; 14:293–303.

100. Coërs C, Telerman-Toppet N, Gerrard JM. Terminal innervation ratio in neuromuscular disease: I. Methods and controls. Arch Neurol 1973; 29:210–214.

101. Coërs C, Telerman-Toppet N, Gerrard JM. Terminal innervation ratio in neuromuscular disease: II. Disorders of lower motor neuron, peripheral nerve and muscle. Arch Neurol 1973; 29:215–222.

102. Ermino F, Buchthal F, Rosenfalck P. Motor unit territory and muscle fiber concentration in paresis due to peripheral nerve injury and anterior horn cell involvement. Neurology 1959; 9:657–671.

103. Stålberg EV. Capability of motor unit sprouting in neuromuscular disorders. AAEE Didactic Program 1987; 33–39.

104. Weddell G, Feinstein B, Pattle RE. The electrical activity of voluntary muscle in man under normal and pathological conditions. Brain 1944; 67:178–257.

105. Yahr MD, Herz E, Moldover J. Electromyographic patterns in reinnervated muscle. Arch Neurol Psych 1950; 63:728–738.

106. Lindsley DB. Myographic and electromyographic studies of myasthenia gravis. Brain 1935; 58:470–480.

107. Kugelberg E. Electromyography in muscular dystrophies. J Neurol Neurosurg Psychiatry 1949; 12:129–136.

108. Trojaborg W. Quantitative electromyography in polymyositis: A reappraisal. Muscle Nerve 1990; 13:964–971.

109. Woolf AL. The theoretical basis of clinical electromyography. Part II. Am J Phys Med Rehabil 1962; 6:241–266.

110. Rudel R. The pathophysiological basis of the myotonias and the periodic paralyses. In: Engel AG, Banker BQ, eds. Myology, vol 1. New York: McGraw-Hill, 1986; 1297–1307.

111. Hoefer PFA, Putnam TJ. Action potentials of muscles in spastic conditions. Arch Neurol Psychiatry 1940; 43:1–22.

112. Goldkamp O. Electromyography and nerve conduction studies in 116 patients with hemiplegia. Arch Phys Med Rehabil 1967; 48:59–63.

113. Bhala RP. Electromyographic evidence of lower motor neuron involvement in hemiplegia. Arch Phys Med Rehabil 1969; 50:632–637.

114. Nepomuceno C, McCutcheon M, Miller JM III, et al. Differential analyses of EMG findings in motor neuron lesions. Am J Phys Med 1977; 56:1–11.

115. Johnson EW, Denny ST, Kelly JP. Sequence of electromyographic abnormalities in stroke syndrome. Arch Phys Med Rehabil 1975; 56:468–473.

116. Spielholz NI, Sell GH, Goodgold J, et al. Electrophysiologic studies in patients with spinal cord lesions. Arch Phys Med Rehabil 1972; 53:558–562.

# Chapter 12
# Evoked Potentials

YASOMA CHALLENOR
ERWIN GONZALEZ
ARMINIUS CASSVAN

Evoked potentials are minute electrical responses, often less than 1 μV in amplitude, recorded in response to an appropriate stimulus. The potential that is evoked by the stimulus is time locked to the stimulus, in contrast to random spontaneous electrical fluctuations such as electroencephalographic activity or other electrical "noise." Synchronous nerve action potentials ascending via sensory pathways generate the earliest response components, while longer latency components of the evoked potential are thought to be generated by postsynaptic potentials of cortical neurons.[1,2] Recording electrodes placed at nonequipotential sites can record evoked potentials. The electrode montages developed over the last decades of investigation of evoked potential techniques represent a compromise between the desirability of having one electrode placed as directly over the generator source as possible (with the reference electrode far away enough to give a maximum potential difference) and the need to reduce distance between electrodes in order to minimize electromyographic (EMG) and electrocardiographic (ECG) contaminants. The scalp electrode "sees" the electrical volley generated by an electrical stimulus from relatively far away, and records multiple peaks as the volley traverses various anatomic structures in this far-field recording, in contrast to the immediacy of the triphasic, near-field response obtained with electrodes sitting directly over a nerve conducting a nerve action potential.[3]

In 1887, Caton noted changes in brain electrical activity in response to visual and somatosensory stimuli.[4,5] There was no photographic record of such animal experiments until 1913.[6] In the early 1940s, Dawson used photographic superimposition of faint oscilloscope traces, with 50 successive somatosensory stimuli, to produce the first reported somatosensory evoked potentials (SSEPs) recorded from the scalp in humans. Fortuitously, his patient had myoclonic seizures, a condition known to cause enlarged SSEPs. In the same report, however, Dawson found recordable SSEPs in 12 of 14 normal subjects, though the response amplitudes were 10% to 20% smaller than the myoclonic patients'.[7] In the 1950s, Dawson personally designed and built an electromagnetic averager.[8] This averager was later used by Giblin to further explore the features of SSEPs.[9–11] At the time of Giblin's explorations, in the 1960s, W.T. Liberson, a physiatrist, was developing techniques for surface recording of SSEPs over the cervical spinal area.[12,13] Liberson also had the foresight, in the 1960s, to explore the relationship of evoked potentials to cognitive events.[14] Currently, in the decade designated *the decade of the brain,* we see significantly wider application of evoked potential studies, in attempts to predict the outcome of CVA cerebrovascular accidents.[15–17] Similarly, evoked potentials have been used to try to predict future physical deficits of infants suspected to have suffered asphyxia or children who clearly did.[18–20] In head injury patients, evoked potentials have been used to titrate modalities of acute medical management[21] as well as to predict outcome.[22–26] Evoked potentials may be divisible into exogenously elicited ones such as those mentioned above and those that are endogenously stimulated by the person's reaction to or attitude toward the stimulus. The latter type of response usually has a longer latency (300 msec or more) than exogenously evoked potentials and has found wide application in clinical, developmental, and neuropsychological research.[27,28]

The introduction into electrodiagnostic units of microprocessors and digital processors has led to rapid escalation in the development of techniques for more efficacious acquisition, analysis, and display of data. Electrical and magnetic stimulation techniques have evolved to study motor pathways, in addition to the amply explored somatosensory, visual, and auditory pathways. Enhanced filtering and averaging techniques are making it possible to obtain reliable evoked responses in increasingly "electrically noisy" environments.[29] Dynamic time-warping algorithms are making it possible to study quantitatively SSEP morphology.[30] Tomorrow we may see the "three-sweep," or perhaps even the "single-sweep," evoked potential![31]

Evoked potentials have focused on evaluation of electrical responses in the brain; however, electrical current flow is associated with an electrically generated magnetic field. Brain electrical activity generates a magnetic field in the space around the head. These neuromagnetic signals are being studied, and may be useful in the future for estimating the number of neurons that contribute to magnetic fields generated by somatosensory, visual, or auditory stimuli.[32–38] Modern developments in brain imaging, such as computed tomography and magnetic resonance imaging, are revealing the mysteries of brain structure. Evoked potential studies have become an increasingly valuable tool for exploring the mysteries of the brain's neurophysiologic function at a finer level than structure. Clearly, evoked potentials are a valuable tool for the continued exploration of neurophysiologic function that researchers would like to promote; for "as long as our brain is a mystery, the universe, the reflection of the structure of the brain, will also be a mystery."[39]

# References

1. Arezzo JC, Legatt AD, Vaughn HG Jr. Topography and intracranial source of somatosensory evoked potentials in the monkey. I. Early components. Electroencephalogr Clin Neurophysiol 1979; 46:155–172.
2. Artezzo JC, Legatt AD, Vaughn HG Jr. Topography and intracranial sources of somatosensory evoked potentials in the monkey. II. Cortical components. Electroencephalogr Clin Neurophysiol 1981; 51:1–18.
3. Kimura J, Kimura A, Ishida T, et al. What determines the latency and amplitude of syationary peaks in far-field recordings? Ann Neurol 1986; 19:479–486.
4. Caton R. The electrical currents of the brain. Br Med J 1875; 2:278–281.
5. Caton R. Description of a new form of recording apparatus for the use of practical physiological classes. J Anat Physiol 1887; 22:103–106.
6. Pravdich-Neminsky VV. Einige elektrische Erscheinungen in Zentralnervensystem bei *Rana temporaria*. Arch Anat Physiol 1913;321–324.
7. Dawson GD. Cerebral responses to electrical stimulation of the peripheral nerve in man. J Neurol Neurosurg Psychiatry 1982; 10:133–141.
8. Dawson GD. A summation technique for the detection of small evoked potentials. Electroencephalogr Clin Neurophysiol 1954; 6:65–69.
9. Giblin DR. The effects of lesions of the nervous system on cerebral responses to peripheral nerve stimulation. Electroencephalogr Clin Neurophysiol 1960; 12:262–265.
10. Giblin DR. Comparison of evoked potentials from cortex and scalp in man. Electroencephalogr Clin Neurophysiol 1962; 14:291–296.
11. Giblin, DR. Somatosensory evoked potentials in healthy subjects and patients with lesions of the nervous system. Ann NY Acad Sci 1964; 112:93–97.
12. Liberson WT, Kim KC. The mapping out of evoked potentials elicited by the stimulation of the median and peroneal nerves. Electroencephalogr Clin Neurophysiol 1963; 15:721–726.
13. Liberson WT, Gratzer M, Zalis A, et al. Comparison of conduction velocities of motor and sensory fibers determined by different methods. Arch Phys Med 1966; 47:17–23.
14. Liberson WT. Study of evoked potentials in aphasics. Am J Phys Med 1966; 45:135–142.
15. Pavot AP, Ignacio D, Lightfoote WE. Prognostic value of multimodality evoked potential studies in cerebrovascular accidents. Presented at the Fifth

Annual Conference of the American Society Clinical Evoked Potentials, White Plains, NY, 1983.

16. Chester CS, McLaren CE. Somatosensory evoked response and recovery from stroke. Arch Phys Med Rehabil 1989; 70:520–525.

17. Papanicolaou AC, Moore BD, Levin HS, et al. Evoked potential correlates of right hemisphere involvement in language recovery following stroke. Arch Neurol 1987; 44:521–524.

18. Frank LM, Furgiuele TL, Etheridge JE. Prediction of chronic vegetative state in children using evoked potentials. Neurology 1985; 35:931–934.

19. Görke W. Somatosensory evoked cortical potentials indicating impaired motor development in infancy. Dev Med Child Neurol 1986; 28:633–641.

20. Whyte HE, Taylor MJ, Menzies R, et al. Prognostic utility of visual evoked potentials in term asphyxiated neonates. Ped Neurol 1986; 2:220–223.

21. Taylor MJ, Houston BD, Lowry NJ: Recovery of auditory brain-stem responses after a severe hypoxic ischemic insult. N Engl J Med 1983; 309:1169–1170.

22. Mackey-Hargadine JR, Hall JW. Sensory evoked responses in head injury. Cent Nerv Sys Trauma 1985;187–206.

23. Shin DY, Ehrenberg B, Whyte J, et al. Evoked potential assessment: Utility in prognosis of chronic head injury. Arch Phys Med Rehabil 1989; 70:189–193.

24. Hume AL, Cant BR. Central somatosensory conduction after head injury. Ann Neurol 1981; 10:411–419.

25. Cant BR, Hume AL, Judson JA, et al. The assessment of severe head injury by short-latency somatosensory and brain-stem auditory evoked potentials. Electroencephalogr Clin Neurophysiol 1986; 65:188–195.

26. Anderson DC, Bundlie S, Rockswold GL. Multimodality evoked potentials in closed head trauma. Arch Neurol 1984; 41:369–374.

27. Courchesne E, Elmasian R, Yeung-Courschense R. Electrophysiological correlates of cognitive processing: P3b and Nc, basic, clinical, and developmental research. In: Halliday AM, Butler SR, Paul R, eds. A Textbook of Clinical Neurophysiology. New York: John Wiley & Sons, 1987;645–676.

28. Zapulla RA. Fundamentals and applications of quantified electrophysiology. In: Zapulla RA, LeFever FF, Jaeger J, et al., eds. Windows on the brain–neuropsychology's technological frontiers. Ann NY Acad Sci 1991; 620:1–21.

29. Sgro JA, Emerson RG, Stanton PC. Advanced techniques of evoked potential acquisition and processing. In: Chiappa KH, ed. Evoked Potentials in Clinical Medicine, ed 2. NY: Raven Press, 1990;609–629.

30. Eisen A, Roberts K, Lawrence PD. Morphological measurement of the SEP using a dynamic time warping algorithm. Electroencephalogr Clin Neurophysiol 1986; 65:136–141.

31. Madhaven GP, deBruin H, Upton ARM. Single Stimulus Evoked Potential. : Departments of Medicine, Electrical and Computer Engineering, McMaster University, 1985. (Internal report No.:BMSP-EP 03-85.)

32. Brenner D, Williamson SJ, Kaufman L. Visually evoked magnetic fields of the human brain. Science 1975; 190:480–482.

33. Kaufman L, Okada Y, Brenner D, et al. On the relation between somatic evoked potentials and fields. Int J Neurosci 1981; 15:223–239.

34. Okada Y, Kaufman L, Brenner D, et al. Modulation transfer functions of the human visual system revealed by magnetic field measurements. Vision Res 1982; 22:319–333.

35. Swinney KR, Wikswo JP. A calculation of the magnetic field of a nerve action potential. Biophys J 1980; 32:719–731.

36. Wikswo JP. Recent developments in the measurement of magnetic fields from isolated nerves and muscles. J Appl Physiol 1981; 52:2554–2559.

37. Williamson SJ, Kaufman L. Evoked cortical magnetic fields. In: Erne SN, Halbohn H-D, Lubbig H, eds. Biomagnetism. Berlin: Walter de Gruyter, 1981.

38. Williamson SJ, Kaufman L. Analysis of neuromagnetic signals. In: Gevins AS, Redmand A, eds. Methods of Analysis of Brain Electrical and Magnetic Signals. Elsevier Science, 1987;217–230.

39. Strauss MB, ed. Familiar Medical Quotations. Boston: Little, Brown, 1968.

# Visual Evoked Potentials

YASOMA CHALLENOR

Visual stimuli that evoke the electrical response that we record for purposes of clinical electrophysiologic evaluation enter the visual system by way of a specific visual field of reference. Next they traverse the cornea, aqueous humor, pupil, lens, vitreous humor, retina, optic disc and nerve, and then the optic chiasm and tracts, lateral geniculate bodies, and the optic radiations, which terminate in the complexities of the visual cortex. Because temporal retinal fibers enter the ipsilateral optic tract and nasal retinal fibers cross the chiasm to enter the contralateral optic tract, visual input from the right visual field enters the left visual tract, and vice versa. As the optic radiations continue posteriorly into the occipital lobes, their fibers curve medially around the posterior horns of the lateral ventricles, to terminate in the primary visual cortices. Each of these structures and pathways may cause changes in the characteristics of the electrical events recorded over the scalp. In general, the electrodiagnostician needs to be sure of the integrity of structures anterior to the optic disc, to interpret test results properly.[1]

The earliest experience with visual evoked potential (VEP) testing involved the use of stroboscopic flash responses. These strobe- or flash-elicited VEPs still offer some clinical utility in revealing whether visual pathways from the retina to the visual cortex are intact in patients in coma or under general anesthesia. The large variation in waveform characteristics between subjects, as well as the relative insensitivity of this type of testing

to visual pathology of peripheral or central etiology, has made it less meaningful than the pattern-reversal stimulus, which has supplanted the flash.[2] A reversible black-and-white checkerboard pattern evokes potentials whose waveform and latencies show substantially less variability and smaller standard deviation than the corresponding components of the flash-evoked response.[3] The checkerboard pattern-reversal maintains constant stimulus luminance throughout, with reversal rates usually at two or three per second. Monocular full-field stimulation for each eye allows interocular comparison of latency and amplitude. Half-field stimulation may also be used. Because of the anatomic characteristics described earlier, a VEP abnormality recorded on stimulating one eye only must be caused by a problem anterior to the chiasm. If symmetric abnormalities are found, the crossed nature of the visual pathways does not permit localization of the lesion except to the areas posterior to the chiasm.

## Test Procedure

The test subject is seated comfortably, preferably with a headrest on the chair to help relax the paracervical, facial, and scalp muscles. The jaw must also be relaxed, to minimize synergistic paracervical muscle use. The pattern-reversal generator, usually a television screen, is placed with the center of the test pattern at a horizontal distance

286

of 1 m from the subject's nasion. If the subject wears corrective lenses, they should be used during the examination unless the uncorrected visual acuity is 20/50 or better. Some electrodiagnosticians accept uncorrected vision up to 20/100, but there is an inverse relationship between better acuity and the latency of the major potential, and a direct relationship between better acuity and the amplitude of the major potential obtained.[4] The subject is instructed to maintain visual fixation on the center of the screen no matter what may be happening nearby. A small dot or cross placed at the center of the screen aids fixation. The clinician observes the patient throughout the test run, to see that he or she maintains fixation. *Recording electrodes* are placed on the scalp at $O_z$ (or at 2 cm above the inion referred to $C_z$), and additional channels are recorded from $O_1$, $O_2$, and $P_z$ referred to $C_z$ (Figure 12A-1) The ground may be at $F_z$ or may be linked ear electrodes, if multimodality studies are being done. Additional electrodes spanning laterally across the occipital area ($L_5$, $L_{10}$, $R_5$, $R_{10}$) may be applied if half-field stimulation is being used. Half-field stimulation requires a high degree of cooperation to sustain fixation (even a small shift in fixation defeats the half-field input), so some electrodiagnosticians feel that the technique is less useful than careful perimetry.[1]

*Test parameters* for the examination include amplification greater than 20,000; in fact, as much as 100,000 may be needed. Filters are set 0.8 to 2 Hz low cutoff and 100 to 300 Hz high cutoff. The filter setting used in standardization of norms for a given laboratory should then be used consistently, as the latency of the major potential ($P_{100}$) may be altered by a change in filter setting.[5] The averager is set to analyze at least 300 msec, and at least 100 stimuli should be averaged. Each trial should be repeated to show consistency of the waveforms. The luminance or contrast adjustment from the television screen and the light in the laboratory should be noted during standardization of norms and maintained consistently thereafter. The $P_{100}$ latency is inversely related to the luminance from the screen, and the amplitude varies directly with changes in luminance. Pupil size affects how much light reaches the retina, and miotic pupils may prolong latency of the $P_{100}$. In routine testing, miotic or mydriatic pupils should not be compared to normal ones.

Test runs should include both large and small checks. Small checks subtending 20′ of or less visual arc represent an optimal challenge to the foveal area, accounting for up to 80% of the VEP amplitude (Figure 12A-2).[6] This correlates with the projection of the fibers from the central 3 to 6 degrees of the visual field to the surface of the occipital lobes. Surface recording electrodes are placed on the scalp directly over this area. In contrast, large checks stimulate parafoveal areas optimally[7]; fibers from the peripheral (parafoveal) retina give projections that end deep in the calcarine fissure (Figure 12A-3). The pattern-reversal rate should be 2 to 3 Hz; at faster rates the waveforms become less distinct. Age has been observed to have little effect on VEP latency until after the fifth decade, when there is a slight, steady increase in latency. Female gender is associated with shorter mean latencies than male gender[9] so laboratory norms may be established according to gender groups. The dominant eye tends to have a slightly larger potential, but, more significantly, the latency for the dominant eye is shorter. Thus, normal values for interocular differences should be included in standardization of norms. Each eye is tested with large and small check sizes, usually expressed as the size of visual arc subtended by one check.

*The waveform* obtained in response to the pattern-reversal stimulus has an initial negative deflection followed by the major positive deflection, commonly called the $P_{100}$ potential. It is this larger positive deflection, which is obtainable in 100% of normal subjects, whose latency is measured (Figure 12A-4). Amplitude is measured from the peak of the initial negative to the peak of the $P_{100}$ potential.

## Clinical Applications of Visual Evoked Potentials

VEPs can be used to distinguish retinal disease from disorders occurring at the optic nerve and beyond, by recording abnormalities of latency and amplitude on focal macular stimulation (smallest check size) and preservation of normal responses to whole-field stimulation by larger checks. In some instances, latency may be minimally prolonged, but the waveform amplitude may be di-

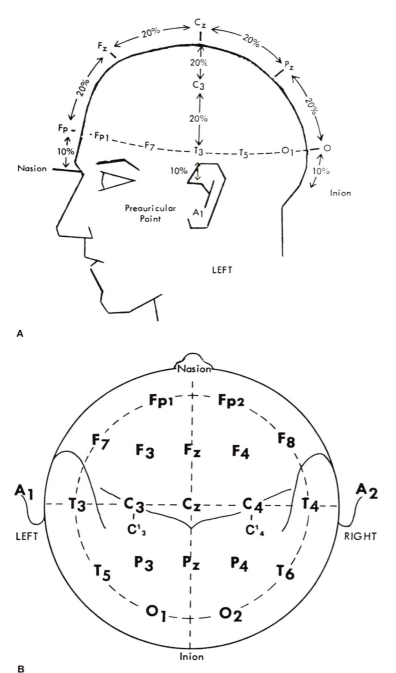

**Figure 12A-1.** (*A*) Standard landmarks in the International 10-20 system of electrode placement: lateral view. (*B*) Standard electrode locations in the International 10-20 System: view from above. (From Rinzler G. The 10-20 system booklet.)

minished.[1,6] *Glaucoma* has been reported to show abnormalities in both latency and amplitude, but these abnormalities are not always present.[10,11] *Optic nerve lesions,* whether induced by ischemia, toxins, inflammation, compressive mass, or de-

myelination, may produce delays in latency or distortions in waveform or amplitude. Ischemia, toxins, and compressive lesions may decrease amplitude and distort waveform to a greater extent than they prolong latency.[12-17] In contrast, inflam-

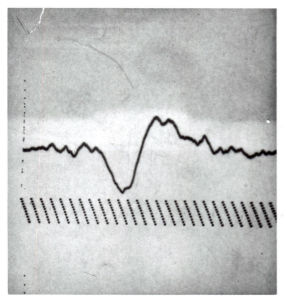

**Figure 12A-2.** Normal VEP obtained from bilateral stimulation with small checks reversal; each check subtends 43′ of visual arc. Each staircase = 10 msec. The height of each staircase = 5μV; normal amplitude 9 μV mean (2.5–20μV).

97% of patients satisfying the McAlpine criteria for definite M S as showing abnormalities in the VEP, with 100% of probable MS and 92% of possible MS showing VEP abnormality, for an overall occurrence of abnormality in MS patients of 92%.[29,30] Other observers have reported overall abnormality in MS varying from 50% to 88% (Figure 12A-5, 6).[28]

Carroll and coworkers[31] performed serial VEPs over a mean interval of 28 months on 116 patients with MS and optic neuritis (19 with optic neuritis; 64, 28, and five patients with, respectively, clinically definite, probable, and possible MS). They found the final overall incidence of VEP abnormality to be 91%. Of note, 53 of the MS patients were visually asymptomatic, yet 36% of them showed VEP abnormalities. This suggested that VEP could be used as a means of detecting subclinical lesions.[31] Chiappa reported the incidence of clinically unsuspected lesions of visual pathways in patients with MS to be 36% for probable MS and 9% for possible MS.[32] More strict criteria for test performance and interpretation may in-

mation, thyroid ophthalmopathy, subacute combined degeneration, sarcoidosis, and demyelination cause predominantly a delay in latency.[18–22] Quite early in VEP testing optic neuritis was noted to cause delays in latency as well as a variety of abnormalities described in the literature.[1,23]

The amplitude of the response obtained in the presence of isolated optic neuritis seems to improve with clinical gains; latency change does not.[24]

In general, a high contrast pattern reversal VEP causes delay in latency in approximately 80% of patients with *multiple sclerosis* (MS), whether or not there is a history of optic neuritis.[25,26] MS patients with *normal vision* and no history of optic neuritis show delays in latency 38% of the time, with the diagnostic yield increasing if the stimulus contrast is lowered.[27] A somewhat different percentage of abnormality observed by different authors may, in part, be due to differences in examining technique.[28] On the other hand, the protean pattern of plaque formation and demyelination in MS may also be responsible, in part, for differences in VEP results. Halliday has reported

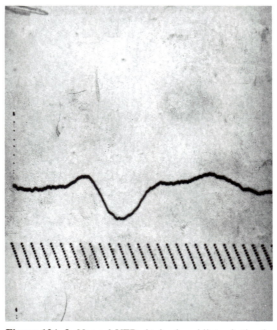

**Figure 12A-3.** Normal VEP obtained on bilateral stimulation with large check reversal: each check subtends 172′ of visual arc. Calibration as for Figure 12A-2.

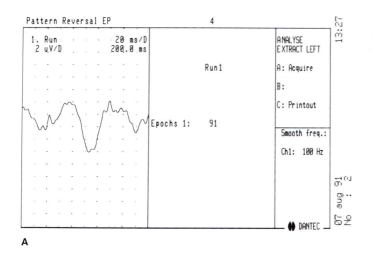

A

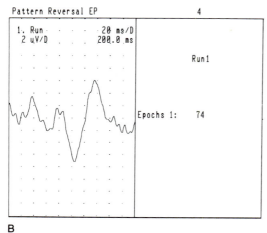

B

**Figure 12A-4.** (*A*) Normal VEP from the left eye of a healthy 28-year-old volunteer. $P_{100} = 108$ msec. (*B*) Right eye of same volunteer. $P_{100} = 105$ msec.

crease the yield of abnormalities in the "possible MS" group.[27,33,34]

As with any new diagnostic modality, many pathologic conditions have been explored with VEPs, and many conditions have been found to be associated with changes in VEP amplitude, latency, or morphology. Dominant optic atrophy, Leber's optic atrophy, and optic nerve hypoplasia have reportedly shown prolongations in VEP latency, with marked diminution in amplitude.[35–38] Papilledema[39,40] and pseudotumor cerebri[41] may show moderate prolongations in latency. Ischemic optic neuropathy affects VEP amplitude earlier and more severely than latency.[42,43] Vitamin $B_{12}$ deficiency, which causes demyelination, prolongs VEP latency[21,44], as may chronic inflammatory demyelinating polyneuropathy.[21] Parkinson's dis-

ease has been shown to produce VEP abnormality, which appears to be correlated with the severity of the condition.[46,47] A number of heredofamilial degenerative disorders, such as Huntington's disease,[48, 49] Friedreich's ataxia,[50,51] and hereditary spastic ataxia,[52] have been reported to show amplitude changes in the VEP, and Friedreich's ataxia also shows significant increased VEP latency. A wide variety of other conditions screened by VEP testing have associated abnormalities,[1,7,53] and no doubt many more will be listed in the future.

*Cortical blindness* has been defined as loss of appreciation of light and dark, loss of optokinetic nystagmus, loss of all reported visual sensation with preserved pupillary responses, extraocular motility, and normal findings on retinal examination.[54] Children with cortical blindness have been

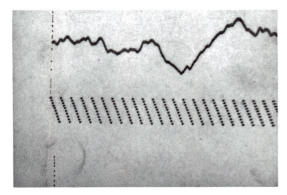

**Figure 12A-5.** A 27-year-old woman had a history of left sixth cranial nerve palsy, and both horizontal and vertical nystagmus for 6 weeks. Subjective gait unsteadiness was felt, without any clear clinical ataxia on neurologic examination. VEP for the left eye (check size subtends 43') was 128 msec. The right eye was normal. MRI showed small plaques scattered throughout the frontal lobes, pons, and midbrain, findings compatible with MS.

are usually used, but they were able to either decrease the amplitude or obliterate the response (four of 15 subjects). This is not an isolated observation,[61] but it does raise issues relating to techniques for conducting the examination. The examiner usually places her or himself in such a way that the patient's fixation of gaze can be observed. Theoretically, voluntary defocusing should also be observable, as long as check size is not made excessively small.[62] In order to eliminate factors implicated in voluntary alteration of potentials, Kupersmith suggested that patients suspected of malingering first be given mydriatic drops, then fitted with the correction that direct refraction (in the ophthalmology or neuroophthalmology testing suite) reveals to be appropriate. The resulting evoked potential may then be interpreted with more certainty.[1] Alternatively, the presence of a later $P_{300}$ potential in a patient who states that she

reported to have abnormalities in VEPs less than half of the time, unless cortical mapping techniques are used, in which case the rate of abnormality is 100%.[55] This may reflect the widespread arrangement of the visual primary and association cortices over the occipital lobes; the primary cortex may sustain a significant loss with preservation of the association cortex, and vice versa. The percentage of abnormality on routine VEP testing is said to increase if small checks are used[56] or if sinusoidal grating, rather than the checkerboard reversal stimulus, is used.[57] It has also been reported that large areas of occipital cortex may be lost, with preservation of the electrical volley approaching the missing area via the optic radiations, to give a preserved though morphologically simplified VEP response.[58] Celesia has suggested that both preservation of VEP responses and residual clinical vision depend on whether or not portions of cortical area 17 are preserved.[59] One corollary of these observations is that use of VEPs to distinguish real from *factitious visual loss* requires testing with small checks that subtend less than 20' of visual arc. Even then, it has been observed that experimental subjects can apparently maintain fixation on the checkerboard pattern while meditating, daydreaming, or focusing beyond the screen, to "avoid perceiving the stimulus."[60] These subjects were challenged with smaller check sizes than

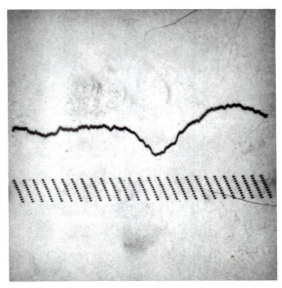

**Figure 12A-6.** A 42-year-old woman who had a history of intermittent diplopia for 2 years had not sought medical attention. She vaguely recalled one episode of visual disturbance described as impaired color perception in one eye lasting a week, which disappeared before she could schedule a physician appointment. She complained of left hemisensory deficit of 2 months' duration, although clinical testing of light touch, pinprick, vibration position, and temperature perception were normal, but deep tendon reflexes were noted to be bilaterally hyperactive in arms and legs, with flexor plantar responses. The VEP was 153 msec on the left (illustrated) and 107 msec on the right.

or he cannot see is indicative of functional vision loss,[63] because the $P_{300}$ is elicited by unpredictable or infrequent stimuli and cannot be voluntarily suppressed by a patient who is concentrating on a task. Using randomly timed stimuli of an ON-OFF checkerboard may make it more difficult to use deceptive strategems.[64]

The development of electrodiagnosis has been a steady extension of neurophysiologic examinations cephalad along the neuraxis, starting with electrical stimulation of muscle, to nerve stimulation for conduction velocity determinations, to sensory pathway stimulation for determination of evoked potentials. Now that sensory evoked potential capacity is extending in time to include later potentials that may reflect aspects of cortical processing, this exciting area of investigation will be of considerable use in the future.

# References

1. Kupersmith MJ. Visual evoked potentials: Enhancing utility. Semin Neurol 1986; 6:217–230.
2. Kooi KA, Güvener AM, Bagchi K. Visual evoked responses in lesions of the optic pathways. Neurology (Minneap) 1965; 15:841–854.
3. Halliday AM. The visual evoked potential in healthy subjects. In: Halliday AM, ed. Evoked Potentials in Clinical Testing. London: Churchill Livingstone, 1982;71–120.
4. Sokol S, Moskowitz A. Effect of retinal blur on the peak latency of the pattern evoked potential. Vision Res 1981; 21:1279–1286.
5. Yiannikas C, Walsh JC. Recording variables affecting the pattern reversal visual evoked potential. Part B—Bandpass. Am J EEG Technol; 1983.
6. Yiannikas C, Walsh JC. The variation of the pattern shift visual evoked potential with the size of the stimulus field. Electroencephalogr Clin Neurophysiol 1983; 55:427–435.
7. Chiappa KH. Pattern-shift visual evoked potentials: Methodology. In: Chiappa KH, ed. Evoked Potentials in Clinical Medicine, ed 2. NY: Raven Press, 1990;75–76.
8. Stockard JJ, Hughes JF, Sharbrough FW. Visually evoked potentials to electronic pattern reversal: Latency variations with gender, age and technical factors. Am J EEG Technol 1979; 19:171–204.
9. Celesia GG, Kaufman D, Cone S. Effects of age and sex on pattern electroretinograms and visual evoked potentials. Electroencephalogr Clin Neurophysiol 1987; 68:161–171.
10. Towle VL, Maskowitz A, Sokol S, et al. The visual evoked potential in glaucoma and ocular hypertension. Ophthalmol Vis Sci 1983; 24:175–183.
11. Huber C, Wagner T. Electrophysiologic evidence for glaucomatous lesions in the optic nerve. Ophthalmic Res 1978; 10:22–29.
12. Wilson WB. Visual evoked response differentiation of ischemic optic neuritis from the optic neuritis of multiple sclerosis. Am J Ophthalmol 1978; 86:530–535.
13. Cox TA, Thompson HS, Hayreh SS, et al. Visual evoked potentials and pupillary signs. Arch Ophthalmol 1982; 100:1603–1607.
14. Ikeda H, Tremain KE, Sanders MD. Neurophysiological investigation in optic nerve disease: Combined assessment of the visual evoked response and electroretinogram. Br J Ophthalmol 1978; 62:227–239.
15. Kupersmith MJ, Weiss PA, Carr RE. The visual evoked potential in tobacco, alcohol and nutritional amblyopia. Am J Ophthalmol 1983; 95:307–314.
16. Halliday AM, Halliday E, Kriss A, et al. The pattern-evoked potential in compression of the anterior visual pathways. Brain 1976; 99:357–374.
17. Feinsod M, Selhorst JB, Hoyt WF, et al. Monitoring optic nerve function during craniotomy. J Neurosurg 1976; 44:29–31.
18. Streletz LJ, Chambers RA, Bae SH, et al. Visual evoked potentials in sarcoidosis. Neurology (NY) 1891; 31:1545–1548.
19. Carroll WM, Mastaglia FL. Leber's optic neuropathy, a clinical and visual evoked potential study of affected and asymptomatic members of a six generation family. Brain 1979; 102:559–580.
20. Wijgaarde R, Van Lith GHM. Pattern EPS in endocrine orbitopathy. Doc Ophthalmol 1979; 48:327–332.
21. Troncoso J, Mancall EL, Schatz NJ. Visual evoked responses in pernicious anemia. Arch Neurol 1979; 36:168–169.
22. Bodnis-Wollner I, Korczyn AD. Dissociated sensory loss and visual evoked potentials in a patient with pernicious anemia. Mt Sinai J Med 1980; 47:579–582.
23. Halliday AM, McDonald WI, Mushin J. Delayed visual evoked response in optic neuritis. Lancet 1972; 1:1982–1985.
24. Halliday AM, McDonald WI, Mushin J. Delayed pattern evoked responses in optic neuritis in relation to visual acuity. Trans Ophthalmol Soc U K 1973; 93:315–324.
25. Sharokhi F, Chiappa FKH, Young RR. Pattern shift

visual evoked responses. Arch Neurol 1978; 35:65–71.

26. Zeese JA. Pattern visual evoked responses in multiple sclerosis. Arch Neurol 1977; 34:314–316.
27. Kupersmith MJ, Nelson JI, Seiple WH, et al. The 20/20 eye in multiple sclerosis. Neurology (Cleve) 1983; 33:1015–1020.
28. Halliday AM. The VEP in the investigation of diseases of the optic nerve. In: Halliday AM, ed. Evoked Potentials in Clinical Testing. London: Churchill Livingstone, 1982;209–210.
29. Halliday AM, McDonald WI, Mushin J. Visual evoked responses in the diagnosis of multiple sclerosis. Br Med J 1973; 4:661–664.
30. McAlpine D, Lumsden CE, Acheson ED, eds. Multiple Sclerosis—A Reappraisal, ed 2. London: Churchill Livingstone, 1972.
31. Carroll WM, Halliday AM, Barrett G, et al. Serial VEPs and visual pathway demyelination: A study of 116 patients with multiple sclerosis and isolated optic neuritis. In: Nodar RH, Barber C., Evoked Potentials II. Boston: Butterworths, 1984;310–318.
32. Chiappa KH. Pattern shift evoked potentials—interpretation. In: Chiappa KH, ed. Evoked Potentials in Clinical Medicine, ed 2. New York: Raven, 1990;111–134.
33. Carroll WM, Halliday AM, Kriss A. Improvements in the accuracy of pattern evoked potentials in the diagnosis of visual pathway disease. Neuroophthalmology (Amsterdam) 1982; 2:237–253.
34. Oishi M, Yamada T, Dickins S, et al. Visual evoked potentials by different check sizes in patients with multiple sclerosis. Neurology 1985; 35:1461–1465.
35. Kline LB, Glaser JS. Dominant optic nerve atrophy: The clinical profile. Arch Ophthalmol 1979; 97:1680–1682.
36. Carroll WM, Mastaglia FL. Leber's optic neuropathy: A clinical and visual evoked potential study of affected and asymptomatic members of a six-generation family. Brain 1979; 102:559–580.
37. Dorfman LJ, Nikoskelainen E, Rosenthal AR, et al. Visual evoked potentials in Leber's hereditary optic neuropathy. Neurology 1977; 1:565–568.
38. Sprague JB, Wilson WB. Electrophysiologic findings in bilateral optic nerve hypoplasia. 1977; 99:1028–1030.
39. Onofrij M, Bodnis-Wollner I, Mylin L. Visual evoked potential latencies in papilledema and hydrocephalus. Neuroophthalmology 1981; 2:85–91.
40. Kirkham TH, Coupland SG. Abnormal electroretinograms and visual evoked potentials in chronic papilledema using time-difference analysis. Can J Neurol Sci 1981; 8:243–248.
41. Sorensen PS, Trojaborg W, Gjerris F, et al. Visual evoked potentials in pseudotumor cerebri. Arch Neurol 1985; 42:150–152.
42. Glaser JS, Laflamme P. The visual evoked response: methodology and application in optic nerve disease. In: Thompson HS, ed. Topics in Neuro-ophthalmology. Baltimore: Williams & Wilkins, 1979;199.
43. Ikeda H, Tremain KE, Sanders MD. Neurophysiological investigation in optic nerve disease: Combined assessment of the visual evoked response and electroretinogram. Br J Ophthalmol 1978; 62:227–239.
44. Hennerici M. Dissociated foveal and parafoveal visual evoked responses in subacute combined degeneration. Arch Neurol 1985; 42:130–132.
45. Pakalnis AB, Drake ME, Barohn RJ, et al. Evoked potentials in chronic inflammatory demyelinating polyneuropathy. Arch Neurol 1988; 45:1014–1016.
46. Bodnis-Wollner I, Yahr M, Thornton J. Interocular VEP latency differences and the effect of treatment in Parkinson's disease. Electroencephalogr Clin Neurophysiol 1980; 50:220–228.
47. Kupersmith MJ, Shakin E, Siegel IM, et al. Visual system abnormalities in patients with Parkinson's disease. Arch Neurol 1982; 39:284–286.
48. Ellenberger C, Petro DJ, Ziegler SB. The visually evoked potential in Huntington's disease. Neurology 1978; 28:95–97.
49. Oepen G, Goerr M, Theoden U. Visual (VEP) and somatosensory (SSEP) evoked potentials in Huntington's chorea. Electroencephalogr Clin Neurophysiol 1981; 51:666–670.
50. Carroll WM, Kriss A, Baraitser M, et al. The incidence and nature of visual pathway involvement in Friedreich's ataxia: A clinical and visual evoked potential study of 22 patients. Brain 1980; 103:413–434.
51. Kirkham TH, Coupland G: An electroretinal and visual evoked potential study in Friedreich's ataxia. Can J Neurol Sci 1981; 8:289–291.
52. Livingstone IR, Mastaglia FL, Edis R, et al. Visual involvement in Friedreich's ataxia and hereditary spastic ataxia. Arch Neurol 1981; 38:75–79.
53. Sokol S. Visual evoked potentials. In: Aminoff MJ, ed. Electrodiagnosis in Clinical Neurology. London: Churchill Livingstone, 1986;441–466.
54. Marquis DG. Effects of removal of visual cortex in mammals with observations on the retention of light discrimination in dogs. Proc Assoc Res Nerv Mental Dis 1934; 13:558–592.
55. Whiting S, Jan JE, Wong PKH, et al. Permanent cortical visual impairment in children. Devel Med Child Neurol 1985; 27:730–739.
56. Chiappa KH, Ropper AH. Evoked potentials in

clinical medicine. N Engl J Med 1982; 306:1140–1150.

57. Chiappa KH. Pattern shift visual evoked potentials: Interpretation. In: Chiappa KH, ed. Evoked Potentials in Clinical Medicine, ed 2. New York: Raven Press, 1990;147–148.

58. Bodnis-Wollner I, Atkin A, Raab E, et al. Visual association cortex and vision in man: Pattern evoked potentials in a blind boy. Science 1977; 198:629–631.

59. Celesia GG, Bushnell MD, Cone T, et al. Cortical blindness and residual vision. Neurology 1991; 41:862–869.

60. Baumgartner J, Epstein CM. Voluntary alteration of VEPs. Ann Neurol 1982; 12:475–478.

61. Cohen SN, Syndulko K, Tourtelotte WW, et al.: Volitional manipulation of visual evoked potential latency. Neurology 1982; 32 (part A):A209.

62. Chiappa KH, Yiannikas. Voluntary alteration of evoked potentials? Ann Neurol 1982; 12:496–497.

63. Towle VL, Sutcliffe E, Sokol S. Diagnosing functional visual deficits with the $P_{300}$ component of the visual evoked potential. Arch Ophthalmol 1985; 103:47–50.

64. Sokol S. Visual evoked potentials. In: Aminoff MJ, ed. Electrodiagnosis in Clinical Neurology. London: Churchill Livingstone, 1986.

# Auditory Evoked Potentials

ARMINIUS CASSVAN

In the 1980s evoked potential studies emerged as invaluable clinical tools for identifying central nervous system lesions. Using noninvasive procedures, these studies not only provide an objective measurement of different sensory functions, but also help to pinpoint the site of cortical and subcortical lesions, at times with striking accuracy.

The brain stem auditory evoked potentials (BAEPs) are just one of the auditory evoked potential (AEP) modalities. BAEPs are of much utility in accurate diagnosis of brain stem tumors and in the particular case of acoustic neuromas may be able to establish the diagnosis. In addition, BAEPs are very helpful in predicting whether coma is metabolic (as a rule reversible) or structural (irreversible) and in the diagnosis of MS.

AEP studies are important in rehabilitation medicine, as clinicians often treat patients with major functional deficiencies such as incoordination and deep sensory involvement, as well as ataxia and balance problems.

## Classification

Because several varieties of AEPs have been identified, discussion of these electrical events should start with an overview of their wide spectrum. The most useful classification is based on latencies. The early (short and very short) AEPs are recorded in the first 10 msec and include the most clinically useful, BAEPs. In addition, the early AEPs include the very short electrocochleogram (ECochG) components and the similarly short frequency-following response (FFR), both at present discussed mostly in research papers.

The middle latency AEPs are not used routinely in clinical practice, though they have some relevance in cortical deafness[1] or coma.[2] They range from 10 to 60 msec and include the neurogenic middle latency responses (MLR) and the myogenic or sonomotor responses. Unless the subject is completely relaxed, as a rule MLRs are masked by the myogenics.

The long- and very long latency AEPs range from 60 msec to a few seconds. Of the various long-latency components, the $P_{300}$, known also as $P_3$, processing potential or cognitive potential, is by far the most important clinically. Its applications in neurology, psychiatry, and psychology are increasing in number. According to a recent study, long-latency responses seem also to help in diagnosing chronic alcoholism.[3]

Late or long latency AEPS (more than 60 msec) also include the vertex or slow cortical potential. Other potentials, of less than 1.5 second latency, are known as *contingent negative variation* and the *sustained potential*. A very late potential is the *galvanic skin response*.

The entire spectrum of early, middle, and long latency AEPs is presented in Table 12B-1. A more recent classification of the AEPs describes 27 waves in terms of site and origin, designation, abbreviation, and significance (Table 12B-2).

**Table 12B-1.** Characteristics of Auditory Evoked Potentials

| Classification | Latency | Evoked Response | Abbreviations | DC Potential | Waveform Nomenclature | Unaffected by level of arousal |
|---|---|---|---|---|---|---|
| Early | <10 msec | Electrocochleo-gram | ECochG | Yes (SP) | Cochlear micro-phonic (CM) | |
| | | | ECoG | | Summating poten-tial (SP) | + |
| | | | | | Component I or N$_1$ and N$_2$ | + |
| | | Brainstem evoked potential | BSEP BAEP | | Components or waves I-VII | + |
| | | Frequency follow-ing response | FFR | | | |
| Middle | 10–60 msec | Myogenic | | – | | |
| | | Sonomotor | | – | | |
| | | Postauricular muscle response | PAM | | | |
| | | Central nervous system responses | | | N$_0$, P$_\phi$, N$_a$, P$_a$, N$_b$, P$_1$ | + |
| Late | >60 sec | Vertex | | | N$_1$-P$_2$-N$_2$ | |
| | | K complex | | | | |
| | | P300 | | | P$_3$ | |
| | <1.5 sec | Contingent nega-tive variation | CNV | Yes | | |
| | | Sustained potential | | Yes | | |
| | 1.5–4.5 sec | Galvanic skin response | GSR | | | |

(From Halliday AM. Evoked Potentials in Clinical Testing. Edinburgh: Churchill Livingstone, 1982.)

AEPs may also be conveniently divided into exogenous and endogenous components (Table 12B-3). The nomenclature is not the same for Table 12B-1 and Tables 12B-2 and 12B-3, particularly for the late and very late potentials. Although at present the brainstem auditory evoked potentials (BAEPS) are the only evoked potentials used in most clinical practice situations, it will be useful to discuss the entire spectrum of responses (potentials) and to provide some answers to questions such as why these potentials occur and what is their relevance in rehabilitation medicine.

## Anatomic-Physiologic Basis

Mechanical sound waves are transformed into action potentials within the ear. Different nerve fibers and cells, part of the auditory pathway, are responsible for producing the various component waves.

The cochlea, which consists of a system of canals and membranes, converts sounds into action potentials (Fig. 12B-1). The sound travels toward the footplates of the stapes, located at the upper region of the cochlea. The cochlear duct is located between the scala vestibuli and the scala tympani. These anatomic structures communicate through the helicotrema. The basilar membrane hosts the organ of Corti and contains sensory cells known as *hair cells*. The cilia (sensory hairs) emanate from hair cells, which are covered by basilar membrane.

The locus theory of hearing[5] refers to oscillations that take place in the inner ear. According to this theory, high frequencies are reproduced in the region of the oval window and low frequencies at the tip of the cochlea. The footplate of the stapes

**Table 12B-2.** Survey of the Currently Most Important Auditory Evoked Potential Components; 27 Waves in Order of Site and Nature of Origin

| Number | Site and Nature of Origin | Designation | Abbreviation | Latency (msec) | Significance |
|---|---|---|---|---|---|
| | | *Electrocochleography* | | | |
| 1 | Presynaptic, inner ear | Microphone potential | CM (Cochlear microphonics) | 0 | Experimental audiology |
| 2 | | Summation potential | SM (Summating potential) | 0 | |
| 3 | Postsynaptic, acoustic nerve | Summation action potential | SAP | 1–2<br>1–2 | Audiology-auditory threshold determination |
| | | *Auditory evoked potentials (Postsynaptic)* | | | |
| 4–10 | Acoustic nerve, medulla, pons, and midbrain | Brainstem auditory evoked potential | BAEP waves I–VII and VIII | 1–8 | Auditory threshold determination<br>Topologic diagnosis |
| 11–16 | Area between midbrain and cortex | Middle auditory evoked potential | MAEP waves | | Auditory threshold<br>Topologic diagnosis |
| | | | No (N10) | 8–9 | |
| | | | Po (P12) | 12 | |
| | | | Na (N16) | 16 | |
| | | | Pa (P25) | 25 | |
| | | | Nb (N30) | 36 | |
| | | | Pb (P50) | 50 | |
| 17 | | 40 Hz response | | | Auditory threshold in low tone area |
| | Nuclear musculature myogenic composition | Sonomotor reflex response | SMRA | 7.4–30 | Unclear and doubtful |
| 18 | Postauricular musculature | | | Negative wave 11.8 ± 0.8<br>Positive wave 16.4 ± 0.7 | |
| 19 | Temporal musculature | | | Negative wave 17.2 ± 1.9<br>Positive wave 16.4 ± 0.7 | |
| 20 | Neck musculature | | | Beginning (7.4)<br>Negative waves 11.3 ± 0.2 and 24.6 ± 1.5<br>Positive waves 16.8 ± 2.4 and 33.8 ± 0.5 | |
| 21 | Frontal musculature | | | Variable, approx 30 | |
| 22–25 | Cortex | Late auditory evoked potential | LAEP waves P1 | 50–75 | Auditory threshold determination |
| | | | N1 | 100–150 | Neurologic and |
| | | | P2 | 175–200 | Neurophysiologic |
| | | | N2 | 200–250 | Research |
| 26 | Cortex and cortical projections | Processing potential | P300 | 280–360 | Psychiatry and Neuropsychology |
| 27 | | Anticipation wave | CNV (contingent negative variation) | Variable | |

(From Maurer K, et al. Evoked Potentials. Toronto: BC Decker, 1989.)

**Table 12B-3.** Division of AEP into Exogenous and Endogenous Parts

| |
|---|
| Exogenous potentials |
| ECochG |
| BAEP |
| MAEP |
| LAEP |
| 40 Hz response |
| |
| Endogenous potentials |
| CNV |
| P300 |
| Stand-by potential |
| Processing negativity |

(From Maurer K, et al. Evoked Potentials. Toronto: BC Decker, 1989.)

is the area where the oscillations start; they are then amplified by the middle ear. The external ear directs the sound while the middle ear serves to amplify the pressure and provides noise protection through muscle action. The oscillations are transmitted as traveling waves toward the canals and then to the basilar membrane of the organ of Corti. Condensation occurs when the footplate of the stapes moves inward while the basilar membrane moves downward toward the scala tympani. Rarefaction implies the reverse phenomenon, as the

**Figure 12B-1.** Maurer K, Lowitzsch K, Stohr M. Evoked Potentials. Toronto-Philadelphia: BC Decker Inc. 1989. Figure 1-2:5.

footplate moves outward and the basilar membrane upward toward the scala vestibuli. The equalization of pressure takes place through the round window.

The oscillations involve not only the basilar membrane but the organ of Corti as well, producing a shearing motion between the tectorial membrane and the cilia of the hair cells. As a result, metabolic, and consequently ionic, changes take place inside the sensory cells. When an appropriate stimulus with an adequate synchronizing potential such as a click acts at the interface of sensory cell and afferent nerve endings, individual action potentials above the threshold stimulus level unite in a volley of action potentials. Saltatory conduction, characteristic for myelinated fibers, directs these potentials along the acoustic nerve toward the central nervous system. If amplitude is sufficiently large, these potentials are recorded as wave N1, near-field technique (ECochG) and wave I, far-field technique (BAEP). Near-field recordings refer to the proximity of the recording site to the presumed neural generator, such as the skull for the visual evoked potentials and also most of the somatosensory evoked potentials and the external ear for ECochG. Far-field recordings deal with brain stem generators, generally.

## Auditory Evoked Potentials Other Than BAEPs

### Electrocochleography

ECochG is the recording of electrical potentials originating from the cochlea and cochlear nerve fibers following acoustic stimulation. Historically, the discovery of bioelectrical potentials in animals[6] was followed by the recording of the negative action potential in nerves.[7] The first published evoked potential recording[8] then led to the EEG, the recorded brain electrical potentials from the human scalp.[9] The year 1930 marked the discovery of electrical potentials of the cochlea[10] known as the *Wever-Bray effect* or *cochlear microphonia* (CM), which was initially thought to be generated by the auditory nerve. In the mid-1930s, Fromm and others[11] further studied cochlear potentials in humans. A technique that involved the insertion of a wire electrode through tympanic membrane perforations successfully recorded the CM from the niche of the round window and promontorium. In 1939, Andreev and coworkers[12] noted that the CM amplitude was too variable and that the potential could not be obtained in subjects with a hearing threshold above 50 dB.

ECochG reflects the electrical potentials of the cochlea and the acoustic nerve; in addition to the CM, a summating potential is also present. The CM and SP are not really of much help for hearing assessment, though they may contribute to the detection of the underlying pathologic condition. Conversely, the acoustic (eighth) nerve action potential is a reliable measure of the cochlear threshold and can be confidently used to estimate hearing (Figure 12B-2).

ECochG is currently of limited use. The technique involves placement of electrodes either through the tympanic membrane (transtympanic) or within the external auditory meatus (extratympanic). The latter technique is more widely used in clinical settings.[13–15] This extratympanic method increases the amplitude of wave I of the BAEP (neurally generated by the eighth nerve), which is advantageous in cases of moderate to severe hearing deficit when wave I cannot ordinarily be identified.[16] Wave I is discussed later in this chapter.

In 1984, the American Electroencephalographic Society recommended a two-channel recording montage when recording an ECochG. The montage consists of channel 1 connecting the mastoid ($M_i$) or earlobe ($A_1$) to the ipsilateral external auditory canal; channel 2 deals with the vertex ($C_z$) referenced to the ipsilateral mastoid ($M_i$) or earlobe ($A_1$). The above recording montage allows for the simultaneous recording of wave $N_1$ (same as wave I) of the ECochG and waves II to VII of the BAEPs, discussed later in this chapter.

### Frequency Following Response

The FFRs or potentials are electrical events that can be recorded directly or with surface electrodes (vertex to ipsilateral mastoid) from the brain stem of animals and humans. They have a fundamental frequency equal to that of the sinusoidal stimulus that elicits them. The latency of these responses is $5.5 \pm 1$ msec and they are superimposed on a slower component of about 10 msec latency (Figure 12B-3). The FFR can be elicited by tone bursts of frequencies up to 2 kHz. The amplitude decreases as the frequency increases. The FFRs can be obtained with intensities higher than 50 db but not lower than that. They can be elicited in infants, but only with difficulty in people aged 40 years or older.[16]

In practical terms, there are two FFRs. When using vertex ($C_z$) to ipsilateral mastoid ($M_i$) montage, known as V derivation, and ipsilateral mastoid ($M_i$) to contralateral mastoid ($C_e$) montage,

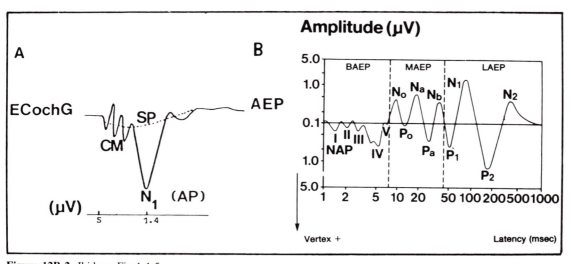

**Figure 12B-2.** Ibidem, Fig 1-1:5.

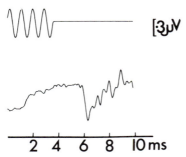

$[3\mu V$

2  4  6  8  10 ms

**Figure 12B-3.** Halliday AM. Evoked Potentials in Clinical Testing. Edinburgh-London-Melbourne-New York: Churchill Livingstone 1982. Fig 10-2:347.

known as H derivation, monaural stimulation with frequencies lower than 0.5 kHz produces two distinct responses: FFR1 and FFR2. The latency difference between them is 1.4 to 1.8 msec. The components are not dependent on the intensity or frequency of the stimulus. There is a correlation between FFR and BAEPs in that the latency difference between $FFR_1$ and $FFR_2$ correlates with the interval between waves III and V of the BAEPs.[17] The evidence points to at least two generators for the FFR, which may be the same generators as for the BAEPs following click stimuli. Using direct depth recordings, it appears that the FFRs represent activity in the superior olivary complex and inferior colliculus. In contradistinction, with surface recordings, only the activity from the inferior colliculus is detected.

Literature on FFRs is not as abundant as that on BAEPs, perhaps because FFR testing is more difficult and requires greater technical skill. The lesser clinical importance of the FFR, as compared to the BAEPs, is another valid reason. The possibility of confusing FFR with the CM should be kept in mind. Both could also be confused with the stimulus artifact.

## Brain Stem Auditory Evoked Potentials

### General Considerations

The BAEPs are five volume-conducted neurogenic potentials (I to V) recorded from the scalp (vertex positive), which originate in the auditory pathway in the brainstem. Together with waves VI and VII, of uncertain origin, these waves occur during the first 10 msec of the spectrum (Figure 12B-4). The stimuli of choice for investigating cochlear nerve and brainstem auditory pathways are abrupt unfiltered clicks delivered through a pair of earphones. While adequate for neurologic studies, they are not recommended for audiologic examination. The clicks contain a wide spectrum of tone frequencies that act mainly through their high-frequency component, whereas in audiology tones with lower frequency are paramount. The click stimuli are generally delivered at a rate of 10 per second, which as a rule results in well-defined evoked potentials. Higher rates may also be used to identify subtle abnormalities.

Two major characteristics differentiate BAEPs from other types of evoked responses. The first can be described as chemical invulnerability, in other words resistance to most of the drugs, to which should be added changes in arousal level or sleep, including reversible comatose states. The second is anatomic specificity. While the validity of the first characteristic is still of value, that of the second appears to be questionable, at least in terms of rigid definition. Indeed, today the one wave–one neural generator theory is seen as obsolete. More recent research suggests that there can be more than one generator for one wave and more than one wave for one generator.[18]

There is general consensus about which BAEPs represent specific neural events. The possible role of the glia as a supportive neural substrate has been discarded in view of a documented too long time constant for glia activation to be directly relevant.[19] The literature has traditionally described neural generators anatomically as follows: the auditory, eighth nerve, for wave I; the cochlear nucleus for wave II; the superior olivary complex for wave III; the lateral lemniscus for wave IV; and the inferior colliculus of the midbrain for wave V (Figure 12B-5). Subsequent work on generator sites has demonstrated that wave II represents a more proximal segment of the eighth nerve rather than the cochlear nucleus[21] while wave V may be generated from the lateral lemniscus rather than at the inferior colliculus level.[22]

Physiologically, graded postsynaptic potentials are elicited in the dendrites or soma at the brain stem auditory pathways level and then electrically transmitted over portions of the postsynaptic cell. Like similar neural elements, postsynaptic poten-

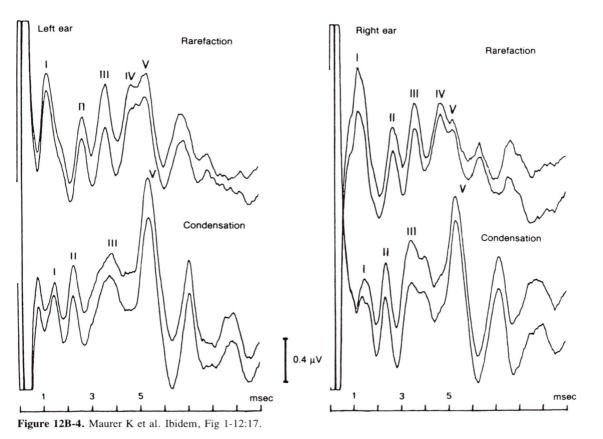

**Figure 12B-4.** Maurer K et al. Ibidem, Fig 1-12:17.

tials (PSPs) are reasonably well localized when compared with all-or-none action potentials generated at the cell body and transmitted along the entire axon. The difference between graded post-synaptic and all-or-none action potentials and between localized and electrical events (those transmitted along the axon) becomes obviously more striking when dealing with long tracts such as the lateral lemniscus for instance. They definitely have different intracellular origins, time constants, fields, and spatial distribution. Only a modest amount of research has addressed the contribution of these responses to BAEPs,[23] and at present it is generally believed that BAEPs reflect the topographically fixed graded PSPs and not the all-or-none traveling wave type of potentials.

This hypothesis has been studied thoroughly by Humphrey,[24] who stated that the distances between current sources (outward membrane current) and sinks (inward membrane current) are greater during peak PSPs than during peak action potentials

activation and that these distances must be considered when assessing the value of voltage at a distant point. Intracellular recordings of PSP-action potential activity with adjacent extracellular recordings support these views.

### Technique

An electrical square wave of 100 to 200 $\mu$sec duration is delivered as a click via audiologic earphones at an usual intensity of 65 to 70 dB. To prevent stimulation of the contralateral ear through bone and air conduction and so achieve monaural stimulation, a "masking noise" of 30 to 40 dB lower intensity than the click stimulus is delivered to the contralateral ear. This is described to the patient as *static* or *ocean noise*.

BAEP testing is best performed with the patient lying supine with the head elevated or sitting in an inclined comfortable chair to reduce neck mus-

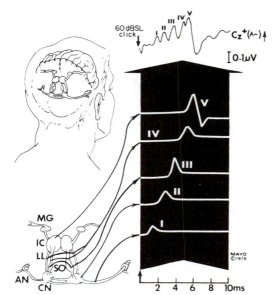

**Figure 12B-5.** Aminoff MJ. Electrodiagnosis in Clinical Neurology. 2nd Edition. Churchill Livingstone. 1986. Fig 15-1:468.

cle activity. The room need not be soundproof but should be quiet. Sedatives are rarely used, except mainly when dealing with children. The amplitudes of the BAEPs are lower than those for other evoked potential modalities. While VEP amplitudes are usually between 5 and 15 and SEPs between 1 and 10 μV, BAEPs are often as low as 0.25 μV. As a consequence, 1000 averaged sweeps are at times necessary to obtain the waves. Each trial is replicated to ensure reproducibility. As noted earlier, the usual click rate is 10 per second, but to detect minor abnormalities not seen at times at lower rates, 20 to 40 per second repetition rates, acting as a sort of stress factor, are also suggested.[25]

Click polarity is defined by the initial movement of the earphone diaphragm, either away from the tympanic membrane (rarefaction) or toward it (condensation). Alternation clicks alternate between rarefaction and condensation. The routine use of rarefaction clicks stems from findings reported in 1978 by Stockard and colleagues,[26] which stated that the amplitude of wave I is higher with this click phase. Wave I recognition is paramount for the clinical interpretation of BAEPs, as two out of three major measurements, namely I–III and I–V interpeak latencies (IPLs), depend

on its presence. The possibility of confusing wave I with the CM should also be kept in mind. Switching polarities to have a better view of wave I also helps differentiate it from the CM. When changing polarity there is no similar change for wave I, though the CM reverses polarity as well (Figure 12B-6). When using the routine surface electrodes placed on the earlobe or mastoid it is not uncommon to find apparent absence of wave I. In this case, a special external ear canal electrode may help (Figure 12B-7). When polarities are reversed, changes may be noted for absolute and interpeak latencies, so in extreme cases this procedure may make a difference between normal and abnormal responses. It is obvious at this point that using more than one repetition rate and one polarity increases the chances of detecting subtle but meaningful abnormalities.[25]

Infants can be subjected to BAEP testing when they are studied for mental retardation or autism related to hearing loss.[27,28] Special caution is necessary in these cases. Testing should proceed at a time when subjects are fed, dry, and asleep. Electrodes of suitable size should be used. When central information is sought, a 10 per second rate is

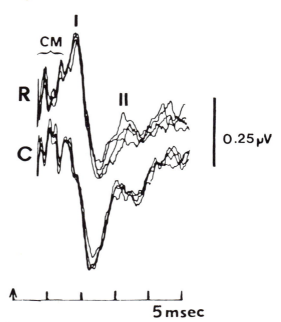

**Figure 12B-6.** Chiappa KH. Evoked Potentials in Clinical Medicine. 2nd Edition. New York: Raven Press. 1990. Fig 4-8:189.

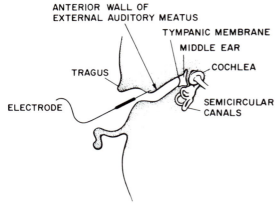

ANTERIOR WALL OF
EXTERNAL AUDITORY MEATUS
TYMPANIC MEMBRANE
MIDDLE EAR
COCHLEA
TRAGUS
ELECTRODE
SEMICIRCULAR
CANALS

**Figure 12B-7.** Ibidem, Fig 4-2:180.

appropriate; when the concern is peripheral hearing, the rate should be increased to 50 to 70 per second. The lowest click intensity at which wave V remains obtainable (wave V recognition threshold) is determined. In subjects devoid of any major hearing problem, wave V is still present at click intensity of 30 to 50 dB.[29]

Besides technical nonpathologic factors already considered, (intensity, masking noise, rate and polarity) individual factors can also affect results of BAEP studies. A substantial body of knowledge is available on the influence of age and gender. While the published papers do not reflect a single view, it is generally agreed that increases in latency from childhood to adult age are rather small, as a rule not affecting normalcy in a mixed-gender laboratory sample.[30] In contradistinction, the difference in BAEP latencies from infancy to adulthood is significant. Ken-Dror and coworkers[31] found the correlation between gestational age and BAEPs central (III–V IPL) and peripheral (I–III IPL) conductions sufficient to provide an estimate of developmental age.

Females have shorter absolute and interpeak latencies than males.[30,32,33] Amplitudes are also generally larger in females.[33–35] Explanations for these findings vary; the most accepted one involves the difference in body size and brain size of males and females.

Increases in both absolute and interpeak latencies occur with gradual decreases in body temperature.[36] Circadian effects on BAEPs are also noted in relation to corresponding changes in body temperature.[37]

Hearing deficiencies are another major patient

factor that affects results of BAEP testing. Hallmark studies[38,39] showed that IPLs were not essentially affected, even in the presence of definite hearing loss. On the other hand, peripheral hearing disorders affect absolute latencies as well as the intensity-latency curve of wave V; both are less important than IPLs.[40] It is no surprise that in cortical deafness BAEPs are as a rule normal while the middle latency responses (MLRs), probably reflecting cortical events, are affected.[1,41]

Pharmacologic agents do not generally prolong the IPLs if body temperature remains normal. Most central nervous system depressants bring about little changes in BAEP values. While the anesthetic agent isoflurane does not affect the BAEP IPLs, in spite of true electrocerebral silence and lack of clinically present central nervous system function in some patients (Figure 12B-8), enflurane, its isomer, is an exception, producing temperature-independent prolongation of IPLs.[42] Other central nervous system depressant or anesthetic agents such as halothane, meperidine, nitrous oxide, barbiturates, or diazepam fail to affect the chemically invulnerable BAEPs.

Some correlation is found between alcoholism and BAEP abnormalities. Prolonged IPLs during acute intoxication is most likely associated with decreased body temperature.[43] The same factor does not account for IPLs abnormalities found in the chronic stage of alcoholism.[44]

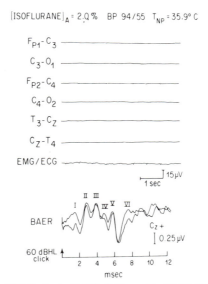

**Figure 12B-8.** Aminoff MJ, Ibidem. Fig 15-10:479.

### Clinical Applications

The multiple clinical applications of the BAEPs are related to the criteria set to define abnormality. In coma, complete absence of all waves is obviously the most ominous. However, premorbid severe hearing loss could explain the disappearance of all waves, since wave I is likely to be absent. Anoxia of the cochlea in a patient with traumatic coma could also result in absence of all waves without affecting the prognosis for recovery. In both cases, a reversible course is still possible. In the absence of all waves except waves I or I and II, which reflect activity in the eighth nerve, the prognosis is poor, with no known exceptions. The third abnormality in terms of severity but one that is more frequent is prolongation of IPLs I–III, III–V, and I–V. Because of their variability, amplitudes are not considered as important as latencies in reflecting lesions and resultant deficits. The amplitude ratio of waves I/V is considered to be a more reliable measure when the click hearing threshold is normal. Even in this circumstance, no conclusion can be reached unless wave V is of very low amplitude and ill-defined.[45] In this context, an absent wave V represents a rather severe abnormality, provided that more than one click polarity, repetition rate, or click intensity is used to verify the findings. Chiappa[46] emphasized the usefulness of decreasing the stimulus intensity, particularly when wave V becomes difficult to identify (Figure 12B-9).

In addition to the abovementioned criteria, prolongation of latency of waves I or III or I–II separation can be seen in disorders such as hereditary motor-sensory neuropathy.[47]

It is well-recognized that BAEPs help detect and localize lesions in the cochlear nerve as well as in the lower and upper brain stem. Their role in monitoring surgical procedures on the brain stem and in the evaluation of conservative therapeutic measures in MS is widely accepted. The contribution of BAEPs to prognosis in coma has already been mentioned. There is no absolute proof that the neural generators for BAEPs are located at the precise sites where they are described, but there is no proof to the contrary either. As the entire brain stem is no longer than 3 to 4 cm, possible errors in localization would seem to have minimal diagnostic consequences. At present, it is not certain if the BAEPs are generated at synapses within gray matter nuclei or by volleys within white matter or by a combination of both. Another hypothesis considers the waveforms to be the result of summation of electrical activity from more than one nucleus.[45]

It is known that, in spite of decussation of most of the auditory pathway at the level of the lateral lemniscus, the findings are, as a rule, ipsilateral rather than contralateral to the stimulated ear. The

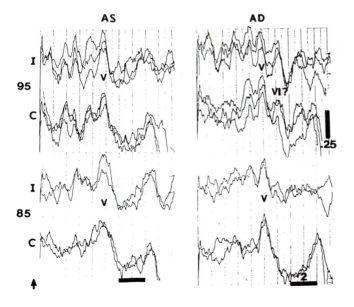

**Figure 12B-9.** Chiappa KH, Ibidem. Fig 4-5:185.

only exception should logically be wave V, which presumably originates above the upper pons, at the levels of lower midbrain or lateral lemniscus (see General Considerations earlier in the chapter). Figure 12B-10 shows a case of pontine glioma with wave V absent on the tumor side but delayed contralaterally.

## Brain Stem Tumors

BAEP studies are of value primarily for diagnosis of cerebellopontine angle (CPA) tumors. No fewer than 600 papers have been published on cases of acoustic neuromas. Wave V latency prolongation or inter-ear differences of wave V latency are used

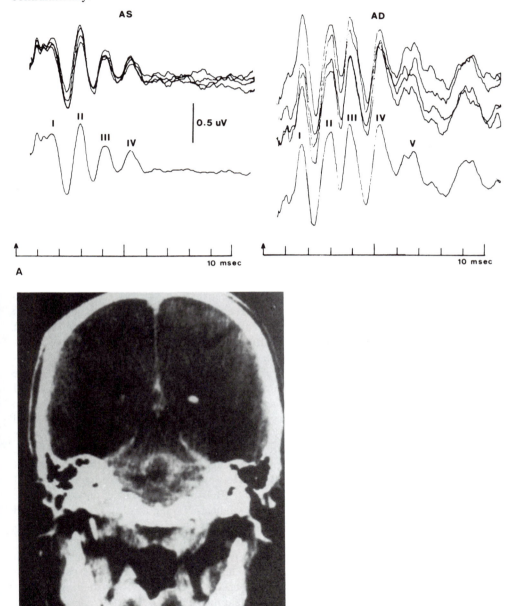

**Figure 12B-10.** Chiappa KH, Ibidem. Fig 5-5:230-231.

frequently as diagnostic criteria.[48–50] One study reported that BAEPs were more sensitive than computed tomography (CT) in detecting acoustic neuromas (41 subjects) and CPA meningiomas (nine cases); CT findings were normal in nine of these patients.[51] In no situation was the reverse found. The most sensitive BAEP abnormalities in acoustic neuromas are delayed I–III IPL and increased inter-ear difference (Figure 12B-11). In a small number of patients with acoustic neuromas wave I is present while all other waves are missing (Figure 12B-12). In exceptional cases, no waves are present and hearing is normal. In patients with large CPA tumors that do not involve the cochlear nerve, CT may detect the lesion before BAEPs do. In these cases, obviously, BAEPs are not as necessary. Magnetic resonance imaging (MRI) did not always prove superior to CT. The high cost of MRI makes BAEP preferable mainly in clinical follow-up studies.[52] In a recent study of 56 acoustic neuroma cases,[53] five patients (11%) had normal BAEPs. There was a significant correlation between the tumor size and III–V IPL.

*Coma and Brain Death*

As mentioned earlier in this chapter, BAEPs are of value in the prognosis of coma or brain death. The differential diagnosis between metabolic (and, therefore, potentially reversible) situations and structural insult to the brain stem is essential for

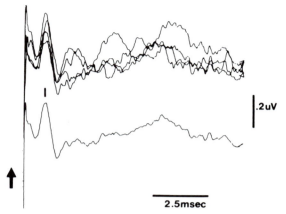

**Figure 12B-12.** Chiappa KH, Ibidem. Fig 5-11:247.

the assessment of prognosis in coma. While the brain stem is resistant to metabolic factors and most central nervous system depressants and anesthetic agents, it is vulnerable to structural damage. Stockard and Sharbrough[54] presented a classic example of reversible metabolic coma, describing a 33-year-old woman in respiratory arrest of unknown origin and duration (Figure 12B-13). The clinical and laboratory findings were compatible with irreversible coma despite normal BAEP studies. She recovered in 4 days. Drug intoxication due to central nervous system depressant overdose was subsequently found, illustrating the value of BAEPs in prognosis. For patients in coma, a normal BAEP study does not always guarantee recovery, as the more rostral structures such as the cortex may be severely damaged. In the case of metabolic coma, a favorable prognosis is often associated with normal BAEPs while abnormal BAEPs are a sure sign of poor outcome. BAEPs are quite accurate in predicting a poor prognosis, given the vital structures in the brain stem. Absent III and IV/V waves with preserved waves I and II (Figure 12B-14) reflect no medullary or pontine activity, indicating brain death. The absence of all the waves, when technical and audiologic problems have been ruled out, has the same significance. Figure 12B-15 shows a typical case of brain death as described by Stockard[55] in a patient with vertebrobasilar thrombosis. The patient underwent manipulation of the neck and lost consciousness. Five hours later, there was a clear discrepancy between a mildly abnormal EEG (Figure 12B-16) and severe BAEP abnormalities, namely absence

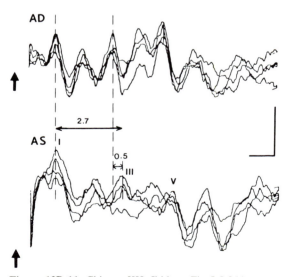

**Figure 12B-11.** Chiappa KH, Ibidem. Fig 5-8:244.

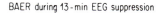

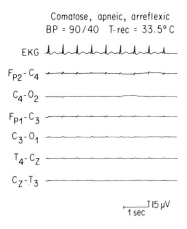

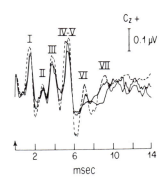

Comatose, apneic, arreflexic
BP = 90/40   T-rec = 33.5° C

BAER during 13-min EEG suppression

**Figure 12B-13.** Aminoff MJ, Ibidem. Fig 15-13:485.

of all the waves. The comatose patient died a day later, and the autopsy revealed a rhombencephalic cause of death.

Goldie and coworkers[56] studied 50 poorly responsive patients with some preserved brain stem and central nervous system functions, reporting no consistent correlation of BAEPs findings with clinical outcome. The patients most unlikely to survive were those with bilaterally absent waves or no wave IV and/or V. Figure 12B-17 illustrates four cases.

*Multiple Sclerosis*

The contribution of BAEP studies in establishing the diagnosis of MS is less significant than the role of VEPs or lower limb SSEPs.[57] The possible finding of an unsuspected lesion in the brain stem while the clinical signs and symptoms are external to it, in the cortex, spinal cord, or optic system, justifies using this procedure. Other reasons to resort to BAEPs for diagnosing MS are equivocal

or uncertain clinical findings, or a need to monitor management measures objectively using sequential BAEP studies. Of a total of more than 1000 cases (all classifications), 46% (466 patients) had abnormal BAEPS, from 21% with possible MS to 55% with definite MS.[45] There is generally much variability in reporting of results in MS, reflecting differences in patient population, technical factors, or even the definition of MS.[45] Logically, BAEP abnormalities are most likely to be found among patients with definite MS or those with clinical signs of brain stem involvement. In the first case, the referring physician already has a diagnosis. In the second, while there is corroboration of clinical findings, a major reason would be to find an unsuspected lesion outside the brain stem. There are papers[58–60] describing cases with probable or possible MS and no clinical evidence of brain stem lesions. The presence of abnormal BAEPs in these cases is more helpful owing to the detection of unsuspected lesions.

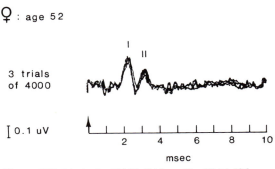

♀ : age 52

3 trials
of 4000

**Figure 12B-14.** Aminoff MJ, Ibidem. Fig 15-14:486.

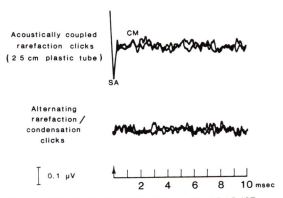

**Figure 12B-15.** Aminoff MJ, Ibidem. Fig 15-15:487.

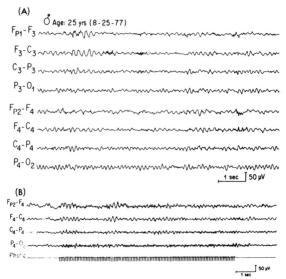

**(A)**

♂ Age: 25 yrs (8-25-77)

Fp1-F3

F3-C3

C3-P3

P3-O1

Fp2-F4

F4-C4

C4-P4

P4-O2

1 sec ⌐ 50 μV

**(B)**

Fp2-F4

F4-C4

C4-P4

P4-O2

Phot

⌐ 50 μV
1 sec

**Figure 12B-16.** Aminoff MJ, Ibidem. Fig 15-16:488.

BAEPs may be used to differentiate between MS, transverse myelitis,[61] and retrobulbar neuritis.[62]

Hearing involvement in MS has been studied extensively.[63] Before the advent of BAEP studies, hearing assessment in MS cases was often complicated by associated vestibular symptoms such as nystagmus and vertigo. Behavioral tests could not differentiate between ear and central nervous system involvement. When BAEP studies were used, the hearing loss could be localized along the entire pathway, from the receptor organ to the upper pons.

Subclinical findings in patients with abnormal BAEPs revealed lesions in clinically silent areas. Finding sites of unsuspected lesions led to changes in diagnosis from probable or possible MS to definite MS. Maurer and Lowitzsch reported on 143 patients whose disease was reclassified as a result.[63]

BAEP abnormalities in MS depend on the location and extent of the demyelinating sites rather than on specific findings. Figures 12B-18 and 12B-19 depict two severe cases, the first affecting the lower pons and the second the upper pons.

*Other Demyelinating Conditions*

Severe BAEP abnormalities are found in congenital demyelinating disorders such as metachromatic leukodystrophy,[64] Pelizaeus-Merzbacher disease,[65] and the rare adrenoleukodystrophy.[66] Central pontine myelinolysis is another demyelinating condition that can show abnormal BAEP findings such as very prolonged I–V IPL up to 8.4 msec, with a decrease in these abnormalities paralleling clinical progress.

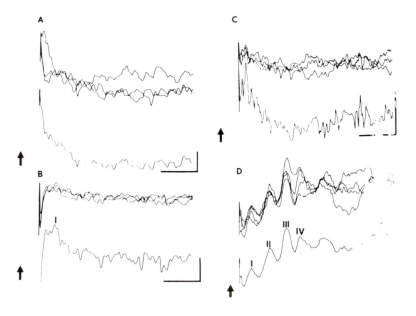

A

B

C

D

I

III   IV

II

I

**Figure 12B-17.** Chiappa KH, Ibidem. Fig 5-17:269.

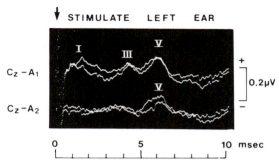

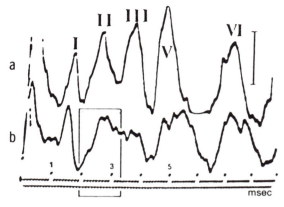

**Figure 12B-18.** Spehlmann R. Evoked Potential Primer. Boston: Butterworth, 1985. Fig 13-1:224.

## Vascular Deficiencies

The rich vascular supply of the brain stem explains the high incidence of vascular brain stem syndromes. BAEPs are abnormal only when the dorsolateral region is involved.[48] The Wallenberg syndrome—thrombosis of the inferior posterior cerebellar artery—usually results in wave changes with an intact wave I (Figure 12B-20) and a correspondence between the clinical picture and electrodiagnosis. Similar changes are seen in Millard-Gubler and Foville's syndrome.

Studies of BAEPs in other types of brain stem vascular conditions have been reported for small series of patients. Brown and coworkers[68] presented 22 patients with intrinsic brain stem lesions, including four with locked-in syndrome, two of them with normal BAEPs. Five subjects with cerebrovascular accidents affecting the brain stem at the pons or at more rostral levels showed BAEPs abnormalities. Kjaer[69] reported that 13 of 15 patients with brain stem infarcts had abnormal BAEPs, but this was found in only one of nine

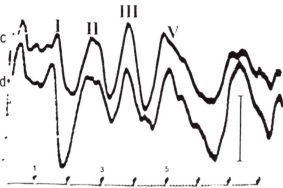

**Figure 12B-20.** Maurer K et al. Evoked Potentials. Toronto-Philadelphia. BC Decker Inc. 1989. Fig 1-42:45.

cases with brain stem TIAs. Conversely, Factor and Dentiger[70] found abnormalities 1 to 16 days after the event in all 8 patients with vertebrobasilar transient ischemic attacks. Physical examination was noncontributory, but the authors found BAEPs to be potentially helpful in differentiating brain stem transient ischemic attacks from syndromes outside the brainstem such as Meniere's syndrome, which, as a rule, is devoid of BAEP changes.[71] An example of BAEPs' role in monitoring management is a case of acute occlusion of the basilar artery[72] in which the BAEP abnormalities returned to normal after selective local thrombocytic therapy with streptokinase (Figure 12B-21).

## Degenerative Disorders

Friedreich's ataxia affects all evoked potential types, across the board. The BAEP abnormalities usually present in this condition[73] enable it to be

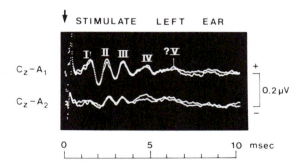

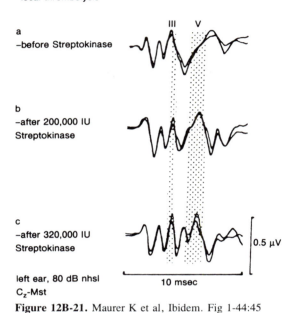

BAEP-Monitoring
Basilar thrombosis
–local thrombolysis–

a
–before Streptokinase

III   V

b
–after 200,000 IU
Streptokinase

c
–after 320,000 IU
Streptokinase

0.5 µV

left ear, 80 dB nhsl
Cz-Mst

10 msec

**Figure 12B-21.** Maurer K et al, Ibidem. Fig 1-44:45

According to Lynn[76] and Nuwer and their coworkers[77] olivopontocerebellar degeneration results in BAEPs abnormalities. BAEPs are also affected at times in Alzheimer's disease,[78] Parkinson's disease,[79] and alcoholism.[80]

*Sudden Infant Death and Apnea Syndromes*

The use of BAEPs in infants at risk for sudden death (SIDS) is questionable. In one case, an infant with normal BAEPs succumbed to crib death.[81] Another study of near-miss SIDs found 11% of infants displayed abnormal BAEPs rostrally.[82] Earlier encouraging papers, reporting BAEP findings in infants at risk for SIDS[83,84] have been contradicted by late studies.[85,86]

In infants affected by apnea syndrome not related to SIDs, a possible correlation exists between apnea and I–V IPL. The number of daily apnea attacks decreased as the I–V IPL decreased, and practically ceased when normal latencies were obtained.[87]

distinguished from other hereditary ataxias with normal BAEPS. This electrophysiologic comparison correlates well with the neuropathologic findings. Cell loss and gliosis are found in the brain stem in association with Friedreich's ataxia[74] but not other ataxias.[75] The BAEP abnormalities (Figure 12B-22) are thought to be secondary to the degeneration of the spiral ganglion, considered to be a homologue of the dorsal root ganglion.[73]

## Middle Latency Auditory Evoked Potentials

### Sonomotor Responses

In 1964, Bickford and coworkers[88] described widespread myogenic responses to auditory stimuli and labeled them *sonomotor responses*. The latencies of these sonomotor potentials ranges from 6 to 50 msec. Since they were recordable with click

**Figure 12B-22.** Aminoff MJ. Electrodiagnosis in Clinical Neurology. 2nd Edition. Churchill Livingstone 1986. Fig 16-13:525.

AGE   DURATION

8     3

10    6

18    8

yr    yr

+0 5 µV

10 ms

stimuli in three patients with sensorineural deafness but normal vestibular function, these potentials were considered to be initiated by the vestibular system. One of the responses, the so-called *inion response,* was shown to increase in amplitude with increased activity of neck muscles. A similar relation between amplitude increase and increased muscle contraction was recorded for other muscles, such as the frontalis and temporalis. The intensity threshold for these potentials is established at 40 dB. While the amplitude of myogenic (sonomotor) responses is affected by muscle tension, the other middle latency components, namely the central nervous system responses, are not influenced by muscle contraction.[89] A component with a 30-msec latency was described[90] in 1965 and considered possibly to originate from a central nervous system structure because of a longer recovery cycle and a different amplitude-intensity function than the sonomotor responses.

Figure 12B-23 shows the difference between rest and neck tension in terms of middle latency myogenic versus central nervous system responses. In Figure 12B-23, the EMG activity, as recorded from the inion is quantified, resulting in an index of muscle activity. The six subjects relax and then contract their neck muscles. When recording at the vertex referred to mastoid, the central nervous system components were more visible with neck muscles relaxed, but these components were gradually attenuated as the recording electrode was moved toward the inion. Conversely, with contraction of the neck muscles the central

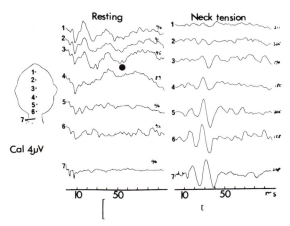

**Figure 12B-23.** Halliday AM. Evoked Potentials in Clinical Testing. Edinburgh-London-Melbourne-New York: Churchill Livingstone 1982. Fig 10-7:369.

nervous system components were contaminated at the vertex channel, and this phenomenon was magnified gradually toward the inion channel ($C_z$ to mastoid for the former and inion to neck for the latter). The conclusions were that both sonomotor and middle latency responses may be obtained from the skull and that they display very different distributions.[91]

In 1963, Kiang and colleagues[92] described another sonomotor component in the latency range of 8 to 50 msec. It was recorded from the postauricular muscle and, in contrast to the inion component, it is mediated through the facial nerve. The threshold for this response is only 10 to 20 dB, in contrast to the inion, frontalis, or temporalis muscle responses, where the threshold was at least 40 dB. The postauricular muscle is vestigial in humans and a response can be obtained in only 70% of patients; in the remaining 30% it is either absent of present only unilaterally. A major characteristic of the postauricular muscle response is that, in contrast to the other myogenics, it is not related to muscle tension. Interference derived from this response has made attempts to identify the components of the central nervous system middle latency responses, especially when abnormal, quite laborious, and restricted. It should be mentioned, however, that some components of the middle latency responses, such as Pa, Nb, and P1, occur after the recorded activity of the postauricular muscle response, so they can still be used efficiently to evaluate the central nervous system rostrally.

Different authors have described motor responses outside the auditory range. They are called *microreflexes,* to differentiate them from muscle artifacts that are not contingent on presentation of a stimulus. The microreflexes include photomotor responses due to tension of neck or forehead muscles, with a positive peak at about 75 msec[93] or photopalpebral reflex to the contraction of the orbicularis oculi muscle to flashing light.[94] Cracco and Bickford[95] reported that in 70% of subjects, somatomotor responses are recorded at the scalp with median nerve stimulation.

In terms of clinical use, the postauricular sonomotor response has some role as a hearing test, because it is elicited through cochlear, but not vestibular, stimulation. Table 12B-4 summarizes the essentials of the sonomotor responses in the middle latency auditory components range.

**Table 12B-4.** Some Myogenic Responses

| Reflex | Description |
|---|---|
| Postauricular muscle response | Diphasic negative/positive wave<br>Latency of positivity 16 msec<br>Much variability between and within subjects<br>Can be bilateral or unilateral<br>Unrelated to muscle tension<br>Recorded on the ipsilateral mastoid |
| Temporalis | Diphasic negative/positive wave<br>Latency of positivity 23 msec<br>Increase with muscle tension<br>Recorded from temporal area |
| Neck muscles | Multiple components<br>Negative waves at 11 and 25 msec<br>Positive waves at 17 and 34 msec<br>Sensitive to muscle tension<br>Recorded from inion |
| Frontalis | Highly variable<br>Mean positive component 30 msec<br>Sensitive to muscle tension |

(From Halliday AM. Evoked Potentials in Clinical Testing. Edinburgh: Churchill Livingstone, 1982.)

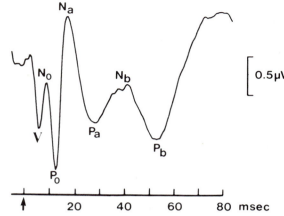

**Figure 12B-24.** Spehlmann R. Evoked Potential Primer. Boston: Butterworth 1985. Fig 14-3:241.

### Middle Latency Responses (Central Nervous System Responses)

Middle latency components, which reflect central nervous system activity, occur between 10 and 50 msec and display amplitudes in the 0.5 to 3.0 μV range (Figure 12B-24 and Table 12B-5). They are generally labeled No, Po, Na, Pa, and Nb, but Pb and P1 are also mentioned in some textbooks. When initially described[96] they were considered "early" auditory evoked responses, but later on their name was changed to the more appropriate *middle latency responses*.[97,98] In terms of presumed neural generators, the earlier ones (No, Po, Na) might arise from the medial geniculate body and polysensory nuclei of the thalamus while the late ones may be generated in wide areas of the association cortex.[96-98] Recordings with electrodes placed on the superior aspect of the temporal lobe during intracranial surgery[99] disclosed a large, positive wave in the latency range of Pa (30 to 45 msec); however, the same latency range corresponds to intense sound activity from the scalp muscles[88,93,97] raising doubts about whether the described wave could be of myogenic origin. In spite of the confusion between neurogenics and myogenics, the evaluation of scalp muscles' contribution[97] and mapping studies[100,101] have shown that these responses are primarily neural in origin. Clinical evidence following bilateral cortex lesions suggests that they do not arise from the primary auditory cortex.[102]

The middle latency components are generally recorded from the vertex (C$_z$) with reference to the mastoid (M) or earlobe (A) with a narrow bandpass filter of 25 to 200 Hz. Compared with tone bursts, click stimuli result in somewhat longer latencies and greater amplitude variations.[103] Repetition rates of 1 to 10 per second do not generally affect the amplitude, though higher rates result in some decrement of amplitude. If it is maintained at moderate intensities neither contralateral masking noise nor binaural stimulation alters the amplitudes.

A few researchers[104,105] report experiencing some difficulty in obtaining well-defined wave-

**Table 12B-5.** Normal Values of Waves V–VII of the BAEP and Waves No, Po, Na, Pa, and Nb of the MAEP Obtained at a Click Intensity of 70 db

| V | VI | VII | No | Po | Na | Pa | Nb |
|---|---|---|---|---|---|---|---|
| 5.4 | 7.0 | 8.6 | 9.6 | 12.5 | 18.1 | 29.4 | 38.5 |
| (0.6) | (1.0) | (0.9) | (4.3) | (3.6) | (7.3) | (8.7) | (9.6) |

From Buettner and Trost. EEG EMG 1985; 16:145.
(From Maurer K, et al. Evoked Potentials. Toronto: BC Decker, 1989.)

forms from neonates; others[106,107] did not report age to be a significant factor.

Shorter latencies and lower amplitudes have been reported in neonates as compared to adults. No activity is recordable beyond 50 msec (Pb, Nc), and the obtainable waves are much clearer with ipsilateral stimulation.[107] Since only the Pa component increases in amplitude with increase in age from 1 to 8 months, this criterion was considered sufficient for audiologic evaluation of young children.[108]

Like BAEPs, the middle latency responses are minimally affected by endogenous factors such as attention or eye closure[109], sleep[110] or sleep deprivation,[111] sedation,[112] and skeletal muscle paralysis.[113] Very deep anesthesia, however, eliminates the middle latency responses[101], even if they are recorded at the surface of the cortex.[99]

The major clinical application of the MLRs is in audiology. The advantages are manifold: it is noninvasive, obtainable during sleep as well as when the subject is awake, recognizable even in early infancy, and displays clear responses at 500 Hz. However, there are disadvantages, of which the major one is relatively poor reliability and thus the necessity to refine the procedure before it is used as an objective measurement technique for hearing evaluation. Galambos and associates[114] described a series of middle latency components obtained with 40-Hz stimulus (40-Hz response), which are considered to be more physiologic and, therefore, more sensitive. The Pa is used for eval-

uation. The 40 Hz is also used in the evaluation of hearing (500 to 1500 Hz range).

The middle latency responses are also used clinically in MS. Robinson and Rudge[115] initially documented changes in middle latency responses amplitude and latency in MS. They subsequently reported[116] a favorable comparison of middle latency responses and BAEPs in the diagnosis of MS, and later on[117] the capacity of using serial middle latency responses recordings to differentiate active from dormant disease. Combined recordings of middle latency responses and BAEPs were used[118] to increase the diagnostic yield of acoustic neuromas. In cortical deafness[1,119] the MLRs are abolished but BAEPs remain. Use of middle latency responses in coma has been mentioned.[2]

## Late Latency Auditory Evoked Potentials

Auditory evoked potentials in the range of 50 or 60 msec to 250 msec are called *late latency components*. The contribution of endogenous factors, very small in the case of middle latency responses, becomes moderate to large in this range, and becomes exclusive from 250 msec on, when dealing with waves such as $P_{300}$, a "cognitive" potential (Table 12B-6, Figure 12B-25).

The four late latency auditory evoked potentials known as $P_1$, at a latency of 50 or 60 to 80 msec, generally used for auditory threshold determina-

**Table 12B-6.** Characteristics of Middle-, Late-, and Long-Latency Auditory Evoked Potentials

| Latency Class | Main Components | Latency Range (msec) | Amplitude Range (μV) | Exogenous Effects | Endogenous Effects |
|---|---|---|---|---|---|
| Middle | No | 8–10 | 0.5–3.0 | Moderate to large | Very small |
| | Po | 11–13 | | | |
| | Na | 16–25 | | | |
| | Pa | 25–35 | | | |
| | Nb | 35–45 | | | |
| Late | P1 | 50–80 | 3.0–15.0 | Moderate | Moderate to large |
| | N1 | 80–120 | | | |
| | P2 | 160–200 | | | |
| | N2 | 200–250 | | | |
| Long | P3 or P300 (CNV, sustained potential, slow wave) | 250–400 | 5.0–20 | Small | Large |

(From Moore EJ. Basis of Auditory Brain-Stem Evoked Responses. New York: Grune & Stratton, 1983.)

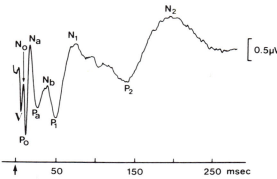

**Figure 12B-25.** Spehlman R, Ibidem. Fig 14-5:244.

tion; $N_1$, latency of 80 to 120 msec; $P_2$, from 160 to 200 msec; $N_2$, from 200 to 250 msec. $N_1$, $P_2$, and $N_2$ waves are mostly used in neurologic and neurophysiologic research. The amplitudes of these potentials are relatively large, in the range of 3 to 15 $\mu$V or more.

These waves are part of a large potential initially described by P.A. Davis[120] in 1930 and in the same year by H. Davis and coworkers,[121] as a result of an analysis of the raw EEG. The potential was named the *slow* or *vertex* potential. Considerable effort and skill were required to isolate this large wave from the random EEG noise. With an amplitude of 15 $\mu$V, it could be seen without an averager, which was nonexistent at that time. Photographic superimposition, such as that done in 1947 by Dawson[122] for the SEPs, helped to identify the component. It was only much later, in the 1960s,[123] that electronic averaging and summating techniques made the slow or vertex potential readily visible. The appellation *vertex potential* has been criticized, since all the AEPs except ECochG are recorded at the vertex. The term should be abandoned.

The exact origin of the slow potential (sum of the four previously described late components) is still unknown. It can also be obtained from the scalp with visual and somatosensory stimuli and here the clear distinction between the three modalities starts to blur. The slow potential was initially thought to arise from the primary auditory cortex or temporoparietal association; neither supposition could be proved.[124] Other studies maintain that $N_1$, $P_2$, and $N_2$ components represent widespread activation of the frontal cortex,[97] while more recently[125] it is suggested that $N_1$ stems from the posterior superior temporal cortex.

The slow potential or the late potentials are obtainable using a vertex-mastoid montage ($C_z$–$M_1,2$) ipsilateral or contralateral. Tone bursts are employed, at a rate of 1 or 2 per second (1 to 2 Hz). A higher rate significantly attenuates the components. A clearly defined averaged response may be obtained after 30 to 64 stimuli. The subject should avoid motion during averaging, lest it blur the display. The filter settings usually employed are 1 to 30 Hz or 1 to 100 Hz. The latency of the $N_1$–$P_2$ components decreases if the intensity of the stimuli increases.[126]

Technical, as well as individual factors need to be considered when discussing the late potentials. The amplitude variability that occurs with changes in rates of stimulation or other stimulus parameters reflects the patient's psychological state and is attributed to the habituation and dishabituation processes. Change in the patient's attention also plays a major role: $N_1$–$P_2$, but mainly the $N_1$ amplitude increases substantially when the patient focuses attention on a specific stimulation element.[128,129] When the patient is in deep sleep, the wave morphology, amplitude, and latency are affected.[130] Age affects the late auditory evoked potential components as well. Decrease in latency from birth to about age 10 years and an increase afterward have been documented. Amplitudes are larger during childhood but then stabilize or decline with age.[131]

In spite of the major current use of late auditory evoked potentials as research tools, they were employed in the past in hearing evaluation procedures and are still used in a number of clinics for the audiologic evaluation of young children, mainly for the detection of possible nonorganic hearing loss. No clear consensus exists about the use of late AEPs in hearing; they should be used only as a supplement to other methods.[132]

The nonaudiometric applications of late auditory evoked potentials are limited. Hyperactive children have been studied and showed smaller attention-dependent changes in late auditory evoked potentials amplitude.[133]

## Long Latency (Cognitive) Auditory Evoked Potentials

Long latency auditory evoked potentials, after 250 msec, are highly variable and subject-dependent expressions of perceptual and cognitive activity.

They comprise different types of waveforms, such as $P_3$ or $P_{300}$, the contingent negative variation (CNV), and the sustained potential.

### The P300 Potential

The $P_3$, $P_{300}$, or late positive component, remains the most extensively studied potential, and it has been the subject of recurrent interest in recent years. Its shape remains similar whether it is elicited by auditory, visual, or somatosensory stimuli. The $P_{300}$ component can be seen with a variety of stimulus presentation conditions, as long as the subject is placed in a task-oriented process. In the case of auditory stimuli, the clinician deals with an "oddball" paradigm, consisting of the subject counting reasonably rare and unexpected occurrences of a target tone buried in more frequently occurring standard tones. Since the target tone may be replaced by moments of silence, obviously it is not the physical difference between the two types of tones that counts but the information supplied to the subject with the occurrence of the target tone.

The $P_{300}$ potential was described in 1965 by Sutton and colleagues[134] who considered the potential's specific task to be the resolution of uncertainty. It is obvious from the initial study that if the subject reads a book, the $P_{300}$ will not be detectable; it becomes apparent as soon as the subject pays attention, for instance in order to slap the thigh at every nonfrequent tone (Figure 12B-26). This event-related potential represents a reflection of mental activity and relates to the degree of task-relevant information contained in the stimulus.

The data suggest that the $P_3$ component is associated with the detection of a task-relevant stimulus event and a memory-updating process related to the decision making.[135] When a very low bandpass cutoff is used, the $P_{300}$ becomes clearly visible after 20 to 30 replications of the relevant target event. The main factors that increase the $P_{300}$ amplitude are the improbability of the stimulus, meaning the difficulty in detecting it, and the fact that the subject is attending to it. Amplitude variations also depend on the subject's feeling that he or she correctly guessed the significance of the stimulus, thus solving the uncertainty about the target stimulus.[136]

Donald and Goff[137] have described an experiment resulting in the differentiation of $P_{300}$ from the contingent negative variation. Subjects were presented with a click, followed after 2 seconds by a tone. They had to respond by pressing a button, which in 75% of the trials produced an unpleasant electric shock. A significant increment in the $P_{300}$ amplitude occurred, but the contingent negative variation did not change.

The origin of the $P_{300}$ component is apparently less controversial than the origin of the late auditory evoked potentials. The available data suggest on one hand that it arises from a much wider area than $N_2$ and on the other that it involves the parietal association areas.[138] Despite opinions expressed in a few papers, the cognitive processes that contribute to generation of the $P_{300}$ remain an unresolved question. As $P_{300}$ latency increases in proportion to the difficulty of a given task while amplitude varies with the degree of unexpectedness of the target tone, the $P_{300}$ is thought to be a complex mixture of at least three waveforms. Together with the preceding $N_1$, $P_2$, and $N_2$ waves,

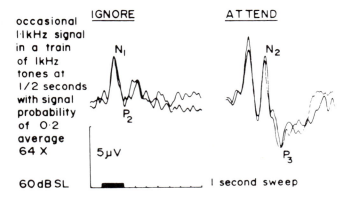

**Figure 12B-26.** Halliday AM. Evoked Potentials in Clinical Testing. Churchill Livingstone 1982. Fig 9-16:337.

these responses probably reflect various aspects of information-processing needed for recognition, retrieval from memory, and judgment about the significance of a signal. $P_{300}$ seems to reflect mental processes that enable us to anticipate significant events in our environment and to react to unexpected changes. Examples of oddball responses occur in everyday life, such as recognition of a known object or familiar face in a crowded room or, respectively, in a crowd or being alerted by a slight change in loudness or rhythm of a familiar sound. It is, therefore, clear that patients suffering from mental disturbances such as dementia, schizophrenia, or depression are prone to show abnormalities of the $P_{300}$ component.[139]

Goodin and colleagues[140] investigated event-related potentials in dementia and compared demented neurologic and psychiatric patients with nondemented ones and normal controls. Using an auditory oddball paradigm, the authors found decreased amplitude and increased latency of the $P_{300}$ in patients with dementia.

The auditory $P_{300}$ recorded in carefully defined demented patients revealed a significant difference between cases of Alzheimer's disease and chronic alcoholics with Korsakoff's syndrome. Delayed latency and reduced amplitude were found in Alzheimer's patients but no abnormalities in Korsakoff's patients or in the control group (1985).[141] In 1986, Goodin and Aminoff[142] studied auditory $P_{300}$ in patients with Alzheimer's disease, Huntington's disease, and dementia associated with Parkinson's disease. In addition to the $P_{300}$, components of the slow cortical potential such as $N_1$, $P_2$, and $N_2$ were also recorded and analyzed. Asymptomatic and "at risk" members of Huntington's families and nondemented Parkinson's patients had normal results. The patients considered to have "subcortical" dementia (Huntington's and Parkinson's patients) revealed a greater degree of $N_2$ and $P_{300}$ delay than the "cortically" demented Alzheimer's cases. This time the patients affected by Huntington's disease showed more abnormalities of $P_2$ latency than did the Parkinson's disease patients. Event-related potentials thus cannot only diagnose but can differentiate three types of dementia. Goodin and colleagues[143] recently studied patients infected with human immunodeficiency virus. More dramatic changes were present in cases with dementia, but 28% of the nondemented patients also showed delayed la-

tency for at least one of the event-related potential components. Auditory evoked potentials have been used for early detection of AIDS dementia, in the selection of patients for different drug treatments, and for serial monitoring of the response to case management measures.

Pfefferbaum and coworkers[144] have compared schizophrenia to dementia of different causes and to depression. Event-related potential studies revealed increased latency and reduced amplitude in the first two conditions, but the results were normal with depression. The abnormal $P_{300}$ response in schizophrenia is used as a physiologic marker and is potentially helpful in defining the clinical spectrum of schizophrenia. Of significance is the fact that $P_{300}$ does not seem to be affected by medication or clinical states: there was no change in patients who were at first definitely psychotic and drug free and then 1 month later free from psychotic symptoms and taking medication.[145] In addition to these advantages, auditory $P_{300}$ studies could be used as a trait marker for schizophrenic families, as they are abnormal in persons with mildly schizoid personality as well as in affected and unaffected pedigrees.[146] Schizophrenia affects not only the $P_{300}$ component but other late and long latency auditory evoked potentials. These findings suggest that a number of aspects of the information process are affected and that $P_{300}$ studies are of certain help in this condition.

### The Contingent Negative Variation and Other Long Latency Auditory Evoked Potentials

The contingent negative variation (CNV) is a slow negative potential shift, described by Walter and coworkers[147] as "an electric sign of sensorimotor association and expectancy in the human brain." The experimental paradigm that most reliably elicits the CNV is made of a warning signal followed after a few seconds by an imperative stimulus to which the patient has to respond (Figure 12B-27). The paradigm used in CNV audiometry consists of an audible stimulus associated with a warning given to the subject that soon after this stimulus a light will come on and will continue to flash rapidly. The subject has to prevent the light from flashing by pressing a button as quickly as possible. The paradigm needs a few trials until the routine is established. A slow negative potential

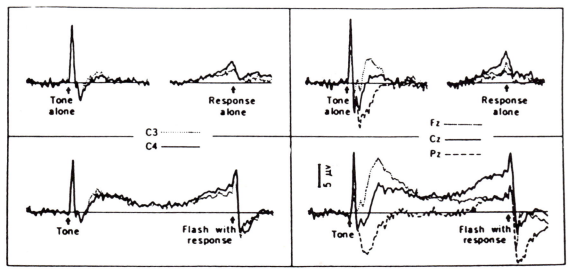

**Figure 12B-27.** Chiappa KH. Evoked Potentials in Clinical Medicine. 2nd Edition. New York: Raven Press 1990. Fig 11-6:579.

(CNV) develops between the auditory potential produced by the warning sound and the visual potential resulting from the flashing light. Afterward, the stimulus intensity of the warning sound is reduced until the patient does not produce a CNV potential because he or she does not hear the sound. The CNV amplitude is dependent not on the intensity of the stimulus but on the subject's expecting the light to flash (*expectancy potential*); thus, there is no change in amplitude even at near-threshold levels.

The CNV potential has to be distinguished from the *Bereitschaft* or readiness potential, which is a type of sustained or DC EEG shift that precedes voluntary movements. The CNV can be obtained without any actual movement. The thought of pressing the button when the light flashes is enough to elicit it.

The CNV can also be confused with potentials generated by eye movements, such as rolling the eyes downward while awaiting the flashing light or any other imperative stimulus. This error can be corrected by asking the subject to focus on a target and to keep the eyes wide open.

The CNV begins about 400 msec after the warning stimulus is presented and ends with the imperative stimulus presentation.[148] It has a very low frequency, less than 1 Hz. It is present bilaterally, and the maximum amplitude is in the midline (15 to 20 $\mu$V). The CNV seems to represent

the summation of two or more waves. A stimulus-related negativity, mostly frontally, possibly related to the orienting response, is followed by a centrally predominant negativity, considered to be related to the premotor potential associated with the motor response.[149] Shorter reaction time increases the amplitude[150]; drowsiness decreases it.[151]

The advantages of the CNV as an audiologic tool are that it is noninvasive, exhibits no change in amplitude with decreased stimulus intensity, is usable with speech stimuli, and has a role in measuring perception (amplitude decreases if, instead of meaningful words, the subject utters meaningless ones). It can be difficult to test young children, as many of them are unable to develop a CNV.

The sustained or DC potential, also called *steady potential,* was initially recognized as a change in the raw EEG recordings, but it can be enforced by averaging.[152] It consists of a negative baseline shift in the EEG that persists between the slow cortex responses marking the onset and offset of a prolonged pure tone stimulus.[153] The exact origin of this potential is unknown, but it is thought to arise mostly over the vertex and frontal regions and probably extends less for posteriorly than the $N_1$ and $P_2$ components of the late auditory evoked potentials. The DC potential decreases in amplitude with the decrease in the stimulus intensity. When the subject fails to pay attention to the stimulus (long-duration pure tone type), there is also a decrease in amplitude. During sleep, the DC potential can still be identified, though it is much smaller.

Methodologic considerations in using the DC potential are similar to those for the other long latency potentials. The electrodes are positioned with the active one at the vertex and the reference on the mastoid process. The bandpass has to accept DC activity. The stimulus is a tone burst of at least 600 msec. At a repetition rate of one per 2 seconds the DC potential has an amplitude of about one-third of the slow cortical potential, and it decreases in amplitude at frequencies over 2 kHz. A clear response is usually obtained after 32 stimuli. At present its clinical use is uncertain.

## Conclusion

The development of brain stem auditory evoked potential studies[19] represented a significant example of far-field potentials invested with solid research attributes. This event delayed work on other early, middle, and late auditory evoked potentials for many years. BAEPs have major clinical applications, the others relatively few. However, the serious student of AEPs should also become acquainted with middle latency responses. These are still neglected, probably at least in part because some are masked by the myogenic, sonomotor responses. The $P_{300}$ cognitive potential can contribute to the psychologic and psychiatric fields where quantification is particularly difficult. Other intermediary waves have some clinical value and can help in extrapolating a diagnosis mainly when recorded together with the $P_{300}$.

Auditory evoked potentials represent an important, relatively new resource in the constellation of noninvasive electrophysiologic diagnostic and prognostic tools helping clinicians explore the central nervous system. As such, it is imperative that further studies continue.

## References

1. Ozdamar O, Kraus N, et al. Auditory brain stem and middle latency responses in a patient with cortical deafness. Electroencephalogr Clin Neurophysiol 1982; 53:224–230.

2. Rosenberg C, Wogensen K, et al. Auditory brainstem and middle- and long-latency evoked potentials in coma. Arch Neurol 1984; 41:835–838.

3. Neiman J, Noldy NE, et al. Late auditory evoked potentials in alcoholics. 1991; 620:73–81.

4. Bloom W, Fawcett DW. A Textbook of Histology, ed 10. Philadelphia: WB Saunders, 1975.

5. Bekesi GV. Experiments in Hearing. New York: McGraw-Hill, 1960.

6. Galvani L. De viribus Electricitatis in Motu Musculari. Commentarius de Bonomens: Scientarium et Artium Instituto atque Academia Commentari. 1791; 7:363–418.

7. du Bois-Raymond E. Untersuchungen uber thierische Elektricitat, vol 1. Berlin: Reimer, 1848.

8. Caton R. The electric currents of the brain. Br Med J 1975; 2:278.

9. Berger H. Uber das Elektrenkephalogram des Menschen. Arch Psychiatrie Nervenkrank 1929; 87:527–570.

10. Wever EG, Bray CW. Auditory nerve impulses. Science 1930; 71:215.

11. Fromm B, et al. Studies in the mechanism of the Wever-Bray effect. Acta Otolaryngol (Stockholm) 1934/35; 22:477–486.

12. Andreev AM, et al. On electrical potentials in the human cochlea. J Physiol (London) 1939; 26:205–212.

13. Yoshie, et al. Nonsurgical recording of auditory nerve action potentials in man. Laryngoscope 1967; 77:76.

14. Salomon G, Elberling C. Cochlear nerve potentials recorded from the ear canal in man. Acta Otolaryngol 1971; 71:319.

15. Montandon PB, et al. Auditory nerve potentials from ear canals of patients with otologic problems. Ann Otol Rhinol Laryngol 1975; 84:164.

16. Coats AC. On electrocochleographic electrode design. J Acoust Soc Am 1974; 56:708.

17. Stillman RD, et al. Components of the frequency following potential in man. Electroencephalogr Clin Neurophysiol 1978; 44:438–446.

18. Spehlmann R. Evoked Potential Primer. Boston: Butterworths, 1985;212.

19. Jewett DL, Williston JS. Auditory evoked far fields averaged from the scalp of humans. Brain 1971; 94:681–696.

20. Sohmer H, Feinmesser M. Cochlear action potentials recorded from the external ear in man. Ann Otol Rhinol Laryngol 1967; 76:427–435.

21. Moller AR, et al. Contributions from the auditory nerve to the brainstem auditory evoked potentials (BAEPs): Results of intracranial recordings in man. Electroencephalogr Clin Neurophysiol 1988; 71:198–211.

22. Moller AR, Jannetta PJ. Interpretation of brain

stem auditory evoked potentials: Results from intracranial recordings in humans. Scand Audiol 1983; 12:125–133.

23. Tsuchitani C. Functional organization of lateral cell groups of the cat superior olivary complex. J Neurophysiol 1977; 40:296–318.

24. Humphrey DR. Re-analysis of the antidromic cortical response. II. On the contribution of cell discharge and PSPs to the evoked potentials. Electroencephalogr Clin Neurophysiol 1968; 25:421–442.

25. Cassvan A, et al. Combined effect of click rate and stimulus polarity on BAEPs latencies. Electromyogr Clin Neurophysiol 1989; 7-8:453–458.

26. Stockard JJ, et al. Nonpathologic factors influencing brain stem auditory evoked potentials. Am J EEG Technol 1978; 18:177–209.

27. Sohmer H, Student M. Auditory nerve and brain stem evoked responses in normal, autistic, minimal brain dysfunction and psychomotor retarded children. Electroencephalogr Clin Neurophysiol 1978; 44:380–388.

28. Tanquay PE, et al. Auditory brain stem evoked responses in autistic children. Arch Gen Psychiatry 1982; 39:174–180.

29. Picton TW, Durieux-Smith A. Auditory evoked potentials in the assessment of hearing. Neurol Clin 1988; 6:791–808.

30. Allison T, et al. Development and aging changes in somatosensory, auditory and visual evoked potentials. Electroencephalogr Clin Neurophysiol 1984; 58:14–24.

31. Ken-Dror A, et al. Auditory brain stem evoked potentials to clicks at different presentation rate: Estimating maturation of pre-term and full-term neonates. Electroencephalogr Clin Neurophysiol 1987; 68:209–218.

32. Beagley HA, Sheldrake JB. Differences in brain stem response latency with age and sex. Br J Audiol 1978; 12:69–77.

33. Jerger J, Hall J. Effects of age and sex on auditory brain stem response. Arch Otolaryngol 1980; 106:387–391.

34. Kjaer M. Recognizability of brain stem auditory evoked potential components. Acta Neurol Scand 1980; 62:20–33.

35. Michalewski HJ, et al. Sex differences in the amplitudes and latencies of the human auditory brain stem potential. Electroencephalogr Clin Neurophysiol 1980; 48:351–356.

36. Markand ON, et al. Effects of hypothermia on brain stem auditory evoked potentials in humans. Ann Neurol 1987; 22:507–513.

37. Marshall NK, Donchin E. Circadian variation in the latency of brain stem responses and its relation to body temperature. Science 1981; 212:356–358.

38. Eggermont JJ, Don M. Analysis of the click-evoked brain stem potentials in humans using high-pass noise masking. II. Effect of click intensity. J Acoust Soc Am 1980; 68:1671–1675.

39. Rosenhammer HJ, et al. On the use of click-evoked electric brain stem responses in audiological diagnosis. III. Latencies in cochlear hearing loss. Scand Audiol 1981; 10:3–11.

40. Galambos R, Hecox K. Clinical applications of the brain stem auditory evoked potentials. Prog Clin Neurophysiol 1977; 2:1–19.

41. Bahls FH, et al. A case of persistent cortical deafness: Clinical, neurophysiologic and neuropathologic observations. Neurology 1988; 38:1490–1493.

42. Jones TA, et al. Temperature-independent alteration of brain stem auditory evoked responses by enflurane. Soc Neurosci Abstr 1978; 4:154.

43. Squires KC, et al. Acute effects of alcohol on auditory brain stem potentials in humans. Science 1978; 102:174.

44. Chu NS, et al. Auditory brain stem potentials in chronic alcohol intoxication and alcohol withdrawal. Arch Neurol 1978; 35:596.

45. Chiappa KH. Evoked Potentials in Clinical Medicine, ed 2. New York: Raven Press, 1990; 237,239,250.

46. Chiappa KH. Utility of lowering click intensity in neurologic applications of brain stem auditory evoked potentials. In: Starr A, Rosenberg C, Don M, et al., eds. Sensory Evoked Potentials. I. An International Conference on Standards in Auditory Brainstem Response Testing, Centro Ricerche e Studi Amplifon, Milan, 1984;131–132.

47. Satya-Murti S, Cacace A. Brain stem auditory evoked potentials in disorders of the primary sensory ganglion. In: Courjon J, Mauguiere F, Revol M, eds. Clinical Applications of Evoked Potentials in Neurology. New York: Raven Press, 1982;219–225.

48. Starr A, Hamilton AE. Correlation between confirmed sites of neurologic lesions and abnormalities of far field auditory brain stem responses. Electroencephalogr Clin Neurophysiol 1976; 41:595–608.

49. House JW, Brackmann DE. Brain stem audiometry in neurotologic diagnosis. Arch Otolaryngol 1979; 105:305–309.

50. Maurer K, et al. Acoustic tumor detection with early auditory evoked potentials and neuroradiological methods. J Neurol 1982; 227:177–185.

51. Parker SW, et al. Brain stem auditory evoked responses in patients with acoustic neuromas and cerebellopontine angle meningiomas. Neurology 1980; 30:413–414.

52. House JW, et al. Magnetic resonance imaging in

acoustic neuroma diagnosis. Ann Otol Rhinol Laryngol 1986; 95:16–20.

53. Grabel JC, et al. Brain stem auditory evoked responses in 56 patients with acoustic neurinoma. J Neurosurg 1991; 74:749–753.

54. Stockard JJ, Sharbrough FW. Unique contributions of short-latency auditory and somatosensory evoked potentials to neurologic diagnosis. In: Desmedt JE, ed. Clinical Uses of Cerebral, Brainstem and Spinal Somatosensory Evoked Potentials. Basel: Karger, 1980;231.

55. Stockard JJ, et al. Nonpathologic factors influencing brain stem auditory evoked potentials. Am J EEG Technol 1978; 18:177.

56. Goldie WD, et al. Brain stem auditory and short-latency somatosensory evoked responses in brain death. Neurology 1981; 31:248–256.

57. Chiappa KH, et al. Brain stem auditory evoked responses in 200 patients with multiple sclerosis. Ann Neurol 1980; 7:135–143.

58. Bartel DR, et al. The diagnosis and classification of multiple sclerosis: Evoked responses and fluid electrophoresis. Neurology 1983; 33:611–617.

59. Fischer C, et al. Diagnostic value of brain stem auditory evoked potentials. Rev Neurol 1981; 137:229–240.

60. Tackmann W, et al. Auditory brain stem evoked potentials in patients with multiple sclerosis: Investigations in patients with different degrees of diagnostic probability. Eur Neurol 1980; 19:396–401.

61. Ropper AH, et al. Absence of evoked potential abnormalities in acute transverse myelopathy. Neurology 1982; 32:80–92.

62. Tackmann W, et al. Multimodality evoked potentials and electrically elicited blink reflex in optic neuritis. J Neurol 1982; 227:157–163.

63. Maurer K, Lowitsch K. Brain stem auditory evoked potentials (BAEP) in reclassification of 143 MS patients. In: Courjon C, Mauguiere F, Revol M, eds. Clinical Applications of Evoked Potentials in Neurology. New York: Raven Press, 1982; 481.

64. Brown FR, et al. Auditory evoked brain stem response and high performance liquid chromatography sulfatide assay as early indices of metachromatic leukodystrophy. Neurology 1981; 31:980–985.

65. Garg BP, et al. Usefulness of BAER studies in the early diagnosis of Pelizaeus-Merzbacher disease. Neurology 1983; 33:955–956.

66. Garg BP, et al. Evoked response studies in patients with adrenoleukodystrophy and heterozygous relatives. Arch Neurol 1983; 40:356–359.

67. Wiederholt WC, et al. Central pontine myelino-

lysis: A clinical reappraisal. Arch Neurol 1977; 34:220.

68. Brown RH, et al. Brain stem auditory evoked responses in 22 patients with intrinsic brain stem lesions: Implications for clinical interpretations. Electroencephalogr Clin Neurophysiol 1981; 51:36P.

69. Kjaer M. Localizing brain stem lesions with brain stem auditor evoked potentials. Acta Neurol Scand 1980; 61:265–274.

70. Factor SA, Dentinger MP. Early brain stem auditory evoked responses in vertebrobasilar transient ischemic attacks. Arch Neurol 1987; 44:544–547.

71. Eggermont JJ, et al. Electrocochleography and auditory brain stem electric responses in patients with pontine angle tumors. Ann Otol Rhinol Laryngol 1980; (Suppl) 89:75.

72. Hacke W, et al. Evoked potential monitoring during acute occlusion of the basilar artery and selective local thrombolytic therapy. Arch Psychiatr Nervenkr 1982; 232:541.

73. Satya-Murty S, et al. Auditory dysfunctions in Friedreich's ataxia: Result of spiral ganglion degeneration. Neurology 1980; 30:1047–1053.

74. Oppenheimer DR. Brain lesions in Friedreich's ataxia. Can J Neurol Sci 1979; 6:173.

75. Strich SJ. Pathological findings in three cases of ataxia-telangiectasia. J Neurol Neurosurg Psychiatry 1966; 24:489.

76. Lynn GE, et al. Olivopontocerebellar degeneration: Effects on auditory brain stem responses. Semin Hear 1983; 4:375–378.

77. Nuwer MR, et al. Evoked potential abnormalities in the various inherited ataxias. Ann Neurol 1983; 13:20–27.

78. Harkins SW. Effects of presenile dementia of the Alzheimer type on brain stem transmission time. Int J Neurosci 1981; 15:165–170.

79. Gawel MJ, et al. Visual and auditory evoked responses in patients with Parkinson's disease. J Neurol Neurosurg Psychiatry 1981; 44:227–232.

80. Begleiter H, et al. Auditory brain stem potentials in chronic alcoholics. Science 1981; 211:1064–1066.

81. Stockard JJ. Brain stem auditory evoked potentials in adult and infant sleep apnea syndromes, including sudden infant death syndrome and near-miss for sudden infant death. Ann NY Acad Sci 1982; 388:443–465.

82. Stockard JJ, Hecox K. Brain stem auditory evoked potentials in sudden infant death syndrome (SIDS), ''near-miss-for-SIDS'' and infant apnea syndrome. Electroencephalogr Clin Neurophysiol 1981; 51:43P.

83. Orlowski J, et al. Abnormal brain stem auditory

evoked potentials in infants with threatened sudden infant death syndrome. Cleve Clin Q 1979; 46:77.

84. Nodar RH, et al. Abnormal brain stem potentials in infants with threatened sudden infant death syndrome. Otolaryngol Head Neck Surg 1980; 88:619.

85. Kileny P, et al. Auditory brain stem responses in sudden infant death syndrome: Comparison of siblings, "near-miss" and normal infants. J Pediatr 1982; 101:225.

86. Gupta PR, et al. Brain stem auditory evoked potentials in near-miss sudden infant death syndrome. J Pediatr 1981; 98:791.

87. Henderson-Smart DJ, et al. Clinical apnea and brain stem neural function in preterm infants. N Engl J Med 1983; 308:353–357.

88. Bickford RG, et al. Nature of averaged evoked potentials to sound and other stimuli in man. Ann NY Acad Sci 1964; 112:204–223.

89. Cody DTR, Bickford RG. Averaged evoked myogenic responses in normal man. Laryngoscope 1969; 79:400–416.

90. Mast TE. Short-latency human evoked responses to clicks. J Appl Physiol 1965; 20:725–730.

91. Robinson K, Rudge P. Centrally generated auditory potentials. In: Halliday AM, ed. Evoked Potentials in Clinical Testing. Edinburgh: Churchill Livingstone, 1982;370.

92. Kiang NY-S, et al. Post auricular electrical response to acoustic stimuli in humans. Quarterly Progress Report No 68. Research Laboratory of Electronics, MIT. Cambridge, Mass: MIT Press, 1963;218–225.

93. Bickford RG. Physiological and clinical studies of microreflexes. Electroencephalogr Clin Neurophysiol 1972; 31 (suppl):93–108.

94. Inanaga K, Yamagushi E. The averaged photopalpebral reflex in man. Electroencephalogr Clin Neurophysiol 1969; 27:665P.

95. Cracco RQ, Bickford RG. Comparison of evoked somatosensory and somatomotor responses in man. Electroencephalogr Clin Neurophysiol 1966; 21:412P.

96. Geisler CD, et al. Extracranial responses to acoustic clicks in man. Science 1958; 138:1210–1211.

97. Picton TW, et al. Human auditory evoked potentials. I. Evaluation of components. Electroencephalogr Clin Neurophysiol 1974; 36:179–190.

98. Davis H. Principles of electric response audiometry. Ann Otol Rhinol Laryngol 1976; 28:1–96.

99. Celesia GG, Puletti F. Auditory cortical areas of man. Neurology 1969; 19:211–220.

100. Goff GD, et al. The scalp topography of human somatosensory and auditory evoked potentials. Electroencephalogr Clin Neurophysiol 1977; 42:57–76.

101. Goff WR, et al. Origins of short-latency auditory evoked response components in man. In: Desmedt JE, ed. Progress in Clinical Neurophysiology, vol 2. Basel: Karger, 1977.

102. Parving A, et al. Middle components of the auditory evoked response in bilateral temporal lobe lesions. Scand Audiol 1980; 9:161–167.

103. Zerlin S, Naunton RF. Early and late averaged electroencephalic response at low sensation levels. Audiology 1974; 13:366–378.

104. Engel R. Early waves of the electroencephalic auditory response in neonates. Neuropaediatrie 1971; 3:147–154.

105. Skinner PH, Glattke TJ. Electrophysiologic response audiometry: State of the art. J Speech Hearing Res 1977; 42:179–198.

106. McRandle CC, et al. Early averaged electroencephalic response to click in neonates. Ann Otol Rhino Laryngol 1974; 83:695–702.

107. Goldstein R, McRandle CC. Middle components of the averaged electroencephalic response to clicks in neonates. In: Hirsh SK, Eldredge DH, Hirsh IJ, et al., eds. Essays Honoring Hallowell David. St. Louis: Washington University Press, 1976.

108. Davis H. Brain stem and other responses in electrical response audiometry. Ann Otol Rhinol Laryngol 1976; 85 (suppl):3–14.

109. Picton TW, Hillyard SA. Human auditory evoked potentials. II. Effects of attention. Electroencephalogr Clin Neurophysiol 1974; 36:191–199.

110. Mendel MI, Goldstein R. Early components of the averaged electroencephalic response to constant level clicks during all-night sleep. J Speech Hearing Res 1971; 14:829–840.

111. Mendel MI, Goldstein R. Stability of the early components of the averaged electroencephalic response. J Speech Hearing Res 1969; 12:351–361.

112. Kupperman GL, Mendel MI. Threshold of the early components of the averaged electroencephalic response determined with tone pips and clicks during drug-induced sleep. Audiology 1974; 13:379–390.

113. Harker LA, et al. Influence of succinylcholine on middle component auditory evoked potentials. Arch Otolaryngol 1977; 103:133–137.

114. Galambos R, et al. A 40-Hz auditory potential recorded from the human scalp. Proc Nat Acad Sci USA 1981; 78:2643–2647.

115. Robinson K, Rudge P. Auditory evoked responses in multiple sclerosis. Lancet 1975; 1:1164–1166.

116. Robinson K, Rudge P. Abnormalities of the au-

ditory evoked potentials in patients with multiple sclerosis. Brain 1977; 100:19–40.

117. Robinson K, Rudge P. The stability of the auditory evoked potentials in normal man and patients with multiple sclerosis. J Neurol Sci 1978; 36:147–156.

118. Terkildsen K, et al. The ABR and MLR in patients with acoustic neuromas. Scand Audiol Suppl 1981; 13:103–107.

119. Graham J, et al. Cortical deafness. A case report and review of the literature. J Neurol Sci 1980; 48:35–59.

120. Davis PA. Effects of the acoustic stimuli on the waking human brain. J Neurophysiol 1939; 2:494–499.

121. Davis H, et al. Electrical reactions of the human brain to auditory stimuli during sleep. J Neurophysiol 1939; 2:500–514.

122. Dawson GD. Cerebral responses to electrical stimulation of peripheral nerve in man. J Neurol Neurosurg Psychiatry 1947; 10:134–140.

123. Davis H, Yoshie N. Human evoked cortical responses to auditory stimuli. Physiologist 1963; 6:164.

124. Kooi KA, et al. Polarities and field configuration of the vertex components of the human evoked response: A reinterpretation. Electroencephalogr Clin Neurophysiol 1971; 31:166–169.

125. Knight RT, et al. The effects of frontal and temporal-parietal lesions in the auditory evoked potential in man. Electroencephalogr Clin Neurophysiol 1980; 50:112–114.

126. Beagley HA, Knight JJ. Changes in auditory evoked response with intensity. J Laryngol Otol 1967; 81:861–873.

127. Picton TW, et al. Habituation and attention in the auditory system. In: Keidel WD, Neff WD, eds. Handbook for Sensory Physiology, vol V, part 3. Heidelberg: Springer-Verlag, 1976.

128. Schwent VL, et al. Selective attention and the auditory vertex potential. I. Effects of stimulus delivery rate. Electroencephalogr Clin Neurophysiol 1976; 40:604–614.

129. Schwent VL, et al. Selective attention and the auditory vertex potential. II. Effects of signal intensity and masking noise. Electroencephalogr Clin Neurophysiol 1976; 40:615–622.

130. Rapin I, et al. Reliability in detecting the auditory evoked response (AER) for audiometry in sleeping subjects. Electroencephalogr Clin Neurophysiol 1972; 32:521–528.

131. Callaway E, Halliday RA. Evoked potential variability. Effects of age, amplitude and methods of measurement. Electroencephalogr Clin Neurophysiol 1973; 34:125–133.

132. Picton TW, Smith AD. The practice of evoked potential audiometry. Otolaryngol Clin North Am 1978; 11:263–282.

133. Zambelli AJ, et al. Auditory evoked potentials in formerly hyperactive adolescents. Am J Psychiatry 1977;134:

134. Sutton S, et al. Evoked potential correlates of stimulus uncertainty. Science 1965; 150:1187–1188.

135. Donchin E, et al. Graded changes in evoked response (P300) amplitude as a function of cognitive activity. Perception Psychophys 1973; 14:319–324.

136. Sutton S, et al. Information delivery and the sensory evoked potential. Science 1967; 155:1436–1439.

137. Donald MW, Goff WR. Attention-related increases in cortical responsivity dissociated from CNV. Science 1971; 172:1163–1166.

138. Picton TW, et al. Evoked potential audiometry. J Otolaryngol (Toronto) 1977; 6:90–119.

139. Blackwood DHR, Muir WJ. Cognitive brain potentials and their application. Br J Psychiatry 1990; 157 (suppl 9):96–101.

140. Goodin DS, et al. Long-latency event-related components of the auditory evoked potential in dementia. Brain 1987; 101:635–648.

141. St. Clair DM, et al. P300 and other long-latency auditory evoked potentials in presenile dementia, Alzheimer type and alcoholic Korsakoff syndrome. Br J Psychiatry 1985; 147:702–706.

142. Goodin DS, Aminoff MN. Electrophysiological difference between subtypes of dementia. Brain 1986; 109:1103–1113.

143. Goodin DS, et al. Long-latency event-related potentials in patients infected with immunodeficiency virus. Ann Neurol 1990; 27:414–419.

144. Pfefferbaum A, et al. Clinical application of the P3 component of event-related potentials. II. Dementia, depression and schizophrenia. Electroencephalogr Clin Neurophysiol 1984; 59:104–124.

145. Blackwood DRH, et al. Changes in auditory P3 event-related potential. Br J Psychiatry 1987; 150:154–160.

146. Blackwood DRH, et al. Auditory P300 and eye tracking dysfunction in schizophrenic pedigrees. Arch Gen Psychiatry 1990;

147. Walter WG, et al. Contingent negative variation: An electric sign of sensorimotor association and expectancy in the human brain. Nature 1964; 203:380–384.

148. Robert CS, Knott JR. The vertex nonspecific evoked potentials and latency of contingent negative variation. Electroencephalogr Clin Neurophysiol 1970; 28:561–565.

149. Sanquist TF, et al. Slow potential shifts of human

brain during forewarned reaction. Electroencephalogr Clin Neurophysiol 1981; 51:639–649.

150. Rockstroh B, et al. The effects of slow cortical potentials on response speed. Psychophysiology 1982; 19:211–217.

151. Yamamoto T, et al. Effects of disturbed sleep on contingent negative variation. Sleep 1984; 7:331–338.

152. Keidel WD. DC potentials in auditory evoked response in man. Acta Otolaryngol 1971; 71:242–248.

153. Picton TW, et al. Human auditory sustained potentials. I. The nature of the response. Electroencephalogr Clin Neurophysiol 1978; 45:186–197.

# Somatosensory and Motor Evoked Potentials

ERWIN G. GONZALEZ

## Somatosensory Evoked Potential

The application of somatosensory evoked potential (SSEP) is a natural extension of the electrodiagnostic medical examination. SSEP testing provides a window for exploring portions of the nervous system that are difficult to study by electromyographic (EMG) and nerve conduction methods. Dawson[1] is credited with the first clinically recorded SSEP. He used simple superimposition of individual responses obtained on the scalp of a patient with myoclonic epilepsy, a condition characterized by large SSEP amplitudes. The limited range and sensitivity of the available instruments hampered initial attempts to record SSEPs in a clinical setting. The last decade, however, has seen major strides in the development and availability of microprocessors, together with the introduction of sophisticated electronic averagers and low-noise amplifier systems, facilitating the utilization of evoked response testing in research and clinical facilities.

### Recording Method

When an appropriate peripheral nerve or dermatome is stimulated, an SSEP is generated along the neuroaxis, progressing to a specific topography in the cortex. These potentials are made up of various components that occur at different latencies. Ideally, the components are labeled according to polarity and latency. In most instances, the mean latency of a particular component is used to identify the potential, no matter what the absolute latency for a given subject. Thus, a component identified as $P_{37}$ may in fact be $P_{38}$, and $N_{45}$ could be $N_{46}$. For this reason, some laboratories simply identify the components based on sequence of appearance, such as $P_1$, $N_1$, $P_2$, $N_2$ (Figure 12C-1). The reader should be aware, however, that polarity may change according to the montage used, and latencies may shift proportionately with the patient's height or arm span.[2-4] The configuration of the SSEP also depends on whether the recording is obtained by unipolar noncephalic (far-field) or bipolar cephalic (near-field) referential techniques.[5,6] In the former case, the reference electrode is placed at a site distant from the spine or scalp, such as the knee or shoulder, whereas in the latter, both recording and reference electrodes are located on the spine or scalp. A change in the recording montage may result in reversal of a particular latency's polarity, but its generator site may not necessarily be the same. For purposes of discussion, in this section I deal only with short-latency potentials (i.e., shorter than 25 msecs and 45 msecs when stimulating the arm and leg, respectively). Though not totally immune, short-latency potentials are more stable and less affected by wakefulness or by light anesthesia. Short-latency potentials are currently of the most interest

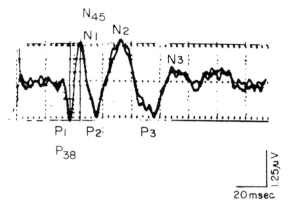

**Figure 12C-1.** Typical example of a normal tibial nerve cortical SSEP. The waveforms are identified according to polarity and mean latency. For individual examinations, absolute latency is reported; thus, $P_{38}$ may in fact be $P_{37}$ or $N_{45}$ could be $N_{46}$. As an alternative, components are labeled according to polarity and their sequence of appearance: $P_1$, $N_1$, $P_2$, $N_2$, etc. (From Gonzalez EG, Hajdu M, Bruno R, et al. Lumbar spinal stenosis: An analysis of pre- and postoperative somatosensory evoked potentials. Arch Phys Med Rehabil 1985; 66:11–14, with permission.)

in clinical SSEP examination.[7,8] The use of long-latency evoked potentials ($P_{300}$) for cognitive evaluation is discussed earlier in this chapter.

The SSEP is mediated primarily via large-diameter peripheral sensory fibers and the dorsal column lemniscal pathways. This assumption is correlated with abnormal SSEPs associated with loss of position sense or experimental destruction of these tracts in animals.[9,10] In cats with experimental dorsal column transection, evidence exists that extralemniscal activity also plays a role, particularly if the stimulus is sufficiently intense.[11] When a mixed nerve is stimulated, group I muscle afferents propagate the impulse, which results in a faster, shorter-latency SSEP, as compared to stimulation of a slower group II cutaneous nerve.[12] Whether excitation of C and delta fibers also produces an SSEP is subject to speculation.[13,14]

A variety of electrodes can be used to record SSEPs. Gold or silver–silver chloride EEG cup electrodes are preferred to platinum needle or clip EEG electrodes because of their lower impedance. Needle and clip electrodes, on the other hand, are quicker to place and secure, particularly in the intraoperative setting. In order to reduce imped-

ance to less than 5 k$\Omega$, the scalp and skin in all electrode placement sites, including the recording, reference, and ground, must be abraded with one of the commercially available gel preparations.

Just about any nerve or dermatome can be stimulated. In upper extremity examinations, mixed nerves like the median and ulnar at the wrist are often used because they yield more consistent and higher-amplitude waveforms.[14,15] Pure sensory fibers can also be stimulated to examine specific segments, as for instance, the forefinger for C-6, the middle finger for C-7, and the little finger for C-8. In the lower extremity, the tibial, peroneal, sural, and saphenous nerves at the ankle or the first web space (L-5), the lateral aspect of the foot (S-1), and the lateral femoral cutaneous nerve or anterolateral aspect of the thigh (L-2) are easily accessible. Table 12C-1 summarizes the different stimulation sites and the normal latencies elicited by segmental sensory examination.[2] Segmental stimulation is discussed further in the section on radiculopathies.

Surface-stimulating electrodes are placed with the cathode proximal to the anode. Wherever the site of stimulation, the intensity is usually three to four times the sensory threshold value or one to two times the motor threshold. The intensity ranges from 10 to 15 mA for constant current or 80 to 120 V for constant voltage stimulator with 0.1 to 0.2 msec pulse duration at a rate of 3 to 4 Hz. In contrast to cortical SSEPs, spinal SSEP latencies and amplitudes are not altered with rates up to 10 Hz. For cortical recordings, however, the optimal compromise between expediency and attenuation is 5 Hz.[16–18]

The recording montage and stimulation sites may vary according to specific components of interest. The standards recommended for recording short-latency SSEPs after upper or lower extremity stimulation, as discussed in this section, follow the guidelines of American Association of Electrodiagnostic Medicine.[19]

Median nerve stimulation at the wrist evokes a cortical response within 25 msec. The analysis time used is 40 msecs from stimulus onset and extended up to 100 msecs if no cortical responses are readily evident. The recommended number of individual trials varies from 250 to 2000. A montage consisting of the following derivations is sug-

**Table 12C-1.** Segmental Sensory Stimulation[2]

| Cutaneous Nerve | Stimulation Site | Segment | Normal Values (msec)* |
|---|---|---|---|
| Musculocutaneous | Forearm | C-5 | $17.4 \pm 1.2$ |
| Median | Thumb | C-6 | $22.5 \pm 1.1$ |
| Median | Fingers 2-3 | C-7 | $21.2 \pm 1.2$ |
| Ulnar | Finger 5 | C-8 | $22.5 \pm 1.1$ |
| Lateral femoral | Thigh | L-2 | $31.8 \pm 1.8$ |
| Saphenous | Knee | L-3 | $37.6 \pm 2.0$ |
| Saphenous | Ankle | L-4 | $43.4 \pm 2.2$ |
| Superficial peroneal | Above ankle | L-5 | $39.3 \pm 1.8$ |
| Sural | Ankle | S-1 | $42.1 \pm 1.4$ |

* $N_{19}$ for upper extremity, $P_{38}$ for lower extremity.

gested for a four-channel recording: (1) $C_{3'}$ or $C_{4'}$ to $F_z$, to record $P_{13-14}$ and $N_{20}$ components; (2) $C3'$ or $C4'$ to Erb's point (EP) (contralateral), to visualize $P_9$, $P_{11}$ $P_{13-14}$, and $N_{20}$; (3) cervical spine (C5S or C2S) to $F_z$, to highlight $N_9$, $N_{11}$, $N_{13}$, and $N_{14}$; and (4) EP (ipsilateral) to EP contralateral to side of stimulation, to record EP potential. Figure 12C-2 demonstrates the typical recordings that result when such a montage is used.

A typical lower extremity examination employs stimulation of the posterior tibial nerve at the ankle. The analysis time spans 60 to 80 msecs and up to 200 msecs before a determination is made that SSEPs are absent. It is suggested that results of 250 to 1000 trials be averaged. A four-channel montage consists of (1) $C_{z'}$ to $F_{pz'}$; (2) T12S to 4 cm rostral to T12S; (3) L3S to 4 cm rostral to L3S; and (4) popliteal fossa to medial surface of the knee. Figure 12C-3 illustrates SSEP recordings obtained following this configuration. For all types of SSEP examinations, a minimum of two averaged acquisitions is necessary to ensure reproducibility of evoked responses.

### Physioanatomic Substrates

Using unipolar recording technique, four early positive potentials with fixed latencies, $P_9$, $P_{11}$, $P_{13}$ and $P_{14}$, are found after median nerve stimulation. They occur independent of recording site, in contrast to the subsequent negative waves, which vary in latency depending on electrode location (Figure 12C-4).[20,21] These far-field potentials represent volume-conducted fields of positivity recorded at some distance from the generator

site and are canceled if the reference site is close to the scalp (Figure 12C-2A).

A relationship exists between scalp-recorded far-field potentials and cervical spine–recorded short-latency potentials whereby polarity is instrumentally inverted (Figures 12C-2B, C). The far-field $P_9$ and cervical $N_9$ are generally thought to arise from the distal part of the brachial plexus and usually precede the negative peak of the EP potential (Figure 12C-2D). The scalp potential $P_{11}$ and cervical $N_{11}$ are thought to arise presynaptically, from the dorsal root entry zone,[23] the dorsal horn,[24] or the dorsal column.[25] Cervical $N_{13}$ appears to be a near-field potential that does not shift from low to high cervical cord, and is thought to arise from the cervical dorsal column.[25,26] The subsequent potentials, $N_{14}$ and $P_{14}$, are much more difficult to record and are thought to arise caudal to the thalamus,[27] perhaps from the brain stem[28] or the medial lemniscus.[29]

The peaks that follow $N_{17}$ are best recorded ipsilaterally; $N_{19}$ appears only contralateral to the site of stimulation. Unlike earlier potentials, $N_{17}$ and $N_{19}$ show progressive latency delay from frontal to parietal electrode placement. $N_{17}$ is believed to arise subcortically from the thalamus[30,31]; $N_{19}$ or $N_{20}$ seems to stem from the primary sensory projection,[32–34] but it is doubtful if this reflects the activity of only a single cortical generator.[35]

There is even less certainty about the generator sources of the posterior tibial nerve SSEP. With electrodes placed over the lower spine, two distinct potentials are recorded. One represents a propagated volley (PV), which increases in recorded latency from caudal to rostral. This represents the afferent volley in the cauda equina at caudal lum-

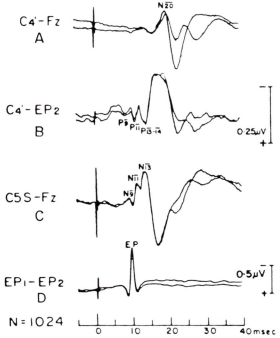

**Figure 12C-2.** Recommended montage using a four-channel recording following left median nerve stimulation at the wrist. (*A*) Cortical unipolar recording using standard EEG 10-20 system. Note $N_{20}$, which is generated from the primary sensory cortex. All of the early far-field potentials are canceled out. (*B*) Unipolar scalp recording referenced to right EP ($EP_2$) shows the early far-field potentials. (*C*) Recording from the fifth cervical spine (C5S) referenced to $F_z$ to record spinal SSEPs. (*D*) Recording at the ipsilateral EP ($EP_1$) referenced to the right EP ($EP_2$). (Redrawn from American Association of Electrodiagnostic Medicine. Guidelines for Somatosensory Evoked Potentials. Rochester, Minn: AAEM, 1984; with permission.)

bar sites and the gracile tract rostrally.[36] This wave is attenuated with bipolar recording; however, a second potential, $N_{22}$, is seen that remains constant in latency though the maximum amplitude is over the T-10–L-1, coinciding with the termination of the conus medullaris at L-1 or L-2 (Figure 12C-5). This probably represents postsynaptic activity in the gray matter of the lumbar cord and is analogous to the $N_{13}$ following median nerve stimulation.[37]

With a scalp far-field or unipolar recording, two widely distributed, low-amplitude responses are recorded, $P_{31}$ and $N_{34}$ (Figure 12C-6). The precise sources of these wavelets are not known. The sim-

ilarity in polarity, temporal, and topographic characteristics to $P_{14}$ and $N_{18}$ potentials after median nerve stimulation imply that they reflect caudal medial lemniscus and subcortical postsynaptic activity in the thalamus or brain stem, or both.[38,39]

In a $C_z$ to $F_{pz}$ configuration, there is cancellation of all earlier waveforms, and the cortical component $P_{38}$ is the first potential visible. $P_{38}$ is most readily recorded posterior to $C_z$ (see Figure 12C-

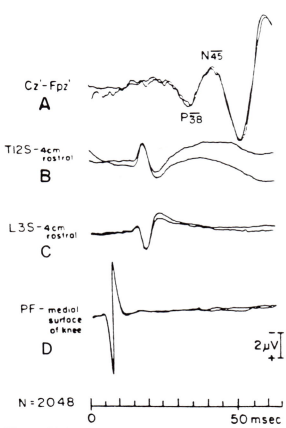

**Figure 12C-3.** A four-channel recording following tibial nerve stimulation at the ankle. (*A*) Bipolar recording using standard scalp recording sites, $C_{z'}$-$F_{pz'}$. Note that the first clearly identifiable wave occurs at $P_{38}$. A small negative potential preceding $P_{38}$ could be barely made out at $N_{34}$. (*B*) Spinal SSEP recorded over the 12th thoracic spine (T12S) referenced 4 cm rostrad. (*C*) Spinal SSEP recorded over the third lumbar spine (L3S) referenced 4 cm rostrad. (*D*) Peripheral sensory recording over the popliteal fossa (PF). (Redrawn from American Association of Electrodiagnostic Medicine. Guidelines for Somatosensory Evoked Potentials. Rochester, Minn: AAEM, 1984; with permission.)

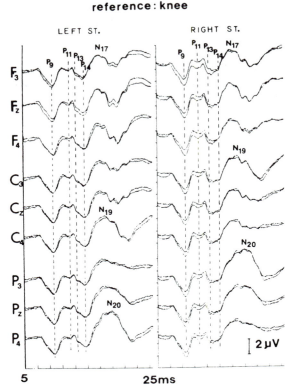

**Figure 12C-4.** Short-latency SSEPs recorded in various scalp locations with reference at the knee. Note the fixed latencies of $P_9$, $P_{11}$, $P_{13}$, and $P_{14}$, regardless of electrode placement. The subsequent negative peaks, on the other hand, shift latency depending on electrode location. (From Yamada T. The anatomic and physiologic bases of median nerve somatosensory evoked potential. Neurol Clin 1988; 6:705–733; with permission.)

3A). In most subjects, when the recording electrode is placed lateral to $C_z$, the maximum amplitude is paradoxically ipsilateral to the side of stimulation. Some authors attribute this phenomenon to representation of the leg and foot primary sensory cortex in the mesial aspect of the postcentral gyrus, within the interhemispheric fissure. $P_{38}$ reflects the ipsilaterally oriented cortical surface positivity, whereas the negative end of this dipole produces a contralateral negative wave.[40–42] It is generally believed that $P_{38}$ results from activation of several regions in the primary sensory area representing the leg and foot.[43] Some researchers contend that the earlier $N_{34}$ reflects the somatosensory cortex instead.[44,45] Table 12C-2 presents a

theoretical comparison of the possible generator sites between median and posterior tibial nerve stimulation.

## Clinical Applications

Although several studies have reported the use of SSEPs to diagnose many diseases of the peripheral and the central nervous system, the fact remains that abnormal SSEPs are not pathognomonic of a specific disease and are commonly considered only in addition to other procedural examinations, including patient history and physical examination.

The clinician faces several problems in interpreting SSEPs. Because of the variation in techniques by which SSEPs are obtained, each laboratory must establish its own normal values. Responses are evaluated by analyzing the absolute latency of the various components. Latency is dependent not only on limb length, height, and type of nerve stimulated, but also on temperature, state of wakefulness, type of recording, and frequency band pass setting, among other variables.[2–4,43, 5–50] Research has demonstrated positive correlation between height and SSEP latency,[3,4] and Figure 12C-7 shows examples of such a relationship. To minimize the effect of temperature upon SSEP values, ambient temperature must be kept between 20° to 22°C.[3] While short-latency SSEPs are relatively unaffected by state of wakefulness, there is nevertheless a drop in amplitude and prolongation of latencies during sleep (Figure 12C-8).[43] This is significant: patients often doze off during the test, and most laboratories administer sedatives prior to a SSEP examination.

Selecting appropriate filter settings is often a juggling act. A common setting is 30 to 3000 Hz. The lower filter setting is a key element in reducing background noise and for the reproducibility of the evoked response. Lowering the filter setting to 1 Hz results in unacceptable SSEP variability, whereas increasing it to 75 Hz markedly reduces the amplitude.[50]

Caution must be exercised when interpreting results in the pediatric age group. It is known that adult values for conduction velocity along the entire somatosensory pathway may not be observed until about age 8 to 12 years,[46,47] and values increase again in elders.[46]

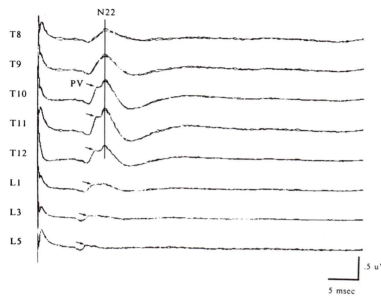

**Figure 12C-5.** Tibial nerve spinal SSEPs recorded over multiple segments of the lumbar and thoracic spines with reference at the iliac crest. Note the propagated volley (PV), which increases in latency from caudal to rostral. PV represents the afferent volley in the cauda equina and gracile tracts. The following wave, $N_{22}$, remains constant, with highest amplitude over the T-10–L-1 spines, which coincide with the termination of the conus medullaris. (From Emerson RG. Anatomic and physiologic basis of posterior tibial nerve somatosensory evoked potential. Neurol Clin 1988; 6:735–749, with permission.

Deviation in latency or interpeak values by more than 3 standard deviations from the norm is regarded as abnormal. Moreover, side-to-side differences in amplitude of more than 50% are also often considered abnormal, though such variation may occasionally occur among normal persons.[51] Waveform morphology is more subjective and difficult to substantiate. The fast Fourier transform technique can be employed to quantitate dispersion of SSEPs.[2]

## Demyelinating Disease

A number of reports have discussed the use of SSEPs in the diagnosis of MS, which is characterized by foci of myelin destruction with relative preservation of the axons and cell bodies. Overall, Chiappa found that 77% of those classified as having definite MS demonstrated abnormalities while only 67% and 49%, respectively, of probable and possible MS patients showed abnormalities.[52] Despite this diagnostic shortcoming, SSEPs are useful in detecting subclinical lesions. Some investigators contend that the diagnostic yield of SEPs for revealing clinically unaffected pathways is higher than that of either VEPs or BAEPs, particularly when a lower extremity nerve is stimulated.[52–55] The sensitivity is further enhanced by hyperthermia.[56] Most laboratories consistently provide multimodality evoked potential testing. As

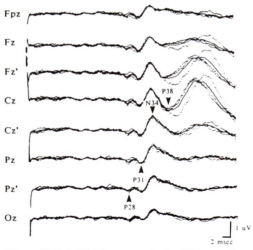

**Figure 12C-6.** Tibial nerve scalp far-field recordings in the sagittal plane using C-5 as reference. Two widely distributed, low-amplitude responses, $P_{31}$ and $N_{34}$, are recorded. The precise generators of these potentials are not known, but they probably reflect activity in the medial lemniscus and thalamus. Note the relative absence of any activity after 35 msec in the $F_{pz}$ recording (*top trace*). (From Emerson RG. Anatomic and physiologic basis of posterior tibial nerve somatosensory evoked potential. Neurol Clin 1988; 6:735–749, with permission.)

**Table 12C-2.** Somatosensory Evoked Potentials and Their Possible Generator Sites Following Median and Tibial Nerve Stimulation

| Median Stimulation | | | Tibial Stimulation | |
|---|---|---|---|---|
| **Spinal EP** | **Cortical EP** | **Generator Site** | **Spinal EP** | **Cortical EP** |
| $N_9$ | $P_9$ | Brachial plexus/cauda equina | PV | – |
| $N_{11-13}$ | $P_{11}$ | Dorsal column | $N_{22}$ | – |
| $N_{14}$ | $P_{14}$ | Medial lemniscus | – | $P_{31}$ |
| – | $N_{17}/N_{18}$ | Thalamus | – | $N_{34}$ |
| – | $N_{19}/N_{20}$ | Primary sensory cortex | – | $P_{38}$ |

previously mentioned, SSEPs have much utility, based upon the length of the white matter tracts involved. The most typical findings are prolongation of absolute and interpeak latencies or loss of components. According to Aminoff,[51,52] after median nerve stimulation it is not unusual to lose the cervical spine potential with preservation of cortical response (Figure 12C-9). Reports differ on the usefulness of SSEPs in following the course of the disease or its response to treatment, including plasmapheresis.[57–60] At present, correlation between clinical and SSEP findings is limited. The advent of MRI, which can detect lesions as small as 3 mm in diameter, has given rise to further doubts about the advantages of SSEPs. SSEPs are more sensitive than MRI in detecting lesions in the posterior fossa.[61] Additionally, other lesions could mimic MRI findings that are frequently associated with MS. A recent study by Turano and others[62] has shown good correlation between MRI

and SSEP findings. Cases in which widespread MRI abnormalities were present despite normal SSEPs were attributed to factors other than demyelination.

*Central Lesions, Strokes, and Brain Injury*

Patients with many types of central nervous system lesions have been subjected to SSEP testing. Lesions in the thalamus and thalamocortical radiation have resulted in loss or attenuation of amplitude and prolongation of latencies. Mesially situated lesions, which primarily affect the lower extremity, show a preferential abnormality in tibial SSEP; lateral lesions, which affect the upper extremity, show median abnormality.[63] Obviously, SSEP abnormalities depend on involvement of the afferent pathways. Thus, patients with Wallenberg's syndrome have normal SSEPs while those with lesions

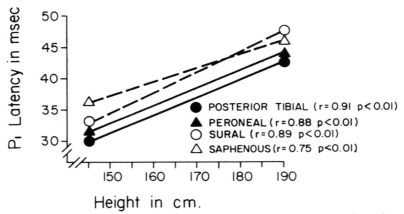

**Figure 12C-7.** Cortical SSEPs as a function of height. The tibial, peroneal, sural, and saphenous nerves were stimulated at the ankle, and SSEPs were recorded using $C_{z'}$ to $F_{z'}$ montage. (From Gonzalez EG, Hajdu M, Bruno R, et al. Lumbar spinal stenosis: An analysis of pre- and postoperative somatosensory evoked potentials. Arch Phys Med Rehabil 1985; 66:11–14, with permission.)

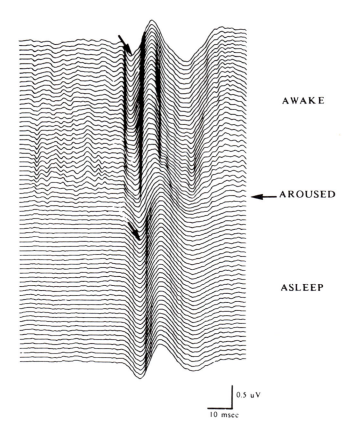

AWAKE

◄— AROUSED

ASLEEP

0.5 uV

10 msec

**Figure 12C-8.** Illustration of SSEP changes in different stages of wakefulness and sleep. Note the drop in amplitude and prolongation of latency. (From Emerson RG. Anatomic and physiologic basis of posterior tibial nerve somatosensory evoked potentials. Neurol Clin 1988; 6:735–749, with permission.)

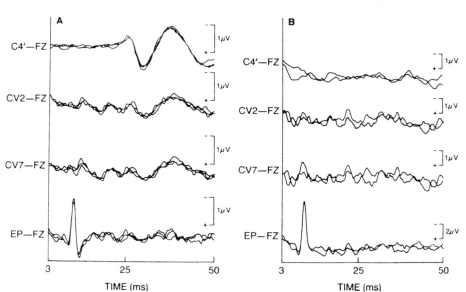

**Figure 12C-9.** SSEPs in two MS patients after median nerve stimulation. (*A*) Well-defined EP (*bottom trace*), ill-defined cervical SSEPs (*middle traces*), and prolonged cortical SSEP (*top trace*). (*B*) No potentials are recognized other than EP. (From Aminoff MJ. The use of somatosensory evoked potentials in the evaluation of the central nervous system. Neurol Clin 1988; 6:809–823, with permission.)

in the medial lemniscus and with locked-in syndrome due to pontine infarction show abnormal SSEPs.[64]

SSEPs among patients with hemispheric strokes have been analyzed to predict functional outcomes.[65–68] A pioneering analysis by Liberson[65] confirmed that SSEPs accurately predict recovery from aphasia. Subsequent reports were encouraging on the value of SSEPs in predicting function. In La Joie and coworkers'[66] series of 42 patients, poor hand function was found among those with abnormal median SSEPs. In another series of 130 patients who had suffered acute strokes, Pavot and colleagues[68] reported that those with normal SSEPs had excellent hand function and 70% were independent in gait and mobility. In contrast, those with absent cortical responses had poor hand function, and 75% were wheelchair bound. The SSEP responses of a small group of 26 patients was compared to other predictor variables, and it was found that the Barthel admission score was a better predictor of functional level but that knowledge of median SSEP and homonymous hemianopsia improve this prediction.[69] Figure 12C-10 shows the interhemispheric SSEP difference in a patient with left hemiparesis. SSEPs in the right hemisphere showed lower amplitude than those in the contralateral side.

Similar applications of SSEPs have been employed to help predict functional outcomes in head injury and coma.[70–74] Sensitivity appears to increase with serial multimodal examination, looking for dynamic trends in the measured parameters. Central conduction time (CCT) as measured by SSEPs has been found by Hume and Cant[70] to be a useful predictor of functional outcome. Some 75% of brain-injured patients with normal CCT achieved good recovery. In contrast, those with absent SSEPs over both hemispheres eventually died, and patients with long-term absence of SSEPs over one hemisphere and consistent CCT abnormalities had residual hemiplegia. In a group of children rendered comatose from various causes those with bilaterally absent SSEPs died or developed severe spastic quadriplegia while those with normal or mild abnormalities eventually were restored to full function.[72] Among adults who suffered cardiac arrest with subsequent anoxic-ischemic coma, those with no recordable SSEPs never recovered cognition; prognosis was less consistent

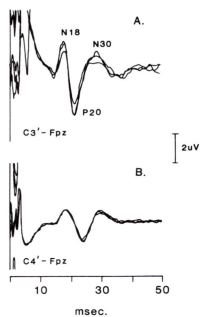

**Figure 12C-10.** Cortical SSEPs obtained in a patient with left hemiparesis. (A) The right median nerve was stimulated at the wrist and recorded over the left hemisphere. (B) The left median nerve was stimulated and recorded over the right hemisphere. Note the lower amplitude in the involved side. (From Chester CS, McLaren CE. Somatosensory evoked responses and recovery from stroke. Arch Phys Med Rehabil 1989; 70:520–525, with permission.)

when SSEPs remained present.[74] The validity of SSEPs in confirming brain death remains controversial.[75,76] In all of the situations just described, SSEPs may provide important prognostic information for groups of patients, though predicting the outcome of individual cases should be tempered with clinical judgment.

*Spinal Cord Injury*

Several studies, including those by Spielholz, Perot, Roweed, and Li and their respective associates have shown that presence of a recordable lower extremity SSEP within 24 to 48 hours after spinal cord injury is usually associated with some clinical improvement.[77–80] This correlates well with clinical experience that those patients with residual sensation tend to regain a certain degree of function. Because SSEPs test only one submodality of somatic sensation, its absence does not necessarily mean a complete lesion, nor does its presence indicate recovery.

### Preventive Monitoring

**Spinal Surgery.** The surgeon's prime concerns during scoliosis and spinal surgery are to provide maximum correction or decompression while preserving neural integrity. To this end, SSEP monitoring has been employed to predict neurologic outcome and minimize postoperative morbidity. SSEPs provide electrophysiologic monitoring under anesthesia that can otherwise be obtained only by clinical examination of a conscious patient. An alternative is a crude examination in a lightly anesthetized patient, as in the *wake-up test*.[81]

A variety of techniques have been reported employing cortical SSEPs, spinal SSEPs, or both.[8,82–87] Preoperative and intraoperative parameters are held constant with a few exceptions. To facilitate placement, needles are used instead of surface cup electrodes, and in an effort to improve spinal recordings, several permutations have been advanced. Nordwall and colleagues[88] used Kirschner wires in the lumbar spine, and while Jones and coworkers[89] utilized epidural recordings. A simpler technique of inserting a needle electrode in the interspinous ligament was reported by Lueders and associates.[90] To overcome the fluctuating skin resistance at the stimulation site, constant current is preferred over constant voltage stimulation. As other operating room equipment tends to interfere with SSEP recordings, it is most important to isolate the SSEP equipment from other power sources and to ensure careful insertion of electrodes.[8,85]

A balanced anesthesia consisting of nitrous oxide plus oxygen, thiopentane, pancuronium, *d*-tubocurarine are the agents of choice.[8,83,84] Halogenated agents are reported to be incompatible with intraoperative SSEPs.[83] Reports to the contrary indicate that controlled doses of halothane, enflurane, and isoflurane are compatible with intraoperative monitoring.[85,91] Bolus injection of any medication is to be avoided during critical periods of monitoring, to minimize compounding variables. SSEP amplitudes are known to become attenuated during hypotension.[83–85,92] Despite this, however, hypotension is often induced during spinal surgery, to reduce blood loss. Gonzalez and coworkers[84]

divided intraoperative monitoring into five periods and found that SSEP values obtained during hypotension provided the best baseline information with which to compare subsequent periods. The surgeon is cautioned if SSEP latency is prolonged by more than 8% to 10% of baseline or when amplitude decrement approaches 50%.[84,85] Figure 12C-11 provides a typical example of normal SSEP recordings during scoliosis surgery; Figure 12C-12 demonstrates a case whereby SSEPs deteriorated during instrumentation, necessitating removal of hardware. The patient woke up paraparetic but recovered completely within 6 months.

It is often believed that SSEPs are transmitted primarily through the posterior columns. Because vascular compromise to the spinal cord is often caused by occlusion of the artery of Adamkiewicz,

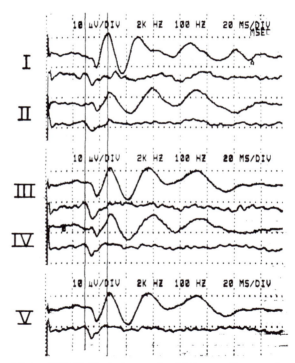

**Figure 12C-11.** Typical example of intraoperative recordings during scoliosis surgery. Each period has two sets of SSEPs, cortical ($C_{z'}$ to $F_{z'}$) is on top, spinal (C7S to $F_{z'}$) at the bottom. Period I is before incision; II, hypotension; III, instrumentation; IV, postinstrumentation; V, closure. Each SSEP was enhanced eight times, gain calibration thus is 1.25μV per division. (From Gonzalez EG, Hajdu M, Keim HA, et al. Quantification of intraoperative somatosensory evoked potentials. Arch Phys Med Rehabil 1984; 65:721–725, with permission.)

C.A. 20y/o Male 78° Thoracic Curve T$_{4-5}$ Hemivertebrae

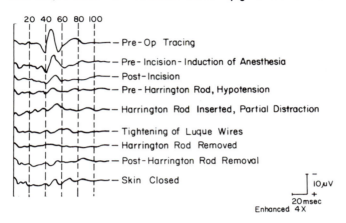

Pre-Op Tracing

Pre-Incision-Induction of Anesthesia

Post-Incision

Pre-Harrington Rod, Hypotension

Harrington Rod Inserted, Partial Distraction

Tightening of Luque Wires

Harrington Rod Removed

Post-Harrington Rod Removal

Skin Closed

10μV

20msec

Enhanced 4X

**Figure 12C-12.** Cortical SSEPs obtained intraoperatively. Note the progressive deterioration of the potentials following instrumentation. SSEPs improved toward the end of the procedure after removal of all hardware. The patient woke up with paraparesis but recovered fully after 6 months. Gain calibration is 2.5μV per division. (From Gonzalez EG, Hajdu M, Keim HA, et al. Quantification of intraoperative somatosensory evoked potentials. Arch Phys Med Rehabil 1984; 65:721–725, with permission.)

only the anterior portion of the cord is likely to be damaged if SSEPs are preserved. There is evidence, however, that the entire transverse diameter is infarcted if occlusion occurs distal to the feeder.[83] The debate continues as to whether SSEP is the appropriate response to monitor. Indeed, there are reports of false negative monitoring,[93,94] but a number of clinical studies continue to demonstrate the usefulness of SEPs.[8,82–87]

Owing to the perceived deficiencies of SSEP monitoring, attention has gradually shifted toward monitoring the motor tracts. New variations have evolved in recent years. Levy[95] introduced transcortical electrical stimulation; Barker[96] and Hess[97] and their coworkers have explored the clinical possibilities of magnetic stimulation.

A more recent application of intraoperative monitoring is in decompressive spinal surgery for narrowed canal syndromes.[98] Spinal stenosis is a condition whereby the anteroposterior or lateral dimensions of the spinal canal are narrowed or abnormally shaped owing to developmental anomaly or degenerative changes. Significant stenosis may cause compression of the nerve roots of the cauda equina in the lateral recess or in one or more foramina. A recent analysis of intraoperative pre- and postdecompression SSEP values among stenosis patients showed a statistically significant improvement in the decompressed nerves.[99] Under these circumstances, monitoring affords the surgeon some guidance to the adequacy of decompression or it may reveal previously unrecognized disease.

In an analysis of pre- and postoperative SSEPs

in 20 cases of spinal stenosis in which a paired two-tailed $t$ test was employed, Gonzalez and colleagues[4] showed significant improvement in latencies of the involved nerves. This improvement is probably attributable to the immediate relief of root compression and the subsequent increase in available numbers of functioning large-diameter myelinated fibers, conversion from conduction block to normal conduction, and perhaps improved axoplasmic flow. Figure 12C-13 typifies pre- and postoperative SSEP findings in a patient with multiple-level spinal stenosis.

SSEP monitoring has also been successfully used during resection of spinal tumors and correction of vascular malformation to assess the extent of cord ischemia during ligation of the feeding vessels.[100,101]

**Aortic Cross-Clamping.** Cross-clamping of the aorta is used to correct aortic coarctation or aneurysm. SSEP monitoring minimizes the inherent risk of cord ischemia—and postoperative paraplegia—during the procedure.[102–105] Any abrupt change in SSEPs during the procedure is considered ominous. Loss of SSEP is usually associated with distal aortic pressure below 40 mm Hg. To prevent cord ischemia, perfusion has to be restored within 15 to 30 minutes.

**Cerebral Hemisphere Monitoring.** The median nerve is a preferred site from which to monitor cerebral function because of the disproportionately large "homunculus" representation of the thumb. SSEP is more specific to the central region of the

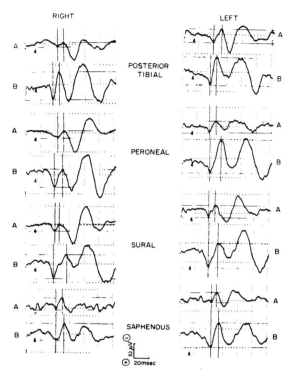

RIGHT  LEFT

POSTERIOR
TIBIAL

PERONEAL

SURAL

SAPHENOUS

20msec

**Figure 12C-13.** Preoperative (A) and postoperative (B) cortical SSEP recordings in a 46-year-old woman, 161 cm tall, with 2-year history of back pain and radiculopathy at the right L-4, L-5, S-1. Note 10-day postoperative improvement in SSEP latencies and amplitudes. (From Gonzalez EG, Hajdu M, Bruno R, et al. Lumbar spinal stenosis: An analysis of pre- and postoperative somatosensory evoked potentials. Arch Phys Med Rehabil 1985; 66:11–14, with permission.)

cortex; EEG covers a wider area. The amplitude of cortical SSEPs decreases whenever cortical blood flow falls below 20 ml per 100 g per minute, and SSEPs are unattainable at 15 ml per 100 g per minute, or a perfusion rate approximately 20% lower than that tolerated by EEG monitoring. This is propitious, as changes in SSEPs are recorded when moderately severe ischemia occurs but before the critical level at which permanent injury results. This results in fewer false positives than with EEGs.[105,106] In most facilities, both EEGs and SSEPs are monitored during carotid endarterectomy, cross-clamping, and cardiopulmonary bypass.

A variation of the procedure is used to localize areas of the motor cortex during neurosurgical pro-

cedures, particularly when the surgical exposure is limited. The technique consists of median nerve stimulation while a strip of platinum or stainless steel disks embedded in flexible silicone sheets or strips is moved around the exposed cortex until potentials are recorded.[87,107] The method can also be adapted to identify other cortical regions representing other body parts.

*Peripheral Nervous System*

Eisen and Aminoff[108] suggested several indications for SSEPs in evaluating peripheral nerve disease: (1) to measure nerve conduction in anatomic sites not routinely accessible by routine studies; (2) to document axonal continuity in the absence of sensory nerve action potentials; (3) to evaluate radiculopathies, particularly when sensory signs or symptoms predominate; and (4) to evaluate plexopathies.

To confirm that abnormal SSEPs are not due to central nervous system disease, Eisen and Aminoff[108] recommend calculating the CCT, which can be obtained by subtracting cortical SSEP latencies from the cervical or lumbar spine potential. CCT should not exceed 7.5 msec in the arm or 22.5 msec in the leg.

**Neuropathies and Nerve Injury.**  The phenomenon of central amplification occurs in normal states and with disease.[109] This amplification can be used to advantage in evaluating the degree of regeneration after nerve injury and in assessing the extent of neuropathy, as in Charcot-Marie-Tooth disease and other hereditary and metabolic neuropathies where routine peripheral nerve conduction studies may not be possible. The phenomenon is secondary to the ability of the cortex to operate as an integrator capable of evoking a sizable response in spite of synaptic delay and severely desynchronized afferent input. Thus, SSEP responses are a direct measure of sensory conduction. In conditions such as Guillain-Barré syndrome, proximal sensory slowing may be difficult to demonstrate with peripheral nerve conduction studies but is readily documented by SSEP examination.

**Radiculopathies.**  New imaging techniques such as CT and MRI have greatly facilitated anatomic localization of root lesions but remain inadequate for defining the physiologic changes that ensue. CT and MRI provide no information on severity or prognosis. Persons older than 50 years often show CT and MRI findings consistent with degenerative disc disease but have no clinical manifestations.

The standard electrophysiologic examinations in radiculopathy are EMG and nerve conduction studies (see Chapters 10 and 11) Specific findings delineating radicular involvement in a specific myotome are the presence of fibrillations or positive waves in the paraspinal muscles, suggesting nerve damage. The limitations are twofold: (1) these potentials occur only after at least a week, and (2) they are absent in neuropraxia. Interpretation of recruitment patterns is subjective at best, and computerized analysis awaits refinement. By definition, radiculopathy occurs proximal to the dorsal root ganglion and, therefore, the conventional sensory conduction velocities are normal. The amplitude of M response has been used by some to define severity,[110] but routine motor nerve conduction velocities are likewise unrevealing. The use of F waves[111] and H reflex[112] were initially heralded as major breakthroughs but have not fulfilled their promise. F waves require stimulation of mixed nerves with supramaximal intensity, so as to cause multisegmental activation. This in essence masks disease in a single root. Consequently, F waves are frequently normal with radiculopathy. On the other hand, H reflex is limited to the gastrosoleus (S-1 sensory root), though it could be facilitated in other muscles by voluntary contraction.[113]

The predominant presenting signs and symptoms of radiculopathy are sensory. In these circumstances, type Ia afferent and type II cutaneous fibers are most likely to be affected.[3] This provides a rationale for why SSEPs have been employed to evaluate radiculopathy. Several methods have been explored in efforts to determine the best technique to identify and isolate the involved root(s). For the same reasons that F waves have a low yield, mixed nerve stimulation to elicit an SSEP is often unproductive, with the possible exception of cases of cervical myelopathy due to spondylosis.[114-116]

Recording of spinal SSEPs is often hampered by technical difficulties. Latency is the only parameter that can be measured with consistency, and that is not likely to be abnormal. This is particularly true in the lower extremity because of the length of the afferent pathway from point of stimulation to recording site. Normally conduction in the distal segment could potentially cancel out slowing in the spinal nerve root, which is, comparatively, a very short segment. Unlike the upper extremity, there is no reliable counterpart for EP recording where interpeak latency with the cervical spine SSEP can be calculated, implying proximal conduction including the roots.

Segmental studies, which include cutaneous nerve, dermatome, and motor point stimulation, appear to be promising, as the inherent problems associated with mixed nerve stimulation are minimized.[107,117-119] The simplest method, stimulation of cutaneous nerves, results in cortical and spinal SSEPs almost comparable to those obtained after mixed nerve stimulation, though the latencies are longer and the amplitudes lower.[119] Disparate involvement between the early and late SSEP potentials in radicular syndromes has been observed.[120] In many instances, the early potentials tend to be prolonged, or sometimes absent, while the later waves fall within normal limits. This behavior is akin to that found in tourniquet paralysis, pointing to the possible roles of both ischemia and compression.

A stimulus of 1.0 msec duration through a needle electrode in the motor point activates type Ia muscle afferents and produces consistently reproducible evoked potentials. This method can likewise be helpful in evaluating radiculopathy, though it cannot isolate a single nerve root.[108]

The ability of dermatomal SSEP to pinpoint specific nerve root involvement, particularly in lumbosacral radiculopathy, has been hailed as a major stride in the clinical application of SSEP recording. However, there are drawbacks in the technique, which requires a large stimulating electrode strip over "signature areas" (Figure 12C-14). Pulses as great as 2.5 times the sensory threshold value are required to excite the cutaneous afferents. The resultant evoked response is smaller and more dispersed, but relatively consistent. With this technique, almost any dermatome can potentially be examined. Proponents believe this method to be an advantageous, noninvasive diagnostic and

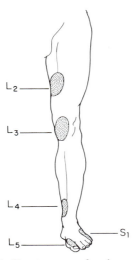

**Figure 12C-14.** Signature areas for placement of stimulating electrodes in dermatomal segmental SSEP determinations in lumbosacral radiculopathy. (Redrawn from Katifi HA, Sedgwick EM. Evaluation of the dermatomal somatosensory evoked potentials in the diagnosis of lumbosacral root compression. J Neurol Neurosurg Psychiatry 1987; 50:1204–1210, with permission.

prognostic tool whose results are reproducible.[121,122] At this time, many other investigators remain skeptical.[123]

**Plexopathies.** It is important to establish the presence of axonal continuity and the absence of root avulsion after traumatic injury to the brachial plexus, in order to decide on the need for a microneurosurgical grafting procedure, the likelihood of success of such grafting, and the prospect for possible spontaneous recovery. For these purposes, myelography, EMG, and NCV studies have been used extensively. The presence of an SSEP despite evidence of meningocele or electrophysiologic findings consistent with root avulsion (fibrillations in the paraspinal muscles, normal sensory nerve action potential, absent M responses, and a positive histamine test result) is still regarded as indicating a favorable prognosis. Unlike EMG, abnormal SSEPs can be noted soon after injury. Which trunks or cords of the brachial plexus are involved can be inferred by stimulating various nerves in the arm.[124–128] For instance, the musculocutaneous nerve gives information on the up-

per trunk and lateral cord; the radial nerve is traced back to the middle trunk and posterior cord; and the ulnar nerve reflects the status of the lower trunk and medial cord. Because of its wide origin from the upper and lower trunks and both medial and lateral cords, median nerve testing can be used as a screen.

Abnormal SSEPs have also been reported in nontraumatic brachial plexopathy, a condition that can follow median sternotomy or brachial plexitis.[129–131]

**Thoracic Outlet Syndrome.** The various clinical entities associated with thoracic outlet syndromes have been elusive to common electrophysiologic examinations. Proximal ulnar nerve conduction and F wave slowing can be found, but often these are not obtained reliably in most clinical settings. To complement these studies, SSEPs have been added to the diagnostic armamentarium.[132,133] One method uses a dynamic approach to evaluate the syndrome. Absolute and interpeak latencies of EP and C7 were determined with the arm in a relaxed anatomic and a dynamic position of abduction and external rotation. In six of 14 symptomatic patients, $N_{13}$ was normal in the anatomic position, but the potential disappeared in the dynamic position.[134]

**Individual Nerve Application.** SEP testing can be used to evaluate various other nerves that are inaccessible by conventional electrodiagnostic techniques. One example is the lateral femoral cutaneous nerve in patients with meralgia paresthetica. This nerve is easily stimulated in the anterolateral aspect of the proximal thigh, even in obese patients.[108,119] Study of the dorsal nerve of the penis or clitoris, a branch of the pudendal nerve, used in conjunction with electrical bulbocavernosus reflex, can provide valuable information in the evaluation of sacral nerve root or plexus injuries and bowel, bladder, or sexual dysfunction.[135] Trigeminal nerve SSEPs have been studied in cases of trigeminal neuralgia.[136] Other cutaneous nerves can also be evaluated, such as the lateral and medial antebrachial cutaneous, dorsal cutaneous branch of the ulnar nerve, and the intercostal and dorsal primary rami.

**Functional Versus Organic Sensory Complaints.** A frequent dilemma in clinical practice is establishing whether a sensory complaint has an organic basis. The medicolegal implications are obvious, particularly when insurance and disability income issues loom large. For the most part, a normal SSEP and peripheral sensory examination would indicate whether or not sensory symptoms have a pathologic basis. This conclusion, however, should be weighed carefully, for, indeed, there are exceptions to the rule. One such example is the presence of normal SSEPs in pure sensory stroke secondary to lacunar infarcts.[137]

**Special Application in Pediatrics.** SSEP recordings are valuable for evaluating a multitude of neurologic diseases because of their inherent objectivity. This is particularly helpful in pediatrics, since the neurologic evaluation of children is often difficult. All the clinical applications mentioned previously apply to the pediatric age group and are of special use in monitoring coma, detecting preclinical abnormalities, and localizing lesions.[138] Research indicates that various leukodystrophies have unique multimodality evoked potential findings.[139,140] Patients with hypotonia and ill-defined neurologic signs often have abnormal SSEPs, indicating the need for further investigation. Abnormalities in SSEPs have been demonstrated in the early course of Huntington's disease, and it may be possible to detect people at risk who carry the gene.[141] Other diseases for which SSEP recording is potentially of value are delayed myelopathy, hemiplegic cerebral palsy, and achondroplasia; it is also valuable in establishing or ruling out organicity of vague sensory complaints.

## Motor Evoked Potentials

Neurophysiologists have now began to explore the previously untapped efferent limb of the central loop. Current motor evoked potential (MEP) methods are derived from techniques tried as early as the late 1800s and early 1900s.[142] In 1954, when electrical stimulation of the unexposed motor cortex became possible, Gualterotti and Patterson tried the technique in baboons and humans.[143] The procedure was too painful to sustain clinical interest. Almost 30 years elapsed before Merton and

Morton refined the technique.[144] Since then, transcranial cortical stimulation (TCS) has evolved as a new medium for investigation, but in a more tempered path than that applied to sensory evoked potentials. The pioneering work of Cowan and associates,[145] and Mills and Murray[146] in applying the test to MS, and by Levy[95] to neurosurgical procedures had barely penetrated the clinical community when Barker and coworkers[96] described a newer method of TCS by magnetic stimulation, which then swept the world of neurophysiology. Thereafter, electrical TCS rapidly fell into disfavor.

The U.S. Food and Drug Administration's classification of transcranial magnetic stimulation as "experimental" has hampered the growth of clinical research. The safety of the procedure needs to be definitively established. In any event, the electrical, thermal, and magnetic energies after TCS are less than, if not comparable to, those of electroconvulsive therapy and MRI. A major concern is the possibility of inducing an epilepsy attack due to electrical stimulation (kindling). To date, no such event has been recorded in normal subjects. Goddard and colleagues[147] indicated that such kindling is unlikely if the stimulus is less than 3 Hz, and in TCS the maximum rate is no greater than 0.3 Hz. Apart from transient headaches and memory lapse, no adverse effects have been reported among subjects.[148,149] Using a pendulum model, Katz and coworkers[150] showed that a minuscule amount of energy is imparted onto metallic fixation devices by the magnetic coil, but no significant paraspinal activity could be detected among healthy volunteers following TCS. Researchers feel that the initial safety concerns are likely to prove unfounded; however, it is prudent to respect the following contraindications: history of seizures, head injury severe enough to cause unconsciousness, or of cranial surgery, or a cardiac pacemaker or other biomedical device.[151]

### Stimulation Techniques

Two types of electrical TCS are employed, bifocal and unifocal. In the former, two stimulators are placed about the cortical motor strip; in the latter, several interconnected pericranial electrodes and one stimulating electrode are used. With either type, anodal stimulation is preferred because a lower threshold is required to elicit an MEP.[148] Of the two types, unifocal stimulation requires less current, because the electrode layout causes a parallel-flowing path, which preferentially penetrates the radially oriented large pyramidal cells, dendrites and axons.[152]

In magnetic stimulation, a high-energy capacitor bank is charged from a high-voltage source through a copper coil, producing a brief magnetic field pulse. Unlike electrical fields, magnetic fields penetrate biologic structures without significant attenuation. The electric field travels in an annular fashion; the intensity is highest under the coil's circumference.[148]

In all types of TCS, surface electrodes are placed over a target muscle to record the MEP. It has been observed that placing the active recording electrode over the motor end-plate and the reference electrode at a distant site results in higher-amplitude MEPs.[151]

The locations of optimal cortical sites for electrical stimulation correlate well with the "motor strip." Thus, Rossini[148] found the lowest threshold for eliciting MEP in the hand is in the contralateral side, lateral to the vertex and slightly frontal to the line connecting the earlobes. Stimulation of the vertex on the other hand results in bilateral MEPs in the lower extremities. The best way to apply the magnetic coil is still subject to research.

Tangential application of the coil over the scalp, with the center just anterior to the vertex, commonly results in hand or arm and leg MEP. If no response is elicited, the coil is moved slightly contralaterally.[151] Cervical[153] and lumbar[154] spine stimulation are achieved with relative ease using magnetic stimulation.

### Physioanatomic Substrate

It is extremely attractive to accept the notion that a single shock TCS causes a synchronous depolarization of groups of cortical motor neurons, which in turn produces a single efferent volley that is propagated down their axons to spinal motor neurons, depolarizing the alpha motor neurons, and after a short synaptic delay results in the eventual activation of the muscle. However, the process is more complex, and it is highly unlikely that only the pyramidal tracts are activated.[142]

Voluntary contraction of the target muscle shortly before or during TCS lowers the excitability threshold of the central motor tracts, with a resultant more robust MEP amplitude (Figure 12C-15). The phenomenon may be due to facilitation of a large population of spinal motor neurons through group I afferent activity from muscles and tendons and enhanced firing of descending corticospinal tracts.[148] Patton and Amassian[155,156] have

**MAGNETIC STIMULATION**

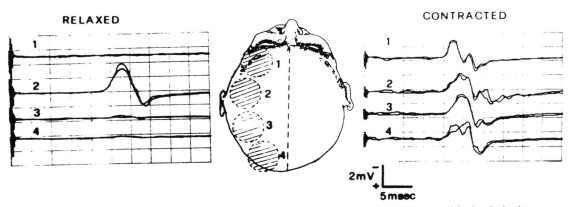

RELAXED                                                          CONTRACTED

2 mV

5 msec

**Figure 12C-15.** MEPs recorded fron the right thenar muscle after magnetic TCS. MEPs are elicited only in the area over the hand motor strip when muscle was relaxed (*left*). In the contracted state (*right*), MEPs were evoked in a wider area of the cortex. (From Rossini PM. The anatomic and physiologic bases of motor evoked potential. Neurol Clin 1988; 6:751–769, with permission.)

observed two types of pyramidal tract responses, a stable early direct wave (D wave), which results from direct excitation of pyramidal neurons, followed by a series of variable deflections (indirect or I waves). I waves are thought to arise from indirect excitation of pyramidal neurons relayed though cortical interneurons. Researchers at present believe that during relaxation, the D and I waves gradually drive a small proportion of spinal motor neurons to their firing threshold and that during contraction, fringe motor neurons that are already close to threshold are fired up to excitation upon arrival of D and I waves. To enhance excitability Rossini has employed prestimulus voluntary contraction of the target muscle, continuous vibration of the tendon, or scalp stimulation with paired shocks.[148,157,158] Facilitation by background voluntary contraction occurs optimally at 15% to 25% of maximum isometric contraction.[148,151,159] Similar effects were also described by Hufnagel and coworkers[160] with nonspecific maneuvers such as sticking out the tongue and counting out loud. Ackerman and associates[159] proposed a different mechanism during postural facilitation. In contrast to results recorded in voluntary contraction, they found an increase in amplitude without decrease in latency in the anterior tibial and soleus MEPs when their subjects were tested standing upright. Whether the difference lies in cortical mechanisms, different descending systems, the spinal circuitry, or a combination of these factors remains unknown.

MEPs in the hand are larger in amplitude than in the leg or foot muscles, perhaps owing to the deeper location of the lower extremity homunculus in the interhemispheric fissure. The fact that, compared to the rest of the spinal cord, the cervical cord receives a relative abundance of pyramidal tract fibers undoubtedly also plays a role.[161,162]

Day,[163] Cracco,[149] Mills,[164] and their coworkers have observed that MEP latency was longer after magnetic stimulation than after electrical stimulation. It is possible that the extra delay is consumed in the central motor pathways and that the types of transcortical stimulation have different modes of eliciting a response. One possible hypothesis is that magnetic stimulation excites the corticospinal neurons transsynaptically whereas electrical stimulation excites them directly.[163]

### Central Motor Pathway Conduction Time

Applying the principles used in determining peripheral motor nerve conduction may not necessarily be appropriate for CCT. In the strictest sense, to measure nerve conduction, the same fibers must be stimulated at two different sites, a single impulse in each fiber must be responsible for the recorded response, and the responses from the two sites must be nearly identical in configuration.[142] In measuring CCT, the spine MEP latency is subtracted from scalp MEP latency (Figure 12C-16). Kadanka and coinvestigators[165] tried to decipher the site of motor pathway excitation during cervical spine stimulation. They compared the motor conduction time in the fastest fibers after spinal stimulation with F and H wave values and concluded that the conduction time after spinal stimulation corresponds with activation of the alpha motor neuron axon near the cell bodies. Without a doubt, spine stimulation is contaminated by noncentral elements such as the axon hillocks or the ventral roots. Realizing this, the reason for the caveat given above becomes obvious. It is therefore appropriate to define such conduction time as latency rather than conduction velocity.

### Clinical Application

The same clinical conditions studied with the different SSEPs are potentially subject to scrutiny with TCS. The lack of extensive clinical experience mandates caution in using the technique to

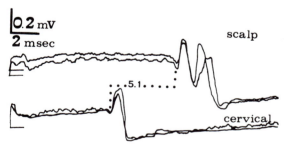

**Figure 12C-16.** MEPs after electrical stimulation of the cortex and cervical region. CCT is calculated at 5.1 msec. (From Rossini PM. The anatomic and physiologic bases of motor evoked potential. Neurol Clin 1988; 6:751–769, with permission.)

"diagnose" specific disorders. Like SSEPs, several factors come into play in deciphering what is normal and abnormal. Because laboratories differ in their methods, no unified normative values are universally applicable. As with SSEPs, there is a strong positive correlation between arm length and height and MEP latency.[150,151] Side-to-side comparison may be more difficult to apply in TCS MEP than with SSEPs. It has been observed that a difference in latency commonly occurs even in healthy subjects[151] and that a statistically significant difference in amplitude has been reported, particularly in the lower extremity.[150] It may be safe to assume that a 50% amplitude difference can be considered abnormal. To avoid such variability, amplitude can be expressed as a percentage of maximum peripheral M response, which is almost always never less than 20%. A value less than 10% is considered abnormal.[151]

In assessing the maturation of the corticospinal tracts, Koh and Eyre[166] observed incremental sensitivity to magnetic stimulation between ages 8 and 11 years and concluded that adult values are reached by age 11. MEP latency increases with age, which is a reflection not only of slowed peripheral conduction but also to central motor delay.[151]

Patients with MS show slowing of CCT as well as reduction of MEP amplitude. Mills and coworkers[146] studied eight clinically definite MS cases and found normal cord-to-axilla conduction times, though CCTs were either markedly prolonged or absent. Whether the technique offers unique advantages over other diagnostic tests remain unanswered. Hess and associates[167] studied 83 patients with MS and correlated their findings with clinical signs. In 72% of cases, CCT was abnormal and correlated well with brisk finger flexor jerks. Among patients with weakness of the abductor digiti quinti, CCT was abnormal in 79% of cases. They found greater sensitivity with the technique compared to visual, somatosensory, or brain stem auditory evoked potentials. Patients with motor neuron disease showed normal CCT, but some exhibited slowing of peripheral conduction as measured by magnetic stimulation.[148,151] In a study of a variety of patients suffering from sensorimotor disturbances, Caramia and colleagues[168] suggested combining the use of MEPs

and SEPs to reveal central propagation abnormalities that may be coupled with peripheral nerve involvement.

In patients with parkinsonism, it is curiously easy to elicit an MEP, and there is reduced CCT, particularly over the more rigid muscles. The same physiologic basis may pertain for such a facilitation as seen with a contracted normal muscle. It is also possible that this phenomenon is due to spinal disinhibition (readily repetitive firing of motor neurons).[151]

In an effort to quantitatively evaluate hemiparesis, Xing and associates[169] used magnetic stimulation and expressed relative amplitude, latency, and threshold of response on the paretic side as a function of responses elicited from the intact side. They concluded that the technique provided a sensitive measure of mild hemiparesis but was of little value for dense paralysis because of the difficulty of eliciting reproducible responses. Dominkus and colleagues subjected a group of 33 patients to TCS 3 days after onset of stroke, and reexamined 23 of them 2 months later.[170] The data demonstrated that motor function changes correlated well with MEP results. Patients who showed normal or prolonged CCT regained function; those with absent CCT did not recover.

Both SSEPs and MEPs were employed in a study of 28 patients with nontraumatic coma by Zentner and Ebner.[171] They hoped to determine if the addition of MEPs increased the prognostic value of SSEPs and concluded that the use of MEPs cannot be recommended for prognostic evaluation of coma of nontraumatic causes.

Dvorak and colleagues[172] performed measurement of MEPs using magnetic TCS in 268 patients with cervical spine disorders. Their data suggest that the method has great sensitivity in detecting compression of the neural structure, particularly among patients with degenerative changes. They also found a high incidence of abnormal CCTs among patients with whiplash injuries, despite absence of a major motor deficit. The same researchers previously established their normative data after cervical spine and plexus stimulation in the axillary region. They hailed the technique as a major advance in spinal cord diagnostics and motor root compression in the intervertebral foramen or canal.[173]

A group of spinal cord–injury patients were investigated by Gainutsos and colleagues,[174] who employed TCS to assess the completeness of the lesions. In all patients, latencies to muscles whose innervation originated above the lesion were normal whereas latencies to muscles innervated below the lesion showed abnormalities. The study also demonstrated that patients deemed to have clinically "complete" lesions possess nerve fibers that descend through the lesion and are capable of conveying impulses leading to muscle contraction. Robinson and Little[175] considered measurement of CCT via TCS, and cervical spine stimulation was deemed a useful diagnostic and follow-up tool in post-traumatic syringomyelia.

TCS holds promise for intraoperative monitoring. Levy[176] recently reviewed his extensive experience with the technique among 98 patients who underwent supratentorial, posterior fossa, and spinal cord procedures. He found that peripheral nerve or EMG responses were substantially more sensitive than the spinal cord responses to injury and hypotension. Reversal of abnormalities did not result in any deficit, but their failure to recover could warn of postoperative motor defect. Spinal cord recording was found to be less reliable. In contrast, however, Kitagawa and colleagues[177] recorded MEP from an epidural electrode and found the technique to be a satisfactory predictor of outcome in a small group of patients undergoing cervical spine surgery. In addition to epidural recording, Preston and coworkers[178] improved upon the method by adding MEP recordings subpially and obtained larger, more consistent amplitudes. At present, the routine clinical use of magnetic stimulation in the operating room milieu is held in abeyance until further research and experience prove the efficacy and safety of the procedure.

The use of magnetic stimulation to evaluate the peripheral nervous system is enticing, particularly because of the relative ease with which proximal and deeply situated nerves can be stimulated. For this reason, the technique has been employed among patients with Guillain-Barré syndrome and brachial plexopathy.[151] The restricted focusing of the currently available magnetic coils limits the usefulness of the technique for stimulating peripheral nerves. Its main value in the peripheral nervous system evaluation may rest in its ability to evaluate the proximal segments of peripheral motor nerves through TCS and spinal stimulation.

## Conclusion

Rapid advances have occurred in electroneurophysiology. The surge in new methods employed to assess the nervous system comes at a time when the overutilization of advanced technologies is under siege. For clinicians, the exploration of previously untapped venues remains tempting; however, the ultimate value of these techniques must be vigorously and conscientiously assessed and the welfare and benefit of patients placed first. A new technique should not be employed, simply because it is new.

## References

1. Dawson GD. Investigations in a patient subject to myoclonic seizures after sensory stimulation. J Neurol Neurosurg Psychiatry 1947; 10:141–162.
2. Eisen A. The somatosensory evoked potentials. Can J Neurol Sci 1982; 9:65–97.
3. Alonso JA, Hajdu M, Gonzalez EG, et al. Cortical somatosensory evoked potentials: Effects of positional changes. Arch Phys Med Rehabil 1989; 70:194–198.
4. Gonzalez EG, Hajdu M, Bruno R, et al. Lumbar spinal stenosis: Analysis of pre- and postoperative somatosensory evoked potentials. Arch Phys Med Rehabil 1985; 66:11–14.
5. Kimura J, Mitsudome A, Beck DO. Field distribution of antidromically activated digital nerve potentials: Model for far-field recording. Neurology 1983; 33:1164–1169.
6. Kimura J, Mitsudome A, Yamada T. Stationary peaks from a moving source in a far-field recording. Electroencephalogr Clin Neurophysiol 1984; 58:351–361.
7. Abrahamson HA, Allison T, Goff WR, et al. Effects of thiopenthal on human cerebral somatic evoked potential. Anesthesiology 1963; 24:650–657.
8. Grundy BL. Monitoring of sensory evoked potentials during neurosurgical operations: Methods and applications. Neurosurgery 1982; II:556–575.
9. Giblin DR. SEP in healthy subjects and in patients with lesions of the nervous system. Ann NY Acad Sci 1964; 122:93–142.

10. Halliday AM. Changes in the form of cerebral evoked responses in man associated with various lesions of the nervous system. Electroencephalogr Clin Neurophysiol 1967; 25:178–192.

11. Martin HF, Katz S, Blackburn JG. Effects of spinal cord lesion on somatic evoked potentials altered by interactions between afferent inputs. Electroencephalogr Clin Neurophysiol 1980; 50:186–195.

12. Burke D, Skuse NF, Lethlean AK. Cutaneous and muscle afferent components of cerebral potential evoked by electrical stimulation of human peripheral nerves. Electroencephalogr Clin Neurophysiol 1981; 51:579–588.

13. Alpsan D. The effect of selective activation of different peripheral nerve fiber groups on the somatosensory evoked potentials in the cat. Electroencephalogr Clin Neurophysiol 1981; 51:589–598.

14. Simpson RK, Blackburn JG, Martin HS, et al. Peripheral nerve fiber and spinal cord pathway contributions to the somatosensory evoked potentials. Exp Neurology 1981; 73:700–715.

15. Yamada T, Kimura J, Young S, et al. Somatosensory evoked potentials elicited by bilateral stimulation of the median nerve and their clinical application. Neurology 1978; 28:218–223.

16. Yamada T. The anatomic and physiologic bases of median nerve somatosensory evoked potentials. Neurol Clin 1988; 6:705–733.

17. Pelosi L, Balbi P, Caruso G. The effect of stimulus frequency on spinal and scalp somatosensory evoked potentials to stimulation of nerves in the lower limb. Electroencephalogr Clin Neurophysiol 1990; 41:149–152.

18. Nuwer M, Dawson E. Intraoperative evoked potential monitoring of the spinal cord: A restricted filter. Scalp method during Harrington instrumentation for scoliosis. Clin Orthop 1984; 183:42–50.

19. American Association of Electrodiagnostic Medicine. Guidelines for Somatosensory Evoked Potentials. Rochester, Minn: 1984.

20. Jones SJ. Short latency potentials recorded from the neck and scalp following median nerve stimulation in man. Electroencephalogr Clin Neurophysiol 1977; 43:853–863.

21. Yamada T, Kimura J, Nitz DM. Short latency somatosensory evoked potentials following median nerve stimulation. Electroencephalogr Clin Neurophysiol 1980; 48:367–376.

22. Cracco RQ, Anzizka B, Cracco JB. Short latency somatosensory evoked potential to median and peroneal nerve stimulation in normal subjects and patients with neurologic diseases. Ann NY Acad Sci 1982; 388:412–415.

23. Lueders H, Lesser R, Hahn J. Subcortical somatosensory evoked potentials to median nerve stimulation. Brain 1983; 106:341–372.

24. Sedgwick EM, El-Negamy E, Frankel H. Spinal cord potentials in traumatic paraplegia and quadriplegia. J Neurol Neurosurg Psychiatry 1980; 43:823–830.

25. Desmedt JE, Cheron G. Central somatosensory conduction in man: neural generators and interpeak latencies of far-field components recorded from neck and right or left scalp and ear lobes. Electroencephalogr Clin Neurophysiol 1980; 50:382–403.

26. Lesser RP, Lueders H, Hahn J, et al. Early somatosensory potentials evoked by median nerve stimulation: Intraoperative monitoring. Neurology 1983; 31:1519–1523.

27. Goff WR, Rosner BS, Allison T. Distribution of cerebral somatosensory evoked responses in normal man. Electroencephalogr Clin Neurophysiol 1962; 14:697–713.

28. Jacobson GP, Tew JM. The origin of the scalp-recorded P14 following electrical stimulation of the median nerve: Intraoperative observation. Electroencephalogr Clin Neurophysiol 1988; 71:73–76.

29. Hashimoto I. Somatosensory evoked potentials from human brainstem: Origins of short latency potentials. Electroencephalogr Clin Neurophysiol 1984; 57:221–227.

30. Tsuji S, Shibasaki H, Kato M, et al. Subcortical, thalamic and cortical somatosensory evoked potentials to median nerve stimulation. Electroencephalogr Clin Neurophysiol 1984; 59:465–476.

31. Yamada T, Graff-Radford NR, Kimura J, et al. Topographic analysis of somatosensory evoked potentials in patients with well-localized thalamic infarction. J Neurol Sci 1985; 68:31–46.

32. Allison T. Scalp and cortical recordings of initial somatosensory cortex activity to median nerve stimulation in man. Ann NY Acad Sci 1982; 388:671–678.

33. Desmedt JE, Cheron G. Somatosensory evoked potentials to finger stimulation in octogenarians and in young adults: Wave forms, scalp topography and transit time of parietal and frontal components. Electroenceph Clin Neurophysiol 1980; 50:404–425.

34. Hume AL, Cant BR. Conduction time in central somatosensory pathway in man. Electroencephalogr Clin Neurophysiol 1978; 45:361–375.

35. Eisen A, Roberts K, Low M, et al. Questions

regarding the sequential neural generator theory of the somatosensory evoked potential raised by digital filtering. Electroencephalogr Clin Neurophysiol 1986; 63:384–388.

36. Seyal M, Gabor AJ. The human posterior tibial somatosensory evoked potential: Synapse dependent and synapse independent spinal components. Electroencephalogr Clin Neurophysiol 1985; 62:323–331.

37. Emerson RG, Seyal M, Pedley TA. Somatosensory evoked potentials following median nerve stimulation. 1. The cervical components. Brain 1984; 107:169–182.

38. Desmedt JE, Cheron G. Non-cephalic reference recording of early somatosensory potentials to finger stimulation in adult or aging normal man: Differentiation of widespread $N_{18}$ and contralateral $N_{20}$ from the prerolandic $P_{22}$ and $N_{30}$ components. Electroencephalogr Clin Neurophysiol 1981; 52:553–570.

39. Mauguiere F, Desmedt JE, Courjon J. Neural generators of $N_{18}$ and $P_{14}$ far-field somatosensory evoked potentials studied in patients with lesions of thalamus or thalamocortical radiations. Electroencephalogr Clin Neurophysiol 1983; 56:283–292.

40. Goff WR, Allison T, Vaughan HG Jr. The functional neuroanatomy of event related potentials. In: Callaway E, Tueting P, Koslow SH, eds. Event-Related Brain Potentials in Man. New York: Academic Press, 1978;1–79.

41. Cruse R, Klem G, Lesser, RP, et al. Paradoxical lateralization of cortical potentials evoked by stimulation of posterior tibial nerve. Arch Neurol 1982; 39:222–225.

42. Seyal M, Emerson RG, Pedley TA. Spinal and early scalp-recorded components of the somatosensory evoked potential following stimulation of the posterior tibial nerve. Electroencephalogr Clin Neurophysiol 1983; 55:320–330.

43. Emerson RG. Anatomical physiologic basis of posterior tibial nerve somatosensory evoked potentials. Neurol Clin 1988; 6:735–749.

44. Tsumoto T, Hirose N, Nonaka S, et al. Analysis of somatosensory evoked potentials to lateral popliteal nerve stimulation in man. Electroencephalogr Clin Neurophysiol 1972; 33:379–388.

45. Dorfman LJ. Indirect estimation of spinal cord conduction velocity in man. Electroencephalogr Clin Neurophysiol 1977; 42:26–34.

46. Dorfman LJ, Bosley TM. Age-related changes in peripheral and central nerve conduction in man. Neurology 1979; 29:38–44.

47. Mutoh K, Hojo H, Mikawa H. Maturation study of short latency somatosensory evoked potentials after posterior tibial nerve stimulation in infants and children. Clin Electroencephalogr 1989; 20:91–102.

48. Gonzalez EG, Berman WS, Hajdu M. Influence of height and type of lower extremity nerve tested on $P_1$ somatosensory evoked potential latency. Arch Phys Med Rehabil 1983; 64:502.

49. Jones SJ, Small DG. Spinal and subcortical evoked potentials following stimulation of posterior tibial nerve in man. Electroencephalogr Clin Neurophysiol 1978; 44:299–306.

50. Rossini PM, Cracco RQ, Cracco JB, et al. Short latency somatosensory evoked potentials to peroneal nerve stimulation: Scalp topography and effect of different frequency filters. Electroencephalogr Clin Neurophysiol 1981; 52:540–552.

51. Aminoff MJ. The use of somatosensory evoked potentials in the evaluation of the central nervous system. Neurol Clin 1988; 6:809–823.

52. Chiappa KH. Use of evoked potentials for diagnosis of multiple sclerosis. Neurol Clin 1988; 6:861–880.

53. Purves SJ, Low MD, Galloway J, et al. A comparison of visual, brainstem auditory, and somatosensory evoked potentials in multiple sclerosis. Can J Neurol Sci 1981; 8:15–19.

54. Khoshbin S, Hallett M. Multimodality evoked potentials and blink reflex in multiple sclerosis. Neurology 1981; 31:138–144.

55. Green JB, Price R, Woodbury SG. Short-latency somatosensory evoked potentials in multiple sclerosis: Comparison with auditory and visual evoked potentials. Arch Neurol 1980; 37:630–633.

56. Phillips KR, Putrin AR, Syndulko K, et al. Multimodality evoked potentials and neurophysiological tests in multiple sclerosis. Effects of hyperthermia on test results. Arch Neurol 1983; 40:159–164.

57. Matthews WB, Small DG. Serial recording of visual and somatosensory evoked potentials in normal man and patients with multiple sclerosis. J Neurol Sci 1979; 40:11–21.

58. Nuwer MR, Packwood JW, Myers LW, et al. Evoked potentials predict the clinical changes in a multiple sclerosis drug study. Neurology 1987; 37:1754–1761.

59. Davis SL, Aminoff MN, Panitch HS. Clinical correlates of serial somatosensory evoked potentials in multiple sclerosis. Neurology 1985; 35:359–365.

60. Weiner HL, Dawson DM. Plasmapheresis in multiple sclerosis. A preliminary study. Neurology 1980; 30:1029–1033.

61. Cutler JR, Aminoff MJ, Brant-Zawadzki M. Evaluation of patients with multiple sclerosis by

evoked potentials and magnetic resonance imaging: A comparative study. Ann Neurol 1986; 20:645–650.

62. Turano G, Jones SJ, Miller DH, et al. Correlation of somatosensory evoked potentials abnormality with brain and cervical cord magnetic resonance imaging in multiple sclerosis. Brain 1991; 114:663–681.

63. Chu N-S. Median and tibial somatosensory evoked potentials. Changes in short- and long-latency components in patients with lesions of the thalamus and thalamo-cortical radiations. J Neurol Sci 1986; 76:199–219.

64. Noel P, Desmedt JE. Somatosensory cerebral evoked potentials after vascular lesions of the brain stem and diencephalon. Brain 1975; 98:113–128.

65. Liberson WT. Study of evoked potentials in aphasics. Am J Phys Med 1966; 45:135–142.

66. La Joie WJ, Reddy NM, Melvin JL. Somatosensory evoked potentials: their predictive value in right hemiplegia. Arch Phys Med Rehabil 1982; 63:223–226.

67. Allen CMC. Predicting the outcome of acute stroke: A prognostic score. J Neurol Neurosurg Psychiatry 1984; 47:475–480.

68. Pavot AP, Ignacia DR, Kutavanish A, et al. Prognostic value of somatosensory evoked potentials in cerebrovascular accidents. Electromyogr Clin Neurophysiol 1986; 26:333–340.

69. Chester CS, McLaren CE. Somatosensory evoked response and recovery from stroke. Arch Phys Med Rehabil 1989; 70:520–525.

70. Hume AL, Cant BR. Central somatosensory conduction after head injury. Ann Neurol 1981; 10:411–419.

71. Rappaport M. Brain evoked potentials in coma and the vegetative state. Head Trauma Rehabil 1986; 1:15–29.

72. De Meirleir LJ, Taylor MJ. The prognostic utility of somatosensory evoked potentials in comatose children. Pediatri Neurol 1987; 3:78–82.

73. Houlden DA, Li C, Schwartz ML, et al. Median nerve somatosensory evoked potentials and the Glasgow scale as predictor of outcome in comatose patients with head injuries. Neurosurgery 1990; 27:701–707.

74. Brunko E, Zegers de Beyl D. Prognostic value of early cortical somatosensory evoked potentials after resuscitation from cardiac arrest. Electroencephalogr Clin Neurophysiol 1987; 66:15–24.

75. Anziska BJ, Cracco RQ. Short latency somatosensory evoked potentials in brain-dead patients. Arch Neurol 1980; 37:222–225.

76. Belsh JM, Chokroverty S. Short-latency somatosensory evoked potentials in brain-dead patients. Electroencephalogr Clin Neurophysiol 1987; 68:75–78.

77. Spielholz NI, Benjamin MV, Engler G, et al. Somatosensory evoked potentials and clinical outcome in spinal cord injury. In: Popp AJ, ed. Neural Trauma. New York: Raven Press, 1979; 217–222.

78. Perot PL Jr, Vera CL. Scalp-recorded somatosensory evoked potentials to stimulation of nerves in the lower extremities and evaluation of patients with spinal cord trauma. Ann NY Acad Sci 1982; 388:359–368.

79. Rowed DW. Value of somatosensory evoked potentials for prognosis in partial cord injuries. In: Tator CH, ed. Early Management of Acute Spinal Cord Injury. New York: Raven Press, 1982;167–180.

80. Li C, Houlden DA, Rowed DW. Somatosensory evoked potentials and neurological grade as predictor of outcome in acute spinal cord injury. J Neurosurg 1990; 72:600–609.

81. Vauzelle C, Stagnara P, Jouvinroux P. Functional monitoring of spinal cord activity during spinal surgery. Clin Orthop 1973; 93:173–178.

82. Brown RH, Nash CL. Current status of spinal cord monitoring. Spine 1979; 4:466–470.

83. Engler GL, Spielholz NI, Bernhard WN, et al. Somatosensory evoked potentials during Harrington instrumentation for scoliosis. J Bone Joint Surg 1978; 60:528–532.

84. Gonzalez EG, Hajdu M, Keim HA, et al. Quantification of intraoperative somatosensory evoked potential. Arch Phys Med Rehabil 1984; 65:721–725.

85. Gonzalez, EG, Hajdu M, Keim HA, et al. Intraoperative somatosensory evoked potential monitoring. Orthop Rev 1984; 13:47–52.

86. Nuwer MR. Use of somatosensory evoked potentials for intraoperative monitoring of cerebral and spinal cord function. Neurol Clin 1988; 6:881–897.

87. Nuwer MR. Evoked Potential Monitoring in the Operating Room. New York: Raven Press, 1986.

88. Nordwall A, Axelgaard J, Harado Y, et al. Spinal cord monitoring using evoked potentials recorded from vertebral bone in cat. Spine 1979; 4:486–494.

89. Jones SJ, Edgar MA Ransford AO, et al. System for electrophysiological monitoring of spinal cord during operations for scoliosis. J Bone Joint Surg 1983; 65:134–139

90. Lueders H, Gurd A, Hahn J, et al. New technique for intraoperative monitoring of spinal cord function: Multichannel recording of spinal cord and

subcortical evoked potentials. Spine 1982; 7:110–115.

91. Pathak CS, Amaddio MD, Scoles PV, et al. Effects of halothane, enflurane, and isoflurane in nitrous oxide on multilevel somatosensory evoked potentials. Anesthesiology 1989; 70:207–212.

92. Grundy BL, Nash CL, Brown RH. Deliberate hypotension for scoliosis surgery. Anesthesiology 1979; 51:578.

93. Ginsburg HH, Shetter AG, Raudzens PA. Postoperative paraplegia with preserved intraoperative somatosensory evoked potentials. J Neurosurg 1985; 63:296–300.

94. Lesser RP, Raudzens P, Luders H, et al. Postoperative neurological deficits may occur despite unchanged intraoperative somatosensory evoked potentials. Ann Neurol 1986; 19:22–25.

95. Levy WJ. Spinal evoked potentials from the motor tracts. J Neurosurg 1983; 58:38–44.

96. Barker AT, Jalinour R, Freeston, IL. Non-invasive magnetic stimulation of the human motor cortex. Lancet 1985; 1:1106–1107.

97. Hess CW, Mills KR, Murray MF. Responses in small hand muscles from magnetic stimulation of the human brain. J Physiol 1987; 388:397–419.

98. Keim H, Hajdu M, Gonzalez EG. Somatosensory evoked potential as a diagnostic aid in the diagnosis and intraoperative management of spinal stenosis. Spine 1985; 10:338–344.

99. Hajdu M, Gonzalez EG, Michelsen C. Somatosensory evoked potential as an intraoperative measure of lumbar nerve root decompression. Arch Phys Med Rehabil 1986; 67:618.

100. Macon JB. Polleti CE, Sweet WH, et al. Spinal conduction velocity measurement during laminectomy. Surg Forum 1980; 31:453–455.

101. Nuwer M, Dawson E. Intraoperative evoked potential monitoring of the spinal cord: A restricted filter, scalp method during Harrington instrumentation for scoliosis. Clin Orthop 1984; 183:42–50.

102. Kaplan BJ, Friedman WA, Alexander JA, et al. Somatosensory evoked potential monitoring during repair of aortic coarctations. J Neurosurg 1986; 19:82–90.

103. Krieger KH, Spencer FC. Is paraplegia after repair of coarctation of the aorta due principally to distal hypotension during aortic cross-clamping? Surgery 1985; 97:2–7.

104. Laschinger JC, Cummingham JN, Catinella FP, et al. Detection and prevention of intraoperative spinal cord ischemia after cross-clamping of the thoracic aorta. Use of somatosensory evoked potentials. Surgery 1982; 92:1109–1117.

105. Lesnick JE, Michele JJ, Simeone FA, et al. Alteration of somatosensory evoked potentials in response to global ischemia. J Neurosurg 1984; 60:490–494.

106. Hyman SA, Skelley CC, Arendall R, et al. Median nerve somatosensory evoked potentials as an indicator of ischemia in a case involving an aneurysm of the internal carotid artery. Neurosurgery 1987; 21:391–393.

107. Lueders H, Lesser RP, Hahn J, et al. Cortical somatosensory evoked potentials in response to hand stimulation. J Neurosurgery 1983; 58:885–894.

108. Eisen A, Aminoff MJ. Somatosensory evoked potentials. In: Aminoff MJ, ed. Electrodiagnosis in Clinical Neurology, ed 2. New York: Churchill Livingstone, 1986; 532–573.

109. Eisen A, Purves S, Hoirch M. Central nervous system amplification: Its potential in the diagnosis of early multiple sclerosis. Neurology 1982; 32:359–364.

110. Johnson EW, Melvin JL. Value of electromyography in lumbar radiculopathy. Arch Phys Med Rehabil 1971; 52:239–243.

111. Kimura J. F-wave velocity in the central segment of the median and ulnar nerves. A study in normal subjects and in patients with Charcot-Marie-Tooth disease. Neurology 1974; 24:539–546.

112. Braddom RL, Johnson EW. Standardization of H reflex and diagnostic use in S1 radiculopathy. Arch Phys Med Rehabil 1966; 55:161–166.

113. Eisen A, Hoirch M, White J, et al. Sensory group Ia proximal conduction velocity. Muscle Nerve 1984; 7:636–641.

114. El Negarny E, Sedgwick EM. Delayed cervical somatosensory potentials in cervical spondylosis. J Neurol Neurosurg Psychiatry 1979; 42:238–246.

115. Ganes T. Somatosensory conduction times and peripheral cervical and cortical evoked potentials in patients with cervical spondylosis. J Neurol Neurosurg Psychiatry 1980; 43:683–689.

116. Yiannikas C, Shahani BT, Young RR. Short latency somatosensory evoked potential from radial, medium, ulnar and peroneal nerve stimulation in the assessment of cervical spondylosis. Arch Neurol 1986; 43:1264–1271.

117. Jorg J, Dullberg W, Koeppen S. Diagnostic value of segmental somatosensory evoked potentials in cases with chronic progressive para- or tetraspastic syndromes. In: Courjon J, Mauguiere F, Revol M, eds. Clinical Applications of Evoked Potentials in Neurology. New York: Raven Press, 1982;347–358.

118. Eisen A. Electrodiagnosis of radiculopathies. Neurol Clin 1985; 3:495–510.

119. Eisen A, Hoirch M, Moll A. Evaluation of radiculopathies by segmental stimulation and soma-

tosensory evoked potentials. Can J Neurol Sci 1983; 10:178–182.

120. Gonzalez EG, Hajdu M. Disparate involvement of short and long latency somatosensory evoked potentials in nerve root decompression. Arch Phys Med Rehabil 1983; 64:494.

121. Green J, Gildenmeister R, Hazelwood C. Dermatomally stimulated somatosensory cerebral evoked potentials in the clinical diagnosis of lumbar disc disease. Clin Electroencephalogr 1983; 14:152–160.

122. Katifi HA, Segwich EM. Evaluation of the dermatomal somatosensory evoked potential in the diagnosis of lumbo-sacral root compression. J Neurol Neurosurg Psychiatry 1987; 50:1204–1210.

123. Aminoff MJ, Goodin DS, Barbaro NM, et al. Dermatomal somatosensory evoked potentials in unilateral lumbosacral radiculopathy. Ann Neurol 1985; 17:171–176.

124. Jones SI, Wynn Parry CB, Landi A. Diagnosis of brachial plexus traction by sensory nerve action potentials and somatosensory evoked potentials. Injury 1981; 12:376–382.

125. Synek VM. Somatosensory evoked potentials from musculocutaneous nerve in the diagnosis of brachial plexus injury. J Neurol Sci 1983; 61:443–452.

126. Synek VM, Cowan JC. Somatosensory evoked potentials in patients with supraclavicular brachial plexus injuries. Neurology 1982; 32:1347–1352.

127. Yiannikas C. Shahani BT, Young RR. The investigation of traumatic lesions of the brachial plexus by electromyography and short latency somatosensory potentials evoked by stimulation of multiple nerves. J Neurol Neurosurg Psychiatry 1983; 46:1014–1022.

128. Zverina E, Kredba J. Somatosensory cerebral evoked potentials in diagnosing brachial plexus injuries. Scand J Rehabil Med 1977; 9:47–54.

129. Hanson MR, Breuer AC, Furlan AJ, et al. Brachial plexus lesions following open-heart surgery: A prospective analysis and possible new mechanism of injury. Neurology 1980; 30:441.

130. Morin JE, Long R, Elleker MG, et al. Upper extremity neuropathies following median sternotomy. Ann Thorac Surg 1982; 34:181–185.

131. England JD, Sumner AJ. Neuralgic amyotrophy: An increasingly diverse entity. Muscle Nerve 1987; 10:60–68.

132. Glover JL, Worth RM, Bendick PJ, et al. Evoked responses in diagnosis of thoracic outlet syndrome. Surgery 1981; 89:86–93.

133. Yiannikas C, Walsh JC. Somatosensory evoked responses in the diagnosis of thoracic outlet syndrome. J Neurol Neurosurg Psychiatry 1983; 46:234–240.

134. Chodorff G, Lee DW, Honet JC. Dynamic approach in the diagnosis of thoracic outlet syndrome using somatosensory evoked responses. Arch Phys Med Rehabil 1985; 66:3–6.

135. Haldeman S, Bradley WE, Bhatia N, et al. Pudendal evoked responses. Arch Neurol 1982; 39:280–283.

136. Bennett MH, Jannetta PJ. Trigeminal evoked potentials in humans. Electroencephalogr Clin Neurophysiol 1980; 48:517–526.

137. Robinson RL, Richey ET, Kase CS. Somatosensory evoked potentials in pure sensory stroke and related conditions. Stroke 1985; 16:818–823.

138. Fagan ER, Taylor MJ, Logan WJ. Somatosensory evoked potentials: Part II. A review of clinical applications in pediatric neurology. Pediatric Neurol 1987; 3:249–254.

139. Garg BP, Markand ON, DeMyer WE, et al. Evoked response studies in patients with adrenoleukodystrophy and heterozygous relatives. Arch Neurol 1983; 40:356–359.

140. Tobimatsu S, Fukui R, Kato M, et al. Multimodality evoked potential in patients and carriers with adrenoleukodystrophy and adrenomyeloneuropathy. Electroencephalogr Clin Neurophysiol 1985; 62:18–24.

141. Noth J, Engel L, Friedemann HH, et al. Evoked potentials in patients with Huntington's disease and their offspring. 1: Somatosensory evoked potentials. Electroencephalogr Clin Neurophysiol 1984; 59:134–141.

142. Young RR, Cracco RQ. Clinical neurophysiology of conduction in control motor pathways. Ann Neurol 1985; 18:606–609.

143. Gualtierotti J, Paterson AS. Electrical stimulation of the unexposed cerebral cortex. J Physiol 1954; 125:278–291.

144. Merton PA, Morton HB: Stimulation of the cerebral cortex in the intact human subject. Nature 1980; 285:227.

145. Cowan JMA, Dick JPR, Day BL, et al. Abnormalities in central motor pathway conduction in multiple sclerosis. Lancet 1984; 2:304–307.

146. Mills KR, Murray NMF. Corticospinal tract conduction time in multiple sclerosis. Ann Neurol 1985; 18:601–605.

147. Goddard GV, McIntyre DC, Leech CK. A permanent change in brain function resulting from daily electrical stimulation. Exp Neurol 1969; 25:295–330.

148. Rossini PM. The anatomic and physiologic bases of motor-evoked potentials. Neurol Clin 1988; 6:751–769.

149. Cracco RQ. Evaluation of conduction in control motor pathways: Technique, pathophysiology and clinical interpretation. Neurosurgery 1987; 20:199–203.

150. Katz RT, Vanden Berg C, Weinberger D, et al. Magnetoelectric stimulation of human motor cortex: Normal values and potential safety issues in spinal cord injury. Arch Phys Med Rehabil 1990; 71:597–600.

151. Eisen AS, Shtybel W. Clinical experience with transcranial magnetic stimulation. Muscle Nerve 1990; 13:995–1011.

152. Bement SL, Ranck JB Jr. A quantitative study of electrical stimulation of central myelinated fibers with monopolar electrodes. Exp Neurol 1969; 24:147–170.

153. Cres D, Chiappa KH, Gominak S, et al. Cervical magnetic stimulation. Neurology 1990; 40:1751–1756.

154. Booth KR, Streletz LJ, Raab VE, et al. Motor evoked potential and central motor conduction: Studies of transcranial magnetic stimulation with recording from the leg. Electroencephalogr Clin Neurophysiol 1991; 81:57–62.

155. Patton HD, Amassian VE. Single and multiple unit analysis of cortical stage of pyramidal tract activation. J Neurophysiol 1954; 17:345–363.

156. Patton HD, Amassian VE. The pyramidal tract: its excitation and functions. In: Field J, ed. Handbook of Physiology-Neurophysiology. Vol. 237–861. Washington, DC: American Physiological Society, 1960.

157. Rossini PM, Caramia MD, Zarola F. Mechanisms of nervous propagation along central pathways: Noninvasive evaluation in healthy subjects and in patients with neurological disease. Neurosurgery 1987; 20:183–191.

158. Rossini PM, Zarola F, Stalberg E, et al. Premovement facilitation of motor evoked potentials in man during transcranial stimulation of the central motor pathways. Brain Res 1988; 458:20–30.

159. Ackerman H, Scholz E, Koehler W, et al. Influence of posture and voluntary background muscle action potentials from anterior tibial and soleus muscle following transcranial magnetic stimulation. Electroencephalogr Clin Neurophysiol 1991; 81:71–80.

160. Hufnagel A, Jaeger M, Elger CE. Transcranial magnetic stimulation: Specific and nonspecific facilitation of magnetic motor evoked potentials. J Neurol 1990; 237:416–419.

161. Lassek AM. The human pyramidal tract. II. A numerical investigation of the Betz cells of the motor area. Arch Neurol Psychiatry 1940; 44:718–724.

162. Lassek AM. The pyramidal tract of the monkey. A Betz cells and pyramidal tract enumeration. J Comp Neurol 1941; 74:193–202.

163. Day BL, Thompson PD, Dick JP, et al. Different sites of action of electrical and magnetic stimulation of the human brain. Neurosci LeHers 1987; 75:101–106.

164. Mills KR, Murray NM, Hess CW. Magnetic and electrical transcranial brain stimulation. Physiological mechanisms and clinical applications. Neurosurgery 1987; 20:164–168.

165. Kadanka Z, Bednarik J, Cerny L. Site of motor pathway excitation during cervical spinal stimulation. Activitas Nervosa Superior 1990; 32:250–256.

166. Koh TH, Eyre JA. Maturation of corticospinal tracts assessed by electromagnetic stimulation of the motor cortex. Arch Dis Child 1988; 63:1347–1352.

167. Hess CW, Mills KR, Murray NM, et al. Magnetic brain stimulation: Central motor conduction studies in multiple sclerosis. Ann Neurol 1987; 22:744–752.

168. Caramia MD, Bernardi G, Zarola F, et al. Neurophysiological evaluation of the central nervous impulse propagation in patients with sensorimotor disturbances. Electroencephalogr Clin Neurophysiol 1988; 70:16–25.

169. Xing J, Katayama K, Yamamoto T, et al. Quantitative evaluation of hemiparesis with corticomyographic motor evoked potential recorded by transcranial magnetic stimulation. J Neurotrauma 1990; 7:57–64.

170. Dominkus M, Grisold W, Jelinak V. Transcranial electrical motor evoked potentials as a prognostic indicator for motor recovery in stroke patients. J Neurol Neurosurg Psychiatry 1990; 53:745–748.

171. Zentner J, Ebner A. Prognostic value of somatosensory and motor evoked potentials in patients with non-traumatic coma. Eur Arch Psych Neurol Sci 1988; 237:184–187.

172. Dvorak J, Hordmann J, Janssen B, et al. Motor evoked potentials in patients with cervical spine disorders. Spine 1990; 15:1013–1016.

173. Dvorak J, Hordmann J, Theiler R. Magnetic transcranial brain stimulation: Painless evaluation of central motor pathways. Normal values and clinical application in spinal cord diagnostics: Upper extremities. Spine 1990; 15:155–160.

174. Gianutsos J, Eberstein A, Ma D, et al. A noninvasive technique to assess completeness of spinal cord lesions in humans. Exp Neurol 1987; 98:34–40.

175. Robinson LR, Little JW. Motor evoked potentials reflect spinal cord function in post-traumatic syr-

ingomyelia. Am J Phys Med Rehabil 1990; 6:307–310.

176. Levy WJ. Clinical experience with motor and cerebellar evoked potential monitoring. Neurosurgery 1987; 20:169–182.

177. Kitagama H, Itoh T, Takano H, et al. Motor evoked potential monitoring during upper cervical spine surgery. Spine 1989; 14:1078–1083.

178. Preston B, Zgur T, Polenc VV. Epidural and subpial cortico-spinal potentials evoked by transcutaneous motor cortex stimulation during spinal cord surgery. Electroencephalogr Clin Neurophysiol 1990; 41:348–351.

# Chapter 13

# Human Thermoregulation

JOHN A. DOWNEY
DANIEL E. LEMONS

"La fixité du milieu intérieur est la condition de la vie libre." Thus Claude Bernard emphasized the biologic significance of the constancy of internal conditions in the body, and he clearly recognized that temperature control was a factor in this constancy. Fever, or elevated body temperature, had been recognized since biblical times as an indication of illness, but not until the development of the thermometer in the 18th century could accurate temperature measurements be made. This led to a more definitive understanding of its significance and control. It is now clear that, in humans and other warm-blooded animals, deep body temperature is regulated to a fine degree most of the time, despite exposure to wide extremes of environmental temperature. This phenomenon is labeled *homeothermy*, in contrast to *poikilothermy*, variation of body temperature with the environmental temperature. Humans with certain neurologic and other medical conditions may lose the regulation of body temperature and become effective poikilotherms.

The skin is exposed to wide variations of ambient temperature, and skin temperature changes as a consequence. Body temperature was once thought to be regulated as a response to change in skin temperature alone, but experiments have shown that some internal temperature changes produce much greater thermoregulatory responses. Central body temperature, $T_b$, is sensed, and when $T_b$ changes, appropriate corrective responses are initiated. This is not to deny that skin temperature

influences the thermoregulatory response; it does, but core temperature changes of equal size produce far greater responses.

## Temperature Measurement

### Skin

Skin temperature varies over the body because of exposure to the environment and change in the circulation of the blood due primarily to thermoregulatory responses. The temperature of the fingers and toes varies most (up to 30°C) and that of the proximal part of the limbs and the trunk less (3° to 4°C). (Temperatures will be expressed as centigrade measurements throughout the chapter.)

### Central or Deep Body Temperature

Ideally, we would like to measure the temperature of the mixed venous blood as it returns to the heart or the temperature at specific sites in the body (particularly the anterior hypothalamus) where evidence suggests the principal central regulators of temperature are located. As it is not possible to measure there, some less ideal site must be selected. Traditionally, temperature measured rectally has been the most reliable and constant. This is true when the body is in thermal balance, whether at rest, during exercise, or with a fever, but rectal temperature does not accurately reflect rapid changes in body heat. When, for example, hot saline is injected into a vein to cause a rise in oral temperature, a compensatory vasomotor reaction occurs in the skin and rectal temperature shows little or no response (Figure 13-1). The rectal temperature is usually about 0.3°C higher than the temperature of the aortic blood.[1] When temperature is measured in the rectum it is important to insert the thermometer the same distance on each occasion and to leave it in place at least 3 minutes. Vaginal temperature and bladder temperature (the latter is measured by thermistor within an indwelling catheter, as during surgery) also accurately reflect the body temperature when it is constant or slowly changing, but they do not reflect rapid changes in central temperature. Oral temperature more accurately reflects the temperature of the blood, owing to the dense vascular supply to the undersurface of the tongue. It is easy to obtain but it is also easily distorted, particularly if the patient has eaten or drunk recently or if breathing through the mouth while the thermometer is in place. Probably the best approximation of the deep body temperature and its changes are in the lower end of the esophagus, where the heart lies close to the

esophagus. Taking a temperature there however, is unpleasant for most patients, who will tolerate it only under exceptional circumstances. In experimental situations temperature has been measured at the eardrum, or by a catheter in the bloodstream itself with specially designed thermistors.

When body temperature is measured by thermometer, at whatever site, it is necessary to do it properly. This means first shaking the thermometer down to the very bottom of the column, to avoid missing states of hypothermia. The thermometer must be placed accurately, protected from distortion by such things as breathing through the mouth, and left in place long enough.

### Normal Body Temperature

Humans' body temperature is remarkably constant when measurements are taken under standard circumstances. Ivy[2] measured the oral temperatures of 276 medical students in class between 8:00 and 9:00 A.M. and found mean body temperature to be 36.7 ± 0.2°C. Small but significant changes in body temperature are related to factors such as time of day, age, sexual activity, and the like.

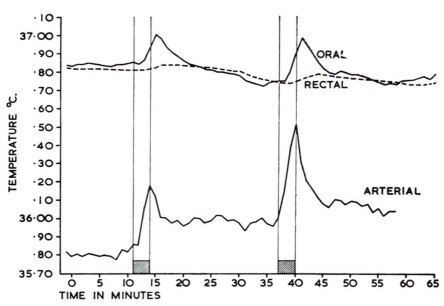

**Figure 13-1.** Oral, rectal, and central arterial temperatures prior to and after two intravenous injections of hot saline. Vertical bars mark the injection periods.

Studies of these factors have increased our understanding of the general subject of temperature regulation.

### Diurnal Changes

Body temperature varies throughout the day, being minimal (about 36.1°C) in the early morning (4:00 to 6:00 A.M.) and maximal (37.4°C) in the later afternoon (Figure 13-2).[3] This variation is one manifestation of the circadian rhythms that are recognized in several areas of physiology, which are affected by sleeping, eating, and light and are regulated by a complex of hormonal changes that are only recently being elucidated.[4] The cycle changes with travel; for example, when a person flies east to west for 8 to 10 hours the cycle readjusts slowly over 3 to 4 days to the new time. Similarly, when workmen change shifts from day to night or work very long hours, as medical students and residents do, their diurnal rhythms are disrupted and they can be adversely affected.

### Age

Regulation of body temperature is different in newborns than in adults, owing in part to the immaturity of the infant's nervous system. Obviously, the effect is even more pronounced in premature infants. Babies have a relatively higher ratio of surface area to mass than adults, and they have difficulty thermoregulating, in both hot and cold environments, because heat exchange with the environment is more rapid. Babies rarely shiver; rather they use the special characteristics of their highly calorigenic brown fat to produce large amounts of heat. Their sweat glands are immature and largely localized on the face and head. Premature babies, especially those born more than 8 weeks before term, do not sweat at all at birth. At the time of delivery many babies are washed in cool water and exposed to (for them) cool environments and are in danger of developing hypothermia. The ideal room temperature for a baby that is well-wrapped is somewhere between 25° and 27°C, and it this should even be warmer for very small infants. Conversely, if children are kept wrapped in too heavy blankets and exposed to heat they can suffer heat stroke.[5]

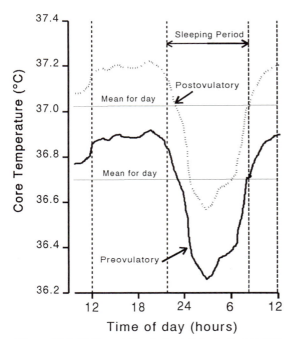

**Figure 13-2.** Daily variation in (rectal) body temperature. The lower curve was obtained in the first (preovulatory) half of the menstrual cycle, the upper curve in the second (postovulatory) half (values represent mean of eight subjects). Shaded area is the sleeping period. (From Brück. Human Physiology. Berlin: Springer-Verlag, 1989, with permission.)

### Elderly Persons

There is increasing evidence that thermoregulatory control is less effective in elders because of both changes in the neurologic system and modifications of behavior. Elderly persons seem less able to sense changes in skin temperature,[6] and then may not respond appropriately to them. There is evidence, too, that elders have abnormal autonomic nervous system responses that are manifested in control of blood pressure and circulation in general, as well as in thermoregulation. This is evidenced by reduced shivering[7] and sweating,[6] though some, but not all, of this may be explained by lack of acclimatization. In addition, older people may take any of several medications for hypertension, gastrointestinal complaints, anxiety, or insomnia, among other conditions. Such medications can seriously affect the sensitivity of the thermoregulatory system. Because elders frequently have abnormal thermoregulation, they account for a large proportion of persons who develop hypothermia and heat stroke. In the context of associated medical conditions, either can prove lethal.

### Gender

Preovulatory women have the same oral temperature as men, but at ovulation the body temperature tends to rise 0.2° to 0.5°C, and remains at that level through the remainder of the cycle. Several hormones, including pregnenolone and pregnanediol, are involved in this rise in temperature. The special circumstances of abnormal thermoregulation in women during menopause (hot flashes) are discussed in Chapter 25. Men and women respond to thermal stresses in somewhat different ways. In the heat, sweating begins in women at a higher skin temperature than in men and women sweat less profusely. In the cold, women have a lower skin temperature than men and lose heat about 10% more slowly.

This phenomenon is due in part to more effective vasoconstriction in women, and to thicker subcutaneous tissues.[8] Some of these differences in thermoregulation between men and women, especially in the heat, may be due to different states of acclimatization and can be abolished by appropriate training and exposure.[9]

### Race

Certain primitive non-Caucasians respond differently to thermal stress than Caucasians do. With whole-body exposure to moderate cold, the metabolic rate of urban Caucasians rises markedly and deep body temperature falls. The metabolic rate of Australian aborigines starts near the same basal level but decreases while rectal and skin temperatures fall to levels well below that of urban Caucasians. On the other hand, Alacaluf natives of southern Chile have a higher resting metabolic metabolism, and it declines slightly on cold ex-

posure, as does the rectal temperature, but the rectal temperature goes no lower than that of a Caucasian. Other groups have responses intermediate to these, but the reasons for the variations are not known. Urbanized men of different races respond in the same way to cold,[10] so this would indicate that at least some of the reactions are not genetic in origin but are manifestations of habituation and acclimatization.

## Regulation of Body Temperature

Body temperature is maintained at a constant level by a balance between heat production and heat loss. The afferent, or sensory, side of this balance involves temperature-sensitive structures in both superficial and deeper central regions of the body.

### Skin Receptors

Neural structures in the skin that appear as undifferentiated nerve endings respond specifically to changes in temperature. These structures, though they appear to be morphologically similar, respond differently to heating and cooling. Neurophysiologic studies[11] indicate there are three types of receptors. One receptor responds to heating with a burst of electrical activity and with an increase in the static neural discharge that is proportional to the steady-state absolute temperature. Another responds to cooling with a burst of activity and an increase in static discharge. Again, the static discharge is proportional to the absolute temperature in the steady state. The third type responds to several stimuli, including warming, with a continuous barrage of activity (Figure 13-3). It would appear that the temperature receptors in the skin send messages to the central nervous system that reflect (1) the absolute temperature of the skin of various areas of the body, (2) the direction of temperature change, and (3) the rate of change of the temperature. By integrating this information, the central nervous system gains an indication of the overall thermal exposure.

Temperature receptors are present throughout the skin and superficial areas of the body, but they vary in density. There are more in the fingers, the

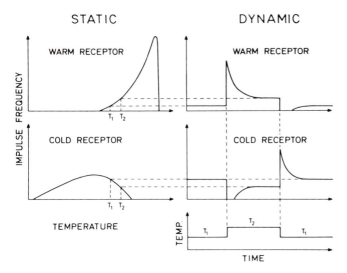

## STATIC    DYNAMIC

WARM RECEPTOR    WARM RECEPTOR

COLD RECEPTOR    COLD RECEPTOR

IMPULSE FREQUENCY

TEMPERATURE

TEMP.

TIME

**Figure 13-3.** Diagram of the firing response of the cold and warm receptors of the skin. The left side shows the static response to steady temperature changes. The right side shows the dynamic response to rapid increases and decreases in temperature. (From Hensel Handbook of Sensory Physiology II, The somatosensory system. Berlin: Springer-Verlag, 1973, with permission.)

face, and the genitalia, and fewer in the proximal part of the extremities and in the trunk, particularly on the back. In total, the neural activity from skin receptors gives an indication of the overall thermal exposure and serves as an early warning to the central nervous system of potential changes in body heat so that appropriate, though short-term, physiologic responses can be initiated to minimize any perturbation.

Research on homeothermic animals employing ablation techniques and the warming or cooling of selected areas of the brain have clearly indicated that there are temperature-sensitive structures in the anterior preoptic region of the hypothalamus and that temperature changes of as little as 0.1°C can initiate appropriate peripheral thermoregulatory responses.[12,13] Microelectrode recording techniques from single nerve cells in the hypothalamus have demonstrated both cells that respond selectively to cooling or heating with changes in electrical firing activity and cells that do not change their activity with temperature.[14,15] These populations of hypothalamic cells, working together, may be the central thermostat that senses and integrates body temperature information and coordinates the responses that hold body temperature at the desired level.[16]

Direct studies of hypothalamic function are not possible in humans, but there is good evidence that central thermoregulatory structures are present and that they respond in a manner similar to those in other mammals. The return of warm or cool blood from an extremity to the central regions of the body causes peripheral vasomotor responses.[17] Intravenous infusion of measured amounts of hot or cold saline produced the appropriate vasomotor response in the hand of normal humans and showed a sensitivity in the central receptors to changes of as little as 0.1°C. Extensive studies of patients with spinal cord transection in our laboratory confirmed the responses to central temperature change. For example, when central temperature was caused to fall to approximately 35.6°C, shivering occurred in the innervated muscles above the level of spinal cord transection, even when the sentient skin of the body was not cooled (and, therefore, there was no peripheral sensory input of cooling). In like manner, warming of the central regions of the body induced sweating above the level of 37.4°C, even when the sentient skin was cool. There was a synergistic relationship between the temperature of the skin and the central temperature: When both central and peripheral cooling took place, the responses occurred earlier and appeared more vigorous than with cooling of either skin or central temperature alone. The same thing happened on the warm side of the response. The most likely location for the temperature-sensitive structures in the central nervous system is in the anterior preoptic hypothalamus; injuries in this region can cause disorders of temperature regulation (Figure 13-4).

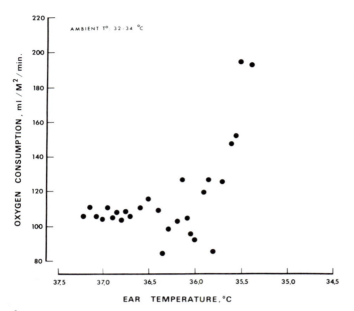

A

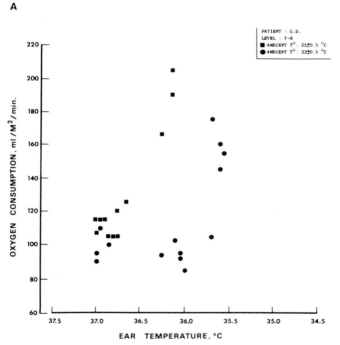

B

**Figure 13-4.** (*A*) Metabolic response of patients with spinal cord transection to a decrease in core temperature. Shivering increases oxygen consumption and causes additional heat production. (*B*) Metabolic response of patients with spinal cord transection to a decrease in core temperature. The lower ambient temperature causes shivering to begin at a significantly higher core temperature; the threshold for the response is altered by the skin temperature.

## *Extracranial Receptors*

There is evidence in animals and humans of temperature-sensitive sites in structures in other regions of the body, including the proximal great veins, the pulmonary vessels,[18] the heart,[19] and the abdominal viscera.[20] In particular, there is evidence in both animals[21] and humans[22] of thermosensitive structures in the spinal cord, though these tend to be rather less sensitive than those in other areas of the central nervous system and the responses they induce are sluggish. They may contribute to the amount of residual thermoregulatory ability of spinal cord–injured patients, as will be discussed later.

### Thermoregulatory Responses

Thermoregulatory mechanisms available to homeotherms include behavioral and postural adjustments and vasomotor changes—peripheral vasodilation or vasoconstriction, piloerection, sweating and panting, and shivering and nonshivering thermogenesis. These are not used equally, but are a hierarchy of responses that can be sequentially activated as the thermal stress increases.

### Environmental Selection and Posture

In animals, as in humans, the most primitive response to externally applied heating or cooling is to seek a better thermal environment or a more advantageous posture. This behavior is also seen in animals such as fish, amphibians, and reptiles, whose major mechanism of body temperature control is selection of an appropriate thermal environment.

Modern humans attempt to avoid extremes of temperature by modifying either their dress or their environment, the environment being modified by such means as central heating or air conditioning. These modifications are so effective that even people living in extremely cold climates may experience only short-term and limited cold stress. Postural changes—curling up in a ball when cool or extending arms and legs when warm—may significantly alter heat exchange with the environment, and they occur even during sleep.

### Regulation of Body Temperature in a Neutral Ambient Temperature

#### Vasomotor Responses

Control of blood flow to the skin regulates the flow of heat between the central or core regions of the body and the periphery. When ambient temperature is "normal" (comfortable), increased skin circulation raises skin temperature, reducing the gradient of heat from central to peripheral areas and increasing the thermal gradient between the skin and environment, thus augmenting heat loss from the skin by radiation and convection. In the heat, blood flow to the skin may increase dramatically. This is accomplished by both redistribution of blood flow from other regions to the skin (Figure 13-5) and increased cardiac output (CO; Figure 13-6).

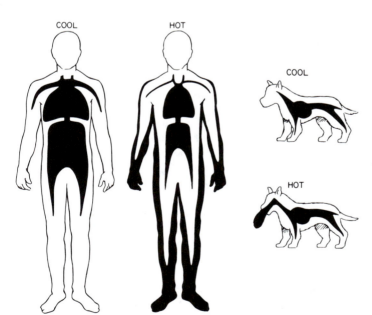

**Figure 13-5.** Schematic illustration of altered distribution of blood volume in heat-stressed humans and dogs. In the human, heat is most efficiently dissipated from the skin of the extremities, but in a furred animal such as a dog heat release occurs most efficiently from the tongue, where panting produces a high rate of evaporation from the surface. (From Rowell. Thermal stress. In: Shepherd J.T., Abboud, F.M., eds. The Handbook of Physiology. : American Physiological Society, 1983, with permission.)

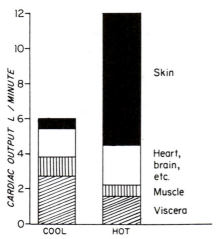

**Figure 13-6.** (*Left*) Estimated distribution of cardiac output between skin and other major organs at rest in normothermia; (*right*) expected distribution during hyperthermia ($T_b > 39°C$). (From Rowell. Thermal stress. In: Shepherd JT, Abboud FM, eds. The Handbook of Physiology, American Physiological Society, 1983, with permission.)

If the ambient temperature is greater than the skin temperature, increased skin circulation actually hastens the onset of hyperthermia by carrying additional heat into the body core. Decreased skin circulation reduces heat loss or gain in the periphery.

The peripheral circulation is controlled through the autonomic nervous system, and not all peripheral vascular beds respond in the same way to thermal stress. The circulation of the skin of the fingers and toes, for example, is under much greater thermoregulatory control than that of the trunk, and only the skin circulation takes part in thermoreflexes. The blood flow to the muscles remains relatively constant unless the muscles are actually heated or cooled. The primary means of fine adjustment of body temperature is variation of blood flow to the skin, and in an ambient temperature of approximately 24° to 32°C, most, if not all, of the heat balance of a naked human at rest is achieved through skin circulatory changes.

### Regulation of Body Temperature in a Warm Ambient Temperature

When the body is exposed to temperatures above 30°C there is progressive cutaneous vasodilatation,

which enhances heat loss to the environment. When this loss is not effective and body temperature begins to rise, panting or sweating begins.

The high heat of evaporation of water (approximately 0.5 to 0.6 kcal/g) affords a potent method of eliminating heat from the body when regulation demands much heat loss. The avenues of evaporative heat loss are the lungs and respiratory passages and sweating onto skin surfaces. The air expired from the lungs is saturated with water vapor taken up by evaporation from the respiratory passages. In many vertebrates, increased ventilation (*panting*) serves as an effective way to increase heat loss. (This is why the dog in the heat in Figure 13-5 increases blood flow to the tongue and nasal area instead of to the skin.) In humans this mechanism is relatively less important, even though respiratory rate is significantly increased by fever or by body heating.

In humans, heat loss by evaporation occurs mostly through sweat excreted on the skin. There are two types of sweat glands. *Eccrine sweat glands* secrete a dilute solution containing sodium chloride, urea, lactic acid, and several trace elements. They are distributed over the whole body and are under the control of the sympathetic cholinergic nerves. Their production of sweat is abolished by atropine.[2] *Apocrine glands,* which are found in association with hair follicles, particularly in the axillae, nipples, and pubic region, secrete a creamy substance that gives rise to body odor. The apocrine glands respond to adrenergic transmitters, and their activity is not abolished by atropine.

The eccrine glands are stimulated by heating and may produce as much as 15 kg of sweat per day; thus the body can lose large amounts of heat.[23] Central body temperature, mean skin temperature, and local skin temperature all can influence the rate of sweating.[24] Humans who lack sweat glands (anhydrosis) are unable to tolerate heat stress.

### Regulation of Body Temperature in a Cool Environment

#### Piloerection

The raising of hair follicles on the skin by contraction of piloerector muscles (''goose or duck bumps'') results in trapping of air on the skin and increases surface insulation. This is effective for hairy animals but not for humans.

*Thermogenesis*

The body's basal metabolic activity (basic metabolic rate) is the means by which it produces heat to maintain its relatively high internal temperature. At an ambient temperature of 26° to 30°C the fine adjustment of body temperature is largely accomplished by vasomotor adjustment, which alters heat loss from the skin. Such a thermal environment is called the *thermoneutral zone*. When the ambient temperature is below the thermoneutral temperature, vasoconstriction occurs. If this is not enough to prevent body heat loss, increased heat production is initiated through shivering.

Shivering is the involuntary, rhythmic contraction of muscles. Initially invisible, it may take the form of muscle tensing. With colder temperatures the muscle contractions are visible. Often, they start in the patient's shoulders, and ultimately they extend to all muscles of the body. Shivering is a potent source of increased heat production by which oxygen consumption can be increased as much as 500% for short periods and as much as 200% to 300% for longer periods. It is mediated by the somatic nerves and requires an intact spinal cord and posterior hypothalamus. No shivering occurs below the level of a spinal cord transection or in limbs paralyzed by poliomyelitis.

Body heat production can also be increased by eating, or exercising, or by the secretion of calorigenic hormones such as norepinephrine. In acclimatized animals there is evidence of nonshivering thermogenesis, particularly in association with increased amount of adrenergic and thyroid hormones, but nonshivering thermogenesis has not been demonstrated as clearly in adult humans. In fact, in the cold, totally paralyzed humans exhibited no increased heat production over at least several hours.[25] The recently discovered human $\beta_3$-adrenergic receptor seems to be specifically involved in activating cellular thermogenesis.[26]

### *Activation of Thermoregulatory Responses*

Appropriate thermoregulatory reflexes can be activated by heating or cooling only the skin, well before any changes in central deep body temperature take place. Warming[27] or cooling[28] the skin in one part of the body causes vasodilatation or vasoconstriction elsewhere so quickly that these reactions can be mediated only by neurologic reflex. These reflex human responses are transient unless there is a fall or rise in central temperature, at which time the vasomotor changes continue and are enhanced (Figure 13-7).[28]

Sudden, extreme cooling of the whole body can initiate shivering, which often produces a rise in central temperature, owing to the concomitant vasoconstriction and increased heat production. Skin

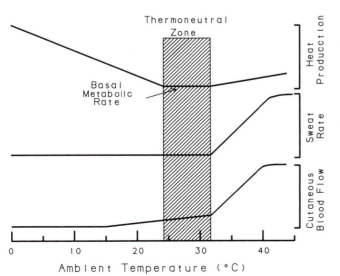

**Figure 13-7.** Schematic of physiologic responses to ambient temperature changes. Between approximately 24° and 32°C, the *thermoneutral zone* or TNZ, neither increased heat loss by sweating nor increased heat production is required; the adjustment of cutaneous blood flow is sufficient to maintain thermal homeostasis. Below this range, intense cutaneous vasoconstriction and increased metabolism increase conservation and production of heat. Above the TNZ, skin blood flow increases dramatically and sweating increases to enhance heat loss at the surface. Heat production also increases slightly because of the increased cardiac work required to sustain the increased blood flow to the skin.

cooling alone produces shivering for only a few minutes that does not resume until the central temperature falls below the basal level. If central temperature continues to fall, the intensity of the shivering progressively increases.

Heating of an area of the skin can cause sweating elsewhere in the body, also before central temperature rises.[29] When the central body temperature increases the sweating induced by skin heating is enhanced and continues as long as the central rise continues.

Central heating or cooling without changes in skin temperature, as occurs in laboratory studies and some clinical situations, causes the appropriate peripheral response, but often only after a significant fall or rise in central temperature. When both peripheral and central heating or cooling occur there is a synergistic response with an earlier and more vigorous reaction.[30–32] In summary, it appears that there is a high degree of control of central body temperature whereas skin temperature varies greatly. Extensive studies have been performed and calculations made so as to represent regulation of the body temperature in a mathematical fashion that would allow prediction of responses to thermal stress.

A more complete understanding of normal thermoregulation will give greater insight into abnormal conditions, particularly those seen in rehabilitation medicine, when, for example, there is disruption of the nervous system, absence of effector organs, (e.g., congenital absence of sweat glands), or a change in the skin (e.g., burns), or when drugs render the body incapable of mobilizing the normal mechanisms. In addition, it is important in all aspects of medicine, particularly rehabilitation medicine, to recognize that the competing regulatory systems in the body can diminish the efficiency of any one system. For example, exercise, which increases heat production and changes the distribution of cardiac output to the exercising muscle, can significantly load the thermoregulatory system with excess heat to be lost, and this can lead to thermal collapse (hyperthermia), especially in a hot environment. Regulation of blood pressure by adjustment of the circulatory system to ensure adequate perfusion of the brain and the vital body organs can likewise be compromised by exposure to heat. An enormous amount of blood must be shifted to the skin to speed heat loss. Sweating can also significantly

deplete the circulating blood volume, interfering with the regulation of body fluid volume.

## Regulation of Body Temperature During Exercise

Exercise causes a rise in body temperature that is proportional to the metabolic work performed and to the independent ambient temperatures over wide extremes.[33] This rise in body temperature with exercise may be due to an adjustment of the set point of body temperature and not simply to overload of the body's heat loss mechanisms. However, in extremes of temperature, as marathon running in the heat or in cold, wet climates, the system can be overloaded and hyper- or hypothermia can occur.

When exercise is terminated the temperature returns toward normal, but it takes as long as 45 to 60 minutes to return to basal level. Consequently, temperature measurements taken shortly after exercise do not accurately reflect basal body temperature. The rise in temperature during exercise cannot be abolished with antipyretic drugs such as aspirin.[34]

### Fever

The most commonly recognized abnormality of human body temperature is fever resulting from infections or inflammation. The rise in body temperature during fever is due to setting of the thermoregulatory system to a new set point and not to a breakdown of thermoregulation or overload of the system. At the onset of fever, after an infection or injection of a pyrogen, the body acts as if it were too cool and sharp cutaneous vasoconstriction occurs, causing conservation of heat followed by shivering (chill), which increases heat production. These continue until a new higher level of body temperature is reached. When the body temperature reaches the higher level it remains constant, and the thermoregulatory system responds to heating or cooling quantitively, in the same fashion as before the fever. This indicates that the sensitivity of the regulation of body temperature is as precise in fever as at normal levels.[35] When the cause of the fever is removed or the fever is abolished by antipyretics that act on the central nervous system, the body mobilizes heat loss mechanisms: behavioral (casting off covers or clothing, Figure 13-8), vasodilatation, and sweating, and temperature is reduced to its pre-fever levels. The pyrogen acts in the central nervous system, inducing a change in the set point of the hypothalamus, as outlined in Figure 13-8.

Fever occurs under a great variety of clinical circumstances, but it appears that the pathophysiology of the fever is common to all. The entrance of a bacterial pyrogen into the body causes phagocytic cells of the body to synthesize and release into the circulation interleukin 1 (IL 1), which in the central nervous system causes alterations in the thermoregulatory system. The production of IL 1 can be initiated by bacteria, fungi, viruses, or immune reactions, but it seems to be produced primarily by the monocytes in the blood and the macrophages in the tissue. The lymphocytes also produce lymphokine, which acts on the monocytes and macrophages to enhance production of IL 1. IL 1 has many actions[36] and probably acts via at least two intermediaries, which in turn act on the central nervous system. One of these substances is a prostanoid derived from arachidonic acid released from the brain, metabolized to the prostaglandin endoporoxide, and then converted to prostaglandin, prostacyclin, and thromboxane. This reaction can be blocked by use of a nonsteroidal, antiinflammatory drug such as aspirin or synthetic agents.

Cortisone is also antipyretic, but its action is to prevent arachidonic acid release from the brain membrane phospholipids.[37,38] When a patient is febrile, it is important to recognize that body temperature is regulated at the new, higher, level. If it is desirable to reduce the temperature, it is important to use antipyretic agents to reset the body's thermostat and then to use physical means to enhance heat loss. Attempting to lower a fever with ice baths or ice blankets alone produces the same rather violent reaction in the body as an attempt to reduce a normal body temperature from 37° to 36°C, and the increased physiologic stress could well be detrimental.

Whether in infection fever is beneficial or should be abolished is not clear. In some ectotherms infected with pathogens, survival is enhanced by allowing fever to persist, but this is not so in others.[39] In rabbits infected with *Pasteurella multocida,* survival was greatest in those that had a febrile response of 1.5° to 2.25°C,[40] and death rates were high when fever was abolished.[41] Other studies were inconsistent. In humans no studies have shown a clear benefit for abolishing fever. Hyperpyrexia can cause complications such as febrile convulsion in children, and the increased metabolism and hyperpnea can be harmful to patients with cardiopulmonary disease. Until studies are performed, it would seem to be logical to reduce fever to a comfortable level (ca. 38.0-38.5°) with antipyretics but not to strive to abolish it altogether.

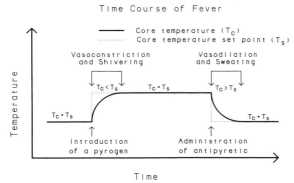

**Figure 13-8.** Schematic diagram of the change in body temperature before, during, and after onset of fever. Note that during the time when there is a difference between the set point of body temperature (*dotted line*) and the actual body temperature (*solid line*), the appropriate thermoregulatory effectors are activated to make the actual body temperature approach the set point.

### Spinal Cord–Injured Patients

Spinal cord–injured patients may have abnormal body temperature regulation or may be less able to respond effectively to changes in ambient temperature, particularly during other physiologic stresses. The amount of impairment depends on the level and completeness of the lesion. With high spinal injury, when a very large portion of the skin is insentient, the patient may be especially insensitive to changes in heat or cold, particularly if the sentient skin is clothed. For example, in a cold environment a patient wearing a warm jacket and mitts may become seriously hypothermic if the lower part of the body is inadequately clothed and yet may not be aware of hypothermia until the warm sentient skin is cooled by the cool recirculating blood.[42] In like fashion, a patient may be in a very warm bath and not be aware of the changes in the central body temperature, particularly if the sentient skin is relatively cool until core temperature has risen significantly.

On the output side of the thermoregulatory system, some of the effector mechanisms are lost. Patients do not shiver below the level of their lesion, so the heat increase so produced is very limited. With a high spinal injury, heat production may increase by only 10% to 15% over resting levels, placing the patient at risk of hypothermia in a cold environment.

Vasomotor control of the lower body may also be seriously impaired when sympathetic outflow is damaged. Because of this, heat would be neither conserved nor lost in response to central temperature changes. Some slow, sluggish, and relatively ineffectual vasomotor control appears to occur at the spinal cord level, and sweating is equally ineffectual below the level of the spinal lesion.[43]

In spinal cord–injured patients it is relative thermal stability, not relative poikilothermy, that is remarkable, and many questions remain as to how this is accomplished. In managing or guiding patients, particularly those with a high spinal lesion, the physician should recommend appropriate adjustment of the environment with air conditioning and heating to help regulate body temperature. Laboratory studies are needed to determine what extremes of temperature are tolerated well. In addition, thermoregulation should be studied in fully rehabilitated spinal-injured patients, particularly those who are in the workforce or who engage in strenuous physical activity such as Olympic-style athletics. Appropriate guidelines and adjustments should then be made based on these studies.

Conditions like skin disease, burns, and amputations may well compromise the ability either to sense temperature changes or to alter blood flow to the skin or sweating rate.

Drugs can modify thermoregulatory effectiveness, too. Any anesthetic agent can reduce the sensitivity of the central nervous system, inducing a state of poikilothermia. This effect can last for some time after consciousness begins to return, leaving patients hyperthermic or hypothermic, depending on the environment and how well-clothed they are.

Alcohol is a central nervous system depressant that reduces the sensitivity of the thermoregulatory system and a direct peripheral vasodilator that increases heat loss. The two effects together can be particularly dangerous in the cold, but they also impair regulation in the heat. Drugs such as tranquilizers, sleeping pills, and antihypertensives, also affect the central nervous system and thus may be particularly damaging to elders.

Narcotics, especially "street drugs," can either be sedatives (e.g., heroin, morphine) and make the user susceptible to hypothermia in the cold, or stimulants (e.g., cocaine, a metabolic stimulant). A massive cocaine overdose can cause serious, sometimes life-threatening, hyperthermia.

## Summary

Body temperature is a tightly regulated physiologic variable and is essential to health. Regulation is effected by achieving a balance between heat production and heat loss, a balance brought about by an intricate system of thermosensitive structures in skin, brain, and probably many other regions of the body, that cause appropriate adjustments in the peripheral regions of the body. The response of humans to activity, environment, stress, and illness can be understood and predicted with knowledge of the basic systems of physiologic controls.

## References

1. Cooper KE, Kenyon JR. A comparison of temperature measured in the rectum, oesophagus, and on the surface of the aorta during hypothermia in man. Bri J Surg 1957; 44:616–619.
2. Ivy AC. What is normal or normality? Q Bull Northwestern Univ Med School 1944; 18:22–32.
3. Pembry MS. Animal heat. In: Schafer, ed. Textbook of Physiology. Edinburgh: Pentland, 1898.
4. Arendt J. Melatonin. Clin Endocrinol 1988; 29:205–229.
5. Goodyear JE. Heat hyperpyrexia in an infant. Med Sci Law 1979; 19:208–209.
6. Robertshaw D. Man in extreme environments, problems of the newborn and elderly. In: Cena K, Clark, JA, eds. Bioengineering, Thermal Physiology and Comfort. Amsterdam: Elsevier, 1981.
7. Paton BC. Accidental hypothermia. Pharmacol Ther 1983; 22:331–377.
8. Hardy JD, DuBois EF. Differences between men

and women in their response to heat and cold. Proc Nat Acad Sci US 1940; 26:389–398.

9. Fox RH, Lofstedt BE, Woodward PM, et al. Comparison of thermoregulatory function in men and women. Appl Physiol 1969; 26:444–453.

10. Hammel HT. Terrestrial animals in cold: Recent studies of primitive man. In: Field J, ed. Handbook of Physiology. Washington, DC: 1964.

11. Hardy JD. Physiology of temperature regulation. Physiol Rev 1961; 41:521–606.

12. Hammell HT. Regulation of internal body temperature. Annu Rev Physiol 1968; 30:641–710.

13. Jessen C. Independent clamps of peripheral and central temperatures and their effects on heat production in the goat. Annu Rev Physiol 1981; 311:11–22.

14. Boulant JA. Hypothalamic control of thermoregulation. Neurophysiological basis. In: Morgane PT, Panksepp J, eds. Handbook of the Hypothalamus. New York: 1980.

15. Heller HC. Hypothalamic thermosensitivity in mammals. In: Giradier L, Seydoux J, eds. Effectors of Thermogenesis. Basel: Experientia, 1978.

16. Hardy JD, Hellon RF, Sutherland K. Temperature-sensitive neurones in the dog's hypothalamus. J Physiol (Lond) 1964; 715:242–253.

17. Pickering GW. The vasosmotor regulation of heat loss from the human skin in relation to external temperature. Heart 1932; 16:115–135.

18. Bligh J. The receptors concerned in the respiratory response to humidity in sheep at high ambient temperature. J Physiol (Lond) 1963; 168:747–763.

19. Downey JA, Mottram RF, Pickering GW. The location by regional cooling of central temperature receptors in the conscious rabbit. J Physiol (Lond) 1965; 170:415–441.

20. Rawson RO, Quick KP. Evidence of deep body thermoreceptor response to intraabdominal heating of the ewe. J Appl Physiol 1970; 28:813.

21. Simon E, Rautenberg W, Jessen C. Initiation of shivering in unanesthetized dogs by local cooling within the vertebral canal. Experentia 1965; 21:476–477.

22. Downey JA, Chiodi HP, Darling RC. Central temperature regulation in the spinal man. J Appl Physiol 1967; 22:91–94.

23. Kuno Y. Human Perspiration. Springfield, Ill: Charles C Thomas, 1956.

24. Nadel ER, Mitchell JW, Saltin B, et al. Peripheral modifications to the central drive for sweating. J Appl Physiol 1971; 31:828–833.

25. Johnson RH, Smith AC, Spalding JMK. Oxygen consumption of paralyzed men exposed to cold. J Physiol (Lond) 1963; 169:584–591.

26. Emorine LJ, Marullo S, Briend-Sutren MM, et al. Molecular characterization of the human beta₃adrenergic receptor. Science 1989; 245:1116–1121.

27. Kerslake DM, Cooper KE. Vasodilation in the hand in response to heating the skin elsewhere. Clin Sci 1950; 9:31–47.

28. Pickering GW. The vasomotor regulation of heat loss from the human skin in relation to external temperature. Heart 1932; 16:115–135.

29. Randall WC, Rawson RO, McCook RD, et al. Central and peripheral factors in dynamic thermoregulation. J Appl Physiol 1963; 18:61–64.

30. Benzinger TH. Heat regulation: Homeostasis of central temperature in man. Physiol Rev 1969; 49:671–759.

31. Downey JA, Chiodi HP, Darling RC. Central temperature regulation in the spinal man. J Appl Physiol 1967; 22:91–94.

32. Downey JA, Miller JM, Darling RC. Thermoregulatory responses to deep and superficial cooling in spinal man. J Appl Physiol 1969; 27:209–212.

33. Nielsen M. Die Regulation der Korpertemperatur bei Muskelarbeit. Skand Arch Physiol 1938; 79:193–230.

34. Downey JA, Darling RC. Effect of salicylates on elevation of body temperature during exercise. J Appl Physiol 1962; 17:323–325.

35. Cooper KE, Cranston WI, Snell ES. Temperature regulation during fever in man. Clin Sci 1964; 27:345–356.

36. Atkins E. Fever: The old and the new. J Infect Dis 1984; 149:339–348.

37. Cranston WI, Hellon RF, Mitchell D, et al. Intraventricular injections of drugs which inhibit phospholipase A₂ suppress fever in rabbits. J Physiol (Lond) 1983; 339:97–105.

38. Gill W, Wilson S, Long WB III. Steroid hypothermia. Surg Gynecol Obstet 1978; 146:944–946.

39. Bernheim HA, Kluger MJ. Fever and antipyresis in the lizard *Dipsosaurus dorsalis*. Am J Physiol 1976; 321:198–203.

40. Kluger MJ, Vaughn LK. Fever and survival in rabbits infected with *Pasteurella multocida*. J Physiol (Lond) 1978; 282:243–251.

41. Vaughn LK, Veale WL, Cooper, KE. Antipyresis: Its effect on mortality rate of bacterially infected rabbits. Brain Res Bull 1980; 7:175–180.

42. Downey JA, Miller JM, Darling RC. Thermoregulatory responses to deep and superficial cooling in spinal man. J Appl Physiol 1969; 27:209–212.

43. Secendorf R, Randall WC. Thermal reflex sweating in normal and paraplegic man. J Appl Physiol 1961; 16:796–800.

# Chapter 14

# Control of the Circulation in the Limbs

DANIEL E. LEMONS
JOHN A. DOWNEY

The peripheral circulation is usually thought of as a mass transport system that moves gasses such as oxygen and carbon dioxide, and other molecules such as glucose and amino acids throughout the body to serve each tissue's metabolic needs. To understand the control of the circulation it is important to broaden this view to include at least two other important functions, which serve systemic needs rather than local ones. First, the peripheral vascular system is a primary effector in the regulation of systemic blood pressure (BP) through its ability to alter the distribution of blood flow and thereby buffer systemic pressure fluctuations. Second, it is the most important pathway for the transport of heat from the central body to the surface, where it can be lost. Without this pathway, humans, along with the other mammals and birds, would be unable to sustain their high rate of metabolism without rapidly overheating. As we will see later, the local metabolic needs and the systemic baro- and thermoregulatory demands on blood flow cannot always be met simultaneously and compromises must often be made.

Blood flow to the limbs varies over a wide range, depending on the need for its three primary functions—mass transfer in support of limb metabolism, regulation of systemic BP, and heat transfer for systemic thermoregulation. At rest, in a neutral temperature environment, the circulation

to the forearm may be 2 to 4 ml per 100 ml of tissue per minute, but in the heat this may rise to 15 ml per 100 ml per minute. The major portion of this increase occurs in the skin, where as much as 50% of the cardiac output (CO) may be directed during heat stress. During exercise the muscle blood flow may increase from the resting value of 2 or 3 to nearly 250 ml per 100 ml of tissue per minute. The vascular, hormonal, and neural elements that permit this range of flows and the circumstances under which they occur are covered in this chapter.

## Hemodynamic Fundamentals of Blood Flow

### Pressure and Other Physical Factors Affecting Blood Flow in Vessels: Simple Circuits

To understand limb circulatory control it is necessary to consider the relationship between pressure, viscosity, geometry, and flow in vessels. The name for this area of study is *rheology,* the study of the flow and deformation of matter. The Poiseuille-Hagen equation below describes the role of the critical physical factors that influence blood flow through a single vessel.

$$V = (P_1 - P_2) \frac{\pi r^4}{8Ln} \tag{1}$$

In this equation, V is the volumetric blood flow, and it is determined directly by the pressure dif-

Dr. Lemons was supported by NIH Grant HL26090-07, NSF CBT-8702582 and the Vidda Foundation.

ference from one end of the vessel to the other, $(P_1 - P_2)$, and the radius of the vessel raised to the fourth power. As the radius and/or the pressure difference increases, so does the flow. V is inversely related to the vessel length, L, and the viscosity of the blood, $n$, so that increases in these parameters decrease the flow through the vessel. The single most important determinant of blood flow is the radius of the vessel. When the radius of a vessel doubles while all other parameters remain the same, flow through the vessel increases 16-fold, because the flow depends on the fourth power of the radius. Consequently, when the vessels of a vascular bed dilate together, as happens during exercise, blood flow through the bed can increase enormously.

The last term in equation 1, which includes the variables of vessel radius and length and blood viscosity, can be thought of as the conductance of the vessel to blood flow. The greater the conductance, the more readily blood will flow through the vessel. Equation 1 may then be simplified as follows:

$$V = (P_1 - P_2) \times K \tag{2}$$

where K is the conductance. As in electrical circuits, the inverse of the conductance, K, is the resistance, R. The greater R the less blood will flow at a given perfusing pressure. The product of 1/R or K and the pressure difference yields the same result:

$$V = (P_1 - P_2)/R \tag{3}$$

This of course is directly analogous to Ohm's law of electrical current flow, which states that current flow equals the voltage difference across an element divided by the electrical resistance.

Even though R is partially determined by vessel length and blood viscosity, it is generally assumed the changes in R are due mostly to changes in vessel radius. This is because vessel length does not usually vary, and viscosity, though somewhat flow dependent, does not change a great deal for a given vessel. As will be discussed later, the vascular resistance of a tissue or of the entire peripheral circulation is a useful index of the functioning of the intact autonomic nervous system. However, R is not measured directly, but rather is calculated according to the rearrangement of equation 3 thus:

$$R = (P_a - P_v)/V \tag{4}$$

In this equation, $P_a$ and $P_v$ are, respectively, the arteriolar inlet and the venular outlet pressures for a vascular bed. In humans, the inlet pressure is usually the systemic pressure, $P_a$, and V may be measured invasively or noninvasively. The outlet pressure of the bed is usually taken to be close to central venous pressure, which may be either measured or, more likely, assumed to be a value from 0 to 5 mm Hg. R for a vascular bed is usually calculated with $P_v$ ignored because it is small, and thus, equation 4 simplifies to

$$R = P_a/V \tag{5a}$$

or,

$$V = P_a/R \tag{5b}$$

Often studies on humans report only limb blood flow measurements and then ascribe blood flow changes to alternations in vascular diameter or tone. As can be seen in equation 5b, $P_a$ also determines flow, and if changes in this driving pressure are not accounted for changes in blood flow cannot be accurately interpreted. Limb blood flow may change because the systemic pressure has changed and not because vascular tone has been altered.

### Blood Flow in Vascular Beds Arranged in Series and in Parallel

The entire circulatory system can be thought of as two primary circulations, the systemic, which is sustained by the left side of the heart, and the pulmonary, which is sustained by the right side; each includes many vessels connected in parallel. Figure 14-1 shows this generalized view. This entire circulation, or components of it, can be analyzed in the same way that electrical circuits can, with resistive, capacitive, and pressure-producing components. Figure 14-2 shows the circulation diagrammed according to this scheme. The batteries represent the right and left sides of the heart, producing a potential difference around the circuit that produces the flow.

As with resistors in an electrical circuit, the total resistance of vessels connected in series equals the sum of the resistances of each of the

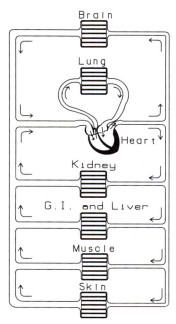

**Figure 14-1.** Schematic view of the human circulatory system. The total circulation passes through the right side of the heart and the lungs, then returns to the left side of the heart, where it is distributed by the arterial system to the organs. The blood passes through many parallel pathways to the various regions and through many more parallel pathways within each organ.

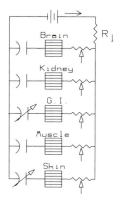

**Figure 14-2.** Electrical equivalent of the human circulatory system. The heart is represented by the battery at the top. Resistor $R_1$ represents the resistance of the distributing arterial system, while the variable resistors before each vascular bed represent the arteriolar resistances, which are the main components of peripheral resistance. The capillaries are parallel conductance pathways of low resistance. All venous beds are represented as capacitors because they can expand to store blood, but the cutaneous and splanchnic beds are represented as variable capacitors because they have the greatest range of capacity and can pool large amounts of blood under certain conditions.

vessels. Thus, the total resistance down the arterial tree from the aorta to a given precapillary arteriole equals the sum of the resistance to flow at each vessel generation. The small radii of the terminal arterioles of the microcirculation produce the highest resistance to flow, and consequently, they are the principal vessels that control total peripheral resistance.

Because the circulation is comprised mostly of many vessels in parallel, it is necessary to understand how total resistance is determined by the resistance in parallel elements. For vascular beds arranged in parallel, the reciprocal of the total vascular resistance equals the sum of the reciprocal of the resistances of the parallel vascular beds:

$$1/R_t = 1/R_{hrt} + 1/R_{br} + 1/R_{kid} + 1/R_{spl} + 1/R_1 \quad (6)$$

where $R_t$, $R_{hrt}$, $R_{br}$, $R_{kid}$, $R_{spl}$ and $R_1$ are, respectively, the total heart, brain, kidney, splanchnic, and limb circulation resistances.

When resistances are in series, the total resistance of the circuit changes in direct proportion to the resistance change in any of the series elements. Thus, if the resistance in one element increased by 10 arbitrary resistance units (RU) the total resistance would also increase by 10 RU. In a parallel circuit, an increase in 10 RU of one parallel element would increase the reciprocal of total resistance by 1/10 RU or $1/R_t + 1/10$. In this case the total resistance is much less affected by the resistance change in a single parallel element. Table 14-1 illustrates this point by showing the result of increasing limb resistance from 40 to 140 RU.

**Table 14-1.** Series and Parallel Vascular Resistances

| Vascular Bed | Series Resistance | Parallel (1/R) | Series Resistance | Parallel (1/R) |
|---|---|---|---|---|
| Heart | 10 | 0.100 | 10 | 0.100 |
| Brain | 10 | 0.100 | 10 | 0.100 |
| Kidney | 20 | 0.050 | 20 | 0.050 |
| Splanchnic | 20 | 0.050 | 20 | 0.050 |
| Limbs | **40** | 0.025 | **140** | 0.007 |
| Sum | 100 | 0.33 | 200 | 0.31 |
| Total resistance | 100 | 3.08 | 200 | 3.26 |
| % Increase | | | **100** | **5.8** |

If these circulations were connected in series, the result would be a 100 RU increase in $R_t$, or a 100% change. In a parallel arrangement, the 100 RU increase in limb resistance results in only a 5% increase in total resistance.

When the (CO), which produces the driving pressure, remains the same, and one of the parallel vascular beds dilates so that its resistance to flow decreases, such as the skin during heat stress, then the entire vascular resistance falls, reducing the pressure drop across the circuit and thus reducing systemic pressure. This is more easily seen when equation 5a is applied to the entire circulation and rearranged as below:

$$P_a = CO \cdot R_t \qquad (7)$$

When $R_t$ falls, then $P_a$ must also fall, unless there is an increase in cardiac output.

In order to maintain systemic pressure when one vascular bed is dilated, it is necessary to increase the resistance to flow in one of the parallel vascular beds and/or to increase cardiac output, thus preventing a change in $P_a$. This is what occurs during heat stress, when the splanchnic bed may constrict as the cutaneous beds dilate so that $P_a$ remains unchanged.

## Features of Arteries and Veins

### Compliance of the Vessel Wall

The adjustment of peripheral vascular resistance depends on the ability of individual vessels to change their diameter, which is determined by the internal pressure and the distensibility of the vessel wall, or its compliance. Arteries and veins differ significantly in their compliance. Figure 14-3 shows compliance curves for an artery and a vein, revealing the relationship between their internal pressure and their diameter. Veins increase their volume to a much greater degree than arteries as the internal pressure increases; thus they have much greater compliance than arteries. For this reason veins are often called the capacitance vessels of the circulation.

Compliance is not a static property of a vessel. In Figure 14-3 the middle compliance curve is for the same vein at a higher level of sympathetic tone. As sympathetic activity increases, the

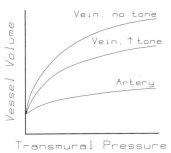

**Figure 14-3.** Relationship between transmural pressure and volume for arteries and veins. Arteries have little change in volume with pressure because their walls are muscular and stiff. Veins have relatively little smooth muscle and expand easily as the transmural pressure increases. Veins that are innervated become stiffer and exhibit a reduced volume-pressure curve when there is sympathetic activity, as shown by the middle curve.

smooth muscle in the vessels contracts and the walls become less compliant, so the relationship between pressure and diameter is altered.

Compliance is a consequence of an active component, the smooth muscle, which contracts and relaxes, and a passive connective tissue component, which stretches as external forces are applied to it. Vessels have varying proportions of smooth muscle and connective tissue collagen and elastin. Elastin is more distensible than collagen, and vessels such as the aorta and its major branches have a large amount of elastin, giving them highly elastic, distensible properties. Small arteries consist mostly of smooth muscle and are consequently highly inelastic. Veins have little smooth muscle, thus their greater compliance.

Because the small arteries and arterioles (vessels smaller than 1 mm) are inelastic but well-endowed with smooth muscle, they provide most of the resistance to flow in the vascular system. For this reason, these vessels are called the *resistance vessels*. Their diameters are determined almost entirely by the contractile state of their smooth muscle, and consequently their resistance can vary over a very wide range. The plot in Figure 14-4 of the intravascular pressure from the left ventricle to the right atrium reveals that the greatest pressure change occurs in the arteriolar resistance vessels. Because of the great resistance of the terminal arterioles, the pressure at the entrance of the capillary circulation is only 8 to 15 mm Hg.

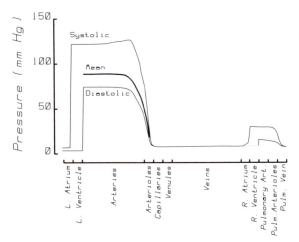

**Figure 14-4.** Systolic, diastolic, and mean pressure distribution in the heart and vascular system. The major drop in pressure occurs in the small distributing arterioles of the systemic and pulmonary circulation, which are referred to as the *resistance vessels*. Venous pressures are low.

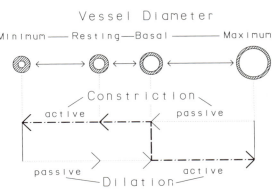

**Figure 14-5.** Resting and basal vascular tone. At a given perfusing pressure, and in the absence of neural, hormonal, and local influences, a vessel has a *basal* diameter. Increases or decreases from this diameter (shown in heavy horizontal lines, - · -) require *active* processes like sympathetic nerve activity, hormones, or local metabolites, while the return to the basal diameter (shown in dotted horizontal lines) requires only the removal of these influences, and is thus called *passive vasoconstriction* or *passive vasodilatation*. Under normal circumstances, most arteries have some tonic sympathetic tone maintaining their *resting* diameter. Further increases in constrictor influence diminishes the diameter until the vessel either is closed or at its minimum diameter. This constriction is termed *active vasoconstriction*. The return from the maximally constricted to the resting or basal state is called *passive vasodilatation* because it requires only the removal of constrictor influences. To increase beyond the basal diameter, dilator nerves, hormones, or local factors are required, and such increases are termed *active vasodilatation*. The return from the maximum diameter requires only the removal of the active vasodilator influences and is termed *passive vasoconstriction*.

## Passive and Active Changes in Vessel Size

Because each vessel segment and vascular bed has different intrinsic properties, nomenclature has been developed to distinguish the mechanisms that produce diameter changes. In the absence of sympathetic input, each vessel has an intrinsic diameter called its *basal* or *intrinsic diameter*. This diameter is the result of the passive, or connective tissue, and active, or smooth muscle, properties of the vessel. At a constant perfusion pressure, increases or decreases from this intrinsic or basal diameter are due to active processes that modify the contractile state of the smooth muscle. Figure 14-5 shows changes from the basal diameter (vertical dashed line) as horizontal dash-dot lines. When sympathetic nerves are present and they are tonically active, the vessel diameter is smaller than its basal diameter; this diameter, which is called the *resting diameter*, is achieved by *active vasoconstriction* via the sympathetic nerves. Constriction of the vessel beyond its resting diameter is also an active process that requires additional sympathetic or hormonal input. Dilatation of the vessel from the constricted state to resting or basal levels is called *passive vasodilatation*, because it requires only the withdrawal of sympathetic vasoconstrictor tone or constrictor hormones. In Figure 14-5 this process is indicated by horizontal dotted lines.

Dilatation of arterioles beyond their basal level is possible when substances such as epinephrine, acetylcholine (Ach), or bradykinin are released, or local metabolites such as lactate or carbon dioxide are present. In some tissues such as skeletal muscle there are also sympathetic vasodilator nerves. As indicated in Figure 14-5, dilatation beyond the basal diameter is called *active vasodilatation* because it is due to added extrinsic stimulation; the return to the basal diameter is a passive process called *passive vasoconstriction* which requires only the withdrawal of the dilator nerve activity or hormone. Active dilatation of the veins has not yet been demonstrated.

## Cellular Aspects of Vessel Function

### Mediators of Vascular Smooth Muscle Contractile State

Because vascular resistance is determined almost entirely by the diameter of the resistance vessels, and the diameter changes from the resting diameter in all vessels depend on the contractile state of the smooth muscle, it is important to briefly review the factors that influence smooth muscle contractile function. The role of the sympathetic nerves has already been mentioned and the release of norepinephrine (NE), and in some cases Ach, and other neurotransmitters by these nerves is for most limb vessels the most important means of controlling vascular tone. The sympathetic nerve and smooth muscle cell are diagrammatically represented in Figure 14-6.

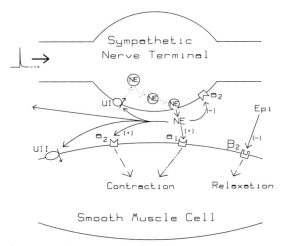

**Figure 14-6.** Synapse between the sympathetic nerve terminal and the smooth muscle cell. Action potentials traveling down the nerve initiate the release of NE from synaptic vesicles into the cleft. NE may traverse the synaptic cleft and bind to $\alpha_{-1}$, $\alpha_{-2}$, or $\beta_2$-receptors, causing either contraction or relaxation. Ultimately, NE may be taken back into the nerve or muscle via active uptake, UI or UII respectively, or it may be degraded or diffuse away from the synapse. Presynaptic $\alpha_{-2}$ receptors mediate negative feedback to the release of NE from the nerve. A ($+$) indicates that the pathway shown increases vascular tone and a ($-$) the opposite. The $\beta_2$-receptors are usually extrajunctional and respond mostly to circulating epinephrine.

### The Sympathetic Nerves

**Nerve-Muscle Synapse.** In contrast to the junction between somatic nerves and striated muscle, where the axons end in a terminal button with a very narrow cleft separating it from the muscle, the sympathetic nerve has enlargements called varicosities along its length, where neurotransmitters are released. These are not always closely apposed to each smooth muscle cell. The cleft between nerve and muscle is typically 5 to 50 nm wide, so considerable diffusion time is often required for NE to reach the smooth muscle cell after it is released from the nerve. Because not all the cells in the muscle are close to the nerve varicosities, either the transmitter must diffuse to the distant cells, or the depolarization induced in the nearby cells must spread electrotonically to the other cells via gap junctions.

The time course of smooth muscle activation is slower than that of the somatic nerve–striated muscle synapse. Inactivation of the response is also slower, and is the result of three simultaneous processes: (1) enzymatic breakdown of the NE by catechol-*o*-methyl transferase (COMT) in the cleft, (2) sodium-potassium-adenosine triphosphatase–dependent reuptake into the sympathetic nerve (reuptake I, UI), or into the smooth muscle cell (reuptake II, UII), and (3) diffusion into the interstitial space, and ultimately into the capillaries. Because some NE released from the nerve finds its way into the bloodstream, plasma NE gives an indication of the level of sympathetic activity. An increase in sympathetic activity results in a rise in plasma NE, which lags behind the onset of activity by 2 to 3 minutes.

The NE that is released from the sympathetic nerves is synthesized by the nerve from tyrosine, which is first converted to dopamine in the nerve's cytoplasm. The dopamine is then packaged in 40 to 60 nm synaptic vesicles, which also contain the enzyme dopamine-$\beta$-hydroxylase, which converts dopamine to NE. When action potentials traveling down the nerve arrive at the nerve varicosity, an inward $Ca^{2+}$ current raises the intraneuronal $Ca^{2+}$ concentration, initiating the fusion of vesicles with the membrane. After fusion with the membrane, the vesicles rupture, releasing their contents into the junctional cleft.

The synaptic vesicles of the nerve contain vasoactive substances besides NE, including adenosine triphosphate (ATP) and an assortment of peptides, depending on where the nerve is located.[1] These substances are coreleased along with NE into the cleft and also affect the contractile state of the smooth muscle cell. The presence of these substances has only recently become known, and their precise role in the regulation of vascular tone is not clear.

**Nerve and Smooth Muscle Cell Membrane Receptors for Vasoactive Agents.** The concept of cellular receptors was postulated long before it was known what the cellular components were. Receptors traditionally have been defined by pharmacologic means, using various drugs found to be either agonists (initiators) or antagonists (inhibitors) of a given effect. Using such techniques it has been possible to establish the existence of several major categories of receptor (adrenergic, muscarinic, dopaminergic, histaminergic), each of which has two to many subtypes. Many of these membrane receptors have now been isolated, sequenced, and cloned.[2] Occupancy of these receptors by the appropriate agent or ligand activates a many-stepped intracellular pathway leading to constriction or dilatation of vessels. Vessels usually have receptors for more than one type of substance; some cause constriction and others dilatation.

Figure 14-6 shows that sympathetic nerves have $\alpha_2$-receptors, usually referred to as *presynaptic receptors*. These receptors bind NE that the nerve releases and mediate feedback inhibition of the release of neurotransmitter, regulating the amount of neurotransmitter released into the cleft. Sympathetic nerves may have muscarinic, purinergic ($P_1$), neuropeptide Y (NPY), and other receptors that are also involved in inhibition of NE release.

*Adrenergic Pathways and the G Proteins*

The adrenergic receptors (AR) have been divided into two major subclasses, $\alpha$-AR and $\beta$-AR, based on the ability of drugs like isoproterenol ($\beta$-AR) or phenylephrine ($\alpha$-AR) to activate or propranolol ($\beta$-AR) or phentolamine ($\alpha$-AR) to block them. There are at least two or three distinct forms of each of these receptor subclasses, $\alpha_1$-AR, $\alpha_2$-AR,

$\beta_1$-AR, $\beta_2$-AR, and $\beta_3$-AR, three of which ($\alpha_1$-AR, $\alpha_2$-AR, $\beta_2$-AR) are found in the vessels of the limb. Both of the $\alpha$-ARs cause constriction when activated, and the $\beta_2$-AR causes dilatation. Table 14-2 lists these receptors, their location in the various vascular beds of the limbs, their agonist and antagonist ligand, their actions when activated, and the intracellular second messenger systems they activate.

When an agonist binds an AR, the receptor interacts with a membrane resident G protein, so called because of its guanosine triphosphatase activity, which in turn mobilizes one or more multistepped intracellular effector pathways.[3–5] There are many forms of the G protein involved in the transmembrane signaling of receptor systems. The G protein that is coupled to the $\beta_2$-AR, $G_s$, activates the membrane-bound enzyme adenylate cyclase (AC). AC catalyzes the production of cyclic adenosine monophosphate (cAMP), which initiates other cytosolic processes leading ultimately to smooth muscle relaxation.

The $\alpha_1$-AR and the $\alpha_2$-AR both cause vasoconstriction but they use different intracellular pathways to do so. The $\alpha_2$-ARs interact with a G protein called $G_i$ which inhibits adenylate cyclase causing a reduction in cAMP levels in the cell. This leads to vasoconstriction via the removal of some tonic cAMP-mediated smooth muscle cell relaxation. Recently, some workers have suggested that other effector pathways might also be activated by $G_i$, which could also lead to smooth muscle cell contraction.[6] $G_i$ may, for instance, directly affect $K^+$ ion channels in the membrane.

The $\alpha_1$-AR appears to act through a G protein that has been designated $G_p$[7] to initiate phospholipase C (PLC)–mediated hydrolysis of membrane phosphatidylinositol 4,5-bisphosphate ($PIP_2$) into two components. The first, inositol, 1,4,5-trisphosphate ($IP_3$) releases calcium from intracellular stores (the sarcoplasmic riticulum [SR]), and the second, diacylglycerol (DAG), directly activates protein kinase C (PKC), which may affect contractile state through a separate mechanism.

*Activation of the Contractile Proteins*

The mechanism of smooth muscle contraction is similar to the sliding filament cross-bridge model

**Table 14-2.** Vascular Endothelial and Smooth Muscle Cell Membrane Receptors That Mediate Vascular Tone*

| Receptor type | Tissues | Agonists | Antagonist | Action | Coupling System | Intermediate Enzyme | Second Messengers | References |
|---|---|---|---|---|---|---|---|---|
| **Adrenergic** | | | | | | | | |
| $\alpha_1$ | most VSM | NE>Epi>>Iso | Prazosin | Vasoconstriction | $G_p$ | PLC | $IP_3$,DAG | 3,4 |
| $\alpha_2$ | Peripheral vein VSM, small arterioles VSM, sympathetic nerves | NE>Epi>>Iso | Yohimbine | Vasoconstriction; ↓NE release | $G_i$, $G_k$ (?) | ↓AC, ↑$g_k$ | ↓cAMP | 3,4,6 |
| $\beta_1$ | SA node, ventricles | Iso>Epi>NE | Propranolol | ↑Rate, ↑contractility | $G_s$ | AC | cAMP | 3,4 |
| $\beta_2$ | Skeletal muscle VSM | Iso>Epi>>NE | Atenolol | Vasodilatation | $G_s$ | AC | cAMP | 3,4 |
| **Cholinergic** | | | | | | | | |
| $M_1$(?) | VSM, endothelium, sympathetic nerves | Ach,carbachol | Pirenzepine, atropine, PTX? | Vasoconstriction, vasodilatation, ↓NE release | $G_p$(?) EDRF | PLC GC | $IP_3$ cGMP | 11,70 71 |
| $M_2$(?) | VSM, endothelium, sympathetic nerves, SA node, AV node | Ach,carbachol | AF-DX116, | Vasoconstriction, vasodilatation, ↓NE release, ↓Rate, ↓conduction | $G_i$(?) EDRF | ↓AC GC | ↓cAMP cGMP | 11,70 71 11 |
| $M_3$(?) | VSM, endothelium, sympathetic nerves | Ach,carbachol | PTX,atropine P-fluorohexa-hydroisol | Vasoconstriction, vasodilatation, ↓NE release | $G_k$(?) $G_p$(?) EDRF | $I_{k,Ach}$ PLC GC | $IP_3$ cGMP | 11,70 71 |
| **Purinergic** | | | | | | | | |
| $P_{2x}$ | VSM | ATP->AMP>adenosine | $ANAPP_3$ | Vasoconstriction | ROC-($Ca^{2+}$) | | | 14 |
| $P_{2y}$ | Endothelium | ATP->AMP>adenosine | $ANAPP_3$ | Vasodilatation | EDRF | | | 14 |
| **Adenosine** | | | | | | | | |
| $A_1$ | VSM | Adenosine,ATP(?) | | Vasodilatation | $G_i$ | AC | cAMP | 15 |
| $A_2$ | VSM | Adenosine,ATP(?) | | Vasodilatation | $G_s$ | AC | cAMP | 15 |
| **Histaminergic** | | | | | | | | |
| $H_1$ | Postcapillary venule endothelium, endothelium | 2-methylhistamine, histamine | Pyrilamine | ↑Capillary permeability | $G_p$ | PLC | $IP_3$ | 72,73 |
| $H_2$ | VSM | 4-methylhistamine, histamine | Burimamide | Vasodilatation Vasodilatation | EDRF GC | GC | cGMP | 72,73 |

| Receptor | Tissue | Agonist | Antagonist | Response | Coupling | Enzyme | Second messenger | Ref. |
|---|---|---|---|---|---|---|---|---|
| **Serotinergic** | | | | | | | | |
| $5HT_{1c}(?)$ | VSM | GR-43175,5-HT | | Vasoconstriction | $G_p(?)$ | PLC | $IP_3$ | 18–20 |
| $5HT_{1b}(?)$ | Endothelium | α-methyl-5-HT, 5-HT | Methysergide | Vasodilatation | EDRF | GC | cGMP | 18–20 |
| $5HT_{1a}(?)$ | VSM | 5-carboxyamido-tryptamine,5-HT | | Vasodilatation | $G_s(?)$ | AC | cAMP | 19 |
| $5HT_2$ | VSM | 5-HT | Ketanserin | Vasoconstriction | $G_p(?)$ | PLC | $IP_3$ | 18–20 |
| $5HT_3$ | Sensory nerve | 5-HT | | | ROC | | | 18 |
| **Peptidergic** | | | | | | | | |
| SP | Endothelium | SP | | Vasodilatation | EDRF | GC | cGMP | 74,75 |
| NPY | VSM | NPY | | Vasoconstriction | | | | 76 |
| VIP | VSM | VIP | | Vasodilatation | | AC | cAMP | 77 |
| **ADH (Vasopressin)** | | | | | | | | |
| $V_1$ | VSM | ADH | | Vasoconstriction | | PLC | $IP_3$ | |
| **ANF(ANP)** | | | | | | | | |
| B | VSM(0.5%) | ANF | | Vasodilatation | | GC | cGMP | 76 |
| C | VSM(95%) | ANF | | ANF clearance | | | | |
| **AII** | | | | | | | | |
| AII | VSM | AII | | Vasoconstriction | $G_?;$ | PLC | $IP_3$, DAG | |

* Abbreviated agonists are NE, norepinephrine; Epi, epinephrine; ISO, isoproterenol; Ach, acetylcholine; ATP, adenosine triphosphate; AMP, adenosine monophosphate; 5-HT, 5-hydroxy triptamine or serotonin; SP, substance P; NPY, neuropeptide Y; VIP, vasoactive intestinal polypeptide; ADH, antidiuretic hormone; ANF, atrial natriuretic factor and AII, angiotensin II. The antagonist PTX is pertussis toxin and $ANAPP_3$ is arylazido aminopropionyl-ATP. Coupling systems are G-protein ($G_x$), ROC-receptor operated ion channel or EDRF—endothelium dependent relaxing factor. Intermediate enzymes are PLC, Phospholipase C; AC, adenylate cycalse or GC, guanylate cyclase. Second messengers are $IP_3$, inositol trisphosphate; cAMP, cyclic adenosine monophosphate; cGMP, cyclic guanosine monophosphate and DAG, diacylglycerol. Not all receptor types are known and uncertainty about the specific type is indicated by a ''(?)''. Intracellular pathways are known only for some receptor systems and those which are as yet undetermined are left blank.

of skeletal muscle, but in smooth muscle the regulation of cross-bridge formation is more complex. As in skeletal muscle, intracellular calcium is one of the most important initiators of smooth muscle contractile activity, but only a transient increase in cytosolic calcium is required to initiate a sustained contraction of the muscle. The calcium that activates the muscle comes predominantly from the sarcoplasmic reticulum (SR), and it is rapidly taken up again after its release. Calcium-dependent calmodulin catalyzes the phosphorylation of myosin light chain kinase (MLK), which in turn phosphorylates the myosin light chain, which forms the cross-bridge with actin, producing contraction. All pathways that increase cytosolic free calcium increase smooth muscle tone, and conversely most pathways that cause smooth muscle relaxation do so at least in part by reducing cytosolic free calcium. There are other pathways that may sensitize or desensitize the contractile proteins to calcium and so cause an increase or a decrease in cross-bridge formation with no change in intracellular calcium. The β-AR vasodilatory pathway may both decrease intracellular calcium and phosphorylate MLK at a site that reduces its activity, thus causing relaxation by two mechanisms.[8]

## Hormones and Other Vasoactive Influences on Smooth Muscle Tone

Many substances and physical factors modify vascular tone. Some are tonic influences that are usually present at some level; others occur only under certain conditions such as exercise, stress, or hemorrhage. Table 14-2 lists the membrane receptors for a number of important vasoactive substances along with their actions in the cardiovascular system and the mechanisms by which they modify tone, if known.

### Acetylcholine

Ach causes vasodilatation of most vascular smooth muscle via activation of muscarinic receptors. The cholinergic vasodilator system of the limbs, particularly the limb muscle, is controlled by the higher brain centers, which increase their activity during fight-or-flight responses or psychological stress.[9,10] Before the discovery of endothelium-derived relaxing factor (EDRF), Ach was thought to dilate smooth muscle directly, but now it is known that the vascular endothelium must be present and that if it is not Ach is a vasoconstrictor. There are five known subtypes of muscarinic receptors, designated $M_1$ to $M_5$, but only the first three are pharmacologically identified, (so far $M_4$ and $M_5$ are known only because of cloning studies[11]). Their amino acid sequences are highly homologous with those of the AR family.[12] It is not clear which receptors are found in the peripheral vessels. Like the ARs, the muscarinic receptors are coupled to G proteins (see Table 14-2). There are also muscarinic receptors on the sympathetic nerves, and when occupied they inhibit the release of NE by the nerve.

### Purines

ATP causes vasoconstriction when applied to smooth muscle, but when the endothelium is present and it is applied inside the vessel lumen it causes vasodilatation.[13] The vasodilatation occurs via EDRF. ATP is a cotransmitter with NE in many sympathetic nerves, and the sympathetic nerves of some small arterioles seem to release mostly or only ATP and thus are sympathetic-purinergic nerves.[14] The receptors for ATP found in the vessels are named $P_{2x}$ and $P_{2y}$; the $P_1$ receptor is found elsewhere.

Adenosine receptors are treated as a separate receptor group with two subtypes, $A_1$ and $A_2$. Though adenosine is a purine, it is far more potent at these receptors than is ATP, adenosine diphosphate (ADP), or AMP, and it is far less potent at the $P_{2x,y}$ receptors. Both subtypes are found in the heart,[15] but the $A_2$ receptors appear to be the ones that mediate vasodilatation.

### Histamine

Histamine is a potent vasodilator found in the walls of mammalian arteries and veins[16] and in mast cells, from which it is released during the inflammatory process. NE appears to exert a tonic inhibitory influence on histamine release from either neuronal or nonneuronal stores; a decrease in NE results in an increase in histamine release. The importance of histamine in circulatory control is not clear.[17] The vasodilatation to histamine in some tissues is dependent on an intact endothelium but receptors on the smooth muscle also mediate vasodilatation. Both $H_1$ and $H_2$ receptors are found in the vessels, and the vasodilatation mediated by $H_1$ receptors is endothelium dependent.

### Serotonin

Serotonin, which is named for the *serum,* from which it was originally isolated, and its vasoconstrictor action, has both vasodilator and vasoconstrictor activity. There are thought to be at least five receptor subtypes, some of which are structurally related to the adrenergic receptors.[18] Most circulating serotonin is contained in platelets, and its action on smooth muscle depends on whether there is an intact endothelium. If the endothelium is present, serotonin binds to receptors on the luminal side and causes the formation of endothelium-derived relaxing factor (EDRF), which then causes vasodilation. If no endothelial cells are present, 5-HT binds to smooth muscle and, depending on the tissue and vessel type, may cause either vasodilatation or vasoconstriction.[19] Serotoninergic nerve fibers have been found in some vascular beds, but none are reported in the vessels of the limbs.[20]

### Angiotensin II

Angiotensin II (AII) is a far more potent vasoconstrictor, on a molar basis, than NE. AII is produced in the circulation from the parent molecule, $\alpha_2$-globulin or renin substrate, a protein circulating in the plasma. The juxtaglomerular cells release the enzyme renin into the circulation when sympathetic activity to the juxtaglomerular cells of the kidney is increased, plasma sodium is decreased, or arterial pressure of the renal artery is diminished. Renin catalyzes the conversion of $\alpha_2$-globulin to angiotensin I (AI). When AI passes through the lung and some other organs it is converted by converting enzyme (CE) of the endothelial cells into AII. AII then binds to specific receptors in the arterioles, causing vasoconstriction. So far, AII has not been shown to cause venoconstriction.

### Vasopressin

Vasopressin or antidiuretic hormone (ADH) is released by the posterior pituitary in response to reductions in plasma osmolality or volume. Perhaps its primary function is the stimulation of the distal and collecting tubules of the kidney to increase their permeability to water, resulting in increased reabsorption, but it is also a potent vasoconstrictor of arterioles. ADH may be important during hemorrhage in augmenting the vasoconstriction in muscle and other peripheral beds to preserve central blood volume.[21]

### Neuropeptides (Coreleased with NE by Sympathetic Nerves)

A variety of vasoactive peptides may be coreleased with NE from the sympathetic nerves, including neuropeptide Y (NPY), vasoactive intestinal protein (VIP), somatostatin, dynorphan (DYN), and galanan (GAL).[1] The significance of these peptides for normal blood flow regulation is not known, but they may be modulator substances that produce effects that persist for some time (30 minutes) after their release. Usually, they are released only at high rates of sympathetic nerve activity, and they may be important during times of high stress or pathologic states.

### Endothelium-Derived Relaxing Factor

Ach, ATP, histamine, serotonin, substance P, and some other substances normally cause vasodilatation but have the opposite effect when the endothelium has been removed.[22] These substances cause vasodilatation by first binding to the endothelial cells, which then release a diffusible factor, EDRF, which causes the smooth muscle cells to relax. There is a tonic release of EDRF by most vessels that partially dilates those vessels, and if EDRF production is pharmacologically inhibited, systemic BP rises. Physical factors like stretch and flow velocity (shear stress) causes EDRF to be released, and platelets are able to cause release of EDRF. Thus, an intact endothelium prevents the constriction caused by platelets and the factors (such as serotonin) that they release, while the absence of endothelium favors vasoconstriction in the presence of platelets. EDRF also inhibits platelet aggregation and adhesion to the vessels.

EDRF dilates the smooth muscle cells by causing them to raise their level of cyclic GMP (cGMP), which through an unknown mechanism then causes smooth muscle cell relaxation. It is now thought that nitric oxide (NO) is EDRF, because it is able to reproduce the effects of EDRF and is inhibited by the same agents that inhibit EDRF. L-Arginine appears to be the source of NO in the endothelial cell.[23]

### Endothelium-Derived Contracting Factor and Endothelin

Endothelial cells also may produce a constricting factor or factors in response to stretch—endothelium-derived contracting factor (EDCF)—which seems to involve a prostanoid, and some endothelia produce a 21–amino acid peptide vasoconstrictor called *endothelin*. The roles of EDCF and endothelin are even less well-characterized than that of EDRF.

### Atrial Natriuretic Factor

Atrial natriuretic factor or atrial natriuretic peptide (ANF or ANP) is released from the atrium in response to stretch and *in vitro* is a vasodilator peptide in large doses. In humans its major physiologic role appears to be to elevate renal blood flow and stimulate greater fluid reabsorption by the kidney tubules. ANF does not appear to be important in the regulation of limb blood flow in humans.

### Local Metabolic and Thermal Influences

During muscle exercise local pH falls and local metabolites increase, directly dilating the arterioles. Microcirculatory studies have shown that the smallest arterioles, those which regulate the level of capillary perfusion, are the most sensitive to pH.[24]

The microvessels as well as some of the large superficial veins have an enhanced response to NE at temperatures lower than 37°C, and these same vessels have many adrenergic receptors of the $\alpha_2$-AR subtype. The response of the $\alpha_2$-AR pathway is inversely related to temperature, so cooling enhances the vasoconstriction due to NE or epi. This is not true of the $\alpha_1$-AR pathway, whose response is directly related to temperature. The inverse thermal response of the $\alpha_2$-AR pathway may be an important local mechanism that helps adjust blood flow to the appropriate level. During exercise, the constrictor effect of sympathetically released NE would be diminished in the terminal arterioles of muscle, as elevated temperature along with local metabolite accumulation and low pH would dilate arterioles, helping to increase muscle perfusion. The cutaneous vessels with many $\alpha_2$-ARs would have an enhanced response in the cold to the sympathetically released NE, further reducing skin blood flow and, consequently, heat lost from the body.

## Systemic Elements of Circulatory Control

### Blood Pressure Regulation

#### The Baroreflex System

Systemic BP is regulated within limits by a very effective negative feedback baroreflex system that monitors pressure in the great vessels and attempts to minimize change by adjusting cardiac output and vascular resistance via the autonomic nervous system. The role of the arterial, or high-pressure, baroreceptors in the baroreflex system was first investigated in 1836,[25] and nearly 100 years later, Cramer[26] showed that there are also baroreceptors in the great veins, atrium, and pulmonary vessels. Both sets of baroreceptors respond to stretch with an increase in firing rate, which increases their tonic inhibition of the medullary sympathetic outflow and their excitation of vagal outflow.

The high- and low-pressure baroreceptors appear to have distinct roles in the regulation of BP. The high-pressure baroreceptor nerves, located in the carotid sinus and the aortic arch, enter the medulla oblongata via the cranial nerves IX and X (see Figure 4-1) and mediate the very rapid responses to fluctuations of systemic arterial pressure. When systemic pressure rises by a few millimeters of mercury there is increased stretch in the walls of the aortic arch and carotid body, which cause the baroreceptor nerves to increase their firing rate. Because these nerves have an inhibitory effect on the medullary sympathetic center, the result of increased arterial pressure is decreased sympathetic outflow to the blood vessels and the heart, causing a decrease in peripheral resistance and cardiac output and a lowering of systemic arterial pressure.

The low-pressure, cardiopulmonary baroreceptors located in the atrial and ventricular walls and in the lung also increase their rate of firing as pressure increases. These nerves also inhibit the medullary sympathetic center, but their pattern of activity during stretch and relaxation is very different from that of the arterial baroreceptors. These receptors do not sense the beat-to-beat variation in systemic arterial pressure and do not respond as rapidly as the high-pressure baroreceptors to pressure change. It seems their role is not rapid correction of BP but rather long-term regulation. They also are important in mediating the adjustments to orthostatic stress via vasoconstriction of some vascular beds.

The difference between the two pressure-sensing pathways has been revealed by studies that eliminate just one or both. When the high-pressure baroreceptor nerves are cut, systemic pressure initially rises but then returns to the same average value, exhibiting wide fluctuations about that value. When the low-pressure baroreceptors are also denervated the average BP increases.[27,28] This indicates that the low-pressure sensors are necessary for maintaining the absolute level of average BP pressure. The high-pressure baroreceptor pathway operates not around an absolute pressure set-point, but rather around a set-point established by some other system, perhaps the cardiopulmonary receptor pathway. The arterial baroreceptor set-point appears to be changed in conditions such as some forms of hypertension in which the regulated pressure is much higher than normal or during exercise, when the regulated pressure is temporarily increased.

### The Chemosensors

The arterial chemosensors located in the carotid and aortic bodies serve as sensory elements for both cardiovascular and pulmonary feedback control. They increase their firing rate when $Po_2$ and pH fall and when $Pco_2$ rises. Stimulation of these receptors during hypoxia may result in increased CO, heart rate, vasoconstriction, venoconstriction, as well as increased ventilation. In contrast to the baroreflex system, however, the chemoreceptor influence on blood flow is not entirely clear and may be far less important under normoxic conditions than during hypoxemia.[29]

### Thermoregulation

The circulation probably first evolved to transport gases and important biologic molecules and cells, but in birds and mammals it is also important for the regulation of heat dissipation. Until recently, the mechanisms by which the blood transports heat were poorly understood. For many years it was thought that heat entered and left the circulation much as oxygen does and that the primary exchange site was the capillaries.[30] It is now clear that heat, being much more diffusible than oxygen, is not carried by vessels as small as capillaries, because their rate of flow is slower than the diffusion of heat through the tissue. Recent experimental and theoretical studies have shown that most heat enters and leaves the circulation in vessels that are 40 $\mu$m or larger.[31,32] This means that by the time arterial blood from the warm core reaches small arterioles in a limb it is thermally equilibrated with the surrounding tissue and no longer carries any heat. Blood velocity is so fast in the large arteries and veins (those larger than 1 mm) that very little heat is lost or gained from them, so they function mainly as conduit vessels, just as they do for oxygen.

Later, the precise way in which the circulatory patterns are altered to facilitate heat loss will be discussed. It is sufficient for now to point out that blood flow to the skin may be very high, as much as 8 L/min, and only a very small fraction of that flow serves a nutritive function. The large capacity for blood flow to the skin is entirely for the purpose of regulating body temperature by increasing heat dissipation at the surface.

## Distribution of the Limb Circulation

The four principal types of limb tissue that receive blood flow are skin, adipose tissue, muscle, and bone. Blood flow to the adipose tissue and bone is the least variable and least important for the systemic functions already mentioned.

### Bone

Bone blood flow serves both to sustain the bone cells and to facilitate ion exchange, particularly calcium.[33] The main vessels run in the cavity of the bone, and branches feed the marrow and the intricate system of channels in the bone. The difficulty of measuring bone blood flow noninvasively has limited the data available for humans, but radioactive microsphere measurements in dogs revealed that cortical and cancellous bone, respectively, received 2.5 and 38.3 ml per 100 ml of tissue per minute, or more than 9% of CO.[34]

### Adipose Tissue

The adipose tissue, which in the limb is mostly distributed subcutaneously, requires an adequate circulatory supply for gas exchange and nutritive exchange plus the transport of free fatty acids (FFAs) released from fat cells. The vessels in adipose tissue are innervated by sympathetic fibers, and they constrict when sympathetic nerves are stimulated. These vessels do not appear to participate in the systemic baroreflex or thermoregulation, but they do dilate during prolonged exercise, suggesting that they facilitate FFA delivery under such conditions.[35]

### Skin

#### Anatomy

The skin is organized into two layers, the epidermis, a layer of keratinized squamous epithelial cells, and the dermis, which contains the blood vessels as well as the glands of the skin, the nerves, and the hair follicles. A recent review of the skin circulation was written by Sparks.[36] Figure 14-7 shows the vascular organization. The main supply vessels to the skin are feeder arteries and veins that branch from the major vessels of the subcutaneous tissue. After they enter the dermal layer these vessels connect to the deep cutaneous plexus (SCP), a plexus of larger countercurrent arteries and veins. From this deep cutaneous plexus arise perpendicular riser vessels that feed the more superficial and much smaller arteriolar plexus (AP). Arterioles rising from this plexus feed the capillary loops near the upper layer of the dermis. After the blood passes through the capillary loops it enters the superficial venous plexus (VP), which has a very high capacity to pool blood and has been mistakenly assumed to be an important site of heat transfer from the blood that passes through the capillaries.[37] The capillary loops of the human nailfold can be visualized noninvasively,[38] and most of the information on human capillary function is derived from such studies.

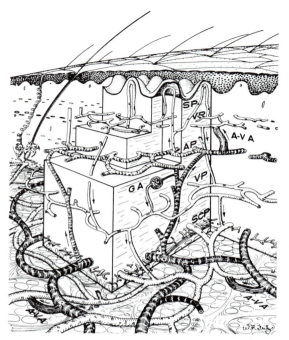

**Figure 14-7.** Arrangement of cutaneous blood vessels combining features normally characteristic of specific regions. Key: SP, subpapillary plexus layer; VP, venous plexus; AP, arteriolar plexus; SCP, cutaneous plexus; AVA, arteriovenous anastomosis; GA, arteriovenous glomus. (From Sparks HV. Skin and muscle. In: Johnson PC, ed. Peripheral Circulation. New York: John Wiley & Sons, 1978; 193–230, with permission.)

In some skin areas of the extermities a very special vascular element called the arteriovenous-anastomosis (AVAs) connects the rising precapillary arteriole to the venous plexus bypassing the capillaries. These highly muscular and richly innervated vessels provide an alternate route for blood from the arteriole to the venular side of the circulation. The greatest density of AVAs is in the tips of the digits, and there are very few in forearm skin.[39] When they are opened, as they are during heat stress, a much higher volume of blood can pass through the skin than would be possible if the blood had to pass through the capillary circulation. Even though the skin comprises only about 5% of the body volume, blood flow through the AVAs may be so great that the skin receives 50% of the CO. Blood that passes through the AVAs into the superficial venous plexus may transfer its heat in the later vessels, though no experiments have yet proven such a phenomenon.

## Nerve Supply

The control of the skin blood flow in the hand and foot is different from that of the forearm, upper arm, calf, and thigh, hereafter designated the proximal limb regions. In the hand and foot there is a high resting level of sympathetically maintained vascular tone, whereas in the proximal limb skin resting sympathetic tone is slight. Figure 14-8 compares the blood flow responses of the hand and the forearm to nerve block and deep body cooling and heating. Virtually all of the dilatation and constriction in the hand is due to decreases or increases in sympathetic constrictor nerve activity, but the forearm skin vessels contain both vasocon-

strictor and vasodilator nerves (see Figure 14-8). The active dilator nerves are important in heat-induced thermoregulatory vasodilatation of proximal limb skin, and these can be blocked by atropine, suggesting that they are cholinergic nerves. When sweating begins there is a further increase in blood flow, which is due mostly to the local release with the sweat of vasoactive substances such as bradykinin.

The proximal limb vasodilator nerves do not seem to play a role in the baroreflex, but the vasoconstrictor nerves to the extremities and proximal limb do.

## Muscle

The skeletal muscle of the limbs accounts for 40% of the total body mass, and can receive a large percentage of the cardiac output during exercise. The blood vessels in skeletal muscle of the limbs have a large range of tone, and the basal flow rate of 2 to 5 ml per 100 ml per minute can increase to 240 ml per 100 ml per minute during heavy exercise. The large increase from the basal level is possible partially because the capillaries are not all perfused at rest[40] and are recruited as the intensity of work increases the demand for oxygen.

### Anatomy

Figure 14-9 shows the microvasculature (vessels smaller than 60 to 80 $\mu$m in diameter) of the cat tenuisimus and biceps femoris muscles.[41] The arteries and veins travel through the tissue as countercurrent pairs from the main limb vessels until the final branching of the terminal arterioles that feed the capillaries. The secondary vessels run parallel to the muscle fibers, like the capillaries. Terminal vessels, which are perpendicular to the muscle fibers, connect the capillaries to the secondary vessels. Myrhage and Erikkson have suggested that the arrangement of these vessels forms a fundamental vascular unit in skeletal muscle, shown in Figure 14-9 as a cylinder.

### Nerve Supply

The muscle vessels contain sympathetic vasoconstrictor nerves, and possibly sympathetic vasodilator nerves, the latter being difficult to demon-

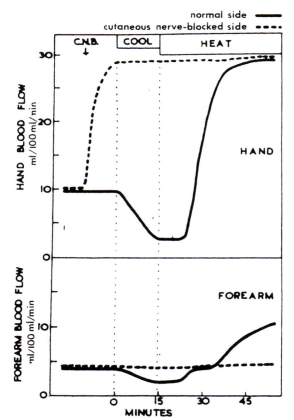

**Figure 14-8.** Schematic representation of changes in blood flow in normal and nerve-blocked hand and forearm during body cooling and heating. At cutaneous nerve block, on one side vasomotor nerves to the hand and forearm skin were blocked with local anesthetic solution. (From Roddie I.C. Circulation to skin and adipose tissue. In: Shepherd JT, Abboud FM, eds. Handbook of Physiology, sec 2, vol 3, pt 1. Bethesda, Md: American Physiological Society, 1983: 285–318, with permission.)

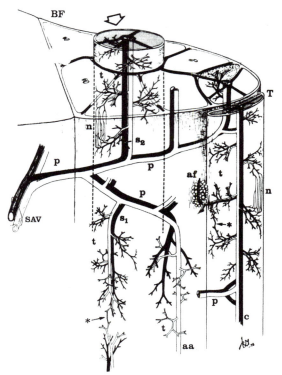

**Figure 14-9.** The vascular arrangement in the thin cat tenuissimus muscle (T) and in the thicker biceps femoris muscle (BF). The terminal arterioles and venules (t) branch in a two-dimensional pattern in the thin muscle and three-dimensionally, within a cylinder ("basic unit", *large arrow*) of muscle fibers, in the thick muscle. Key: SAV, supplying artery and vein; p, primary vessel; $s_1$ and $s_2$, secondary vessels; c, central vessel; n, capillary network; aa, arterial anastomosis connecting ends of primary arteries; af, fascia containing adipose tissue adjacent to the tenuissimus muscle; *, arterial anastomosis. (From Myrhage R, Eriksson E. Arrangement of the vascular bed in different types of skeletal muscles. In: Hammersen F, Meissner K, ed. Skeletal Muscle Microcirculation. Cambridge University Press.)

strate directly. The $\alpha$-ARs on the smooth muscle are innervated but the $\beta_2$-ARs are not, suggesting that they respond mostly to circulating epinephrine released from the adrenals. When the sympathetic nerves to muscles are cut there is a two- to three-fold increase in blood flow, indicating that, in comparison to the skin, there is less sympathetically mediated resting tone. The increase in flow (up to 100-fold) is due, not to sympathetic withdrawal, but rather to active vasodilatation of the muscle vascular bed by neuronal, hormonal, or local mechanisms.

## Functional Regulation of Blood Flow

Now that the fundamental cellular and systemic elements of blood flow regulation have been discussed it is possible to consider how these work in commonly encountered situations of postural change, exercise, thermal stress, and psychological stress.

### *Orthostatic Adjustment*

The basic cardiovascular challenge is to maintain adequate perfusion to the organs of the body. The brain is the preeminent organ with regard to perfusion, and given its inability to function without a constant supply of oxygenated blood and its position above heart level in many vertebrates, rapid adjustments must be made to maintain adequate perfusion pressure during postural change.

Figure 14-10 summarizes the cardiovascular events during movement from prone to upright posture. The normal sequence is as follows: (1) pooling of blood in the organs below heart level due to gravity, (2) reduction of central venous return and a fall in central venous pressure (panel 5, central blood volume), (3) reduction of cardiac filling because of reduced venous return to the right heart (panel 2, right atrial pressure falls; panel 4, stroke volume declines), and consequent fall in CO via the Frank-Starling mechanism (panel 3, CO), (4) sensing of the fall in central venous pressure or right atrial pressure by the low-pressure, cardiopulmonary baroreceptors, which reduce their firing rate and thereby (a) disinhibit the medullary sympathetic centers, causing sympathetic activity to increase with ensuing peripheral vasoconstriction (panels 7 and 8, decreases in forearm, splanchnic, and renal blood flow) and (b) reduce input to the vagal nucleus decreasing vagal outflow and thus allowing heart rate to increase (panel 6, heart rate), (5) reduction of arterial systolic BP because of the reduced CO (panel 1, arterial pressure), and (6) sensing of the fall of systolic BP by the carotid body an aortic arch baroreceptors, which also reduce their rate of firing and disinhibit the sympathetic centers and stimulate the vagal centers of the medulla.

As the right side of Figure 14-10 shows, walking activates the venous pump or "second heart," which facilitates return of venous blood and of

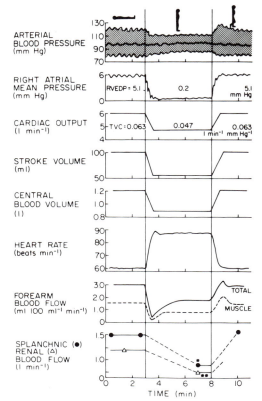

ARTERIAL BLOOD PRESSURE (mm Hg)

RIGHT ATRIAL MEAN PRESSURE (mm Hg)
RVEDP = 5.1    0.2    5.1 mm Hg

CARDIAC OUTPUT (l min⁻¹)
TVC = 0.063    0.047    0.063 l min⁻¹ mm Hg⁻¹

STROKE VOLUME (ml)

CENTRAL BLOOD VOLUME (l)

HEART RATE (beats min⁻¹)

FOREARM BLOOD FLOW (ml 100 ml⁻¹ min⁻¹)    TOTAL    MUSCLE

SPLANCHNIC (●) RENAL (△) BLOOD FLOW (l min⁻¹)

TIME (min)

**Figure 14-10.** Normal cardiovascular responses to upright posture (middle panel) and activation of muscle pumping by gently contracting leg muscles without movement (right panel). Numbers in panel 2 (right atrial pressure) show right ventricular end-diastolic pressure (RVEDP). Numbers in panel 3 (CO) show total vascular conductance (TVC). Time courses for changes in CO and derived variables and for splanchnic and renal flows are approximate. (From Rowell LB. Human Circulation. New York: Oxford University Press, 1986, with permission.)

central venous pressure to its supine value. As a result, all of the parameters return to their original supine values.

## Exercise

As with most of the previous discussion, it is not possible to discuss the limb circulation in isolation from circulation to other parts of the body or the functioning of the heart. This is particularly true in the case of exercise, when almost all of the increase in blood flow occurs in the muscles of the working limbs but at the expense of blood flow to other organs and increased work by the heart.

Exercise, therefore, is dealt with in a systemic fashion, as are circulatory adjustments to thermal stress in the following section. For detailed reviews of exercise physiology the reader is referred to references 42 through 45.

### Pattern of Cardiovascular Responses to Exercise

There is a very predictable cardiovascular response to exercise depending on the fitness of the person and the intensity of the exercise, as well as the state of hydration, ambient temperature, age, and disease.

**Cardiac Function.** Figure 14-11 shows the response of three classes of individuals of differing fitness to graded increases in oxygen uptake resulting from increasing workload. The three classes represent a range of work capacity as measured by their maximal oxygen uptake capacity, $Vo^2$ max, from very low for the patients with mitral stenosis (MS) to very high for "elite" endurance athletes (ATH). CO increases in a more or less linear fashion almost to the point that $Vo^2$ max is reached. The resting CO of around 6 L/min is similar in all three groups, but the maximum attainable value is much greater in the athletes, who can reach a CO greater than 40 L/min. Maximum heart rate is similar for all groups, but the most fit have a much lower resting rate, owing to both lower sympathetic activity and higher resting vagal tone. The initial increase in heart rate is thought to be produced primarily via withdrawal of vagal tone, whereas increases above 100 beats/min are the result of increased sympathetic activity to the heart.[46]

Interestingly, stroke volume does not change significantly as $Vo^2$ increases, partly because of the decreased filling time that results from the increase in heart rate. Stroke volume is much greater in fit persons, and for this reason athletes are able to maintain a given level of CO at a much lower heart rate than untrained persons. The reasons for the increased stroke volume in athletes are ill-understood, but it appears that their end-diastolic volume is increased[47] and ventricular dimensions are increased.[48] It has also been suggested that there is an increase in cardiac contractility with conditioning, but most reviewers do not support this hypothesis.[42,49,50]

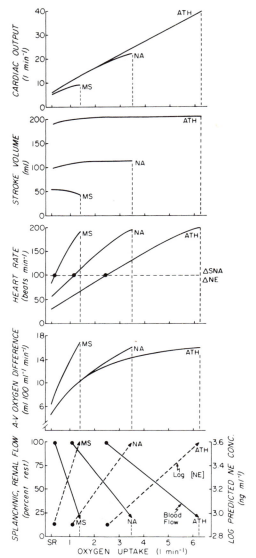

**Figure 14-11.** Representative cardiovascular responses to graded dynamic exercise in three groups of persons whose levels of $Vo_2$ max are very low (patients with "pure" mitral stenosis [MS]), normal (normally active subjects [NA], or very high (elite endurance athletes [ATH]). The dashed vertical line shows the $Vo_2$ max for each group. The horizontal dashed line in the third panel shows the heart rate where plasma NE ($\Delta$NE) and sympathetic nerve activity ($\Delta$SNA) increase. These solid circles are transferred to the splanchnic and renal blood flow and the NE-oxygen axes in the bottom panel. They show that in each group splanchnic and renal flows begin to fall when heart rate reaches 100 beats per minute, and that plasma NE concentration also begins to rise rapidly at this heart rate. (From Rowell LB. Human Circulation. New York: Oxford University Press, 1986, with permission.

**Sympathetic Nerve Activity.** The horizontal dashed line in the heart rate panel of Figure 14-11, which intersects the ordinate at 100 beats per minute, is to indicate that at this heart rate there is an increase in sympathetic nerve activity that serves both to increase heart rate and to increase vasoconstriction in nonexercising vascular beds such as the renal and splanchnic ones. The bottom panel of the figure shows the decrease in splanchnic and renal blood flow as a percentage change from control values. At the same time that vasoconstriction begins an increase in circulating NE is due to the overflow of sympathetically released NE into the circulation.

**Systemic Blood Pressure.** In the section on hemodynamics of blood flow it was pointed out that, if systemic BP is not to fall, increases in vascular conductance of a vascular bed must be matched either by a similar reduction in conductance of another bed, or by an increase in CO, or both. From this discussion it is clear that both of these mechanisms are used to maintain BP during exercise. The reduction in blood flow to renal, splanchnic, and other nonexercising beds contributes to the maintenance of systemic BP while the vascular conductance is increasing dramatically in the working muscles. These regional flow reductions alone are not sufficient, however, to maintain BP, and an increase in CO is essential. Actually, the increase in CO and vascular resistance in some vascular beds more than compensates for the decreased vascular resistance in the exercising muscle, and BP may actually rise.

The observed rise in BP with exercise suggests that there is resetting of the baroreceptor set-point during exercise. Rowell[42] recently reviewed the arguments for and against baroreflex resetting and concluded that unquestionably blood pressure is regulated as tightly during exercise as at rest and appears to be regulated at a higher level, but the sensitivity of the response to systemic pressure changes is unaltered.

*Increases in Muscle Perfusion and the Redistribution of Regional Blood Flow During Exercise*

As muscular contractions begin, the demand for oxygen and for metabolite removal increases rapidly, and there is a need for increased blood flow. Muscle has a remarkable ability to increase its blood flow[51] from the resting value of 3 to 5 ml per 100 ml per minute to greater than 240 ml per 100 ml per minute. Blood flow in exercising muscle of rats may exceed 340 ml per 100 ml per minute and it is not clear what the actual limit to vascular conductance in humans is. How is muscle blood flow increased by such a dramatically large amount? First, there is a large increase in the number of capillaries that are perfused. During rest, microcirculatory studies show that only a part of the available capillaries are perfused at any given time; the precapillary arterioles open and shut periodically.[40] The control of this microcirculatory behavior is not clear, but evidence points to local metabolic factors, including pH, $Po_2$, $Pco_2$, $K^+$, ATP, adenosine, osmolarity, and temperature.[17] These factors may cause the precapillary arterioles to dilate or constrict as their concentrations or levels wax and wane.[52] As exercise becomes intense and capillarity has reached its maximum, oxygen delivery may not be adequate to sustain aerobic metabolism. At such a point there is a constant maximal local vasodilatory stimulus at the precapillary arterioles and a strong systemic cardiovascular response, which results in both increased CO and redistribution of blood flow to exercising muscle and away from nonexercising tissues.

In humans there is vasoconstriction in the visceral organs and nonexercising muscle—and initially in the skin—to help meet increasing demand for blood flow in working muscle. While it is difficult to measure regional blood flow changes in humans, a study in baboons, where radiolabeled microspheres were used to quantify blood flow changes, revealed that all regions measured except the spinal cord had reduced blood flow (see Figure 14-12).[53] The largest decreases were in the skin, nonexercising muscle, adipose tissue, and the liver. To gain a better quantitative sense of how flow reductions in these beds increases the blood flow available to the exercising muscle Rowell[42] compared the blood flow distribution at rest and at maximal exercise in the same three groups of subjects shown in Figure 14-11. Figure 14-13 demonstrates that although blood flow reductions in renal, hepatic, gastrointestinal tract, and other organs are significant, they account for only a small part of the total increase in flow to the work-

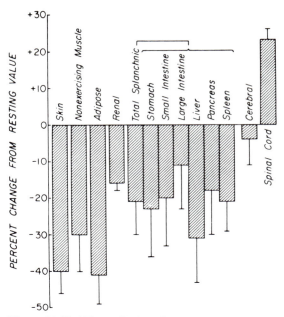

**Figure 14-12.** "Humanlike" redistribution of blood flow during mild dynamic exercise (cycling) in conscious baboons as measured by the distribution of radioactive microspheres. (From Rowell LB. Human Circulation. New York, Oxford University Press, 1986, with permission.)

ing muscle, and that the additional blood flow must come from an increase in CO.

Despite the relatively small contribution of flow redistribution to the increase in blood flow to exercising muscle, it is not negligible, particularly in the MS group, who have a limited ability to increase CO and where the redistributed flow represents about 30% to 40% of the total increase in flow to the exercising muscle. In the untrained normals and the athletes the redistribution of flow accounts for only 12% to 17% and 6% to 10% of the total increase in flow to exercising muscle.

### Increased Oxygen Extraction During Exercise

In addition to increased flow to exercising muscle, the muscles are better able to extract oxygen, increasing the arteriovenous oxygen gradient. The efficiency of oxygen extraction is expressed as the arterial-venous (A-V) oxygen difference. During rest the A-V oxygen difference of muscle is around 4.5 ml per 100 ml, or about 23% extraction (see the fourth panel of Figure 14-11). As $Vo_2$ max is approached, this value reaches 17 to 18 ml per

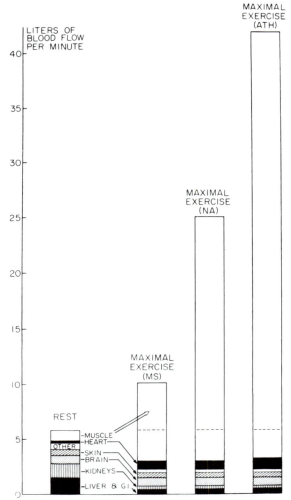

**Figure 14-13.** Total CO and its distribution during rest and brief exercise requiring $Vo_2$ max in three groups depicted in Figure 14-11. During exercise, blood flow to nonexercising regions, except the heart, was almost the same in all three groups. The higher coronary flow in athletes reflected the greater tissue mass; the volumetric blood flow should have been the same. (From Rowell LB. Human Circulation. New York: Oxford University Press, 1986, with permission.)

tion gradient from the capillary to the muscle is much greater. The geometry of the capillaries is also changed during muscle contraction, from a relatively straight tube when the muscle is relaxed to a highly curved, serpentine configuration that greatly increases the capillary-muscle fiber surface area ratio.[40]

The oxygen extraction of nonexercising tissue is also increased owing to the decreased flow velocity through them. At rest, when flow is faster, these tissues have a very low oxygen extraction efficiency, and during exercise they can extract the same amount of oxygen from much less blood because the blood transit time is increased.

*Effects of Chronic Exercise on Muscle Blood Flow*

Figure 14-11 shows the physiologic result of long-term training. The maximum heart rate is not increased, but stroke volume is, and consequently, CO is much improved. In the limbs, the principal change in the vascular system is the increase in muscle capillarity. This increase is not the dynamic increase seen in all individuals as muscle work begins, but rather is an increase in the maximum number of capillaries available for exchange. One study[54] found that sedentary persons had 329 capillaries per square millimeter and that after 8 weeks of training they had 395 per square millimeter. In the same study, the number of capillaries per muscle fiber increased from 1.36 to 2.00.

*Competition for Blood Flow Between Thermoregulation and Muscle Metabolism*

In the next section the limb vascular responses to heat stress are discussed in detail; for now it is sufficient to say that blood flow to the skin is a critical mechanism by which mammals lose the excess heat they continually produce. Even in a cool environment prolonged muscle exercise generates a great deal of excess heat, which must be lost to the environment if overheating is not to occur. As we have seen above, exercising muscle increases its blood flow as much as 100-fold and can create a demand for blood flow that exceeds the maximum CO of the heart. At the same time, the skin, which is at first vasoconstricted during

100 ml, or about 85% extraction. The greater extraction of oxygen from the blood is due to several factors. First, the perfusion of more capillaries both shortens the average oxygen diffusion distance and increases the diffusion area from the capillary to the muscle fiber.[52] Transit time of the blood through the capillary may also increase somewhat, and, of course, the oxygen concentra-

exercise, must soon begin to dilate to allow the blood to carry heat to the surface, where it can be lost. Thus, the competing drives for thermoregulation, BP maintenance, and maintenance of muscle metabolism, which together exceed CO, must somehow be reconciled.

When the skin begins to dilate after prolonged exercise in a cool environment, blood pools in the cutaneous veins, and this ultimately reduces central venous volume, cardiac filling pressure, and stroke volume. This is a gradual change that has been called *cardiovascular drift*. To compensate for the drop in stroke volume and to maintain cardiac output, heart rate increases.[55] After a time of exercise, especially in the heat, the renal, hepatic, and splanchnic beds are further constricted, and the cutaneous blood flow is reduced. Thus, body temperature is allowed to rise so the working muscle can continue to be perfused. In the hierarchy of systems, maintenance of muscle flow and systemic pressure are more important than maintenance of a constant body temperature.

### Heat and Cold Stress

In endotherms the vascular system facilitates the necessary removal of the large excess of centrally produced heat in neutral and warm environmental conditions. In this section the precise nature of the circulatory responses to heat and cold are discussed; a complete discussion of thermoregulation can be found in Chapter 13.

In thermoneutral conditions (26° to 28°C for nude humans), the only active thermoregulatory mechanism is regulation of skin blood flow and thermoneutrality is called the *zone of maximum vasomotor instability*. Waxing and waning of skin blood flow in the extremities provides the minute-to-minute variation in heat loss and conservation in the thermoneutral state, where metabolic heat production is least. In such a state about 70% of body heat is produced in the viscera, heart, and brain, centrally located areas, and it must somehow escape to the surface. The importance of circulation in transferring this heat to the surface is illustrated in Figure 14-14, where a simulation of the human thermal balance is shown for a situation in which no heat transfer by the blood is allowed. The simulation shows that if the heat produced in these central areas could escape only by molecular diffusion through the tissues, the body core temperature ($T_b$) would not reach steady state until it about 80°C. A lethal temperature would be reached in only 3 hours.

### Centrally Mediated Response to Skin or Body Cooling

When the skin is cooled there is rapid vasoconstriction that is partly central in origin. Cutaneous thermal sensors relay information to the spinal cord and hypothalamus, where all thermosensory information is integrated, and an increase in sympathetic drive to the cutaneous vessels causes the vasoconstriction. This initial response is transient,

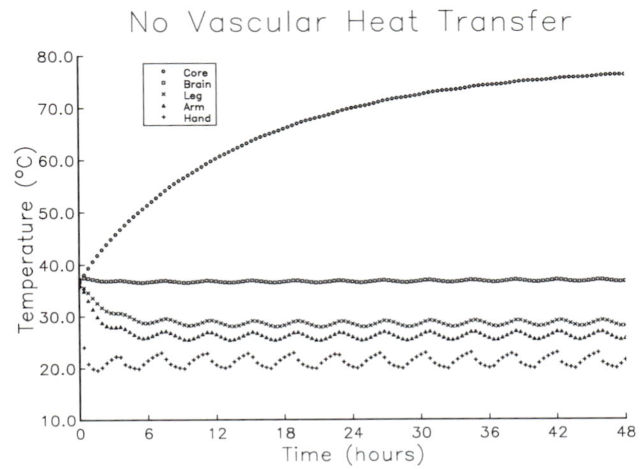

**Figure 14-14.** Simulation of human body temperature change at rest in a thermoneutral environment. The model assumed that the circulation functioned normally except that it did not carry any heat. It also assumed that metabolic heat production was constant. The core body temperature (open circles) rose slowly, reaching a lethal temperature of 42°C after about 3 hours. It did not reach a steady-state temperature until 48 hours. Leg, arm, and hand temperatures fell because their resting heat production is low and their heat loss is high. Under normal conditions their temperatures are maintained because they receive warm blood from the body core.

and BF returns to resting values unless the recirculating blood from the limb produces some central body cooling that activates a more persistent thermoregulatory response. During intense cutaneous vasoconstriction the minimally perfused skin, along with the underlying subcutaneous fat, provides a layer of insulation, and the temperature gradient from the skin surface into the muscle becomes almost linear,[56] yielding the least possible heat transfer from the body.

*Local Vascular Response to Cooling*

Temperature also has a direct effect on the vascular smooth muscle and the sympathetic nerves. Falling temperature directly enhances the response of the $\alpha_2$-AR pathway, and in the skin veins and terminal muscle arterioles, where there are many $\alpha_2$-ARs, moderate local cooling causes further constriction when some sympathetic tone is present.[57–59]

**Cold-Induced Vasodilatation, CIVD.** Long ago, Sir Thomas Lewis observed a curious response to low temperature in the blood flow to human fingers (Figure 14-15).[60] He found that when the hand is immersed in ice water there is an initial intense vasoconstriction that reduces blood flow to a minimum. After 30 to 40 minutes of continued immersion, blood flow increases, raising the finger temperature, and then decreases again. This oscillating blood flow to the finger continues with a frequency of one cycle of constriction and dilatation every 30 to 40 minutes or less. This *Lewis* or *hunting reaction* is thought to be a tissue-protective feature of hand blood flow, which minimizes the loss of body heat to the cold water by vasoconstricting and allowing the hand to become very cold and then periodically warms the hand to prevent freezing and tissue damage. Such an explanation is appealing, and it may or may not be correct, but the mechanism behind this phenomenon is now understood.

During the initial rapid cooling of the hand, the central and local response is to constrict the blood vessels via increased sympathetic outflow and a cooling-induced increase in $\alpha_2$-AR responsiveness, respectively. This much reduces blood flow and so reduces heat transfer to the hand from the central body, causing hand temperature to fall quickly. After 10 to 20 minutes, the hand temperature becomes so low that sympathetic neurotransmission and the $\alpha$-AR receptor pathway are blocked,[61] and NE concentration eventually falls owing to the circulation and to reuptake and me-

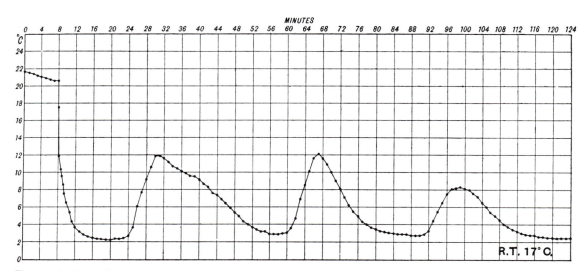

**Figure 14-15.** Cold-induced vasodilatation (CIVID). Skin temperature of the index finger cooled in crushed ice. The periodic increases in skin temperature were also called the *hunting* or the *Lewis reaction*. (From Lewis T. Observations upon the reactions of the vessels of human skin to cold. Heart *Clinical Science.* 1930; 15: 177–208, with permission.)

tabolism. The smooth muscle–contractile mechanisms are probably partially paralyzed also. The vessels then begin to relax and receive warm blood from the central body, and they and the surrounding tissue, including the sympathetic nerves are rewarmed. When the sympathetic nerves have warmed sufficiently, they begin to release NE again, which causes renewed vasoconstriction. This cycle is repeated until cooling of the hand ceases. Animal experiments[62] have confirmed that this is the mechanism by which CIVD occurs.

### Centrally Mediated Vascular Response to Heat

When humans enter a hot environment, thermal sensors in the skin relay the information to the hypothalamus and spinal cord, and the first response is the dilatation of cutaneous vessels. If exposure to heat is prolonged and the heat intense enough to increase $T_b$, then skin blood flow eventually reaches its maximum level of 7 to 8 L/min. Sweating much increases the ability of the skin to dissipate heat, and without it the large blood flow to the skin would be insufficient for effective body cooling. The increase in skin blood flow is achieved through both redistribution of blood flow away from splanchnic regions and muscle and increased CO.[42]

During whole-body heating in humans forearm blood flow immediately begins to rise, followed by an increase in blood flow to the feet and legs.[37] This increased blood flow is largely in the skin, because even though much of the muscle mass is near the surface, there is no evidence that its blood flow increases during heat stress. About the time forearm blood flow begins to increase, sweating also begins. With a sustained rise in $T_b$ there is a persistent increase in forearm blood flow, and to support such a large flow increase, CO increases by 6 to 7 L/min. A simultaneous decrease in splanchnic, renal, and muscle blood flow, contributes about 1 L/min more to skin blood flow and allows an increase in skin blood flow of 7 to 8 L/min. The increased vascular resistance of the splanchnic, renal, and muscle beds and the increased CO together do not completely compensate for the large increase in vascular conductance of the skin, so arterial pressure falls for the first 30 to 40 minutes of heat exposure, after which it slowly returns to normal. Increased pooling of blood in the cutaneous veins cause right arterial mean pressure to fall slowly throughout the period of heat exposure, until it approaches 0.5 mmHg. Stroke volume increases, as does heart rate, in order to raise CO.

The vasoconstriction in viscera and muscle, and the increase in CO are sympathetically mediated but are not initiated by the baroreflex system. The response seems to be driven solely by the thermoregulatory centers, as raising arterial pressure back to normal by elevating and then occluding the legs does not reduce either the vasoconstriction or the heart rate response.

**Local Vascular Responses to Heating.**   Directly applied heat dilates cutaneous vessels that have some vasoconstrictor tone, and this has often been interpreted as an important local mechanism of thermoregulation and heat loss. Cutaneous veins contract less well to applied NE when they have been warmed to 39°C from 34°C, and if they have been partially constricted with NE they dilate when warmed.[63] Heating reduces the $\alpha_2$-AR response to NE, and in vessels such as terminal arterioles and cutaneous veins, where such receptors may predominate, heat has a major effect on blood flow. The effect of heat on other receptor-mediated constrictor and dilator pathways is not known.

Heating with diathermy, ultrasound, or hotpacks is a common practice in physical medicine and rehabilitation, and one of the therapeutic goals of these treatments is to increase blood flow (see reference 64 for an extensive review of the use of therapeutic heat). In animals, where intense local heating of muscle is possible, there is a critical temperature between 41° and 44°C beyond which pronounced vasodilatation may occur. The physiologic basis of this dilatation is not known. One study showed that temperature oscillation of the heated dog thigh occurred after 30 to 40 minutes, with a pattern similar to CIVD.[65] The temperature oscillations appeared to be due to the primary effect of heat on the vessels, which caused them to dilate, followed by the cooling effect of the increased blood flow, which caused them to return somewhat to their original diameters. If heating was intense enough there was sometimes a long-lasting temperature oscillation.

Heating does not always cause vessels to dilate, and one study demonstrated that moderate heating constricts the small arterioles of skeletal muscle.[66] A recent study in humans[67] found that ultrasound applied to the calf at the maximal allowed clinical dose of 3 w/cm$^2$ slightly increased vascular resistance. It is quite likely that heating of soft tissues to less than the critical temperature for vasodilatation either has no effect on blood flow or diminishes it slightly. However, increasing temperature, like decreasing temperature, has a complex effect on limb blood flow that depends on the intensity and duration of the heating.

### Psychological Stress

Subjects exposed to psychological stress have increased blood flow to forearm skeletal muscle via a cortical pathway mediated by sympathetic cholinergic nerves.[68] Neither the skin nor the calf muscles appear to respond to stress with vasodilatation.[10] Severe stress does not have much effect on the cutaneous vessels. Mild stress such as a taxing intellectual task or unexpected loud noise cause transient vasoconstriction of the skin vessels via the sympathetic nerves. Such stimuli are used to test the integrity of the autonomic nervous system and the cutaneous vascular sympathetic responses.

### Diving

The diving reflex is present in many species and, from an evolutionary viewpoint, is retained in humans. The response includes parasympathetically mediated bradycardia and sympathetic vasoconstriction of some vascular beds, including renal, splanchnic, and muscular. Water or cold on the face, which is sensed by trigeminal afferents, initiate the response. In diving mammals and birds, where diving is an important part of day to day survival, the diving reflex is similar to that in humans, but it may be more dramatic, producing nearly complete cessation of blood flow to muscle.[69] Diving bradycardia is a useful test of vagal integrity, and it is less pronounced or absent in patients with some degree of parasympathetic failure.

## References

1. Gibbons IL. Morphological evidence for regional diversification of autonomic cotransmission in different parts of the cardiovascular system. Proc XVII IUPS Cong 1989; 1:28.
2. Kobilka BK, Matsui J, Kobilka TS, et al. Cloning, sequencing, and expression of the gene coding for the human platelet alpha$_2$-adrenergic receptor. Science 1987; 238:650–656.
3. Levitzki A. Beta-adrenergic receptors and their mode of coupling to adenylate cyclase. Physiol Rev 1986; 66:819–854.
4. Weiss ER, Kelleher DJ, Woon CW, et al. Receptor activation of G proteins. FASEB J 1988; 2:2841–2848.
5. Robishaw JD, Foster KA. Role of G proteins in the regulation of the cardiovascular system. Ann Rev Physiol 1989; 51:229–244.
6. Limbird LE. Receptors linked to inhibition of adenylate cyclase: Additional signaling mechanisms. FASEB J 1988; 2:2686–2695.
7. Fain JN, Wallace MA, Wojcikiewicz RJH. Evidence for involvement of gunine nucleotide-binding regulatory proteins in the activation of phospholipases by hormones. FASEB J 1989; 2:2569–2574.
8. Kamm KE, Stull JT. Regulation of smooth muscle contractile elements by second messengers. Ann Rev Physiol 1989; 51:299–313.
9. Abrahams VC, Hilton SM, Zbrozyna AW. The role of active muscle vasodilation in the altering stage of the defense reaction. J Physiol (Lond) 1964; 171:189–202.
10. Rusch NJ, Shepherd JT, Webb RC, et al. Different behavior of the resistance vessels of the human calf and forearm during contralateral isometric exercise, mental stress and abdominal respiratory movements. Circ Res 1981; 48(pt 2):I118–I130.
11. Lechleiter J, Peralta D, Clapham D. Diverse functions of muscarinic acetylcholine receptor subtypes. Trends Pharmacol Sci 1989; (suppl):34–38.
12. Dohlman HG, Caron MG, Lefkowitz RJ. A family of receptors coupled to guanine nucleotide regulatory proteins. Biochemistry 1987; 26:2657–2664.
13. Kennedy C. Possible roles for purine nucleotides in perivascular neurotransmission. In: Burnstock G, Griffith SG, eds. Nonadrenergic Innervation of Blood Vessels, vol I, Putative Neurotransmitters. Boca Raton, Fla: CRC Press, 1988; 65–76.
14. Burnstock G. Sympathetic purinergic transmission in small blood vessels. Trends Pharmacol Sci 1989; 9:116–117.
15. Romano F, MacDonald SG, Dobson JG Jr. Adenosine receptor coupling to adenylate cyclase on rat

ventricular myocyte membranes. Am J Physiol 1989; 257:H1088–H1095.

16. Howland RD, Spector S. Disposition of histamine in mammalian blood vessels. J Pharm Exp Ther 1972; 182:239–245.

17. Shepherd JT. Circulation to skeletal muscle. In: Shepherd JT, Abboud FM, eds. Handbook of Physiology, sect 2, The Cardiovascular System, vol III, Peripheral Circulation and Organ Blood Flow, part 1. Bethesda, Md: American Physiological Society, 1983; 319–370.

18. Hartig PR. Molecular biology of 5-HT receptors. Trends Pharmacol Sci 1989; 10:64–69.

19. Angus JA. 5-HT receptors in the coronary circulation. Trends Pharmacol Sci 1989; 10:89–90.

20. Griffith SG. Serotonin (5-HT) as a neurotransmitter in blood vessels. In: Burnstock G, Griffith SG, eds. Nonadrenergic Innervation of Blood Vessels, vol. I, Putative Neurotransmitters. Boca Raton, Fla: CRC Press, 1988;27–40.

21. Cowley AW JR. Vasopressin and cardiovascular regulation. In: Guyton AC, Hall JE, eds. Cardiovascular Physiology IV. International Review of Physiology vol 26. Baltimore: University Park Press, 1982;189–242.

22. Furchgott RF, and Vanhoutte PM, Endothelium-derived relaxing and contracting factors. FASEB J 1989; 3:2007–2018.

23. Moncada S. Biosynthesis of nitric oxide from L-arginine: A path for the regulation of cell function and communication. Biochem Pharmacol 1989; 38:1709–1715.

24. McGillivray KM, Faber JM. Selective effect of metabolic control on $\alpha_2$-adrenergic mediated contraction of microvascular smooth muscle. FASEB J 1988; 2:A1873.

25. Cooper A. Some experiments and observations on tying the carotid and vertebral arteries, and the pneumogastric phrenic and sympathetic nerves. Guy's Hosp Rep 1836; 1:457–472.

26. Cramer W. On the action of veratrum viride with some remarks on the interrelationship of the medullary centres. J Pharmacol 1915; 7:63–82.

27. Persson PB, Ehmke H, Kirchheim H. Cardiopulmonary-arterial baroreceptor interaction in control of blood pressure. News Physiol Sci 1989; 4:56–59.

28. Persson PB. Cardiopulmonary receptors in "neurogenic hypertension." Acta Physiol Scand 1988; 570 (suppl):1–54.

29. Eyzaguirre C, Fitzgerald RS, Lahiri S, et al. Arterial chemoreceptors. In: Shepherd JT, Abboud FM, Geiger SR, eds. Handbook of Physiology, sect 2, The Cardiovascular System, vol III Peripheral Circulation and Organ Blood Flow, part 2. Be-

thesda, Md: American Physiological Society, 1983; 557–622.

30. Pennes HH. Analysis of tissue and arterial blood temperatures in the resting human forearm. J Appl Physiol 1948; 1:93–122.

31. Lemons DE, Chien S, Crawshaw LI, et al. The significance of vessel size and type in vascular heat transfer. Am J Physiol 1987; 253:R128–R135.

32. Weinbaum S, Jiji LM, Lemons DE. Theory and experiment for the effect of vascular microstructure on surface tissue heat transfer—part I: Anatomical foundation and model conceptualization. ASME J Biomech Eng 1984; 106:321–330.

33. Kelley PJ. Pathways of transport in bone. In: Shepherd JT, Abboud FM, eds. Handbook of Physiology, sect 2, The Cardiovascular System, vol III, Peripheral Circulation and Organ Flow, part 1. Bethesda, MD: American Physiological Society, 1983;371–396.

34. Morris MA, Kelly PJ. Use of tracer microspheres to measure blood flow in conscious dogs. Calicif Tissue Int 1980; 32:69–76.

35. Bulow J, Madsen J. Adipose tissue blood flow during prolonged heavy exercise. Pflugers Arch 1976; 363:231–234.

36. Sparks HV. Skin and muscle. In: Johnson PC, ed. Peripheral Circulation. New York: John Wiley & Sons, 1978; 193–230.

37. Roddie IC. Circulation to skin and adipose tissue. In: Shepherd JT, Abboud FM, eds. Handbook of Physiology, section 2, The Cardiovascular System, vol III, Peripheral Circulation and Organ Blood Flow, part 1. Bethesda, Md: American Physiological Society, 1983;285–318.

38. Fagrell B. Microcirculation of the skin. In: Mortillaro NA, ed. The Physiology and Pharmacology of the Microcirculation. New York: Academic Press, 1984;133–180.

39. Clark ER. Arteriovenous anastomoses. Physiol Rev 1938; 18:229–247.

40. Groom AC. Skeletal and cardiac microcirculation. In: Tsuchiya M, Asano M, Mishima Y, et al. Microcirculation: An Update, vol 1. Amsterdam: Elsevier, 1987;83–98.

41. Myrhage R, Eriksson E. Arrangement of the vascular bed in different types of skeletal muscles. In: Hammersen F, Messmer K, eds. Skeletal Muscle Microcirculation. Basel: S Karger, 1984;1–14.

42. Rowell LB. Human Circulation. New York: Oxford University Press, 1986.

43. Astrand P-O, Rodahl K. Textbook of Work Physiology. New York: McGraw-Hill,1977.

44. Marshall RJ, Shepherd JT. Cardiac Function in Health and Disease. Philadelphia: WB Saunders, 1968.

45. Wade OL, Bishop JM. Cardiac Output and Regional Blood Flow. Oxford: Blackwell, 1989.

46. Christensen NJ, Brandsborg O. The relationship between plasma catecholamine concentration and pulse rate during exercise and standing. Eur J Clin Invest 1973; 3:299–306.

47. Rerych SK, Scholz PM, Sabiston DC, et al. Effects of exercise training on left ventricular function in normal subjects: A longitudinal study by radionuclide angiography. Am J Cardiol 1980; 45:244–252.

48. Morganroth J, Maron BJ, Henry WL, et al. Comparative left ventricular dimensions in trained athletes. Ann Intern Med 1975; 82:521–524.

49. Sjostrand T. The regulation of the blood distribution in man. Acta Physiol Scand 1952; 26:312–327.

50. Blomqvist CG, Saltin B. Cardiovascular adaptations to physical training. Annu Rev Physiol 1983; 45:169–189.

51. Andersen P, Saltin B. Maximal perfusion of skeletal muscle in man. J Physiol (Lond) 1985; 366:233–249.

52. Granger HJ, Borders JL, Meininger GA, et al. Microcirculatory control systems. In: Mortillaro NA, ed. The Physiology and Pharmacology of the Microcirculation. New York: Academic Press, 1983;209–236.

53. Hohimer AR, Hales JR, Rowell LB, et al. Regional distribution of blood flow during mild dynamic leg exercise in the baboon. J Appl Physiol 1983; 55:1173–1177.

54. Andersen P, Henriksson J. Capillary supply of the quadriceps femoris muscle of man: Adaptive response to exercise. J Physiol (Lond) 1977; 270:677–691.

55. Ekelund L-G. Circulatory and respiratory adaptation during prolonged exercise. Acta Physiol Scand 1967; 292 (suppl):1–38.

56. Bazett HC. Temperature sense in man. In: Temperature: Its Measurement and Control in Science and Industry. New York: Reinhold, 1941;489–501.

57. Faber JE. Effect of local tissue cooling on microvascular smooth muscle and postjunctional $alpha_2$-adrenoceptors. Am J Physiol 1988; 255:H121–H130.

58. Flavahan NA, Vanhoutte PM. Effect of cooling on $alpha_1$- and $alpha_2$-adrenergic responses in canine saphenous and femoral veins. J Pharmacol Exp Ther 1986; 238:139–147.

59. Vanhoutte PM, Flavahan NA. Effects of temperature on alpha adrenoceptors in limb veins: Role of receptor reserve. Fed Proc 1986; 45:2347–2354.

60. Lewis T. Observations upon the reactions of the vessels of the human skin to cold. Heart 1930; 15:177–208.

61. Rusch NJ, Shepherd JT, Vanhoutte PM. The effect of profound cooling on adrenergic neurotransmission in canine cutaneous veins. J Physiol (Lond) 1981; 311:57–65.

62. Gardner CA, Webb RC. Cold-induced vasodilation in isolated, perfused rat tail artery. Am J Physiol 1986; 251:H176–H181.

63. Cooke JP, Shepherd JT, Vanhoutte PM. The effect of warming on adrenergic neurotransmission in canine cutaneous vein. Circ Res 1984; 54:547–553.

64. Lehmann JF, DeLateur BJ. Therapeutic heat. In: Lehmann JF, ed. Therapeutic Heat and Cold. Baltimore: Williams & Wilkins, 1982; 404–562.

65. Roemer RB, Oleson JR, Cetas TC. Oscillatory temperature response to constant power applied to canine muscle. Am J Physiol 1985; 249:R153–R158.

66. Hogan RD, Franklin TD, Avery KS, et al. Arteriolar vasoconstriction in rat cremaster muscle induced by local heat stress. Am J Physiol 1982; 242:H996–H999.

67. Snortum AL. Blood Flow Responses to Ultrasound Dosage and Direct Surface Cooling as Measured by Venous Occlusion Plethysmography. M.S. Thesis. Columbia University, 1989.

68. Blair DA, Glover WE, Greenfield ADM, et al. Excitation of cholinergic vasodilator nerves to human skeletal muscles during emotional stress. J Physiol (Lond) 1959; 148:633–647.

69. Blix AS, Folkow B. Cardiovascular adjustments to diving in mammals and birds. In: Shepherd JT, Abboud FM, Geiger SR, eds. Handbook of Physiology, sect 2, The Cardiovascular System, vol III, Peripheral Circulation and Organ Blood Flow, part 2. Bethesda, Md: American Physiological Society, 1983;917–946.

70. Ashkenazi A, Peralta EG, Winslow JW, et al. Functional diversity of muscarinic receptor subtypes in cellular signal transduction and growth. Trends Pharmacol Sci 1989; (suppl):16–22.

71. Duckles SP, Acetylcholine. In: Burnstock G, Griffith SG, eds. Nonadrenergic Innervation of Blood Vessels, vol I, Putative Neurotransmitters. Boca Raton, Fla: CRC Press, 1988;15–26.

72. Carson MR, Shasby SS, Shasby MD. Histamine and inositol phosphate accumulation in endothelium: cAMP and G protein. Am J Physiol 1989; 257:L259–L264.

73. Tsuru H. Histamine receptors in the cardiovascular system. In: Vanhoutte PM, Vatner SF, eds. Vasodilator Mechanisms. New York: S Karger, 1983;70–80.

74. Burnstock G. Nonadrenergic innervation of blood vessels—some historical perspectives. In: Burnstock G, Griffith SG, eds. Nonadrenergic Innervation of Blood Vessels, vol I, Putative Neurotransmitters. Boca Raton, Fla: CRC Press, 1988;1–14.

75. Owman C. Role of neural substance P and coexisting calcitonin gene–related peptide (CGRP) in cardiovascular function. In: Burnstock G, Griffith SG, eds. Nonadrenergic Innervation of Blood Vessels, vol I, Putative Neurotransmitters. Boca Raton, Fla: CRC Press, 1988;77–100.

76. Polak JM, Bloom SR. Atrial natriuretic peptide (ANP), neuropeptide Y (NPY) and calcitonin gene–related peptide (CGRP) in the cardiovascular system of man and animals. In: Burnstock G, Griffith SG, eds. Nonadrenergic Innervation of Blood Vessels, Vol. I, Putative Neurotransmitters. Boca Raton, Fla: CRC Press, 1988;127–144.

77. Edvinsson L, Uddman R. Vasoactive intestinal polypeptide (VIP): A putative neurotransmitter in the cardiovascular system. In: Burnstock G, Griffith SG, eds. Nonadrenergic Innervation of Blood Vessels, vol I, Putative Neurotransmitters. Boca Raton, Fla: CRC Press, 1988;101–126.

# Chapter 15
# Exercise and Fatigue

JONATHAN R. MOLDOVER
JOANNE BORG-STEIN

Exercise is a cornerstone of rehabilitation medicine's therapeutic armamentarium, but as such it must be well conceived and highly specific. In prescribing exercise, both the specificity of training and the therapeutic goal must be considered. The rehabilitation medicine clinician must clearly understand the physiologic response to exercise, the biophysical properties of connective tissue, and the alterations and limitations imposed by the pathomechanics and pathophysiology of various disease states. In this chapter we review the biochemical and neuromusculoskeletal response to exercise, with emphasis on clinical applications.

Exercise may be defined as "activity that requires physical or mental exertion, especially when performed to develop or maintain fitness."[1] In rehabilitation medicine, exercise is prescribed to develop strength, endurance (stamina), coordination, range of motion, and flexibility, in order to restore and to enhance function.

The human body exhibits an elegant and predictable response to the various forms of exercise that will be reviewed, including the immediate physiologic responses to exercise and the longer-term adaptations to regular training that allow it to enhance its performance. These predictable physiologic changes are the rationale for many of our therapeutic programs.

## General Principles of Exercise

### Acute Response to Exercise

#### Energy Production

A limiting factor in exercise is energy production. At the cellular level, adenosine triphosphate (ATP), a high-energy phosphate compound, is the major source of available energy. Phosphocreatine (PC) in the muscle cell is another high-energy compound that is available in very limited quantities and serves to regenerate ATP in the following reaction that also involves adenosine diphosphate (ADP):

$$ATP + Creatine \leftrightarrow ADP + PC$$

Because the available PC is consumed in several seconds, ATP needs to regenerated in other ways during continued exercise. This can be done aerobically in the mitochondria, through the oxidation of glucose, glycogen, fatty acids, or amino acids. These enter as acetyl coenzyme A (aCoA) in the Krebs cycle and yield ATP in the electron transport chain (Figure 15-1). Alternatively, ATP may be regenerated anaerobically through the process of glycolysis, which occurs in the cytoplasm. During glycolysis, glucose (six carbons) is broken down

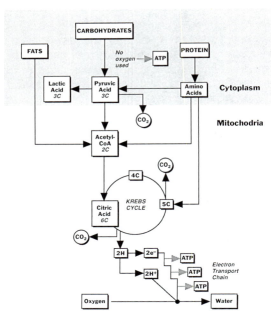

**Figure 15-1.** The production of ATP by means of anaerobic metabolism in the cytoplasm or aerobic metabolism in the mitochondria. (Adapted from Åstrand P-O, Rodahl K. Textbook of Work Physiology, ed 3. New York: McGraw-Hill, 1986.)

to pyruvate (three carbons) and ATP is generated. In the presence of an adequate supply of oxygen the resulting pyruvate may be converted to acetyl CoA (two carbons) and transported to the mitochondria, where it can continue through the Krebs cycle and electron transport chain. In the absence of sufficient oxygen, pyruvate is reduced to lactate. Lactate enters the venous blood and subsequently is reoxidized in the liver and muscle during the postexercise recovery period, when sufficient oxygen is present. The lactate level is a measure of anaerobic metabolism or oxygen debt.

There are three stages of energy production during exercise. During the first few seconds of heavy exercise, energy is obtained anaerobically from the already stored high-energy compounds PC and ATP. This is referred to as the *alactic phase*. As activity continues over the next 5 to 10 seconds, stored muscle glycogen and glucose are broken down anaerobically to lactate via glycolysis. This is the *anaerobic, or glycolytic, phase*. As oxygen becomes available through increased pulmonary ventilation and circulatory changes, ATP can be generated aerobically through the ox-

idation of glycogen, glucose, fat, and protein (Figure 15-2). This is the *aerobic phase*. During light exercise the aerobic supply may be sufficient to sustain activity, but if the exercise is strenuous the anaerobic contribution may continue and lactic acid accumulates. The major limiting factor to prolonged exercise is intolerance to the accumulation of lactate. During the recovery period, lactate is reoxidized, phosphocreatine and ATP are replenished, and, oxygen consumption gradually decreases.

## Cardiopulmonary Response

During exercise with large muscle groups, the cardiovascular system responds with an increase in heart rate and a rise in cardiac output. Simultaneously, blood flow is preferentially increased to the exercising muscles as a result of local vasodilatation and is shunted away from nonexercising regions such as the splanchnic and renal beds. The pulmonary minute ventilation increases with exercise, allowing increased oxygen uptake and clearance of carbon dioxide. Chapter 7 provides a detailed discussion of the cardiopulmonary response to exercise.

## Endocrine Response

Catecholamines are released into the circulation in increased quantities during exercise, stimulating

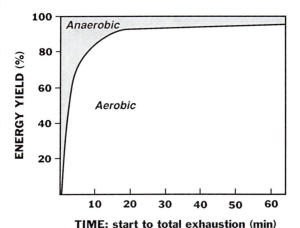

**Figure 15-2.** The temporal relationship of anaerobic and aerobic metabolism during exercise. (Adapted from Åstrand P-O, Rodahl K. Textbook of Work Physiology, ed 3. New York: McGraw-Hill, 1986.)

glycogenolysis and lipolysis, thus making available ble glucose and free fatty acids for use as energy sources. Growth hormone levels rise and insulin levels fall, further contributing to the increased availability of glucose. These mechanisms, as well as hepatic gluconeogenesis (synthesis of glucose in the liver), are counterbalanced by increased sensitivity to insulin and increased glucose utilization by muscle cells,[2] the net result being the maintenance of normal serum glucose concentrations.[3]

### Hematologic Response

During exercise there is an acute increase in fibrinolysis as well as an increase in platelets, but platelet function is unchanged.[4,5] During strenuous exercise circulatory blood volume decreases as a result of fluid shifts and losses from sweating, but the effect of regular physical exercise is to cause an increase in red cell mass and circulating plasma volume. A disproportionate increase in plasma volume can cause pseudoanemia in athletes.[6]

### Renal Response

During vigorous exercise, acute hemoconcentration occurs, owing to sweating, and decreases renal blood flow and the glomerular filtration rate. Urine output therefore decreases. Serum potassium concentration is transiently increased, owing to release from exercising muscle cells.[7]

### Psychological Effects

Perhaps the best-known acute psychological effect of aerobic exercise is an increase in the plasma level of β-endorphin,[8] an opiate-like substance associated with mild euphoria. Short-term alleviation of stress is also reported.[9]

## Principles of Training

Before considering specific issues clinicians should address in prescribing exercise intended to develop flexibility, strength, or endurance, it is useful to provide a brief review of the basic principles of training that underlie all exercise. The specifics vary much, depending on the type of training and the desired functional outcome. The term *training effect* refers to a series of predictable biochemical and neurophysiologic adaptations to the chronic performance of physical exercise that, in turn, will improve the efficiency of energy utilization, muscle physiology, and coordination in the patient, resulting in a higher level of physical performance.

### Specificity

A key concept in training is that the biophysical adaptations and improved performance of muscle are specific to the training stimulus used, both the type of exercise and the specific muscle groups exercised. The basis for this lies in the differences in the biochemical and morphologic adaptations that result from aerobic (versus anaerobic) training.[10] Furthermore, there is specificity of training, related to motor learning, that enhances the skilled performance of a specific task and is best accomplished by practicing that task.[10]

### Overload

To continue increasing a patient's strength or endurance, the required training stimulus must be increased periodically, in either intensity or duration of work, to ensure an "overload," or taxing of the musculoskeletal system. As the enzyme systems involved adapt to the increased demand, each task is performed with greater biochemical efficiency. No training effect occurs unless the appropriate systems are stressed beyond the usual daily requirements or beyond the level to which they have become adapted. For any type of training to be effective, a certain minimum amount of exercise (frequency and duration) must be performed at a specified minimum intensity.

### Intensity

*Intensity* refers to the level at which the work will be performed. How intensity is expressed depends on the nature of the exercise being prescribed. When training for endurance (aerobic capacity), intensity may be measured as a percentage of maximum oxygen consumption, maximum heart rate, or perceived rate of exertion. Training for strength may be prescribed in terms of either absolute or relative load. These terms are discussed further in appropriate sections of this chapter.

## Duration

*Duration* may be expressed in units of time for aerobic training or isometric holding, or as the number of repetitions of a dynamic strength or endurance training activity. As a rule, the higher the intensity of an activity, the shorter the duration needed to achieve a training effect, and vice versa, but duration must be long enough at the given intensity to result in overload. For most forms of exercise, there is no generally accepted agreement on minimal or optimal duration.[11]

## Frequency

In prescribing exercise it is important to state the required frequency. Because a training effect often requires overload resulting in a catabolic response in the muscle followed by an anabolic response that overshoots the baseline, daily exercise is not desirable when the goal is high-intensity strength or endurance training. Lower-intensity training may require daily doses of exercise to achieve a training response.[11] On the other hand, for neuromuscular reeducation the frequency of training may have to be more than once a day to produce carryover. Stretching exercises usually need to be performed at least once a day to produce a good response. Thus, to decide on the frequency of training required to achieve the desired physiologic response in the patient, the clinician needs to consider the type of exercise, its relative intensity, and the duration.

## Interval Training

*Interval training* is exercise performed intermittently, alternating periods of high work intensity with periods of less intense work or rest. This method has several clinical applications. For a very deconditioned person with low exercise tolerance, interval training extends the total time and amount of work that can be done.[12] Another application is training for short-duration–high-intensity exercise, such as sprint racing, where anaerobic conditioning is desirable. Anaerobic training occurs if relatively high loads are used during short work intervals, whereas if the exercise stimulus is of submaximal intensity over longer periods, aerobic enzyme systems are utilized and trained. The intensity of the stimulus and duration of the work ultimately determine which system is preferentially trained.[10]

## Specific Types of Exercise

### Exercise for Range of Motion

Each joint has a physiologic range of motion, and there is some variation among individuals. The clinician may prescribe range-of-motion exercises to prevent loss of range in an immobilized hospital patient, to increase range where limitations already exist, or as stretching for a seasoned athlete. The act of stretching causes tension in both muscle and associated connective tissues. The effects on the connective tissues are detailed below.

### Anatomy and Physiology of Connective Tissue

Connective tissue is composed of collagen fibers within a proteoglycan matrix. Loose connective tissue is a relatively disorganized collection of collagen fibers that lines opposing mobile surfaces.[13] It may become fibrotic, contracted, and shortened when subjected to immobilization, resulting in joint capsule contractures and limited range of motion (see Chapter 17). Tendons and ligaments are made of organized connective tissue and have a linear arrangement of collagen fibers that is determined and maintained by regular deforming forces such as muscle tension. The rate of collagen turnover varies between tissues: injured tissues have the highest rate of turnover, and tendon and skin relatively slow turnover.[14]

The joint capsule and ligaments provide an important contribution to the stabilization of joints. The capsule consists primarily of collagen and elastin, discounting the 70% that is water.[15]

Another large contribution to joint stability derives from the surrounding musculature. Adaptive shortening occurs in muscles as well. A muscle immobilized in a shortened position demonstrates muscle belly shortening within a week. After 3 weeks in this position, the loose connective tissue in the muscle becomes dense connective tissue, and a fixed muscle contracture develops.[16]

Synovial fluid bathes the articular cartilage and

is necessary to maintain lubrication and mobility of the joint. Boundary lubrication and a hydrostatic mechanism provide lubrication for the articulating cartilaginous surfaces. Boundary lubrication reduces friction by preventing the two articular surfaces from actually coming in contact, and it occurs through the binding of a glycoprotein to the cartilage surfaces.[17] The hydrostatic mechanism functions by squeezing water out of the cartilage by pressure, which coats the cartilage surface, providing lubrication.[18] This mechanism predominates at heavy loads. Hyaluronate provides boundary lubrication for the synovial tissues.[19] Immobility of the normal joint results in reduction in water (up to 6%), hyaluronic acid (40%), and other glycosaminoglycans, with a resultant loss of lubrication efficiency.[20]

*Exercise to Maintain Range of Motion*

For a healthy person, everyday use is all that is required to maintain a functional range of motion. If illness or surgery interferes with this, slow, sustained stretch and range-of-motion exercises should be performed two or three times daily. Quick, jerky stretching is to be avoided, as it stimulates the muscle spindle of the intrafusal muscle fibers, causing the muscle to contract reflexively. On the other hand, slower sustained stretching causes firing of the Golgi tendon organs, which lie in series with extrafusal muscle fibers, and results in muscle relaxation (see Chapter 6).[21] Extra caution must be observed after surgery or in the presence of joint inflammation. Range-of-motion exercises may be performed by the patient actively, with partial assistance, or passively using another extremity, a therapist, or a continuous passive range-of-motion (CPM) machine. Proper positioning to encourage passive stretching is another important technique in maintaining range of motion.

*Exercise to Increase Range of Motion (Stretching)*

Stretching applies physiologic principles similar to those discussed in the preceding section. Tendons demonstrate nonlinear deformation in response to stress (Figure 15-3). In the first phase, little force is required for elongation, as the collagen fibers undergo straightening and the elastic fibers elon-

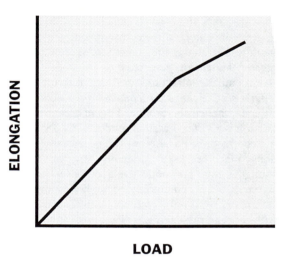

**LOAD**

**Figure 15-3.** The relationship between load and elongation of a tendon under stretch.

gate. The second phase of elongation is characterized by breaking crosslinks in the tendon and by disruption of some smaller collagen fibers. The second stage requires greater force per increment of elongation. If sufficient force is applied, a third phase of elongation, characterized by tendon failure, ensues.

The deformation of tendons is also time dependent. Application of a smaller force over a prolonged period will result in tendon *creep*—irreversible elongation of the tendon.

Stretching techniques are used in the treatment of myofascial pain syndromes. Application of superficial heat and ultrasound has been shown to facilitate tendon and muscle stretching,[22] and neuromuscular facilitation techniques have been used to relax involved muscles.

*Exercise for Strength*

*Types of Muscle Contraction*

**Isotonic Contraction.** By definition, isotonic exercise occurs when the tension or torque generated by the muscle is constant throughout the movement. In practice this is very difficult to accomplish, and a better term is *dynamic contraction,* which may be subdivided into several types of contractions: concentric, eccentric, and isokinetic.

Concentric contractions are also known as *shortening* or *positive contractions.* As the muscle shortens, less force is generated; thus, the force generated is not uniform throughout the arc of motion. The slower the velocity of shortening, the greater the tension generated.

Eccentric contractions are also referred to as *lengthening* or *negative contractions*. At a given velocity, the tension produced by an eccentric contraction is greater than that produced by a concentric contraction. For this reason, eccentric contractions may be used efficiently as part of a strengthening program. Delayed-onset muscle soreness, which commonly occurs 24 to 48 hours after exercise, is more common with eccentric than with concentric exercise. The possible mechanisms for exercise-induced delayed-onset muscle soreness were reviewed by Armstrong,[23] who proposed a model beginning with structural damage in the muscle fiber caused by high tension resulting in disruptive of calcium homeostasis caused by damage to cell membranes. This process leads to necrosis, which peaks about 2 days after exercise. Products of the ensuing macrophage activity and inflammation cause the sensation of soreness.

**Isokinetic Contraction.**   Isokinetic contraction, as produced by the Cybex machine and other devices, is performed at a constant angular velocity, torque being generated against a preset device that controls speed of contraction.[24] *Torque* is defined as the product of force multiplied by the distance between the center of rotation and the point where the force is applied. This form of exercise is defined by the equipment used for the exercise, as such contractions do not exist in nature. Most isokinetic devices utilize concentric contraction, but some of the newer machines, such as the KIN-COM, can produce eccentric isokinetic contractions. These exercise machines are useful for providing a relatively safe dynamic training program after trauma or surgery. Most of them produce elaborate printouts with tabulations of objective data. Such data may be useful for following trends during a rehabilitation program, but caution must be observed in extrapolating from the information to predict function in the real world. Hageman reviewed several issues that may influence the reliability and validity of isokinetic testing.[25] Factors such as positioning in the machine, length of the lever arm, stabilization of the subject, calibration of the machine, speed of contraction, and the effect of gravity are important. In addition, poor correlation among torque values reported by the various currently available machines makes it impossible to compare norms or data of individual patients when they are obtained on different brands of machines. Correlations of printout data with patients' functional outcome has been poor, both for orthopedic and neurologic rehabilitation. The principles of specificity of training and testing suggest that it might be difficult to estimate functional work capacity from the results of isokinetic testing.

**Isometric Contraction.**   *Isometric, or static, exercise* occurs when force is exerted against an immovable or relatively immovable object. *Isometric exercise* is defined as muscle contraction without movement of the joint(s) crossed by the active muscle(s). The intensity of isometric contraction is usually expressed as a percentage of the maximum force of contraction. Isometric exercise elevates both heart rate and blood pressure. The resulting increase in myocardial oxygen demand may precipitate angina in susceptible persons (see Chapter 7).

Isotonic training is the best preparation for isotonic tasks, such as lifting; similarly, isometric training is most appropriate for isometric tasks such as holding or gripping. There is, however, some crossover effect between the two types of training (Figure 15-4).[26]

*Determinants of Strength*

*Strength* represents the maximal force that a muscle can produce. There are several major determinants of strength.

**Cross-Sectional Area.**   Strength is proportional to the cross-sectional area of a muscle, which is measured at right angles to the direction of the parallel muscle fibers.[27]

**Recruitment.**   Recruitment of motor fibers in a coordinated, properly sequenced fashion also determines strength. Proper sequencing of agonist and antagonist activity is necessary for maximum voluntary contraction. The degree to which motor units fire simultaneously to produce maximum tension, the *synchronization ratio*, is one determinant of motor unit recruitment. Another factor in recruitment is the frequency of firing.[10,28] Smaller

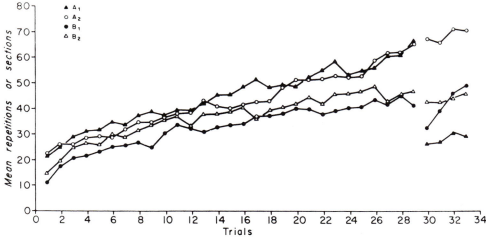

**Figure 15-4.** Comparison of isotonic and isometric training. Groups A1 and A2 underwent isotonic training; groups B1 and B2 had isometric training. Groups A1 and B1 switched training regimens on day 30. (From DeLateur BJ, Lehmann JF, Stonebridge J, et al. Isotonic versus isometric exercise: A double-shift transfer of training study. Arch Phys Med Rehabil 1972; 53:212–216.)

motor units have a lower threshold for discharge and are recruited with low-force activities. As the need for increased force arises, these smaller motor units increase the frequency of discharge and additional (larger) motor units are recruited. These larger motor units in turn increase their discharge rate in response to increasing demand (Figure 15-5). Thus, both recruitment of new motor units and increasing frequency of firing (rate coding) are determinants of maximal strength.

**Length-Tension and Force-Velocity Relationships.** The greatest total tension that a muscle can develop depends on both active and passive tension at any given length. *Equilibrium length* is defined as the length of an unstimulated, unattached muscle. Maximal force is generated by a muscle at 120% of its equilibrium length, corresponding ultrastructurally with the length at which there is maximum single overlap between actin and myosin (see Chapter 5 for a detailed discussion).[10] Anatomic limitations of joint motion restrict muscle length to between 70% and 120% of their equilibrium length, allowing the muscle to generate its maximum force at its maximum anatomic length.

The velocity of muscle contraction also affects the maximum strength that can be developed. For a given contractile force, less energy and decreased muscle activation (as assessed on electro-

myography) are required during eccentric contraction than during concentric contraction. Rapid concentric contraction produces less tension than slow concentric contraction, whereas rapid eccentric contraction produces more tension than slow eccentric contraction. Accordingly, the greatest force is developed during a rapid eccentric contraction, and the least force with a rapid concentric contraction (Figure 15-6).[27,29] These characteris-

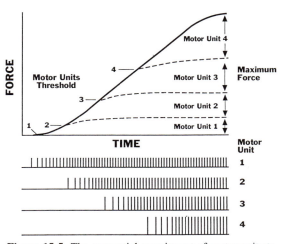

**Figure 15-5.** The sequential recruitment of motor units to provide increasing force of contraction. (Adapted from Åstrand P-O, Rodahl K. Textbook of Work Physiology, ed 3. New York: McGraw-Hill, 1986.)

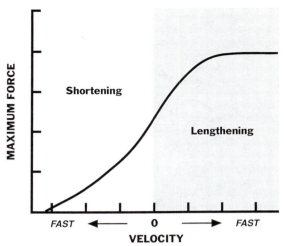

**Figure 15-6.** The relationship between speed of contraction and maximum force generated for shortening (concentric) and lengthening (eccentric) contractions. The 0 velocity point represents an isometric contraction. (Adapted from Knuttgen HG. Neuromuscular Mechanisms for Therapeutic and Conditioning Exercise. Baltimore: University Park Press, 1976.)

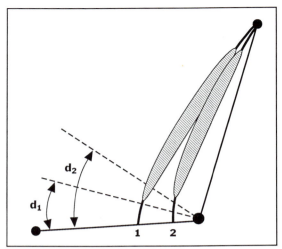

**Figure 15-7.** The relationship between the point of insertion of a muscle and the maximum arc of rotation. Insertion closer to the center of rotation allows a greater arc but a lower maximum force. (Adapted from DeLateur BJ. Exercise for strength and endurance. In: Basmajian JV, ed. Therapeutic Exercise, ed 4. Baltimore: Williams & Wilkins, 1984.)

tics can be used in the design of strengthening programs.

**Psychological Factors.** Neuropsychological factors may play a role in the measurement and development of strength. Motivation at any given time is important as is overall motivation to pursue a training regimen. Åstrand discusses the positive and negative effects of psychological stress on athletic performance.[10] Visual input, perceptual ability, and proprioceptive feedback are also necessary for optimal strength.

**Kinesiology.** The geometry of the origin and insertion of the muscle relative to the joint line that will serve as the center of the axis of rotation is important in determining torque. When the muscle inserts close to the center of the axis of rotation, less force can be exerted at the distal end but a larger arc is generated. When the insertion is farther from the center of rotation, the converse is true; that is, greater force is exerted over a shorter arc (Figure 15-7). The position of the muscle is also important, as the maximum force is generated at a muscle length approximately 1.2 times the equilibrium length. The maximum tension that can

be generated depends on the lever arm and the relative length at the time of contraction.

**Fiber Types.** Each human muscle is a mosaic of type I and type II fibers; the relative proportions vary, depending on the general demands made of the muscle. Type I fibers are the slow oxidative fibers and are generally derived from smaller motor neurons, responding to demands of low, sustained force. The type II fibers (which have two subtypes, IIa and IIb) are recruited later and respond to demands requiring higher forces generated over shorter periods. The maximum force generated by a muscle depends on the relative proportions of type I and type II fibers that make up the muscle and how this compares with the task being asked of it (see Table 5-1).

### Standard Training Programs

#### Progressive Resistive Exercise

Progressive resistive exercise (PRE) describes dynamic strengthening exercise that involves using weights or resistance for a specified number of repetitions. As training progresses, resistance is increased. Two techniques of PRE have been popularized in the literature: DeLorme and Oxford.[30,31] In 1945, DeLorme first described his techniques, based on the 10 repetition maximum (10 RM). A *repetition maximum* is the maximum weight that can be moved through the joint's full range of motion against gravity a given number of times. Thus, the 10 RM is the load that can be lifted 10 times through the full range. Based on a new 10 RM determined each week, the training sessions consist of 10 repetitions each at 50%, 75%, and 100% of the 10 RM. As the patient's strength increases, the 10 RM is increased accordingly. One potential disadvantage of the technique is that the patient may become fatigued toward the end of the session, just when the highest load is to be lifted.

The Oxford technique is similar to the DeLorme technique, except that each session starts with 10 repetitions of 100% 10 RM, followed by 10 reps each of 75% and 50% of 10 RM. The fact that patients report less fatigue with the Oxford method may make this a less effective form of training than the traditional DeLorme technique.[32] Another disadvantage of the Oxford technique is that the muscle is not warmed up before maximal effort is exerted. Disadvantages of both techniques are that they are time consuming, require assistance from a physical therapist or trainer, and use a constant load. Another issue in designing these programs is the number of repetitions.

Atha reviewed a number of studies and concluded that the most effective strength training uses a five or six RM schedule.[11] The torque generated by a muscle at any point during the arc of motion varies and is determined by the factors discussed previously—length of the muscle, angle of insertion of the tendon, patient's effort. Because the torque generated is variable but the resistance constant, the net effective training load varies at different points in the range of motion and is thus submaximal at points where the greatest torque is generated. To increase the strength of the muscle, the patient may progressively increase the weight lifted or the rate at which a given weight is lifted.

### Eccentric Training

One popular technique for eccentric muscle training utilizes equipment manufactured by Nautilus.

The Nautilus system of training has as its unique feature a cam that superficially resembles a nautilus shell. This cam variably adjusts the resistance throughout the range of motion to approximate the average torque that is produced for a given muscle group. Because of this specialized cam design, separate devices are necessary to train each muscle group. Resistance is provided for both the concentric and eccentric contractions of each muscle group, adding to the efficiency of this strengthening regimen. Other machines are also available, including some that provide eccentric isokinetic contractions. Eccentric training can also be accomplished with simple weights, with assistance during the concentric phase provided by an attendant or the other limb, followed by a controlled eccentric contraction to lower the weight. Atha provides a thorough analysis of articles comparing eccentric and concentric training in his excellent review of strengthening exercise.[11]

### Isokinetic Training

Isokinetic exercise requires special equipment, now produced by a number of manufacturers, to provide a constant velocity (measured in degrees per second) during muscle contraction. The machine allows the individual to exert maximum force throughout the range of motion and provides a corresponding resistance to maintain the velocity of contraction. A particularly useful feature of several of these machines is a printout or graphic documentation of a subject's progress. One unique concern of isokinetic training is the specificity of the velocity of training: velocity chosen for training should correspond to the velocity required for the ultimate (functional) activity. The maximal torque for concentric isokinetic contractions decreases with increasing velocity,[33] whereas the reverse is true for eccentric isokinetic contraction.[34] The speeds selected for training should reflect the need to generate an appropriate loading force and the anticipated functional requirements of the patient.

### Isometric Training

Isometric exercise may be performed for strength training; the recommended duration of each contraction is 6 seconds. Müller described an isometric program with a 1-second maximal contraction per muscle per day.[35] Although this seems attractive in its simplicity and efficiency, most clinicians find that programs of multiple contractions lasting 6 seconds (to prevent the exaggerated cardiac response) are more effective. The strength gains are specific to the angle at which the exercise is performed, and this limits its general applicability.[10] The major utility of isometric exercise is for patients whose joint range of motion is either very limited or, owing to inflammation or surgery, uncomfortable when the clinician wants to prevent significant atrophy.

*Mechanisms of Strength Gain*

The major mechanisms of strength gains that underlie all strengthening programs are hypertrophy of fibers (cross-sectional area) and neural factors.[36] Moritani and de Vries found that during the first 1 to 2 weeks of training the major contribution to strength gain was from neural factors.[37] Hypertrophy becomes the dominant factor in increased strength after 3 to 5 weeks. The mechanisms underlying the early phase of training appear to be better synchronization and more effective recruitment of motor units. The relative proportion of type I and II fibers remains constant, but considerable changes can occur within each fiber type (and between type IIa and IIb) with training.[38,39] The mechanism of strength gain does not appear to change with aging: even nonagenarians have been shown to respond to a strengthening program with increased strength and muscle hypertrophy.[40]

Which type of strengthening exercises to prescribe for a patient depends on the desired goal. Because the expected results are specific to the

training modality, it makes the most sense to tailor the training regimen to the patient's needs and the dynamics of the activity. At all times, it must be remembered that the patient must be "overloaded" and the training tasks must exceed the demands of everyday activity. The clinician must regularly reassess and upgrade the prescription if strength gain is to continue.

### *Exercise for Endurance*

In discussing endurance training the distinction must first be made between training for muscle endurance and training for total body endurance (aerobic capacity).

### *Training Muscle Endurance*

*Muscle endurance* must be defined operationally for each situation. It may refer to the holding time for an isometric contraction, the number of repetitions of a brief isometric contraction, or the number of repetitions of a dynamic contraction (concentric, eccentric, or isokinetic). Research shows that isometric and isotonic endurance can be trained preferentially.[26] It is equally important to consider the force of the contraction as a percentage of the maximal strength of that muscle. Figure 15-8 demonstrates the relationship between strength and endurance for both dynamic and static work. This relationship clearly indicates that increasing the strength of a muscle increases the endurance for any given absolute submaximal load by making it a smaller percentage of the maximum contraction.

The DeLorme axiom states that muscle endur-

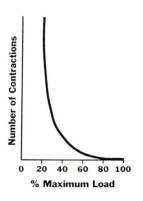

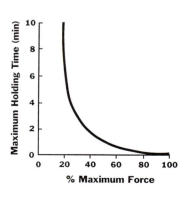

**Figure 15-8.** (*A*) The relationship between endurance (number of contractions) and relative load for dynamic work. (Adapted from Knuttgen HG. Neuromuscular Mechanisms for Therapeutic and Conditioning Exercise. Baltimore: University Park Press, 1976.) (*B*) The relationship between endurance (holding time) and relative load for static work. (Adapted from Kottke FJ, Stillwell GK, Lehmann JF, eds. Krusen's Handbook of Physical Medicine and Rehabilitation, ed 3. Philadelphia: WB Saunders, 1987.)

ance can be trained by using relatively low loads for high numbers of repetitions (as opposed to high-load low-repetition training for strength). This concept was called into question by DeLateur, in a study that demonstrated that loads in a fairly broad range (30% to 100% of maximum) had similar effects on strength and endurance if the exercises were performed to the point of fatigue.[32] Prolonged exercise with lighter loads as well as the muscle training that takes place during aerobic conditioning have a different effect than strength training on histologic and biochemical changes in muscle. With endurance training there is a decrease in the size of type I fibers instead of the hypertrophy of type II fibers with strength training. This decrease in the cross-sectional area of the type I fibers is accompanied by increases in capillary density and in the myoglobin content of the fibers, thus increasing the cells' ability to transport oxygen to the mitochondria. There is also an accompanying increase in the number and size of the mitochondria and in the concentration of oxidative enzymes within the mitochondria, thus increasing the cells' capacity for aerobic metabolism.

*Training for Aerobic Capacity*

Aerobic training programs increase the maximum oxygen consumption ($VO_2max$).[41,42] The changes in the cardiac response to exercise following such a program are discussed in Chapter 7. These changes have been interpreted as suggesting that there is actually some training or strengthening of the heart itself. This is not the case, however, as is demonstrated by the fact that the cardiac response to exercise only changes for exercise performed by muscle groups involved in the training. Thus, training on a treadmill changes the cardiac response to lower extremity work but has no effect on the cardiac response to upper extremity work, and vice versa.

The benefits of aerobic training are due to a combination of the changes in the type I skeletal muscle fibers noted above and an increase in the blood volume. The peripheral muscle changes reduce the need to shunt blood from other vascular beds to the working muscle, thus reducing the peripheral resistance and, consequently, the afterload on the left ventricle. The muscle changes also make each absolute exercise load a smaller percentage of the maximum capacity, thus reducing the activation of the sympathetic nervous system and reducing the increase in circulating catecholamines associated with exercise. The increased blood volume that has been demonstrated with these training programs results in increased venous return. This combines with the bradycardia to produce greater diastolic filling, and thus a larger stroke volume, which produces a higher maximum cardiac output, resulting in larger maximum oxygen consumption (aerobic capacity).

Typical aerobic training programs use dynamic exercise of large muscle groups. Owing to the specificity of training it is necessary to include all groups that the patient needs for vocational and avocational uses. The usual exercises include walking, running, swimming, rowing, cycling, aerobic calisthenics, and arm ergometry. The intensity of exercise is usually expressed as a percentage of the maximum heart rate, but absolute loads on a calibrated ergometer can also be used. Although training at 75% of any person's age-determined maximum heart rate (see Chapter 7) is usually considered ideal, training can be achieved with intensities in the range of 40% to 60% of maximum, if a wider margin of safety is needed because of coronary artery disease or if the patient is too debilitated to tolerate a more strenuous program.

A relatively strenuous program ought to include warm-up and cool-down phases. During a warm-up of less intense activity, induction of the aerobic enzymes and stretching of the soft tissues occurs, making the exercise more efficient and less likely to cause injury. A cool-down phase of gradually decreasing intensity exercise reduces the risk of postural hypotension and cardiac arrhythmia. The duration of training is usually 20 to 30 minutes, including the warm-up and cool-down phases. Lower-intensity programs may need a longer duration which to be tolerable may require interval training at first. Frequency of training is usually three times a week, though with a very low-intensity program more frequent sessions may be needed to achieve a training effect. A significant increase in aerobic capacity (reflected in lower heart rate at the same submaximal loads) should be evident within 4 to 6 weeks. At the beginning of the program the patient should be advised that all of the improvements in work capacity and cardiac response to exercise will be lost in a short time unless a maintenance program is followed after the end of the formal training period.

### Training for Cardiopulmonary Rehabilitation

The changes in the cardiopulmonary response to exercise that occur with aerobic training programs can be utilized to design rehabilitation programs for cardiac and pulmonary disease patients. Such programs can increase the work capacity of these patients even though there is no change in the coronary circulation and no change in lung volumes or gas exchange (see Chapter 7).

Cardiac rehabilitation after a myocardial infarction begins in the cardiac care unit. In an uncomplicated case the goal is to provide a gradual increase in exercise intensity, progressing from bed rest to stair climbing over a 10- to 14-day period.[43] After discharge from the hospital the patient usually goes through a 6- to 8-week convalescent phase, during which the intensity of exercise remains constant but duration is gradually increased. The next phase involves aerobic training (described in Chapter 7). The advantage of training for the cardiac patient is based on the change in myocardial oxygen consumption. Thus, even though there is no change in the anginal threshold, more work can be accomplished within that limit.

Rehabilitation for pulmonary disease patients has largely the same rationale. (The improved efficiency of ventilation that follows an aerobic training program is also described in Chapter 7.) In addition to the improved ventilatory mechanics, the pulmonary patient who has been inactive for some time may actually realize a decrease in oxygen consumption for submaximal activities, owing to the improved mechanical efficiency that results from improved movement skills.[44] Overall, however, the usual result of training is increased physical work capacity with little or no change in lung volume, flow rate, or arterial blood gases.

### Exercise for Neuromuscular Reeducation

For rehabilitation of patients with impaired voluntary motor control due to central nervous system (CNS) disease such as cerebral palsy, cerebrovascular accident, traumatic brain injury, or brain tumor, the focus of the exercise program becomes acquisition or reacquisition of controlled, coordinated voluntary movement rather than of strength per se. *Control* is the ability to carry out a chosen activity with the proper intensity and to start and stop that activity at will. Coordination is the ability to execute a properly timed, sequenced, and manipulated purposeful movement in a smooth manner. In training for coordination, the patient develops a motor engram after many repetitions of the same activity sequence (an engram is the neuronal representation in the central nervous system of a specific preprogrammed pattern of muscle performance). As coordination develops through repetition and practice, the patient can perform the same activity with greater efficiency and fluidity. Millions of repetitions are necessary to develop maximum performance of a new motor activity.[45,46]

The development of an engram requires facilitation of the desired activity and inhibition of undesired movements. All of the various systems for neuromuscular reeducation use either facilitative or inhibitory techniques to modify primitive and advanced postural reflexes for the purpose of enhancing movement, increasing coordination, controlling abnormal tone, or enhancing stretching in normal muscles. The clinical applications include preexercise stretching, normalization of tone, and enhancement of function in patients with cerebral palsy, head injury, stroke, or spinal cord injury. Before discussing the major techniques for neurofacilitation, it is useful to review the underlying neurophysiologic reflexes.

### Reflexes Used in Neuromuscular Reeducation Programs

The primitive postural reflexes are defined as those that are coordinated in the spinal cord or medulla. They include the flexion reflex,[47] the long spinal reflex, and the crossed extension-flexion reflex.[48] With the exception of the stretch reflex, which is normally present in adults, these reflexes are present at birth and normally disappear early in infancy, reappearing only in the presence of abnormal cortical development, as in cerebral palsy, or acquired higher CNS dysfunction such as stroke or head injury (see Chapter ?).

The stretch reflex (also known as the *myotatic reflex*) is routinely tested during the neurologic examination. It is a simple reflex with the afferent input resulting from change in muscle length received via the muscle spindle and transmitted by the Ia afferents. Monosynaptic excitement of the alpha motorneurons that supply the stretched muscle results in muscle contraction. Full details are presented in Chapter 6.

In normal infants, pressure on the palm or distal plantar surface of the foot results in gross extension of the arm or leg, respectively. This positive supporting reaction disappears at about 2 months of age, but it may resurface after cortical injury.

The tonic labyrinthine reflex is stimulated by the position of the head in space and is strongest at an angle of 45 degrees to the horizontal. Extensor tone predominates in the supine position, and flexor tone in the prone position.

The asymmetric tonic neck reflex (ATNR), which occurs in response to turning or tilting the head to one side, is extension of the limbs on the side the chin is facing, and flexion on the side of the occiput. In the symmetric tonic neck reflex, neck flexion results in arm flexion and leg extension; the opposite effects result from neck extension. Both the symmetric and asymmetric tonic neck reflexes should be integrated by age 6 to 7 months.

The physiologic (advanced) postural responses include the righting reflexes, the equilibrium reactions, and the protective extension response. The righting reflexes help maintain the correct head alignment in space by responding to visual, vestibular, tactile, and proprioceptive stimuli. The equilibrium reactions and the protective extension response serve to readjust posture and extend the extremity to maintain balance and prevent falling. These reflexes normally emerge at various stages of development in early childhood and are then present throughout life. They help maintain (1) proper orientation of the head and body in space and (2) balance.

## Control of Muscle Tone

A certain amount of tone (resistance to passive stretch) is present in normal resting muscle. Diseases that affect the lower motor neuron reduce tone, making the limb floppy. The conditions that are treated with neuromuscular reeducation techniques usually involve damage to the upper motor neuron, where there is increased tone or spasticity. The hallmark of spasticity is increased resistance to passive stretch, which becomes greater when the speed of stretching is increased and is associated with increased deep tendon reflexes and clonus. In general terms, spasticity is the result of reduced higher-level regulatory influence on the spinal reflexes and decreased inhibition of the Ia motor neurons from descending cortical influence. (For a detailed discussion, see Chapter 6.) The typical hemiplegic limb demonstrates impaired isolated joint movement; instead, movement patterns are crude and synergistic.[49] There are typical extension and flexion synergy patterns in the lower and upper extremities that become important in the discussion of the different neurofacilitation techniques that follows.

## Neurofacilitation and Inhibition Techniques

Now we discuss four commonly used neurofacilitation methods with their physiologic rationale and clinical applications. Though all are in common clinical use and most therapists use an eclectic approach, there is little hard evidence that any of these techniques alters the natural history of recovery from the conditions for which they are used. The methods are useful, however, in providing compensatory techniques, making transfers, bed mobility, stretching, and even ambulation safer and rendering patients better able to perform them with less assistance.

**Proprioceptive Neuromuscular Facilitation.** Proprioceptive neuromuscular facilitation (PNF) utilizes resistance to facilitate movement. The therapist provides maximal resistance to the stronger muscle components of specific spiral and diagonal patterns, thus facilitating the pattern's weaker components. The amount of resistance must be limited for patients with spasticity, so as not to further increase the tone. For that reason, PNF is best applied for supraspinal lesions with hypotonia to promote normalization of tone.[50,51]

**Brunnstrom.** Twitchell described six stages of motor recovery, which progress from complete flaccidity and paralysis through the appearance of spasticity and gross synergistic movements to the disappearance of spasticity and the return of isolated joint movements and coordinated activity.[49] The Brunnstrom techniques use resistance, associated reactions, and primitive postural reactions to facilitate gross synergistic movement and return of muscle tone, especially in the early stages of recovery.[52] During later stages of recovery, development of isolated movement and control are emphasized. Like the PNF technique, the Brunnstrom method is advocated to help normalize tone in a hemiplegic patient with persistent flaccidity.

**Bobath or Neurodevelopmental Techniques (NDT).** In contradistinction to the PNF and Brunnstrom methods, the neurodevelopmental techniques (NDT) developed by the Bobaths emphasize normalization of increased tone using certain reflex inhibitory movement patterns (RIPs).[53] These RIPs are generally opposite to the typical hemiplegia synergy patterns and are performed without resistance. In addition, NDT incorporates the use of advanced postural reactions to help stimulate recovery. It has been claimed that NDT facilitates motor recovery and reduces hypertonicity.

*Rood*

The Rood method uses tactile stimuli such as fast brushing, quick stroking, or icing of the skin, ostensibly to facilitate specific groups of muscles to promote functional activity.[54,55] The selection of muscle groups depends on which stage of development or recovery the patient has achieved. Rood described four stages of neurophysiologic mobility: (1) development of functional mobility, (2) development of stability, (3) development of stability and mobility, and (4) development of skilled movement.[56] Level 1 involves activities such as rolling over. Levels 2 and 3 incorporate the development of stability, which prepares the body for weight bearing, including positions such as quadruped and standing. Last, level 4 involves development of skilled movements, such as walking. The Rood techniques are reversible and can be used either to stimulate activity in a patient with hypotonia or to decrease spasticity in a patient with hypertonia.

*Exercise for Development of Proprioception and Coordination*

Frenkel's exercises are commonly used for impairment of proprioception due to CNS pathology or incoordination due to cerebellar dysfunction. Exercises of progressive complexity begin with the patient in a supine position, followed as the patient improves by sitting and standing. Precise coordination and motion is stressed, as well as accurate performance of each task. Repetition and visual feedback help the patient reinforce the acquired skills.[57]

## Fatigue

### Definition

The first problem encountered in discussing fatigue is the definition. In physiology, the term is often used in relation to isolated nerve-muscle preparations with its original meaning: diminished response to an unchanging stimulus or requirement of a larger stimulus to produce the same response. When the whole person is considered, however, the definition inevitably becomes intertwined with the various subjective sensations associated with fatigue, such as tiredness, exhaustion, aching or soreness of muscles, or shortness of breath. As Dill pointed out,"...The various unmistakably disagreeable sensations commonly referred to by the word *fatigue* are in fact the accompaniments of a great variety of different physiological conditions, which have in common only this, that the physiological equilibrium of the body is somewhere breaking down."[58] Darling has warned against confusing the symptoms of fatigue with fatigue itself.[59] Distinctions between generalized fatigue and local muscle fatigue are considered below.

### Generalized Fatigue

For the purposes of this discussion, *generalized fatigue* is defined as the state that occurs when the aerobic systems of an organism have been taxed to the degree that the physiologic equilibria involved begin to break down. Associated subjective symptoms range from weariness to exhaustion; objective signs may include decreased speed, accuracy, or coordination. The duration of exercise needed to produce generalized fatigue varies with the relative intensity of the exercise for the individual. Most authorities acknowledge that in the industrial setting an intensity greater than 30% to 40% of the individual's maximum aerobic capacity cannot be sustained for an 8-hour day without producing generalized fatigue.[10,60] Intensities greater than 50% of maximum cannot be tolerated longer than 2 hours. Depending on the type of exercise and its intensity, the limiting factor may be the buildup of metabolic products such as lactic acid, the exhaustion of metabolic substrate such as glycogen, or a decrease in arousal generated by the reticular activating system.[61]

The relationship of generalized fatigue to the relative intensity of exercise is extremely important in rehabilitation medicine. People with disabilities must deal with a combination of higher than usual energy requirements for most activities (owing to the poor mechanical efficiency of abnormal gait patterns and assistive devices) and lower than normal maximum oxygen consumption. Often, rehabilitation professionals assume that people with disabilities are "fit" because their activities are generating high cardiac or metabolic responses, but it must be remembered that fitness is relative to the individual's needs. Thus, a person with a disability should be trained to two to three times the energy requirement of the usual form of mobility to be considered personally fit. Because they rarely are, most people with disabilities avoid generalized fatigue by limiting their activities and lifestyles.

## Muscle Fatigue

Muscle fatigue refers to a process that is closer to the original physiologic definition of a diminished response to the same stimulus. It may be associated with the subjective symptoms of muscle soreness, stiffness, or pain. Objective signs include decreased rate or rhythm of exercise, substitution of other muscles, and decreased precision of performance. The mechanism of muscular fatigue varies with the type, intensity, and duration of muscle contraction. Except in myasthenia gravis or dosing with curariform drugs, fatigue is not the result of failure of neuromuscular transmission. With isometric contraction, the limiting factor appears to be local ischemia due to the decreased circulation produced by the contraction. With isotonic, and presumably isokinetic, contractions there may be a combination of central and peripheral factors, including depletion of intracellular potassium, depletion of glycogen, accumulation of lactic acid and other metabolites, reduced pH, reduction of calcium ion release from the sarcoplasmic reticulum, or undefined CNS factors.

The onset of muscle fatigue with isometric contraction varies with the relative intensity of the work performed. A maximal contraction can be sustained for a few seconds, 50% maximum for a minute or so, and a 15% maximum contraction for more than 10 minutes. A similar phenomenon is seen with isotonic contractions.[10] The decrease in time to fatigue is exponential in relation to the maximum contraction. Though the exponential rise noted in most studies begins at 15% to 20% of maximum, there is evidence that this value decreases when applied to a full working day. In the industrial workplace, even loads less than 10% of maximum may produce local muscle fatigue. In the rehabilitation setting, again the emphasis is on relative load for the individual muscles involved. For example, the upper extremity muscles do more work than "normal" when a patient walks with an ambulation aid or propels a wheelchair, and if these muscles are not trained to a high higher level they fatigue prematurely.

The fatigue is reversible with rest. It is a normal phenomenon; indeed, it is necessary for training to occur. Of concern to clinicians is the possibility of irreversible damage resulting from extreme overwork. Though this is most likely to occur in patients with lower motor neuron weakness (best exemplified by the postpolio syndrome), it has been described in people with apparently normal neuromuscular systems.

### Neuromuscular Exhaustion Syndrome

Nielsen described four cases of severe muscle wasting following a period of overwork.[62] He termed this syndrome the *generalized neuromus-*

*cular exhaustion syndrome*. All four patients had no evidence of neuromuscular disease before the onset. One patient was a 37-year-old worker in a sugar warehouse who stacked a thousand 100-pound bags (50 tons) per shift. His problems started the day after working a double shift. Another was an executive with a type A personality who played in a company baseball game "covering the whole field." The third was a 17-year-old girl with anorexia nervosa who was forced to participate in a vigorous gymnastics program to improve her appetite. The fourth was a 55-year-old restaurateur who for several days worked all day in his restaurant and all night remodeling it. In each case the period of muscle overwork was followed by the sudden onset of restlessness, fasiculations, and rapid muscle atrophy. Even after a period of rest and gradual remobilization these patients did not recover their previous strength. Though the mechanism of this phenomenon is not clear, these cases are significant because they demonstrate what can happen when overload is carried to the extreme, causing irreversible muscle fatigue. These patients apparently ignored the usual warning symptoms of muscle fatigue, owing to psychological problems or intense motivation. As such they probably represent the extreme case in normal healthy persons of a phenomenon that can occur more easily in people with motor unit disease, which is best exemplified by the postpolio syndrome.

*The Postpolio Syndrome*

Bennett and Knowlton defined overwork weakness as "... a prolonged decrease in both the absolute strength and in the endurance of a muscle subsequent to a period or periods of work."[63] They wrote of the concept of performance improvement versus performance deterioration, depending on the intensity and duration of exercise for a given muscle. They argued that while too little exercise leads to atrophy and more exercise to improvement, still more exercise can lead to deterioration (Figure 15-9). They felt that most of the population is so far down at the *disuse* end of the curve that any training will lead to improvement; this makes it difficult for many people to conceive of further increases in intensity leading to decreased strength. The authors pointed out that this tendency is not unique to diseased motor units and

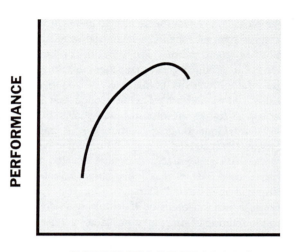

**INTENSITY OF TRAINING**

**Figure 15-9.** The relationship between performance and intensity of training. Note that a point is reached at which further increased intensity results in a performance decrement. (Adapted from Knowlton GC, Bennett RL. Overwork. Arch Phys Med Rehabil 1957; 38:18–20.)

that normal persons can suffer the same consequences if pushed far enough.

Reviewing 246 polio patients, Bennett and Knowlton found four cases of lasting, functionally significant decreased strength following unsupervised increased activity.[64] Sharrard found a low incidence of overwork weakness in reviewing 142 polio patients treated with a carefully supervised DeLorme program.[65] Overwork weakness has also been reported in muscular dystrophy patients.[66]

The mechanism of this phenomenon is not clear. Lundervold and Seyffrath suggested that the damage is caused by the friction of inactive denervated muscle fibers rubbing against actively contracting fibers, damaging the motor nerve endings.[67] Bennett and Knowlton stated that overwork weakness occurs when repeated demands on a muscle equal or exceed the maximal strength and endurance of that muscle.[63] They noted four situations that can lead to such overload. The first is when the maximum work output of the muscle does not challenge the muscle circulation. They pointed out that persons with motor unit disease have a decreased number of active motor units working in muscles that have a normal capillary supply, thus reducing local anoxia, acidosis, and accumulation of metabolites. This relatively high circulation reduces the sense of local muscle fatigue, allowing the person to overwork. The second is when a person is conditioned to tolerate great disparity between innervation effort and extent of response. The authors believed that part of the normal sense of fatigue is produced by proprioceptive input from active muscle. When the amount of motor activation needed to produce a movement doubles, normal persons feel too tired to continue. Bennett and Knowlton hypothesized that patients with a reduced number of innervated motor units who are exposed to a training program may learn to tolerate this sensation and override the inhibitory input. The third is when the initial innervation effort is so great that incremental increases are smaller than the least detectable differences. The fourth is when motivation for performance is so great as to negate the sensation of fatigue. This factor seems especially important in polio patients who were taught that they could increase strength and throw away their braces by pushing themselves to exercise harder. Throughout their lives the successful ones responded to fatigue and decreased function by trying to push themselves harder. This resulted in further decreased strength, atrophy, and various other musculoskeletal sequelae of polio.

Electromyographic studies of patients who suffered increasing weakness long after the original polio infection show increased motor unit size, increased insertional activity, increased fiber density, and increased jitter (see Chapter 11).[68,69] There is no difference in electrodiagnostic findings between those patients with stable strength and those with progressive weakness and fatigue. The findings do emphasize the heavy demand being placed on the residual anterior horn cells, which may contribute to their tendency to fatigue and drop out with time. Another possibility is that at least part of the problem relates to the normal aging process with loss of anterior horn cells, the effect being exaggerated by the large number of muscle fibers lost with each motor cell.

Thus, it appears that the overwork fatigue syndromes seen in polio patients and others with diseases of the lower motor neurons are part of a continuum that includes "normal" persons who perform relatively excessive exertion. The lessons clinicians are learning from the polio population must be kept in mind when working with persons with other disabilities who throughout their lives will be exposed to abnormal physical stresses as a result of rehabilitation programs.

## Conclusion

Therapeutic exercise is likely to remain a cornerstone of the rehabilitation armamentarium. Reasonable, functionally significant goals must be developed before the exercise prescription is written. Only then can the clinician choose the proper form of exercise and prescribe the proper dose. Suitable rest periods must be considered to avoid the pitfalls of fatigue. Determination of appropriate outcome measures depends on an intelligent understanding of the effects of exercise and the selection of the proper exercise for the established goals.

## References

1. American Heritage Dictionary. Boston: Houghton Mifflin, 1981.
2. Richter EA, Garetto CP, Goodman MN, et al. Muscle glucose metabolism following exercise in the rat: Increased sensitivity to insulin. J Clin Invest 1982; 69:785.
3. Richter EA, Ruderman NB, Schneider SH. Diabetes and exercise. Am J Med 1981; 70:201.
4. Simon HB. Exercise, health, and sports medicine. In:, ed. Scientific American Medicine. 1988; 8.
5. Warlow CP, Ogston D. Effect of exercise on platelet count, adhesion and aggregation. Acta Haematol 1974; 52:47.
6. Oscal LB, Williams BT, Hertig BA. Effect of exercise on blood volume. J Appl Physiol 1968; 24:622.
7. Costill DL. Sweating: Its composition and effects on body fluids. Ann NY Acad Sci 1977; 301:160.
8. Howlett TA, Tomlin S, Ngahfoong L, et al. Release of beta-endorphin and met-enkephalin during exercise in normal women's response to training. Br Med J 1984; 288:1950.
9. Morgan WP. Affective beneficence of vigorous physical activity. Med Sci Sports Exerc 1985; 17:94.
10. Åstrand P-O, Rodahl K. Textbook of Work Physiology, ed 3. New York: McGraw-Hill, 1986.
11. Atha J. Strengthening muscle. Exerc Sport Sci Rev 1981; 9:1–73.
12. Smoldaka VN. Interval training in rehabilitation medicine. Arch Phys Med Rehabil 1973; 54:428–431.

13. Kottke FJ. Therapeutic exercise to maintain mobility. In: Kottke FJ, Stillwell GK, Lehmann JF, eds. Krusen's Handbook of Physical Medicine and Rehabilitation, ed 3. Philadelphia: WB Saunders, 1987.

14. Nimni ME. Collagen: Structure, function, and metabolism in normal and fibrotic tissues. Semin Arthritis Rheum 1983; 13:1–86.

15. McCarty: Arthritis and Allied Conditions, ed 11. Philadelphia: Lea & Febiger, 1989.

16. Halar EM, Bell KR. Contractures and other deleterious effects of immobility. In: Delisa JA, ed. Rehabilitation Medicine: Principles and Practice. Philadelphia: JB Lippincott, 1988.

17. Swann DA, Radin EL. The molecular basis of articular lubrication I: Purification and properties of a lubricating fraction from bovine synovial fluid. J Biol Chem 1972; 274:8069–8083.

18. Linn FC, Sokoloff L. Movement and composition of interstitial fluid of cartilage. Arthritis Rheum 1965; 8:481–493.

19. Swann DA, et al. Role of hyaluronic acid in joint lubrication. Ann Rheum Dis 1974; 33:318–326.

20. Akeson WH, Amiel D, Abel MS, et al. Effects of immobilization on joints. Clin Orthop 1987; 219:28–35.

21. Wolf SE. Morphological and functional considerations for therapeutic exercises. In: Basmajian JV, ed. Therapeutic Exercise, ed 4. Baltimore: Williams & Wilkins, 1984.

22. Lehmann JF, DeLateur BJ. Therapeutic heat. In: Lehmann JF, ed. Therapeutic Heat and Cold, ed 3. Baltimore: Williams & Wilkins, 1982.

23. Armstrong RB. Mechanisms of exercise-induced delayed onset muscular soreness: A brief review. Med Sci Sports Exerc 1984; 16:529–538.

24. Thistle HG, Hislop HJ, Moffroid M, et al. Isokinetic contraction: A new concept of resistive exercise. Arch Phys Med Rehabil 1967; 48:279–282.

25. Hageman PA. Concentric and eccentric isokinetic testing of the extremities. Crit Rev Phys Rehabil Med 1990; 2:49–63.

26. DeLateur BJ, Lehmann JF, Stonebridge J, et al. Isotonic versus isometric exercise: A double-shift transfer of training study. Arch Phys Med Rehabil 1972; 53:212–216.

27. DeLateur BJ. Exercise for strength and endurance. In: Basmajian JV, ed. Therapeutic Exercise, ed 4. Baltimore: Williams & Wilkins, 1984.

28. Sale DG. Influence of exercise and training on motor unit activities. Exerc Sport Sci Rev 1987; 15:95–151.

29. Dillingham MF. Strength training. Phys Med Rehabil State of the Art Rev 1987; 1:555–568.

30. DeLorme TL, Watkins AL. Technics of progressive resistance exercise. Arch Phys Med 1948; 29:263–273.

31. Zinorieff AN. Heavy resistance exercises: The "Oxford technique." Br J Phys Med 1951; 14:129–132.

32. DeLateur BJ, Lehmann JF, Fordyce WE. A test of the DeLorme axiom. Arch Phys Med Rehabil 1968; 49:245–248.

33. Prietto CA, Caiozzo VJ. The in-vivo force-velocity relationships of the knee flexors and extensors. Am J Sports Med 1989; 17:607.

34. Griffen JW. Differences in elbow flexion torque measured concentrically, eccentrically, and isometrically. Phys Ther 1987; 67:1205.

35. Müller EA. Influence of training and inactivity on muscle strength. Arch Phys Med Rehabil 1970; 51:449–462.

36. Sale DG. Neural adaptation to resistance training. Med Sci Sports Exerc 1988; 20(suppl):S135–S145.

37. Moritani T, De Vries HA. Neural factors versus hypertrophy in the time course of muscle strength gain. Am J Phys Med 1979; 58:115–130.

38. Jolesz F, Sreter FA. Development, innervation, and activity-pattern–induced changes in skeletal muscles. Ann Rev Physiol 1981; 43:531–552.

39. Buchthal F, Schmalbruch H. Motor unit of mammalian muscle. Phys Rev 1980; 60:90–142.

40. Fiatarone MA, Marks EC, Ryan ND, et al. High-intensity strength training in nonagenarians. Effects on skeletal muscle. JAMA 1990; 263:3029–3034.

41. Saltin B, Blomqvist G, Mitchell JH, et al. Response to exercise after bed rest and after training. Circulation 1968; 38(suppl 7):1–50.

42. Karnoven MJ, et al. The effect of training on heart rate. A longitudinal study. Ann Med Exp Biol Fenn 1957; 35:305.

43. Wenger NK. Physiological basis for early ambulation after myocardial infarction. Cardiovasc Clin 1978; 9:107–115.

44. Paez PN, Phillipson EA, Masangkay M, et al. The physiologic basis of training patients with emphysema. Am Rev Respir Dis 1967; 95:944–953.

45. Kottke FJ. From reflex to skill: The training of coordination. Arch Phys Med Rehabil 1980; 61:551–561.

46. Crossman ER. Theory of acquisition of speed-skill. Ergonomics 1959; 2:153–166.

47. Marie P, Foix C. Reflexes d'automatisme medullaire et reflexes dits de defense. Le phenomene des raccourcisseurs. Semaine Med 1913; 33:505–508.

48. Sherrington CS. The Integrative Action of the Nervous System, ed 2. New Haven: Yale University Press, 1947.

49. Twitchell TE. The restoration of motor function following hemiplegia. Brain 1951; 74:443–480.
50. Kabat H. Studies on neuromuscular dysfunction, XI. New principles of neuromuscular reeducation. Permanente Found Med Bull 1947; 5:111.
51. Kabat H. Proprioceptive facilitation in therapeutic exercise. In: Licht S. Therapeutic Exercise, ed 2. New Haven, 1965.
52. Brunnstrom S. Movement Therapy in Hemiplegia. New York, 1971.
53. Bobath K, Bobath B. Treatment of cerebral palsy based on analysis of patients' motor behavior. Br J Phys Med 1952; 15:107–117.
54. Rood MS. Neurophysiological reactions as a basis for physical therapy. Phys Ther Rev 1954; 34:444–449.
55. Stockmeyer SL. An interpretation of the approach of Rood to the treatment of neuromuscular dysfunction. Am J Phys Med 1967; 6:900–955.
56. Dewald JP. Sensorimotor neurophysiology and the basis of neurofacilitory therapeutic techniques. In: Brandstater ME, Basmajian JV, eds. Stroke Rehabilitation. Baltimore: Williams & Wilkins, 1987.
57. Frenkel HS. Treatment of Tabetic Ataxia by Means of Systematic Exercises. Philadelphia: 1902.
58. Dill DB. The Harvard Fatigue Laboratory: Its development, contributions, and demise. Circ Res 1967; 20(suppl 1):I161–I170.
59. Darling RC, Fatigue. In: Downey JA, Darling RC, eds. Physiological Basis of Rehabilitation Medicine. Philadelphia: WB Saunders, 1971.
60. Work Practices Guide for Manual Lifting. DHHS, Publ No. 81-122. National Institute for Occupational Safety and Health, 1981.
61. Grandjean E. Fatigue: Its physiological and psychological significance. Ergonom 1968; 11(5):427–436.
62. Nielsen JM. A subacute generalized neuromuscular exhaustion syndrome. JAMA 1944; 126(13):801–806.
63. Knowlton GC, Bennett RL. Overwork. Arch Phys Med Rehabil 1957; 38:18–20.
64. Bennett RL, Knowlton GC. Overwork weakness in partially denervated skeletal muscle. Clin Orthop 1958; 12:22–29.
65. Sharrard WJW. Muscle recovery in poliomyelitis. J Bone Joint Surg 1955; 37B:63–79.
66. Johnson EW, Braddom R. Overwork weakness in facioscapulohumeral muscular dystrophy. Arch Phys Med Rehabil 1971; 52:333–336.
67. Lundervold A, Seyffarth H. Electromyographic investigations of poliomyelitic paresis during the training up of the affected muscles, and some remarks regarding the treatment of paretic muscles. Acta Psychiatr Neurol Scand 1942; 17:69–87.
68. Einarsson G, Grimby G, Stålberg E. Electromyographic and morphological functional compensation in late poliomyelitis. Muscle Nerve 1990; 13:165–171.
69. Ravits J, Hallett M, Baker M, et al. Clinical and eletromyographic studies of postpoliomyelitis muscular atrophy. Muscle Nerve 1990; 13:667–674.
70. Knuttgen HG. Neuromuscular Mechanisms for Therapeutic and Conditioning Exercise. Baltimore: University Park Press, 1976.

# Chapter 16
# Energy Expenditure During Ambulation

ERWIN G. GONZALEZ
PAUL J. CORCORAN

The intricacies involved in the seemingly simple process of walking are never considered until problems occur. As a child attempts to take the first steps, two natural forces, inertia and gravity, make the child stumble forward and fall. But soon enough, the child learns to defy these forces and begins to walk with the fluidity of an adult.[1] Persons with disabilities face similar challenges during the process of regaining their ability to ambulate after an injury or disease that hampers this well-syncopated motion.

Medical rehabilitation requires active participation and work on the part of the patient seeking to regain the capability of ambulating. An effective rehabilitation program must attempt to increase the patient's ability to perform work and concurrently decrease the amount of work required. The former goal is achieved through exercise and rehabilitation training; the latter by judicious use of adaptive devices or environmental manipulation.

## Normal Gait

To comprehend the energy requirements of normal and abnormal ambulation requires an understanding of its basic physiology and biomechanics. Recourse can be made to the classic works by Saunders,[2] Inman,[3] and Eberhart and their coworkers,[4] and by others[5,6] who discuss the major determinants of normal and pathologic gait. Simply put, all the determinants of normal gait result in mini-mizing inertial changes and the vertical and horizontal displacement of the center of gravity. The net effect is a smooth, sinusoidal translation of the center of gravity through space along a path that requires the least energy expenditure. (Ee).

During gait, two main events occur in which energy is consumed. One is in controlling forward movement during deceleration toward the end of swing phase and for shock absorption at heel strike, and the other is in propulsion during push-off, when the center of gravity is propelled up and forward.[7,8] Ironically, more energy is expended to control forward movement than to propel forward.

The fine articulations characteristic of the intact human leg result in a normal gait pattern. If movement occurs only at either end, as in a stick, "compass gait" results, marked by abrupt acceleration and deceleration and unnecessary vertical excursion of the center of gravity by about 3 inches. The six determinants of gait, as described by Saunders and coworkers,[2] explain how cost-efficient ambulation is achieved. *Pelvic rotation, pelvic tilt,* and *knee flexion* all act to flatten the arc through which the center of gravity is translated, with a resultant total amplitude less than 2 inches. Maximal *pelvic rotation* occurs when both legs are on the ground, called the *period of double support*. At this point, the center of gravity drops to its lowest level. With pelvic rotation of 4 degrees in either direction the limbs are essentially lengthened, and the lowest point of the center of gravity pathway is elevated, or its vertical downward excursion is reduced by 3/8 inch. As one limb swings forward (*swing phase*), *pelvic tilt* or drop of 4 degrees occurs on the same side and carries the center of gravity along with it, since it is located midway between the hips, a few centimeters in front of the second sacral vertebra. This results in 3/16 inch reduction of the arc during *midstance* on the opposite leg when the path is at its highest point. The same effect occurs with a 15-degree knee flexion at midstance, which reduces the leg length, reducing the peak of the path by 7/16 inch. These three determinants add up to a 1-inch reduction of the total amplitude, which is less than 2 inches, compared to 3 inches in compass gait. Considering that the path taken by the center of gravity reflects the total body mass or body weight, the energy saving is quite significant.

The fourth and fifth determinants, *knee* and *foot motions,* help minimize the abrupt inflections at the point of intersections of the up-and-down path taken by the center of gravity, producing a smooth, sinusoidal curve instead of an arched pattern. The sixth determinant defines the motion of the *center of gravity in the horizontal plane.* As one moves forward and stands on one leg, the center of gravity shifts to a position over the supporting foot, thus providing stability. If human legs were sticks, to do this, the center of gravity would shift 6 inches to one side and then to the other. Producing this excursion wastes energy. Because of the natural valgus aligment at the knees, however, the feet are closer to the midline. As a result, the center of gravity shifts only 2 inches. The arc in the horizontal plane is also a smooth, sinusoidal curve. In three-dimensional perspective, the vertical and horizontal arcs simulate the figure 8.[3] Figure 16-1 illustrates the path of the center of gravity as it translates through space during ambulation. The more these determinants assume abnormal states, as in locomotor disabilities, the less efficient ambulation becomes, resulting in greater energy expenditure.

Examination of peak muscle activity during ambulation shows that, though muscles contract concentrically, the predominant activities occur during eccentric contraction. As examples, the dorsiflexors lengthen to prevent foot slap, the quadriceps absorb shock and contract eccentrically to allow the knee to bend, and the hamstrings decelerate the limb during the swing phase.[9–11] Eccentric

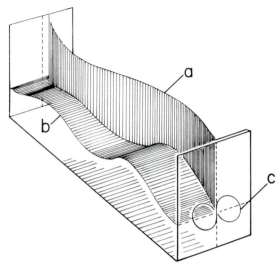

**Figure 16-1.** Path taken by the center of gravity during normal ambulation. Note the sinusoidal curves in both vertical and horizontal planes. In a three-dimensional perspective, the two curves define a figure 8. (Redrawn from Inman VT, Ralston HJ, Todd F. Human Walking. Baltimore, Williams & Wilkins, 1981, with permission.)

contraction is more energy efficient than concentric contraction and demonstrates how the human body has developed kinetically and kinematically to minimize energy cost.

## Energy Sources and Metabolism

Physical activity requires expenditure of energy. Oxygen consumption is most commonly used as a measure of Ee during extended activity such as walking, primarily because the principal energy for such types of activities is supplied through aerobic metabolic pathways.[12] After working about 2 minutes at a constant submaximal level, the body reaches *steady state*. At this point, the level of oxygen consumption meets tissue demands, and the heart beat and respiratory rate become constant. The level of oxygen consumption at steady state closely reflects actual energy cost. The only source of energy that the human body can use is the chemical energy contained in complex food molecules.[13] Oxidation of these to simple substances such as water and carbon dioxide is an exothermic reaction:

$$C_6H_{12}O_6 + 6\,O_2 = 6\,CO_2 + 6\,H_2O +$$
$$686 \text{ K cal/mole} \qquad (1)$$

This overall chemical reaction is the sum of multiple steps, some of which are coupled in the body to other reactions, that produce chemical or physical work. The upper limit of efficiency is determined by the proportion of these steps that can be 'usefully coupled. The real efficiency is actually less than this, as some energy is converted to heat rather than to useful work. At rest, the available work energy is spent to purchase the displacements from equilibrium that are necessary to sustain life. During physical exertion, muscle efficiency rarely exceeds 25% and on average is closer to 20% for level walking, so much of the energy consumed is lost to heat and the rest is used to do external work.

During activity there is interplay between aerobic and anaerobic mechanisms. In *aerobic oxidation* (Krebs' citric acid cycle), carbohydrates and fats provide the primary fuels. These substrates are oxidized through a series of reactions leading to the production of adenosine triphosphate (ATP). Oxygen is the final hydrogen acceptor, and water is formed. The net equation for this cycle, which also involves adenosine diphosphate (ADP), is this:

$$\text{Glucose} + 36\,ADP + 36\,P_1 + 36\,H^+ + 6\,O_2 \rightarrow$$
$$6\,CO_2 + 36\,ATP + 42\,H_2O \qquad (2)$$

The availability of oxygen is not required in the second type of oxidative reaction. In *anaerobic metabolism* (glycolytic pathway) glucose is converted to pyruvate and then to lactic acid (lactate), which is the final hydrogen acceptor. The net equation for this cycle is:

$$\text{Glucose} + 2\,P_1 + 2\,ADP \rightarrow 2\,\text{Lactate} +$$
$$2\,ATP \qquad (3)$$

For activities that require less than 50% of maximal aerobic capacity ($V_{O_2}$ max), the aerobic mechanisms are usually sufficient to supply the energy. For strenuous exercise, however, both mechanisms are called into play. The anaerobic system yields much less energy per unit of glucose than the aerobic mechanism, and its use is limited by a person's tolerance to the resultant lactic acidosis. In daily life, the anaerobic system is used for sudden and short bursts of activity, making it possible for the body to achieve a higher rate of energy production than can be achieved by aerobic oxidation alone. An understanding of the foregoing concepts is a necessary first step to understanding the energy demands ambulation places on persons with disabilities.

## Energy Measurement

### Terminology

*Work* is equal to the product of force and distance. In walking, the *forces* are primarily gravity and friction, plus the inertia of acceleration and deceleration. The *distance* is the up-and-down and side-to-side motions of the body's center of gravity and the separate body segments. To diminish the work required for a task such as walking, the force may be decreased (e.g., using a lighter prosthesis), or the distance may is shortened (e.g., providing knee flexion in a prosthesis to decrease the vertical excursion of the center of gravity). *Power,* on the other hand, is the *rate* of doing work— (force × distance)/time. In handicapped and normal activities, the rate of Ee can be kept tolerable if force and/or distance is decreased, or if the time spent on the task is increased (e.g., by walking more slowly).[13]

Though these concepts are practical, the use of the two terms can be confusing when applied to ambulation. The *work* required for walking is not at all the same as the *Ee per unit distance* of ambulation (kilocalories per meter). Similarly, equating *power* as *Ee per unit time (kilocalories per minute)* is inappropriate, because kilocalories per minute is a measure of energy input per minute of metabolic function, not mechanical force times distance divided by time.[14]

### Units of Measurement

A review of the literature is often confusing, because different authors use different units of measurement. Table 16-1 presents conversion factors for some of the more frequently used units of measure. In this chapter, Ee per unit time is expressed as kilocalories per minute per kilogram and Ee/unit distance is analyzed in terms of kilo-

**Table 16-1.** Equivalent Units of Speed, Energy Expenditure per Unit of Time and Distance

*Units of speed*
1 m/min
= 3.28 ft/min
= 0.037 mph
= 0.06 km/hr
= 0.055 ft/sec
= 0.017 m/sec

*Units of Ee/unit distance (work\*)*
1 kcal (kilocalorie)
= 1000 cal (gram calorie)
= 3086 ft lbs
= 427 kg m
= 3.988 BTU
= 0.00156 hp hr
= 0.00116 kw hr

*Units of Ee/unit time (power\*)*
1 kcal/min
= 1000 cal/min
= 3086 ft lbs/min
= 427 kg m/min
= 69.733 watts (joules sec)
= 3.968 BTU/min
= 0.0935 hp
= 0.0697 kw

\* Though the term is not appropriate for expressing calorie expenditure during ambulation, equivalent values are given for readers' reference. These units are occasionally used in the literature.

**Table 16-2.** Energy Cost of Light Activities in Adults (kcal/min/70 kg)

| Activity | Ee (kcal/min/70 kg) |
|---|---|
| Sleeping | 0.9 |
| Lying quietly | 1 |
| Lying quietly doing mental arithmetic | 1.04 |
| Sitting at ease | 1.2–1.6 |
| Sitting, writing | 1.9–2.2 |
| Standing at ease | 1.4–2.0 |
| Walking, 1 MPH (27 m/min) | 2.3 |
| Standing, washing, and shaving | 2.5–2.6 |
| Standing, dressing, and undressing | 2.3–3.3 |
| Light housework | 1.7–3.0 |
| Heavy housework | 3.0–6.6 |
| Office work | 1.3–2.5 |
| Typing, electric typewriter | 1.13–1.39 |
| Walking 2 mph (54 m/min) | 3.1 |
| Light industrial work | 2.0–5.0 |
| Walking 3 mph (80 m/min) | 4.3 |

## Methods of Measuring Energy Expenditure

### Indirect Calorimetry

Estimation of Ee by measurement of oxygen consumption was introduced by Atwater at the end of the 19th century. Though precise computation of oxygen consumption and carbon dioxide production is not feasible, the technique is the one method most frequently employed in Ee studies. The procedure rests on the knowledge that, after an average diet, a subject at rest in a postprandial steady state generates about *4.83 kcal of energy for every liter of oxygen consumed.*[13] This varies slightly, depending on the specific food in question, as for instance, 5.05 kcal for carbohydrates, 4.74 for fats, 4.46 for proteins, and 4.86 for ethyl alcohol. However, the use of the standard average value of 4.83 kcal/L results in inaccuracies no greater than a few percent in a subject who eats a mixed diet.

Measurement of the oxygen consumption rate under specified resting conditions constitutes the BMR test, formerly used as an index of thyroid function. At rest, body surface area is the body dimension that correlates most accurately with Ee. Surface area is easily predicted from nomograms of height and weight; however, most activities in rehabilitation involve moving all or parts of the

calories per minute per kilogram. For a 70-kg human in normal health the basal metabolic rate (BMR) is approximately 1 kcal/min. This unitary value is convenient for comparing values during various activities for an average-sized adult, which then may be read directly as multiples of the basal rate. In exercise physiology and cardiac rehabilitation, the BMR is sometimes referred to as a metabolic unit, or MET. For untrained persons, an Ee greater than 5 kcal/min, or five times the BMR, results in anaerobic metabolism, which leads to oxygen debt and accumulation of lactic acid. The maximum that a person can sustain for several hours is about 5 kcal/min. This physiologic fact probably sets the limit on ''light'' industrial work or *comfortable walking speed* (CWS). Table 16-2 lists different types of light activities. Several excellent studies, including those of Passmore and Durnin,[15] Brown and Brengelmann,[16] and Gordon,[17] address energy metabolism and units.

body against gravity. During exercise, there is better correlation with the total weight of the subject, plus clothing and adaptive devices worn or carried, than with surface area. Therefore, in this chapter oxygen consumption is expressed per unit of body weight.

In most systems used to measure human oxygen consumption, the expired air is collected and its volume is measured. The concentration of expired oxygen is determined, and the expired volume of oxygen is subtracted from the oxygen in the inspired ambient air, which is 20.93% unless it is altered by environmental changes. The volume is corrected to conditions of standard temperature (37°C), pressure (760 mm Hg), and relative humidity (zero or dry), otherwise referred to as STPD (Figure 16-2).

The simplest method of collecting expired air is in a large floating bell spirometer if the patient is stationary, or in a rubber-impregnated canvas such as the Douglas bag or a neoprene or other nonporous plastic bag if the patient is moving about. The bell spirometer provides a direct read-ing of gas volume. If a bag is used, its contents are later passed through a gas meter to determine the expired volume, and the air is analyzed for oxygen content by chemical or physical means. To avoid variation caused by the specific dynamic action (SDA) of food, metabolic studies are customarily performed on fasting subjects.

Investigators at the Max Planck Institute in Germany in the 1940s developed a small portable respirometer that could be carried on the patient's back like a knapsack. It stored an aliquot of the total expired air in a rubber bladder. This and other similar respirometers permitted many studies of Ee in actual field situations in industry, athletics, and at home.[18,19] Computerized metabolic carts are now available for on-line measurement of oxygen consumption.

Carbon dioxide production also correlates with Ee, but the relationship varies more with dietary differences. In addition, the body's bicarbonate buffer system allows significant amounts of carbon dioxide to be stored during exercise or hypoventilation, causing variations in carbon dioxide output that are unrelated to the instantaneous metabolic level. For this reason, oxygen consumption is simpler to use than carbon dioxide production as an indirect measure of Ee.

### Heart Rate

Heart rate (HR) bears a linear relationship to oxygen consumption and correlates with work measurements such as speed of walking, running, or bicycling in an ergometer. Measurement of HR is simple and requires no special equipment. Though less precise than oxygen consumption determination, HR has often been used as an index of energy consumption in studies in which a large number of observations are more important than accuracy.[12,20–22] Measurement of HR has been suggested as a routine procedure whenever elderly, debilitated, or cardiac patients are given therapeutic exercise.[23] However, in clinical medicine the usefulness of HR as an index of Ee is limited because data upon which the norms are based were derived from studies of high work rates among healthy people, trained athletes, or laborers.

Astrand's nomogram makes possible the prediction of a person's maximum oxygen consump-

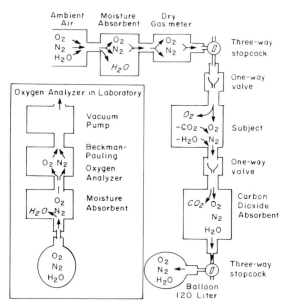

**Figure 16-2.** System used in most oxygen consumption determination (see text). (From Corcoran PJ Brengelmann GL. Oxygen uptake in normal and handicapped subjects, in relation to speed of walking beside velocity-controlled cart. Arch Phys Med Rehabil 1970; 51:78–87, with permission.)

tion for lower extremity exercise. Astand's method is based on heart rate and oxygen consumption during submaximal exercise, multiplied by an age correction factor.[12] In a group of sedentary adults, however, the extrapolation underestimated actual maximum oxygen consumption by 27%[24] The inaccuracy is more remarkable for the smaller workloads that disabled persons typically bear.

At low work levels, HR can vary independently of Ee, being affected by such factors as cardiac disease, drugs, fatigue, emotion, postprandial state, total circulating hemoglobin, hydration, ambient temperature, posture, body build, and percentage of body fat. Thus, HR is of limited value in Ee research, though it does offer a convenient clinical tool, as when one subject's resting and exercise HR are compared to estimate the intensity of exercise or work.

Both HR and blood pressure show a greater increase when a given rate of work is performed by the upper extremities as in crutch walking than with lower extremity activity such as normal walking. This phenomenon is probably due to the fact that when a muscle contracts with a given percentage of its maximum force, the effect on blood pressure is approximately the same as during the same percentage of contraction of any other muscle.[25] Thus, the smaller arm muscles contract more markedly and stimulate the cardiovascular system more than the larger leg muscles doing the same work. This should be borne in mind when patients who have cardiovascular disease are considered for training with hand-held ambulation aids, wheelchair,[26] or any forceful arm and hand exercises. Sustained isometric or static exercise similarly produces a disproportionate cardiovascular response as compared to dynamic or isotonic contraction.[27]

### Pulmonary Ventilation

The pulmonary ventilation rate correlates fairly closely with energy cost at medium workloads, if a predetermined regression line is used for each subject.[28] For long-term recording of pulmonary ventilation to estimate caloric expenditure, a simple flow meter mounted on a face mask can be used.[29] Like heart rate, ventilation rate is useful mainly when the need for simplicity outweighs the need for accuracy.

## Energy Expenditure in Normal Persons

### Rest

The BMR, or resting metabolism per unit of body size, is low at birth, reaches its peak around age 2 years, and declines by 30% during the growing years and by another 10% during adulthood.[30,31] At every age, females tend to have about a 10% lower metabolic rate, whether at rest or during activity. The metabolic rate also increases about 10% for every 1°C rise in body temperature above normal. Cooling the body initiates shivering and also increases BMR, as the body attempts to restore or maintain normal temperature. Extreme shivering can increase the metabolic rate to as much as 6 kcal/min for short periods.[13]

During sleep, the metabolic rate is 5% to 10% lower than BMR, or slightly less than 1 kcal/min for a 70-kg human; sitting and standing at rest require slightly more than 1 kcal/min (see Table 16-2).

### Ambulation

During the past few decades several studies on the energy cost of walking have produced surprisingly similar data (Table 16-3). In 1961, McDonald[32] reviewed world literature for the period 1912 to 1958 and analyzed and tabulated the Ee of walking. Fisher and Gullickson[14] published a similar study in 1978, which also included a tabulation of disabled ambulation. In the same year, Waters and co-workers[33] summarized their experience among normally capable persons and those with disabilities. McDonald's review[32] revealed that the gross Ee at speeds of 60 to 80 m/min varied only slightly. At 80 m/min, the Ee was 0.067 and 0.061 kcal/min/kg for males and females, respectively. The least energy was spent at speeds approximating 80 m/min, or 3 miles per hour (mph), which is the average CWS. The average Ee per unit distance at 80 m/min was $0.830 \text{ kcal} \times 10^{-3}$/m/kg for males and $0.760 \text{ kcal} \times 10^{-3}$/m/kg for females.

**Table 16-3.** Energy Expenditure: Normal Ambulation (Literature) vs Equation 4*

| Author/Year | N | Comment | Speed (m/min) Subject | Difference (%) (normal 80m/min) | Ee/unit time* (kcal/min/kg) Subject | Normal NSSS | Difference (%) | Ee/unit distance (kcal × 10⁻³ /m/kg) Subject | Difference (%) (NCWS 0.786 kcal × 10⁻³/m/kg) |
|---|---|---|---|---|---|---|---|---|---|
| Ralston, 1958 | 19 | M/F CWS | 74 | −8 | 0.058 | 0.0580 | 0 | 0.784 | 0 |
| Bobbert, 1960 | 2 | M† | 81 | 1 | 0.063 | 0.0638 | −1 | 0.778 | −1 |
| McDonald, 1961 | 333 | Review/M | 80 | 0 | 0.067 | 0.0629 | 6 | 0.838 | 7 |
| McDonald, 1961 | 58 | Review/F | 80 | 0 | 0.061 | 0.0629 | −3 | 0.763 | −3 |
| Corcoran, 1970 | 32 | M/F CWS | 83 | 4 | 0.063 | 0.0655 | −4 | 0.759 | −3 |
| Ganguli, 1973 | 16 | M† | 50 | −38 | 0.044 | 0.0423 | 4 | 0.880 | 12 |
| McBeath, 1974 | 10 | M/F CWS | 72 | −10 | 0.066 | 0.0565 | 17 | 0.917 | 17 |
| Imms, 1976 | 8 | Servicemen | 88 | 10 | 0.065 | 0.0700 | −7 | 0.739 | −6 |
| Waters, 1976 | 25 | M/F CWS | 82 | 3 | 0.063 | 0.0646 | −3 | 0.768 | −2 |
| Huang, 1979 | 25 | M/F CWS | 80 | 0 | 0.074 | 0.0629 | 18 | 0.925 | 18 |

\* Equation 4: Ee(kcal/min/kg) = (29 + 0.0053 $V^2$)/1000. [V = Velocity in m/min]
† Speed selected by researcher
NSSS = Normal, same speed as test subjects
NCWS = Normal, CWS of 80m/min
CWS = Comfortable walking speed
Key: M, male; F, female.

Heavy persons use more energy walking at a given speed, but when corrected for their weight plus that of clothing and any equipment carried, their metabolic rate is similar to that of normal-weight subjects. Age and height have no effect, but in most studies females usually show about 10% less Ee at a given speed. Ralston,[34] however, did not find significant difference between the sexes, and Waters[33] found the reverse.

The energy cost of walking rises more steeply as speed increases. This relationship is curvilinear (Figure 16-3B). At higher speeds, a given increment in speed necessitates a greater increase in oxygen consumption than at slower speeds. Ralston[34] derived an equation to calculate energy cost of ambulation (V = velocity in meters per minute):

$$Ee \ (kcal/min/kg) = (29 + 0.0053 \ V^2) / 1000 \quad (4)$$

Given this equation, Ee can be easily calculated per unit time or unit distance, and the results vary only slightly from those quoted by other authors (see Table 16-3) Similar second-order regression equations have been published by Bobbert[35] and by Corcoran and Brengelmann.[36] In this chapter,

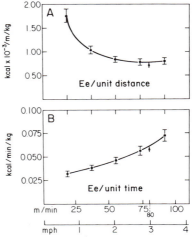

**Figure 16-3.** Ee per unit distance (A) decreases to a minimum at about 80 m/min, the normal average CWS. However, the energy expenditure per unit time (B) increases steadily as walking speed increases. Both curves express the relationship: speed = Ee per unit time/Ee per unit distance. The normal values shown in these curves, and used in this chapter, are derived from equation 4: (29 + 0.0053 $V^2$)/1000. The normal values at the CWS of 80 m/min = 0.063 kcal/min and 0.000786 kcal/m. The dumbells indicate one standard deviation above and below the mean.[36]

equation 4 is be used for comparative purposes; it produces these normal values for Ee at CWS:

$$\text{Speed (80 m/min)} = \frac{\text{Ee/unit time (0.063 kcal/min)}}{\text{Ee/unit distance (0.000786 kcal/m)}} \quad (5)$$

The Ee per unit distance is greater at very slow speeds than at ordinary walking speeds and greater again at faster speeds. Figure 16-3A shows once again that the calorie cost of walking a given distance is lowest at around 80 m/min, the CWS.

The biomechanical and physiologic explanations for the most efficient speed of ambulation are not entirely clear. It seems that human neuro-musculoskeletal development has evolved a CWS at which the major determinants of gait are most effective, whereas the metabolic apparatus chooses one with the most economical calorie cost, which does not exceed the 5 kcal/min limit for sustained work without going into oxygen debt. The level of Ee is approximately equal when Ee values per unit time are compared for a person with disability walking at a slower speed and a normally capable person walking at normal CWS (NCWS) of 80 m/min. This implies that in order to remain within the 5 kcal/min limit, a person with disability compensates by walking slower. The Ee per unit time and Ee per unit distance are frequently greater in such a person than in a *normal* person who is walking at the *same speed* as the *subject* with disability (*NSSS*). Because the harsh reality of life is that the world does not slow down for people with disabilities, it is impractical to use this type of comparison, though it is commonly used in the literature.

Most investigators believe that *Ee per unit distance* walked is the *true net energy cost* and the best basis for comparing gait efficiency between normal and abnormal ambulation.[34,37,38] This is particularly true if the Ee per unit distance at the speed chosen by a person with disability is matched against the Ee per unit distance calculated at the NCWS. With this approach, the magnitude of difference between normal and disabled walking can be fully appreciated. For example, the total amount of calories consumed by a person with disability who walks a total distance of 30 m at a speed of 60 m/min can be compared with the calorie consumption of an intact person who walks

the same distance but at a normal CWS of 80 m/min. Under this circumstance, the Ee for disabled ambulation is almost always greater than that for normal walking. Like their able-bodied counterpart, persons with disabilities also tend to select a walking speed at which the work of walking a given distance is minimal.[13] This optimal speed may not be achievable if the disability is very severe so that the energy cost exceeds 5 kcal/min, or if cardiovascular or respiratory capacity is diminished.[38]

The upper limit of normal walking speed is 5 to 6 mph or 135 to 160 m/min. At speeds in excess of 135 m/min the energy cost of running is less than that of walking. At slower speeds, walking requires less energy than running.[39] The curve of the energy cost of running at various speeds, if superimposed on the nonlinear curve for walking in Figure 16-3A, intersects the walking curve near the speed of approximately 135 m/min (Figure 16-4). Having patients run on a speed-controlled treadmill provides a way to administer precise doses of work for a cardiovascular reconditioning program.

The energy cost of walking on a 10% to 12% grade is approximately twice the Ee of walking on level ground. On a 20% to 25% upgrade, the cost is tripled. On downgrades the Ee is lowest at a

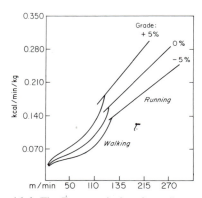

**Figure 16-4.** The Ėe per unit time for ordinary walking rises sharply at speeds faster than approximately 135 m/min, and running becomes less demanding than walking. Note that the relationship of Ee to speed is nearly linear for running. The limit to running speeds is set by the maximum aerobic capacity that the subject can attain. (After Margaria R, et al. Energy cost of running. J Appl Physiol 1963; 18:367–370, with permission.)

10% grade and rises again on steeper down slopes.[39]

Adding extra body weight, clothing, or adaptive devices to the subject causes a linear increase in the energy cost of walking. Added loads are carried most efficiently on the head, somewhat less efficiently on the back, still less so in the hands, and least efficiently on the feet.[40] The addition of 2-1/2 lbs to shoe weight can increase the Ee by 5% to 10%. This may be due to the gravitational force exerted during the up-and-down excursion of the feet during the gait cycle and to the greater mass that must be accelerated and decelerated at the end of the limb. The implications for prosthetic and orthotic design are obvious.[13] Soft or uneven ground can increase energy demands by 40% or more, and wearing 3-inch high heels by 10% to 15%.

## Levels of Activity Measured by Magnitude of Energy Cost

The energy demands placed on a person during different levels of activity and during ambulation require discussion. This topic is important because of the frequent coexistence of deconditioning and cardiovascular disease among people with disabilities who are undertaking rehabilitation. A semi-quantitative continuum from light to hard work is useful in rehabilitation.[17] Such a frame of reference for energy consumption for the patients provides the physician basic guidelines upon which to make decisions on activity levels. Metabolic demands of more than 5 kcal/min are impossible for an average-sized, untrained adult to sustain without intervals of rest. This level is equivalent to oxygen uptake of 1 to 1.25 L/min. Table 16-4

lists the grades of work as proposed by Christensen.[41] This classification is based on intermittent work, which is more realistic in real-life situations. More than 55 years ago, the League of Nations developed criteria for continuous activities.[42] The energy cost in this classification is only about half that recommended by Christensen. Figure 16-5 defines the levels of physical activity as well as the functional and therapeutic cardiac classifications plotted against the rate of Ee in normal ambulation, an experience most persons can relate to. The graph can be used to plot the Ee of ambulation for different types of disabilities, providing a sensible perception of what patients go through when ambulating. This is particularly relevant because in many disabilities deconditioning and cardiovascular disease are often associated factors.

## Energy Expenditure with Disability

It would be ideal if all the information provided in this section were precise; however, the search of the literature and our experience in the laboratory indicate that, at best, the values quoted are approximations. Clearly, there is inherent difficulty in studying a large cohort of subjects with disabilities who can ambulate at a constant speed for at least 4 minutes. The actual values given by researchers will be quoted with reference to speed of ambulation and oxygen consumption, with units of energy expenditure recalculated as kilocalories per minute per kilogram and kilocalories per meter per kilogram. Despite obvious shortcomings, for the sake of uniformity, comparison of Ee with normally capable subjects will be calculated in keeping with equation 4:[34]

$$Ee \ (kcal/min/kg) = (29 + 0.0053 \ V^2) \ / \ 1000 \quad (4)$$

**Table 16-4.** Work (Intermittent) Classification by Magnitude of Energy Cost[15,17]

| Classification | Ee (kcal/min/70kg) | Example |
|---|---|---|
| Light | 2.6–4.9 | Mixing cement |
| Moderate | 5.0–7.5 | Shovelling 8-kg load |
| Heavy | 7.6–10.0 | Splitting wood |
| Very heavy | 10.1–12.5 | Carrying 20 lbs upstairs |
| Extraordinarily heavy | ≥12.5 | Carrying 60 lbs upstairs |

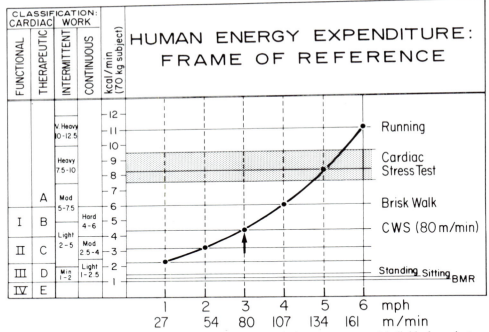

**Figure 16-5.** A frame of reference compares the Ee per unit time among normal individuals against levels of work and cardiac classification. The diagram can be used to plot the level of energy expenditure of walking and other activities among disabled and normal persons.

where V is velocity in meters per minute. This equation yields the closest approximate Ee value across several reported studies (see Table 16-3). The NCWS is considered at 80 m/min. If comparisons are made between *normally capable subjects* at the *same speed* as *subjects* with disabilities, these are indicated as *NSSS*.

### Immobilization of Body Segments

Immobilization and deformity of the joints of the trunk and lower extremities interfere with the harmonious movements of gait. Ralston[43] studied the effects of immobilizing various body segments during locomotion and when the arms were taped to the sides. He found no significant change. The Ee per unit time increased by a factor of 6% when one ankle was immobilized, rising to 9% when both were immobilized and the subject walked at a CWS of 73 m/min. The major role played by the knee joint is emphasized by the disproportionate increase of 37% in Ee when the knee was

restricted at 135 degrees. Keeping the joint at 180 degrees resulted in 13% rise in Ee. In the optimal angle of immobilization of 165 degrees, the added demands rose by only 10%. Immobilization of the hip at 180 degrees also resulted in a 13% rise in Ee, but at 150 degrees this dropped to 6%. Torso immobilization caused an increase of 10% over a wide range of speeds.

Waters and coworkers[44] immobilized 20 young, healthy subjects with a plaster cast on the predominant limb. All were placed in a long-leg cast, and 10 each in a cylinder or a short-leg cast. Although no significant increases in the average rate of Ee were noted between types of casts when the subjects walked with bearing full weight without crutches, the velocity of ambulation significantly decreased in proportion to the extent of immobilization. While the Ee per unit time became progressively higher in proportion to the level of immobilization, the differences were not statistically significant when compared to NSSS, despite a 14% to 34% increase. The net energy cost was consistently higher than NCWS, by 17% and 49%.

The increase in HR with all types of casts was also significantly higher than would be expected in normal walking.

### Lower Extremity Amputations

More knowledge is available on the energy cost of ambulation with lower extremity amputations than for any other type of disability. Though published data vary in the number of subjects, speed of ambulation, types of prosthesis worn, and technique of Ee determination, adequate information is available to make valid conclusions about the energy demands resulting from amputations.

This disability is unique in the sense that a body part is actually missing and replaced by an external device. Despite innovative approaches in the design of prosthetic replacements, the muscles that supply the power and the joints that sense position and load in the limb are no longer present. The higher the level of amputation, the more gait deviations occur, with resultant rises in energy cost.

### Symes' Amputation

Waters and coworkers[38] studied 15 vascular Symes' amputees and found their CWS to be 54 m/min, or 33% slower than normal. The Ee per unit time was 24% greater than for NSSS, while the work per unit distance was 30% greater at the amputees' slower speed, as compared to NCWS. These results are not significantly different from those of below-knee (BK) amputees.

### Below-Knee Amputation

Sufficient information exists in the literature to allow reasonable assumptions to be made regarding the energy demands imposed by BK amputation (Table 16-5). In 1955, Reitmeyer[45] reported his findings on two subjects who reportedly walked an average of 60 m/min, or 25% slower than an average person. The calculation for Ee per unit time and distance could be in error, as the values derived were unexpectedly lower than normal. Ralston[37] also studied two patients whom he directed to walk at the rate of 49 m/min. At this speed the Ee was 0.055 kcal/min/kg, which is slightly less than the Ee at NCWS. This rate of walking was less efficient, though: Ee per unit distance was higher by 43%. Molen[46] and Ganguli and coworkers[47] chose to walk their traumatic BK volunteers at a speed of 50m/min, and their Ee findings were in close agreement with Ralston's.[37]

Gonzalez and associates[48] determined oxygen

**Table 16-5.** Energy Expenditure: Below-Knee Amputation

| Author/Year | N | Comment | Speed (m/min) Subject | Difference (%) (normal 80m/min) | Ee/unit time* (kcal/min/kg) Subject | Normal NSSS | Difference (%) NSSS | NCWS (80m/min) | Ee/unit distance (kcal × 10⁻³/m/kg) Subject | Difference (%) (NCWS 0.786 kcal × 10⁻³/m/kg) |
|---|---|---|---|---|---|---|---|---|---|---|
| Reitmeyer, 1955 | 2 | Trauma | 60 | −25 | 0.035 | 0.0481 | −27 | −44 | 0.583 | −26 |
| Ralston, 1971 | 2 | BK | 49 | −39 | 0.055 | 0.0417 | 32 | −13 | 1.122 | 43 |
| Molen, 1973 | 54 | Trauma | 50 | −38 | 0.066 | 0.0423 | 56 | 5 | 1.320 | 68 |
| Ganguli, 1973 | 20 | Trauma | 50 | −38 | 0.060 | 0.0423 | 42 | −5 | 1.200 | 53 |
| Gonzalez, 1974 | 9 | Trauma/PVD | 64 | −20 | 0.062 | 0.0507 | 22 | −2 | 0.969 | 23 |
| Waters, 1976 | 13 | PVD | 45 | −44 | 0.056 | 0.0397 | 41 | −11 | 1.244 | 58 |
| Waters, 1976 | 14 | Trauma | 71 | −11 | 0.074 | 0.0557 | 33 | 17 | 1.042 | 33 |
| Pagliarulo, 1979 | 15 | Trauma/congen | 71 | −11 | 0.074 | 0.0557 | 33 | 17 | 1.042 | 33 |
| Huang, 1979 | 6 | BK | 48 | −40 | 0.048 | 0.0412 | 16 | −24 | 1.000 | 27 |
| Nielsen, 1989 | 2 | FlexFoot | 80 | 0 | 0.078 | 0.0629 | 24 | 24 | 0.975 | 24 |
| Waters, 1976 | 15 | Vascular Symes' | 54 | −33 | 0.055 | 0.0445 | 24 | −13 | 1.019 | 30 |

\* Equation 4: Ee(kcal/min/kg) = (29 + 0.0053 $V^2$)/1000. [V = Velocity in m/min]
Key: PVD, peripheral vascular disease; congen, congenital amputation.

consumption among nine BK amputees whose average age was 58 years. They measured the length of the residual limb and found a negative correlation between length and energy cost, but none with speed of ambulation. The average self-selected CWS was 64 m/min, 20% slower than normal. At this speed, the Ee per unit time (0.062 kcal/min) was practically equal to NCWS but 22% higher than for NSSS (Figure 16-6). Similarly, the Ee per unit distance was higher by a factor of 23% than that for NCWS. Like that of their normal counterparts, the CWS of BK amputees coincided with the speed of maximum efficiency (Figure 16-7). The authors emphasized the importance of preserving residual limb length in order to minimize the rise in Ee.

Waters and colleagues[38] investigated 13 vascular and 14 traumatic BK amputees. The vascular group, whose average age was 63 years, chose to walk 44% slower; the "traumatic BKs," who were considerably younger, walked only 11% slower than normal. At their chosen CWS, their rate of oxygen consumption per minute remained within normal range for the vascular and traumatic groups, though the Ee per unit distance in comparison with NCWS rose 58% and 33%, respectively. Pagliarulo and colleagues[49] elaborated further on these traumatic BK amputees and reiterated

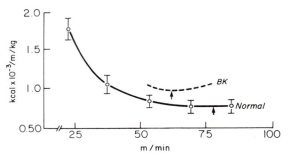

**Figure 16-7.** Comparison of Ee *per unit distance* between normal and BK amputees. The dumbells indicate one standard deviation. The arrows indicate CWSs, which coincide with speed of maximum efficiency for both normal subjects and amputees. (Redrawn from Gonzalez EG, et al. Ee in below-knee amputees: Correlation with stump length. Arch Phys Med Rehabil 1974; 55:111–118, with permission.)

the importance of allowing amputees to choose their own speed. They also found a significant rise in HR and Ee per unit time when comparing ambulation with axillary crutches without prosthesis and prosthesis walking. Huang[50] also reported findings approximately similar to those of the studies cited here.

**Stair Climbing and Load Carrying with a Below-Knee Prosthesis.** All of the studies previously mentioned were performed on level ground. Ganguli and coworkers[47,51–53] studied a group of young BK amputees as they climbed 127 steps with 14.2 cm risers for a vertical ascent of 18 m. Normal control subjects spent 0.0776 kcal/min/kg; the subjects spent 9% more. The same group applied similar technique to studying the effect of load carrying on a cohort of five left-side BK amputees. The subject and control groups carried loads of 7.5 kg on level ground and up stairs. As expected, the subjects consumed more energy than the controls—47% more. Contrary to what might be expected, the side on which the load was carried did not make any statistically significant difference in Ee. The effect of asymmetry, however, appears to be a factor in the rise in energy cost: BK subjects fare better carrying a load in each hand. The results of stair climbing were difficult to assess in view of the varying rates of ascent. This study is important in demonstrating that BK amputees can perform work levels of up to 6.5 kcal/min, a mod-

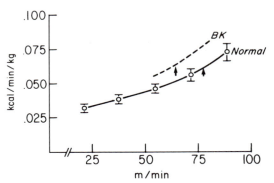

**Figure 16-6.** A comparison of curves of Ee *per unit time* between normal subjects and BK amputees. The dumbells indicate one standard deviation. The arrows indicate CWS. Note that the energy cost at these two speeds are approximately equal, meaning that a BK amputee spends as much energy walking at a slower speed as normal subjects do at the CWS of 80 m/min. (Redrawn from Gonzalez EG, et al. Energy expenditure in below-knee amputees: Correlation with stump length. Arch Phys Med Rehabil 1974; 55:111–118, with permission.)

erate level of intermittent work. This information is useful in vocational rehabilitation.

**Prosthesis Design.** Despite myriad traditional as well as technologically advanced designs in prosthetic components, very little is known about their effects on energy cost of ambulation. Cummings and coauthors[54] studied the Ee difference between the use of supracondylar cuff suspension and the thigh corset among 17 newly amputated, untrained subjects. They found no statistically significant difference in Ee, disproving the commonly held notion that the lighter weight of the cuff suspension, or the more secure suspension provided by the thigh corset, reduces the energy demand. Half the subjects were retested after a week of prosthetic training. As anticipated, speed of ambulation increased while Ee decreased.

In a recent report, Nielsen and coworkers[55] compared energy cost and gait efficiency during ambulation in BK amputees using the SACH foot and in three active, physically fit amputees using the Flex-Foot. Seven other subjects, briefly mentioned in the study, walked at 71.4 and 77.8 m/min, using the SACH and the dynamic foot, respectively. Of particular interest in this study is the lower Ee observed with higher walking velocities using the Flex-Foot. The decrease was most noticeable at speeds of 70 to 80 m/min and was negligible at slower speeds. MacFarlane and coworkers[56] attributed the difference in performance using the dynamic foot to the increase in the time subjects were willing to spend in single support, which resulted in smoother vertical trunk motion and greater biomechanical efficiency. The study done by Wagner and colleagues[57] is the only one that does not report any difference in speed of ambulation between subjects using the Flex-Foot and the SACH foot.

*Above-Knee Amputation*

Surgeons who are less willing to risk the morbidity of delayed wound healing often opt for above-knee (AK) amputation. While this may prove most efficacious in the short term, the long-term ambulatory consequence is a gamble, particularly for aged and more debilitated patients.

Encouraging reports were published between the 1950s and early 1970s on the walking speed and energy cost of ambulation among AK amputees. Muller and Hettinger,[58] and Erdman[59] and Inman and their colleagues[60] reported the slower speed selected by their subjects but recorded lower than normal Ee. This would lead to the unlikely conclusion that it becomes easier to walk after losing a leg. More recent studies have not supported this supposition (Table 16-6). Bard and Ralston[61] studied six amputees but elaborated on only one case. In a subsequent report, Ralston[37] elected to study one subject walking at 49 m/min and found a 27% increase in Ee per unit distance versus NCWS, though the rate of oxygen consumption was within normal range.

Later studies were more consistent with what is apparent in the clinical setting. Ganguli and coworkers[62] studied six young amputees and reported on four who completed the study. The researchers chose the speed of 50 m/min, and the recorded caloric cost of 0.088 kcal/min/kg was 108% higher than NSSS, and 40% higher compared to an intact person walking at the usual CWS. The Ee per unit distance rose by 124% when compared to NCWS. These values are somewhat high, and the subjects fell into oxygen debt sooner than anticipated.

Waters,[38] Huang,[50] Bard and Ralston,[61] Traugh,[63] James,[64] and Otis[65] all reported in their studies that the Ee per unit time fell within the normal range. In other words, their subjects chose to ambulate at a slower speed at which the rate of Ee was more or less equivalent to NCWS (0.063 kcal/min/kg). The Ee per unit distance, the index of efficiency, reveals an increase of between 52% and 116%.

**Locked versus Unlocked Prosthetic Knee.** Traugh and coworkers[63] studied nine middle-aged or elderly AK amputees in an effort to determine the mode of ambulation that required the least energy. They found the CWS among the amputees to be 51% slower. The Ee per unit time was 65% higher than NSSS (Figure 16-8). Like other disabled ambulators, the subjects apparently chose to walk more slowly to keep their rate of Ee close to NCWS (0.063 kcal/min/kg). Compared to NCWS, however, the Ee per unit distance rose by 99%, and the subjects were not able to walk fast enough to achieve the most efficient speed (Figure 16-9).

**Table 16-6.** Energy Expenditure: Above-Knee Amputation

| Author/Year | N | Comment | Speed (m/min) | | Ee/unit time* (kcal/min/kg) | | | | Ee/unit distance (kcal × 10⁻³ /m/kg) | |
|---|---|---|---|---|---|---|---|---|---|---|
| | | | Subject | Difference (%) (normal 80m/min) | Subject | Normal NSSS | Difference (%) NSSS | NCWS (80m/min) | Subject | Difference (%) (NCWS 0.786 kcal ×10⁻³/m/kg) |
| Muller, 1952 | 2 | AK | 70 | −13 | 0.053 | 0.0550 | −4 | −16 | 0.757 | −4 |
| Muller, 1952 | 1 | AK | 40 | −50 | 0.023 | 0.0375 | −39 | −63 | 0.575 | −27 |
| Bard/Ralston, 1959 | 6 | AK | 68 | −15 | 0.061 | 0.0535 | 14 | −3 | 0.897 | 14 |
| Erdman, 1960 | 9 | AK | 47 | −41 | 0.035 | 0.0407 | −14 | −44 | 0.745 | −5 |
| Inman, 1961 | 1 | AK | 62 | −23 | 0.017 | 0.0494 | −66 | −73 | 0.274 | −65 |
| Ralston, 1971 | 1 | AK | 49 | −39 | 0.049 | 0.0417 | 17 | −22 | 1.000 | 27 |
| James, 1973 | 37 | Trauma | 51 | −36 | 0.061 | 0.0428 | 43 | −3 | 1.196 | 52 |
| Ganguli, 1974 | 6 | Lock free | 50 | −38 | 0.088 | 0.0423 | 108 | 40 | 1.760 | 124 |
| Traugh, 1975 | 9 | AK | 39 | −51 | 0.061 | 0.0371 | 65 | −3 | 1.564 | 99 |
| Waters, 1976 | 13 | PVD | 36 | −55 | 0.061 | 0.0359 | 70 | −3 | 1.694 | 116 |
| Waters, 1976 | 15 | Trauma | 52 | −35 | 0.062 | 0.0433 | 43 | −2 | 1.192 | 52 |
| Huang, 1979 | 6 | AK | 47 | −41 | 0.062 | 0.0407 | 52 | −2 | 1.319 | 68 |
| Isakov, 1983 | 3 | Free knee | 66 | −18 | 0.088 | 0.0521 | 69 | 40 | 1.333 | 70 |
| Isakov, 1983 | 3 | Lock knee | 61 | −24 | 0.081 | 0.0487 | 66 | 29 | 1.328 | 69 |
| Otis, 1985 | 5 | AK-tumor | 52 | −35 | 0.069 | 0.0433 | 59 | 10 | 1.327 | 69 |

* Equation 4: $Ee(kcal/min/kg) = (29 + 0.0053 \, V^2)/1000$. [V = Velocity in m/min]
Key: Lock free, locked and free prosthetic knee; PVD, peripheral vascular disease.

Values obtained using crutches without prosthesis were about the same, though HR was faster. No statistical difference was found between ambulating with a locked and an unlocked knee; however, a significant reduction (7%) was noted when subjects walked with the knee setting they customarily preferred. On the other hand, wheelchair propulsion imposed an increase only of 9% above NSSS.

Isakov and colleagues[66] elaborated further on the differences in Ee in ambulation with a locked and an unlocked knee. A total of 14 vascular amputees older than 50 years and three young traumatic amputees were studied. In both groups, ambulation with a locked knee resulted in a smaller increase in heart rate. The older group walked faster with the locked knee, whereas the younger group fared better with the unlocked knee. Oxygen consumption was determined only among the younger group. Despite the higher metabolic cost of ambulating with an unlocked knee, the younger group preferred the setting owing to their better physical condition, which enabled them to walk faster, and thus more efficiently.

**Traumatic versus Vascular Amputation.** James[64] reported on the metabolic cost of ambulation among 37 traumatic amputees and reported an average CWS of 51 m/min, or a 36% reduction in speed. However, the Ee per unit distance was 52% greater than NCWS, though the rate of oxygen consumption at the slower speeds fell within the normal range. Among six similarly young amputees, Huang's group[50] reported the same results, except that the Ee/unit distance was 68% higher. James' values[64] were replicated by those obtained by Waters and colleagues[38] in their study of 15 young traumatic amputees. However, in a group of 13 older vascular amputees, speed slowed to 36 m/min, or 55% slower, while the Ee per unit distance rose 116% relative to NCWS. Waters and colleagues[38] also calculated the *relative energy cost* (rate of oxygen uptake divided by the subject's maximum aerobic capacity). The relative cost among the vascular amputees was found to be 63%, in contrast to 35% among the younger subjects. The authors emphasized the fact that activity requiring greater than 50% of maximum

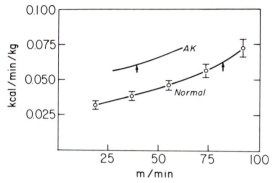

**Figure 16-8.** Comparative curves of Ee *per unit time* between normal and AK subjects. The dumbells indicate one standard deviation. The arrows indicate CWS. The energy cost at these CWSs are approximately equal, meaning that an AK amputee spends as much energy walking at a slow pace as normal subjects do at the CWS of 80 m/min. (Redrawn from Traugh G, et al. Energy expenditure of ambulation in patients with above-knee amputation. Arch Phys Med Rehabil 1975; 56:67–71, with permission.)

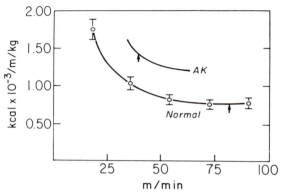

**Figure 16-9.** Ee *per unit distance* for normal subjects and AK amputees. The dumbells indicate one standard deviation. The arrows indicate CWSs, which coincide with speed of maximum efficiency for normal persons. Note that the amputees could not comfortably walk fast enough to reach their most efficient speed. (Redrawn from Traugh G, et al. Energy expenditure of ambulation in patients with above-knee amputation. Arch Phys Med Rehabil 1975; 56:67–71, with permission.)

aerobic capacity results in anaerobic metabolism and resulting loss of endurance. They noted that this finding is corroborated by their clinical experience that fewer than 10% of such patients were initially fitted with a prosthesis and fewer than 50% of those fitted walk enough to qualify for their study.

## Resection En Bloc and Knee Replacement versus AK Amputation.

Emphasis on the importance of restoring lower extremity function in patients with tumor about the knee has been enhanced by the 80% 3-year disease-free survival rate for patients with osteogenic sarcoma.[65] Otis and coworkers[65] examined 14 patients treated with complete surgical resection of the sarcomatous knee (en bloc resection) and knee replacement as well as twelve who underwent AK amputation for osteogenic sarcoma. Those with en bloc resection walked significantly faster (14%) than their AK counterparts. The en bloc resection group also did better than the AK amputees with regard to Ee per unit distance and relative energy cost. Five subjects from each group were tested early (6 to 12 months postoperatively) and again later (18 to 30 months postoperatively). The en bloc patients reached an early plateau of maximum performance

after 6 months; the AK subjects improved slowly for up to 2.5 years, perhaps as a result of continued experience and training in the use of the prosthesis. At their best, the en bloc resection group had a 50% increase in Ee per unit distance, as compared to 69% increase among the AK amputees. A distinct difference between this group of young amputees and those with traumatic amputation is their lower maximal aerobic capacity (and, thus, higher relative energy cost) which is perhaps attributable to the effect chemotherapy has on the myocardium. The study advocated the en bloc procedure, in view of the short-term superior performance along with the psychological and cosmetic advantages over AK amputation.

**Load Carrying.**  In a study of six young trauma amputees, Roy and collaborators[67] tested their subjects walking on level ground at a speed of 50 m/min, with and without extra loads on their shoulders of 5, 10, and 15 kg. As expected, oxygen consumption, peak heart rate, and pulmonary ventilation values were higher in the test group. From an ergonomic viewpoint, the authors found what might ordinarily be considered as light work becomes hard or very hard work among AK amputees and encroached much on their physical reserves. For instance, a load of 5 kg caused a mean Ee of 0.089 kcal/min/kg, or 6.23 kcal/min for a 70-kg man; this falls in the category of moderately hard intermittent work. A load of 15 kg increases the Ee to 0.118 kcal/min/kg (8.26 kcal/min for an average-sized person), which falls in the classification of heavy work. The energy cost for the same task for nonamputees was within the category of light intermittent work. The vocational implications are self-evident.

## Hip Disarticulation and Hemipelvectomy Amputation.

Eight patients with hip disarticulation (HD) and 10 with hemipelvectomy (Hp) were investigated by Nowroozi and coworkers.[68] The HD group walked 41% slower than the average 80 m/min and the Hp amputees 51% slower. At this speed, the Ee per unit time rose 30% and 47% for HD and Hp, respectively, as opposed to NSSS. The Ee per unit distance rose 43% and 75% for HD and Hp, respectively, as compared to NCWS. The study also demonstrated that for this group of patients, prosthesis use was more demanding than the use of axillary crutches without a prosthesis. The fine performance of this group of patients, as compared to the AK subjects in the study of Otis and colleagues[65] could be attributed to their physical fitness and to the fact that none had been receiving chemotherapy or radiotherapy for at least 6 months before the study.

### Bilateral Amputations

**Bilateral Below-Knee Amputation.** Meager information is available on Ee among bilateral amputees (Table 16-7). In an unpublished work, Corcoran and associates,[69] (cited by Gonzalez's group[48]) reported a 20% reduction in speed of ambulation (64 m/min) and a 41% rise in Ee per unit distance among a group of bilateral BK (BK-BK) amputees. Like the unilateral BK subjects, they chose the most efficient CWS. At this CWS, the BK-BK subjects spent slightly more Ee per unit time than NCWS.

DuBow and others[70] investigated six elderly BK-BK patients. Their subjects chose a CWS of 40 m/min, a 50% reduction from the norm; however, their own control group walked only an average of 62.5 m/min and thus reported a 36% reduction in speed. At 40 m/min, the test group consumed exactly the same amount of calories as would NSSS at 0.037 kcal/kg. The rise in Ee per unit distance, compared to their normal controls' CWS of 62.5 m/min, was reported at 123%. This inordinate increase could be attributed to an error in technique or to a miscalculation. Clinical experience also disproves the reported 123% rise. If this were true, most BK-BK amputees would be functionally worse off than unilateral AK amputees, yet most bilateral BK patients outperform them. If a comparison had been made against nor-

**Table 16-7.** Energy Expenditure: Double Amputation and Other Levels

| Author/Year | N | Comment | Speed (m/min) Subject | Speed (m/min) Difference (%) (normal 80m/min) | Ee/unit time* (kcal/min/kg) Subject | Ee/unit time* (kcal/min/kg) Normal NSSS | Ee/unit time* Difference (%) NSSS | Ee/unit time* Difference (%) NCWS (80m/min) | Ee/unit distance (kcal × 10⁻³ /m/kg) Subject | Ee/unit distance Difference (%) (NCWS 0.786 kcal × 10⁻³/m/kg) |
|---|---|---|---|---|---|---|---|---|---|---|
| Gonzalez, 1974 | 5 | BK-BK | 64 | −20 | 0.071 | 0.0507 | 40 | 13 | 1.109 | 41 |
| Dubow, 1983 | 6 | BK-BK, PVD | 40 | −50 | 0.037 | 0.0375 | −1 | −41 | 0.925 | 18 |
| Huang, 1979 | 4 | AK-AK | 23 | −71 | 0.065 | 0.0318 | 104 | 3 | 2.826 | 260 |
| Corcoran, 1971 | 2 | AK-AK | 32 | −60 | 0.072 | 0.0344 | 109 | 14 | 2.250 | 186 |
| Corcoran, 1971 | 2 | AK-BK | 35 | −56 | 0.060 | 0.0355 | 69 | −5 | 1.714 | 118 |
| Nowroozi, 1983 | 8 | HD, Tumor | 47 | −41 | 0.053 | 0.0407 | 30 | −16 | 1.128 | 43 |
| Nowroozi, 1983 | 10 | Hp, Tumor | 40 | −50 | 0.055 | 0.0375 | 47 | −13 | 1.375 | 75 |

* Equation 4: $Ee(kcal/min/kg) = (29 + 0.0053 V^2)/1000$. [V = Velocity in m/min]
Key: PVD, peripheral vascular disease

mal values obtained from equation 4, the rise in Ee per unit distance would have been 18%; however, this value is unusually low. The authors commented on the poor physical status of their test group, reporting that most died or became nonambulatory within a year of the study. They also noted technical difficulties with their automated equipment.

**Above-Knee–Below-Knee Amputation.** Corcoran's group[69] studied a small group of AK-BK patients and found their CWS to be 35 m/min or 56% slower than 80 m/min norm, and they observed a 69% rise in calorie expenditure and 118% increase in net cost compared to NCWS. There are no published papers on AK-BK amputation to verify the information.

**Bilateral Above-Knee Amputation.** Huang's group[50] reported findings on four bilateral AK amputees (AK-AK), three of whom completed the study. The speed chosen by the subjects was 23 m/min, 71% slower than normal. At this speed, the Ee per unit distance is 260% higher than for NCWS. Findings of this study compared favorably with those of Corcoran's group,[69] who reported that their subjects slowed their pace by 60% but increased the Ee per unit distance by only 186%.

A single AK-AK amputee subject was examined by Crouse and others[71] to determine the cardiac and metabolic response in ambulating with regular long-leg prostheses (LLPs) as opposed to short-leg prostheses (SLPs or "stubbies"). The subject and three controls were exercised on a treadmill at increasing velocities of 38 to 80 m/min at 0% elevation for a total of 12 minutes. The subject was able to exercise for a longer period (27%) while using the SLPs. The mean energy cost was 23% higher for the LLPs than for the SLPs, and 80% higher than the cost recorded for the normal controls. Compared to the Ee rate recorded for the normal subjects, the amputee's rate of Ee was higher by 45% with the stubbies. With both types of prosthesis, the patient's heart rate rose above normal: 33% higher with SLPs and 52% higher with LLPs. Despite advantages of the SLP, the patient preferred the LLPs because they offered greater social acceptance.

*Crutch Walking for Amputees*

The question often arises why an amputee should walk with a prosthesis when crutches are available as an alternative. Several studies[38,59,63,68,72] have compared the metabolic demands of using crutches with and without a prosthesis to those of normal ambulation (Table 16-8). In general, these authors found that amputees walking with crutches but without a prosthesis chose to walk slower than normal (39 to 71 m/min) but the energy consumption per unit time was more or less equal or somewhat lower when compared to the rate of expenditure at NCWS. A distinct exception was a group of young traumatic BK amputees in the study by Waters' group,[38] who walked at 71 m/min and spent considerably more energy than any other group. As expected, at the amputees' slower speed, the Ee per unit distance was less efficient than normal. Table 16-8 shows that the subjects could have adjusted their speed to coincide with the maximum level of efficiency.

Interesting insights come to light when crutch walking without a prosthesis is compared to walking with a prosthesis. Waters and colleagues[38] found that crutch walking led to a significant increase in the heart rate and the rate of oxygen consumption in all groups except vascular AK amputees, as compared to using a prosthesis. In their study, all AK amputee subjects walked faster with crutches alone, while the reverse was true for the BK amputees, except the traumatic BK amputees, who walked at the same speed with either crutches or prostheses. Bard and Ralston[61] found their AK subjects walked slower and spent more energy when they walked with forearm crutches. Traugh and colleagues,[63] on the other hand, reported 7% less Ee while walking with crutches, when compared to the energy consumption of those using prosthesis with the preferred knee setting. Erdman and coworkers[59] did not report any difference in either mode of ambulation, though the heart rate was consistently faster and took longer to recover to baseline when patients walked with crutches alone. Ganguli and colleagues[72] reported a 35% reduction in Ee per unit time in a group of AK amputees who used crutches alone. In contrast to other studies, however, they found no difference in heart rate. Nowroozi and associates[68] found that

**Table 16-8.** Energy Expenditure: Crutch Ambulation in Amputation

| Author/Year | N | Comment | Speed (m/min) | | Ee/unit time* (kcal/min/kg) | | | | Ee/unit distance (kcal × 10⁻³ /m/kg) | |
| | | | Subject | Difference (%) (normal 80m/min) | Subject | Normal NSSS | Difference (%) NCWS NSSS | (80m/min) | Subject | Difference (%) (NCWS 0.786 kcal × 10⁻³/m/kg) |
|---|---|---|---|---|---|---|---|---|---|---|
| Bard/Ralston, 1959 | 6 | AK, forearm | 58 | −28 | 0.069 | 0.0468 | 47 | 10 | 1.190 | 51 |
| Inman, 1961 | ? | AK, forearm | 45 | −44 | 0.065 | 0.0397 | 64 | 3 | 1.444 | 84 |
| Erdman, 1960 | 9 | AK, axill | 47 | −41 | 0.038 | 0.407 | −7 | −40 | 0.809 | 3 |
| Ganguli, 1974 | 10 | AK, axill | 50 | −38 | 0.065 | 0.0423 | 54 | 3 | 1.300 | 65 |
| Traugh, 1975 | 9 | AK, axill | 39 | −51 | 0.059 | 0.0371 | 59 | −6 | 1.513 | 92 |
| Waters, 1976 | 13 | AK, PVD, axill | 48 | −40 | 0.072 | 0.0412 | 75 | 14 | 1.500 | 91 |
| Waters, 1976 | 15 | Trauma, AK, axill | 65 | −19 | 0.076 | 0.0514 | 48 | 21 | 1.169 | 49 |
| Waters, 1976 | 13 | PVD, BK, axill | 39 | −51 | 0.070 | 0.0371 | 89 | 11 | 1.795 | 128 |
| Waters, 1976 | 14 | Trauma, BK, axill | 71 | −11 | 0.108 | 0.0557 | 94 | 71 | 1.521 | 94 |
| Waters, 1976 | 15 | PVD, Syme, axill | 39 | −51 | 0.062 | 0.0371 | 67 | −2 | 1.590 | 102 |
| Nowroozi, 1983 | 8 | Tumor, HD, axill | 56 | −30 | 0.052 | 0.0456 | 14 | −17 | 0.929 | 18 |
| Nowroozi, 1983 | 10 | Tumor, Hp, axill | 53 | −34 | 0.050 | 0.0439 | 14 | −21 | 0.943 | 20 |

* Equation 4: Ee(kcal/min/kg) = (29 + 0.0053 V²)/1000. [V = Velocity in m/min]
Key: Forearm, forearm / Loftstrand crutches; Axill, axillary crutches; PVD, peripheral vascular disease

Hp and HD subjects walked faster and consumed less energy while using crutches. Available research does not indicate with any consistency what mode of ambulation the subjects preferred. Factors such as upper extremity maximum aerobic capacity, general fitness, and motivation all play a role, but these investigations confirm that crutch walking is an effective alternative to using a prosthesis. Additionally, the old dictum that the ability to crutch walk is a good indicator that the same patient can walk with a prosthesis seems to hold true.[59] The caveat is the cardiovascular stress imposed by this activity. In most clinical settings, both physician and patient opt for the prosthesis, except when prosthetic ambulation is not feasible

## Summary

Barring other complications, BK amputees frequently achieve a high level of ambulatory performance, owing to the relatively low level of extra demand on oxygen consumption. At their CWS, the rate of calorie expenditure equals that of normal persons walking at 80 m/min. Like able-bod-

ied persons, BK amputees choose a CWS that is the most efficient in terms of energy cost. The speed of ambulation has no correlation with length of the residual limb. The level of fitness and physical activity, along with age, appear to play a more important role; however, residual limb length has a direct bearing on the subsequent rise in Ee. Amputation should be performed at the lowest level allowed by tissue integrity and blood supply. Under the right circumstances, such amputees can be vocationally rehabilitated and become able to do manual labor that requires a moderate level of intermittent work.

A single AK amputation dramatically curtails functional ambulation, particularly for aged or sedentary patients. The importance of preserving the knee joint is highlighted by the finding that a BK-BK amputee walks better than a unilateral AK amputee. Given the fact that 35% of dysvascular amputees lose the remaining limb within 3 to 5 years, it becomes even more urgent that the knee joint be saved.[73] The limited physical activity typical of AK patients severely reduces their maximum aerobic capacity, and thus the relative energy cost exceeds the bounds of what can be tolerated for extended periods. These amputees perform better with their preferred knee setting, which should not be changed casually simply for the sake of esthetics. The use of crutches offers a practical alternative, since oxygen demands are similar, but the fact that the cardiovascular stress is consistently greater must be considered, particularly with dysvascular patients.

Training for strength and endurance should be an integral part of amputee rehabilitation. The amputee's ability to choose the most efficient CWS, for which the Ee is similar to that of able-bodied persons at their normal CWS, is a prerequisite for success.

Higher levels of unilateral and bilateral amputations impose exponential increases in energy requirement that dramatically reduce the amputees' ability to cover even short distances. In these cases, a good argument can be made for a wheelchair, even though this may produce cardiovascular stress from increased upper extremity work.

The choice among the technologically advanced prosthetic components, in terms of their influence upon reducing energy expenditure, still remains to be determined objectively. A summary of our experience in the laboratory is presented in Figure 16-10.

## Hemiplegia

The variations in gait characteristics among hemiplegics depend on the extent of neurologic deficit. The degree of gait deviation reflects directly on the metabolic demands of walking (Table 16-9). The earliest study that attempted to quantify the energy requirements of hemiplegic ambulation was published in 1959 by Bard and Ralston,[61] who reported on three subjects walking at varying slow speeds as they spent as much or more Ee per unit distance than Ee at NCWS. In a later study of 15 hemiplegics, Bard[74] reported a nearly normal Ee rate per unit time, and a 37% rise in Ee per unit distance compared to NCWS.

Corcoran and others[75] studied the effects of plastic and metal leg braces on speed and energy cost of hemiparetic ambulation. Unlike previous investigators, the authors consistently found that for their test group ambulation required more energy cost than for normal subjects walking at the same slow speeds. With no brace, the CWS was 42 m/min, 48% slower than the 80 m/min norm, and averaged 62% greater than normal oxygen consumption for that speed. The use of either the conventional metal short-leg brace or the plastic solid ankle-foot orthosis (AFO) in ambulation re-

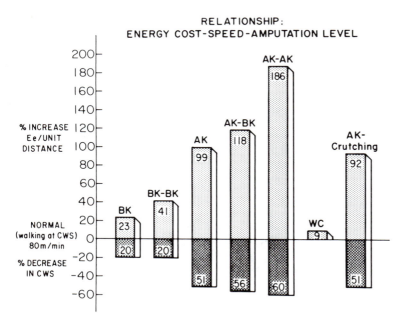

**Figure 16-10.** Summary of increase in Ee *per unit distance* and reduction of velocity among amputees as compared to normal subjects at the comfortable walking speed of 80 m/min. The values have been derived from various studies performed by the authors and other collaborators.[48,63,69]

**Table 16-9.** Energy Expenditure: Hemiplegia

| Author/Year | N | Comment | Speed (m/min) Subject | Speed (m/min) Difference (%) (normal 80m/min) | Ee/unit time* (kcal/min/kg) Subject | Ee/unit time* (kcal/min/kg) Normal NSSS | Ee/unit time* (kcal/min/kg) Difference (%) NCWS NSSS | Ee/unit time* (kcal/min/kg) Difference (%) NCWS (80m/min) | Ee/unit distance (kcal × 10⁻³ /m/kg) Subject | Ee/unit distance (kcal × 10⁻³ /m/kg) Difference (%) (NCWS 0.786 kcal × 10⁻³/m/kg) |
|---|---|---|---|---|---|---|---|---|---|---|
| Bard, 1963 | 15 | CVA | 41 | −49 | 0.044 | 0.0379 | 16 | −30 | 1.073 | 37 |
| Corcoran, 1970 | 15 | No brace | 42 | −48 | 0.062 | 0.0383 | 62 | −2 | 1.476 | 88 |
| Corcoran, 1970 | 15 | Plastic AFO | 49 | −39 | 0.067 | 0.0417 | 61 | 6 | 1.367 | 74 |
| Corcoran, 1970 | 15 | Metal AFO | 49 | −39 | 0.067 | 0.0417 | 61 | 6 | 1.367 | 74 |
| Lehneis, 1976 | 2 | Metal AFO | 22 | −73 | 0.056 | 0.0316 | 77 | −11 | 2.545 | 224 |
| Lehneis, 1976 | 2 | Spir/Hemi AFO | 22 | −73 | 0.054 | 0.0316 | 71 | −14 | 2.455 | 212 |
| Gersten, 1971 | 15 | Free ankle | 17 | −79 | 0.041 | 0.0305 | 34 | −35 | 2.412 | 207 |
| Gersten, 1971 | 15 | Rigid ankle | 17 | −79 | 0.042 | 0.0305 | 38 | −33 | 2.471 | 214 |
| Hash, 1978 | 19 | CVA | 30 | −63 | 0.056 | 0.0338 | 66 | −11 | 1.867 | 137 |

\* Equation 4: Ee(kcal/min/kg) = $(29 + 0.0053\ V^2)/1000$. [V = Velocity in m/min]
Key: CVA, cerebrovascular accident; AFO, ankle-foot orthosis; Spir/Hemi, spiral and hemispiral.

sulted in a significant increase in speed (49 m/min) and reduction in Ee, over ambulation with no brace. There was, however, no statistically significant difference between Ee with the two types of orthoses, which was 61% higher than in NSSS. At the subjects' CWS, the slope of oxygen consumption was greater than normal, indicating the higher price they have to pay to achieve small increments in speed. At their CWS, the rate of oxygen consumption per unit time among the hemiparetic subjects was approximately the same as NCWS (Figure 16-11). When energy cost was expressed per unit distance, it was found that hemiparetic patients cannot comfortably walk fast enough to achieve minimum oxygen consumption per meter walked. The rise in Ee per unit distance was 74% using an AFO, but 88% with no brace (Figure 16-12). Wearing either type of brace, the subjects' ability to ascend and descend stairs was significantly better than when they wore no brace at all.

Corcoran and colleagues[75] were emphatic about the importance of accurate speed control when studying the metabolic cost of ambulation, since patients use up savings in energy to achieve faster speeds. If speed is not measured accurately or maintained at a constant rate, small variations caused by different sets of conditions may be ob-

scured, as may have happened in some studies involving other disabilities.

Gersten and Orr[76] measured in 15 hemiparetic patients the external work of walking at the very slow speed of 17 m/min. They compared the results of a rigid ankle metal brace and one that allowed some dorsiflexion and plantar flexion. They found no significant difference in work per unit distance but indicated that whenever the dif-

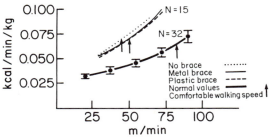

**Figure 16-11.** Polynomial regression curves of average energy cost at various walking speeds for hemiparetic patients and normal subjects. The dumbells indicate one standard deviation. Ee *per unit time* for both groups is approximately equal at their comfortable walking speeds, as indicated by an arrow. (Redrawn from Corcoran PJ, et al. Effects of plastic and metal leg braces on speed and energy cost of hemiparetic ambulation. Arch Phys Med Rehabil 1970; 51:69–77, with permission.)

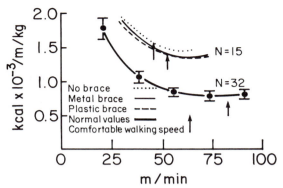

**Figure 16-12.** Ee *per unit distance* among hemiparetic and normal subjects. The dumbells indicate one standard deviation. Note that, unlike normal subjects, the hemiparetic group falls short of the theoretically optimal speed at which calorie expenditure would be minimal. (Redrawn from Corcoran PJ, et al. Effects of plastic and metal leg braces on speed and energy cost of hemiparetic ambulation. Arch Phys Med Rehabil 1970; 51:69–77, with permission.)

ference was greater than 7% the subjects invariably chose the orthosis with lower energy cost.

Lehneis and colleagues[77] analyzed the effect of an advanced plastic lower limb orthosis and that of conventional metal braces. Among eight subjects, two were hemiparetic patients who were fitted with a conventional orthosis and with the spiral and hemispiral orthosis. The study noted a reduction in Ee per unit distance of 12% when the advanced orthoses were used.

## Paraplegia

Loss of the major determinants of gait is more pronounced in paraplegia than in amputation or hemiplegia. From a pragmatic point of view, it is immediately apparent that the patient with spinal cord injury (SCI) or impairment that leads to loss of locomotor capability must expend an enormous amount of energy to regain some semblance of walking. SCI patients and clinicians alike face the emotional tug of war in deciding whether to invest considerable time and effort in an activity that may eventually prove expensive and functionally unproductive. To this end, in search of a rational

approach, several researchers have evaluated the energy requirements of ambulation for paraplegics (Table 16-10). Long and Lawton[78] determined that patients with lesions at T1–T11 do not become functional ambulators, whereas those with lesions at T12 and below usually succeed. This was later confirmed by Rosman and Spira.[79]

### Conventional Ambulation

The pioneering work led by Gordon[80,81] while at Columbia University set the direction for subsequent studies on the energy expenditure of paraplegic walking. In his study of 11 subjects with paraplegia of various causes, he found the speed of ambulation to be 66% slower than normal. The rate of expenditure per unit time was 162% to 174% higher than NSSS, and the net cost per unit distance was 317% more than for NCWS. He concluded that ambulation seemed to be an impractical solution and offered the wheelchair as an alternative for most, but not all, patients. He demonstrated that continuous paraplegic crutch walking with a swing-through gait was as exhausting as a 400-meter run. Clinkingbeard's group[82] reported similarly dismal findings.

Waters and Lunsford[83] provided an extensive look at energy requirement in a large cohort of young paraplegic patients, 67 of whom were able to ambulate. For the group, the average CWS was 27 m/min, or 66% slower than the norm, while the Ee per unit time was 113% higher compared to that of NSSS. When analyzed against NCWS, the Ee per unit distance was 230% higher. The results indicate that the test group walked slower to keep their Ee down to tolerable levels, but as a result, they were unable to cover much distance. The study also looked into the effects produced by high- and low-level lesions. As expected, the lower the level of the lesion, the faster the speed, and the lower the rise in metabolic requirement. In a later study, Waters and coworkers[84] focused on the determinants of gait performance among a group of 36 spinal cord–injury (SCI) patients. The subjects were classified according to type of orthotic prescription, AFO versus knee-AFO (KAFO), assistive devices (cane, crutches, walker), and ambulatory motor index (AMI). The AMI was based on a manual muscle test of the

**Table 16-10.** Energy Expenditure: Paraplegia

| Author/Year | N | Comment | Speed (m/min) Subject | Speed Difference (%) (normal 80m/min) | Ee/unit time* (kcal/min/kg) Subject | Normal NSSS | Difference (%) Normal NSSS | NCWS NSSS (80m/min) | Ee/unit distance (kcal × 10⁻³ /m/kg) Subject | Difference (%) (NCWS 0.786 kcal × 10⁻³/m/kg) |
|---|---|---|---|---|---|---|---|---|---|---|
| **General** | | | | | | | | | | |
| Gordon, 1956 | 11 | Various causes | 27 | −66 | 0.086 | 0.0329 | 162 | 37 | 3.185 | 305 |
| Gordon, 1956 | 3 | Thoracic | 27 | −66 | 0.090 | 0.0329 | 174 | 43 | 3.333 | 324 |
| Clinkingbeard, 1974 | 4 | Thoracic | 4 | −95 | 0.043 | 0.0291 | 48 | −32 | 10.750 | 1268 |
| Clinkingbeard, 1974 | 3 | Lumbar | 20 | −75 | 0.048 | 0.0311 | 54 | −24 | 2.400 | 205 |
| Cerny, 1980 | 11 | T12–L2 | 32 | −60 | 0.098 | 0.0344 | 185 | 56 | 3.063 | 290 |
| Chantraine, 1984 | 3 | Parallel bars | 15 | −81 | 0.043 | 0.0302 | 42 | −32 | 2.867 | 265 |
| Chantraine, 1984 | 3 | Crutches | 23 | −71 | 0.079 | 0.0318 | 148 | 25 | 3.435 | 337 |
| Waters, 1985 | 67 | All levels | 27 | −66 | 0.070 | 0.0329 | 113 | 11 | 2.593 | 230 |
| Waters, 1985 | 10 | T1–T9 | 18 | −78 | 0.058 | 0.0307 | 89 | −8 | 3.222 | 310 |
| Waters, 1985 | 57 | T10 & below | 28 | −65 | 0.072 | 0.0332 | 117 | 14 | 2.571 | 227 |
| Waters, 1989 | 36 | SCI ambulators | 41 | −49 | 0.072 | 0.0379 | 90 | 14 | 1.756 | 123 |
| Yakura, 1990 | 10 | All levels | 59 | −26 | 0.075 | 0.0474 | 58 | 19 | 1.271 | 62 |
| **Orthotic Types** | | | | | | | | | | |
| Merkel, 1984 | 8 | SC walker | 9 | −89 | 0.059 | 0.0294 | 100 | −6 | 6.556 | 734 |
| Merkel, 1984 | 8 | Conv walker | 6 | −93 | 0.061 | 0.0292 | 109 | −3 | 10.167 | 1193 |
| Merkel, 1984 | 8 | SC crutches | 18 | −78 | 0.067 | 0.0307 | 118 | 6 | 3.722 | 374 |
| Merkel, 1984 | 8 | Conv crutch | 15 | −81 | 0.089 | 0.0302 | 195 | 41 | 5.933 | 655 |
| Huang, 1979 | 8 | SC crutches | 14 | −83 | 0.053 | 0.0300 | 76 | −16 | 3.786 | 382 |
| Ragnarsson, 1975 | 11 | Conventional | 21 | −74 | 0.064 | 0.0313 | 104 | 2 | 3.048 | 288 |
| Ragnarsson, 1975 | 14 | Pnuematic | 27 | −66 | 0.067 | 0.0329 | 104 | 6 | 2.481 | 216 |
| Nene, 1989 | 10 | ParaWalker | 13 | −84 | 0.043 | 0.0299 | 44 | −32 | 3.308 | 321 |
| Marsolais, 1988 | 2 | FNS | 15 | −81 | 0.095 | 0.0302 | 215 | 51 | 6.333 | 706 |

\* Equation 4: Ee(kcal/min/kg) = (29 + 0.0053 $V^2$)/1000. [V = Velocity in m/min]
Key: SCI, spinal cord injury; SC, Scott-Craig orthosis; Conv, conventional braces; FNS, functional neuromuscular stimulation.

lower limbs and was found to be a reliable index of functional mobility that correlated significantly with energy expenditure.

*Effects of Long-Term Bracing*

Chantraine[85] and Yakura[86] and their coworkers have studied the effects of long-term bracing and the changes in ambulation parameters. Chantraine and coworkers[85] collected energy metabolism data on seven male paraplegic patients with complete lesions at T9–L1. Of these, four patients had recently undergone rehabilitation while three were seasoned walkers. The cost of walking on a treadmill with a swing-through gait between parallel bars was 50% less for trained subjects than for new ambulators. Yakura's group[86] performed a longitudinal study among 10 SCI patients. At 1 year follow-up, the patients walked significantly faster and more efficiently, had lower HR, and required less axial load on their upper extremities. The authors concluded, however, that, despite the significant training effect of continued brace walking, the cardiovascular stress and energy demands of walking remain considerable.

*Advanced Orthotic Ambulation*

Researchers have turned to a variety of orthotic designs in search of ways to lower the metabolic demands of ambulation. The hope was to bring walking within the reach of most paraplegics.

Lehman and coworkers[87] noted that the double–ankle stop type of joint requires significantly less vertical lifting of the center of gravity, thus requiring less acceleration to carry the center of gravity forward, which in turn results in less mechanical work. Merkel and coworkers[88] studied eight complete motor paraplegic subjects with lesions at T10 and below to determine the efficiency of the conventional single-stopped KAFO (SS-KAFO) as opposed to the Scott-Craig KAFO (SC-KAFO). The latter orthosis is a double upright, with offset knee joint, bail lock, adjustable anterior and posterior ankle pin stops, a crossbar at the level of the ankle joint and sole plate extending beyond the metatarsal heads. They found no significant difference in Ee for a standing subject between the two types of braces. When subjects ambulated with a walker, the SC-KAFO was 31% more energy efficient than the SS-KAFO, but the difference between the two types of orthoses was not statistically significant. While crutch walking, however, the SC-KAFO required significantly less energy per unit distance than the SS-KAFO (Figure 16-13). The fact remains, however, that the energy required for ambulation remains as much as 382% more per meter compared to NCWS. Miller

and colleagues[89] made similar comparisons during the subjects' negotiation of architectural barriers such as stairs, turns, and ramps and found no significant difference between the two braces in terms of Ee. Huang's group[90] likewise looked into the energy cost of ambulation among SCI patients using the SC-KAFO. The rate of ambulation reflected the patients' preferred CWS, which averaged 14 m/min, or 83% slower than normal. At that speed, the energy cost was roughly equivalent to that of normal persons ambulating at their own CWS, but the Ee per unit distance was almost 382% more.

Nene and coinvestigators[91] found almost similar results with paraplegics ambulating with a hip guidance orthosis or the ParaWalker, previously described by Patrick and McClelland.[92] In comparing their results with those in the literature, Nene's group[91] were encouraged to find that the device resulted in more efficient walking than did conventional long leg braces. They believed that the energy demands required in walking with the ParaWalker were within sustainable limits and challenged the traditional advice to paraplegics to opt for wheelchair mobility.

In the hope that a lightweight device would

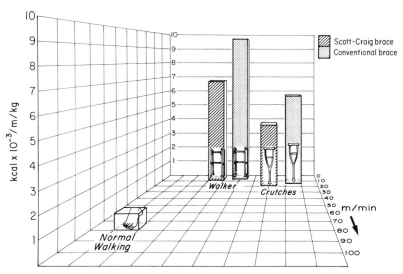

**Figure 16-13.** Energy efficiency-cost per meter of ambulation among paraplegic subjects using either Scott-Craig KAFO or single-stopped KAFO and either walker or crutches. Subjects walked at their own comfortable walking speed. (After Merkel KD, et al. Energy expenditure of paraplegic patients standing and walking with two knee-ankle-foot orthoses. Arch Phys Med Rehabil 1984; 65:121–124, with permission.)

increase the use of braces, researchers developed the pneumatic OrthoWalk. Ragnarsson and colleagues[93] studied 14 paraplegics, two of whom were in the pediatric age group. All except three subjects used the OrthoWalk as well as conventional long-leg metal braces. When using the pneumatic orthosis, the subjects covered more ground at a CWS of 27 m/min. The Ee per unit distance was statistically less than with use of conventional braces. The article did not specify the results per kilogram, but assuming an average weight of 70 kg, the subjects demonstrated approximately the same Ee per unit time as NCWS, but 216% higher Ee per unit distance. Ragnarsson and colleagues[93] doubt if use of the OrthoWalk alters the fact that only the most exceptional patients will continue to pursue the exhausting task of ambulating with orthoses.

*Functional Neuromuscular Stimulation*

The increased oxygen consumption of patients while ambulating with long-leg braces occurs primarily during the swing phase and is disproportionately less during the stance phase. In addition, the nonreciprocating gait pattern is dynamically discontinuous and loses the advantage provided by momentum as the speed increases. As a consequence, the patient is required to lift all of the body weight with each step or swing-through. The recently introduced technique of functional neuromuscular stimulation (FNS) is now being applied to respond to these shortcomings (see Chapter 23). Marsolais and Edwards[94,95] reported on the energy cost of ambulation using FNS. In an initial inquiry,[94] they studied four paraplegics, reported the results from two subjects, and compared the values with those reported in other studies. The mean Ee per unit time Marsolais and Edwards[94,95] reported with FNS was 0.095 kcal/min/kg, compared to 0.058 kcal/min/kg reported for the conventional LLB. Despite this, however, the authors were encouraged because of an accompanying 75% increase in working muscle mass due to inclusion of the hip and leg muscles. The net result was a decrease in the intensity of energy use relative to working muscle mass. The anaerobic component of FNS also appeared to be less. Unlike LLB and normal walking, the Ee/unit time theoretically decreases as the FNS walking speed increases. Unfortunately, the fastest speed a subject achieved

with FNS was 34 m/min, and no subject was able to walk more than 300 m because of fatigue or perceived exertion. This is understandable, as the aerobic cost of the activity is approximately six times a patient's BMR. While normal sedentary persons are able to sustain muscle activity at or below 50% of maximum aerobic capacity, the FNS anaerobic component probably occurs at or below that level, owing to the synchronized stimulation of motor neurons and muscle fibers. Additionally, FNS tends to recruit the large superficial motor neurons (fast twitch) more than the deeper, smaller (slow twitch) motor neurons. In a follow-up report[95] on four complete paraplegic patients, two of whom also participated in the first study, Marsolais and Edwards[94,95] measured the metabolic requirement of FNS ambulation. They also sought to determine whether the use of an open-loop FNS could significantly increase the maximum aerobic capacity and tolerance to lactic acid accumulation when combined with arm ergometry training. Their data suggest that paraplegic subjects could develop sufficient aerobic and anaerobic capacity to walk several hundred meters with FNS and a rolling walker, while maintaining a cardiopulmonary reserve. The problem of local muscle fatigue (probably due to ischemia) continued to plague the subjects. With modern technology and experience, FNS holds the potential to advance beyond its present status and offers the future possibility of a reasonable alternative to conventional orthosis.

Clinicians as well as paraplegic patients and their families all perceive walking as a worthy goal, or even as the *sine qua non* of successful rehabilitation. Crutch walking often does play a useful role in the initial rehabilitation of a paraplegic patient: it strengthens the upper body, develops balance and aerobic capacity, and imparts a sense of accomplishment, of having made a comeback. Few successful paraplegic ambulators maintain the demanding, and sometimes dangerous, skill for long; and its principal value may be in building a positive attitude toward the wheelchair as a liberating rather than confining device.

### Wheelchair Propulsion

If humans had wheels instead of legs and feet, the efficiency of ambulation would be much improved. The horizontal and vertical excursions of the center of gravity would follow a straight line; thus less work. As academic as this notion may appear, the following discussion validates the argument.

Several studies have been made of patients engaged in wheeling (Table 16-11). Waters and Lunsford[83] determined the energy consumption of wheelchair locomotion among 124 paraplegic subjects. The speed of wheeling was only very slightly slower than normal and the energy consumed was within the normal range. The elevated HR associated with wheeling, in comparison with normal walking, was attributed to the fact that the great majority of the work is done by the upper extremities.

Cerny and colleagues[96] investigated the use of wheelchairs as an alternative to ambulation. Their study included 11 patients, eight who regularly used a wheelchair and three who routinely ambulated. Not unexpectedly, the authors concluded that wheeling was significantly less difficult than walking with braces. On level ground, their subjects were able to keep up with able-bodied persons as they wheeled at 75 m/min. They spent no more Ee per unit time and consumed only 9% more Ee per unit distance than NCWS. Data compiled by Cerny's group[96] suggested that the wheelchair is destined to be the primary mode of ambulation for those who require two KAFOs, unless they are willing to work under anaerobic condi-

**Table 16-11.** Energy Expenditure: Wheelchair Propulsion

| Author/Year | N | Comment | Speed (m/min) Subject | Speed Difference (%) (normal 80m/min) | Ee/unit time* (kcal/min/kg) Subject | Normal NSSS | Difference (%) NSSS | NCWS NSSS (80m/min) | Ee/unit distance (kcal × 10⁻³ /m/kg) Subject | Difference (%) (NCWS 0.786 kcal × 10⁻³/m/kg) |
|---|---|---|---|---|---|---|---|---|---|---|
| Hildebrandt, 1978 | 29 | Polio/other Front/rear wheel | 67 | − 16 | 0.037 | 0.0528 | − 30 | − 41 | 0.552 | − 30 |
| Hash, 1978 | 14 | CVA | 37 | − 54 | 0.048 | 0.0363 | 32 | − 24 | 1.297 | 65 |
| Cerny, 1980 | 8 | Paraplegia | 75 | − 6 | 0.064 | 0.0588 | 9 | 2 | 0.853 | 9 |
| Wolfe, 1978 | 10 | Normal, cncrt | 57 | − 29 | 0.056 | 0.0462 | 21 | − 11 | 0.982 | 25 |
| Wolfe, 1978 | 10 | Decon, cncrt | 53 | − 34 | 0.062 | 0.0439 | 41 | − 2 | 1.170 | 49 |
| Wolfe, 1978 | 15 | Paraplegia, cncrt Hard Tire, WC | 83 | 4 | 0.075 | 0.0655 | 14 | 19 | 0.904 | 15 |
| Wolfe, 1978 | 15 | Paraplegia, cncrt Pneum tire, WC | 80 | 0 | 0.075 | 0.0629 | 19 | 19 | 0.938 | 19 |
| Wolfe, 1978 | 10 | Normal, carpet | 43 | − 46 | 0.060 | 0.0388 | 55 | − 5 | 1.395 | 78 |
| Wolfe, 1978 | 10 | Decon, carpet | 37 | − 54 | 0.067 | 0.0363 | 85 | 6 | 1.811 | 130 |
| Wolfe, 1978 | 15 | Paraplegia Carpet Hard tire | 65 | − 19 | 0.081 | 0.0514 | 58 | 29 | 1.246 | 59 |
| Wolfe, 1978 | 15 | Paraplegia Carpet Pneum tire | 64 | − 20 | 0.082 | 0.0507 | 62 | 30 | 1.281 | 63 |
| Waters, 1985 | 124 | Paraplegia All levels | 72 | − 10 | 0.055 | 0.0565 | − 3 | − 13 | 0.764 | − 3 |
| Waters, 1985 | 55 | T1–T9 | 68 | − 15 | 0.053 | 0.0535 | − 1 | − 16 | 0.779 | − 1 |
| Waters, 1985 | 69 | T10–Below | 76 | − 5 | 0.057 | 0.0596 | − 4 | − 10 | 0.750 | − 5 |
| Hilbers, 1987 | 9 | Sports chair | 67 | − 16 | 0.044 | 0.0528 | − 17 | − 30 | 0.657 | − 16 |
| Hilbers, 1987 | 9 | Regular chair | 67 | − 16 | 0.053 | 0.0528 | 0 | − 16 | 0.791 | 1 |

* Equation 4: Ee(kcal/min/kg) = $(29 + 0.0053 \ V^2)/1000$. [V = Velocity in m/min]

Key: Polio, poliomyelitis; CVA, cerebrovascular Accident; cncrt, concrete Floor; carpet, carpeted Floor; WC, Wheelchair.

tions and are able to achieve a velocity of 54 m/min or faster.

Several studies have addressed factors that influence the performance of wheelchairs (Figure 16-14). Hildebrandt and colleagues[97] found that steering accuracy, net energy cost, and load on the circulatory system were significantly less with standard rear wheel–drive chairs than with front wheel–drive chairs. Hilbers and White[98] compared the sports chair with conventional-design wheelchairs and found that the energy cost of propelling the former was about 17% less than for the latter, and they attributed the greater efficiency of the sports chair to its design rather than its lighter total mass. Wolfe and others[99] examined the effects of floor carpeting and the type of tires on wheelchairs used by 10 normal, 10 deconditioned, and 15 low-level paraplegic subjects. In all three groups, the velocity of wheeling was significantly slower on carpeted floors than on hard surfaces. Among the paraplegic subjects, the speed was almost equal

with pneumatic and with hard tires. All groups had higher oxygen consumption on carpeting than on hard floors, but the difference was not statistically significant except among paraplegic subjects who used pneumatic tires, when the Ee per unit distance on carpeted floors was significantly higher than on concrete floors. These findings should be borne in mind by designers of homes and institutions where wheelchairs will be in common use.

To provide independent mobility at NCWS for patients with restricted cardiopulmonary reserve, clinicians should not be reluctant to prescribe electrically powered wheelchairs or scooters. Table 16-2 data suggest that the energy cost of using a power wheelchair is similar to that of "sitting at ease" (1.2 to 1.6 kcal/min/70kg). The energy cost of using a scooter, which provides less back and arm support, is probably similar to that of "sitting, writing" (1.9 to 2.2 kcal/min/70 kg). The effect of increasing speed is probably negligible, though comparative data are lacking and research is needed.

Persons with disabilities who walk short distances with difficulty (e.g., multiple sclerosis patients), or who propel a manual wheelchair slowly and laboriously (e.g., cerebral palsy patients), can enhance their lifestyle by using a power wheelchair or scooter. Clinicians may advocate withholding power mobility aids from any patient who can propel a manual wheelchair, however awkwardly, in the belief that their stamina would regress if a powered wheelchair were provided. We found no data to support this notion, but the question requires careful research.

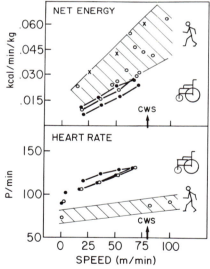

**Figure 16-14.** Ee *per unit time* and heart rate during level wheelchair driving compared with corresponding values for walking drawn from the literature. While this particular study shows lower Ee for propelling a wheelchair on a smooth, level surface than for normal walking, different sets of variables could increase the rate of expenditure. (Redrawn from Hildenbrant G, et al. Energy cost of propelling wheelchairs at various speeds: Cardiac response and effect on steering accuracy. Arch Phys Med Rehabil 1970; 51:131–136, with permission.)

### Crutch Ambulation in Various Disabilities

Many patients require assistive devices such as crutches during and after rehabilitation, and clinicians are always concerned to ensure that prescribed devices meet the patient's needs as much as possible. For example, a patient's choices between different types of gait patterns are influenced by locomotor skills, cardiovascular fitness, and specific needs relevant to the disability. Crutch walking alters the natural movement of the extremities and requires greater lift of the body to swing the legs through. Muscle groups that ordinarily play little or no role in walking are recruited, contributing further to the increased energy expenditure (Table 16-12). Many factors, therefore, must be considered in prescribing mobility aids as basic as crutches. Crutch walking as an alternative for amputees has already been discussed (see Table 16-8).

*Crutch Walking Among Healthy Volunteers*

Several studies have reported what happens when an otherwise healthy person is forced to walk with crutches. Shoup[100] and Wells[101] studied the kinematics and energy variation of the swing-through gait and found them to depend upon speed and degree of disablement. The trunk serves to conserve approximately half the energy that could be expended. McBeath and colleagues[102] tested a group of 10 volunteers between ages 22 and 32 years. The subjects used axillary as well as forearm crutches as they walked with the following gait patterns: partial and non–weight-bearing (NWB), two-point, and swing-through. The self-selected velocity was less than for normal walking,

**Table 16-12.** Energy Expenditure: Crutch Walking

| Author/Year | N | Comment | Speed (m/min) Subject | Difference (%) (normal 80m/min) | Ee/unit time* (kcal/min/kg) Subject | Normal NSSS | Difference (%) NCWS NSSS | NCWS (80m/min) | Ee/unit distance (kcal × 10⁻³ /m/kg) Subject | Difference (%) (NCWS 0.786 kcal × 10⁻³/m/kg) |
|---|---|---|---|---|---|---|---|---|---|---|
| **Normal Subjects** | | | | | | | | | | |
| McBeath, 1974 | 10 | Cane | 60 | −25 | 0.062 | 0.0481 | 29 | −2 | 1.033 | 31 |
| McBeath, 1974 | 10 | PWB, axill | 55 | −31 | 0.051 | 0.0450 | 13 | −19 | 0.927 | 18 |
| McBeath, 1974 | 10 | 2 pt, axill | 57 | −29 | 0.061 | 0.0462 | 32 | −3 | 1.070 | 36 |
| McBeath, 1974 | 10 | ST, axill | 58 | −28 | 0.070 | 0.0468 | 49 | 11 | 1.207 | 54 |
| McBeath, 1974 | 10 | PWB, forearm | 55 | −31 | 0.054 | 0.0450 | 20 | −14 | 0.982 | 25 |
| McBeath, 1974 | 10 | 2 pt, forearm | 59 | −26 | 0.058 | 0.0474 | 22 | −8 | 0.983 | 25 |
| McBeath, 1974 | 10 | ST, forearm | 55 | −31 | 0.061 | 0.0450 | 35 | −3 | 1.109 | 41 |
| McBeath, 1974 | 10 | NWB, forearm | 53 | −34 | 0.067 | 0.0439 | 53 | 6 | 1.264 | 61 |
| Fisher, 1981 | 8 | 3 pt, NWB, axil | 30 | −63 | 0.052 | 0.0338 | 54 | −17 | 1.733 | 121 |
| Fisher, 1981 | 8 | 3 pt, NWB, axil | 40 | −50 | 0.066 | 0.0375 | 76 | 5 | 1.650 | 110 |
| Fisher, 1981 | 8 | 3 pt, NWB, axil | 50 | −38 | 0.071 | 0.0423 | 68 | 13 | 1.420 | 81 |
| Fisher, 1981 | 8 | 3 pt, NWB, axil | 60 | −25 | 0.087 | 0.0481 | 81 | 38 | 1.450 | 84 |
| Fisher, 1981 | 8 | 3 pt, NWB, axil | 70 | −13 | 0.095 | 0.0550 | 73 | 51 | 1.357 | 73 |
| Fisher, 1981 | 8 | 3 pt, NWB, axil | 80 | 0 | 0.118 | 0.0629 | 88 | 87 | 1.475 | 88 |
| **Post–fracture and cast** | | | | | | | | | | |
| Imms, 1976 | 3 | Fx, LLC, crutch | 57 | −29 | 0.082 | 0.0462 | 77 | 30 | 1.439 | 83 |
| Imms, 1976 | 11 | Fx, crutches | 65 | −19 | 0.074 | 0.0514 | 44 | 17 | 1.138 | 45 |
| Imms, 1976 | 10 | Fx, 2 canes | 69 | −14 | 0.072 | 0.0542 | 33 | 14 | 1.043 | 33 |
| Waters, 1976 | 20 | Normal, LLC, ST | 51 | −36 | 0.096 | 0.0428 | 124 | 52 | 1.882 | 139 |
| Waters, 1976 | 10 | Normal, CC, ST | 52 | −35 | 0.098 | 0.0433 | 126 | 56 | 1.885 | 140 |
| Waters, 1976 | 10 | Normal, SLC, ST | 61 | −24 | 0.104 | 0.0487 | 113 | 65 | 1.705 | 117 |

* Equation 4: Ee(kcal/min/kg) = (29 + 0.0053 V²)/1000. [V = Velocity in m/min]
Key: PWB, partial weight bearing; 2 pt, = Two-point gait; 3 pt, Three-point gait; ST, Swing-through gait; NWB, non–weight bearing; FX, fracture; LLC, long-leg cast; SLC, short-leg cast; CC, cylinder cast; axill, axillary crutches; forearm = forearm/Loftstrand crutches.

and the energy used was greater than for normal gait for either type of crutch. Walking with two-point alternating and three-point partial weight-bearing (PWB) gaits with either cane or crutches required approximately 18% to 36% more energy per unit distance than NCWS. Swing-through and three-point NWB gaits required an increase of 41% to 61% in net energy cost.

Fisher and Patterson[103] tested eight normal volunteers as they ambulated with axillary and forearm crutches and likewise found no difference in Ee with either type of crutches. Oxygen consumption rose twofold (Figure 16-15). The high energy cost of crutch walking was underscored with the finding that, even at the slow speed of 30 m/min, oxygen consumption was 40% of that for the maximum upper extremity stress test. At 80 m/min, Ee per unit distance rose to 88%, which is clearly above the anaerobic threshold. Though the investigation did not clarify the most efficient speed, crutch walking at 40 to 50 m/min was suggested as being tolerable. The Ee/unit time at this speed is about the same as the normal Ee at NCWS (see Figure 16-15). The authors provided further insights into the cardiovascular stress of crutch walking.[104] Heart rate for crutch walking was significantly higher than that for walking, and the slope versus oxygen consumption for crutch walking parallels that of an upper extremity stress test.

In a study of young, healthy volunteers, Waters and colleagues[44] immobilized their subjects in long-leg casts, cylinder casts, and short-leg casts, and asked them to use crutches with a NWB swing-through gait. The degree of oxygen consumption and the physical exertion recorded during crutch walking was above the anaerobic threshold and could be categorized as continuous hard or intermittent moderate work.

*Crutch Walking Following Fracture and Hip Replacement*

Imms and colleagues[105] followed the energy cost of ambulation among 13 patients who were recovering from fractures. Those who ambulated with LLC and crutches spent considerably more energy than persons who walked normally. These patients recovered efficient ambulation as they progressed from crutches to canes, and finally to no assistive device, but they ambulated only at slower speeds. Pugh[106] noted a similar sequence of events as he followed the course of one patient after hip replacement. Brown[107] and collaborators studied the energetics of walking pre- and postoperatively in a group of patients who had undergone total hip replacement. Those who had unilateral hip disease did quite well and improved their speed of ambulation with a concomitant decrease in Ee per unit distance. Of the patients with bilateral hip disease, those with two hip replacements fared considerably better than those with only one. The evidence presented confirms that it is prudent to

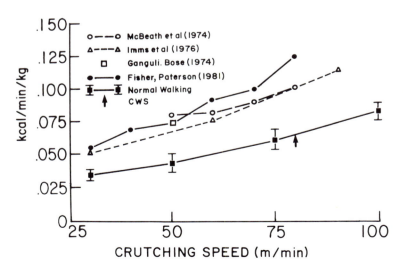

**Figure 16-15.** Relationship between crutch-walking speed and Ee among normal subjects as drawn from the literature. (Redrawn from Fisher S, Paterson R. Energy cost of ambulation with crutches. Arch Phys Med Rehabil 1981; 62:250–256, with permission.)

ensure that patients engage in upper extremity endurance training before they begin to ambulate with crutches.[103,104]

### Effect on Energy Expenditure of Stairs and Ramps

Corcoran and Templer[108] found that both normal and crutch ambulators perform better on stairs than on ramps, in terms of energy cost per vertical rise. The steeper the ramp or stairs, the greater the advantage of stairs in total energy cost; however, if horizontal movement is also considered, the 5% ramp is less taxing. In situations like those in most transportation terminals, where people need to ascend 10 meters while progressing 200 meters horizontally, stairs require 29% more energy than a 5% ramp, and 45% more time. Fisher and Patterson[103] and Ganguli and Bose[109] also performed experiments on patients' performance on stairs and noted a nearly twofold increase in the net energy cost for those ambulating with crutches.

The metabolic cost of stair climbing can be predicted from a simple nomogram if the height of step or riser and step frequency are known (Figure 16-16).[108] If a subject's weight and the riser height are known, the nomogram indicates the step frequency needed to achieve any desired rate of Ee. This nomogram makes it possible to use any stairway as a precise ergometer for aerobic conditioning.

Descending stairs requires only 23% of the energy needed for ascending the same staircase. Because coming down stairs does not exceed light work levels, the process is useless for aerobic conditioning. Ascending one flight of stairs at the usual speed takes only 10 to 15 seconds but requires a burst of 12 to 14 kcal/min/70 kg of energy. This makes stair climbing the most strenuous activity of the day for most people.

### Other Disabilities

The literature describing the effects of other disabilities on energy requirements of ambulation is scant. Bearing in mind the dynamic changes that occur in the gait pattern among the pediatric age group, the metabolic differences between them and adults, and the inherent difficulty of engaging them in experiments, children are nevertheless underrepresented in this type of study. Cooper[22] and Rose[110] and their associates noted that among normal children the relationship between heart rate and oxygen uptake was linear throughout a wide range of walking speeds. The same relationship was found in children with cerebral palsy, which offered the possibility of using this parameter as a simple means of evaluating energy costs in pediatric rehabilitation. As with adults, however, the caveat remains that heart rate varies considerably, particularly at lower work intensities. Rose and

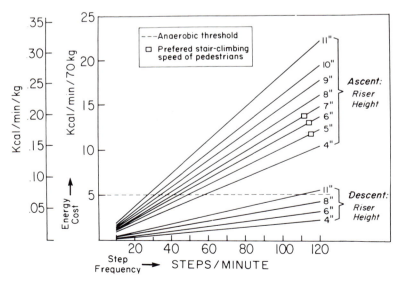

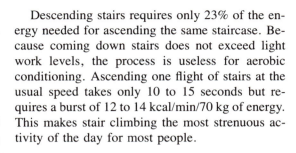

**Figure 16-16.** Relationship between the height of each step (riser), the step frequency, and the energy cost of ascent or descent. The nomogram can be used to predict the energy expenditure for subjects who can use stairs for exercise.

associates[111] further examined 18 normal and 13 children with cerebral palsy. The most efficient speed among normal children approximated the adult velocity of 80 m/min, while those for cerebral palsy patients averaged 51 m/min. The energy cost of walking for those with hemiplegic cerebral palsy compared favorably with that of their normal counterparts, but those with diplegia expended 200% more energy.

Olgiati and colleagues[112] found a twofold increase in the energy cost of walking among patients with multiple sclerosis (MS). These patients had very slow pace and frequently experienced dyspnea and leg fatigue. In an effort to define the roles of spasticity, ataxia, and weakness, the same authors studied 33 MS patients who did not suffer from cardiopulmonary disease.[113] Their findings showed a 65% rise in Ee per unit distance and indicated that lower extremity spasticity, rather than weakness, accounted for at least 40% of the variability.

The effects of a progressive activity program on the physiologic work performance of chronic low back pain patients was examined by Thomas and coworkers.[114] Fifteen chronic low back pain sufferers participated twice daily in mat exercises, bicycling, and walking. Before treatment, the average CWS was 55 m/min with an expenditure rate of 0.056 kcal/min/kg; after the program, the CWS increased to 74 m/min, with Ee of 0.064 kcal/min/kg. The small posttreatment increase in rate of oxygen consumption, coupled with a faster CWS, resulted in enhanced efficiency. The authors pointed out that LBP patients frequently regress to a lifestyle that eventually reduces their fitness level and stressed the importance of reversing the phenomenon with a proper exercise regimen.

## Conclusion

Rehabilitative therapy can have a dramatic impact on the physiologic responses of persons with disabilities, just as a potent pharmacologic agent can. The multiplicity of factors that affect the ultimate outcome can be carefully sorted if the process is based on scientific data. Much remains to be explained clinically. The prescription of ambulation aids demands knowledge that is more far reaching than is commonly appreciated. Persons with disabilities walk slower to minimize the rate of calorie expenditure, but at the price of increased net cost and reduced efficiency. The choices between types of ambulatory aids, devices, and gait patterns should be based not on a predetermined protocol but rather on analysis of each individual's unique abilities or disabilities.

## References

1. Morton DJ, Fuller DD. Human Locomotion and Body Form: Study of Gravity and Man. Baltimore: Williams & Wilkins, 1952.
2. Saunders JB, Inman VT, Eberhart HD. The major determinants in normal and pathological gait. J Bone Joint Surg 1953; 35A:543–558.
3. Inman VT, Ralston HJ, Todd F. Human Walking. Baltimore: Williams & Wilkins, 1981.
4. Eberhart HD, Inman VT, Bresler B. Principal elements in human locomotion. In: Klopsteg PE, Wilson PD, eds. Human Limbs and Their Substitutes. New York: McGraw-Hill, 1964;437–471.
5. Cavagna GA, Margaria R. Mechanics of walking. J Appl Physiol 1966; 21:271–278.
6. Eftman H. Forces and energy changes in leg during walking. Am J Physiol 1939; 125:339–356.
7. Klopsteg PE, Wilson PD, eds. Human Limbs and Their Substitutes. New York: McGraw-Hill, 1954.
8. Inman VT. Conservation of energy in ambulation. Arch Phys Med Rehabil 1967; 47:484–488.
9. Cavagna GA, Saibene FP, Margaria R. External work in walking. J Appl Physiol 1963; 181:1–9.
10. Margaria R. Positive and negative work performances and their efficiencies in human locomotion. Int Z Angew Physiol 1968; 25:339–351.
11. Eftman H. Function of muscles in locomotion. Am J Physiol 1939; 125:357–366.
12. Astrand P-O, Rodahl K. Textbook on Work Physiology. New York: McGraw-Hill, 1970.
13. Corcoran PJ. Energy expenditure during ambulation. In: Downey JA, Darling RD. Physiological Basis of Rehabilitation Medicine. Philadelphia, WB Saunders, 1971;185–198.
14. Fisher SV, Gullickson G Jr. Energy cost of ambulation in health and disability: A literature review. Arch Phys Med Rehabil 1978; 59:124–133.
15. Passmore R, Durnin JVGA. Human energy expenditure. Physiol Rev 1955; 35:801–840.
16. Brown AC, Brengelmann G. Energy metabolism. In: Ruch TC, Patton HD, eds. Physiology and Biophysics, ed 19. Philadelphia, WB Saunders, 1965; 1030–1049.

17. Gordon E. Energy costs of activities in health and disease. Arch Intern Med 1958; 101:702–713.
18. Muller EA, Hettinger T. Effect of the speed of gait on the energy transformation in walking with artificial legs. Germ Ztrschr Orthop 1953; 83:620–627.
19. Montoye HJ, van Huss WD, Reineke EP, et al. An investigation of the Muller-Franz calorimeter. Int Z Angew Physiol 1958; 17:28–33.
20. Master AM, Oppenheimer ET. A simple exercise tolerance test for circulatory efficiency with standard tables for normal individuals. Am J Med Sci 1929; 177:223–243.
21. Ganguli S, Datta SR. A new method for prediction of energy expenditure from heart rate. J Industrial Engineering 1978; 58:560–561.
22. Cooper DM, Weiler-Ravell D, Whipp BJ, et al. Growth-related changes in oxygen uptake and heart rate during progressive exercise in children. Pediatr Res 1984; 18:845–851.
23. Anderson AD. The use of the heart rate as a monitoring device in an ambulation program: A progress report. Arch Phys Med Rehabil 1964; 45:140–146.
24. Rowell LB, Taylor HL, Wang Y. Limitations to prediction of maximal oxygen intake. J Appl Physiol 1964; 19:919–927.
25. Lind AR. Cardiovascular responses to static exercise. (Isometrics anyone?) Circulation 1970; 41:173–176.
26. Hildebrandt G, Voigt E-D, Bahn D, et al. Energy costs of propelling wheelchair at various speeds: Cardiac response and effect on steering accuracy. Arch Phys Med Rehabil 1970; 51:131–136.
27. Darling RC. Exercise. In: Downey JA, Darling RC. Physiological Basis of Rehabilitation Medicine. Philadelphia, WB Saunders. 1971;167–183.
28. Ford AB, Hellerstein HK. Estimation of energy expenditure from pulmonary ventilation. J Appl Physiol 1959; 14:891–893.
29. Bloom WL. A mechanical device for measuring human energy expenditure. Metabolism 1965; 14:955–958.
30. DuBois EF. Basal Metabolism in Health and Disease, ed 3. Philadelphia, Lea & Febiger, 1936.
31. Boothby WM, Berkson J, Dunn AL. Studies of the energy metabolism of normal individuals. Am J Physiol 1936; 116:468.
32. McDonald I. Statistical studies of recorded energy expenditure of man. Part II, Expenditure on walking related to weight, sex, height, speed and gradient. Nutr Abstr Rev 1961; 31:739–762.
33. Waters RL, Hislop HJ, Perry J, et al. Energetics: Application to the study and management of locomotor disabilities energy cost of normal and pathologic gait. Orthop Clin North Am 1978; 9:351–77.
34. Ralston HJ. Energy-speed relation and optimal speed during level walking. Int Z Angew Physiol Einschl Arbeitsphysiol 1958; 17:277–283.
35. Bobbert AC. Energy expenditure in level and grade walking. J Appl Physiol 1960; 15:1015–1021.
36. Corcoran PJ, Brengelmann GL. Oxygen uptake in normal and handicapped subjects, in relation to speed of walking beside velocity-controlled cart. Arch Phys Med Rehabil 1970; 51:78–87.
37. Ralston HJ. Dynamics of the human body during locomotion: The efficiency of walking in normal and amputee subjects. Final Report, SRS Grant RD 2849-M, Aug, 1971. Berkeley: Biomechanics Laboratory, University of California, San Francisco, 1971.
38. Waters RL, Perry J, Antonelli D, et al. Energy cost of walking of amputees: Influence of level of amputation. J Bone Joint Surg 1976; 58A:42–46.
39. Margaria R, Cerretelli P, Aghemo P, et al. Energy cost of running. J Appl Physiol 1963; 18:367–370.
40. Soule RG, Goldman RF. Energy cost of loads carried on the head, hands or feet. J Appl Physiol 1969; 27:687.
41. Christensen EH. Physiological valuation of work in the Nykroppa Iron Works. Presented at the Ergonomics Society Symposium on Fatigue, Leeds, London, 1953.
42. League of Nations, Technical Commission. Report on the Physiologic Basis of Nutrition. Publication II, Economic and Financial. 1936.
43. Ralston HJ. Effects of immobilization of various body segments on energy cost of human locomotion. In: Proceedings of Second International Congress on Ergonomics, Dortmund, 1964. Ergonomics 1965; 12:(suppl)53–60.
44. Waters RL, Campbell J, Thomas L, et al. Energy cost of walking in lower-extremity plaster cast. J Bone Joint Surg 1982; 64A:896–899.
45. Reitmeyer H. Energy consumption and gait characteristics in walking and bicycling in unilateral below-knee amputees. Z Orthop 1955; 86:571–589.
46. Molen NH. Energy/speed relation of below-knee amputees walking on motor-driven treadmill. Int Z Angew Physiol 1973; 31:173–185.
47. Ganguli S, Datta SR, Chatterjee BB, et al. Performance evaluation of amputee-prosthesis system in below-knee amputees. Ergonomics 1973; 16:797–810.
48. Gonzalez EG, Corcoran PJ, Reyes RL. Energy expenditure in below-knee amputees: Correlation

with stump length. Arch Phys Med Rehabil 1974; 55:111–119.

49. Pagliarulo, MA, Waters RL, Hislop HJ. Energy cost of walking of below-knee amputees having no vascular disease. Phys Ther 1979; 59:538–542.

50. Huang C-T, Jackson JR, Moore NB, et al. Amputation: Energy cost of ambulation. Arch Phys Med Rehabil 1979; 60:18–24.

51. Ganguli S, Datta SR. Studies in load carrying in below-knee amputees with a PTB prosthesis system, J Med Eng Tech 1977; 57:151–154.

52. Roy AK, Ganguli S, Datta SR, et al. Performance evaluation of BK amputees through graded load carrying test. Acta Orthop Scand 1977; 48:691–695.

53. Ganguli S, Datta SR, Chatterjee BB, et al. Performance evaluation of amputee-prosthesis system in below-knee amputees. Ergonomics 1973; 16:797–810.

54. Cummings V, March H, Steve L, et al. Energy costs of below-knee prostheses using two types of suspension. Arch Phys Med Rehabil 1979; 60:293–297.

55. Nielsen PH, Schurr DG, Golden JC, et al. Comparison of energy cost and gait efficiency during ambulation in below-knee amputees using different prosthetic feet. A preliminary report. J Prosthet Orthot 1989; 1:24–31.

56. MacFarlane PA, Nielsen DN, Schurr DG, et al. Gait comparison for below-knee amputees using a Flex-Foot versus a conventional prosthetic foot. J Prosthet Orthot 1991; 3:150–161.

57. Wagner J, Sienko S, Supan T, et al. "Motion analysis of SACH vs Flex-Foot in moderately active below-knee amputees." Clin Prosthet Orthot 1987; 11:55–62.

58. Muller EA, Hettinger TH. Arbeitsphysiologische Untersuchungen verschiedener Oberschenkel-Kunstbeine. Z Orthop 1952; 81:525–545.

59. Erdman WJH, Hettinger Th, Saez F. Comparative work stress for above-knee amputees using artificial legs or crutches. Am J Phys Med 1960; 39:225–232.

60. Inman VT, Barnes GH, Levy SW, et al. Medical problems of amputees. Calif Med 1961; 94:132–138.

61. Bard G, Ralston HJ. Measurement of energy expenditure during ambulation, with special reference to evaluation of assistive devices. Arch Phys Med Rehabil 1959; 40:415–420.

62. Ganguli S, Bose KS, Datta SR, et al. Ergonomics evaluation of above-knee amputee–prosthesis combinations. Ergonomics 1974; 17:199–210.

63. Traugh GH, Corcoran PJ, Reyes RL. Energy expenditure of ambulation in patients with above-knee amputations. Arch Phys Med Rehabil 1975; 56:67–71.

64. James U. Oxygen uptake and heart rate during prosthetic walking in healthy male unilateral above-knee amputees. Scand J Rehabil 1973; 5:71–80.

65. Otis JC, Lane JM, Kroll MA. Energy cost during gait in osteosarcoma patients after resection and knee replacement and above-knee amputation. J Bone Joint Surg 1985; 67A:606–611.

66. Isakov E, Susakz, Becker E. Energy expenditure and cardiac response in above-knee amputee while using prosthesis with open and locked knee mechanisms. Scand J Rehab Med 1985; 12(suppl):108–111.

67. Roy AK, Datta SR, Chatterjec BB, et al. Ergonomic study on above-knee prosthetic rehabilitees carrying graded loads. Ergonomics 1976; 19:431–440.

68. Nowroozi F, Saronelli ML, Gerber LH. Energy expenditure in hip disarticulation and hemipelvectomy. Arch Phys Med Rehabil 1983; 64:300–303.

69. Corcoran PJ, Reyes RL, Gonzalez EG. Energy cost of ambulation in bilateral leg amputees. Presented at the 48th Annual Session, American Congress of Rehabilitation Medicine, San Juan, Puerto Rico, Nov 10, 1971.

70. DuBow LL, Witt PL, Kadaba MP, et al. Oxygen consumption of elderly persons with bilateral below-knee amputations: Amputation vs wheelchair propulsion. Arch Phys Med Rehabil 1983; 64:255–259.

71. Crouse SF, Lessard CS, Rhodes J, et al. Oxygen consumption and cardiac response of short-leg and long-leg prosthetic ambulation in a patient with bilateral above-knee amputation: Comparisons with able-bodied men. Arch Phys Med Rehabil 1990; 71:313–317.

72. Ganguli S, Bose KS, Datta SR, et al. Biomechanical approach to functional assessment of use of crutches for ambulation. Ergonomics 1974; 17:365–374.

73. The Geriatric Amputee: Principles of Management. Proceedings of a Workshop on the Geriatric Amputee, Washington, DC, June 9-10, 1969. Washington: National Academy of Sciences, National Research Council, 1971.

74. Bard B. Energy expenditure of hemiplegic subjects during walking. Arch Phys Med Rehabil 1963; 44:368–370.

75. Corcoran PJ, Jebsen RH, Brengelmann GL, et al. Effects of plastic and metal leg braces on speed and energy cost of hemiparetic ambulation. Arch Phys Med Rehabil 1970; 51:69–77.

76. Gersten JW, Orr W. External work of walking in

hemiparetic patients. Scand J Rehabil Med 1971; 3:85–88.

77. Lehneis HR, Bergofsky E, Frisina W. Energy expenditure with advanced lower limb orthoses and with conventional braces. Arch Phys Med Rehabil 1976; 57:20–24.

78. Long CH, Lawton EB. Functional significance of spinal cord lesion level. Arch Phys Med Rehabil 1955; 36:249–255.

79. Rosman N, Spira E. Paraplegic use of walking braces: Survey. Arch Phys Med Rehabil 1974; 55:310–314.

80. Gordon EE. Physiological approach to ambulation in paraplegia. JAMA 1956; 161:686–688.

81. Gordon EE, Vanderwalde H. Energy requirements in paraplegic ambulation. Arch Phys Med Rehabil 1956; 37:276–285.

82. Clinkingbeard JR, Gersten JW, Hoehn D. Energy cost of ambulation in traumatic paraplegic. Am J Phys Med 1964; 43:157–165.

83. Waters RL, Lunsford BR. Energy cost of paraplegic locomotion. J Bone Joint Surg 1985; 67A:1245–1250.

84. Waters RL, Yakura JS, Adkins R, et al. Determinants of gait performance following spinal cord injury. Arch Phys Med Rehabil 1989; 70:811–818.

85. Chantraine A, Crielaard JM, Onkelinx A, et al. Energy expenditure of ambulation in paraplegics: Effects of long-term use of bracing. Paraplegia 1984; 22:173–181.

86. Yakura JS, Waters RL, Adkins RH. Changes in ambulation parameters in spinal cord injury individuals following rehabilitation. Paraplegia 1990; 28:364–370.

87. Lehmann JF, DeLateur BJ, Warren CG, et al. Biomechanical evaluation of braces for paraplegics. Arch Phys Med Rehabil 1969; 50:179–188.

88. Merkel KD, Miller NE, Westbrook PR, et al. Energy expenditure of paraplegic patients standing and walking with two knee-ankle-foot orthoses. Arch Phys Med Rehabil 1984; 65:121–124.

89. Miller NE, Merritt JL, Merkel KD, et al. Paraplegic energy expenditure during negotiation of architectural barriers. Arch Phys Med Rehabil 1984; 65:778–779.

90. Huang C-T, Kuhlemeier KV, Moore NB, et al. Energy cost of ambulation in paraplegic patients using Craig-Scott braces. Arch Phys Med Rehabil 1979; 60:595–600.

91. Nene AV, Patrick JH. Energy cost of paraplegic locomotion with the Orlau ParaWalker. Paraplegia 1989; 27:5–18.

92. Patrick JH, McClelland, MR. Low–energy cost reciprocal walking for adult paraplegic. Paraplegia 1985; 23:113–117.

93. Ragnarsson KT, Sell GH, McGarrity M, et al. Pneumatic orthosis for paraplegic patients: Functional evaluation and prescription considerations. Arch Phys Med Rehabil 1975; 56:479–483.

94. Marsolais EB, Edwards BG. Energy costs of walking and standing with functional neuromuscular stimulation and long leg braces. Arch Phys Med Rehabil 1988; 69:243–249.

95. Edwards BG, Marsolais EB. Metabolic responses to arm ergometry and functional neuromuscular stimulation. J Rehab Res Rev 1990; 27:107–114.

96. Cerney K, Waters R, Perry J. Walking and wheelchair energetics in persons with paraplegia. Phys Ther 1980; 60:1133–1139.

97. Hildenbrandt G, Voigt E-D, Bahn D, et al. Energy costs of propelling wheelchair at various speeds: Cardiac response and effect on steering accuracy. Arch Phys Med Rehabil 1970; 51:131–136.

98. Hilbers PA, White TP. Effects of wheelchair design on metabolic and heart rate responses during propulsion by persons with paraplegia. Phys Ther 1987; 67:1355–1358.

99. Wolfe GA, Waters R, Hislop HJ. Influence of floor space on the energy cost of wheelchair propulsion. Phys Ther 1977; 57:1022–1026.

100. Shoup TE, Fletcher LS, Merrill BR. Biomechanics of crutch locomotion. J Biomechanics 1974; 7:11–20.

101. Wells RP. The kinemetrics and energy variations of swing-through crutch gait. Biomechanics 1979; 12:579–585.

102. McBeath AA, Bahrke M, Balke B. Efficiency of assisted ambulation determined by oxygen consumption measurement. J Bone Joint Surg 1974: 56A:994–1000.

103. Fisher S, Patterson R. Energy cost of ambulation with crutches. Arch Phys Med Rehabil 1981; 62:250–256.

104. Patterson R, Fisher SV. Cardiovascular stress of crutch walking. Arch Phys Med Rehabil 1981; 62:257–260.

105. Imms FJ, MacDonald ID, Prestidge SP. Energy expenditure during walking in patients recovering from fractures of the leg. Scand J Rehabil Med 1976; 8:1–9.

106. Pugh LG. The oxygen intake and energy cost of walking before and after unilateral hip replacement, with some observations on the use of crutches. J Bone Joint Surg 1973; 55B:742–745.

107. Brown MB, Batten C, Porell D. Efficiency of walking after total hip replacement. Orthop Clin North Am 1978; 9:364–367.

108. Corcoran PJ, Templer JA. Stair climbing for cardiovascular reconditioning. Presented at the 37th Annual Assembly, American Academy of Physical

Medicine and Rehabilitation, Atlanta, Georgia, Nov. 19, 1975.

109. Ganguli S, Bose KS. Biomechanical approach to functional assessment of use of crutches for ambulation. Ergonomics 1974; 17:365–374.

110. Rose J, Gamble JG, Madeiros J, et al. Energy cost of walking in normal children and in those with cerebral palsy: Comparison of heart rate and oxygen uptake. J Pediatr Orthop 1989; 9:276–279.

111. Rose J, Gamble JG, Burgos A, et al. Energy expenditure index of walking for normal children and for children with cerebral palsy. Dev Med Child Neurol 1990; 32:333–340.

112. Olgiati R, Jacquet J, di Prampero PE. Energy cost of walking and exertional dyspnea in multiple sclerosis. Am Rev Respir Dis 1986; 134:1005–1010.

113. Olgiati R, Burgunder J-M, Mumenthaler M. Increased energy cost of walking in multiple sclerosis: Effect of spasticity, ataxia, and weakness. Arch Phys Med Rehabil 1988; 69:846–849.

114. Thomas LF, Hislop HJ, Waters RL. Physiological work performance in chronic low back disability. Phys Ther 1980; 60:407–411.

# Chapter 17

# Physiologic Changes Associated with Bed Rest and Major Body Injury

ROBERT JOHN DOWNEY
CHARLES WEISSMAN

Despite the variety of disorders and procedures seen on a surgical service, experience teaches that postoperative recovery often follows a predictable course. Operations are traumas visited on a patient; common to both operative and accidental trauma is a period of recovery marked, to varying degrees, by reduced activity, recumbency, and mobilization of the body's resources to effect healing. It is our goal in this chapter to describe the features of recovery that most healing patients have in common and the changes that form the pathophysiologic substrate upon which the unique aspects of each disease process and corrective operation are superimposed.

# Physiology of Bed Rest

ROBERT J DOWNEY

Bed rest is routinely, and often casually, prescribed for a wide variety of pathophysiologic states, the rationale being to reduce functional demands on a diseased body. Earlier in this century prolonged bed rest was much more widely recommended than it is today, particularly after myocardial infarction.[1,2] With recognition of the unfavorable effects of prolonged inactivity, emphasis shifted toward more rapid remobilization, particularly in the early postoperative period. Nevertheless, almost all hospitalized patients are subjected to some period of reduced activity, and therefore the physiologic alterations that occur as a result of decreased activity and changes in posture form the basis on which all other pathophysiologic processes of illness are superimposed.

## Cardiovascular and Fluid Alterations

Many studies, utilizing a wide variety of experimental subjects and of protocols, have been undertaken to examine the cardiovascular effects of prolonged immobilization. For example, Dietrick and colleagues[3] examined physiologic and metabolic changes in four healthy young males immobilized in pelvic and leg-casts for 6 weeks. Graveline and coworkers[4] examined primarily hemodynamic parameters in four males immersed up to 24 hours in water, to simulate weightlessness. Miller[5] and Vogt[6] and their coworkers focused primarily on the fluid shifts associated with bed rest in groups of young males, for 28 and 10 days, respectively. Saltin's group[7] measured exercise tolerance in five young males by following maximal oxygen uptake during 21 days' bed rest followed by 8 weeks' recuperative activity. The only two studies of subjects other than young males were performed by Gaffney and associates,[8] who examined short-term effects of head-down tilt on middle-aged men, and by Convertino and colleagues,[9] who examined the hemodynamic alterations associated with exercise following 10 days' bed rest in twelve 50-year-old men. Combining elements of several such studies provides an overview of the cardiovascular changes that accompany bed rest.

The veins of the lower extremity are part of the postcapillary blood pool, which comprises approximately 70% of the overall intravascular volume. Contraction of the gastrocnemius and soleus muscles during normal ambulation compresses sinusoids contained within each muscle and propels venous blood toward the heart. Reflux during muscle relaxation is prevented by the presence in the veins below the common iliac vein of delicate but strong bicuspid valves. These mechanisms are imperfect; with standing, approximately 500 ml of blood shifts from the upper body to the lower and venous pressures stabilize at approximately 80 to 100 mm. Hg.[10] "Modest" levels of lower extremity activity transiently lower this pressure head to approximately 25 mm Hg, but the shift of blood out of the thorax largely persists. When a person

448

is lying down, the blood can more readily leave the lower extremities and acts to augment venous return centrally, causing increased stretching of baroreceptors in the right atrium, the walls of the carotid artery, and the aortic arch, which initiates vasodepressor responses—decreased heart rate and contractility, peripheral vasodilatation, increased renal blood flow, diuresis (Table 17-1).

Blomqvist and colleagues[11] studied the effects of a head-down tilt on 10 healthy men over 24 hours. Here, a marked central fluid shift led to elevation of central venous pressure and increases in the left ventricular end-diastolic volume and stroke volume, but because of reflex compensatory decrease in heart rate there was no increase in cardiac output. These changes were transient; all values returned to levels similar to the upright position after 24 hours. However, these subjects did demonstrate diminished orthostatic tolerance, increased heart rate, and decreased stroke volume during submaximal exercise, and, overall, decreased maximal exercise capacity when they returned to the upright position. More recently, Lathers and associates[12] measured cardiovascular responses to degrees of downward tilt to $-5$ degrees and found, during the first 2 to 3 hours, decreased mean thoracic fluid index, suggesting increased intrathoracic fluid (principally blood sequestered in the lungs[8]) leading to decreased heart rate, stroke volume, pulse pressure, and cardiac output. These findings conflict, to some degree with those cited previously.

With this central fluid shift while lying down and increased effective intravascular volume, initially diuresis occurs; the average decrease in plasma volume after 24 hours is 5%. This continues and reaches 10% in 6 days, and 20% after 14 days.[13] The volume loss exceeds the net return in fluid from the lower extremities and may occur by mechanisms other than renal response to central volume receptors, such as alterations in atrial natriuretic factor.

**Table 17-1.** Cardiovascular Alterations with Bed Rest

Early increased central blood volume with diuresis
Increased resting heart rate
Exaggerated increase in pulse with exercise
Decreased maximal cardiac output with exercise

Many investigators have noted orthostatic intolerance after prolonged bed rest. They attributed this, in part at least, to the intravascular volume depletion noted above, possibly compounded by an increase in venous pooling in the lower extremities because of increased venous compliance after bed rest. In addition to the changes in intravascular volume and venous tone, prolonged recumbency blunts cardiac responsiveness to rapid changes in posture. Bed rest increases the resting pulse from 4 to 15 beats per minute, and after bed rest there is a more pronounced increase in heart rate with exercise. For example, normal volunteers experienced an increase in pulse to approximately 129 beats per minute during submaximal exercise, whereas after bed rest the same exercise demand drove the heart rate to approximately 165 beats per minute.[7,16] Similarly, Chobanian and coworkers[17] found that bed rest exaggerated the increase in heart rate in response to movement from supine to upright: control subjects experienced an increased heart rate of 13%, whereas experimental subjects demonstrated increases of 32% after 3 days' bed rest, 62% after 7 days', 89% after 21 days'. This exaggerated increase in heart rate does not seem to translate into increased cardiac output: in fact, the increases in both stroke volume and cardiac output to maximal exercise are reduced by about 25% following prolonged bed rest, perhaps suggesting a poorly defined myocardial depressant factor.[7,17,18] On the basis of echocardiographic studies, Hung and colleagues[19] suggested that left ventricular ejection fraction increased normally during both supine and upright exercise but the resting left ventricular end-diastolic volume decreased by 16%, consistent with a decrease in venous return rather than depressed myocardial function. The observed alterations in the cardiovascular system's ability to accommodate to changes in body position and distribution in intravascular volume may be due to alterations in autonomic function. It has been suggested[20] that the tachycardia that follows bed rest is related to either decreased vagal tone, decreased sensitivity to vagal stimulation, increased sympathetic tone, or insensitivity to sympathetic stimulation. Subjects given atropine to block vagal tone had a significantly higher heart rate after bed rest than during control periods, and Robinson's group[21] and Melada's[22] found the vasovagal manifestations of orthostatic intolerance following bed rest could be attributed to increased β-adrenergic activity, as symptoms could be blocked by propranolol.

## Respiration

Oxygen uptake and carbon dioxide elimination occur through the ventilation of alveoli in contact with circulating blood. A certain inefficiency is built into the system, as portions of the airway are ventilated but not perfused (dead space) and portions are perfused but not well-ventilated (shunt). These mismatches normally are small in adults, but in postoperative and bedridden patients ventilation and perfusion are badly mismatched.

The normal respiratory cycle of inspiration and expiration occurs as a balance of the opposing tendencies of the elastic lung parenchyma to collapse and the stiffer chest wall to expand. The volume of the lung at rest, following a normal expiration when these forces are balanced, is called the *functional residual capacity* (FRC). In a normal erect man during a spontaneous breath, distribution of ventilation and blood flow are uneven. The amount of perfusion of blood to each area of the lung is a function of the perfusion pressure (pulmonary artery and venous pressures) and the pressures in the surrounding tissues (airway pressure and hydrostatic pressures due to gravity). Based on the varying relationship between these pressures, the isolated lung can be divided into three regions: zone I (apical), where the alveolar pressure exceeds both pulmonary arterial and venous pressure so that perfusion theoretically does not occur; zone II (middle); where the alveolar pressure is less than pulmonary arterial pressure but still more than pulmonary venous pressure, so that blood flow is dependent on the pulmonary artery–alveolar pressure gradient; and zone III (basilar), in which pulmonary venous pressure exceeds alveolar pressure and blood flow is dependent on the pulmonary artery–venous pressure gradient.[23] Any body position other than upright increases the proportion of the lung subject to zone III conditions. The supine position causes posterior lung segments from base to apex to move increasingly into zone III, and either lateral position increases the extent of zone III in the dependent lung.[24] In zone III areas there is a tendency

to increasing distension of the pulmonary vasculature and the accumulation of pulmonary interstitial fluid (Figure 17-1).

Gravity causes pleural pressure to become progressively more negative from the lung base to its apex, primarily because of the weight of the basilar lung tissue pulling down on the tissue in the apex. Thus, the airway-distending pressure is most effective at the apex, and at rest the apical alveoli are more distended than the basilar alveoli. If a breath is initiated from the FRC, the change in transpulmonary pressure at the apices and the base is equal, but because the apical alveoli are already distended and higher on the alveolar pressure-volume curve, the volume change in the lung with

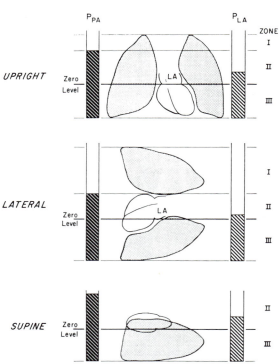

**Figure 17-1.** The effects of changes in body position on zonal distribution of blood flow. We have assumed that the absolute values for $P_{PA}$, $P_{ALV}$ and $P_{LA}$ remain constant in all positions (see heights of respective columns). In the lateral position, an entire lung may be in zone III. Intrapleural pressure is more positive around the *down* lung than the *up* lung, owing to the gravitational effect. Therefore, alveoli in the down lung are smaller and more prone to collapse. Thoracotomy in the patient with heart disease ($P_{LA}$ high) requires ventilation with end-expiratory pressure to prevent terminal airway collapse in the down lung.

each unit of pressure change is less at the apices. Therefore, the basilar lung segments are ventilated preferentially.[25,26]

At some point during expiration, as lung volumes are reduced, alveoli close while being perfused and are not available for ventilation. The point at which these alveolar closures begin to occur is called the *closing volume,* and it is normally below the FRC, meaning that at the end of expiration the alveoli have not yet begun to close (Figure 17-2).[27] In certain circumstances this may not be true; for example, obese persons have decreased expiratory reserve volume and smokers have increased closing volume, so in each situation alveolar closure begins at a point above the end-tidal point, causing alveoli to be perfused with blood but not ventilated and rendering them ineffective for gas exchange.

The closing volume has been shown to be rel-

atively independent of posture; however, the FRC decreases by about 20% in the supine position.[28] This may be sufficient to place the closing volume above the end-tidal point, which closes the basilar alveoli. These alveoli remain closed for the initial portion of the next inhalation, and the ventilation is shunted to the open apical alveoli. Blood continues to flow through the poorly ventilated or unventilated basilar segments, and the apical segments receive ventilation in excess of blood flow, all of which tends to decrease arterial oxygenation.

Placing a normal person in a recumbent position leads to changes in all lung volumes except the tidal volume (TV). Craig and colleagues[29] found that changing a normal human from upright to a supine position resulted in a loss of 2% of the vital capacity, 7% of the total lung capacity, 10% of the closing volume, 19% of the residual volume, 46% of the expiratory reserve volume, and 30% of the functional residual capacity. (Changes to positions other than the supine lead to small losses of volume: normal subjects had a decrease in FRC of only 17% when moved from the upright to the lateral decubitus position.[30]) Interestingly, these changes might be *less* pronounced in patients with chronic pulmonary disease: Marini and coworkers[30] also reported that patients with chronic airflow obstruction exhibited change in FRC of only 3.5% on moving from an upright to a supine position, and a decrease of only 1.9% on moving to the lateral decubitus position. Furthermore, this study found a significant decrease in arterial oxygen saturation in supine normal subjects, but not in patients with significant airflow obstruction.

The actual degree to which the described physiologic changes affect respiration has been studied only partially. Cardus' group[31] found in normal young males that after 10 days of bed rest there was a mean decrease in $PaO_2$ of 9 mm Hg, an increase of 10 mm Hg in $P(A-a)O_2$, but no change in the mean arterial carbon dioxide concentration. Such changes probably would not be important in these normal young men.

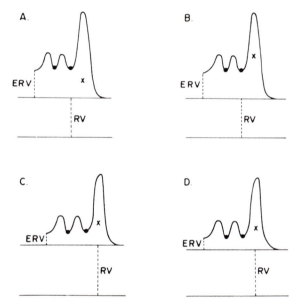

**Figure 17-2.** Relationship between closing volume (CV) and expiratory reserve volume (ERV), with ( ) representing the end-tidal point, and (X), the CV. (*A*) Normal CV less than ERV and below the end-tidal point. (*B*) Smoker has increased CV that is larger than the normal ERV and is above the end-tidal point. (*C*) Obese patient with decreased ERV. (*D*) Postoperatively, normal patient has decreased ERV; even a normal CV becomes larger than ERV and is above the end-tidal point. In the postoperative period, the CV would be even farther above ERV in obese patients, smokers, and patients with airway disease. Key: RV, residual volume.

## Muscle Disuse

Multiple studies have demonstrated that muscle strength, size, and stamina are all affected by a lack of activity and that this weakening process affects all aspects of muscle function and structure. Booth[32] provides a more comprehensive discussion of muscle disuse.

Disuse causes a progressive decrease in muscle strength associated with a decrease in cross-sectional area of the muscle fibers. In healthy humans, MacDougall and colleagues[33] described a 5% decrease in arm circumference with a 35% decrease in elbow extension strength following 5 weeks' immobilization. Witzman and coworkers[34] demonstrated in rats that both twitch and tetanic tension (expressed as either the product of whole muscle or unit cross-sectional area) was diminished in chronically shortened soleus or extensor digitorum muscle and that this occurs whether the immobilized muscle was stretched, neutral, or shortened.[35]

The decline in maximal attainable tension[32] and loss of muscle weight[35] occur rapidly, reaching a new steady state 5 to 10 days after immobilization. Booth[36] found that after an initial lag period of slow weight loss during the first day or two, 50% of the eventual loss had occurred by the 8 to the 10th day. The muscle wasting is thought to be the result of decreased muscle protein synthesis rather than increased protein breakdown.[37] Because the cellular content of mRNA for actin remained unchanged for 3 days while the synthesis of actin had decreased by the 6th hour,[35] the control was felt to be exerted at some step in the translation or elongation sequence. Muscle collagen synthesis is also reduced, though the rate of decrease in formation is less than that of the noncollagen proteins, resulting in a transient increase in collagen concentration despite absolute collagen content.[38] The change in contractile properties may also be due to qualitative changes in muscle protein composition, as well as the quantitative changes in protein levels: Reiser and colleagues[39] noted a 30% increase in the mean maximal shortening velocity of fibers of immobilized rat soleus muscles, which they attributed to a relative increase in the amount of fast-to-slow myosin isoenzymes.

As mass and maximal attainable tension decrease, fatigability during work increases. The peak tension from pulse train stimulation is less in the soleus muscle of rats immobilized 6 weeks than in that of controls. Before the stimulation exercise the immobilized muscles were found to have decreased levels of adenosine triphosphate (ATP) and glycogen stores[32,36] and more rapid depletion of both those stores and accumulation of lactic acid during exercise than in immobilized.[33] Also contributing to rapid fatigability is apparently decreased capability on the part of the immobilized muscle to utilize fatty acids[40] as compared to the trained state, in which the muscle uses fat more rapidly and carbohydrates more slowly.[41]

## Calcium Metabolism

Maintaining a skeleton capable of resisting the mechanical forces applied during activity depends on the intermittent application of these same forces. When a stress is applied to a bone, as in normal activity or exercise, the strain is sensed, and subsequently, changes in osteoclast and osteoblast cellular activity result.[42,43] If no force is applied to the skeleton, either because of plaster immobilization, strictly enforced bed rest, paralysis, or the weightlessness of space flight, bone mineral is lost because the rate of bone formation drops below the rate of bone mineral absorption. A review of the literature shows that decreased mobility is associated with early rapid bone mineral loss, which later leads to less but stable bone mass.

Bone mineral loss was first measured in convalescing patients, but similar losses occur in healthy subjects, owing to either prolonged bed rest[44] or conditions of weightlessness.[45] After 84 days' weightlessness aboard *Skylab* 4, daily stool and urine calcium losses averaged 18 g for the three crewmen; the 3.9% rate of loss was higher from the calcaneus than from the radius, suggesting that the calcaneus is more susceptible, either because of a proportionately greater reduction in weight bearing or because it is composed of trabecular bone.

In a study of five healthy men at bed rest for as long as 36 weeks,[46] a consistent pattern of change was seen: urine calcium increased at a rate of 12% per week until a peak level of excretion was reached at 100 mg per day above control levels after about 16 weeks. Net losses of total body calcium in urine, sweat, and feces averaged 0.5% per month. There were parallel losses in phosphorus and hydroxyproline, and total body phosphorus declined an average of 150 mg per day below controls. Urinary hydroxyproline excretion was also increased to a level of 10 mg per day above baseline controls by the 6th week. The rate of calcium loss is different for different bones of the body: the rate of loss from the calcaneus averaged 5% per month—ten times the rate of loss from the body as a whole—and the mineral content of the radius revealed no change throughout the 10-week study, suggesting that during bed rest, mineral loss occurs only from bones that normally bear weight.[46] One study found that bone mineral loss from the vertebral bodies of normal males put at strict bed rest was not significant over a 5-week period.[47]

When healthy subjects resumed ambulation, calcium and phosphorus balances begin to return toward the positive side, but slowly, becoming positive only after 4 weeks.[44] The increase in phosphorus balance was much more rapid, suggesting phosphate uptake into tissues other than bone, such as muscle. This study found that with ambulation remineralization occurred at a rate similar to the rate of loss with immobility and that all subjects had reached or exceeded initial values by the 36th week. Other studies,[48] which examined disuse osteopenia in patients with fractures, suggested that bone mineral content might not be completely regained even after as long as 14 years of activity.

Illness or disease enhances the rate of bone mineral loss beyond that of immobilization alone. The rate of loss for 139 patients confined to bed because of either leg fracture or herniated discs was found to approximate 2% of total calcium per month.[49] Spinal cord injury with paralysis causes osteopenia in the bones below the level of the lesion, and total bone volume decreases rapidly over the first months after an injury, stabilizing at approximately 70% of baseline, a rate of decrease approximately 100 times greater than that associated with aging.[50]

## Gastrointestinal Alterations

Gastrointestinal function is altered with bed rest.[51] Nonviscous boluses, but not viscous materials, pass through the esophagus more rapidly when the subject is upright rather than supine[52]; this in-creased rate of transit in the upright position is associated with increased velocity of the esophageal wave and shortening of lower esophageal sphincter relaxation time. The transit time of a bolus through the stomach is as much as 66% slower when the subject is lying down as when standing, though[53,54] gastric acidity is increased owing to activation of the sympathetic system and inhibition of gastric bicarbonate secretion.[55] Small bowel motility is reduced by inactivity,[56] and defecation is certainly altered by a change in body position: the forces generated during straining after stool in the sitting position are threefold those generated when squatting.[57]

## Hormone Alterations

Bed rest causes multiple alterations in the endocrine system, mostly the result of the reduced level of activity, and, to a lesser extent, to changes in posture. The affected hormones, other than those related to the changes in intravascular volume discussed previously, are of two axes: insulin and glucose, and adrenocortical steroids. Blotner[58] first noted that ill patients whose treatment included prolonged bed rest demonstrated reduced glucose tolerance, and Dietrick and colleagues[3] demonstrated that this decreased tolerance was in part due to bed rest, independent of intercurrent disease. Hyperinsulinemia accompanied this hyperglycemia,[59] with reduction in peripheral glucose uptake.[60] Owing to inactivity, muscle develops insulin resistance and exogenous insulin administered to subjects on bed rest results in significantly smaller decreases in blood glucose levels when compared to pre–bed rest control values.[61] This intolerance occurs as soon as 3 days after immobilization, with peripheral glucose uptake decreasing by 20%, and by 14 days by 50%. There does not seem to be an accompanying alteration in hepatic glucose production[62] or in the insulin responsiveness of muscle protein breakdown,[63] suggesting that the defect in insulin action is not generalized.

Changes in circulating glucocorticoids closely related to the changes in insulin levels and responsiveness are observed. Vernikos-Danellis and colleagues[64] showed that circadian rhythmicity of cortisol blood levels persists but the amplitude of the cycle diminishes. In the same patients, bed rest destabilized thyroid hormone rhythms, as evidenced by elevation of the triiodothyronine ($T_3$) level, and, as noted in a separate study,[64] circulating growth hormone levels decreased following 10 days' inactivity, and subsequently rose by day 20. Catecholamine and methoxamine (dopamine) levels appear to be unchanged by bed rest[65]; the effect of inactivity on glucagon level is not known. Taken together, these findings suggest that the alteration in glucose homeostasis that occurs with bed rest may result from both decreased muscle responsiveness and alterations in hypothalamic-pituitary axis function.

## Bed Rest and Venous Thrombosis

Thrombosis may occur in any venous tract of the body, but it is most frequent in the veins of the legs and pelvis, especially in the deep veins of the calf.[66] Estimates of the incidence of deep venous thrombosis (DVT) range from 29% for postoperative general surgical patients to 44% following surgery for hip fractures.[67] Schlosser[68] performed meta-analysis of publications, attempting to estimate the prevalence of fatal post-operative pulmonary embolism. He found it to be approximately 0.2% to 1.2%. About 600,000 cases of pulmonary embolism occur annually among medical and surgical patients in the United States, and a third prove fatal.[69] In one autopsy series, Havig[70] reported that pulmonary embolism contributed to death in about 20% of cases. The natural history of a thrombosed vein is eventual recanalization; however, in some patients, thrombosis may result in the destruction of the venous valve system and, particularly if the thrombosis involves the popliteal veins[71] and the ankle-perforating veins,[72] may lead over a period of years to severe chronic edema and ulcerations.

Since the time of Virchow, clinicians have appreciated that decreased venous blood flow contributes to the creation of thrombis, but stasis alone is not enough. In fact, Hewson[73] described blood static between two ligatures on a dog's jugular vein that remained fluid for as long as 3 hours. Stasis, therefore, is a *permissive* factor: it promotes but is not sufficient to cause, thrombosis.

There are many theories to explain the additional factors that cause a static pool of blood to thrombose. Thrombi probably arise simultaneously from several sites within a single venous system, usually valve cusps. Sevitt[74] showed that the nidus of origin is located in the valve pocket near the normal endothelium of the vein wall and is composed primarily of red blood cells and fibrin, platelets being restricted to the growing portion of the thrombus. Karino and Motomiya[75] found a stagnant area in the deepest portion of the valve pocket; this may serve as a "trap" for cellular aggregates. Stasis may generate local areas of hypoxia, which may damage the underlying endothelium, rendering the area thrombogenic.[76]

Even in the absence of direct vessel wall damage, stasis alone probably leads to the generation of the enzyme thrombin, which can lead to platelet aggregation and thrombin deposition,[77] and thrombin may also lead to damage of the endothelial surface.[78] Alterations in fibrinolysis may play a role: most surgical procedures seem to be followed by a period of depressed fibrinolytic activity lasting a little more than a week.[79]

It is likely, therefore, that no single factor is responsible for venous thrombosis but that decreased flow in the deep veins of the legs secondary to inactivity allows the factors responsible for intravascular coagulation to have maximal effect on a concentrated area. Flow in the iliac vein is reduced by about 50% during a period of anesthesia in the supine position[80] and this decrease may be due in part to a decrease in arterial inflow. Bird[81] demonstrated that calf arterial flow was only 58% of normal following a period of general anesthesia. The profound effect of inactivity on the incidence of DVT is confirmed by the observation of increased prevalence in the paralyzed extremities of hemiplegics.[82]

In summary, bed rest alone causes generalized deconditioning of healthy subjects involving most of the physiologic system of the body, including the cardiovascular, pulmonary, gastrointestinal, hormonal, and skeletal systems. When the patient not only is at bed rest but has been injured or has undergone a serious medical or surgical intervention, the consequences can be severe. It is necessary now to review the effects of injury or trauma on the bodily systems.

# An Overview of the Response to Injury

CHARLES WEISSMAN

Major body injury, surgical or accidental, provokes reproducible metabolic, hormonal, and hemodynamic responses[83] characterized by altered protein homeostasis,[84] hypermetabolism,[85] altered carbohydrate metabolism,[86] sodium and water retention,[87] and increased lipolysis.[88] The abnormal carbohydrate metabolism includes increased endogenous hepatic glucose production (gluconeogenesis) and reduced glucose clearance (insulin resistance), which results in hyperglycemia. The major body fuel becomes fat; therefore, lipolysis is increased and lipogenesis retarded.[89] Protein abnormalities are manifested by negative nitrogen balance, reflecting accelerated net protein breakdown (catabolism).[90] The magnitude of these changes is essentially proportional to the extent of injury (Table 17-2).[91]

## Mediators of the Response

### The Neuroendocrine Axis

All mechanisms that initiate, regulate, and sustain response to major body injury have not yet been identified. One area of particular interest has been the neuroendocrine axis. It has long been recognized that injured patients have elevated levels of "counterregulatory," or antiinsulin, hormones—cortisol, glucagon, catecholamines.[92] The insulin level is usually elevated, but not enough to prevent the universally observed hyperglycemia.[93] In ad-

dition, growth hormone (GH),[94,95] aldosterone,[96] and vasopressin[97] values are elevated. The mechanism for these elevations is thought to be at least in part neurally mediated.[98] Afferent impulses stimulate secretion of hypothalamic releasing factors (e.g., corticotropin-releasing factor (CRF)[99] and vasoactive intestinal peptide[100]) that, in turn, stimulate the pituitary to release proopiomelanocortin,[101] prolactin,[102,103] vasopressin,[97] and GH.[95,103] Plasma vasopressin concentrations are elevated following a variety of stresses, including surgery,[104–107] pneumonia,[108] myocardial infarction with or without left ventricular failure,[109,110] and electroconvulsive therapy.[111] Plasma vasopressin concentrations increase following the start of surgery and often remain elevated for days after its completion.

The magnitude and duration of the plasma vasopressin level increases are proportional to the degree of stress.[106,107,112,113] CRF, acting synergistically with vasopressin, stimulates secretion of proopiomelanocortin from the pituitary gland.[111,114,115] Proopiomelanocortin is metabolized to adrenocorticotropic hormone (ACTH), and β-endorphin, thus, the link between the endogenous opiod and the hypothalamic pituitary-adrenal axis.[101] Stimulation of adrenomedullary release of catecholamines and enkephalins by CRF is another linkage between the two. Pituitary prolactin secretion is thought to be mediated at least partially by vasoactive intestinal peptide, though other mediators may be operative,[116–118] but the role of pro-

**Table 17-2.** Alterations That Follow Injury

| Ebb Phase | Flow Phase |
|---|---|
| Blood glucose elevated | Glucose normal to elevated |
| Normal glucose production | Glucose production increased |
| Free fatty acids elevated | Free fatty acid flux increased |
| Serum insulin low | Serum insulin normal to elevated |
| Catecholamines elevated | Catecholamines normal to elevated |
| Glucagon elevated | Glucagon elevated |
| Blood lactate elevated | Blood lactate normal |
| $O_2$ consumption depressed | $O_2$ consumption normal |
| Cardiac output low | Cardiac output increased |
| Core temperature decreased | Core temperature elevated |

lactin in the response to stress is unclear. Levels of thyroid-stimulating hormone (TSH), follicle-stimulating hormone (FSH), and leuteinizing hormone (LH) change little during surgery,[105] but LH and FSH decrease on the first postoperative day.[119] Hume and colleagues[98] demonstrated that division of the afferent input from an area of injury can reduce secretion of ACTH. Others have demonstrated that subarachnoid and epidural local anesthetic blockade of the neurogenic stimuli from the area of surgery can attenuate the increases in plasma concentrations of catecholamines,[120] ACTH,[121] aldosterone,[121] cortisol,[122] renin,[121] GH,[119] prolactin,[123] and antidiuretic hormone.[121] Large doses of narcotics (4 mg/kg morphine, 100 μg/kg fentanyl) can also attenuate the increase in the levels of cortisol and catecholamines, presumably by suppressing central nervous system output.[124,125]

### Catecholamines

Catecholamines exist in the circulation both free and as the sulphur conjugate that accounts for 60% to 90% of the total catecholamines.[126] The serum levels of the catecholamines norepinephrine,[127] epinephrine,[128] and dopamine,[127] have been observed to increase after a variety of stresses, including anxiety, hypotension,[129] hypothermia, hypercarbia, and accidental injury.[130] In critical

illness the proportions of free and total (free plus conjugated) catecholamines remain constant.[126] Epinephrine is secreted by the adrenal medulla in response to sympathetic nervous system activation, whereas norepinephrine spills over into the plasma after being released from the sympathetic nerve endings. The sympathetic nervous system, in turn, is controlled by the hypothalamus, the area of the brain responsible for the excretion of releasing factors (e.g., CRF) that initiate the secretion of other endocrine hormones. Plasma levels of epinephrine and norepinephrine do not necessarily increase concurrently.[131] A study of major accidental injury found that plasma epinephrine concentrations increased for only about 48 hours whereas norepinephrine levels remained elevated as long as 8 to 10 days.[132] Abdominal[133] and cardiac[134] surgery produce increases in both hormones, whereas pelvic surgery increases mainly epinephrine.[132] Importantly, in both abdominal[135] and pelvic[122,132] surgery the greatest plasma epinephrine concentration was observed in the immediate post-surgery period. Halter and colleagues[135] found that during abdominal surgery the initial adrenergic activation occurred during the time of the actual surgery and not between the induction of anesthesia and the skin incision. The type of anesthesia has a major influence on the amount of catecholamine secretion during surgery.[120]

The plasma epinephrine level reflects adrenomedullary secretion, and the plasma norepinephrine level is an index of sympathetic nervous system activity. It is important to realize that most of the norepinephrine released by sympathetic ganglia is removed from the synapse by reuptake into the nerve ending.[136] Thus, only the norepinephrine that "spills" over into the plasma is assayed.[137] Plasma levels are determined by the relationship between spillover rate and plasma clearance rate. Studies of norepinephrine kinetics after cholecystectomy demonstrated that plasma norepinephrine increased considerably during the postoperative period because of an increase in the appearance (spillover) rate while neither plasma clearance[138] nor forearm extraction of norepinephrine differed from preoperative values.[139] Christensen and colleagues[139] noted that, despite elevated postoperative plasma norepinephrine levels, there was no change in blood pressure, probably reflecting decreased sensitivity to norepinephrine.

Epinephrine in physiologic doses results in glycogenolysis, increased hepatic gluconeogenesis with mobilization of gluconeogenic precursors from peripheral tissues, inhibition of insulin release, peripheral insulin resistance, and lipolysis.[140,141] Epinephrine is a very potent stimulator of gluconeogenesis. During starvation, the ability of epinephrine to stimulate gluconeogenesis decreases, in contradistinction to glucagon, whose gluconeogenic ability is less in starved subjects than in fed ones.[142]

### Glucocorticoids and Other Steroids

Cortisol has many actions, including stimulation of gluconeogenesis, increasing proteolysis[143] and alanine synthesis, sensitizing adipose tissue to the action of lipolytic hormones (GH and catecholamines), and antiinflammatory action. In addition, it causes insulin resistance by decreasing the rate at which insulin activates the glucose uptake system, probably because of post–insulin receptor block.[144,145] Increased pituitary production of ACTH stimulates increased glucocorticoid production. Glucocorticoids have a negative feedback effect on ACTH production and can also stimulate adrenomedullary secretion of catecholamines. The administration of 500 mg cortisol sodium succinate at the time of surgical incision attenuated the rise in plasma ACTH.[146] ACTH release is itself stimulated by CRF, as well as by catecholamines, vasopressin, and vasoactive intestinal peptide.[147]

Cortisol production is increased by stress and is thought to be a major mediator of the response, as adrenalectomized animals and patients with Addison's syndrome fare poorly when stressed. This was well-demonstrated by the increased mortality observed following use of etomidate to sedate critically ill patients.[148] It was later found that etomidate blocks adrenal steroidogenesis by inhibiting 11-β-hydroxylation and 17-α-hydroxylation.[149,150] Cortisol is thought to be a vital hormone because it diverts utilization from muscles to the brain, facilitates the action of catecholamines, and prevents overreaction of the immune system to injury.[151] Facilitating catecholamine action and secretion helps maintain cardiovascular stability during surgical stress.

In general, the magnitude and duration of both

intraoperative and postoperative ACTH and cortisol levels correlate well with the degree of surgical trauma.[152] A recent study demonstrated that patients undergoing neck exploration (a mild degree of trauma) under isoflurane–nitrous oxide anesthesia had an elevated plasma concentrations of ACTH, cortisol, and epinephrine, but only on emergence from anesthesia.[153] The increase in ACTH secretion during surgery is often far greater than that required to produce a maximal adrenocortical response.[122] This was demonstrated by the observation that administration of exogenous ACTH during surgery did not increase plasma cortisol concentration.[122] The circadian rhythm of cortisol excretion (maximum levels at 6:00 to 8:00 AM with a subsequent decrease) is altered but not abolished after surgery.[154] The rhythm may, however, be shifted in time by as much as 6 hours after major surgery. Studies with labeled cortisol demonstrated that during and after surgery, calculated volume of distribution increased about 175% and metabolic clearance rate about 130%.[155] During surgery, cortisol binding to albumin, but not transcortin, decreased, and postoperatively the reverse was true.[156] Thus, in both situations, free cortisol increased more than was reflected by measurement of total serum cortisol alone. The increased free cortisol seen following surgery is due to an increase in total plasma cortisol, as well as a decrease in cortisol-binding capacity.[157] Barton and colleagues[158] found a constant but nonlinear relationship between free and total plasma cortisol and concluded that measurement of total plasma cortisol was an adequate measure of cortisol response in surgical and trauma patients.

In trauma patients Barton and associates[159] observed that, within 2 hours of injury, the plasma cortisol value of patients with moderate injury was increased in proportion to the severity of the insult. In those with more severe trauma, the plasma cortisol level fell, both in relation to ACTH and in absolute terms, a situation associated with poor chance of survival. The authors felt this may be due at least partially to limited response of the adrenal cortex to ACTH.[159]

The production of other steroid hormones is also altered by injury. Parker and colleagues[160] observed that though the cortisol value increased after burn injury, production of the adrenal androgen and dehydroepiandrosterone sulfate decreased.

Decreased plasma testosterone levels have been observed after surgery[161,162] and after myocardial infarction.[163] Woolf and associates[164] observed that critically ill men and women have decreased plasma concentrations of respectively, testosterone and estradiol. The latter explains the amenorrhea seen during such stress. The exact cause is not clear, but it may be decreased or altered secretion of intrapituitary and suprapituitary substances (e.g., FSH and LH)[119] or decreased response of the pituitary to gonadotropin-releasing hormone, or both.[165]

### Glucagon and Insulin

Glucagon and insulin are both secreted by the pancreas, the former by alpha cells and the latter by beta cells. These endocrine secretions enter the portal vein, so the liver is exposed to high concentrations of both. Glucagon increases hepatocyte cyclic adenosine monophosphate (cAMP) and promotes gluconeogenesis[166]; insulin has the opposite effect: it decreases intracellular cAMP concentration and prevents gluconeogenesis. In addition, glucagon increases glycogenolysis, lipolysis, and ketogenesis in the liver during starvation or diabetic ketoacidosis. The receptor mechanism that increases cAMP levels is not the same as that used by adrenergic mediators.[167] Stimulators of glucagon secretion include hypoglycemia, protein ingestion, amino acid infusion, endorphins, exercise, GH, epinephrine, and glucocorticoids.[168,169] Suppression of glucagon secretion can be achieved by infusion or ingestion of glucose, somatostatin, and insulin.[170]

Insulin is an anabolic hormone with a multitude of effects. In addition to its role in increasing glucose transport across the cell membranes of adipose tissue and muscle, it stimulates glycogen production, inhibits lipolysis in adipose tissue, inhibits hepatic ketogenesis, and increases the rate of amino acid transport and protein synthesis in muscle, adipose tissue, and liver. The glucagon-insulin ratio is the major determinant of the degree of gluconeogenesis. During starvation, the ratio is increased (increased glucagon and decreased insulin levels), and gluconeogenesis is promoted; in the fed state the reverse is true. After most (but not all[120]) types of major surgery[170] there is a rise in the plasma glucagon level, though in some[120]

the value peaks later than that of cortisol, some 18 to 48 hours after injury or surgery.[170] As in starvation, there is an increased glucagon-insulin ratio. Insulin levels decrease during surgery,[171] possibly owing to suppression of secretion by elevated levels of catecholamines[171,172] or increased urinary losses.[173] This suppression can be abrogated by α-adrenergic blockade.[174] The hormonal milieu of low insulin with elevated counterregulatory hormones is thought to be a stimulus to gluconeogenesis. In septic patients this mechanism may fail and cause hypoglycemia, a situation associated with poor survival rates.[175] Postoperatively, the insulin level is increased, and this is thought to be due to increases in both plasma glucose and epinephrine-induced β-adrenergic stimulation. Unlike with starvation, however, the plasma insulin concentrations are often markedly increased above the basal value, though they are inappropriately low for the prevailing level of glycemia.

Recent treatment protocols in burn patients have employed somatostatin, a hormone found in the pancreatic D cells and the hypothalamus that suppresses release of GH, insulin, and glucagon.[175,176] When somatostatin was infused into these patients, the rate of glucose production decreased, as did the rate of clearance. If insulin is also infused into patients receiving somatostatin, the rate of glucose clearance returns to basal level, normalizing glucose kinetics. It thus appears that glucagon is a major mediator of gluconeogenesis. The lesser role of the catecholamines in the abnormal glucose metabolism of burn patients was demonstrated when propranolol failed to reduce the rates of glucose production or glucose cycling.[177] It is likely that catecholamines and glucagon work synergistically: either one, infused alone into normal subjects, causes only transient elevation in gluconeogenesis; when they are infused simultaneously gluconeogenesis is more prolonged.[178]

### Growth Hormone

GH is a polypeptide secreted by the anterior pituitary. Hypothalamic GH–releasing factor stimulates its secretion; somatostatin inhibits it. GH is important in the regulation of growth during the prenatal and neonatal periods and childhood.

Many of its actions are indirect, mediated by somatomedins or insulin-like growth factors (IGFs).[179] Somatomedin C (IGF-I) and somatomedin A (IGF-II) are two of these factors; the former is produced by the liver.[180]

GH also has unique metabolic effects: initial exposure (2 to 3 hours) may produce insulin-like effects (likely due to the release of insulin), but after longer exposure counterregulatory and anabolic effects appear.[181] GH causes glucose intolerance; the mechanism includes insulin resistance, probably owing to an insulin postreceptor defect in both hepatic and extrahepatic tissues.[182] Another cause of the observed hyperglycemia may be a reduction in splanchnic retention of glucose (i.e., decreased hepatic uptake or increased intestinal absorption).[183] GH infusion increases lipolysis, as evidenced by increases in glycerol and non-esterified fatty acid concentrations.[184] GH increases the incorporation of amino acids into protein.[185]

After injury, burns, and surgery, concentrations of GH in the blood are elevated,[103,186] the increase being roughly proportional to the degree of trauma. Frayn and coworkers[187] noted that immediately after musculoskeletal injury plasma GH levels rose sharply, but they rapidly returned to normal. Interestingly, plasma somatomedin activity was depressed for 2 to 3 days after injury, indicating a dissociation between GH and somatomedin. Instead, somatomedin activity was more closely related to insulin concentrations; somatomedin activity may reflect nutritional state and insulin may play a role in its regulation (thus the name, *insulin-like growth factor*). Somatomedin C concentrations are reduced in malnourished children and hospital patients.[188] In studies of critically ill patients, serum somatomedin C concentration consistently and positively correlated with nitrogen balance measurements.[189]

Investigators who have studied the effects of GH infusion in postoperative and burn patients have noted increases in nitrogen retention, nitrogen turnover, metabolic rate, and fat oxidation.[190] Whether GH infusions are useful therapeutically is still under investigation.

### Thyroid Hormones

Even in acute illnesses that do not involve the thyroid there are profound alterations in thyroid homeostasis. Most frequently, the *sick euthyroid syndrome* is produced, and this includes a reduction in serum $T_3$ level, low or normal thyroxine ($T_4$), normal free $T_4$, and elevated reverse $T_3$ ($rT_3$) whereas TSH is normal.[191] $T_3$ resin uptake is often increased. In critically ill postoperative patients, Zaloga and coworkers[192] observed that, though the serum TSH response to thyrotropin-releasing hormone (TRH) was normal after surgery, the maximal TRH-induced increase in serum TSH and the integrated serum TSH response to TRH were suppressed in the early postoperative period. Postoperative TSH suppression correlated with elevated dopamine level.[193] There is also evidence that the TSH released may have altered glycosylation and may be less potent a stimulator of $T_4$ release into the blood.[194] The increased conversion of $T_4$ to $rT_3$ has been observed in severe systemic disease, including cerebrovascular disease,[190] hepatic disease,[121,195] malnutrition, starvation fasting,[196–199] myocardial infarction,[200] after surgery,[201] during treatment with corticosteroids,[202] and in high catecholamine states such as burns.[203] Smallridge and colleagues[204] observed that serum angiotensin-converting enzyme levels, which parallel thyroid hormone levels, were reduced after surgery, as was $T_3$. Some investigators have noted an increase in severity of illness[205] and in mortality rate[206] among patients with significantly decreased $T_3$ and $T_4$ levels and elevated $T_3$ RU and $rT_3$ values.

Administered intravenously to normal subjects dopamine decreases basal TSH levels, inhibits the TSH response to TRH, and decreases serum levels of $T_4$ and $T_3$.[207] Similar observations have been made in critically ill patients receiving dopamine infusions,[207] which likely prolongs and aggravates the characteristic low $T_4$ state.

The most intriguing aspect of thyroid metabolism in the critically ill patient is that, despite low $T_3$ and $T_4$, many of these patients are hypermetabolic.

### Counterregulatory Hormone Interactions

The interaction of the counterregulatory hormones (glucagon, catecholamines, cortisol) in the response to injury is of much interest. Cortisol, glucagon, and the catecholamines are called *counterregulatory* hormones because they oppose the effects of insulin and act synergistically to increase hepatic glucose production. Shamoon's group[178] explored the short-term effects of combined infusion into normal subjects of hydrocortisone, glucagon, and epinephrine designed to simulate the plasma levels that result from moderate injury. They observed increased glucose production (gluconeogenesis) and decreased glucose clearance; the effect was more pronounced when all three hormones were administered together than when they were infused individually or in groups of two, suggesting that they act synergistically.[207] One possible explanation for this synergism is the fact that glucagon increases intracellular cAMP, especially in the liver, by a non–β-receptor mechanism.[166] It could thus amplify the actions of epinephrine.

Cortisol has been reported to act synergistically with epinephrine and other beta agonists (an action employed in the treatment of asthma). Mechanisms proposed include cortisol-induced inhibition of catechol-*o*-methyl transferase and blockade of catecholamine reuptake.[208,209] More recent studies have proposed that cortisol increases β-receptor mRNA, and thus presumably increases the number of β-receptors.[210] In other studies, infusion of the three hormones caused significant negative nitrogen and potassium balances, glucose intolerance, hyperinsulinemia, insulin resistance, sodium retention, and peripheral leukocytosis.[211,212] In only one of the studies was significant sustained hypermetabolism observed.[211] The nitrogen losses appear to be due mainly to the effects of cortisol, since nitrogen balance during cortisol infusion was similar to that seen during infusion of all three hormones. The nitrogen losses were also not of the magnitude observed after accidental injury. Gelfand and colleagues[212] observed no significant alterations in leucine flux or oxidation and only small increases in 3-methyl histidine excretion, indicating little muscle breakdown. Therefore, other mediators must cause the proteolysis and massive nitrogen loss observed in patients. Also, normal subjects were not febrile and did not have increased acute phase–reactant proteins and decreased serum iron. Treatment protocols in which the pyrogenic steroid etiocholanolone[213] was injected into normal subjects resulted in fever, leukocytosis, and hypoferremia without elevations in the counterregulatory hormones, hyperglycemia, or negative nitrogen balance. Infusion of the coun-

terregulatory hormones plus etiocolanolone simulated more of the features of the response to injury than when they were administered individually.[214] Thus, both endocrine and inflammatory mediators appear to be active in the response to injury and sepsis.

### The Immune System Connection: Cytokines

An explosion of knowledge has occurred about nonendocrine factors that may figure prominently in the response to stress. Many insights have been gained from increased understanding of the immune system. Watters and colleagues observed after etiocholanone injections an increase in the plasma activity of interleukin 1 (IL 1),[213] a substance released by activated human monocytes and macrophages in response to various antigenic stimuli. Also called *endogenous pyrogen* or *leukocyte endogenous factor,* it modulates many of the tissue responses to inflammation. It induces hepatocytes to synthesize and release acute-phase reactants (e.g., macroglobulin, complement, immunoglobulins),[215] makes endothelium adhesive for monocytes,[215] promotes fibroblast growth,[216] causes fever,[217] and may be involved in muscle breakdown (Figure 17-2).[218] Baracos and colleagues[219] reported that a biologic extract rich in IL 1 simulated skeletal muscle proleolysis in vitro via protaglandin $E_2$ (Pg$E_2$) formation. Clowes and coworkers[220] identified a polypeptide from the serum of septic patients that also caused muscle proteolysis in vitro.

Whether IL 1 or a related substance is involved in proteolysis is still unclear (see Protein Metabolism). IL 1 also activates the expression of granulocyte colony–stimulating factor (G-CSF), granulocyte macrophage–colony stimulating factor (GM-CSF), and B cell–stimulating factor 2 (BSF-2, also called IL 6) in endothelial cells, helper T cells, bone marrow stroma cells, and fibroblasts.[221–223] These factors in turn activate marrow progenitor cells, and leukocytosis results.[224] Luger and colleagues[225] observed decreased IL 1 activity in patients with fatal sepsis, but in those who survived the levels were normal. One explanation is that the elevated plasma concentrations of catecholamines suppress monocytic IL 1 production. Another monokine, hepatocyte-stimulating factor (also called BSF-2 and IL 6), has been shown to induce fibrinogen synthesis in hepatocytes.[226,227] It is also produced by human endothelial cells in response to IL 1 tumor necrosis factor (TNF), and to bacterial liposaccharide stimulation.[228]

Cachectin, or TNF,[229] is another important cytokine that appears to have metabolic effects. This protein is secreted by macrophages in response to exposure to endotoxin[230] and *Candida albicans* organisms.[231] Administration of TNF to animals results in most of the manifestations of septic shock: hypotension, metabolic acidosis, hemoconcentration, hyperglycemia, hyperkalemia, hemorrhagic lesions of the gastrointestinal tract, and acute tubular necrosis.[232] Waage and colleagues[233] noted a correlation between TNF levels, degree of septic shock, and subsequent death in patients with meningiococcemia. In addition, TNF causes fever by direct action on the hypothalamus and by inducing IL 1 secretion.[234,235] The latter substance then mediates many of the changes described above. In a recent study, Michie and colleagues[236] infused normal subjects with endotoxin and found that serum levels of TNF peaked after 90 to 180 minutes. Associated with this peak were increases in plasma ACTH and epinephrine concentrations, body temperature, and heart rate. Pretreatment with ibuprofen did not affect the increase in TNF level but did suppress the increase in body temperature and ACTH. It has also been shown that TNF can dramatically decrease the synthesis and activity of lipogenic enzymes in cultured adipocytes, thus the name *cachectin*.[237] This mirrors the decreased lipogenesis observed with whole body measurements in septic and injured patients. Lymphotoxin, also called TNF-β, is a product of activated T cells and has biologic activity similar to that of cachectin.[238–240]

IL 2 (T-cell growth factor), another cytokine that may participate in the metabolic response to stress, is secreted by T cells in response to stimuli such as IL 1 and causes generation and proliferation of antigen-specific cytotoxic and helper T cells required for cell-mediated immunity. IL 2 production is reduced in injured patients, and the volume of production is inversely correlated with the severity of injury.[241] This decreased IL-2 synthesis is likely due to excessive $PgE_2$ output by inhibitory monocytes.[242] $PgE_2$ is associated with reduced lymphokine production,[243] inhibited lymphocyte-mediated cytolysis, and inhibition of lymphocyte mitogenesis.[243] Partial restoration of IL 2 synthesis can occur by blocking the cyclooxygenase pathway with indomethacin.[242] Burn patients exhibit not only decreased IL 2 synthesis but also inability to effect expression of high-affinity functional IL 2 receptors.[244] The duration of reduced IL 2 production may be as long as 60 days after the burn injury, and it correlates with the severity of the burn.[242] Also, septic burn patients produce less IL 2 than nonseptic ones. These alterations in IL 2 homeostasis may be one mechanism of postinjury depression of cell-mediated immunity.

One of the main interests in IL 2 is its use in cancer immunotherapy.[245] The complications of such therapy (when given in large doses) constitute a response similar to that seen after injury and sepsis: weight gain due to fluid retention, noncardiogenic pulmonary edema, hyperpyrexia, nephrotoxicity, and hepatotoxicity.[246,247] It is still unclear whether this response is due to a pharmacologic effect or a physiologic one; and whether it is due to stimulation of other mediators or is just an effect of IL 2 itself. In patients receiving IL 2 infusions, the levels of ACTH, cortisol, GH, and interferon gamma (IFN-γ) in the blood have been shown to be elevated.[248–251]

IFN-γ, a glycoprotein released by stimulated T lymphocytes, is another mediator of the immune stress response.[252] It activates macrophages to release IL 1, TNF,[253] G-CSF, M-CSF, and BSF-2,[223] increases IL 2 receptors on monocytes, and reduces release of $PgE_2$[254] and urokinase-type plasminogen activator.[253] It reduces immune suppressor activity by inhibiting $PgE_2$ release as well as inhibiting viral replication. Elevated serum levels of IFN-γ have been observed in patients with pelvic inflammatory disease.[255] Platelet-activating factor, a phospholipid product of activated macrophages, may also be active,[256] especially in the response to endotoxin.

### Other Mediators

Other substances have been implicated in the metabolic response to stress. Bradykinin is a vasoactive substance that stimulates intracellular prostaglandin production and is released by hypoxia and ischemia. When small doses (2.0 and 4.0 μg/kg/

hr) of bradykinin were infused into patients after abdominal surgery, there was a decrease in glucose production and arterial glucose concentrations.[257] It is postulated that the bradykinin-induced increase in hepatic prostaglandins causes inhibition of glucagon-induced cAMP formation, thus inhibiting hepatic gluconeogenesis.[257,258] Preliminary reports indicate that such bradykinin infusions may increase nitrogen retention.[259]

## The Endocrine–Immune System Interaction

It has long been recognized that pharmacologic doses of glucocorticoids suppress cellular immunity. Glucocorticoids cause release of neutrophils from the bone marrow, reduction in circulating monocytes and macrophages, and sequestration of T cells in the bone marrow; they cause lysis of immature T cells, inhibit IFN-γ, IL 1,[229] and IL 2 production, and block phospholipase $A_2$ (responsible for prostaglandin and leukotriene production) and the action of certain proteases involved in inflammation.[260] There are glucocorticoid receptors on leukocytes; peripheral leukocytes have also been observed to secrete ACTH when infected by a virus or exposed to endotoxin.[261] Recent observations have identified many more links between the endocrine and immune systems.

A number of studies have demonstrated the ability of IL 1 to stimulate ACTH[262,263] and CRF release.[263] Brown and coworkers demonstrated that IL 1 and IL 2 enhance the expression of the mRNA to proopiomelanocortin.[264]

Controversy exists as to whether IL 1 directly stimulates ACTH secretion by pituitary cells or directs the release of CRF from hypothalamic cells.[265] (It is possible that this depends on the type of IL 1, alpha or beta.) It has also been observed that IL 1 and IFN-γ[266] stimulate release of ACTH-like substances (and endorphins) from peripheral white blood cells. Hepatocyte-stimulating factor can also cause ACTH secretion from pituitary cells via a leukotriene mechanism.[267] There is evidence that IL 1 can stimulate insulin and glucagon secretion.[267] IL 1 may thus be an important mediator activating the endocrine response to stress. Platelet-activating factor, another activated monocyte product, increases gluconeo-

genesis.[268] The endocrine system may also play a role in the regulation of monokine production.

IFN-γ increases serum cortisol levels when infused into cancer patients for 20 minutes (60 MU/m²).[269] This elevated cortisol level persists at least 24 hours and may explain the impaired immune responsiveness observed after IFN-γ infusion. Whether IFN-γ has direct corticotropic action or induces ACTH-like activity is unclear, because with brief infusions the level of ACTH is only minimally elevated.

β-Endorphin is another stress-induced substance that can affect immune function. Levy and associates[270] observed a temporal association between β-endorphin levels and depressed immune function after trauma. In vitro, β-endorphin enhances natural killer lymphocyte activity in a dose-related fashion, an effect that is reversed with naloxone. Other natural opioid substances also have immunomodulating effects.[272–273] For example, morphine has profound effects on neutrophil function. It can decrease chemotaxis, increase bactericidal activity for *Staphylococcus aureus*, and increase resting and zymosan-stimulated neutrophil oxygen consumption.[274]

Other endocrine substances besides glucocorticoids appear to have immune function. β-Adrenoreceptors seem to regulate the function of human natural killer lymphocytes,[275] while studies in vitro with stress hormones (cortisol, epinephrine, norepinephrine, glucagon) have shown modulation of neutrophil and lymphocyte activity.[276] Recently, somatotropin has been shown to prime mononuclear phagocytes (macrophages) to augment production of reactive oxygen metabolites, restore the T-cell proliferative response and IL 2 synthesis, augment the activity of cytolytic delayed hypersensitivity and natural killer T cells, and increase antibody synthesis in response to T cell–dependent mitogen.[277] It thus appears that the endocrine and immune systems interact on many levels.

## Immune-Mediated Changes Following Injury

Patients have been found to have significant abnormalities of cellular immunity following surgery.[278] This is manifested as anergy in response to skin testing and has been correlated with increased risk of sepsis and mortality in surgical patients.[279,280] Results of tests of lymphocyte and macrophage function in vitro, such as mixed lymphocyte culture reaction, response to lymphokines, generation of cytotoxic T cells, and proliferative reaction to PPD, are normal in such patients.[278] Thus, it is the physiologic environment that contributes to the anergic state. Suppressor T cells are increased in number. A major cause of this immune suppression appears to be failure to produce IL 2.[281] Humoral immunity is also decreased in surgical patients. It has been observed[282] that there is failure to produce specific antibodies (i.e., those to tetanus toxoid) but not total failure of immunoglobulin G (IgG) synthesis. Patients with depressed cellular immunity have the most depressed humoral immunity and elevated $PgE_2$ production. Elevated $PgE_2$ supresses IL 1, IL 2, and IFN-γ, a situation that may be present as long as 7 to 10 days after injury.[243] Indomethacin, an inhibitor of $PgE_2$ production, results in restoration of blood monocyte response to antigenic stimulation. Also, addition of lymphokines abrogates the anergic response to antigenic stimulation.[283] It thus appears that the lymphokines are involved in multiple (metabolic, immune-mediated, and hematopoietic) aspects of the response to stress.

## Biochemical Changes Following Injury and Sepsis

### Carbohydrate Metabolism

The major fuel source for healthy humans is glucose. It enters the circulation either from endogenous sources (glycogenolysis and gluconeogenesis) or from external ones (via the digestive tract or intravenously). It can then be (1) metabolized to carbon dioxide, water and energy, (2) converted and stored as glycogen, or (3) converted to fat. Insulin facilitates glucose uptake by cells, promotes glycogen synthesis, and opposes gluconeogenesis. Catecholamines and glucagon stimulate glycogenolysis and hepatic gluconeogenesis; cortisol also stimulates the latter.

A prominent feature of the response to injury or sepsis is hyperglycemia, initially to the mobi-

lization of liver glycogen. The hyperglycemia persists beyond exhaustion of the glycogen supply, owing to a marked increase in hepatic glucose production plus reduced glucose clearance. This increase in glucose production is due to hepatic gluconeogenesis, which uses amino acids, lactate, pyruvate, and glycerol as substrates. The lactate and pyruvate arise from glycogenolysis and glycolysis in peripheral tissues, especially muscle. The amino acids arise from the breakdown of muscle, the glycerol from the metabolism of triglycerides (fat).

The rise in hepatic glucose production is marked. In normal subjects about 200 g of glucose is produced every day. Noninfected burn patients may produce 320 g per day and infected ones 400 g per day. Black and colleagues,[284] using a glucose clamp technique, demonstrated that trauma patients have a decreased maximal glucose clearance rate. Insulin clearance was twice normal, and insulin resistance appeared to occur in peripheral tissues such as skeletal muscle. They ascribed resistance to a postreceptor problem. Some investigators[285] have suggested that insulin levels are inadequate to maintain normoglycemia because of the suppression of insulin secretion by high epinephrine concentrations as well as increased insulin turnover resulting in increased insulin clearance.[286]

Studies of patients undergoing cholecystectomy demonstrate a small increase in hepatic glucose production with markedly decreased peripheral utilization.[287] These effects are associated with increases in hepatic uptake and peripheral production of lactate, glycerol, and alanine. In addition, the linear relationship between arterial glucose and insulin levels that existed before surgery was no longer present afterward. A major mediator is epinephrine: infusion into postabsorptive normal subjects results in increased splanchnic release of glucose (i.e., enhanced gluconeogenesis) and reduced peripheral tissue uptake of glucose.[284] Cortisol infusion produces similar effects, but whereas after the start of the epinephrine infusion they appear almost immediately, they are delayed with cortisol infusion.[288] Epinephrine, but not cortisol, inhibits insulin secretion, an action that enhances glucagon's actions. The mechanism for this inhibition appears to be inhibition of insulin exocytosis, which can be reversed with α-adrenergic blockade.[289] β-Adrenergic activity, on the other hand, is responsible for the increased hepatic glucose production.[290]

Infusion of somatostatin, the histamine $H_2$ receptor antagonists ranitidine and naloxine failed to alter glucose kinetics in postoperative patients, but the prostaglandin antagonists diclofenac and dipyridamole increased insulin levels and decreased the rate of glucose turnover, implying that prostaglandins may play a role in glucose kinetics.[291] The increased gluconeogenesis plus insulin resistance results in poor utilization of both endogenous and exogenous carbohydrates in stressed patients. In fact, administration of exogenous glucose or other nutrients, which in normal subjects reduces hepatic gluconeogenesis,[292,293] partially decreases it in injured and septic patients.

### Fat Metabolism

Fat can be either utilized as an immediate energy source or stored. Ingested as well as endogenous long-chain triglycerides are metabolized into free fatty acids and glycerol. The free fatty acids can be metabolized as fuel or can be reesterified back to triglycerides. In the fed (high-insulin) state reesterification predominates and lipolysis is inhibited[294]; in the starved state, with a high glucagon-insulin ratio, fat is metabolized to free fatty acids (lipolysis) and then oxidized as fuel, with the associated production of ketone bodies by the liver mitochondria. The ketone bodies are then transported to other organs to be used as fuels. The oxidation of exogenous lipids blocks the lipolysis of endogenous fat. It appears that fat mobilization, with the increase in free fatty acids, impairs muscle glucose uptake and oxidation.[295]

Glucagon and epinephrine increase the rate and degree of lipolysis; which is potentiated by cortisol owing to activation of hormone-sensitive lipase, the enzyme that controls adipocyte lipolysis. This enzyme is stimulated by $\beta_1$-adrenergic agonists and inhibited by $\alpha_2$-adrenergic stimulation.[296] It is inhibited by insulin, which promotes lipogenesis. Forse and coworkers[296] surmised that the lipolysis seen in sepsis and trauma is due to increased $\beta_1$-activity, decreased $\alpha_2$-activity, or both, because infusion of epinephrine stimulated lipolysis in only four of seven burn patients.[297] The

fact that some were not stimulated is not due to adrenergic receptor desensitization, as adrenergic blockage (with propanolol) markedly decreased lipolysis. This continued responsiveness to catecholamines despite long-term exposure has also been observed in vitro: adenylate cyclase from burned rat adipose tissue retained responsiveness to chronic isoproterenol stimulation, unlike that from tissue of unburned rats, which became unresponsive.[298] Chronic adrenergic stimulation in the setting of burn injury may not cause desensitization (down regulation) like that observed in normal subjects but may be due to the synergistic effects of the eliminated glucagon, cortisol, and other mediators. A lack of down-regulation may help explain the prolonged period of catabolism seen after major trauma. The effects of prolonged stress on the cellular response to catecholamines require further examination. `

Trauma patients exhibit increased lipolysis and utilize fat as the major fuel source.[175] Plasma glycerol and free fatty acid levels are elevated, fatty acid and glycerol turnover are accelerated,[299-301] and lipid oxidation is increased. Lipoprotein lipase is the capillary endothelium membrane-bound enzyme that hydrolyzes triglycerides (bound to very-low density lipoproteins and chylomicrons) to glycerol and fatty acids. Heparin releases this enzyme into the bloodstream,[302] causing an immediate increase in the intravascular hydrolysis of lipids. Following trauma, muscle lipoprotein lipase activity is increased but adipose tissue lipoprotein lipase is decreased.[303] In sepsis, muscle lipoprotein lipase activity is decreased. Thus, there appears to be a difference between trauma and sepsis.[303] Studies with labeled ($^{14}C$) palmitate and labeled Intralipid have demonstrated increased oxidation and clearance.[304,305] It is also interesting to note that, in severely injured and burn patients the ratio of the rate of appearance of free fatty acids to the rate of appearance of glycerol increases, indicating that rate of reesterification is greater in adipose tissues. This apparently "futile" cycle in adipose tissue may be one of the causes of hypermetabolism in these patients. Treatment with propranolol decreased the rate of appearance of glycerol and FFA in burn patients; this process thus appears to be mediated adrenergically.[306] The increase in lipolysis also increases the amount of glycerol available for gluconeogenesis.

During the period of stress following surgery and trauma and during infection, the plasma levels of ketones remain low, even during calorie deprivation.[307,308] This is surprising, given the increased availability of blood-borne free fatty acid caused by lipolysis. Studies of patients after elective surgery have demonstrated a two- to threefold increase in ketones 3 hours after surgery; thereafter levels decreased toward normal.[309] Forearm extraction of β-hydroxybutyrate and acetoacetate decreases immediately after surgery. The cause of this reduced ketone production and utilization has been ascribed to the elevated plasma insulin and alanine concentrations and the increased uptake and β-oxidation of free fatty acids.[310]

Traumatized and septic patients appear to have reduced lipogenicability. This becomes especially apparent when such patients are given large glucose loads, with the resultant reduced ability to raise their respiratory quotient much above 1.0.[311] One cause of this may be TNF, which can block lipogenesis in isolated adipocytes (by decreasing lipoprotein lipase activity) and has been implicated as the mediator of cachexia in neoplastic and parasitic diseases.[96,123,312] IL 1-β may have similar but less potent effects,[313] as may PgE$_2$.[314]

Metabolic abnormalities observed in patients with cancer command much interest. Patients with weight-losing gastrointestinal cancers have a greater ability to oxidize glucose than normal subjects.[315] These patients may also have enhanced gluconeogenesis and muscle wasting. The latter is associated with an elevated cortisol and a reduced insulin level, a status conducive to catabolism. They may also have a higher rate of lipolysis but impaired ability to oxidize free fatty acids and infused fat emulsion. The latter is in contradistinction to septic and injured patients, who have a markedly increased ability to oxidize fat plus accelerated lipolysis.[316]

### Protein Metabolism

Injury (surgical, traumatic, burn) and sepsis accelerate protein breakdown,[317] which effect is manifested in increased urinary nitrogen loss, increased peripheral release of amino acids, and inhibited muscle amino acid uptake with sepsis.[318]

The amino acids originate from both injured tissue and uninjured skeletal muscle and are transported to the liver for conversion to glucose (gluconeogenesis) and for protein synthesis. The negative balance observed in such patients represents the net result of breakdown and synthesis: breakdown is increased and synthesis either increased or diminished.[319] Jahoor and colleagues[320] observed in burned children that the volume of protein breakdown was elevated to the same degree during the acute and convalescent phases but synthesis increased in the latter phase, to create a positive nitrogen balance. Different muscle groups respond differently to injury and sepsis, some undergoing more proteolysis than others.[321] Amino acid uptake by the liver is enhanced, which causes increased gluconeogenesis. Also, hepatic protein synthesis of selected proteins (acute-phase reactants) increases, while that of others decreases. The acute-phase reactants include fibrinogen, complement, C-reactive protein, haptoglobin, α$_1$-acid glycoprotein, α$_1$-antitrypsin, α$_1$-antichymotrypsin, ceruloplasmin, ferritin, and serum amyloid A.[322] The degree of acute-phase response is proportional to the level of tissue injury.[320] Proteins whose synthesis is decreased include transferrin, albumin, retinols, and prealbumin. Stimulators of the acute-phase reactants include cytokines such as IL 1 and IL 6, TNF, and IFN-γ[323–326]; neuroendocrine mediators (specifically glucocorticoids); and possibly toxic products such as bacterial lipopolysaccharides. It has been observed that after IL 1 stimulation the total amount of protein synthesized does not increase; rather, synthesis of the acute-phase proteins is favored.

The mediators of muscle breakdown may be many. Adrenergic activity may be involved in catabolism since α-adrenergic blockage reduces nitrogen loss. Glucagon and cortisol also have catabolic activity,[290] but the degree of nitrogen loss observed during the infusion of the counterregulatory hormones (glucagon, epinephrine, cortisol) into normal subjects is less than that observed after injuries that cause comparable increases in the counterregulatory hormones.[212] Recent studies have indicated that TNF may be the principal catabolic monokine and that IL 1 potentiates skeletal muscle proteolysis.[327] Initial reports indicated that in vitro proteolysis could be blocked by cyclooxygenase inhibitors, leading to the hypothesis that catabolism was mediated by prostaglandins, specifically $PgE_2$.[219] More recent studies in vivo of burned and septic rats indicate that indomethacin is unable to block proteolysis,[328,329] which implies that prostaglandins may not be the mediators of proteolysis. Ason and coworkers[330] note that administration of indomethacin postoperatively to gastrectomy patients reduced fever, attenuated cortisol and catecholamine increase, and reduced protein loss, though they do not clarify whether only the reduction of fever (central cyclooxygenase inhibition) or another action of the indomethacin such as peripheral cyclooxygenase inhibition is operative. Muscle breakdown does require lysosomal proteolytic enzyme.[331] Studies of patients after abdominal surgery have indicated that infusion of somatostatin, ranitidine, or naloxone significantly decreased the rate of net protein catabolism, whether patients received 5% dextrose or TPN.[291] The contribution of the various mediators of stress to proteolysis is still unclear.

The metabolism of the individual amino acids, especially glutamine, is drawing much interest. Glutamine is the most abundant amino acid in blood. Glutamine levels in muscle and blood decrease markedly following injury and sepsis, and it is consumed rapidly by replicating cells such as fibroblasts, lymphocytes, and intestinal endothelial cells. Glutamine and alanine transport two thirds of the circulating amino acid nitrogen, and in the postabsorptive and injured state comprise more than 50% of the amino acids released by muscle.[332] In persons in the stressed state, the glutamine released by muscle is taken up by the intestinal tract, where some is converted to alanine, which is then converted by the liver to glucose. It is likely that a good portion of the alanine converted by hepatic gluconeogenesis is supplied by the intestine. Glutamine is also metabolized to ammonia by the gut. The ammonia is then transported by the portal vein directly to the liver for disposal via the urea cycle. In the stressed state, it appears that glutamine can replace glucose as a fuel.[332] Similar observations have been made during glucocorticoid administration.[333] It is possible that the use of glutamine may decrease protein catabolism in the intestine and elsewhere and may prevent the gut atrophy associated with starvation and parenteral feeding.[332]

## Energy Metabolism

In most instances, stressed patients have an increase in metabolic rate. After elective surgery, the increase is about 10% to 15%. The peak occurs around the third postoperative day, and patients with sepsis have a larger increase (20% to 40%), whereas those with burns experience the greatest increases (up to 120%, essentially the increase is proportional to the extent of the burn).[334] This increase in energy expenditure is probably mediated by the change in metabolic milieu. Catecholamines infused into normal subjects increase the metabolic rate,[335] and this increase is even greater when cortisol, glucagon, and catecholamines are infused together.[336] IL 1 and TNF both have been reported to increase energy expenditure.[327] Some researchers have ascribed the increased energy expenditure associated with the injured state to the increase in protein metabolism, particularly increased protein synthesis.[337] Yet this may not always be the case. Lowry and colleagues[338] noted that after elective surgery there was only modest change in energy expenditure, despite an increase in protein turnover. This implied there was little relation between the two. The other metabolic process that may contribute to the increase in energy expenditure is the substantial increase in carbohydrate and fat "futile cycling," a situation that causes a major increase in energy expenditure. The teleologic reason for this increase in futile cycling is that it affords these patients the flexibility to adapt quickly to changes in energy substrate demands.[306]

Various environmental factors may also affect energy expenditure. Elevated ambient temperature (and humidity) have been shown to reduce the energy expenditure of burn patients by reducing evaporative losses and, in turn, reducing the need to generate increased energy to maintain body temperature.[339]

## Nutritional Support

An understanding of response to stress is important in planning the nutritional support of an injured or septic patient. Nutritional support provides exogenous substrate utilization, because injured and septic patients do not respond to nutrients as postabsorbtive or starved subjects do. The underlying disordered metabolism makes it difficult to design a support regimen.

Administering glucose to a starved subject decreases gluconeogenesis and lipolysis, but in stressed patients exogenous glucose does not produce these effects to the same degree.[340] Thus, in stressed, hypermetabolic, and hypercatabolic patients with disordered glucose tolerance, administration of carbohydrates must be approached carefully. Though it is necessary to provide some glucose calories to achieve some degree of protein sparing (by stimulating increased secretion of the anabolic hormone insulin) and to reduce gluconeogenesis, an excessive glucose load should be avoided.[341] Excess glucose is metabolized to carbon dioxide and converted to glycogen, but it is not as readily converted to fat, owing to a block in net lipogenesis.[311] Administration of a large glucose load to such patients may result in further increases in energy expenditure associated with further rises in norepinephrine.[311] This rise in metabolic rate (oxygen consumption), along with increased carbon dioxide production, requires increased minute ventilation. It is thus recommended that glucose intake for such patients be limited to less than 6 mg/kg/min.[342,343] Inability to utilize glucose has prompted interest in using other carbohydrates; fructose, xylitol, and glycerol have been or are being studied.[344]

Critically ill, stressed (trauma, sepsis) patients often derive as much as 80% of their energy requirement from fat. Fat emulsions containing polyunsaturated long-chain triglycerides are administered intravenously. Most patients readily clear and oxidize these, but a small portion with severe sepsis are unable adequately to clear and to oxidize fat.[345] Stressed patients used fat to provide as much as 50% of nonprotein calories. Jeejeebhoy and colleagues[346] have compared nutritional formulations containing carbohydrate (glucose) as their sole nonprotein source to those containing approximately equal amounts of glucose and fat. They found that the two formulations are equally nitrogen sparing.[346]

The provision of protein to stressed patients is an important aspect of nutritional support. Adequate nonprotein calories (from lipid and carbohydrates) must be provided, so that the infused amino acids can be used as substrate for protein synthesis rather than as an energy substrate to alleviate nitrogen losses. The catabolic state of burn injury, trauma, and sepsis markedly impairs efficient utilization of exogenous nitrogen. This has sparked much interest in what is the optimum nonprotein calorie-nitrogen intake ratio and what amount and type of protein are required. Controversy exists over the use of branched-chain enriched amino acid solutions to improve overall nitrogen balance. Some studies have demonstrated better nitrogen retention with the branched-chain enriched solutions than with conventional solutions[347,348]; others have not.[349,350] There is continued interest in further modifying the composition of amino acid solutions to improve nitrogen retention.

In summary, recent investigation has demonstrated that the response to surgical and infectious stress is mediated by complex interactions between nervous, endocrine, immune, and hematopoietic systems. Not only is the neuroendocrine system operative, but monokines and lymphokines such as IL 1, IL 6, and TNF also play important roles. The discovery of these mediators and of macrophage-derived substances that operate at the local wound level (such as epidermal growth factors[351]), coupled with advances in molecular biology, portend much for the future. The ability to alter endocrine response with techniques such as epidural anesthesia,[352,353] the ability to block specific aspects of the response (e.g., with adrenergic and prostaglandin antagonists), and the ability to synthesize potential beneficial mediators with recombinant DNA techniques (e.g., GH[354]) may allow modulation of the response to decrease debility and complications. It is also important to remember that some information in this review may be dated, owing to the rapid advances and discoveries being made in this and related areas.

## References

1. Mallory GK, White PD, Salcedo-Salgar J. The speed of healing of the myocardial infarction: A study of the pathologic anatomy in seventy-two cases. Am Heart J 1939; 18:47–671.

2. Jetter WW, White PD. Rupture of the heart in patients in mental institutions. Ann Intern Med 1944; 21:783–802.

3. Dietrick JE, Whedon GD, Shorr E. Effects of immobilization upon various metabolic and physiologic functions of normal men. Am J Med 1948; 4:3–36.

4. Graveline DE, Barnard GW. Physiological effects of a hypodynamic environment: Short-term studies. Aerospace Med 1964; 35:1194–1200.

5. Miller PB, Johnson RL, Lamb LE. Effects of four weeks of absolute bed rest on circulatory functions in man. Aerospace Med 1964; 35:1194–1200.

6. Vogt FB, Johnson PC. Plasma volume and extracellular fluid volume change associated with 10 days bed recumbency. Aerospace Med 1967; 38:21–25.

7. Saltin B, Blomqvist G, Mitchell JH, et al. Response to exercise after bed rest and after training: A longitudinal study of adaptive changes in oxygen transport and body composition. Circulation 1968; 38(suppl 7):1–55.

8. Gaffney FA, Nixon JV, Karlsson ES, et al. Cardiovascular deconditioning produced by 20 hours of bedrest with head-down tilt (−5 degrees) in middle-aged men. Am J Cardiol 1985; 56:634–638.

9. Convertino V, Hung J, Goldwater D, et al. Cardiovascular responses to exercise in middle-aged men after 10 days of bedrest. Circulation 1982; 65:134–140.

10. Flye MW. Disorders of veins. In: Sabiston DC, ed. Textbook of Surgery. Philadelphia: WB Saunders, 1986;1709–1730.

11. Blomqvist CG, Nixon JV, Johnson RL, et al. Early cardiovascular adaptation to zero gravity stimulated by head-down tilt. Acta Astronaut 1980; 7:543–553.

12. Lathers CM, Diamandis PH, Riddle JM, et al. Acute and intermediate cardiovascular responses to zero gravity and to fractional gravity levels induced by head-down or head-up tilt. J Clin Pharmacol 1990; 30:494–523.

13. Johnson PC, Driscoll TB, Carpenter WR. Vascular and extravascular fluid changes during six days of bedrest. Aerospace Med 1971; 42:875–878.

14. Henricksen L, Sjersen P. Effect of ''vein pump'' activation upon venous pressure and blood flow in human subcutaneous tissue. Acta Physiol Scand 1977; 100:14–21.

15. Thompson FJ, Barnes CD, Wald JR. Interactions between femoral venous afferents and lumbar spinal reflex pathways. J Auton Nerv Syst 1982; 6:113–126.

16. Taylor HL, Henschel A, Brozek J, et al. Effects

17. Chobanian AV, Lille RD, Tercyak A, et al. The metabolic and hemodynamic effects of prolonged bed rest in normal subjects. Circulation 1974; 49:551–559.

18. Hyatt KH, Kamenetsky LG, Smith WM. Extravascular dehydration as an etiologic factor in postrecumbency orthostatism. Aerospace Med 1969; 40:644–650.

19. Hung J, Goldwater D, Convertino V, et al. Mechanics for decreased exercise capacity after bedrest in normal middle-aged men. Am J Cardiol 1983; 51:344–348.

20. Goldberger AL, Goldwater D, Bhargava V. Atropine unmasks bed-rest effect: A spectral analysis of cardiac interbeat intervals. J Appl Physiol 1986; 61:1843–1848.

21. Robinson BF, Epstein Se, Beiser GD, et al. Control of heart rate by the autonomic system. Studies in man on the interrelation between baroreceptor mechanism and exercise. Circ Res 1966; 19:400–411.

22. Melada GA, Goldman RH, Luetscher JA, et al. Hemodynamics, renal function, plasma renin and aldosterone in man after 5 to 14 days of bedrest. Aviat Space Environ Med 1975; 46:1049–1055.

23. West JB. Ventilation—Blood Flow and Gas Exchange, Ed 3. Philadelphia, JB Lipincott, 1977.

24. Laver MB, Hallowell P, Goldblatt A. Pulmonary dysfunction secondary to heart disease: Aspects relevant to anesthesia and surgery. Anesthesiology 1970; 33:161–192.

25. Macklem PT. Respiratory mechanics. Ann Rev Physiol 1978; 40:157–184.

26. Minh VD, Kurihara N, Friedman PJ, et al. Reversal of pleural pressure gradient during electrophrenic stimulation. J Appl Physiol 1974; 37:496–504.

27. Tisi GM. Preoperative evaluation of pulmonary function. Am Rev Respir Dis 1979; 119:293–310.

28. Lumb PD. Perioperative pulmonary physiology. In: Sabiston DC, Spencer FC, eds. Surgery of the Chest, ed 5. Philadelphia: WB Saunders, 1990.

29. Craig DB, Wahba WM, Don HF. Airway closure and lung volumes in surgical positions. Can Anaesth Soc J 1971; 18:92–99.

30. Marini JJ, Tyler ML, Hudson Ld, et al. Influence of head-dependent positions on lung volume and oxygen saturation in chronic airflow obstruction. Am Rev Respir Dis 1984; 129:101–105.

31. Cardus D. Oxygen alveolar-arterial tension differences after ten days recumbency in man. J Appl Physiol 1967; 23:934–967.

32. Booth FW. Physiologic and biochemical effects of

immobilization on muscle. Clin Orthop 1987; 219:15–20.

33. MacDougall JD, Ward Gr, Sale DG, et al. Biochemical adaptation of human skeletal muscle to heavy resistance training and immobilization. J Appl Physiol 1977; 43:700–703.

34. Witzmann FA, Kim DH, Fitts RH. Effect of hindlimb immobilization on the fatigability of skeletal muscle. J Appl Physiol 1983; 54:1242–1248.

35. Watson PA, Stein JP, Booth FW. Changes in actin synthesis and alpha-actin mRNA content in rat muscle during immobilization. Am J Physiol 1984; 247:C39–44.

36. Booth FW, Seider MJ. Recovery of skeletal muscle after three months of hindlimb immobilization in rats. J Appl Physiol 1979; 47:435–439.

37. Goldspink DF. The influence of immobilization and stretch on protein turnover of rat skeletal muscle. J Physiol (Lond) 1977; 264:267–282.

38. Savolainen J, Vaanen K, Vihko V, et al. Effect of immobilization on collagen synthesis in rat skeletal muscles. Am J Physiol 1987; 252:R883–R888.

39. Reiser PJ, Kasper CE, Moss RL. Myosin subunits and contractile properties of single fibers from hypokinetic rat muscles. J Appl Physiol 1987; 63:2293–2300.

40. Rifenberick DH, Max SR. Substrate utilization by disused rat skeletal muscles. Am J Physiol 1974; 226:295–297.

41. Holloszy JO, Booth FW. Biochemical adaptations to endurance exercise in muscle. Physiol Rev 1976; 38:273–291.

42. Rubin CT, Lanyon LE. Regulation of bone formation by applied dynamic loads. J Bone Joint Surgery 1984; 66A:397–402.

43. Whedon GD: Disuse osteoporosis: Physiological aspects. Calcif Tissue Int 1984; 36 (suppl 1): S146–S150.

44. Donaldson CL, Hulley SB, Vogel JM, et al. The effect of prolonged bed rest on bone mineral. Metabolism 1970; 19:1071–1084.

45. Smith MC, Rambaut PC, Vogel JM, et al. Bone mineral measurement—experiment M078. In: Johnston RS, Dietlein LF, eds. Biomedical Results from Skylab. Cited in: LeBlanc A, Schneider V, Krebs J, et al. Spinal bone mineral after 5 weeks of bed rest. Calcif Tissue Int 1987; 41:259–261.

46. Hulley SB, Vogel JM, Donaldson CL, et al. The effect of supplemental oral phosphate on the bone mineral changes during prolonged bed rest. J Clin Invest 1971; 50:2506–2518.

47. LeBlanc A, Schneider V, Krebs J, et al. Spinal bone mineral after 5 weeks of bed rest. Calcif Tissue Int 1987; 41:259–261.

48. Nilsson BER. Post-traumatic osteopenia. Acta Orthop Scand 1966; 91:1–55.

49. Rose GA. Immobilization osteoporosis. Br J Surg 1966; 53:769–774.

50. Minaire P, Meunier P, Edouard C, et al. Quantitative histological data on disuse osteoporosis: Comparison with biological data. Calcif Tissue Res 1974; 17:57–73.

51. Moses FM. The effect of exercise on the gastrointestinal tract. Sports Med 1990; 9:159–172.

52. Dooley CP, Schlossmacher B, Valenzuela JE. Modulation of esophageal peristalsis by alterations of body position: Effect of bolnus viscosity. Dig Dis Sci 1989; 34:1662–1667.

53. Moore JG, Datz FL, Christian PE, et al. Effect of body posture on radionuclide measurements of gastric emptying. Dig Dis Sci 1988; 33:1592–1595.

54. Mojaverian P, Vlasses PH, Kellner PE, et al. Effects of gender, posture, and age on gastric residence time of an indigestible solid: Pharmaceutical considerations. Pharm Res 1988; 5:639–644.

55. Sjovall H, Forssell H, Haggendal J, et al. Reflex sympathetic activation in humans is accompanied by inhibition of gastric $HCO_3$-secretion. Am J Physiol 1988; 255(6 pt 1):G752–G758.

56. Evans DF, Foster GE, Harcastle JD. Does exercise affect small bowel motility in man. Gut 1989; A1012.

57. Sikirov B-A. Etiology and pathogenesis of diverticulosis coli: A new approach. Med Hypoth 1988; 26:17–20.

58. Blotner H. Effect of prolonged physical inactivity on tolerance of sugar. Arch Intern Med 1945; 75:39–44.

59. Pawlson LG, Field JB, McCally M, et al. Effects of two weeks of bedrest on glucose, insulin and human growth hormone in response to glucose and arginine stimulation. Aerospace Med Abstr 1968;105.

60. Lipman RL, Schnure JJ, Bradley Em, et al. Impairment of peripheral glucose utilization in normal subjects by prolonged bed rest. J Lab Clin Med 1970: 76:221–230.

61. Altman DF, Baker SD, McCally M, et al. Carbohydrate and lipid metabolism in man during prolonged bedrest. Clin Res 1969; 17:543.

62. Stuart CA, Shangraw RE, Prince MF, et al. Bedrest–induced insulin resistance occurs primarily in muscle. Metabolism 1988; 37:802–806.

63. Shangraw RE, Stuart CA, Prince MF, et al. Insulin responsiveness of protein metabolism in vivo following bedrest in humans. Am J Physiol 1988; 255:E548–E558.

64. Vernikos-Danellis J, Leach CS, Winget CM, et

al. Changes in glucose, insulin and growth hormone levels associated with bedrest. Aviat Space Environ Med 1976; 47:583–587.

65. Pequinot JM, Guell A, Gauquelin G, et al. Epinephrine, norephrine and dopamine during a 4-day head-down bed-rest. J Appl Physiol 1985; 58:157–163.

66. Stamatakis JD, Kakkar VV, Lawrence D, et al. Failure of aspirin to prevent postoperative deep vein thrombosis in patients undergoing total hip replacement. Br Med J 1978; 1:1031.

67. Bergqvist D, Efsing HO, Hallbrook T, et al. Thromboembolism after elective and post-traumatic hip surgery—a controlled prophylactic trial with dextran 70 and low-dose heparin. Acta Chir Scand 1979; 145:213–218.

68. Schlosser V. Klinik, Prophylaxe und Therapie der Lungenembolie aus chirurgischer Sicht. Med Klin 1977; 72:1947, cited in Bergqvist D. Postoperative Thromboembolism: Frequency, Etiology, Prophylaxis. New York: Springer-Verlag, 1983.

69. Dalen J, Alpert J. Natural history of pulmonary embolism. Prog Cardiovasc Dis 1975; 17:259.

70. Havig O. Deep vein thrombosis and pulmonary embolism. An autopsy study with multiple regression analysis of possible risk factors. Acta Chir Scand Suppl 1977;478.

71. Shull KC, Nicholaides AN, et al. Significance of popliteal reflux in relation to ambulatory venous pressure and ulceration. Arch Surg 1979; 114:1304–1306.

72. Haimovici H. Pathophysiology of postphlebitic syndrome with leg ulcer. In: Haimovici H, ed. Haimovici's Vascular Surgery: Principles and Techniques. Norwalk, Conn: Appleton and Lange, 1989;971–978.

73. Hewson W. Experimental inquiries. 1. An inquiry into the properties of the blood, with some remarks on some of its morbid appearances, and an appendix relating to the discovery of the lymphatic system in birds, fish and the animals called amphibians. London: T Cadell, 1771. In Bergqvist D. Postoperative Thromboembolism: Frequency, Etiology, Prophylaxis. New York: Spring-Verlag, 1983;41.

74. Sevitt S. The structure and growth of valve-pocket thrombi in femoral veins. J Clin Path 1974; 27:517–528.

75. Karino T, Motomiya M. Vortices in the pockets of a venous valve. Microvasc Res 1981; 21:247.

76. Malone PC, Hamer JD, Silver IA. Oxygen tension in venous valve pockets. Thromb Haemost 1979; 42:230.

77. Hume M, Sevitt S, Thomas LP. Venous thrombosis and pulmonary embolism. Cambridge: Harvard University Press, 1970.

78. Lough J, Moore S. Endothelial cell injury induced by thrombin or thrombi. Lab Invest 1975; 33:130–135.

79. Mansfield A. Alterations in fibrinolysis associated with surgery and venous thrombosis. Br J Surg 1972; 59:754–757.

80. Clark C, Cotton LT. Blood flow in deep veins of legs. Recording technique and evaluation of methods to increase flow during operation. Br J Surg 1968; 55:211–214.

81. Bird AD. Effect of surgery, injury, and prolonged bedrest on calf blood flow. Aust NZ J Surg 1972; 41:374–379.

82. Warlow C, Ogston D, Douglas AS. Deep venous thrombosis of the legs after strokes. Part I: Incidence and predisposing factors. Br Med J 1976; 1:1178–1183.

83. Buckingham JC. Hypothalamo-pituitary responses to trauma. Br Med Bull 1985; 41:203–211.

84. Cuthberson DP. The disturbance of metabolism produced by bony and non-bony injury with notes on certain abnormal conditions of bone. Biochem J 1930; 24:1244–1263.

85. Kinney JM, ed. The application of indirect calorimetry to clinical studies. Assessment of Energy Metabolism in Health and Disease. Columbus, Oh: Ross Laboratories, 1980;42–45.

86. Imamura M, Clowes GHA Jr, Blackburn GL. Liver metabolism and gluconeogenesis in trauma and sepsis. Surgery 1975; 77:868–880.

87. Lequesne LP, Cochrane JPS, Feldman NR. Fluid and electrolyte disturbances after trauma: The role of adrenocorticol and pituitary hormones. Br Med Bull 1985; 41:212–217.

88. Meguid MM, Brennan MF, Aoki TT, et al. Hormone-substrate interrelationships following trauma. Arch Surg 1974; 109:776–783.

89. Frayn KN. Substrate turnover after injury. Br Med Bull 1985; 4:232–239.

90. Oppenheim WL, Williamson DH, Smith R. Early biochemical changes and severity of injury in man. J Trauma 1980; 20:135–140.

91. Chernow B, Alexander HR, Smallridge RC, et al. Hormonal responses to graded surgical stress. Arch Intern Med 1987; 147:1273–1277.

92. Frankenhaesur M, Rauste-von Wright M, Collins A, et al. Sex differences in psychoneuroendocrine reactions to examination stress. Psychosomat Med 1978; 46:334–343.

93. Kuntscher FR, Galletti PM, Hahn C, et al. Alterations of insulin and glucose metabolism during cardiopulmonary bypass under normothermia. J Thorac Cardiovasc Surg 1985; 89:97–106.

94. Goschke H, Bar E, Girard J, et al. Glucagon, insulin, cortisol, and growth hormone levels following major surgery: Their relationship to Human

prolactin and growth hormone release during surgery and other conditions of stress. J Clin Endocrinol Metab 1972; 35:840–851.

95. Newsome HH, Rose JC. The response of adrenocorticotrophic hormone and growth hormone to surgical stress. Horm Metab Res 1978; 10:465–470.

96. Korpassy A, Stoekel H, Vecsec P. Investigations of hydrocortisone secretion and aldosterone excretion in patients with severe prolonged stress. Acta Anaesthesiol Scand 1972; 16:161–168.

97. Cochrane JP, Forsling ML, Gow NM, et al. Arginine vasopressin release following surgical operations. Br J Surg 1981; 68:240–213.

98. Hume DM, Egdahl RH. The importance of the brain in the endocrine response to injury. Ann Surg 1959; 150:697–712.

99. Rivier C, Plotsky P. Mediation by corticotropin-releasing factor (CRP) of adenohypophyseal hormone secretion. Annu Rev Physiol 1986; 48:475–498.

100. Crozier TA, Drobnick L, Stafforst D, et al. Opiate modulation of the stress-induced increase of vasoactive intestinal peptide (VIP) in plasma. Horm Metab Res 1988; 20:352–356.

101. Reisine T. Neurohumoral aspects of ACTH release. Hosp Pract 1988; 23:77–96.

102. Arnetz BB. Endocrine reactions during standardized surgical stress: The effects of age and methods of anaesthesia. Age Ageing 1985; 14:96–101.

103. Noel GL, Suh HK, Stone JG, et al. Human prolactin and growth hormone release during surgery and other conditions of stress. J Clin Endocrinol Metab 1972; 35:840–851.

104. Breslow MJ, Jordan DA, Christopherson R, et al. Epidural morphine decreases postoperative hypertension by attenuating sympathetic nervous system hyperactivity. JAMA 1989; 261:3577–3581.

105. Chan V, Wang C, Yeung RTT. Pituitary-thyroid response to surgical stress. Acta Endocrinol 1978; 88:490–498.

106. Von Bormann B, Weidler B, Dennhardt R, et al. Influence of epidural fentanyl on stress-induced elevation of plasma vasopressin after surgery. Anesth Analg 1983; 62:727–732.

107. Cochrane JPS, Forsling ML, Gow NM, et al. Arginine vasopressin release following surgical operations. Br J Surg 1981; 68:209–213.

108. Dreyfuss D, Leviel F, Paillard M, et al. Acute infectious pneumonia is accompanied by a latent vasopressin-dependent impairment of renal water excretion. Am Rev Respir Dis 1988; 138:583–589.

109. McAlpine HM, Cobbe SM. Neuroendocrine changes in myocardial infarction. Am J Med 1988; 84 (suppl 3A):61–66.

110. McAlpine HM, Morton JJ, Leckie B, et al. Neuroendocrine activation after acute myocardial infarction. Br Heart J 1988; 60:117–124.

111. Widerlov E, Ekman R, Jensen L, et al. Arginine vasopressin, but not corticotropin-releasing factor, is a potent stimulator of adrenocorticotropic hormone following electroconvulsive treatment. J Neural Transm 1989; 75:101–109.

112. Moran WH, Mittenberger FW, Shuayl WA, et al. Relationship of anti-diuretic hormone secretion to surgical stress. Surgery 1964; 56:99–107.

113. Wu WH, Zbuzek VK. Vasopressin and anesthesia and surgery. Bull NY Acad Med 1982; 58:427–442.

114. Salata RAM, Jarrett DB, Verablis JG, et al. Vasopressin stimulation of adrenocorticotropin hormone (ACTH) in humans. J Clin Invest 1988; 81:66–74.

115. Gaillard RC, Riondel AM, Ling N, et al. Corticotropin releasing factor activity of CRF 41 in normal man is potentiated by angiotensin II and vasopressin but not desmopressin. Life Sci 1988; 43:1935–1944.

116. Lightman SL, Unwin RJ, Graham K, et al. Vasoactive intestinal polypeptide stimulation of prolactin release and renin activity in normal man and patients with hyperprolactinemia: Effects of pretreatment with bromocriptine and dexamethazone. Eur J Clin Invest 1984; 14:444–448.

117. Falsetti L, Zanagnolo V, Gastaldi A, et al. Vasoactive intestinal peptide (VIP) selectively stimulates prolactine release in healthy women. Gynceol Endocrinol 1988; 2:11–18.

118. Rolandi E, Raggiani E, Franceschini R, et al. Prolactin release induced by physical exercise is independent from peripheral vasoactive intestinal polypeptide secretion. Ann Clin Res 1988; 20:428–430.

119. Crane-Chartens AC, Odell WB, Thompson JC. Anterior pituitary function during surgical stress and convalescence. Radioimmunoassay measurement of blood, TSH, LH, FSH, and growth hormone. J Clin Endocrinol 1969; 29:63–71.

120. Engquist A, Fog-Moller F, Christiansen C, et al. Influence of epidural analgesia on the catecholamine and cyclic AMP response to surgery. Acta Anaesthesiol Scand 1980; 24:17–21.

121. Brandt MR, Olguard K, Kehlet H. Epidural analgesia inhibits renin and aldosterone response to surgery. Acta Anaesthesiol Scand 1979; 23:267–272.

122. Engquist A, Brandt MR, Fernandes A, et al. The blocking effects of epidural analgesia on the adrenocortisol and hyperglycemia responses to surgery. Acta Anaesthesiol Scand 1977; 21:330–335.

123. Kehlet H. Epidural analgesia and the endocrine-

metabolism response to surgery: Update and perspectives. Acta Anaesthesiol Scand 1984; 28:25–127.

124. George JM, Reier CE, Lanese RR, et al. Morphine anaesthesia blocks cortisol and growth hormone response to surgical stress in humans. J Clin Endocrinol Metab 1974; 38:736–741.

125. Walsh ES, Paterson JL, O'Riordan JBA, et al. Effect of high dose fentanyl anaesthesia on the metabolic and endocrine response to cardiac surgery. Br J Anaesth 1981; 53:1155–1165.

126. Woolf PD, Hamill RW, Lee LA, et al. Free and total catecholamines in critical illness. Am J Physiol 1988; 254:E287–E291.

127. Davies CL, Malyneuf SG, Newman RJ. HPLC determination of plasma catecholamines in road accident casualties. Br J Clin Pharmacol 1981; 13:283P.

128. Frayn KN, Little RA, Maycock PF, et al. The relationship of plasma catecholamines to acute metabolic and hormonal responses to injury in man. Circ Shock 1985; 16:229–240.

129. Benedict CR, Grahame-Smith DG. Plasma noradrenaline and adrenaline concentrations and dopamine beta-hydroxylase activity in patients with shock due to septicemia, trauma, and hemorrhage. J Med 1978; 185:1–20.

130. Jaattela A, Alho A, Avikainen V, et al. Plasma catecholamines in severely injured patients: A prospective study on 45 patients with multiple injuries. Br J Surg 1975; 62:177–181.

131. Davies CL, Newman RJ, Molyneux SG, et al. The relationship between plasma catecholamines and severity of injury in man. J Trauma 1984; 24:99–105.

132. Nistrup-Madsen S, Fog-Moller F, Christiansen C, et al. Cyclic AMP, adrenaline, and non-adrenaline in plasma during surgery. Br J Surg 1978; 65:191–193.

133. Butler MJ, Britton BJ, Wood WG, et al. Plasma catecholamine concentrations during operations. Br J Surg 1977; 64:786–790.

134. Stanley TH, Berman L, Green O, et al. Plasma catecholamine and cortisol responses to fentanyl-oxygen anesthesia for coronary-artery operations. Anesthesiology 1980; 53:250–253.

135. Halter JB, Pflug AE, Porte D. Mechanism of plasma catecholamine increases during surgical stress in man. J Clin Endocrinol Metab 1977; 45:936–940.

136. Esler M. Assessment of sympathetic nervous function in humans from norepinephrine plasma kinetics. Clin Sci 1982; 62:247–254.

137. Esler M, Jennings G, Korner P, et al. Measurements of total and organ specific kinetics in humans. Am J Physiol 1984; 247:E21–E28.

138. Hilsted J, Christiansen NJ, Madsbad S. Whole body clearance of norepinephrine. J Clin Invest 1983; 71:500–505.

139. Christiansen NJ, Hilsted J, Hegedus L, et al. Effects of surgical stress and insulin on cardiovascular function and norepinephrine kinetics. Am J Physiol 1984; 247:E29–E34.

140. Deibert DC, DeFronzo RA. Epinephrine-induced insulin resistance in man. J Clin Invest 1980; 65:717–721.

141. Waldhaus WK, Gasic S, Bratusch-Marrain P, et al. Effect of stress hormones on splanchnic substrate and insulin disposal after glucose ingestion in healthy humans. Diabetes 1987; 36:127–135.

142. Hendler RG, Sherwin RS. Epinephrine-stimulated glucose production is not diminished by starvation: Evidence for an effect on gluconeogenesis. J Clin Endocrinol Metab 1984; 58:1014–1021.

143. Simmons PS, Miles JM, Gerich JE, et al. Increased proteolysis: An effect of increases in plasma cortisol within the physiologic range. J Clin Invest 1984; 73:412–420.

144. Rizza RA, Mandarino LJ, Gerich JE. Cortisol-induced insulin resistance in man: Impaired suppression of glucose production and stimulation of glucose utilization due to a postreceptor defect of insulin action. J Clin Endocrinol Metab 1982; 54:131–138.

145. Brown AD, Wallace P, Breachtel G. In-vivo regulation of non–insulin mediated and insulin mediated glucose uptake by cortisol. Diabetes 1987; 36:1230–1237.

146. Raff H, Flemma RJ, Findling JW, et al. Fast cortisol-induced inhibition of the adrenocorticotropin response to surgery in humans. J Clin Endocrinol Metab 1988; 67:1146–1148.

147. Axelrod J, Reisine TD. Stress hormones: Their interaction and regulation. Science 1984; 224:452–459.

148. Lendingham IM, Watt I. Influence of sedation on mortality in critically ill multiple trauma patient. Lancet 1983; 1:1270.

149. Wagner RL, White PF, Kan PB, et al. Inhibition of adrenal steroidogenesis by the anesthetic etomidate. N Engl J Med 1984; 310:1415–1421.

150. Moore RA, Allen MC, Wood PJ, et al. Perioperative endocrine effects of etomidate. Anaesthesia 1985; 40:124–130.

151. Ganong WF. The stress response—a dynamic overview. Hosp Pract 1988; 23:155–171.

152. Newsome NH, Rose JC. The response of human adrenocorticotrophic hormone and growth hormone to surgical stress. J Clin Endocrinol 1971; 33:481–487.

153. Udelsman R, Norton JA, Jelenich SE, et al. Responses of the hypothalamic-pituitary-adrenal

and renin-angiotensin axes and the sympathetic system during controlled surgical and anesthetic stress. J Clin Endocrinol Metab 1987; 64:986–993.

154. McIntosh TK, Lothrop DA, Lee A, et al. Circadian rhythm of cortisol is altered in postsurgical patients. J Clin Endocrinol Metab 1981; 53:117–122.

155. Kehlet H, Binder CHR. Alterations in distribution volume and biological half-life of cortisol during major surgery. J Clin Endocrinol Metab 1973; 36:330–333.

156. Kehlet H, Binder C, Engbaek C. Cortisol binding capacity in plasma during anaesthesia and surgery. Acta Endocrinol 1974; 75:119–124.

157. Vozumi T, Manabe H, Kawashima Y, et al. Plasma cortisol, corticosterone and non–protein bound cortisol in extra corporeal circulation. Acta Endocrinol 1972; 69:517–525.

158. Barton RN, Passingham BJ. Effect of binding to plasma proteins on the integration of plasma cortisol concentrations after accidental injury. Clin Sci 1981; 61:399–405.

159. Barton RN, Stoner HB, Watson SM. Relationship among plasma cortisol, adrenocorticotropin and severity of injury in recently injured patients. J Trauma 1987; 27:384–392.

160. Parker RC, Baxter CR. Divergence in adrenal steroid secretory pattern after thermal injury in adult patients. J Trauma 1985; 25:508–510.

161. Cartensen H, Terner N, Thoren L, et al. Testosterone, leutinizing hormone, and growth hormone in blood following surgical trauma. Acta Chir Scand 1972; 138:1–7.

162. Hamanaka Y, Kurachi K, Aono T, et al. Effects of general anesthesia and severity of surgical stress on serum LH and testosterone in males. Acta Endocrinol 1975; 78:258–265.

163. Wang C, Chan V, Tse TF, et al. Effect of acute myocardial infarction on pituitary-testicular function. Clin Endocrinol 1978; 9:249–253.

164. Woolfe PD, Hamill RW, McDonald JV, et al. Transient hypogonadotropic hypogonadism caused by critical illness. J Clin Endocrinol Metab 1985; 66:444–450.

165. Gebhart SSP, Waltt NB, Clark RV, et al. Reversible impairment of gonadotropin secretion in critical illness. Arch Intern Med 1989; 149:1637–1641.

166. Lyengar R, Schwartz TL, Brinbaumer L. Coupling of glucagon receptors to adenylcyclase. J Biol Chem 1979; 254:1119–1123.

167. Farah AE. Glucagon and the circulation. Pharmacol Rev 1983; 35:181–217.

168. Wise JK, Hendler R, Felig P. Influence of glucocorticoids on glucagon secretion and plasma amino acid concentrations in man. J Clin Invest 1973; 52:2774–2782.

169. Unger RH, Orce L. Glucagon and the A cell. N Engl J Med 1981; 304:4518–4575.

170. Russell RCG, Walker CJ, Bloom SR. Hyperglucogonemia in the surgical patient. Br Med J 1975; 1:10–12.

171. Holter JB, Pflug AE. Effects of anesthesia and surgical stress on insulin secretion in man. Metabolism 1980; 29:1124–1127.

172. Unger Rh. Glucagon and insulin:glucagon ratio in diabetes and other catabolic illnesses. Diabetes 1971; 20:834–838.

173. Meguid MM, Aun F, Soeldner JS. The effect of severe trauma on urine loss of insulin. Surgery 1976; 79:177–181.

174. Nakoo K, Miyata M. The influence of phentolamine on adrenergic blocking agent on insulin secretion during surgery. Eur J Clin Invest 1977; 7:41–45.

175. Giovanni I, Boldrini G, Castagneto M, et al. Respiratory quotient and patterns of substrate utilization in human sepsis and trauma. J Parenter Enter Nutr 1983; 7:226–231.

176. Wolfe RR, Burk JF. Somatostatin infusion inhibits glucose production in burn patients. Circ Shock 1982; 9:521–527.

177. Wolfe RR, Herndon DN, Jahoor F, et al. Effect of severe burn injury on substrate cycling by glucose and fatty acids. N Engl J Med 1982; 317:397–402.

178. Shamoon H, Hendler R, Sherwin RS. Synergistic interactions among anti-insulin hormones in the pathogenesis of stress hyperglycemia in humans. J Clin Endocrinol Metab 1981; 52:1235–1241.

179. Baxter RC. The somatomedins: Insulin-like growth factors. Adv Clin Chem 1986; 25:49–65.

180. Underwood LE, D'Ercole AJ, Clemmons DR, et al. Paracrine functions of somatomedins. J Clin Endocrinol Metab 1986; 15:5–77.

181. Felig P, Marliss EB, Cahill GF. Metabolic response to human growth hormone during prolonged starvation. J Clin Invest 1971; 50:411–421.

182. Rizza RA, Mandarino LJ, Gerich JE. Effects of growth hormone on insulin action in man. Diabetes 1982; 31:663–669.

183. Bratusch-Marrain P, Gasic S, Waldhaus WK, et al. Effect of growth hormone on splanchnic glucose and substrate metabolism following oral glucose loading in healthy man. Diabetes 1984; 33:19–25.

184. Keller V, Schnell H, Girard J, et al. Effect of physiological elevation of plasma growth hormone levels on ketone body kinetics and lipolysis in normal acutely insulin deficient man. Diabetologia 1984; 26:103–108.

185. Sonntag WE, Hylka VW, Meites J. Growth hormone restores protein synthesis in skeletal muscle of old male rats. J Gerontol 1985; 40:684–694.

186. Aarimaa A, Gryvalahati E, Viikari J, et al. Insulin, growth hormone, and catecholamines as regulators of energy metabolism in the course of surgery. Acta Chir Scand 1978; 144:411–422.

187. Frayn KN, Price DA, Maycock PF, et al. Plasma somatomedin activity after injury in man and its relationship to other hormonal and metabolic changes. Clin Endocrinol 1984; 20:179–187.

188. Minuto F, Barreca A, Adami GF, et al. Insulin-like growth factor 1 in human malnutrition: Relationship with some body composition and nutritional parameters. JPEN 1989; 13:392–396.

189. Lee HY, Shul J, Pekary AE, et al. Secretion of thyrotropin with reduced concanavalin-A–binding activity in patients with severe non thyroid disease. J Clin Endocrinol Metab 1987; 65:942–945.

190. Ward HC, Halliday D, Sim AJW. Protein and energy metabolism with biosynthetic growth hormone after gastrointestinal surgery. Ann Surg 1983; 206:56–61.

191. Becker RA, Wilmore DW, Goodwin CW, et al. Free $T_4$, free $T_3$ and reverse $T_3$ in critically ill, thermally injured patients. J Trauma 1980; 20:713–721.

192. Zalonga GP, Chernow B, Smallridge RC, et al. A longitudinal evaluation of thyroid function in critically ill surgical patients. Ann Surg 1985; 201:456–464.

193. McLarty DG, Ratcliffe WA, McColl K, et al. Thyroid hormone levels and prognosis in patients with serious non-thyroidal illness. Lancet 1975; 2:275–276.

194. Chopra IJ, Solomon DH, Chopra U, et al. Alterations in circulating thyroid hormones and thyrotropin in hepatic cirrhosis: Evidence for euthyroidism despite subnormal serum triiodothyronine. J Clin Endocrinol Metab 1974; 39:501–511.

195. Nomura S, Pittman CS, Chambers JB Jr. Reduced peripheral conversion of thyroxine to triiodothyronine in patients with hepatic cirrhosis. J Clin Invest 1975; 56:6113–6152.

196. Chopra IJ, Smith SR. Circulating thyroid hormones and thyrotropin in adult patients with protein-calorie malnutrition. J Clin Endocrinol Metab 1975; 40:221–227.

197. Gardner OF, Kaplan MM, Stanley CA, et al. Effect of triiodothyronine replacement on the metabolic and pituitary response to starvation. N Engl J Med 1979; 300:579–584.

198. Spaulding SW, Chopra IJ, Sherwin RS, et al. Effect of caloric restriction and dietary composition on serum $T_3$ and reverse $T_3$ in man. J Clin Endocrinol Metab 1976; 42:197–200.

199. Vagerakis AG, Buiger A, Portray GI, et al. Diversion of peripheral thyroxine metabolism from activating to inactivating pathway during complete fasting. J Clin Endocrinol Metab 1975; 41:191–194.

200. Smith SJ, Bos G, Gerbrandy J, et al. Lowering of serum 3, 3′,5-triiodothyronine–thyroxine ratio in patients with myocardial infarction. Eur J Clin Invest 1981; 8:99–102.

201. Burr WA, Black EG, Griffiths RS, et al. Serum triiodothyronine and reverse triiodothyronine concentrations after surgical operation. Lancet 1975; 2:1277–1279.

202. Degrout LJ, Hoye K. Dexamethasone suppression of serum $T_3$ and $T_4$. J Clin Endocrinol Metab 1976; 42:976–978.

203. Vaughan GM, Becker RA, Unger RH, et al. Non-thyroidal control of metabolism after burn injury: Possible role of glucagon metabolism. Metabolism 1985; 34:637–641.

204. Smallridge RC, Chernow B, Snyder R, et al. Angiotensin-converting enzyme activity: A potential marker of tissue hypothroidism in critical illness. Arch Intern Med 1985; 145:1829–1832.

205. Silberman H, Eisenberg D, Ryan J, et al. The relations of thyroid indices in the critically ill patient to prognosis and nutritional factors. Surg Gynecol Obstet 1988; 166:223–238.

206. Philips RH, Valente WA, Caplan ES, et al. Circulating thyroid hormone changes in acute trauma: Prognostic implications for clinical outcome. J Trauma 1984; 24:116–119.

207. Kaptein EM, Spencer CA, Kamiel MB, et al. Prolonged dopamine administration and thyroid hormone economy in normal and critically ill subjects. J Clin Endocrinol Metab 1980; 51:387–393.

208. Kalsner S. Mechanism of hydrocortisone potentiation of responses to epinephrine and norepinephrine in rabbit aorta. Circ Res 1969; 24:383–395.

209. Geddes BA, Jones TR, Dvorsky RJ, et al. Interaction of glucocorticoids and bronchodilators on isolated guinea pig trachea and human bronchial smooth muscle. Am Rev Respir Dis 1974; 110:420–427.

210. Fraser CM, Potter PC, Chung FZ, et al. Glucocortisoid regulation of human lung beta-adrenergic receptor density occurs at the level of genes transcription. Fed Proc 1987; 1:1463.

211. Bessey PQ, Watters JM, Aoki TT, et al. Combined hormonal infusion stimulates the metabolic response to injury. Ann Surg 1984; 200:264–280.

212. Gelfand RA, Matthews DE, Bier DM, et al. Role of counterregulatory hormones in the catabolic response to stress. J Clin Invest 1984; 74:2238–2248.

213. Watters JM, Bessey PQ, Dinarello CA, et al. The induction of interleukin-1 in humans and its metabolic effects. Surgery 1985; 98:298–305.

214. Watters JM, Bessey PQ, Dinarello CA, et al. Both inflammatory and endocrine mediators stimulate host responses to sepsis. Arch Surg 1986; 121:179–190.

215. Dinarello C. Interleukin 1 and pathogenesis of the acute phase response. N Engl J Med 1984; 311:1413–1418.

216. Schmidt JA, Mizel SB, Cohen D, et al. Interleukin 1: A potential regulator of fibroblast proliferation. J Immunol 1982; 128:2177.

217. Jones PG, Kauffman CA, Bergman AG, et al. Fever in the elderly. Production of leukocytic pyrogen by monocytes from elderly persons. Gerontology 1984; 30:182–187.

218. Saklatvala J, Pilsworth LMC, Sarsfield SV, et al. Pig catabolin is a form of interleukin 1. Biochem J 1984; 224:461–466.

219. Baracos V, Rodeman P, Dinarell CA, et al. Stimulation of muscle degradation and prostaglandin E$_2$ release by leukocytes pyrogen (interleukin 1). N Engl J Med 1983; 308:553–558.

220. Clowes GH, George BC, Villee CA, et al. Muscle proteolysis induced by a circulating peptide in patients with sepsis or trauma. N Engl J Med 1983; 308:544–552.

221. Kaushansky K, Lin N, Adamson JW. Interleukin 1 stimulates fibroblasts to synthesize granulocyte macrophage– and granulocyte colony–stimulating factors. J Clin Invest 1988; 81:92–97.

222. Clark SC, Kame R. The human hematopoietic colony-stimulating factors. Science 1987; 236:1229–1236.

223. Miyajima A, Miyatake S, Schreurs J, et al. Coordinate regulation of immune and inflammatory responses by T-cell–derived lymphokines. FASEB J 1988; 2:2462–2473.

224. Broudy VC, Kaushansky K, Harlan J, et al. Interleukin 1 stimulates human endothelial cells to produce granulocyte colony stimulating factors. J Immunol 1987; 139:464–468.

225. Luger A, Graf H, Schwartz HP, et al. Decreased serum interleukin 1 activity and monocyte interleukin 1 production in patients with fatal sepsis. Crit Care Med 1986; 14:458–461.

226. Northoff H, Andue T, Tran-Thi TA, et al. The inflammation mediators interleukin-1 and hepatocyte-stimulating factor are differently regulated in human monocytes. Eur J Immunol 1987; 17:707–711.

227. Bauer J, Ganter V, Geiger T, et al. Regulation of interleukin-6 expression in cultured human monocytes and monocyte-derived macrophages. Blood 1988; 72:1134–1140.

228. Jirik FR, Podor TJ, Hirano T, et al. Bacterial lipopolysaccharide and inflammatory mediators augment IL-6 secretion by human endothelial cells. J Immunol 1989; 142:144–147.

229. Nathan CF. Secretory products of macrophages. J Clin Invest 1987; 79:319–326.

230. Beutler B, Krochin N, Milsork IW, et al. Control of cachetin (tumor necrosis factor) synthesis: Mechanisms of endotoxin resistance. Science 1986; 232:977–980.

231. Djend JY, Blanchand DK, Richards AL, et al. Tumor necrosis factor induction by *Candida albicans* from human natural killer cells and monocytes. J Immunol 1988; 141:4047–4052.

232. Tracey KJ, Beutler B, Lowry SP, et al. Shock and tissue injury induced by recombinant human cachectin. Science 1986; 234:470–474.

233. Waage A, Halstensen A, Espevik T. Association between tumor necrosis factor in serum and fatal outcome in patients with meningococcal disease. Lancet 1987; 1:355–357.

234. Nawroth PP, Bank I, Handley D, et al. Tumor necrosis factor/cachetin interacts with endothelial cell receptors to induce release of interleukin 1. J Exp Med 1986; 163:1363–1375.

235. Bachwich PR, Chensue SW, Lorrick JW, et al. Tumor necrosis factor stimulates interleukin-1 and prostaglandin E$_2$ production in resting macrophages. Biochem Biophys Res Commun 1986; 136:94–101.

236. Michie HR, Mangue KR, Spriggs DR, et al. Detection of circulating tumor necrosis factor after endotoxin administration. N Engl J Med 1988; 318:1481–1486.

237. Torti FM, Dieckmann B, Beutler B, et al. A macrophage factor inhibits adipocyte gene expression: An in-vitro model of cachexia. Science 1985; 229:867–869.

238. Paya CV, Kenmotsu N, Schoon RA. Tumor necrosis factor and lymphotoxin secretion by human natural killer cells lead to antiviral cytotoxicity. J Immunol 1988; 141:1989–1995.

239. Cavendar DE, Edelbaum D, Ziff M. Endothelial cell activation induced by tumor necrosis factor and lymphotoxin. Am J Pathol 1989; 134:551–560.

240. Kohaleh MB, Smith EA, Soma Y, et al. Effect of lymphotoxin and tumor necrosis factor on endothelial and connective tissue cell growth and function. Clin Immunol Immunopathol 1988; 49:261–272.

241. Abraham E, Regan RF. The effects of hemorrhage and trauma on interleukin 2 production. Arch Surg 1985; 120:1341–1344.

242. Faist E, Meures A, Aker CC, et al. Prostaglandin E$_2$ (PGE$_2$)–dependent suppression of interleukin

alpha (IL-2) production in patients with major trauma. J Trauma 1987; 27:837–848.

243. Faist E, Mewes A, Strasser T, et al. Alteration of monocyte function following major injury. Arch Surg 1988; 123:287–292.

244. Teodorczyk-Injeyan JA, Sparkes BG, Mills GB, et al. Impaired expression of interleukin 2 receptor (IL 2R) in the immunosuppressed burn patient: Reversed by exogenous IL 2. J Trauma 1987; 27:180–187.

245. Rosenberg SA, Lotze MT, Mule JJ. New approaches to the immunotherapy of cancer using interleukin 2. Ann Intern Med 1988; 108:853–864.

246. Lee RE, Lotze MT, Skibber JM, et al. Cardiovascular effects of immunotherapy with interleukin 2 killer cells. J Clin Oncol 1988; 17:51–59.

247. Conant EF, Fox KR, Miller WT. Pulmonary edema as a complication of interleukin-2 therapy. AJR 1989; 152:749–752.

248. Doyle MV, Lee MT, Forg S. Comparison of the biological activities of human recombinant interleukin 2 (125) and native interleukin 2. J Biol Response Mod 1985; 4:96–109.

249. Lotze MT, Matory YL, Ettinghauser SE, et al. In vivo administration of purified human interleukin 2: II. Half-life, immunologic effects and expansion of peripheral lymphoid cells in vivo with recombinant IL-2. J Immunol 1985; 135:2865–2875.

250. Rosenstein M, Ettinghausen SE, Rosenberg SA. Extra vasation of intravascular fluid mediated by the systemic administration of recombinant interleukin 2. J Immunol 1986; 137:1735–1742.

251. Michie HR, Evberlein TJ, Spriggs DR, et al. Interleukin-2–initiated metabolic response associated with critical illness in human. Ann Surg 1980; 208:492–503.

252. Vilcek J. Gray PW, Rinderknecht E, et al. Interferon gamma: A lymphokine for all seasons. Lymphokine Res 1985; 11:1–10.

253. Collort MA, Belin D, Vassalli JD, et al. Gamma interferon enhances macrophage transcription of the tumor necrosis factor/cachectin interleukin 1 and urokinase genes which are controlled by short-lived repressors. J Exp Med 1986; 164:2113–2118.

254. Boraschi D, Censini S, Tagliabue A. Interferon reduces macophage suppressive activity by inhibiting prostaglandin E$_2$ release and inducing interleukin 1 production. J Immunol 1984; 133:764–768.

255. Grifo JA, Jeremias J, Ledger WJ, et al. Interferon-gamma in the diagnosis and pathogenesis of pelvic inflammatory disease. Am J Obstet Gynecol 1989; 160:26–31.

256. Borquet D, Touquit L, Shen TY, et al. Perspectives in platelet–activating factor research. Pharmacol Rev 1987; 39:97–145.

257. Jauch KW, Hartl WH, Georgieff M, et al. Low-dose bradykinin infusion reduces endogenous glucose production in surgical patients. Metabolism 1988; 37:185–190.

258. Jauch KW, Gunther B, Hartl W, et al. Improvement of impaired postoperative insulin action by bradykinin. Biol Chem Hoppe-Seyler 1986; 367:207–210.

259. Wicklmayr M, Dietze G, Gunther B, et al. Improvement of glucose assimilation and protein degradation by bradykinin in maturity onset diabetes and in surgical patients. Adv Exp Med Biol 1979; 120:569–576.

260. Besedovsky H, del Ray A, Sorkin E, et al. Immunoregulatory feedback between interleukin 1 and glucocorticoid hormones. Science 1986; 233:652–655.

261. Buckingham JC. A role for leukocytes in the control of adrenal steroid genesis. J Endocrinol 1984; 114:1–2.

262. Woloski BM, Smith EM, Meyer WJ, et al. Corticotropin releasing activity of monokines. Science 1985; 230:1035–1037.

263. Lumpin MD. The regulation of ACTH secretion by IL-1. Science 1987; 238:452–455.

264. Brown SL, Smith LR, Blalock JE. Interleukin 1 and interleukin 2 enhance prooplomelanocortin gene expression in pituitary cells. J Immunol 1987; 139:3181–3183.

265. Sapolsky R, Rivier C, Yamamoto G, et al. Interleukin 1 stimulates the secretion of hypothalamic corticotropin-releasing factor. Science 1987; 238:522–524.

266. Smith EM, Blalock JE. Human lymphocyte production of corticotropin and endorphin-like substances: Association with leukocyte interferon. Proc Natl Acad Sci USA 1981; 78:7530–7534.

267. George DT, Abeles FB, Mapes CA, et al. Effect of leukocyte endogenous mediators on endocrine pancreas secretory responses. Am J Physiol 1977; 233:E240–E245.

268. Lang CH, Dubrescre C, Bugby GJ, et al. Platelet activating factor (PAF) induces increase in glucose kinetics. Fed Proc 1987; 46:738.

269. Krishran R, Ellinwood EH, Laszlo J, et al. Effect of gamma interferon on the hypothalmic-pituitary adrenal system. Biol Psychiatry 1987; 22:1163–1166.

270. Levy EM, McIntosh T, Block PH. Elevation of circulatory beta-endorphin levels with concomitant depression of immune parameters after traumatic injury. J Trauma 1986; 26:246–249.

271. Simpkins CO, Tate E, Alailima S. Beta-endorphin and lipopolysaccharide interactions with human neutrophils. J Nat Med Assoc 1988; 80:199–203.

272. Shavit Y, Lewis JW, Terman GW, et al. Opioid peptides mediate the suppressive effect of stress on natural killer cell cytotoxicity. Science 1984; 223:188–190.

273. Wybran J, Appelboom T, Famaey JP, et al. Suggestive evidence for receptors for morphine and methion-enkephalin on normal human blood T lymphocytes. J Immunol 1979; 123:1068–1075.

274. Deitch EA, Xo D, Bridges RM. Opioids modulate human neutrophil lymphocyte function: Thermal injury alters plasma beta-endorphin levels. Surgery 1988; 104:41–48.

275. Hellstrand K, Hermodsson S, Strannegard O. Evidence for a beta-adrenoceptor–mediated regulation of human natural killer cells. J Immunol 1985; 134:4095–4099.

276. Deitch EA, McIntyre RB. Stress hormones modulate neutrophil and lymphocyte activity in vitro. J Trauma 1987; 27:1146–1154.

277. Edwards CK, Ghiassudin SM, Schepper JM, et al. Insulin production following injury and sepsis. J Trauma 1987; 27:1031–1038.

278. Tellado-Rodriguez, Christou NV. Clinical assessment of host defense. Surg Clin North Am 1988; 68:41–55.

279. Harvey KB, Moldawer LL, Bistrian BR, et al. Biological measures for the formulation of a hospital prognostic index. Am J Clin Nutr 1981; 34:2013–2022.

280. Johnson WC, Ulrich F, Meguidi MM, et al. Role of delayed hypersensitivity in predicting postoperative morbidity and mortality. Am J Surg 1979; 137:536–539.

281. Wood, JJ, Rodrick ML, Mahony JB, et al. Inadequate interleukin 2 production. Ann Surg 1984; 200:311–320.

282. Nohr CW, Christou NV, Rose H, et al. In vivo and in vitro humoral immunity in surgical patients. Ann Surg 1984; 200:373–380.

283. McLean LD. Delayed type hypersensitivity testing in surgical patients. Surg Gynecol Obstet 1988; 166:285–293.

284. Black PR, Brooks DC, Bessey PQ, et al. Mechanisms of insulin resistance following injury. Ann Surg 1982; 196:420–435.

285. Turinsky J, Saba TM, Scovill WA, et al. Dynamics of insulin secretion and resistance after burns. J Trauma 1977; 17:344–350.

286. Dahn MS, Lange P, Mitchell RA, et al. Insulin production following injury and sepsis. J Trauma 1987; 27:1031–1038.

287. Stjernstrom H, Jorfeldt L, Wiklund L. Interrelationship between splanchnic and leg exchange of glucose and other blood-borne energy metabolites during abdominal surgical trauma. Clin Physiol 1981; 1:59–72.

288. Rizza RA, Mandarino LJ, Gerich JE. Cortisol induced insulin resistance in man: Impaired suppression of glucose production and stimulation of glucose utilization due to a postreceptor defect of insulin action. J Clin Endocrinol Metab 1982; 54:131–138.

289. Nakoo K, Miyata M. The influence of phentolamine, an adrenergic blocking agent on insulin secretion during surgery. Eur J Clin Invest 1977; 7:41–45.

290. Shaw JHF, Hodaway CM, Humberstone DA. Metabolic intervention in surgical patients: The effects of alpha- and beta-blockade on glucose and protein metabolism in surgical patients receiving total parenteral nutrition. Surgery 1988; 103:52–55.

291. Shaw JHF, Wolfe RR. Metabolic intervention in surgical patients. Ann Surg 1988; 207:44–52.

292. Muller MJ, Moring J, Seitz L. Regulation of hepatic glucose output by glucose in vivo. Metabolism 1988; 37:55–60.

293. Shaw JHF, Klein S, Wolfe RR. Assessment of alanine, urea, and glucose interrelationship in normal subjects and in patients with sepsis with stable isotropic tracers. Surgery 1985; 97:551–568.

294. Wolfe RR, Peters EJ. Lipolytic response to glucose infusion in human subjects. Am J Physiol 1987; 252:E218–E223.

295. Rennie MJ, Holloszy JO. Inhibition of glucose uptake and glycogenolysis by availability of substrate in cell-oxygenated perfused skeletal muscle. Biochem J 1977; 168:161–173.

296. Forse RA, Leibel R, Askanazi J, et al. Adrenergic control of adipocyte lipolysis in trauma and sepsis. Ann Surg 1987; 206:744–751.

297. Wolfe RR, Herndon DN, Peters EJ, et al. Regulation of lipolysis in severely burned children. Ann Surg 1987; 206:214–221.

298. Aprille JR, Aikawa N, Bell TC, et al. Adenylate cyclase after burn injury: Resistance to desensitization by catecholamines. J Trauma 1979; 19:812–818.

299. Carpentier YA, Askanazi J, Elwyn DH, et al. Effects of hypercaloric glucose infusion on lipid metabolism in injury and sepsis. J Trauma 1979; 19:649–654.

300. Nordenstrom J, Carpentier YA, Askanazi J, et al. Free fatty acid mobilization and oxidation during total parenteral nutrition in trauma and infection. Ann Surg 1983; 198:725–735.

301. Galster AD, Bier DM, Cryer P, et al. Plasma

palmitate turnover in subjects with thermal injury. J Trauma 1984; 24:938–945.

302. Persson E, Nordenstrom J, Vinnars E. Plasma clearance of fat emulsion during continuous heparin infusion. Acta Anaesthesiol Scand 1987; 31:189–192.

303. Robin AP, Askanazi J, Greenwood MRC, et al. Lipoprotein lipase activity in surgical patients: Influence of trauma and sepsis. Surgery 1981; 90:401–408.

304. Nordenstrom J. Utilization of exogenous and endogenous lipid for energy production during parenteral nutrition. Acta Chir Scand Suppl 1982; 510:1–42.

305. Robin AP, Nordenstrom J, Askanazi J, et al. Influence of parenteral carbohydrate on fat oxidation in surgical patients. Surgery 1984; 195:608–618.

306. Wolfe RR, Herndon DN, Jahoor F, et al. Effect of severe burn injury on substrate cycling by glucose and fatty acids. N Engl J Med 1987; 317:403–408.

307. Smith R, Fuller DJ, et al. Initial effect of injury on ketone bodies and other blood metabolites. Lancet 1975; 1:1–3.

308. Avary JC, Siegel JH, Nakatani T, et al. A biochemical basis for depressed ketogenesis in sepsis. J Trauma 1986; 26:419–425.

309. Schofiel PS, Frent TJ, Sugden MC. Ketone-body metabolism after surgical stress or partial hepatectomy. Biochem J 1987; 241:475–481.

310. Hartl WA, Jauch KW, Kimmig R, et al. Minor role of ketone bodies in energy metabolism by skeletal muscle tissue during the postoperative course. Ann Surg 1988; 207:95–101.

311. Askanazi J, Carpenter YA, Elwyn DH, et al. Influence of total parenteral nutrition on fuel utilization in injury and sepsis. Ann Surg 1980; 191:40–46.

312. Bagby GJ, Corll CB, Thompson JJ, et al. Lipoprotein lipase suppressing mediator in serum of endotoxin-treated rats. Am J Physiol Endocrinol Metab 1986; 251:E470–E476.

313. Beutler B, Cerami A. Recombinant interleukin-1 suppress lipoprotein lipase activity in 3T3 cells. J Immunol 1985; 135:3969–3971.

314. Kather H, Biger W, Michel G, et al. Human fat cell lipolysis is primarily regulated by inhibitory modulators acting through distinct mechanisms. J Clin Invest 1985; 76:1559–1565.

315. Shaw JHF, Wolfe RR. Glucose and urea kinetics in patients with early and advanced gastrointestinal cancer: The response to glucose infusion, surgical resection, and total parenteral nutrition. Surgery 1988; 103:455–461.

316. Shaw JHF, Wolfe RR. Fatty acid and glycerol

kinetics in septic patients and in patients with gastrointestinal cancer. Ann Surg 1987; 205:368–376.

317. Shaw JF, Wildbore M, Wolfe RR. Whole body protein kinetics in severely septic patients. Ann Surg 1987; 205:288–294.

318. Hasselgren PO, James JH, Fischer JE. Inhibited muscle amino acid uptake in sepsis. Ann Surg 1986; 203:360–365.

319. Jahoor F, Wolfe RR. Regulation of protein catabolism. Kidney Int 1987; 82(suppl 22):581–593.

320. Jahoor F, Desai M, Herndon DN, et al. Dynamics of the protein metabolic response to burn injury. Metabolism 1988; 37:330–337.

321. Downey RS, Monafo WW, Karl IE, et al. Protein dynamics in skeletal muscle after trauma: Local and systemic effects. Surgery 1986; 90:265–274.

322. Stahl WM. Acute phase protein response to tissue injury. Crit Care Med 1987; 15:545–550.

323. Castell JV, Gomez-Lechon MJ, David M, et al. Interleukin-6 is the major regulator of acute phase protein synthesis in adult human hepatocytes. FEBS Lett 1989; 24:237–239.

324. Ramadori G, Mitsch A, Rieder H, et al. Alpha- and gamma-interferon but not interleukin 1 modulates synthesis and secretion of beta$_2$-microglobulin by hepatocytes. Eur J Clin Invest 1988; 18:343–351.

325. Perlmutter DH, Dinarello CD, Pupsai PI. Cachectin/tumor necrosis factor regulates hepatic acute phase gene expression. J Clin Invest 1986; 78:1349–1354.

326. Andus T, Geiger T, Hirano T. Action of recombinant human interleukin 6, interleukin 1B, and tumor necrosis factor alpha on the m-RNA reduction of acute phase proteins. Eur J Immunol 1988; 18:739–746.

327. Pomposelli JJ, Flores EA, Bistrian RR. Role of biochemical mediators in clinical nutrition and surgical metabolism. J Parenter Enter Nutr 1988; 12:212–218.

328. Hasselgren PO, Talamini M, Lafrance R, et al. Effect of indomethacin on proteolysis in septic muscle. Ann Surg 1982; 202:557–562.

329. Hasselgren RO, Warner BW, Hummel R, et al. Further evidence that accelerated muscle protein breakdown during sepsis is not mediated by prostaglandin E$_2$. Ann Surg 1988; 207:399–406.

330. Asoh T, Shirosaka C, Uchida I, et al. Effects of indomethacin on endocrine responses and nitrogen loss after surgery. Ann Surg 1987; 206:770–776.

331. Clark AS, Kelly RA, Mitch WE. System response to thermal injury in rats. J Clin Invest 1984; 74:888–897.

332. Souba WW, Smith RJ, Wilmore DW. Glutamine

metabolism by the intestinal tract. J Parenter Enter Nutr 1985; 9:608–617.

333. Souba WW, Wilmore DW. Gut-liver interaction during accelerated gluconeogenesis. Arch Surg 1985; 120:66–70.

334. Turner WW, Ireton CS, Hunt JL, et al. Predicting energy expenditures in burn patients. J Trauma 1985; 25:11–16.

335. Askanazi J, Forse RA, Weissman C, et al. Ventilatory effects of the stress hormones in normal man. Crit Care Med 1986; 14:602–606.

336. Gil KM, Forse RA, Askanazi J, et al. Energy metabolism in stress. In: Garrow JS, Halliday D, eds. Substrate and Energy Metabolism. London: John Libbey, 1985;203–212.

337. Wilmore DW, Aulick LH. Metabolic changes in burned patients. Surg Clin North Am 1978; 58:1173–1187.

338. Lowry SF, Leyaspi A, Jeevanandam M, et al. Body protein kinetics during perioperative intravenous nutritional support. Surg Gynecol Obstet 1986; 163:303–309.

339. Cuthbertson DP, Fell GS, Smith CM, et al. Metabolism after injury 1. Effects of severity, nutrition, and environmental temperature on protein, potassium, zinc, and creatinine. Br J Surg 1972; 59:925–931.

340. Long CL. Energy balance and carbohydrate metabolism in infection and sepsis. Am J Clin Nutr 1977; 30:1301–1310.

341. Shaw JHF, Wolfe RR. Determinations of glucose turnover and oxidation in normal volunteers and septic patients using stable and radio-isotopes: The response to glucose infusion and total parenteral feeding. Aust NZ J Surg 1986; 56:785–791.

342. Wolfe RR, O'Donnell TF, Stone MD, et al. Investigation of factors determining the optimal glucose infusion rate in total parenteral nutrition. Metabolism 1980; 29:892–900.

343. Burke JF, Wolfe RR, Mullany CJ, et al. Glucose requirements following burn injury. Parameters of optimal glucose infusion and possible hepatic and respiratory abnormalities following excessive glucose intake. Ann Surg 1979; 190:274–279.

344. Georgieff M, Moldawer LL, Bistrian BR, et al. Xylitol: An energy source for intravenous nutrition after trauma. J Parenter Enter Nutr 1988; 9:189–199.

345. Lindholm M, Rossner S. Rate of elimination of the intralipid fat emulsion from the circulation in intensive care patients. Crit Care Med 1982; 11:740–747.

346. Jeejeebuoy KN, Anderson GH, Nakhooda AF, et al. Metabolic studies in total parenteral nutrition. J Clin Invest 1976; 52:125–136.

347. Cerra FB, Mazuski J, Teasley K, et al. Nitrogen retention in critically ill patients is proportional to the branched chain acid load. Crit Care Med 1983; 11:775–778.

348. Cerra F, Blackburn G, Hirsch J, et al. The effect of stress level, amino acid formula, and nitrogen dose on nitrogen retention in traumatic and septic stress. Ann Surg 1987; 205:282–287.

349. Bonau RA, Jeevanandam M, Moldawer L, et al. Muscle amino acids flux in patients receiving branched chain amino acid solutions after surgery. Surgery 1987; 101:400–407.

350. Bauer RH, Muggia-Sullam M, Vallgren S, et al. Branched chain amino-acid–enriched solutions in the septic patient. Ann Surg 1986; 203:13–20.

351. Rappolee DA, Mark P, Badna MJ, et al. Wound macrophages express TGF alpha and other growth factors in vivo: Analysis by mRNA phenotyping. Science 1988; 241:708–711.

352. Shaw JHF, Galler L, Holdaway IM, et al. The effect of extradural blockade upon glucose and urea kinetics in surgical patients. Surg Gynecol Obstet 1987; 165:260–265.

353. Simpson PJ, Radford SG, Lockyer JA. The influence of anaesthesia on the acute phase protein response to surgery. Anaesthesia 1987; 42:690–696.

354. Ziegler TR, Young LS, Manson JM, et al. Metabolic effects of recombinant human growth hormone in patients receiving parenteral nutrition. Ann Surg 1988; 208:6–16.

# Chapter 18

# Obesity and Weight Control

ELSWORTH R. BUSKIRK

Overweight and obesity result from a positive energy balance created by relatively greater energy intake or smaller energy expenditure. Because physical activity increases energy expenditure, it is important to consider a physically active lifestyle for both prevention and treatment of obesity. A physically active lifestyle can help improve cardiorespiratory fitness; promote flexibility, mobility, and physical self-confidence; modify risk factors associated with the development of cardiovascular disease and maturity-onset diabetes; allow weight loss with larger food intake that still is nutritionally adequate; and preserve a higher resting metabolic rate than that commonly observed with diet restriction. Development of a regular physical activity regimen can create appreciation of the need for total lifestyle management. Such lifestyle management may well involve choosing foods that help reduce body fat and maintain optimal weight. Thus, the aims of a physically active lifestyle are to increase energy expenditure, preserve muscle and metabolically active tissue mass, provide enjoyment, and emphasize healthy lifestyle awareness. Nevertheless, an obese sedentary person contemplating a more active lifestyle is well-advised to proceed slowly, preferably with competent professional assistance.

## Classification of Obesity

The National Health and Nutrition Examination (NHANES II) survey suggested that approximately 40 million people in the United States are at least 20% overweight. More than 13 million were reported to be at least 40% overweight; persons in this category—and those up to 100% overweight—were regarded as *moderately obese*. Persons more than 100% overweight may be regarded as *severely* or *morbidly obese*.[1]

Overweight is not the same as obesity. *Obesity* refers to excess body fat; *overweight* to excessive body weight relative to standards for height. Though they are often used interchangeably, overweight and obesity do have different meanings. In practice, the NHANES data described a translation of overweight to obesity,

"A higher percentage of women than men are obese. In the age range 20 to 74 years, 14% of the men and 24% of the women are 20% or more overweight. Black women are more likely to be obese than white women, regardless of age or income—a difference that does not hold for men."[2]

Clinicians frequently use the body mass index (BMI = $wt \cdot ht^{-2}$) to define overweight. The normal limits are 20 to 25 for men and 19 to 24 for women. *Overweight* is associated with a BMI between the upper limit of normal and 30, and obesity with a BMI greater than 30.[2,3] BMI is independent of frame size, but there is a direct relationship (i.e., the larger the frame the larger the BMI) among those with equal proportions of body composition components.

Researchers have attempted to use skin fold measurements to classify obesity. Seltzer and Mayer[4] did so using the triceps skin fold. They suggested that at age 12 years in boys a triceps skin fold greater than 18 mm indicates obesity and for girls the value is any greater than 22 mm. The critical thickness increases with age until among those 30 to 50 years, a triceps skin fold of 23 mm for men and 30 mm for women indicates obesity. If one accepts the equivalent fat content calculated from skin fold thicknesses to be acceptable for the classification of obesity, one might accept more than 25% body fat for men and more than 30% for women as the lower limits of obesity. Durnin and Wormersley[5] developed a table of equivalent fat content for men and women and demonstrated that skin fold thickness gradually decreases with age. They summed the thicknesses of four skin folds (biceps, triceps, subscapular, suprailiac) and reported the following approximate sums for four age groups of men: 17 to 29 years, 80 mm; 30 to 39 years, 70 mm; 40 to 49 years, 50 mm; 50 years and older, 45 mm. A similar trend of lower magnitude was reported for women, the values were as follows: 16 to 29 years, 65 mm; 30 to 39 years, 60 mm; 40 to 49 years, 45 mm; 50 years and older, 40 mm.

A variety of other techniques are now available for assessing body fat; however, what percentage of fat constitutes obesity has differed, depending on the purposes of the study, the population, and other variables. Thus, the selection of criteria has varied and there has been no consensus, though it appears possible to select practical guidelines. Body fat in excess of 25% of body weight for men and 30% for women appears to be a reasonable criterion for excessive body fat,[6] while more than 40% body fat for men and 50% for women could define severe or morbid obesity. Considerable debate continues as to what amount of fat constitutes a health risk; to date, no firm decision has been made.[7,8]

Some clinicians suggest that the eye provides a sufficiently useful perception of body fat, but such appraisals provide nothing useful in quantitative terms. Body composition and fatness measurements are recommended for assessment of changes brought about by medical treatment or other therapy, including exercise.

The definition of obesity changes depending on the perspective of the classification scale. For example, if physiologic strain (respiratory, cardiovascular, thermal) serves as a criterion, the respective strains brought about by common stresses such as exercise intensity, environmental conditions such as heat and humidity, hypo- and hyperbaria, and hypoxia could be used for classification purposes. In that case, the 25% body fatness criterion for men and 30% for women may be too high. Similarly, these criteria may be too lax in light of current health attitudes and the emphasis on leanness. Thus, obesity criteria should be not only population specific but also meaningful in terms of health or pathologic or physiologic strain criteria.

Bray[9] has stressed the multiple causes of obesity and has classified obesity anatomically and etiologically. His anatomic classification focuses on fat storage pattern—localized or generalized. The etiologic classification focuses on the type, postulated mechanism, and treatment of obesity. The types of obesity include hypothalamic, endocrine, nutritional, genetic, drug-induced, and sedentary lifestyle–induced. Each group has several subtypes. Though lack of exercise is involved in only one category, exercise interacts with a variety of regulatory and metabolic mechanisms, such as glucose and insulin metabolism, catecholamine metabolism, lipolysis, and peripheral receptor activity.

Classification by volume of adipose tissue cells requires valid and reliable measurements of cell size and total body fatness from which to calculate cell number.[10] Both adipocyte size and number vary among regional fat deposits, in an individual and among individuals. Nevertheless, hypercellular persons are frequently those who had childhood-onset obesity. Those who develop obesity later in life are largely normocellular. Björntorp[11] has suggested that these two types of obesity may respond differently to therapy.

A more recent classification based on regional distribution of body fat depends on girth measurements.[12,13] The critical measure is viewed as the waist-hip circumference ratio. In both men and women sizable ratios have been related to increased risk of cardiovascular disease, including myocardial infarction, angina pectoris, stroke, and death.[13]

## Physiologic Risks

Obesity has been linked to a variety of conditions that adversely affect physiologic function and health status (Table 18-1)—cardiovascular, respi-

**Table 18-1.** Conditions Associated with Obesity

Cardiovascular
    Reduced myocardial function: arrhythmias
    Enlarged heart: congestive heart failure
    Artherosclerosis: coronary heart disease
    Cerebrovascular disease
    Hypertension
    Varicoses
    Hypoxia syndromes: pulmonary hypertension
    Edema

Respiratory
    Reduced pulmonary function: hypoventilation
    Sleep apnea
    Loss of sensitivity to $CO_2$
    Pneumonia
    Dyspnea on exertion

Metabolic
    Diabetes mellitus, type II
    Hyperinsulinemia
    Cirrhosis of the liver
    Gout
    Hyperlipidemia
    Gallbladder disease
    In women, osteoarthritis in weight-bearing joints

Thermoregulatory
    Reduced heat tolerance

Other
    Menstrual and ovarian abnormalities
    Complications of pregnancy
    Appendicitis
    Peptic ulcer
    Endometrial carcinoma, other cancer, leukemia
    Greater risk at surgery
    Poor tolerance for anesthesia
    Compromised mobility: greater risk of accidents
    Greater risk of suicide

(Data from Mann,[95] Garrow,[96] Stunkard,[97] Alexander,[39] Buskirk,[84] and Brownell and Stunkard.[99])

ratory, temperature regulation, and metabolic disturbances.

## Cardiovascular Disease

The association between excessive overweight or obesity and cardiovascular disease has been described for many years as the circulation of obese patients has been studied.[14–18] In two prospective studies of coronary heart disease (CHD) in which skin fold measurements were used to calculate adiposity it was found that the projected increase in coronary disease risk was related to greater fatness in middle-aged men.[19,20] Nevertheless, controversy exists. Keys[19] presented a discussion of the problem and calculated the probability of CHD-related deaths in relation to BMI for men from the Chicago Gas Company study, the U.S. railroad study, and some European studies. The probability of a CHD-related death was increased at the extremes of the BMI distribution (i.e., very low and very high values). Keys concluded that risk of heart disease increases substantially only at the extremes of underweight and overweight or fatness. Bloom and coworkers[21] also found that rates of CHD and cardiovascular disease (CVD) to be higher in the most obese men than in nonobese ones, no matter whether the men were normotensive or hypertensive. These results were obtained in a prospective epidemiologic study of a cohort of Japanese-American men aged 45 to 65 years who were followed for 12 years in the Honolulu Heart Program.

Hypertension is of considerable consequence in obesity because of associated atherosclerosis, arterial wall damage, retinopathy, and renal vascular disease. Bloom's group[21] concluded that for obese persons hypertension is associated with increased risk of CVD. Messerli and colleagues[22,23] postulated that in obese hypertensive persons, the circulating blood volume is large and the relatively greater venous return adds a load to a left ventricle already burdened by high afterload caused by arterial hypertension. They suggested that the double burden on the left ventricle may enhance the long-term risk of congestive heart failure. Messerli's group noted disparate effects of obesity and hypertension on total peripheral resistance and intravascular volume—the former was relatively lower and the latter relatively higher in obese subjects—and the effects partially offset each other. Comparison of obese men with normal blood pressure and with hypertension revealed expansion of extracellular and interstitial fluid in the hypertensive group. The volumes paralleled the degree of obesity.[24]

Obese patients have been found to have greater cardiac output, stroke volume, left ventricular filling pressure, and left ventricular eccentric hypertrophy than normal ones. The drop in arterial pressure with weight loss may well be caused by decreased adrenergic activity leading to decreased cardiac output along with some lowering of vascular resistance. The relatively elevated cardiac output, in hypertensive obese patients, along with relatively restricted arterial capacity, may well be associated with the low vascularity of adipose tissue. Increased blood viscosity may contribute to the elevated arterial pressure in grossly obese persons.[25]

When morbidly obese patients underwent gastric restriction and subsequently achieved substantial weight loss, follow-up echocardiography revealed that the mean left ventricle (LV) dimension in diastole and mean blood pressure were significantly decreased. The conclusions were that cardiac chamber enlargement, LV hypertrophy, and LV systolic dysfunction occur in many morbidly obese patients and that these functions may improve following substantial weight loss (Table 18-2).[26] Similar observations were made by Rubal and Elmesallamy,[27] who compared observations on obese women and control subjects. The obese women had greater mean blood pressure, LV wall thickness, LV end-diastolic volume, LV mass, and left atrial and aortic root dimensions. The investigators concluded that significant structural changes in the myocardium occur in obese subjects, even though they are free of cardiovascular symptoms.

Persons with the obesity-hypoventilation syndrome (pickwickian syndrome) have a relatively larger pulmonary blood volume (pulmonary circulatory congestion), probably because of pulmonary arterial vasoconstriction and hypertension secondary to hypoxia and hypercapnic acidemia.[28] The linking of left- and right-sided heart problems with CHD and hypertension, as can occur in grossly obese persons, severely limits functional cardiovascular and respiratory capacity.

Another risk factor for CHD associated with obesity is hyperlipidemia.[29-32] Serum triglyceride concentrations tend to be more elevated than total cholesterol, and the proportion of high-density lipoprotein cholesterol (HDL) tends to be lower in many obese subjects.[31] Serum lipids have been shown to be elevated after experimental production of obesity via simple overeating of a diet high in carbohydrate.[33]

The pattern of body fat distribution tends to be important: greater risk of developing CHD is as-

**Table 18-2.** Comparison of Cardiac Size, Wall Thickness, and Function of 34 Morbidly Obese Patients Before and After Weight Loss

| Echocardiographic Variable | N | Before Weight Loss (Mean ± SD) | After Weight Loss (Mean ± SD) | P |
|---|---|---|---|---|
| LV internal dimension in diastole (cm) | | | | |
| Normal (3.6–5.5) | 21 | 5.0 ± 0.3 | 4.8 ± 0.3 | NS |
| Enlarged (>5.5) | 13 | 6.0 ± 0.2 | 5.1 ± 0.2 | <0.02 |
| LV internal dimension in systole (cm) | | | | |
| Normal (≤3.7) | 19 | 3.2 ± 0.2 | 3.0 ± 0.2 | NS |
| Enlarged >3.7) | 15 | 4.7 ± 0.2 | 3.5 ± 0.2 | <0.01 |
| LV fractional shortening (%) | | | | |
| Normal (28–44) | 21 | 35 ± 3 | 37 ± 3 | NS |
| Low (<28) | 13 | 22 ± 2 | 31 ± 2 | <0.01 |
| LV posterior wall thickness (cm) | | | | |
| Normal (0.6–1.1) | 16 | 0.9 ± 0.1 | 0.9 ± 0.1 | NS |
| Increased (>1.1) | 18 | 1.3 ± 0.1 | 1.3 ± 0.1 | NS |
| RV internal dimension (cm) | | | | |
| Normal (0.7–2.3) | 24 | 1.8 ± 0.1 | 1.7 ± 0.1 | NS |
| Enlarged (>2.3) | 10 | 2.5 ± 0.1 | 2.3 ± 0.2 | NS |
| Body weight (kg) | 34 | 135 ± 8 | 79 ± 6 | <0.005 |

Key: NS, not significant.
(Adapted from Alpert MA, Terry BA, Kelly DL. Effect of weight loss on cardiac chamber size, wall thickness, and left ventricular function in morbid obesity. Am J Cardiol 1985; 55:783–786.)

sociated with the male or android pattern of distribution,[13,29,34] which consists of a relatively high (>1.0) waist-hip circumference ratio, in contrast to the female or gynecoid pattern, in which body fat is greater around the hips and thighs (ratio <1.0). Relatively higher plasma concentrations of triglycerides and total cholesterol and lower concentrations of high-density lipoproteins have been observed with the male pattern of fat distribution.[34] A further extension of regional distribution analysis has suggested that the relative differences in plasma lipid concentrations associated with a waist-hip circumference ratio greater than 1.0 may be importantly related to a large store of *intraabdominal* fat, including omental and mesenteric, rather than to subcutaneous fat.[35]

Investigation of the children who participated in the Bogalusa Heart Study[36] showed that several risk factors for CHD increased with age, including BMI, total serum cholesterol, and diastolic blood pressure. With increased body fat, especially in boys', total serum cholesterol and triglycerides increased also, particularly low-density and very–low density lipoproteins.[37,38]

In a person at rest blood flows through adipose tissue at a rate of approximately 2 to 3 ml per minute per 100 g of tissue.[39] Alterations in pressure-flow relationships have been observed in the adipose tissue vascular bed in response to changes in oxygen tension, pH, circulating blood volume, mechanical factors, exercise, temperature, sympathetic nerve activity, and several hormones.[40] Since the vascular beds in adipose tissue also serve as blood volume reservoirs, displacement or augmentation of the contained volume has central cardiovascular effects. In general, adipose tissue blood flow is related inversely to fat cell volume but directly to the number of fat cells.[39] Following prolonged fasting and weight loss, which produces a reduction in cardiac output, there is a relatively increased number of fat cells per unit of adipose tissue weight, which is accompanied by a relatively greater blood flow. These changes reduce the total blood flow to the smaller fat cell volume.[41]

## Respiration

Deposition of fat over the thoracic cavity and within and over the abdomen increases the likelihood of regressive changes in pulmonary function; for example, the functional residual volume (FRC) of the lung is decreased with moderate or gross obesity. The smaller FRC is brought about by thoracic cavity squeeze. Both the mass of overlying adipose tissue and an elevated diaphragm contribute to the squeeze.[42–44] The lesser FRC is to a large extent associated with reduction in the expiratory reserve volume (ERV); the residual volume remains relatively unchanged or elevated (Table 18-3).[45] Abnormalities in the ventilation-perfusion distribution of gases and lung mechanics may be associated with the reduction in ERV.

The mechanical work of breathing, reflected in a higher oxygen cost of breathing,[46] is increased in obesity. The intercostal muscles being forced to move the large adipose tissue mass overlying the thorax and the contracting diaphragm work against an enlarged and distended abdomen. As the increased work of breathing occurs at reduced lung volume, a feeling of respiratory distress occurs that reduces the desire and ability to exercise.

Obesity-hypoventilation syndrome occurs in about 5% of severely obese patients. It is characterized by hypoventilation, periodic respiration, somnolence, cyanosis, polycythemia, right ventricular hypertrophy, and heart failure; this constellation was dubbed the pickwickian syndrome by Burwell and coworkers.[47] The ERV and chest

**Table 18-3.** Respiratory Function in Normal and Obese Subjects Categorized by Weight-Height Ratios

| | Weight-Height Ratio (kg × cm$^{-1}$) | |
|---|---|---|
| **Variable** | **Normal (0.60–0.69)** | **Obesity (1.10–1.19)** |
| VC (% P) | 108 ± 5 | 69 ± 14 |
| ERV (L) | 1.35 ± 0.14 | 0.48 ± 0.18 |
| ERV (% P) | 100 ± 8 | 32 ± 11 |
| FRC (% P) | 80 ± 4 | 75 ± 14 |
| RV (% P) | 63 ± 6 | 141 ± 37 |
| MVV (% P) | 102 ± 7 | 61 ± 12 |

Key: VC, vital capacity; % P, percentage of predicted value; ERV, expiratory reserve volume; FRC, functional residual capacity; RV, residual volume; MVV, maximal voluntary ventilation.
(Adapted from Ray CS, Sae DY, Bray G, et al. Effects of obesity on respiratory function. Am Rev Respir Dis 1983; 128:501–506.)

wall compliance are reduced, along with alveolar volume and gas exchange.[39] Shallow breathing at a low lung volume causes small airway closure and regional atelectasis that lead to increased venous admixture, physiologic shunting, nonuniformity of pulmonary capillary perfusion, and increased physiologic dead space.[48] There is decreased respiratory response to hypoxia and hypercapnia. Pulmonary hypertension in the obesity-hypoventilation syndrome has several causes: pulmonary vasoconstriction secondary to hypoxia and acidosis, biventricular hypertrophy, elevated pulmonary venous pressure, and transpulmonary diastolic pressure gradient.[39] When the syndrome does occur, sleep apnea may lead to sudden death. Fortunately, some of the features of the obesity-hypoventilation syndrome can be reversed by weight reduction such as the hypoventilation and the respiratory response to carbon dioxide, but impaired response to hypoxia may persist.[39,49] In some patients a ketogenic diet caused increased carbon dioxide response independent to changes in body weight or pulmonary mechanics.[50]

### Exercise Tolerance

Several respiratory factors have been identified that limit exercise tolerance in obese persons: (1) increased metabolic and associated ventilatory requirements to perform exercise; (2) increased cost of breathing because of the high breathing frequency and the interfering chest wall and abdominal fats; and (3) pulmonary insufficiency related to the heavy work of breathing and lung atelectasis. These changes in pulmonary function exacerbate the ventilatory strain associated with exercise by obese persons, and the high metabolic cost of breathing reduces exercise tolerance and the amount of work accomplished in a given time, thus increasing the imbalance between energy intake and expenditure.

### Sleep Apnea

The syndrome of obstructive sleep apnea in obese persons is caused by increased pharyngeal resistance and decreased airway patency, and both are important determinants in airway collapse or oc-

clusion during sleep. White and colleagues[51] found that both weight and weight-height ratio were significantly related to pharyngeal resistance (r = 0.53 and 0.59, respectively) and indicated that these relationships increase with age. The apnea problem, as it relates to obesity, may also be associated with a markedly reduced total respiratory compliance during recumbency compared to that of normal subjects.[28]

### Temperature Regulation

When exposed to heat or cold, normal persons maintain relatively constant body temperature by a variety of physiologic responses. Exercise causes increased heat production and when it is performed in a hot and humid environment it can strain the body's heat loss capability. Blood flow through the skin is increased during heat stress, to afford greater heat loss by evaporation. During exercise there is competition between the requirements of the working muscle and circulation through the skin. In obese persons, relatively less blood flow is allocated to the skin, to facilitate heat loss, and this compromises heat balance. Thus, obese persons are less tolerant of exposure to heat or exercise in a warm or hot and humid environment than are normal people, often suffering hyperthermia and even shock and collapse. There are several reasons.

First, a fat person is rounder and, so, has a smaller surface area–body mass ratio. As heat exchange with the environment by convection, radiation, and evaporation is proportional to body surface area exposed, a small ratio is associated with less heat exchange per unit mass. Second, the specific heat of fat stored in adipose tissue is lower than that of water or other tissue. Thus, for a given heat load persons with excessive adipose tissue exhibit a greater rise in body temperature per kilogram of body weight. Third, the heat-activated sweat gland density of obese persons is lower owing to stretching of the skin to accommodate the fat mass (Table 18-4), which may compromise evaporative capacity.[52] Fourth, the cardiorespiratory system of obese persons may be taxed at a relatively lower exercise intensity in warm or hot environments because of the necessity to supply blood to working muscle and to the skin for

**Table 18-4.** Average Density and Calculated Total of Heat-Activated Sweat Glands in Obese and Lean Men and Women*[†]

| Subjects (N) | Statistics | HASG · cm$^{-2}$ | SA (Dubois) (m$^2$) | Total HASG (millions) |
|---|---|---|---|---|
| Obese men (3) | $\overline{X}$ | 46.7 | 1.89 | 1.04 |
| | SD | 17.2 | ±0.32 | 0.33 |
| Lean men (6) | $\overline{X}$ | 59.2 | 1.69 | 1.00 |
| | SD | 12.5 | 0.03 | 0.22 |
| Obese women (6) | $\overline{X}$ | 74.5 | 2.00 | 1.48 |
| | SD | 9.9 | 0.11 | 0.19 |
| Lean women (4) | $\overline{X}$ | 99.8 | 1.55 | 1.56 |
| | SD | 11.8 | 0.08 | 0.25 |

* Subjects sat in 47°C ± 1°C dry-bulb, 24°C ± 1.5°C wet bulb environment for 45 minutes before measurements were made.
[†]HASG data were determined from 46 skin sites—18 on the trunk and 28 on the limbs—with a starch-iodine–impregnated bond paper technique.
Key: HASG, heat-activated sweat glands; SA, surface area; $\overline{X}$, mean; SD, standard deviation.
(Adapted from Bar-Or O, Lundegren HM, Magnusson LI, et al. Distribution of heat-activated sweat glands in obese and lean men and women. Hum Biol 1968; 40:235–248.)

effective heat loss.[53] Last, there is a significantly lower volume of skin blood flow in proportion to central body temperature in obese persons who exercise in the heat. The skin blood flow is important to support heat loss to the environment, and the relatively lower flow reduces heat loss (Table 18-5).[54]

In summary, it seems that fatter persons are more susceptible to hyperthermia when exercising in warm or hot environments, particularly, if evaporative cooling associated with sweating is com-

**Table 18-5.** The Average Slope of the Forearm Blood Flow–Deep Body Temperature (Esophageal Temperature, T$_{es}$) Relationship in a Thermoneutral* and a Warm[†] Environment

| Subjects | Statistic | Thermoneutral | Warm |
|---|---|---|---|
| Obese (N = 5) | $\overline{X}$ | 7.35 | 8.92 |
| | SEM | 0.69 | 1.09 |
| Lean (N = 5) | $\overline{X}$ | 10.26** | 12.08** |
| | SEM | 0.78 | 0.54 |

* Thermoneutral environment: T$_{db}$ = 22°C T$_{wb}$ = 14°C
[†] Warm environment:         T$_{db}$ = 38°C T$_{wb}$ = 20°C
**$P < 0.05$ when comparing data from lean and obese subjects.
(Adapted from Vroman NB, Buskirk ER, Hodgson JL. Cardiac output and skin blood flow in lean and obese individuals during exercise in the heat. J Appl Physiol 1983; 55:69–74.)

promised.[55–58] Healthy, young, obese subjects engaged in basic military training or late summer or early fall football practice have suffered heat injury and even death, especially before being effectively heat acclimated.[53]

In a cold environment, subcutaneous fat provides thermal insulation, which is about two to four times as effective as an equivalent amount of lean tissue. In tolerable cold (minimally clothed) an obese person who accomplishes a fixed work task has a lower body surface temperature for a higher deep body temperature than a lean person.[53] The higher deep body temperature in obese persons occurs despite only modest increase in metabolism brought about by shivering or other means of heat production. In lean persons exposure to cold air, and particularly cold water (e.g., 15°C, 59°F), can elevate metabolism two- to threefold, but similar exposure of obese people produces little if any increase in metabolism.[59,60] Body cooling activates a variety of mechanisms (Table 18-6). In general, obese subjects activate fewer physiologic and behavioral mechanisms. Though the perception of thermal comfort among the obese is not much different than among the lean, they tolerate cold considerably better, suffering less physiologic strain.

O'Hara and colleagues[61] introduced an interesting idea in their concept of "treatment" of obesity by exercise in the cold. The investigators exposed six obese men for 10 days to a very cold environment ($-34°C$) in which they performed various types of exercise for about 3.5 hours per day. The mean daily energy expenditure for the exercise was 1242 kcal. Following early cold-induced diuresis of about 1 kg that may also have involved water loss from partially depleted glycogen stores, substantial body fat was also lost, which loss was well-sustained 2 months after completion of the experimental regimen. O'Hara's group[62] cited additional evidence that substantial body fat loss can occur among soldiers who work hard in an Arctic environment. Sheldahl and colleagues[63] attempted to confirm such results among women who exercised at about 36% to 40% of their aerobic power for about 90 min/day five times per week for 8 weeks in cool water ($17°$ to $22°C$; $62°$ to $68°F$). Some women lost a small amount of body weight and fat, but the losses were insignificant. Although the women experienced considerable heat debt and associated calorie turnover (on the order of 500 to 600 kcal/day; see Table 18-7), their appetite, satiety, and associated kcal intake were apparently unaltered. In contrast to the studies of O'Hara's group, who demonstrated effective loss of body weight and fat, Sheldahl and coworkers could not confirm such results, perhaps because the temperature was not as cold and the exposure shorter lived.

**Table 18-6.** Mechanisms Activated by Moderate Body Cooling in Lean and Obese Subjects

| Mechanism | Lean | Obese |
|---|---|---|
| Physiological | | |
| Stimulation of cutaneous thermal receptors | Yes | Yes |
| Cutaneous vasoconstriction | Yes | Yes |
| Increased secretion of epinephrine and norepinephrine | More | Less |
| TSH secretion | More | Less |
| Semiconscious increase in motor activity | More | Less |
| Shivering | More | Less |
| Piloerection | Yes | Yes |
| Behavioral | | |
| Body curling and extremity protection | More | Less |
| Add clothing | More | Less |
| Seek warmer environment | Frequently | Less so |

**Table 18-7.** Mean Daily Heat Debt ($Q_b$), Metabolic Heat Production (M) and Cumulative Caloric Turnover ($Q_b + M$) Incurred by Obese Women ($N = 7$) during 90 Min of Exercise in Cool Water*

| Statistic | $Q_b$ (kcal) | M (kcal) | $Q_b + M$ (kcal) |
|---|---|---|---|
| $\overline{X}$ | 186 | 380 | 566 |
| SEM[†] | ±10 | ±3 | ±13 |
| Range | 135–215 | 305–470 | 496–620 |

* Underwater cycle ergometer in $17°$–$22°C$ water.
† SEM, standard error of the mean.

(Adapted from Sheldahl LM, Buskirk ER, Loomis ER, et al. Effects of exercise in cool water on body weight loss. Int J Obesity 1982; 6:29–42.)

Subsequent to the work on men by O'Hara's group,[61] Murray and coworkers[64] performed a cold exposure experiment on somewhat obese women in a $-20°C$ environment. The women exercised 200 minutes per day at about 30% of their aerobic power for 5 days during the winter months. The women lost about 0.5 kg of fat, a relatively inconsequential change compared to the losses of men and of the women themselves when they exercised in a warmer environment. The investigators gave several possible reasons why exercising in the cold did not produce greater loss of body fat in the women: (1) lower exercise intensity (the most plausible explanation), (2) greater stability of fat stores, (3) avoidance of caffeine (a stimulator of lipolysis), and (4) translocation of fat to deep fat depots.

The perception of thermal "pleasantness" among obese women has been explored. Obese women rated lower deep body and skin temperatures more comfortable than did leaner women. The conclusion was drawn that the setpoint for body temperature perception is lower in obese than in lean women.[65]

### Altered Metabolism

Obese persons have a higher blood concentration of insulin and a decreased rate of hepatic insulin extraction.[66–68] Glucose uptake and utilization by skeletal muscle may also be decreased, but by increasing insulin secretion from the pancreas, a more normal blood sugar level is maintained. The primary increase in pancreatic insulin secretion presumably is mediated by the pancreatic nerves, but excessive carbohydrate intake may also provoke increased insulin secretion. Belfiore and coworkers[69] have suggested that insulin resistance in obesity is due to the failure of key enzyme depression of catabolic pathways.

Patients who are hypertensive as well as obese have higher fasting or glucose-stimulated circulating insulin concentrations than those who are normotensive, even though the nonobese hypertensive patients may also have insulin resistance.[70] This observation reveals the possibility of an important relationship between blood pressure and insulin that does not involve obesity. Diet-induced loss of weight and fat in obese persons restores insulin sensitivity before blood pressure becomes more normal. In obese patients with hypertension, diet and exercise decrease insulin concentrations and increase insulin sensitivity while they lower blood pressure.[68] Thus, regular exercise can be regarded as a useful adjunctive therapeutic measure for obese persons, including those who have diabetes or hypertension. Some common metabolic alterations associated with obesity are listed in Table 18-8; for each, exercise produces a counter effect.

It has been postulated that a gain in body fat (body energy stores) is strongly influenced by overall sympathetic tone, the defect in obesity being associated with a deficiency of circulating norepinephrine (NE) rather than failure to respond to the neurotransmitter.[71] Abnormal hypothalamic neural output is at least partially responsible for any diminished sympathetically released NE in obese persons. Obese subjects may have an inadequate ability to elevate sympathetic tone in the presence of food, which suggests the use of ephe-

**Table 18-8.** Common Metabolic Alterations with Obesity*

Greater insulin secretion
Insulin resistance
   Skeletal muscle
   Adipocytes after hypertrophy
Hyperlipidemia
Growth hormone insensitivity to hypoglycemia

* In each instance regular exercise has a counter effect.

**Table 18-9.** Changes in Metabolism with Sympathomimetics

I. Percentage Increase in Resting Metabolic Rate (RMR) Over 150 minutes in Response to Sympathomimetics and/or a 300-kcal (1.25MJ) Meal in Eight Lean and Eight Postobese Subjects

| Treatments | Lean (%) | Postobese (%) |
|---|---|---|
| Ephedrine | $4.82 \pm 0.97$ | $5.68 \pm 0.87$ |
| Ephedrine/methylxanthines | $10.4 \pm 1.4$ | $10.9 \pm 1.2$ |
| Meal | $15.2 \pm 1.5$ | $5.65 \pm 0.67*$ |
| Meal + both drugs | $22.6 \pm 2.5$ | $16.7 \pm 1.2*$ |

II. Percentage Change in Daily Energy Intake and Expenditure During Treatment with Sympathomimetics

| Group | Intake (%) | E Expend. (%) | Balance (%) |
|---|---|---|---|
| Lean | $0 \pm 2.6$ | $+0.5 \pm 0.6$ | $-0.7 \pm 2.5$ |
| Formerly Obese | $-16.2 \pm 4.0*$ | $+8.1 \pm 2.6*$ | $-24.3 \pm 2.4*$ |

Values: Mean ± standard error (* significant difference between treatments $P<0.02$).

Drug doses: Ephedrine 22 mg; methylxanthines, 30 mg caffeine, and 50 mg theophylline.

Adapted from Dulloo AG, Miller DS: Obesity: A disorder of the sympathetic nervous system. Wld Rev Nutr Diet 1987; 50:1–56.)

drine-methylxanthine mixtures as a metabolic stimulant: the former increases the NE content of sympathetic nerve terminals and the latter inhibits the breakdown of cyclic adenosine monophosphate (AMP) in the tissues and antagonizes the inhibitory effects of adenosine on NE secretion. In obese persons, this drug mixture normalizes the thermogenic response to a meal and increases fasting metabolic rate and 24-hour energy expenditure (Table 18-9).

### Thermogenesis

Thermogenesis, the production of heat by the body, can be induced by a single nutrient (cholesterol, protein, fat) a meal, a meal pattern, exercise, or drugs. The thermic effect of food in obese subjects was found reduced in some,[72,73] but not all,[74,75] studies. Danforth[76] concluded that the decreased heat production is inversely related to the extent of insulin resistance and can partially be restored by weight loss; the thermogenic defect in obesity may be the consequence of a slower carbohydrate storage rate and greater inhibition of gluconeogenesis. It is well known that overfeeding increases the resting metabolic rate (RMR) and underfeeding decreases it in both lean and obese subjects. The respective changes are not exclusively related to changes in fat-free body mass or the metabolically active tissue mass. Generally, lean people have lower RMRs than obese ones,[77] and after weight loss the RMR of obese individuals is reduced.[78,79]

Exercise increases heat production and energy expenditure, though, for most people who are not dedicated athletes, this rarely means more than a 50% increase in RMR over 24 hours. The elevation in energy expenditure with regular exercise is a desirable adjunct to any weight loss regimen, but it is distinctly secondary to restriction of calorie intake. For most people, regulation of food intake appears to be closely related to energy expenditure,[80] except with rather continuous exhausting exercise, when appetite cannot keep up with energy expenditure and body weight is lost.[53] In obese persons the ability to deliver oxygen to working muscle and the rate of its utilization by these muscles (aerobic power, $VO_2max$) may be reduced, depending on age, sex, and history. Thus, their relative fitness to perform hard work is reduced, causing them to limit activity to relatively low exercise intensity and for shorter periods.

It is difficult for obese people to develop the exercise habit, and even if they join a supervised exercise program they generally do not continue to exercise when they leave the program (Table 18-10).[53,81,82] Several reasons for lessening activity were cited, but available time, poor motivation and loss of social support predominated. A list of beneficial effects is presented in Table 18-11; the most important one is increased energy expenditure.

Drugs can stimulate thermogenesis. The sympathomimetic amines have already been mentioned. A special issue of the *International Journal of Obesity* (supplement 3 to volume 11, 1987) was devoted to the topic, and in it Munro provides an overview of drug treatment for obesity.[83]

Several categories of drugs have been evaluated experimentally: those that facilitate appetite reduc-

**Table 18-10.** Obese Subjects' Reasons for Decreased Adherence to Conditioning Program Activities Following Its Termination, and Frequency of Mention*

| Stated Reason | Obese Subjects* (%) |
|---|---|
| Inability to find or make time, job demands, young children and family demands, pressure of university coursework or research, sick relative to care for, and move to new house | 61 (11) |
| Poor self-discipline or motivation, no car for transportation to an exercise program, no parking proximal to exercise facilities, no exercise facilities near home, and hiatus between program termination and availability of other supervised exercise | 44 (8) |
| Loss of social support afforded by the conditioning program group | 33 (6) |
| Another leisure exercise mode with aerobic component pursued | 17 (3) |
| Disappointment with weight loss during program | 6 (1) |

* Percentage of subjects citing reason, with number of subjects citing reason given in parentheses. Many participants cited multiple reasons and all are included.

(MacKeen PC, Franklin Ba, Nicholas WC, et al. Body composition, physical work capacity and physical activity habits at 18 month follow-up of middle-aged women participating in an exercise intervention program. Int J Obesity 1983; 7:61–71.)

tion, those that partially block gastrointestinal absorption, those that reduce central neurotransmission, and those that stimulate β-adrenoreceptors. Hormones have been utilized as well—thyroid-stimulating hormone (THS), triiodothyronene ($T_3$), growth hormone, and glucagon. All elevate the metabolic rate to some extent.[84]

The potential for increasing metabolism by use of thermogenic agents such as sympathomimetic amines is encouraging. Pasquali and colleagues[85] report results using ephedrine hydrochloride and etilefrine hydrochloride in different groups of obese patients. They observed about a three-point drop in BMI when these drugs were administered for 3 months. They concluded that the drugs may be especially valuable for obese patients who are chronically adapted to low-energy expenditure or who have documented thermogenic defects.

Drug therapy is recommended when necessary to satisfy a specific need for weight reduction, such

**Table 18-11.** Beneficial Effects of Regular Exercise for Obese Persons

Physiologic effects
    Increased daily energy expenditure
    Relatively decreased appetite
    Increased or preserved muscle mass
    Reduced body fatness—(aided by dietary restriction)
    Increased functional capacity
    Decreased plasma insulin concentration
    Increased tissue sensitivity to insulin, skeletal muscle
    Decreased serum triglyceride concentration
    Decreased heart rate both at rest and during submaximal exercise
    Decreased systolic blood pressure
    Increased stroke volume
    Decreased peripheral vascular resistance
    Decreased cardiac work, submaximal exercise
    Increased flexibility
    Better motor coordination

Psychological effects
    Reduced fatigue on the job, recreational activities
    Increased self-satisfaction and acceptance
    Improved self-perception, image
    Improved social interactions
    Improved self-esteem and confidence
    More balanced perspective about regular exercise

(Data from Horton,[98] Brownell and Stunkard,[99] and Buskirk.[84])

as that associated with elective surgery. In terms of long-term treatment, it is viewed as unethical to justify such treatment until there is extensive documentation of evidence of both drug efficacy and safety.

## Dietary Regimens

A compendium of dietary regimens has been prepared by Vasselli and coworkers[86] (Table 18-12). Body weight and fat loss can be achieved with dietary (calorie) restriction if energy expenditure is maintained or increased. The problem with dietary restriction, as with exercise, is adherence to the prescribed regimen. The types of diets, together with a rough description and general experience using the diet are included in Table 18-12. Care must be taken to ensure that restricted diets contain all essential nutrients. Many who have worked extensively with obese patients, even though they may initially use specific starter diets, prefer to ''wean'' to a well-balanced diet containing a variety of good foods, with limits on quantity

that are compatible with goals for weight loss or maintenance.

The calorie equivalent of stored body fat (triacylglyceride) is between 9.0 and 9.3 kcal/g. Nevertheless, body weight loss is not comprised of stored fat alone; though it consists largely of fat, it contains water and protein as well. Thus, the calorie equivalent of 6.5 to 8.0 kcal/g of weight is lost. Early during weight loss induced by diet restriction, more water is lost and the calorie equivalent might be as low as 2.5 kcal/g. These values translate to about 1200 kcal/lb of weight lost when starting a weight reduction program and increase to about 3500 kcal/lb as weight loss continues.

## Exercise Programs

To reduce body weight and fat, exercise must involve reasonably high energy expenditure.[84,87] Movement of the body mass is important. This can be accomplished by walking, hiking, stair climbing, lawn mowing, dancing, jogging, or cross-country skiing, among other activities. Table 18-13 lists the approximate calorie turnover associated with several common activities. Values with respect to individual differences in body weight are included. Weight-supported activities include bicycling (or indoor cycle ergometer riding) and particularly swimming. Significant calorie turnover can be generated if the speed of pedaling or stroking is appreciable and sustained.

For obese persons, walking is an effective way to start an exercise program. The pace and distance covered can be regularly increased until an acceptable calorie turnover is achieved. Walking a mile uses essentially as much energy as jogging or running a mile; thus distance covered is important in structuring a simple exercise regimen for an obese person. In addition, a simple lifestyle change is more likely to be continued than a more complex one. A walking regimen can mean less reliance on vehicular transportation, using stairs instead of elevators, parking at a distance from the job, walking to deliver a message rather than phoning. Walking with a companion or as part of a sightseeing or hiking group provides important social support.

Warnold and coworkers[88] structured slow and rapid walking regimens for obese patients who

**Table 18-12.** Categories of Weight Loss Diets

| Type of Diet | Description | Characteristics |
|---|---|---|
| Nutritionally balanced<br>  Unrestricted Calories<br>  Restricted Calories | Liquid homogenate | Monotonous |
|     Varied Items | Mixed low-calorie diet (800–1200 kcal) | Carefully controlled calorie intake, palatable (satisfying)? |
|     Formula | Liquid homogenate | Carefully controlled calorie intake, monotonous |
| Nutritionally unbalanced (may also be calorically restricted)<br>  Altered porportions of macronutrients | 1. High-protein, or high-carbohydrate, low-fat | Less efficient calorie utilization, reduced fat deposition, difficult to compensate for excluded foods |
| | 2. Low-carbohydrate, high-fat or high-protein | Ketosis, decreased appetite, small excretory loss of calories, difficult to compensate for excluded foods |
|   Focus on a specific food item | Grapefruit, kelp, vitamin $B_6$, etc. | Promote lipolysis, reduced efficiency of calorie utilization, monotonous |
| Calorically dilute | High-fiber, low-fat | Slowed ingestion rate (more chewing required), impaired digestion, absorption of nutrients, satiety-inducing |
| Fasting<br>  Very few-calories | Protein or protein-carbohydrate mixture, 300–600 kcal/day | Reduces body fat, spares body protein, ketosis |
|   Total fast | | Reduces body fat and protein, highly ketogenic |

(From Vasselli JR, Cleary MP, Van Itallie TB. Modern concepts of obesity. Nutr Rev 1983; 41:361–373.)

were about 40% body fat. Slow walking ranged from 25 to 42 m/min (0.93 to 1.57 mph) and rapid walking from 45 to 75 m/min (1.68 to 2.80 mph). Each patient started with a slow walk, though even the rapid rate would be regarded as slow by many lean people. We have usually used a similar approach when working with obese subjects (i.e., start with slow walking then go to faster walking and then to other activities). Table 18-14 lists the advantages of walking; Table 18-15 lists additional activities undertaken by obese subjects with whom we have worked.

Unfortunately, most obese people cannot swim well (though most float quite readily) enough to use swimming as a means of regular exercise. Nevertheless, alternative activities can be undertaken in the water—using a kickboard with or without kickfins, kicking while grasping the side of a pool, walking or jogging in waist-deep water, cycling an immersed ergometer, striding in a deeper pool while suspended in a harness or buoyed up by as flotation device. Such exercise in water avoids much weight bearing and reduces strain on joints by using the water to provide buoyancy.[63,89,90] Sheldahl and colleagues[63] showed that women can cycle an ergometer in water for 90 minutes or longer and expend upward of 400 kcal per exercise session and while maintaining "near thermal neutrality." This relatively comfortable in-water exercise for obese persons could logically be extended for longer periods, as many of them find it more tolerable than weight-bearing exercise.

## Exercise and Safety

Goodman and Kenrick[91] noted that, when obese persons participated in a walk-jog program, they

**Table 18-13.** Approximate Calorie Expenditure for 1 Hour of Physical Activity*

| Activity | | Body Weight | | | | |
|---|---|---|---|---|---|---|
| | (kg) | 56.8 | 68.2 | 79.5 | 90.9 | 113.6 |
| | (lbs) | 125 | 150 | 175 | 200 | 250 |
| Sitting, writing, or reading | | 60 | 72 | 84 | 96 | 120 |
| Domestic housework | | 204 | 246 | 282 | 318 | 408 |
| Walking (2 mph)[†] | | 174 | 210 | 240 | 276 | 348 |
| Walking (3 mph) | | 240 | 300 | 360 | 450 | 510 |
| Jogging (5.0 mph) | | 300 | 360 | 420 | 510 | 620 |
| Cycling (6.0 mph) | | 240 | 300 | 360 | 400 | 480 |
| Mowing grass (power) | | 204 | 246 | 282 | 318 | 402 |
| Mowing grass (manual) | | 228 | 270 | 312 | 348 | 444 |
| Bowling (nonstop) | | 240 | 300 | 360 | 430 | 510 |
| Dancing (moderate) | | 210 | 252 | 288 | 330 | 390 |
| Dancing (vigorous) | | 288 | 342 | 396 | 450 | 540 |
| Golf (walking) | | 198 | 240 | 288 | 330 | 408 |
| Skiing (cross-country) (5 mph) | | 312 | 426 | 480 | 530 | 640 |
| Swimming (moderate crawl) | | 240 | 288 | 336 | 378 | 480 |

* Approximate values for activities that can be undertaken by many obese persons. Values vary with rate of exercise and efficiency with which activity is performed. Interpolation and extrapolation can be used for subjects who differ in weight.
† 1 mph = 1.6093 km/hr.
(Data from Brownell and Stunkard[99] and Buskirk.[84])

had a higher incidence of injury than leaner ones. Pollock and colleagues[92] found that for men who participated in a regular exercise program the incidence of injuries was significantly related to their fatness. Franklin and associates[93] found that among 23 middle-aged obese women, seven sustained foot or leg injuries severe enough to force temporary discontinuation or modification of their activity. Most injuries occurred during the first 8 weeks of the program, despite their exercise of extreme caution in undertaking all physical activity gradually and following adequate warm-up and routine stretching. Nevertheless, in a well-orga-

nized and supervised physical activity program the injury rate is acceptably low and the injuries minor. Injury remains something to plan for, but it should not warrant undue concern.

Table 18-16 lists a variety of factors that contribute to a successful exercise program for obese persons. Personal preparation, selection of appropriate apparel and footwear, and foot care all are important. Orthotic devices that provide heel support or compensatory foot pronation may be necessary so that exercise can be undertaken more

**Table 18-14.** Advantages of Walking

Avoids musculoskeletal problems associated with running
Avoids traffic hazards of cycling
Avoids inconvenience of trying to find a swimming pool
  or special recreational facilities
Requires no extraordinary skill
Can be done almost anywhere and at any time
Can produce a training effect
Is inexpensive
Affords socializing with a companion while walking
Affords exercising a pet and sharing the pet's
  companionship

**Table 18-15.** Simple Physical Activities Recommended for Obese Subjects

Walking
Stair climbing
Walk and jog
Selected strength and flexibility exercises
Dancing, with or without partner: aerobic, simple steps to
  music
Distance swimming
Walking purposefully in waist-deep water
Cycling, perhaps on tricycle
Cycling in water
Treading in water with or without flotation device

**Table 18-16.** Factors That Could Enhance
Adherence to an Exercise Program

Select appropriate exercise:
  Emphasize movement of body mass
  Emphasize all opportunities for walking
  Emphasize that all daily activities are exercise
Provide realistic expectations, no miracles:
  Amount of exercise, intensity, and duration
  Time commitment and frequency
  Physiologic and psychological changes
Start slowly
Select convenient hours
Select pleasant surroundings
Provide individual attention
Encourage group activity, socialization
Have highly motivated group leader
Record results, use some self-monitoring
Provide positive feedback about changes in weight, fat-
  ness, exercise capacity, heart rate, blood pressure,
  serum lipids, glucose, insulin, uric acid
Utilize deposit and refund (rewards)
Emphase education: self, family members, close friends
  and companions; gain understanding of energy turnover
  brought about by diet and exercise

safely and more enjoyably. Nevertheless, exercise
can give rise to physiologic and pathologic hazards
(Table 18-17). Careful physical examination and
a complete medical history can obviate many of
these problems.

Complex behavior modifications are likely to
be necessary if a weight reduction regimen is going
to result in permanent beneficial lifestyle changes.

**Table 18-17.** Potential Hazards of Exercise for
Obese Persons

Precipitation of angina pectoris or myocardial infarction
Excessive rise in blood pressure—isometric exercise
Aggravation of degenerative arthritis and other joint
  problems
Ligamentous injuries
Injury from falling
Excessive sweating, chafing
Hypohydration and reduced circulating blood volume to
  the skin
Heat stroke or heat exhaustion
Lower extremity edema

(Data from Horton,[98] Stunkard,[97] and Buskirk.[84])

Table 18-18 lists characteristics of obese persons
who are likely to benefit from an exercise program.

In an attempt to ascertain the successful strategies employed to maintain desirable weight once
weight loss is achieved, Wing and Jeffrey[94] questioned 42 men and 22 women who were originally,
on average, 43% overweight and who had sustained a weight loss of 10 kg (22 lb) or more for
1 year (Table 18-19). These ''successful'' individuals were most concerned about appearance, but
more than half paid attention to diet and exercise.

## Other Considerations

Adipose tissue is a special tissue for energy storage, and it is peculiar because specific progenitor
cell types have not been clearly described. In addition, adipocytes contain receptors that are responsive to neurogenic and hormonal stimulation.
These two aspects of adipose tissue are described
briefly in the following sections.

### Adipocyte Differentiation

That precursor and preadipocyte cells differentiate
is known, but the factors that regulate adipocyte
differentiation are not known. It has been suggested that the condensation of mesenchymal cells
around blood vessels is responsible for development of primitive fat organs. Adipocytes are observed following tissue vascularization. Thus, the
interaction of precursor cells and preadipocytes

**Table 18-18.** Characteristics of Obese Persons
Who Are Most Likely to Benefit from an
Exercise Program

Slightly or moderately obese
Became obese as an adult
Had not previously tried to lose weight
Sincerely desires weight reduction
Psychologically adjusted to pursuit of weight reduction
  goal
Can intelligently follow directions
Has no complicating disease or disability
Is willing to make the commitment
Can find the time and the facilities

**Table 18-19.** Most Popular Strategies of Formerly Obese Persons for Maintaining Weight Loss

| Strategy | Percent Using Strategy |
|---|---|
| Frequent weighing | 75 |
| Reduced snacking | 60 |
| Reduced meal portions | 60 |
| Better food selection | 57 |
| Increased exercise | 55 |

(Data from Wing and Jeffery[94] and Buskirk.[84])

with capillary endothelial cells may be important as are constituents in blood such as growth hormone responsible for adipocyte development. In addition, adipogenic serum activity may also play a role in differentiation; such activity has been demonstrated in serum from last-trimester pregnant women and from umbilical cord blood.[100] The effects of such serum are ascertained by the responsiveness of cell cultures.

### Receptors and Lipolytic Responsiveness

Adipose tissue is innervated by the sympathetic nervous system. The concentration of norepinephrine in adipose tissue is on the order of 40 ng per gram of tissue. Both $\beta$-adrenoreceptors and $\beta$-receptors are present. Although the $\beta_1$-receptor has been thought to be associated with lipolytic activity, there is the possibility that a new $\beta$-adrenoreceptors subtype is responsible. The $\alpha_2$-receptors demonstrate antilipolytic action. In addition to stimulating lipolysis through sympathetic activation of adipocytes, lipolysis may also be stimulated by catecholamines released from the adrenals. Denervation of adipose tissue leads to increased lipid mass; whereas, electrical stimulation leads to fatty acid release. Blocking of sympathetic activity inhibits lipid mobilization.[101]

Regional differences have been observed in adipose tissue lipolysis: lipolytic activity is greater in omental than in subcutaneous tissue. Lesser insulin action and $\alpha_2$-adrenoreceptors antilipolytic activity is thought to be responsible. Catecholamines appear less lipolytic in gluteal and femoral subcutaneous adipose tissue than in similar abdominal

tissue. Perhaps there is enhanced $\alpha_2$-adrenoreceptor responsiveness in the gluteal and femoral tissue. Site variation in receptor distribution, as well as the signals from the receptors, may play a role in regulation. Development of regional forms of obesity such as the protruding abdominal (android) type or the gluteal-femoral (gynecoid) type may depend on regional receptor and signal variations. The android type is predominant in men and the gynecoid in women. The android type has been associated with elevated free fatty acids in the portal system and impaired glucose metabolism by the liver.[13,102]

Sex hormones may also be important in influencing fat distribution: testosterone treatment in women increases the size of upper body adipocytes, and estrogen therapy in men increases fat cell numbers in the thighs.[103] Progesterone appears to increase femoral lipoprotein lipase (LPL) activity in women, which appears to be inhibited by testosterone. Estradiol and testosterone exhibit lipolytic action in adipoytes from the abdominal region. In addition, long-term exposure to corticosteroids might increase femoral LPL activity and decrease abdominal lipolysis.[105]

### Summary

Unfortunately, gross obesity constitutes a disabling condition that compromises physiologic function and leads to, or is associated with, considerable morbidity, particularly chronic disease. The development of cardiovascular, respiratory, and neuromotor problems leads to disability, which then promotes a sedentary lifestyle. Muscle mass is reduced and exercise tolerance becomes low. Grossly obese persons can benefit from a weight reduction program. Multiple interventions are most useful, including attention to identifiable medical problems, the patient's psyche, diet, and exercise.

### References

1. Van Itallie TB. Health implications of overweight and obesity in the United States. Ann Intern Med 1985; 103:983–988.

2. Bray GA. Obesity in America: An overview of the second Fogarty International Center Conference on Obesity. Int J Obesity 1979; 3:363–375.

3. Thomas AE, McKay DA, Cutlip MB. A nomograph method for assessing body weight. Am J Clin Nutr 1976; 29:302–304.

4. Seltzer CC, Mayer J. A simple criterion of obesity. Postgrad Med 1965; 38:A101–A107.

5. Durnin JVGA, Womersley J. Body fat assessed from total body density and its estimation from skinfold thickness measurements on 481 men and women aged 16 to 72 years. Br J Nutr 1974; 32:77–97.

6. Buskirk ER. Obesity: A brief overview with emphasis on exercise. Fed Proc 1974; 33:1948–1951.

7. Fitzgerald FT. The problem of obesity. Annu Rev Med 1981; 32:221–231.

8. Keys A. Overweight, obesity, coronary heart disease and mortality. Nutr Rev 1980; 38:297–307.

9. Bray GA, ed. Comparative Methods of Weight Control. Westport, Conn: Technomic, 1980.

10. Hirsch J, Batchelor B. Adipose tissue cellularity and human obesity. Clin Endocrinol Metab 1976; 5:299–311.

11. Bjorntorp P. The fat cell: A clinical view. In: Bray GA, ed. Recent Advances in Obesity Research II. London: Newman, 1978.

12. Bjorntorp P. Regional patterns of fat distribution. Ann Intern Med 1985; 103:994–995.

13. Buskirk ER, Puhl S. Adipose tissue distribution and metabolic consequences. In: Levander OA, ed. AIN Symposium Proceedings Nutrition 87 Washington, DC: The American Institute of Nutrition, 1987;97–102.

14. Alexander JK. Obesity and the circulation. Mod Concepts Cardiovasc Dis 1963; 32:799–803.

15. Amad KH, Brennan JC, Alexander JK. The cardiac pathology of chronic exogenous obesity. Circulation 1965; 32:740–749.

16. Prodger SH, Dennig H. A study of the circulation in obesity. J Clin Invest 1932; 11:789–806.

17. Robinson SC, Brucer M. Hypertension, body build and obesity. Am J Med Sci 1940; 199:819–829.

18. Terry AH. Obesity and hypertension. JAMA 1923; 81:1283–1284.

19. Keys A, Aravanis C, Blackburn H, et al. Coronary heart disease: Overweight and obesity as risk factors. Ann Intern Med 1972; 77:15–27.

20. Paul O. A longitudinal study of coronary heart disease. Circulation 1963; 28:20–31.

21. Bloom E, Reed D, Katsuhiko Y, et al. Does obesity protect hypertensives against cardiovascular disease? JAMA 1986; 256:2972–2975.

22. Messerli FH, Christie B, DeCarvalho JGR, et al. Obesity and essential hypertension, hemodynamics, intravascular volume, sodium excretion and plasma renin activity. Arch Intern Med 1981; 141:81–85.

23. Messerli FH, Sundgaard-Rise K. Resin E. et al. Disparate cardiovascular effects of obesity and arterial hypertension. Am J Med 1983; 74:802–812.

24. Raison J, Achmastos A, Asmar R, et al. Extracellular and interstitial fluid volume in obesity with and without associated systemic hypertension. Am J Cardiol 1986; 57:223–226.

25. Messerli FH. Cardiovascular effects of obesity and hypertension. Lancet 1982; 1:1165–1168.

26. Alpert MA, Terry BA, Kelly DL. Effect of weight loss on cardiac chamber size, wall thickness and left ventricular function in morbid obesity. Am J Cardiol 1985; 55:783–786.

27. Rubal BJ, Elmesallamy FH. Cardiac adaptations in a group of obese women. J Obesity Weight Reg 1984; 3:236–247.

28. Luce JN. Respiratory complications of obesity. Chest 1980; 78:626–631.

29. Barakat HA, Burton DS, Carpenter JW, et al. Body fat distribution, plasma lipoproteins and the risk of coronary heart disease of male subjects. Int J Obesity 1987; 12:473–480.

30. Garn SM, Bailey SM, Block WD. Relationshps between fatness and lipid level in adults. Am J Clin Nutr 1979; 32:733–735.

31. Kannel WB, Gordon T, Castelli WP. Obesity, lipids and glucose intolerance. The Framingham Study. Am J Clin Nutr 1979; 32:1238–1245.

32. Miettinen TA. Cholesterol production in obesity. Circulation 1971; 44:842–850.

33. Anderson JT, Lawler A, Keys A. Weight Gain from simple overeating. II. Serum lipids and blood volume. J Clin Invest 1957; 36:81–88.

34. Larson B, Svardsudd K, Wein L, et al. Abdominal adipose tissue distribution, obesity and risk of cardiovascular disease and death: 13-year follow-up of participants in the study of men born in 1913. Br Med J 1984; 288:1401–1404.

35. Fujioka S, Matsuzawa Y, Tokunaga K, et al. Contribution of intraabdominal fat accumulation to the impairment of glucose and lipid metabolism in human obesity. Metabolism 1987; 36:54–59.

36. Frericks RR, Webber LS, Srinivasan SR, et al. Relation of serum lipids and lipoproteins to obesity and sexual maturity in white and black children. Am J Epidemiol 1978; 108:486–496.

37. Freedman DS, Burke GL, Harska DW, et al. Relationship of changes in obesity to serum lipid and

lipoprotein changes in childhood and adolescence. JAMA 1985; 254:515–520.

38. Berenson GS, McMahan CA, Voors AW, et al. Occurrence of multiple risk-factor variables for cardiovascular disease in children. In: Berenson, GS, McMahan CA (eds.) Cardiovascular Risk Factors in Children. New York: Oxford University Press, 1980; 311–320.

39. Alexander JK. The heart and obesity. In: Hurst JW, ed. The Heart, Arteries and Veins, ed. 5. New York: McGraw Hill, 1982; 1584–1590.

40. Rosell S, Belfrage E. Blood circulation in adipose tissue. Physiol Rev 1979; 59:1078.

41. Alexander JK, Peterson KL. Cardiovascular effects of weight reduction. Circulation 1972; 45:310–318.

42. Bedell GN, Wilson WR, Seebohm PM. Pulmonary function in obese persons. J Clin Invest 1958; 37:1049–1060.

43. Buskirk ER, Bartlett HL. Pulmonary function and obesity. In: Tobin RB, Mehlman MA, eds. Advances in Modern Human Nutrition, vol I. Park Forest South, Ill: Pathotox, 1980;211–224.

44. Bartlett HL, Buskirk ER. Body composition and the expiratory reserve volume in lean and obese men and women. Int J Obesity 1983; 7:339–343.

45. Ray CS, Sae DY, Bray G, et al. Effects of obesity on respiratory function. Am Rev Respir Dis 1983; 128:501–506.

46. Cherniak RM, Guenter CA. The efficiency of the respiratory muscles in obesity. Can J Biochem Physiol 1961; 39:1215–1222.

47. Burwell CS, Robin ED, Whaley RD, et al. Extreme obesity associated with alveolar hypoventilation—a pickwickian syndrome. Am J Med 1956; 21:811–818.

48. Said SI. Abnormalities of pulmonary gas exchange in obesity. Ann Intern Med 1960; 53:1121–1124.

49. Rochester DF, Enson Y. Current concepts in the pathogenesis of the obesity-hypoventilation syndrome: Mechanical and Circulatory factors. Am J Med 1974; 57:402–420.

50. Fried PI, McClean PA, Phillipson EA, et al. Effect of ketosis on respiratory sensitivity to carbon dioxide in obesity. N Engl J Med 1976; 294:1081–1086.

51. White DP, Lombard RM, Cadieux RJ, et al. Pharyngeal resistance in normal humans: Influence of gender, age and obesity. J Appl Physiol 1985; 58:365–371.

52. Bar-Or O, Lundegren HM, Magnusson LI, et al. Distribution of heat activated sweat glands in obese and lean men and women. Hum Biol 1968; 40:235–248.

53. Buskirk ER, Bar-Or O, Kollias J. Physiological effects of heat and cold. In: Wilson N, ed. Obesity. Philadelphia: FA Davis, 1969;119–139.

54. Vroman NB, Buskirk ER, Hodgson JL. Cardiac output and skin blood flow in lean and obese individuals during exercise in the heat. J Appl Physiol 1983; 55:69–74.

55. Bar-Or O, Lundegren HM, Buskirk ER. Heat tolerance of exercising obese and lean women. J Appl Physiol 1969; 26:403–409.

56. Schvartz E, Saar E, Benar D. Physique and heat tolerance in hot-dry and hot-humid environments. J Appl Physiol 1973; 34:799–803.

57. Wyndham CH. The physiology of exercise under heat stress. Annu Rev Physiol 1973; 35:193–220.

58. Epstein Y, Shapiro Y, Brill S. Role of surface area-to-mass ratio and work efficiency in heat intolerance. J Appl Physiol 1983; 54:831–836.

59. Buskirk ER, Kollias J. Total body metabolism in the cold. Bull NJ Acad Sci 1969; March:17–25.

60. Buskirk ER. Cold stress: A selective review. In: Folinsbee LJ, et al., eds. Environmental Stress. New York: Academic Press, 1978;249–266.

61. O'Hara WJ, Allen C, Shephard RJ. Treatment of obesity by exercise in the cold. Can Med Assn J 1977; 8:773–785.

62. O'Hara WJ, Allen C, Shephard RJ. Loss of body weight and fat during exercise in a cold chamber. Eur J Appl Physiol 1977; 37:205–218.

63. Sheldahl LM, Buskirk ER, Loomis JL, et al. Effects of exercise in cool water on body weight loss. Int J Obesity 1982; 6:29–42.

64. Murray SJ, Shephard RJ, Greaves S, et al. Effects of cold stress and exercise on fat loss in females. Eur J Appl Physiol 1986; 55:610–618.

65. Zaborska-Markiewicz B, Staszkiewicz M. Body temperature set-point and the conscious perception of skin temperature in obese women. Eur J Appl Physiol 1987; 56:479–481.

66. Peiris AN, Mueller RA, Smith GA, et al. Splanchnic insulin metabolism in obesity: Influence of body fat distribution. J Clin Invest 1986; 78:1648–1657.

67. Grey N, Kipnis DM. Effect of diet composition on the hyperinsulinemia of obesity. N Engl J Med 1971; 285:827–831.

68. Landsberg L. Insulin and hypertension: Lessons from obesity. N Engl J Med 1987; 317:378–379.

69. Belfiori F, Ianello S, Rabuazzo AM. Insulin resistance in obesity: A critical analysis at enzyme level. Int J Obesity 1979; 3:301–323.

70. Ferrannini E, Buzzigola G, Bonadonna R, et al. Insulin resistance in essential hypertension. N Engl J Med 1987; 317:350–357.

71. Dulloo AG, Miller DS. Obesity: A disorder of the sympathetic nervous system. Wld Rev Nutr Diet 1987; 50:1–56.

72. Pitlet PL, Chappius PL, Aecheson K, et al. Thermic effect of glucose in obese subjects studied by direct and indirect calorimetry. Br J Nutr 1976; 35:282–292.

73. Swaminathan R, King RFGJ, Holmfield J, et al. Thermic effect of feeding carbohydrate, fat, protein and mixed meal in lean and obese subjects. Am J Clin Nutr 1985; 42:177–181.

74. Felig P, Cunningham I, Levitt M, et al. Energy expenditure in obesity in fasting and postprandial state. Am J Physiol 1983; 244:E45–E51.

75. Segal KR, Gutin B. Thermic effects of food and exercise in lean and obese women. Metabolism 1983; 32:581–589.

76. Danforth E. Diet and obesity. Am J Clin Nutr 1985; 42:1132–1145.

77. James WPT. Elevated metabolic rates in obesity. Lancet 1978; 1:1122–1125.

78. Welle SL, Armatruda JM, Forbes GB, et al. Resting metabolic rate of obese women after rapid weight loss. J Clin Endocrinol Metab 1984; 59:41–74.

79. den Besten C, Vansant G, Westrate JA, et al. Resting metabolic rate and diet-induced thermogenesis in abdominal and gluteal-femoral obese women before and after weight reduction. Am J Clin Nutr 1988; 47:840–847.

80. Mayer J, Roy P, Mitra KP. Relation between caloric intake, body weight and physical work: Studies in an industrial male population in West Bengal. Am J Clin Nutr 1956; 4:169–175.

81. Franklin BA, MacKeen PC, Buskirk ER. Body composition effects of a 12-week physical conditioning program for normal and obese middle-aged women, and status at 18-month follow-up. Int J Obesity 1978; 2:394.

82. MacKeen PC, Franklin BA, Nicholas WC, et al. Body composition, physical work capacity and physical activity habits at 18-month follow-up of middle-aged women participating in an exercise intervention program. Int J Obesity 1983; 7:61–71.

83. Munro JF. Drug Treatment of obesity: An overview. Int J Obesity 1987; (suppl 3):13–15.

84. Buskirk ER. Obesity. In: Skinner JS, ed. Exercise Testing and Exercise Prescription for Special Cases. Philadelphia: Lea & Febiger, 1987;149–173.

85. Pasquali R, Cesari MP, Besteghi L, et al. Thermogenic agents in the treatment of human obesity: Preliminary results. Int J Obesity 1987; 11(suppl 3):23–26.

86. Vasselli JR, Cleary MP, Van Itallie TB. Modern concepts of obesity. Nutr Rev 1983; 41:361–373.

87. Oscai LB. The role of exercise in weight control. In: Wilmore J, ed. Exercise and Sports Sciences Review, Vol. I. New York: Academic Press, 1973;103–123.

88. Warnold I, Carlgren G, Krotkiewski M. Energy expenditure and body composition during weight reduction in hyperplastic obese women. Am J Clin Nutr 1978; 31:750–763.

89. Castronic M. Jog in the pool—no pain. J Phys Ed 1976; 74:8–18.

90. Evans BW, Cureton KJ, Purvis JW. Metabolic and circulatory responses to walking and jogging in water. Res Q 1867; 49:442–449.

91. Goodman CE, Kenrick MM. Physical fitness in relation to obesity. Obesity Bariatr Med 1975; 4:12–15.

92. Pollock ML, Gettman LR, Milesis CA, et al. Effects of frequency and duration of training on attrition and incidence of injury. Med Sci Sports 1977; 9:31–36.

93. Franklin B, Buskirk ER, Hodgson J, et al. Effects of physical conditioning on cardiorespiratory function, body composition and serum lipids in relatively normal-weight and obese middle-aged women. Int J Obesity 1979; 3:97–109.

94. Wing RR, Jeffrey RW. Successful losers: A descriptive analysis of the process of weight reduction. Obesity Bariatr Med 1978; 7:190–191.

95. Mann GV, Obesity, the nutritional spook. Am J Publ Health 1971; 61:1491–1498.

96. Garrow JS. Energy Balance and Obesity in Man, ed. 2. New York: Elsevier, 1978; 243.

97. Stunkard AJ, ed. Obesity. Philadelphia: WB Saunders, 1980.

98. Horton ES. The role of exercise in the prevention and treatment of obesity. In: Obesity in Perspective, vol 2, part 1. DHEW Publ No (NIH)75,708. Washington, DC: U.S. Government Printing Office, 1975;62–66.

99. Brownell KD, Stunkard AJ. Physical activity in the development and control of obesity. In: Stunkard AJ, ed. Obesity. Philadelphia: WB Saunders, 1980;300–324.

100. Kuri-Harcuch W, Carrera-DeLaTorre B, Arkuch-Kuri S, et al. Human adipogenic serum activity increases during pregnancy. Int J Obesity 1985; 9:299–306.

101. Trayhurn P, Ashwell P. Control of white and brown adipose tissues by the autonomic nervous system. Proc Nutr Soc 1987; 46:135–142.

102. Arner P. Role of antilipolytic mechanisms in adipose tissue distribituion and function in man. Acta Med Scand Suppl 1988; 723:144–152.

103. Kissebah AH, Peiris AN, Evans DJ. Mechanisms associating body fat distribution to glucose intolerance and diabetes mellitus: Window with a view. Acta Med Scand Suppl 1988; 723:78–89.

104. Bouchard C. Genetic factors in the regulation of adipose tissue distribution. Acta Med Scand Suppl 1988; 723:135–141.

105. Rebuffe-Scrive M. Steroid hormones and distribution of adipose tissue. Acta Med Scand Suppl 1988; 723:121–134.

# Chapter 19
# Urogenital Physiology

STEVEN A. KAPLAN
JERRY G. BLAIVAS
ANN BREUER

Two of the most important goals in the rehabilitation of patients with neurologic lesions are restoration of voiding and of sexual function. In this chapter the micturition cycle is divided into its two major phases, storage (filling) and emptying (voiding), and relevant lower urinary tract anatomy and neurophysiology are discussed. The lower urinary tract is very well-suited for its primary function, the storage and timely expulsion of urine.[1] The storage function of the bladder is performed largely by its ability to increase volume, up to a point, with little or no change in intravesical pressure. The sphincteric action of both the vesical neck and the proximal urethra maintain continence despite the wide range of intravesical pressures that occurs during ordinary physical activity. Micturition is a complex series of finely tuned and integrated neuromuscular events that involve many neurologic pathways. Final integration of these events occurs in the rostral pons in an area known as the pontine micturition center.[2] As an important relationship exists between the lower urinary tract and sexual function, pertinent male and female anatomy, and the physiology of both erection and female response, are reviewed. Erectile physiology in males and the engorgement of the external genitalia and vaginal lubrication in females involve a complex series of neurologically mediated vascular phenomena within a hormonal milieu. Supraspinal psychological and neurologic factors play an important role in modifying these essentially reflex phenomena. It should be emphasized that much of the experimental work to date has been done in animals, so exact extrapolation to the human model is not possible. In particular, the "human psyche" is difficult to evaluate, qualitatively or quantitatively. This chapter therefore presents the basic mechanisms underlying the physiology of both micturition and sexual function.

## Genitourinary Anatomy

Though no anatomic distinction exists, the lower urinary tract can be thought of as being composed of a bladder and a sphincter. Grossly, the muscle fibers and mucosa of the bladder blend imperceptibly with those of the vesical neck and urethra, and no real "anatomic" sphincter exists that can be seen with the naked eye. Rather, the sphincter is a unique arrangement of smooth and striated muscle interlaced with fibrous and elastic connective tissue that constitutes the "physiologic" sphincter. Of note, the mucosal lining of the urethra is characterized by *inner wall softness,* which keeps the walls coapted and forms a watertight seal.[3]

The bladder is composed of two main components, the body and the base (trigone).[4] The detrusor is composed of interlacing bundles of smooth muscle arranged in a loose network. Individual muscle bundles cross one another; they follow no consistent pattern, but the outer and inner layers tend to be oriented longitudinally, particularly as they approach the vesical neck.[4,5] In addition, a series of detrusor fibers, termed the *fundal ring* originates posteriorly and loops around the trigone and vesical neck.[6] Posteriorly, these fibers are separated from the internal orifice by the trigone: anteriorly, they are in close approximation to the internal urethral orifice. The trigone is a triangular area demarcated superiorly and laterally by the ureteral orifices and inferiorly by the internal urethral orifice. As the ureteral musculature approaches the bladder, it loses its spiral configuration and assumes a longitudinal one. The ureterovesical junction is marked by a condensation of tissue called Waldeyer's sheath, which serves to anchor the ureter to the bladder wall. The intramural ureter traverses the bladder obliquely through a tunnel of approximately 2 cm in length. At the ureteral orifice, the ureteral musculature begins to fan out and meets the musculature from the other side to form the superficial trigone. The superficial trigone muscle continues through the urethra and extends to the verumontanum in males and to the distal third of the urethra in females. Because of the relative thinness of the superficial trigone as compared to the detrusor musculature, it is thought that its only function is to anchor the ureteral orifices so that they are pulled distally and inferiorly during voiding. This movement of the ureter, when coupled with the compression of the ureteral lumen as it courses obliquely through the detrusor, prevents vesicoureteral reflux.[5,7,8]

The musculature of the urethra consists of circularly and longitudinally oriented fibers of both striated and smooth muscle, but the proportion and functional significance of each remains a subject of controversy. Important differences exist between male and female anatomy. It is widely agreed that in both sexes there are longitudinal or helical bundles of smooth muscle that extend from the base of the bladder into the prostatic urethra in the male and almost throughout the entire urethra in the female. In the male there is a rather well-defined, circularly oriented smooth muscle group just below the bladder neck.[7,9] Some researchers believe that this proximal urethral circular smooth muscle is identical to the prostatic

capsule and that this structure is the primary involuntary internal sphincter. Dixon and Gosling, however, deny that this is a urinary sphincter; they believe that it is a "genital" sphincter that serves as a barrier to retrograde ejaculation during sexual intercourse.[5]

The intraurethral rhabdosphincter and periurethral musculature of the pelvic diaphragm comprise the striated voluntary muscle component of the urethra. The intraurethral portion surrounds the middle third of the female urethra and is composed mostly of slow-twitch muscle fibers.[5] The muscle is even more prominent in the male and extends to the vesical neck.[10,11] Some investigators believe this rhabdosphincter constitutes the primary urethral sphincter in both sexes.

In summary, the presence of both circular and longitudinal fibers in both the vesical neck and urethra provide the anatomic substrate for understanding the mechanisms of micturition and urinary continence. Thus, contraction of longitudinal fibers serves to shorten and widen the urethra during voiding, thus opening the urethra for unimpeded flow. Contraction of circular fibers aids in the maintenance of continence; relaxation opens the urethra for micturition.

## Genitourinary Neurophysiology

### Afferent Pathways

Afferent fibers are projections of dorsal spinal root ganglia axons, and in some species there is evidence that some of the afferent fibers are located in the ventral root as well.[12] Afferent fibers establish many synapses after leaving the posterior root ganglion. Some of these synapses include (1) the pelvic nucleus in the anteromedial area, (2) the dorsal horn, which ascends ipsilaterally, and (3) the dorsal horn, which crosses the midline and ascends the contralateral spinothalamic tract. The afferent fibers of the pelvic nerve are thought to initiate voiding, impulses arising from tension receptors in the bladder wall and being transmitted via small diameter A gamma and C fibers.[13] Most bladder afferents contain substance P, vasoactive intestinal polypeptide (VIP), and other neuropeptides.

## Parasympathetic Nerves

The primary parasympathetic nerve involved in micturition is the pelvic nerve. Its primary neurotransmitter is acetylcholine at both the pre- and postganglionic synapse, but recent reports suggest the presence of noncholinergic, nonadrenergic receptors at the postganglionic synapse.[14] The pelvic nerve nucleus is located in the anteromedial cell column of the second, third, and fourth segments of the sacral spinal cord.[15,16]

Detrusor contractions can be caused either by administration of acetylcholine or electrical stimulation of the pelvic nerve.[15,17–20]; however, the bladder contraction induced by electrical stimulation cannot be completely blocked by atropine, unlike the detrusor contraction elicited by administration of acetylcholine.[21,22] Recent evidence suggests that this *atropine resistance effect,* recognized for many years, may be related to a noncholinergic, nonadrenergic neurotransmitter. The effect of acetylcholine and pelvic nerve stimulation on the muscles of the urethra is even less well-understood. Researchers variously reported increased urethral resistance, decreased urethral resistance, or no change.[18,23–26]

The ventral roots of the second through the fourth sacral segments house the efferent parasympathetic fibers. These fibers merge to form the pelvic nerve (nervi erigentes), but the anatomy of this nerve varies considerably from species to species.[20,27] The pelvic nerve plexus is formed by fibers of both the pelvic nerve and the hypogastric nerve. Although it never forms an identifiable nerve trunk, the pelvic nerve plexus does send ''twigs'' of fibers to both bladder and urethra, and then the majority of efferent fibers resynapse in the pelvic ganglia in or near the walls of the bladder and urethra. Elbadawi called these peripheral ganglia *the urogenital short neuron system.*[28] This system connects extensively with sympathetic fibers, which are similarly situated throughout the bladder and urethral wall.

The ganglia of the short neuron system are composed predominantly of three types of cells, adrenergic, cholinergic, and small intensely fluorescent (SIF) neurons.[29,30] The importance of the short neuron system is that it ensures that neurologic lesions do not completely denervate the bladder and urethra. For example, extensive radical surgery, such as abdominoperineal resection of the rectum, does not ablate the short neuronal system. Thus, central or preganglionic neurologic lesions result in decentralization rather than denervation.

## Sympathetic Nerves

The importance of the sympathetic nervous system in voiding is controversial, but recent studies in cats provide new information that may be clinically applicable.[31–34] The cell bodies of the sympathetic nerves lie in the intermedial lateral cell column of T-10 to L-2. After traversing the ventral roots, efferent sympathetic fibers form synapses in the prevertebral ganglia of the lumbar sympathetic chain. At this point, they branch out to form the presacral plexus, which then bifurcates to form the right and left hypogastric nerves. The hypogastric nerve meets the pelvic nerve to form the pelvic plexus. The sympathetic ganglia located in the pelvic plexus and the urethral and bladder wall are part of the urogenital short neuron system. Modulation of reflex activity affecting micturition is an important function of the intramural neuronal network. $\alpha$-Adrenoreceptors of the sympathetic system mediate storage of urine in two ways. The first action is via closure of both the proximal urethra and the bladder neck; the second action is via inhibition of neuronal transmission between the pre- and postganglionic parasympathetic nerve.[34] $\beta$-Adrenoreceptors mediate relaxation of the body of the bladder.[35–39] The sympathetic nervous system has little role in sensory function; in fact, in humans presacral neurectomy has no effect on either afferent urethral or bladder function.[40]

## Somatic Nerves

The striated muscles of the pelvic floor, as well as the rhabdosphincter, are innervated primarily by the pudendal nerve. Histochemical studies employing horseradish peroxidase have demonstrated that the pudendal nerve cell bodies originate in Onufrowicz's (Onuf's) nucleus in the anterior horn of the second through the fourth segments of the sacral spinal cord.[8,41] It is of interest that the cells of Onuf's nucleus are much more resistant to degenerative processes such as amyotrophic lateral sclerosis than other anterior horn cells, though Onuf's nucleus cells are always affected in Shy-Drager syndrome. The pudendal nucleus is located at either S-2 or S-3, which is one segment above the parasympathetic nucleus.[42] Thus, certain neurologic disorders, such as myelodysplasia or multiple sclerosis, may cause disparate lesions of the bladder and striated external urethral sphincter.[43,44]

## Physiology of Voiding

### *Storage of Urine*

#### *Physical Principles*

The behavior of the normal bladder depends on both its active and passive properties. Collagen, elastin, and resting smooth muscle constitute the main tissues responsible for the passive properties of the bladder. In contrast, the active behavior of the bladder is determined by the contractile elements of smooth muscle. *Elasticity* is that property of a material that determines the tendency of the stressed material to return to its unstressed geometric configuration; *viscosity* is that property of a material that tends to retard deformation of the stressed material.[45] On the other hand, *plasticity* refers to the ability of a substance to sustain an irreversible deformation that occurs only after a certain threshold of stress is exceeded.[46] Elasticity can be measured by the change in wall tension as the bladder is stretched. Thus, in a cystometrogram, bladder pressure and volume are measured; when they are plotted against each other the relationship is not linear and thus, indicates that physical properties other than elasticity alone are involved.

The response of the bladder to stretch is dependent on a number of factors, including the duration of stretch, the rate at which the bladder is stretched, and hysteresis.[45,47,48] If the bladder is stretched rapidly, detrusor pressure and wall tension are great, but if it is stretched to a new length and that length is maintained, pressure falls. Thus, during a cystometrogram, the faster the filling rate, the higher the pressure rise. Hysteresis refers to a property of the bladder: the tension-length or pressure-volume relationship is dependent on the conditions that existed prior to the strain (i.e., the degree of filling). Thus, if the bladder is filled and emptied at a constant rate, each phase has a different pressure-volume curve.

The behavior of actin and myosin during bladder filling is not clearly understood, nor is the relative effect of smooth muscle contractions on the volume-pressure curve. Research has demonstrated that some individual smooth muscle cells manifest spontaneous activity during vesical filling and that this may contribute to bladder tone.[49]

*Accommodation* is that property of the bladder that allows it to accept increasing volumes of urine without a concomitant rise in intravesical pressure. Usually, the degree of pressure rise during normal bladder filling is no more than 15 cm $H_2O$. This pressure-volume relationship is defined by the LaPlace equation—$P = 2T/R$—where P is detrusor pressure, T is the wall tension in the bladder, and R is the radius of the bladder. Because the bladder radius is the same for any given bladder volume, the equation can be simply reduced to one that says that pressure is dependent on wall tension. Thus, bladder wall tension is dependent on both the active and passive properties and constituents of the bladder, that is, actin, myosin, collagen, and elastic tissue. As the bladder wall becomes stiffer (thicker or hypertrophic) wall tension increases for a given volume and there is a concomitant rise in detrusor pressure.

*Compliance* is defined as the change in the volume-pressure relationship. Bladder compliance is difficult to assess in the human bladder, for a number of reasons; it is very dependent on the rate of filling, hysteresis, the duration of filling, and smooth muscle activity. In addition, compliance may vary during different parts of the filling curve.

For continence to be maintained, urethral pressure must be higher than intravesical pressure, which is the sum of intraabdominal pressure, inherent detrusor pressure, and the potential (or gravitational) energy that is related to the "height" of urine above the meatus. *Urethral closure pressure* is defined as the difference between intravesical and urethral pressure. The resting urethra has a significantly higher pressure than the bladder, usually in the range of 40 to 80 cm $H_2O$. Both passive and active forces play prominent roles in the maintenance of this relatively high intraurethral pressure. Passive forces result from both the elastic and collagen fibers and also inner wall softness.[3] Active pressure changes are caused by periurethral striated muscles of the pelvic floor and also by intraurethral smooth and striated muscle contractions. In contrast to the bladder, the urethra is cylindrical. The pressure-volume relationship in the urethra is defined by the LaPlace equation for a cylinder: $P = T/R$. In summary, high intraurethral pressure is due, in large part, to its small radius and its dynamic high wall tension when compared to that of the bladder.

### Expulsion of Urine

Voluntary micturition is accomplished by activation of the *micturition reflex,* which is integrated in the pontine micturition center (Figure 19-1). This complex coordinated event is initiated by sudden and complete relaxation of the striated muscle of the urethra and pelvic floor.[2,43] Urethral pressure falls and detrusor pressure rises concomitantly, heralding the detrusor contraction. The reduction in urethral pressure is greatest at the membranous urethra in the male and at the distal urethra in the female. Both the urethra and the bladder neck gradually open and assume their wid-

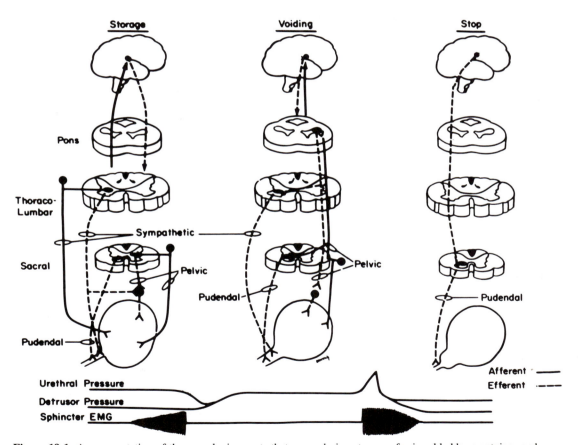

**Figure 19-1.** A representation of the neurologic events that occur during storage of urine, bladder emptying, and during sudden interruption of the voiding stream. Note that during micturition, detrusor (bladder) pressure is greater than urethral pressure with electrical silence of the electromyogram.

est cross-sectional area during peak flow, and bladder and urethra become a single isobaric unit as flow begins.[50–52] The mechanism of the micturition reflex is discussed under Neurologic Considerations.

*Physical Principles*

The active or dynamic component of the bladder muscle wall is comprised of both actin and myosin filaments. Actin (thick) filaments are attached to the cell membrane; myosin (thin) filaments are located in the cytoplasm. Depolarization of the cell, mediated by calcium influx and phosphorylation of myosin, results in muscle contraction. Muscle shortening is secondary to sliding of actin and myosin filaments past each other.[53] When the detrusor muscle contracts, one of two events occurs: muscle shortening or the development of force. The faster the muscle contracts, the less force it generates.

Some individual smooth muscle cells demonstrate spontaneous activity during filling and may act as pacemakers to regulate bladder activity.[49] In addition, at rest, detrusor smooth muscle cells have spontaneous action potentials. When stretched, the action potentials increase, both in frequency and in amplitude while the resting membrane potential decreases.[54] Thus, as the bladder fills there is a gradual increase in the quantity of spontaneous action potentials, resulting in contraction of individual muscle fibers. At a certain level of firing, the detrusor contracts and voiding ensues.

When the expulsive energy of the bladder overcomes the resistance of the urethra, voiding is accomplished. If one applies hydrodynamic principles to the lower urinary tract, the bladder can be conceptualized as a pump and the urethra as a pipe. Urethral resistance determines the flow rate for any given bladder contraction, but the applicability of this mathematical model is limited because the urethra is distensible. There have been a variety of both mathematical and computer-generated indices of bladder function, but to date none has achieved wide clinical applicability.[55]

A more sophisticated approach to expulsion is to study the energy balance during micturition. The energy that the bladder provides to expel urine is derived from three sources: intraabdominal pressure, inherent detrusor pressure, and the potential or gravitational energy, which reflects the level of urine above the meatus. Intravesical pressure is the sum of these three components. The energy provided by the bladder is then converted to either heat, which is dissipated in the urethra, or kinetic energy of the urinary stream.

The dissipated heat energy in the urethra plays little role with respect to voiding; however, there are various theories regarding the mechanism of heat dissipation during micturition. One is dissipation secondary to friction. When fluid passes through a tube, the rate of energy lost as friction depends on the characteristics of the fluid (viscosity); the characteristics of the flow (velocity); and the characteristics of the tube, (length and cross-sectional area).[56] The dissipation of energy increases as friction as the urethra gets longer, narrower, or more irregular; with urine, dissipation increases velocity. Another theory is dissipation secondary to geometric considerations: the preceding considerations about friction assume that the urethra is a rigid tube, but, the characteristic geometric configuration of the urethra is not static. Thus, during a contraction, two potential scenarios may ensue, based on the relative distensibility of the urethral wall proximal to the contraction. If the urethra is relatively nondistensible, flow is constant throughout the contraction. Because the cross-sectional area of the urethral wall at the site of the contraction is reduced, the velocity of the urine increases. Thus, the kinetic energy of the fluid increases. Similarly, if the urethral wall is more distensible, flow rate across the contraction may diminish as does the kinetic energy.

*Neurologic Considerations*

As bladder volume and pressure increase, afferent impulses from the bladder and urethra signal the time to void. Voluntary micturition ensues unless it is consciously suppressed.

The *micturition reflex* (see Figure 19-1) is integrated in the rostral brain stem in an area designated the *pontine micturition center,* which is connected to the *sacral micturition center* via spinal pathways in the posterior and lateral columns.[2,57–59] The micturition reflex is a coordinated interaction between the detrusor muscle and the urinary sphincter. No single stimulus appears to initiate the micturition reflex; rather, multiple neural events exert influence via one or more mechanisms and affect the threshold for voiding. Descending neural influences from the cingulate and frontal cortex, hypothalamus, and medial regions of the pons raise the threshold of micturition. In contrast, the threshold for micturition is lowered by increasing activity of the vesical afferents and the dorsolateral pons and mammillary bodies.[58–61] The first event in the micturition reflex is relaxation of the external urethral sphincter caused by cessation of efferent pudendal nerve firing.[2] At the same time, sympathetic activity is suppressed, which results in cessation of the inhibitory effects of sympathetic stimulation. Then the combination of neural impulses across the pelvic ganglion and efferent postganglionic firing results in a detrusor contraction. Finally, inhibition of vesical neck stimulation allows opening of the urethra (see Figure 19-1).

Spinal cord injury, transverse myelitis, multiple sclerosis, or myelodysplasia can interrupt this *long routed micturition reflex* and usually results in uncoordinated micturition.[2,62,63] Control over the micturition reflex is accomplished by ill-understood neural pathways that connect different parts of the brain with the pontine micturition center. Suprapontine neurologic lesions, such as a cerebrovascular accident, tumor, Parkinson's disease, or normal-pressure hydrocephalus, usually result in loss of control over the micturition reflex.[2]

## Pathophysiology of Lower Urinary Tract Symptoms

Based on urinary tract physiology, it is useful to classify lower urinary tract dysfunction into one of three groups: bladder filling and storage problems, bladder emptying problems, or combinations of the two.[1] Accurate diagnosis of a problem depends on careful assessment of the patient's history, physical examination, laboratory studies, and urodynamic assessment. Bladder symptoms are characterized as either irritative or obstructive. Irritative symptoms include urinary frequency, urgency, urge incontinence, nocturia, dysuria, and a constant feeling of suprapubic discomfort, pain, or urge to void. Obstructive symptoms consist of urinary hesitancy, decreased size and force of the stream, a feeling of incomplete bladder emptying, postvoid dribbling, overflow incontinence, and total urine retention. Symptoms elicited from the patient are often unreliable predictors of underlying disease and should serve only as a guide for directing further diagnostic evaluation.

The most remediable cause of urinary bladder symptoms is urinary tract infection, and no patient should be evaluated further until infection has been excluded by urinalysis and appropriate cultures. If hematuria is noted on routine urinalysis when infection has been excluded, radiologic evaluation of the kidneys and upper tracts, via either intravenous pyelography or ultrasonography, and cystoscopy are mandatory to exclude neoplastic conditions and urolithiasis.

Screening urodynamic evaluation should be performed on most uninfected patients whose persistent bladder symptoms do not respond to empiric treatment. For most patients, an accurate diagnosis can be obtained by cystometry, an estimation of urinary flow rate, postvoiding residual urine volume, and, in selected cases, voiding cystourethrography. More sophisticated studies such as sphincter electromyography, and synchronous video and urodynamic studies are more accurate but necessary only for persistent diagnostic and therapeutic problems.[64] Cystometry is performed by filling the bladder with gas or liquid while recording the detrusor pressure, bladder volume, and sensations of first urge and severe urge to void. Cystometry assesses bladder compliance, sensation, capacity and involuntary bladder contractions (Figure 19-2). Urine flow rate is measured electronically with commercially available flowmeters. Reduced urine flow suggests either bladder outlet obstruction or impairment of bladder contractility.[64]

### *Urinary Filling or Storage Problems*

#### *Involuntary Detrusor Contractions*

The most common cause of irritative voiding symptoms is involuntary detrusor contractions, defined as a sudden nonvolitional rise in bladder pressure. Their numerous causes include neurologic problems and bladder outlet obstruction, but some are idiopathic. Involuntary bladder contrac-

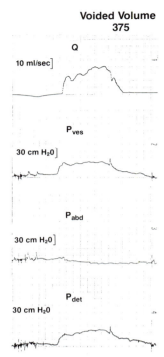

**Voided Volume**
**375**

Q

10 ml/sec]

P$_{ves}$

30 cm H$_2$0]

P$_{abd}$

30 cm H$_2$0]

P$_{det}$

30 cm H$_2$0

**Figure 19-2.** A typical bladder pressure–urinary flow rate curve. Q represents flow, P$_{ves}$ is total vesical or bladder pressure, P$_{abd}$ is abdominal pressure, and finally, P$_{det}$ is the subtracted pressure (P$_{ves}$ − P$_{abd}$), which represents inherent bladder pressure. In this patient, the maximal flow rate was 21 ml/sec and maximal detrusor pressure 50 cm H$_2$O.

tions due to neurologic lesions are categorized as *detrusor hyperreflexia;* in the absence of a neurologic lesion, the condition is termed *detrusor instability.*

Involuntary detrusor contractions are treated according to cause. When involuntary contractions are secondary to bladder outlet obstruction, relief of the obstruction usually results in cessation of the involuntary detrusor contractions. When there is no obstruction, the gold standard of therapy has been anticholinergic medication such as propantheline bromide or oxybutinin; however, these medications are effective for only approximately 50% of patients. Many patients also require intermittent self-catheterization to empty the bladder. Other therapeutic modalities currently being investigated include behavior modification, functional electrical neural stimulation (transcutane-

ously, percutaneously, or by direct stimulation of nerve roots), and surgical "denervation procedures" such as dorsal root section. Augmentation enterocystoplasty is almost always effective, but usually requires self intermittent catheterization.

*Small Bladder Capacity*

Normal bladder capacity is quite variable but usually is smaller >300 ml. Therefore, irritative voiding symptoms occur if the bladder capacity is smaller (i.e., 200 ml or less). The most common causes of a "pathologically" reduced bladder capacity include infection or involuntary detrusor contractions and low compliance.

It is very difficult to distinguish *idiopathic sensory urge* (i.e., urinary frequency, urgency, in the absence of intrinsic lower urinary tract disease) from a pathologically reduced bladder capacity. Both tuberculosis and interstitial cystitis can have characteristic cystoscopic changes; but they are not present in all patients. Repeating the cystoscopic examination under high spinal (above T-6) or general anaesthesia may be useful, as the bladder capacity of patients with detrusor fibrosis remains small, while in those with idiopathic sensory urgency it is normal.

Therapy of symptomatic small-capacity bladders is directed at the underlying lesion. All patients with sensory urge should undergo diagnostic cystoscopy, and any suspicious lesions should be investigated by biopsy, since one of the most important diagnostic entities to rule out is transitional cell carcinoma in situ of the bladder. This condition may be overlooked unless bladder biopsy is routinely obtained, even when there are no overt cystoscopic lesions. Balloon hydrodistension with a specially designed catheter (Helmstein) can be used under anaesthesia to distend a bladder with a capacity of less than 400 ml. The catheter is introduced into the bladder, with the patient under high epidural anesthesia, and the balloon is inflated to whatever volume is needed to attain a balloon pressure equal to systolic blood pressure, usually to volumes of 500 to 1000 ml. The bladder is left 4 hours in this distended state, while fluid is added or removed from the balloon as necessary to maintain the desired pressure. This treatment has proven effective in more than 60% of patients, but there have been reports of intraoperative bladder rupture in 5% of cases. The rupture is usually retroperitoneal and can be treated by leaving an indwelling vesical catheter for 5 to 7 days and administering broad-spectrum antibiotics.

If hydrodistension fails, surgical augmentation cystoplasty may be attempted: its two goals are to increase bladder capacity and lower intravesical pressure. A segment of bowel is isolated with its vascular pedicle intact and an anastomosis to the dome of the bladder is created. In some instances it may be necessary to excise most of the diseased bladder and create the anastomosis of bowel to the remaining trigone. Supravesical diversion should be reserved for patients who are either not good candidates for hydrodistension or augmentation cystoplasty or do not respond to them.

### Sensory Urgency

Sensory urgency describes a constellation of symptoms characterized by urinary frequency and urgency, often accompanied by suprapubic pain and discomfort or the feeling of a constant urge to void, all without any overt urodynamic abnormalities. These symptoms can usually be reproduced at relatively low bladder volumes, and while the symptoms are occurring no bladder contractions are evident on cystometry and bladder capacity is normal under anesthesia. Diagnostic misnomers for this symptom complex have included *urethral syndrome, trigonitis,* and *interstitial cystitis.* Patients with idiopathic sensory urgency void frequently, not because of involuntary detrusor contractions or infection but simply because it it hurts too much if they postpone voiding.

Therapy directed at curing infection or alleviating involuntary bladder contractions is doomed to failure in patients with sensory urgency. In this group of patients other empiric therapy is also unsuccessful, and it may in fact exacerbate the condition. Patients develop secondary psychological symptoms and their symptoms often are thought to have a primary psychiatric cause. In fact, there is no way conclusively to separate patients with primary psychopathology from those who have developed secondary psychiatric symptoms because of their incurable bladder condition. Regardless of the underlying cause, however,

structured behavior modification seems to be the most practical approach for these difficult patients.

### Sphincter Abnormalities

Incontinence which occurs when the patient coughs, sneezes, or strains is *stress incontinence.* It is due to either abnormal descent of the proximal urethra when the patient increases intraabdominal pressure (hypermobility) or to intrinsic sphincter deficiency. In the former the increased intraabdominal pressure is transmitted unequally to the bladder and urethra. Leakage occurs when vesical pressure exceeds urethral pressure. Blaivas has likened this to a hernia of the proximal urethra through the pelvic floor.[65] The sphincter itself is relatively normal; it is capable of maintaining a watertight seal but cannot withstand the effects of increased pressure. Therefore, any operation designed to prevent descent of the proximal urethra (the suspension operations) is almost uniformly successful in effecting a cure. Other procedures that have been described include the injection of substances such as Teflon or collagen around the urethra. Preliminary results have been encouraging, but careful patient selection is required.

*Intrinsic sphincter deficiency* describes a condition in which the sphincter cannot maintain a watertight seal, and therefore leakage occurs with the slightest provocation. The cause of sphincteric failure is almost always either neurologic injury or multiple surgeries.[64,65] The standard procedures described above to alleviate stress incontinence have little role in the management of these patients; however, the creation of a pubovaginal sling has met with a high success rate.[65,66] In males, the insertion of an artificial urinary sphincter has met with some success.

### Bladder Emptying Problems

#### Impairment of Bladder Contractility

Poor bladder emptying is secondary to either bladder outlet obstruction or impaired detrusor contractility. Though poor detrusor contractions may be attributable to myogenic, neurogenic, or psychological causes current tests cannot distinguish between these causes. Most neurologic causes of detrusor abnormalities are associated with other neurologic deficits. For example, a neurologic lesion that affects the second through the fourth segments of the sacral spinal cord usually results not only in detrusor areflexia, but also perianal anesthesia, poor anal tone, absent voluntary control of the anal sphincter, and absence of the bulbocavernosus reflex.

The most effective therapy for this group of patients, regardless of the cause of impaired contractility, is intermittent clean self-catheterization (CIC), timed to regularly empty the bladder and prevent periods of overdistension. A reasonable regimen is to perform CIC approximately every 6 hours; highest priority is given to accomplishing the catheterization on schedule. Despite their widespread use, parasympathomimetics (bethanechol) and α-sympathetic blocking agents (phenoxybenzamine) have not been shown to be effective for these conditions.

*Bladder Outlet Obstruction*

Outlet obstruction due to an enlarged prostate is the most common cause of voiding dysfunction in older males. Approximately 10% to 15% of men aged 50 years require a definitive procedure for prostatism by age 80 years. The pathognomonic diagnosis for bladder outlet obstruction is poor urine flow in the presence of an adequate detrusor contraction (greater than 45 cm $H_2O$).

Relief of the obstruction usually results in resolution of the patient's symptoms. Prostatectomy has traditionally been the primary therapy. The procedure generally is tolerated well (mortality rate 0.2%), but recently there has been an explosion in the urologic literature of alternative methods for relieving bladder outlet obstruction. These include medications, balloon dilatation of the prostatic urethra, hyperthermia, and insertion of intraprostatic coils. They have met with variable success, and long-term studies are needed to assess their efficacy. In women the diagnosis of bladder outlet obstruction is very difficult to make and usually requires sophisticated video and urodynamic techniques to delineate precisely both the site and the nature of the obstruction.[65]

Bladder neck obstruction may be primary or secondary. Primary bladder neck contraction most likely results from either abnormal contraction of the vesical neck during voiding or failure of the vesical neck to open. The bladder neck usually appears normal during cystoscopic visualization, so the diagnosis may be missed. Transurethral bladder neck incision is usually curative. α-Sympathetic blocking agents and urethral dilatation each reportedly have been effective, but this has not been our experience. Secondary bladder neck obstruction almost always is a complication of surgery for incontinence that resulted in scarring; it must be treated surgically.

Urethral meatal stenosis is an uncommon cause of bladder outlet obstruction yet it is "overdiagnosed." Most urethral meatal "strictures" diagnosed by calibrating the size of the meatus at urodynamic testing, are found not to cause obstruction. Empiric urethral dilatation or meatoplasty is a common resort, even though there is no evidence in the literature of efficacy of either. More important is the potential harm that these procedures may cause, since by causing fibrosis of the urethra they may result in either bladder outlet obstruction or urinary incontinence.

### *Urine Storage and Emptying Problems*

*Detrusor–External Sphincter Dyssynergia* (DESD) describes involuntary contraction of the external urethral sphincter during an involuntary detrusor contraction (Figure 19-3). It is seen almost exclusively in patients with neurologic lesions of the suprasacral spinal cord.[2,62] Despite the outlet obstruction caused by the contracting external sphincter, women with this condition, in contrast to men, are at little risk for developing urologic complications unless they are treated with an indwelling catheter.[65] Their main problem is incontinence, which is very difficult to manage. The optimal form of therapy is a combination of relaxation of the detrusor with anticholinergic medication and CIC.

For men who are unable to self-catheterize, the next course of management is external sphincterotomy. This is done by making a transurethral incision through the obstructing sphincter. The procedure renders the patient incontinent and prevents the high intravesical pressures associated

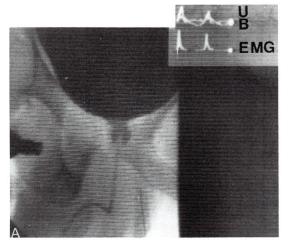

**Figure 19-3.** Urodynamic and radiographic representation of detrusor–external sphincter dyssynergia. Note that during a sustained involuntary bladder contraction (B) there is maximal EMG activity. There is minimal passage of contrast beyond the contracted external urethral sphincter. (U, urethral pressure).

with DESD. If this fails, augmentation cystoplasty with continent vesicostomy and closure of the vesical neck probably offers the best alternative to supravesical urinary diversion.

Patients with areflexia or "low compliant" bladder and sphincteric incontinence usually have

conditions associated with parasympathetic, sympathetic, or pudendal denervation. This may be caused by a variety of conditions, including spinal cord infarction, myelodysplasia, or prior radical pelvic surgery (abdominoperineal resection of the rectum or radical hysterectomy). Treatment for these patients is very difficult. On occasion, CIC suffices if the bladder is emptied often enough so that incontinence does not occur. Patients with bladder neck denervation occasionally respond to α-sympathetic stimulation, either alone or in combination with β-blockade. Once rendered continent, the bladder can be emptied by CIC. On occasion it is necessary to create a pubovaginal sling and to manage the patient with CIC. Figure 19-4 depicts a treatment algorithm for patients with voiding dysfunction.

## Physiology of Sexual Function

As for voiding dysfunction, it is imperative that the health care professional have a clear understanding of normal sexual function, including both physiologic and psychological response, before "disorders" can be treated. We review normal genital anatomy and innervation, male and female sexual response, and sexual function in patients with spinal cord injury.

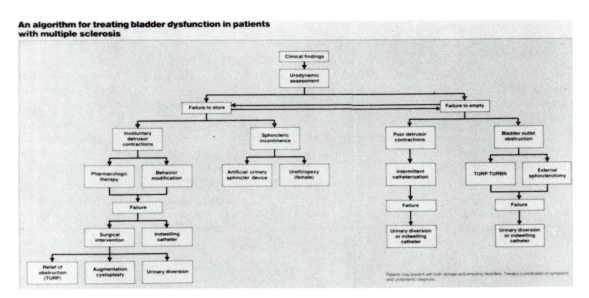

**Figure 19-4.** Treatment algorithm for voiding dysfunction.

## Genital Anatomy

### Males

The physiology of penile erection is dependent on a series of complex interactions involving the vascular, hormonal, and neurogenic systems of the body.[67] The penis is divided into three portions: the root, the body, and the glans. The root, which lies in the superficial perineal pouch, provides fixation and stability. The body consists of three spongy erectile bodies covered by various layers of fascia and skin. The glans is the distal expansion of the corpora spongiosa, which is one of the aforementioned erectile bodies. The skin covering the penis is thin and loosely connected with underlying penile fascia.

The paired corpora cavernosa lie dorsally and are surrounded by a double layer of dense fibrous connective tissue, Buck's fascia. As the corporal cavernosal bodies approach the perineum, they diverge to form the crura of the penis. The corporal bodies are composed of a maze of endothelium-lined spaces invested by smooth muscle. Each crus adheres firmly to the ischial and pubic ramus and is surrounded by the ischiocavernosus muscle. The corpus spongiosum surrounds the urethra and lies ventral and centrally within the penis. Its posterior end is bulbous (the bulbar urethra) and is surrounded by the bulbospongiosus muscle. Its distal ends expands conically to form the glans penis and fits over the rounded end of the paired corpora cavernosa. The urethra opens in the most distal aspect of the glans penis. The three masses of erectile tissue that comprise the body of the penis expand to become rigid when engorged with blood.

The supporting structures of the penis are the fundiform and suspensory ligaments. The fundiform ligament is superficial and runs in continuity from the abdominal fascia to the penis and finally ends within the septa of the scrotum. The suspensory ligament is deep and attaches at the level of the symphysis pubis. The blood supply to the penis arises from the internal pudendal artery, which is a branch of the internal iliac artery. At the level of the urogenital diaphragm, the perineal segment of the internal pudendal artery divides into four terminal branches: (1) the urethral artery, (2) the bulbar artery, (3) the deep penile artery, and (4) the deep dorsal artery. The urethral artery supplies blood to the corpus spongiosum; the bulbar artery sends branches to the bulbospongiosus and the bulbar urethra; the deep penile artery supplies blood to the paired corpora cavernosa; and the deep dorsal artery travels between the layers of the suspensory ligament and lies in close continuity between the paired dorsal veins and nerves of the penis. It supplies the glans penis.

The three main channels of venous outflow are the cavernous veins and the superficial and deep dorsal veins. The corpora cavernosum is drained by the the cavernous vein. The superficial dorsal vein drains the foreskin and empties directly into the external pudendal vein. Finally, the glans penis and a part of the cavernous bodies are drained by the deep dorsal vein complex, which ends in the prostate venous plexus.

### Females

The clitoris is the homologue of the dorsal part of the penis. It consists of two small erectile cavernous bodies. The erectile body consists of two crura clitoridis and the glans clitoridis with overlying skin and prepuce. The glans is situated superiorly at the fused termination of the crura. It is composed of a combination of erectile tissue and a prepuce.

Bartholin's glands lie inferior and medial to the bulbocavernosus muscle. Their secretion is clear, viscid, and alkaline. During sexual activity there is increased secretory activity. In most women the gland become involuted and shrunken after about age 30 years. Other glands associated with secretory activity include Skene's glands, whose openings are close to the urethral meatus.

The nerve supply to the female external and internal genitalia includes a complex integration between somatic and autonomic nerve pathways. The innervation of the pudendum (which includes the mons pubis, labia minora and majora, clitoris, and vagina) consists of branches from the iliohypogastric, ilioinguinal, genitofemoral as well as the sacral plexus. The pudendal nerves carry the somatic sensory fibers. The distribution of nerve endings within the glans clitoris varies from total absence to a rich supply in the prepuce. Obviously, any neurologic injury to the nerve endings to the clitoris takes on clinical significance with respect to potential sexual difficulties during the rehabilitation period.

The uterus and ovaries are innervated by the autonomic nerves, which include branches of the superior and inferior hypogastric plexus. These plexi contain both sympathetic and parasympathetic (nervi erigentes) components, the nervi erigentes being primarily sensory. Somatic afferent nerves synapse at the T-11 and T-12 segments. The nerve supply of the ovaries arises from the lumbosacral sympathetic chain and passes into the ovary along the ovarian artery.

### Neurophysiology of Erection

The hemodynamics of erection can be summarized as an increase in blood flow to the penis with redirection of that blood within the complex and interlacing sinusoids of the cavernosal bodies. While this statement is simplistic, it does serve as the basic model to describe neurophysiologic function. Like the urinary tract, the male genitalia are innervated via both somatic and autonomic nerve fibers. The pudendal nerves mediate penile sensation, and their major role is to provide sensation for the initiation and maintenance of penile erection.[68] The autonomic nervous system provides the major neurologic input to achieve penile erection, specifically the blood vessels in the paired corpora cavernosa. As early as 1863 it was known that electrical stimulation of the pelvic nerve (a parasympathetic nerve) induced an erection in dogs, and it is still thought that the parasympathetic nervous system is the predominant neurostimulator.[69] Neuropeptides may also be important in the initiation or maintenance of erection.

The sympathetic nervous system components that mediate erection originate in the thoracolumbar spinal cord. Investigators noted that ablation of the pelvic parasympathetic nervous system did not totally abolish erectile capability.[70] At present, the role of the adrenergic system in erectile physiology is unclear. Intracavernosal injections of α-adrenergic blocking agents (e.g., papaverine, phentolamine) promote erection. In addition, sympathetic stimulation causes detumescence. It re-

mains to be determined which neurotransmitter modulates this response and at what anatomic site this modulation occurs.

It should be emphasized that there is "higher central" control of penile erection. In monkeys, it has been demonstrated that the anterior medial part of the hypothalamus is a positive locus for erection.[71] In addition, visual stimuli are probably mediated via parts of the subcorticolimbic system (i.e., the mammilary bodies and cingulate gyrus). Electrical stimulation and electroencephalographic studies have demonstrated to be important centers in the limbic lobe of Broca. Lesions of the medial preoptic lobe of the hypothalamus in rats abolish sexual activity.

The efferent pathway from the cerebral cortex to the sacral spinal cord proceeds from the preoptic hypothalamic region, median forebrain bundle, and substantia nigra of the midbrain.[72] These fibers enter the ventrolateral pons and travel through the spinal cords in the reticulospinal tracts.

### Male Sexual Response

The male sexual response consists of erection, ejaculation, emission, and orgasm. The excitement phase consists of erection, which may subside if stimulation is inadequate or ceases. Ejaculation is composed of seminal emission (delivery of semen into the urethra) and propulsion of seminal contents via the glans, with closure of the bladder neck to prevent the entry of seminal fluid into the bladder. Orgasm is a sensory phenomenon occurring in the cerebral cortex in association with the ejaculatory reflex, which involves a complex interplay of somatic and autonomic nervous system pathways. The major motor neurologic stimulus to ejaculation is the sympathetic nervous system, mediated via the hypogastric nerve. This includes stimulation of the peristaltic waves of the smooth muscles of the ampulla, seminal vesicles, and prostate. In addition, the bladder neck is closed during ejaculation via α-adrenergic stimulation. The parasympathetic system serves only to provide stimulation of periurethral and prostatic gland secretion. The somatic nervous system provides penile sensation and contributes to perineal muscle contraction. Finally, cerebral and subcortical centers also influence the ejaculatory reflex with loci identified in the thalamus.[71]

### Female Sexual Response

In females, the initial sexual response includes engorgement and swelling of the labia and clitoris as well as lubrication of the vagina. As stimulation continues, the clitoris becomes increasingly swollen. During orgasm, the clitoris is maximally engorged and the walls of the vagina alternate contraction and relaxation. During the excitement phase, there is also engorgement of the nipples and breasts. The mechanism of this response is a combination of parasympathetic modulation causing vasodilatation as well as inhibition of sympathetic mediated vasoconstrictor tone. In summary, in both men and women, sexual response is a complex interaction of cortical, autonomic, and somatic nervous system events. However, the role of psychosocial phenomena such as performance and orgasmic expression cannot be overemphasized.

### Sexual Response After Spinal Cord Injury

Impotence is defined as the inability to achieve an erection adequate for penetration during sexual intercourse. The incidence of impotence after spinal cord injury approximates 75%.[73] Only 70% of patients with upper motor neuron lesions attempt intercourse and only half of those patients who try are successful.[74] It is interesting to correlate the level of spinal cord injury with the quality of erectile response. The majority of patients (66%) who are injured above T-12 have erections involving all three corporal bodies, in contrast to patients with injury below T-12, who can achieve erectile engorgement of the corpora cavernosa only. This is most likely due to the lack of sympathetic nervous system effect in patients with injury below the level of T-12.[75] Erections occur more frequently in patients with lesions of upper motor neuron origin than in those with lower motor neuron lesions. In addition, the likelihood of achieving erections sufficient for vaginal penetration is greater with an incomplete injury than a complete one.

Erections in the spinal cord–injured patient are conveniently classified as either psychogenic or reflex. Psychogenic erections occur because of stimulation mediated at higher cortical levels, whereas reflex erections are mediated through local stimuli. Interruption of supraspinal pathways results in psychogenic erectile dysfunction. However, many of these patients can achieve reflex erections; unfortunately, these are usually of short duration and are poorly sustained. It should be noted that some 70% of patients with cauda equina lesions are impotent. Because of impairment of pudendal nerve–mediated sensation, these patients do not have reflex erections. The physiology of psychogenic erections in this group of patients is poorly understood.[68]

The management of erectile dysfunction in spinal cord patients should be directed to one of four treatment regimens or a combination of several. The first involves sexual counseling and behavior therapy. In addition to reassurance and assistance in the "information" process, the physician or counselor can help the patient gradually return to being a sexually functioning adult. Basic concepts of bladder management prior to sexual stimulation and the prevention of autonomic dysreflexia during intercourse are invaluable to the patient. This alone may be enough to alleviate the anxieties of the rehabilitating patient.[76]

The second treatment regimen includes penile injection of vasoactive substances, now the most common way to treat patients with sexual dysfunction. The mechanism of erection achieved with intracavernous injection of α-sympatholytic agents such as papaverine and phentolamine has been researched extensively. Of greatest importance is the finding that men with erectile dysfunction secondary to a neurogenic cause respond to a minimal amount of the drug, so the long-term side effects of penile fibrosis and scarring at the injection site are much greatly reduced. The major short-term sequela of intracorporeal injection is priapism. This is easily reversed by intercorporeal irrigation with epinephrine. Thus, careful dose titration cannot be overemphasized.

The third option for treatment includes the use of a vacuum suction device so that negative pressure allows inflow of blood into the penis. The blood is maintained in situ by placing a band around the base of the penis. Contraindications to the use of a vaccum device include patients who are taking anticoagulants or have blood dyscrasias. Finally, use of this device requires bimanual dexterity which may be a limiting factor for some patients.[77] The fourth treatment regimen is a penile prosthesis. Available prostheses include semirigid, self-contained, inflatable and pump-supported models. Obviously, the likelihood of prosthesis failure is increased with the more "exotic" prostheses; however, with the advent of intracorporeal injections, the need for penile prostheses for spinal cord–injured patients has decreased dramatically. This is fortunate, as these patients have special problems because of their increased incidence of urinary tract infection and skin problems and the potential effects of these on a foreign body. It is not advisable to place a prosthesis in a patient who has a "chronic" indwelling Foley or suprapubic catheter because of the potential for infection. Other treatment modalities, such as a yohimbine, have not yet been studied adequately to allow us to comment on their overall efficacy.

Ejaculatory failure in spinal cord–injured patients approaches 80% to 90% of patients. In addition, at least that many patients are anorgasmic. Very few patients with high spinal cord lesions can ejaculate. Preservation of ejaculatory function is greatest in patients with incomplete upper motor neuron lesions. In contrast, ejaculation is preserved in 60% of patients with either cauda equina or conus medullaris injury. This is especially true when the lesion is incomplete.[68] Because of impairment of pelvic muscles, patients usually have a dribbling type of ejaculation. A number of treatment modalities address ejaculatory failure in this group of patients. These include pharmacologic manipulation with either subcutaneous physostigmine or intrathecal neostigmine, which must be carried out in an intensive care unit where blood pressure can be monitored.[73] Vibratory stimulation of the glans penis has resulted in ejaculation rates of 60%, and a number of studies have confirmed resultant pregnancies though the quality of the sperm may be reduced.[78]

The use of electrical ejaculation has increased fertility in spinal cord–injury patients. Depending on the neurologic status of the patient, the procedure can be done with or without anaesthesia. The patient may ejaculate either retrograde or antegrade, though the more viable semen is obtained via the antegrade route. To increase the viability of sperm obtained via retrograde ejaculation, the patient is catheterized before electroejaculation and the bladder is instilled with buffers that help to alkalinize the urine. Then the patient is stimulated and finally recatheterized to recover sperm. Using this modality, pregnancy rates of 50% have been obtained.[79] It should be noted that all these techniques (particularly vibratory stimulation of the glans) are associated with potential autonomic dysreflexia, and care should be used when employing them.

There is very little literature on sexual dysfunction in female spinal cord–injured patients. Vaginal lubrication occurs in response to direct stimulation if the sacral reflex arc is intact and to psychogenic stimuli with lower motor neuron lesions. Hormonally mediated ovulation is not affected by spinal cord injury. Once again, education and reassurance are important. It is noteworthy that autonomic dysreflexia has been reported secondary to labor contractions in patients with high cord lesions. Delivery by cesarean section has been advocated for this group of patients.

## References

1. Wein AJ. Classification of neurogenic voiding dysfunction. J Urol 1981; 125:605.
2. Blaivas JG. The neurophysiology of micturition: A clinical study of 550 patients. J Urol 1982; 127:958.
3. Zinner NR, Sterling AM, Ritter RC. Role of inner wall softness in urinary continence. Urology 1980; 16:115.
4. Woodbourne RT. Anatomy of the bladder. In: Boyarski S, ed. The Neurogenic Bladder. Baltimore: Williams & Wilkins, 1967; 3–17.
5. Dixon J, Gosling J. Structure and innervation in the human. In: Torrens M, Morrison JFB, eds. The Physiology of the Lower Urinary Tract. London: Springer-Verlag, 1987.
6. Uhlenhuth E, Hunter DW Jr, Loechel WF. Problems in the Anatomy of the Pelvis. Philadelphia: JB Lippincott, 1953; 1–157.
7. Hutch JA. Anatomy and Physiology of the Bladder, Trigone and Urethra. New York: Appleton-Century-Crofts, 1972.
8. Tanagho EA, Schmidt RA, Araugo CG. Urinary striated sphincter: What is its nerve supply? Urology 1982; 24:415.
9. Gil Vernet S. Morphology and Function of Vesico-

Prostatourethral Musculature. Treviso: Edizioni Canova, 1968.

10. Hanes RW. The striped compressor of the prostatic urethra. Br J Urol 1970; 41:481.

11. Oerlich TM. The urethral sphincter muscle in the male. Am J Anat 1980; 158:229.

12. Coggehsall RE. Law of separation of function of the spinal roots. Physiol Rev 1980; 60:716.

13. deGroat WC, Kawatani M, Hisamitsu T, et al. The role of neuropeptides in the sacral autonomic reflex pathways of the cat. J Auton Nerv Syst 1983; 7:339.

14. Elbadawi A. Neuromorphologic basis of vesicourethral function. I. Histochemistry, ultrastructure, and function of intrinsic nerves of the bladder and urethra. Neurourol Urodynam 1982; 1:3.

15. Kuru M. Nervous control of micturition. Physiol Rev 1965; 45:425.

16. Yamamoto T, Satomi H, Ise H, et al. Sacral spinal innervation of the rectal and vesical smooth muscles and the sphincteric striated muscles demonstrated by the horseradish peroxidase method. Neurosci Lett 1978; 7:41.

17. Brindley GS. Control of the bladder and urethral sphincters by the surgically implantable electrical stimulators. In: Chisolm GD, Williams DF, eds. Scientific Foundations in Urology, Chicago: Year Book, 1982; 464–470.

18. Creed KE, Tulloch AGC. The effect of pelvic nerve stimulation and some drugs on the urethra and bladder of the dog. Br J Urol 1978; 50:398.

19. Fagge CH. On the innervation of the urinary passages in dogs. J Physiol 1902; 28:304.

20. Langworthy OR. Innervation of the pelvic organs of the rat. Invest Urol 1965; 2:491.

21. Ambache N, Zar MA. Noncholinergic transmission by postganglionic motor neurons in the mammalian bladder. J Physiol (Lond) 1970; 210:761.

22. Taira N. The autonomic pharmacology of the bladder. Ann Rev Pharmacol 1972; 12:197.

23. Graber P, Tanagho EA. Urethral responses to autonomic nerve stimulation. Urology 1975; 6:52.

24. Elliott TR. The innervation of the bladder and urethra. J Physiol 1906–1907; 35:367.

25. Girado JM, Campbell JB. The innervation of the urethra of the female cat. Exp Neurol 1959; 1:44.

26. McGuire EJ, Wagner FC Jr. The effects of sacral denervation on bladder and urethral function. Surg Gynecol Obstet 1977; 144:343.

27. Gruber CM. The autonomic innervation of the genitourinary system. Physiol Rev 1933; 13:497.

28. Elbadawi A, Schenk EA. A new theory of the innervation of the bladder musculature. IV. Innervation of the vesicourethral junction and external urethral sphincter. J Urol 1974; 80:341.

29. Elbadawi A, Schenk EA. Dual innervation of the mammalian urinary bladder. A histochemical study of the distribution of cholinergic and adrenergic nerves. Am J Anat 1968; 119:405.

30. Owman C, Sjostrand NO. Short adrenergic neurons and catecholamine-containing cells in vas deferens and accessory male genital glands of different mammals. Z Zellforsch 1965; 66:300.

31. Blaivas JG, Barbalias GA. Characteristics of neural injury after abdominoperineal resection. J Urol 1983; 128:84–90.

32. deGroat WC, Lalley PM. Reflex firing in the lumbar sympathetic outflow to activation of vesical afferent fibers. J Physiol 1972; 226:289.

33. deGroat WC, Booth AM. Inhibition and facilitation in parasympathetic ganglia of the urinary bladder. Fed Proc 1980; 39:2990.

34. deGroat WC, Kawatani M. Neural control of the urinary bladder: Possible relationship between peptidergic inhibitory mechanisms and detrusor instability. Neurourol Urodynam 1985; 4:285.

35. Benson GS, Wein WJ, Raezer DM, et al. Adrenergic and cholinergic stimulation and blockage of the human bladder base. J Urol 1976; 116:174.

36. Downie JW, Dean DM, Carro-Ciampi G, et al. A difference in sensitivity to alpha-adrenergic agonists exhibited by detrusor and bladder neck of the rabbit. Can J Physiol Pharmacol 1975; 53:525.

37. Ek A, Alm P, Andersson KE, et al. Adrenergic and cholinergic nerves of the human urethra and urinary bladder: A histochemical study. Acta Physiol Scand 1977; 99:34.

38. Nergardh A. The interaction between adrenergic and cholinergic receptor functions in the outlet region of the urinary bladder. Scand Urol Nephrol 1974; 8:108.

39. van Buren GA, Anderson GF. Comparison of the urinary bladder base and detrusor to cholinergic and histaminergic receptor activation in the rabbit. Pharmacology 1979; 18:136.

40. Learmonth JR. A contribution to the neurophysiology of the urinary bladder in man. Brain 1931; 54:147.

41. Morgan C, Nadelhaft I, deGroat WC. The distribution of visceral primary afferents from the pelvic nerve within Lissauer's tract and the spinal gray matter and its relationship to the sacaral prasympathetic nucleus. J Comp Neurol 1981; 201:415.

42. Rockswold GL, Bradley WE, Chou CM. Innervation of the urinary bladder in higher primates. J Comp Neurol 1980; 193:509.

43. Blaivas JG, Labib KB, Bauer SB, et al. A new approach to electromyography of the external urethral sphincter. J Urol 1977; 117:773.

44. Blaivas JG, Scott M, Labib KB. Urodynamic evaluation as a test of sacral cord function. Urology 1979; 9:692.

45. Coolsaet BRLA. Stepwise Cystometry. A New Method to Investigate Properties of the Urinary Bladder. Doctoral thesis, Erasmus University, Rotterdam, 1977.

46. van Duyl WA. A model for both the passive and active properties of urinary bladder tissue related to bladder function. Neurourol Urodynam 1985; 4:275.

47. Klevmark B. Effects of extrinsic bladder denervation on intramural tension and on intravesical pressure patterns. Acta Physiol Scand 1977; 101:176.

48. van Mastrigt R, Coolsaet BLRA, van Duyl WA. The passive properties of the urinary bladder in the collection phase. Med Biol Eng Comput 1978; 16:471.

49. Coolsaet BLRA. Bladder compliance and detrusor activity during the collection phase. Neurourol Urodynam 1985; 4:263.

50. Griffiths DJ: Urodynamics: The Mechanics and Hydrodynamics of the Lower Urinary Tract. Bristol: Adam Hilger, 1980.

51. Woodside JR. Micturitional static urethral pressure profilometry in women. Neuorourol Urodynam 1982; 1:149.

52. Yalla SV, Sharma GVRK, Barsamian EM. Micturitional urethral pressure profile during voiding and the implications. J Urol 1980; 124:649.

53. Brading A. Physiology of smooth muscle. In: Torrens Michael, Morrison JFB, eds. The Physiology of the Lower Urinary Tract. Berlin: Springer-Verlag, 1987.

54. Ursillo RC. Electrical activity of the isolated nerve urinary bladder strip preparation of the rabbit. Am J Physiol 1961; 210:408.

55. Griffiths DJ. The mechanics of micturition. In: Yalla SV, Elbadawi A, McGuire EM, et al. eds. The Principles and Practice of Neurology and Urodynamics. New York: Macmillan, 1988.

56. Sterling AM, Ritter RC, Zinner NR. The physical basis of obstructive uropathy. In: Hinman F Jr, ed. Benign Prostatic Hypertrophy. New York: Springer-Verlag, 1983.

57. Barrington FJF. The effect of lesions of the hind and mid-brain on micturition of the cat. Q J Exp Physiol 1925; 15:181.

58. Barrington FJF. The localisation of the paths subserving micturition in the spinal cord of the cat. Brain 1933; 56:126.

59. Morrison JFB. Bladder control: Role of the higher levels of central nervous system. In: Torrens M, Morrison JFB, eds. The Physiology of the Lower Urinary Tract. London: Springer-Verlag, 1987.

60. Barrington FJF. The central nervous control of micturition. Brain 1928; 51:209.

61. Barrington FJF. The component reflexes of micturition in the cat. Part III. Brain 1941; 64:239.

62. Blaivas JG, Fisher DM. Combined radiographic and urodynamic monitoring: Advances in technique. J Urol 1981; 125:541.

63. McGuire EJ, Brady S. Detrusor-sphincter dyssynergia. J Urol 1979; 121:774.

64. Blaivas JG, Salinas J. Type III stress urinary incontinence. The importance of proper diagnosis and treatment. Surg Forum 1984.

65. McGuire EJ, Woodside JR, Borden TA, et al. Prognostic value of urodynamic testing in myelodysplastic patients. J Urol 1981; 126:205.

66. McGuire EM, Lytton B, Kohorn EI, et al. Value of urodynamic testing in stress urinary incontinence. J Urol 1980; 124:256.

67. Abber JC, Lue TF. Evaluation of Impotence. Prob Urol 1987; 1:476.

68. Siroky MB. Neurophysiology of male sexual dysfunction in neurologic disorders. Semin Neurol 1988; 8:136.

69. Eckhardt C. Untersuchungen uber die Erektion des Penis beim Hund. Beitr Anat Physiol 1863; 13:123.

70. Root WS, Bard P. The mechanism of feline erection through sympathetic pathways with some remarks on sexual behavior after de-afferentation of the genitalia. Am J Physiol 1947; 150:80.

71. Maclean PD, Ploog DW. Cerebral representation of penile erection. J Neurophysiol 1962; 25:29.

72. Siroky MB, Krane RJ. Physiology of male sexual dysfunction. In: Krane RJ, Siroky MB, eds. Clinical Neuro-Urology. Boston: Little, Brown, 1979.

73. Stone AR. The sexual needs of the injured spinal cord patient. Prob Urol 1987; 3:529–536.

74. Talbot HS. The sexual functioning paraplegic. J Urol 1973; 91:1975.

75. Comarr AE. The Total Care of Spinal Cord Injuries. Boston: Little, Brown, 1977.

76. Strasberg PD, Brady SM. Sexual functioning of persons with neurologic disorders. Sem Neurol 1988; 8:141.

77. Witherington R. Mitigating impotence with an external vacuum device. Contemp Urol 1990; 4:44.

78. Brindley GS. Reflex ejaculation under vibratory stimulation in paraplegic men. Paraplegia 1981; 9:299.

79. Bennett CJ, Ayers JW, Randolph JF Jr. Electroejaculation of paraplegic males followed by pregnancies. Fertil Steril 1987; 48:1070.

# Chapter 20

# Autonomic Function in the Isolated Spinal Cord

BRENDA S. MALLORY

The most devastating effects of a complete spinal cord injury (SCI) are the complete loss of sensation and voluntary motor activity below the level of the lesion. In contrast, the basic vital functions such as the circulation, alimentation, defecation, and micturition appear to be grossly maintained though devoid of supraspinal control. Closer observation confirms that significant dysfunction in these basic homeostatic mechanisms are present in all persons with SCI. In this chapter I discuss the autonomic responses associated with upper motor neuron type lesions of the spinal cord. In this situation, organization of the neuronal circuitry subserving a given autonomic response is independent of supraspinal control (except of course via the cranial nerves, which by definition are not involved by SCI). The altered autonomic responses that are described may be organized in either the spinal cord or the peripheral autonomic ganglia.

## Organization of the Autonomic Nervous System

The autonomic nervous system (discussed in Chapter 4) is divided into the parasympathetic and sympathetic nerves. Efferent neuronal cells of the autonomic nervous system, which are located in either the brain stem or the spinal cord are termed *preganglionic neurons*. These cells project preganglionic fibers, which synapse upon postganglionic neurons located in various ganglia and plexuses outside the central nervous system (CNS). The postganglionic neuron in turn projects a postganglionic fiber to a specific target organ or effector tissue.

The sympathetic division of the autonomic nervous system has sympathetic preganglionic neurons (SPNs) located in the intermediolateral (IML) cell column of the thoracic and upper lumbar spinal cord, and these project sympathetic preganglionic fibers to postganglionic neurons in either the paravertebral chain or the various prevertebral plexuses (see Figure 4-2.) Parasympathetic preganglionic neurons are found in the brain stem and the sacral spinal cord. There are four parasympathetic brain stem nuclei: nucleus Edinger-Westphal, superior and inferior salivatory nuclei, and the dorsal vagal complex of the medulla.[1] Sacral parasympathetic preganglionic fibers project to intramural and extramural ganglia of the pelvic viscera. Chapter 4 describes the cranial parasympathetic preganglionic projections.

It is generally assumed that all preganglionic neurons are cholinergic and have nicotinic postsynaptic receptors,[2] but in the cat thoracolumbar intermediate zone there are also neuron cell bodies that are reactive for the peptides enkephalin, neurotensin, somatostatin, and substance P.[3] The presence and release of a variety of substances capable of effecting or modifying neurotransmission has led to the abandonment of the traditional view of "one neurotransmitter for one neuron."[2] Neurotransmitters such as acetylcholine have a duration of action measured in milliseconds, whereas actions of peptides can last minutes.

Most postganglionic sympathetic neurons release norepinephrine (NE) as their primary neurotransmitter.[4] Most of the NE is taken up by the nerve terminal, but some escapes into the plasma, where it can be measured and correlated with activity of sympathetic neurons.[2] Skin sweat glands that subserve thermoregulation are innervated by sympathetic cholinergic postganglionic fibers acting on muscarinic (blocked by atropine) receptors. Postganglionic parasympathetic junctions are also muscarinic cholinergic. Target tissues for postganglionic autonomic fibers include cardiac muscle, sinoatrial and atrioventricular nodes, smooth muscle, secretory glands, and sensory receptors,[1,5,6] fat cells,[7] hepatocytes,[1,8] and lymphoid organs, including thymus, spleen, lymph nodes, and gut-associated lymphoid tissue.[1]

Sympathetic and parasympathetic preganglionic neurons receive afferent fibers from both somatic and visceral sources and projections from the central nervous system. Some autonomic reflexes are complete at the spinal level and others have a supraspinal relay.

## Renovascular Function

Afferent renal nerves (ARNs) contain fibers from: (1) renal mechanoreceptors that are sensitive to alterations in intrarenal pressure produced by ureteral occlusion, renal vein occlusion, increases in renal arterial perfusion pressure, or application of external mechanical stimuli to the kidney, and (2) renal chemoreceptors: R1 chemoreceptors are activated by renal ischemia and R2 chemoreceptors by renal ischemia and changes in the ion composition of the fluid in the renal interstitium.[9] ARNs project to supraspinal structures via two pathways: (1) the dorsal root ganglion and thoracic spinal cord and (2) the vagus nerve to the nodose ganglia. In rats the kidney has more afferent neurons in the nodose ganglia than in the dorsal root ganglia.[10]

Preganglionic neurons to the human kidney are in spinal cord segments T-5 to L-3.[11] The fibers that make up the renal plexus derive from the celiac plexus, the thoracic and lumbar branches of the splanchnic nerves, the superior and inferior mesenteric plexus, the intermesenteric nerves, and the superior hypogastric plexus (also known as the inferior mesenteric ganglion). Renal nerve fibers that enter the kidney come from the renal plexus and course along the renal artery and vein to enter the hilus. Postganglionic adrenergic fibers innervate the arteriolar wall and tubular epithelium in both the proximal and distal tubules.[11]

Decreases in efferent renal sympathetic nerve activity result in decreases in renal tubular solute and water resorption, whereas an increase in renal nerve activity results in increases in solute and water resorption.[11] An increase in efferent renal nerve activity causes renin release via two mechanisms: (1) stimulation of $\beta_1$-adrenoceptors on the juxtaglomerular granular cells or (2) prostaglandin-dependent $\alpha$-adrenoceptor–mediated renal vasoconstriction with subsequent activation of the renal vascular baroreceptor (which responds to changes in afferent arteriole wall tension) and macula densa receptor (which senses changes in the rate of sodium chloride delivery to the distal tubule).[11]

A drop in systemic blood pressure is sensed by the carotid and aortic baroreceptors, and through the vagus nerve to the CNS results in reflex activation of efferent renal nerves.[11] This reflex is lost in SCI, though sympathetic afferent pathways may eventually compensate for lost baroreceptor and vagal pathways that occur following spinal cord transection. Volume expansion decreases efferent renal nerve activity mediated via afferents in the cervical vagus.[11]

SCI has specific effects on urinary excretion of salt and water. Compared to control subjects, quadriplegics have lower urine sodium excretion and lower urine volume[12] but higher urine osmolality. Plasma renin activity and plasma aldosterone levels are higher in both paraplegic and quadriplegic persons than in controls with an intact spinal cord.[12] Paraplegics have greater urinary sodium excretion and urinary potassium excretion and urine osmolality than control subjects or quadriplegics. The cause of the increased sodium and potassium excretion in paraplegic subjects is unknown. Some 5% to 10% of persons with SCI have hypoosmolar hyponatremia, which is generally asymptomatic.[12] The effect of renal mechanisms on blood pressure control is discussed in the following section.

## Cardiovascular Function

Afferent fibers from the heart project via either the sympathetic cardiac nerves or the vagus nerve and are intermingled.[13] Parasympathetic afferent fibers from sensory receptors in the heart have cell bodies in the jugular and nodose ganglia and are conveyed via the cardiac branches of the parasympathetic vagus nerve and project centrally to the nucleus tractus solitarius (NTS). The sympathetic afferents course in the inferior cervical and thoracic sympathetic cardiac nerves, then via white rami communicantes to cell bodies in the dorsal root ganglia (T-1 to T-5). The traditional view is that afferent sympathetic cardiac fibers mediate cardiac nociception and afferent vagal cardiac fibers mediate cardiovascular reflexes.[13] However, vagal afferent fibers may have some role in the mediation of cardiac nociception such as pain referred to the head and neck, and afferent sympathetic fibers may also transmit some cardiovascular reflexes.[13]

Baroreceptors are located in the carotid sinuses and in the walls of the aortic arch. A decrease in arterial blood pressure inhibits firing and a rise in blood pressure increases firing in afferent baroreceptor fibers that are carried in the vagus and glossopharyngeal nerves to the NTS of the medulla.[14] Baroreceptor-mediated sympathoinhibition is predominantly a brain stem reflex mediated via ventral medullary neurons.[15–17] There is also some evidence that baroreceptor inhibition of sympathetic activity can be exerted at the spinal cord level, suggesting that some fibers conveying baroceptor afferent information course directly to the spinal cord.[18,19]

Peripheral chemoreceptors that sense a fall in oxygen or a rise in carbon dioxide are located in the carotid bodies and the aorta and have afferent fibers in the glossopharyngeal and vagus nerves.[14] The brain also has chemoreceptors that sense carbon dioxide. In response to systemic hypoxia, perfusion of vital organs needs to be maintained. Hypoxia results in activation of peripheral chemoreceptors, and hypercapnia results principally in activation of central chemoreceptors.[20] Che-

moreceptor reflexes result in vasoconstriction principally in skeletal muscle vascular beds[21] via activation of the sympathetic adrenergic system.

The medulla oblongata is the most important region in the brain that controls blood pressure.[22] Medullary neurons are critical for: (1) integration of arterial baroreceptor and chemoreceptor reflexes,[23] (2) arterial pressure elevations associated with excitation of somatic afferent fibers in response to pain[24] or to exercise,[25] and (3) the potent increases in sympathetic discharge and arterial pressure produced by either rendering the brain stem ischemic (the cerebral ischemic reflex)[26] or by mechanical distortion (the Cushing reflex).[22,27]

Cardiac preganglionic sympathetic neurons in humans are found in spinal cord segments T-1 to T-4, whereas the preganglionic neurons for the peripheral vasculature are found mainly in spinal cord segments T-1 to L-2.[28] A small proportion of the neurons in the IML column are interneurons.[29] The cholinergic SPNs innervate the adrenal medulla or noradrenergic neurons in sympathetic ganglia, which in turn innervate blood vessels and the heart. The heart is also innervated by three branches of the vagus nerve (superior cervical cardiac, inferior cervical cardiac, thoracic cardiac). Preganglionic efferent parasympathetic axons in these branches form synapses with neurons in the ganglia of the cardiac plexus.

As the autonomic effects associated with increased carbon dioxide are sympathetic responses, quadriplegics would not be expected to show sympathetic responses to increased carbon dioxide because efferent pathways from the brain stem vasomotor center to the SPNs are disruptioned. This supposition is supported by the results of a study of mechanically ventilated quadriplegic subjects.[30] No change in heart rate could be detected in the quadriplegic subjects in response to elevation of carbon dioxide[30]; however, in another study, six quadriplegics with complete lesions above the sympathetic outflow responded to breathing carbon dioxide by increased blood pressure, both in the horizontal and the tilted positions, which suggests either a peripheral or spinal cord effect of hypercapnia.[31]

Disorders of cardiovascular regulation are common following spinal cord injuries that disrupt supraspinal control of thoracic sympathetic outflow. Both hypotension and hypertension can occur, depending on the time after injury and associated complications.

### Mechanisms of Hypotension

After a high spinal cord transection systemic arterial pressure drops,[32] owing to a drop in cardiac output and in total peripheral resistance. Resistances of the muscle and visceral vascular beds is decreased equally.[33] With no connection between the medullary baroreceptor systems and the spinal cord, sympathetic activity cannot be increased to compensate for postural changes.

In contrast to intact subjects, quadriplegics have a lower resting concentration of catecholamines,[34,35] and there is no significant increase in either norepinephrine or epinephrine when quadriplegics change from a lying to a sitting position[34]; this appears to be due to a reduction in norepinephrine release and not to a decrease in norepinephrine clearance.[36] Resting skin blood flow is greater in quadriplegics than in control subjects.[34,37] This is in keeping with observations of diminished resting vasoconstrictor tone and much lower plasma NE levels.

Immediately following cervical spinal cord transection in animals, discharges of cervical, cardiac, hepatic, gastric, adrenal, renal, and lumbar paravertebral chain sympathetic nerves were reduced,[38–42] whereas discharges of mesenteric and splenic nerves were not.[40,42,43] Subsequent removal of afferent input to the spinal cord did not change the rate of the ongoing neural activity, indicating that the spontaneous activity remaining after spinal cord injury was likely generated either within the spinal cord or at ganglionic sites.[44] Pacemaker-type potentials that could produce spontaneous activity have not been observed in SPNs; this suggests that the ongoing activity of SPNs seen after spinal cord transection is instead generated by intraspinal systems extrinsic to the SPN.[29]

The activity in mesenteric sympathetic nerves following acute spinal cord transection in anesthetized cats was not as prominent in decerebrate unanesthetized cats. That suggests that the maintained sympathetic activity noted in the study mentioned previously may have been an artifact of anesthesia,[45] but nevertheless, the level of sympathetic activity that remained after acute spinal cord transection in cats was unable to provide significant vasomotor tone.[44] The firing pattern of mesenteric and other sympathetic nerves, however, changed from a rhythmic, synchronized discharge to a less synchronized one when brain stem descending input was disrupted by spinal cord transection.[41,46,47] It may be that the new desynchronized discharge of SPNs could not support vascular tone adequately, regardless of the magnitude of SPN discharge. A less likely explanation is that the maintained mesenteric nerve activity in anesthetized cats following acute spinal cord transection did not subserve vasomotor functions.[33]

### Mechanisms of Blood Pressure Normalization After Spinal Cord Injury

In humans, orthostatic hypotension occurs after SCI,[48] but after a time the ability to maintain blood pressure in a sitting position improves.[14] Improvement may be due to the development of spinal reflex control of blood pressure or to long-term regulation by renal fluid control. For a recent review, see Cole's.[49]

To investigate the effect of sympathetic activity on blood pressure control, Osborn and coworkers[50] studied spinal cord–transected rats whose (1) sodium and water intake was maintained at pretransection levels, and (2) urine outflow was unobstructed to preserve normal renal function. Arterial pressure was normal by day 9 following the spinal cord transection.[50] Although blood pressure returned to pretransection levels, the heart rate, which had fallen significantly after the spinal lesion, remained low. Two possible explanations for the normalization of arterial pressure are (1) that it is a result of increased vascular sensitivity to a constantly low level of sympathetic activity and (2) that it is due to a steadily increasing level of sympathetic nerve discharge.[50]

To test these hypotheses, Osborn and coworkers recorded changes in arterial pressure in response to injection of phenylephrine into atropinized rats with either cervical spinal cord transection or ganglionic blockade.[50] The results were similar for both groups, indicating that pressor sensitivity at least to exogenous catecholamines does not increase following chronic spinal cord transection in rats. The development of denervation supersensitivity would have increased pressor sensitivity. This lack of increased pressor sensitivity agrees with investigations of adrenergic receptor density in persons with SCI.[51,52] The enhanced pressor response to norepinephrine in humans with cervical SCI reported by Mathias and colleagues[53] may not have been due to denervation sensitivity, as suggested, but may have resulted from the absence of baroreceptor-mediated sympathoinhibition. The lack of denervation supersensitivity following SCI may be due to periodic episodes of sympathetic hyperreflexia.[50]

Before, but not after, spinal cord transection in rats, ganglionic blockade resulted in a profound drop in arterial pressure.[50] This indicates that the normalization of arterial pressure following spinal cord transection in rats cannot be attributed to spinally generated sympathetic activity. Normalization may occur because autoregulatory controllers of blood flow completely dominate within 24 hours following spinal cord transection, with the result that any remaining sympathetic vasoconstrictor activity is without effect. Hypotension following spinal cord transection may therefore be principally the result of a decrease in sympathetic activity to vascular beds with relatively weak autoregulatory properties, such as skin and skeletal muscle.[50]

The development of spasticity may contribute to the recovery of arterial pressure owing to increased central venous volume resulting from enhanced venous return and to physical compression on the arterial side of the skeletal muscle beds, which would increase vascular resistance.[50]

The vasoconstrictor activity of the renin-angiotensin system and arginine vasopressin (AVP), as well as renal sympathetic nerve activity, all may enhance renal retention of sodium and water, which would influence arterial pressure in the longterm. Research findings show that quadriplegic persons have increased plasma renin levels and high normal aldosterone levels,[12,48] probably owing to renin release by the juxtaglomerular cells in response to the decreased renal perfusion that accompanies low arterial pressures.[54] Renin acts on angiotensinogen in the plasma, forming angiotensin, which is converted to angiotensin II, a major vasoconstricting hormone. Increased release

of aldosterone is probably a direct effect of the increased serum renin level.[14]

Over a period as short as 12 to 36 hours following spinal cord transection in dogs, baseline arterial pressure has been shown to be directly related to the level of salt and water intake.[55] Following spinal cord transection, rats were in part dependent on angiotensin II vasoconstrictor activity for maintenance of arterial pressure.[50] Long-term quadriplegics exhibit decreased urinary sodium excretion and expansion of the extracellular fluid compartment.[56,57]

The secretion of AVP by the posterior pituitary gland is predominantly controlled by (1) changes in plasma osmolality, which are sensed by osmoreceptors in the hypothalamus, and (2) changes in blood volume and blood pressure relayed from cardiovascular receptors in the carotid sinus and thorax via the glossopharyngeal and vagal cranial nerves to the NTS and thence to the paraventricular and supraoptic nuclei of the hypothalamus.[58] No differences in resting levels of AVP have been identified between control and quadriplegic subjects.[58] Infusion of hypertonic saline causes plasma AVP to rise in both control and quadriplegic subjects; however, at any given level of plasma osmolality, plasma AVP tended to be higher in the quadriplegics than in the control subjects.[12] Unlike control subjects, quadriplegics demonstrated an increase in mean arterial pressure (MAP) without an increase in heart rate as a result of hypertonic saline infusion. In quadriplegics water loading resulted in normal suppression of urine osmolality but subnormal free water clearance during maximal water diuresis, despite appropriately suppressed levels of plasma AVP.[12] Plasma AVP increased following head-up tilt in both control and quadriplegic subjects, but the increase was significantly greater in the quadriplegic group.[58] These studies indicate that quadriplegics have normal cardiovascular and osmotic control of AVP secretion. The increase in postural release of AVP may be responsible for the oliguria seen in persons with SCI after prolonged sitting.[58]

Infusion of AVP did not change MAP or heart rate in control subjects but did result in a marked rise in MAP and bradycardia in quadriplegics. The bradycardic effect of AVP in quadriplegics was probably the result of baroreflex activation of the intact vagal efferents secondary to the rise in MAP.

The reason for the pressor response is not clear; it may have been due to increased sensitivity to peripheral pressor vascular effects of AVP or because baroreflex-mediated inhibition of sympathetic tone was interrupted by the spinal cord lesion.[58]

In control subjects and in persons with SCI below the L-1 level, blood pressure rises with sitting and is lower when they are recumbent. In quadriplegics, blood pressure is lower when sitting than when lying down.[12] This rise in blood pressure during recumbency has been attributed to fluid shifts into the central compartment and subsequent increased venous return and stroke volume. This expansion of central blood volume after recumbency and the accompanying elevation in blood pressure inhibiting the release of AVP may explain the diuresis associated with recumbency in quadriplegics,[59] an effect that is not observed in either paraplegic persons or intact ones.

### Mechanism of Autonomic Hyperreflexia

Autonomic hyperreflexia (AH, also known as *autonomic dysreflexia*) is manifested by hypertension, sweating, headache, and bradycardia[49,60,61] and is most often associated with SCI at or above the T-6 level. This disorder is reported to affect 30% to 90% of quadriplegics and high paraplegics.[62] In individuals with SCI common sources of afferent stimulation that result in AH include bladder distension, pressure sores, childbirth, and rectal distension.[63] Afferent input enters the spinal cord below the level of the spinal cord lesion and projects to the IML cell column via propriospinal pathways. The spinal sympathetic pathways linking the supraspinal cardiovascular centers with the peripheral sympathetic outflow are interrupted at the level of the injury, but the parasympathetic efferent pathways through the vagus nerve, as well as the afferent arc of the baroreceptor reflex through the glossopharyngeal and vagus nerves, are intact after SCI. Bradycardia results from activation of efferents in the vagus nerve coursing to the sinoatrial node. Descending sympathoinhibitory projections through the spinal cord that would normally result in vasodilatation are disrupted by SCI, and the bradycardia alone is not adequate to reduce blood pressure. Treatment requires that the eliciting cause be eliminated or that pharmacologic treatment be instituted. Pharmacologic treatment is aimed primarily at producing direct vasodilatation (calcium-channel blockers, nitrates, hydralazine, diazoxide) or ganglionic blockade (mecamylamine).[64]

Spinal cord transection sometimes results in increased sympathetic responses to afferent stimulation or in decreased sympathetic responses to a given afferent stimulation.[29] For example, in intact rats nonnoxious stimulation of the chest wall decreased adrenal nerve activity and decreased adrenal catecholamine secretion, whereas noxious stimulation of the chest elicited increases in adrenal nerve activity and adrenal catecholamine secretion. After spinal cord transection both stimuli increased adrenal nerve activity. Spinal cord transection therefore converted a previously sympathoinhibitory response to a nonnoxious stimulus into a sympathoexcitatory one.[29]

Spinal sympathoexcitatory reflexes, which are under such strong supraspinal inhibition that they are not observable in some intact animals, may become evident after spinal cord transection. Studies in rats demonstrated a spinal component of the somatosympathetic reflex in both intact and spinal cord–transected animals. The spinal component of the reflex was sometimes difficult to demonstrate in intact animals, and in fact the spinal component of some sympathetic reflexes appeared to be under tonic inhibition by supraspinal systems.[29] Sympathetic hyperactivity after spinal cord transection may be due as much to disinhibition of sensory pathways as to direct disinhibition of the sympathetic systems themselves.

Research has shown that activation by capsaicin of chemo-and mechanoreceptors in the small intestine, peripheral vasculature, or urinary bladder of rats produces a depressant response in cardiovascular SPNs.[65] However bladder distension or intravesical capsaicin (which activates afferent C fibers[66]) in spinal cord–transected rats activated a reflex excitatory response conveyed by pelvic nerve afferents that probably involved activation of SPNs via propriospinal pathways.[65] Altered reflex responses in SPNs may account for the massive autonomic hyperreflexia displayed by quadriplegic persons, particularly responses to stimuli arising from the rectum and urinary bladder.

There are problems to consider in studying sympathetic regulation organized in a spinal model.[29] Following acute SCI, experimental results may be obscured by spinal shock. In chronic SCI the system the researcher studies may not be the spinal component of normal sympathetic regulation but a new system formed by regeneration and plasticity.[29]

### Other Cardiovascular

Although the most important sequelae of autonomic cardiovascular dysfunction following SCI are related to disorders of blood pressure control,[49] recent studies have identified additional alterations in cardiovascular function in persons with high SCI. Those dysfunctions may be attributed to autonomic nervous system dysfunction. For a recent review of cardiovascular control following SCI see Mathias and Frankel.[67]

In contrast to normal subjects and those with normal variant ST segment elevation, quadriplegic subjects have been found to have significant multilead ST elevation on electrocardiography (ECG)[68] that is not altered by exercise. Persons with acute severe injury to the cervical spinal cord have an increased incidence of ventricular and supraventricular arrhythmias and cardiac arrest, but the arrhythmogenic state does not extend into the chronic injury period.[68] The maximal heart rate during arm exercise has been reported to be significantly lower for quadriplegic than for paraplegic subjects.[69] Significantly lower values for stroke volume, cardiac output, and cardiac index were obtained for both paraplegic and quadriplegic groups when compared to the observed values for the control group without SCI. Quadriplegic subjects have even lower values for stroke volume and cardiac output than paraplegic ones. These differences may have been due to reduced sympathetic stimulation, but other factors resulting from a lower metabolic rate and smaller active skeletal muscle mass are probably involved.[70]

## Pulmonary Function

Pulmonary problems are common following SCI. They are secondary to impairments in inspiratory and expiratory function, with associated abnormalities in gas exchange that are largely the result of ineffective cough mechanisms. The muscles of respiration are of three groups: (1) the diaphragm, (2) the intercostals and accessory muscles of respiration, and (3) the abdominal muscles.[71] The diaphragm is innervated by the phrenic nerve (C-3 to C-5) and is the principal muscle of respiration. The intercostal muscles are innervated from the corresponding thoracic segments of the spinal cord. Secondary respiratory muscles are the muscles attached to the ribs, such as sternocleidomastoid and the scalene, that do not usually function in respiration but are called upon to provide for hyperventilation in normal subjects or ventilation in subjects with cardiorespiratory dysfunction. Abdominal muscles are predominantly expiratory as far as respiratory function is concerned.

Following SCI, the supraspinal respiratory centers in the brain stem continue to function normally, so that impairment in respiratory function is largely determined by the level of the SCI. In acute quadriplegia, inspiratory capacity is decreased about 40%, and diminished expiratory capacity results in severe impairment of coughing.[72] Long-term quadriplegics have been found to have significantly lower values for tidal volume, forced vital capacity (FVC), forced expiratory volume in 1 second ($FEV_{1.0}$), and maximum breathing capacity than either paraplegics or control subjects in response to maximal arm exercise.[70]

The effect of afferent input on parameters of respiration has been investigated in SCI subjects. Normally, ventilatory drive is increased by hypercapnia (primarily via central chemoreceptor stimulation) and hypoxia (primarily via peripheral chemoreceptor stimulation).[20] In quadriplegics, the central respiratory centers appear to respond normally to hypercapnia and hypoxia. The control of a range of ventilatory responses—tidal volume, respiratory frequency, inspiratory and expiratory durations, and mean inspiratory airflow—does not appear to require afferent pathways from the rib cage and intercostal muscles.[73] Sensory input from the mouth, lung, or diaphragm has been shown to be sufficient to modulate the duration, intensity, and timing of the phrenic nerve discharge during the first loaded breath in quadriplegic subjects.[73] A group of ventilated quadriplegics detected changes in tidal volume of as little as 100 ml just as well as did a group of ventilated control subjects.[74] The sensory information that allowed the quadriplegic group to detect changes in lung volume probably arose from visceral lung afferents that project to the CNS in the vagus nerve. Sensation of the need to cough and of congestion has been reported to remain after high cervical spinal cord lesions.[74] It has also been shown that ventilated quadriplegic subjects can reliably perceive an increase in $P_{CO_2}$ in the physiologic range as an uncomfortable sense of "air hunger."[30] Quadriplegics describe the sensation of air hunger as coming from the chest.[30]

## Temperature Regulation

The classical cold and warm sensors are located in the hypothalamus and the skin; however, there is evidence of mesencephalic, medullary, spinal, and intraabdominal temperature sensors.[75] Afferent fibers from peripheral warm and cold receptors with cell bodies in the dorsal root ganglia enter the spinal cord and ascend contralaterally to the medial lemniscus and thalamus and have further projections to the hypothalamus.[76] The preoptic area of the hypothalamus is implicated as the generator of the thermal set-point and central integrator of thermoregulatory responses.[76] Efferents from the hypothalamus control thermoregulatory vasomotor and sudomotor tone as well as nonshivering and shivering thermogenesis via descending noradrenergic and cholinergic fibers. These exit the spinal cord below C-7.[76]

Impairment of temperature regulation is a recognized hazard for persons with SCI.[77] The failure of temperature regulation following SCI occurs because of deficits in the balancing mechanisms of heat production and heat loss. These mechanisms consist of peripheral and central control systems (see Chapter 13 for details of normal human temperature control).

Cooling the skin—regardless of whether central body temperature changes—causes increased heat production via shivering.[78] In paraplegics, deep or central temperature receptors sensitive to cold are also able to initiate shivering above the level of the SCI, and these receptors can act independently of the temperature of the skin above the SCI.[78] Researchers have postulated that in normal humans these central cold receptors may be a backup mechanism that comes into play if there is a loss

or diminution of skin cold receptor reflex activity.[78] In humans shivering does not occur below the level of a complete SCI, and therefore shivering is thought not to be a spinal reflex.[79] In dogs that had high spinal cord transections, a clearly visible shiverlike muscle tremor was induced below the level of spinal cord transection by spinal cord cooling, but the tremor was less intense in the spinal cord–transected dog than in the pretransection state.[76] This suggests that spinal cord cold sensors are present in this species and are activated when there is sufficient cooling.

An important mechanism controlling heat transfer from the body core to the surface is the adjustment of cutaneous blood flow.[75] Cooling of peripheral or central areas results in a reduction of skin blood flow and a simultaneous increase in flow to central vascular regions.[75] In control subjects, cooling or warming of one hand elicits a cutaneous vasomotor response of the contralateral hand and both legs.[80] Several investigations have failed to observe a similar cutaneous vasomotor response below the level of SCI.[80–83]; others have observed vasomotor responses below the level of SCI in both primates and humans.[83–85] Tsai and coworkers[83] reported that all vasomotor responses to cooling or warming in the paraplegic lower extremities of men were absent following acute SCI (T-5 to T-11). The vasomotor responses in the intact upper extremities were not altered. By 4 months after injury the ipsilateral local vasomotor responses to warming and cooling in the paraplegic lower extremities returned to normal, and by 18 months after injury, the crossed vasomotor reflex to cooling and warming recovered to normal.

The most important mechanisms of heat loss in humans are vasodilatation, sweating, and behavioral aspects—choice of posture, amount of clothing, altering ambient temperature. Conscious control of behavior depends on sensory appreciation of temperature. In one study, paraplegic subjects did feel hot as their oral temperature was raised 1° to 1.5°C by heating insensate skin.[86] However, in the case of one T-8 paraplegic, researchers reported that a fall in central temperature to 36.2°C was not associated with a conscious appreciation of cold.[87] The perception of warm and cold after SCI appears to depend on the temperature of the sentient skin.

The primary and principal stimulus that elicits the thermoregulatory sweating response is a change in core temperature.[88] Sweat glands receive dual innervation by both cholinergic and adrenergic fibers and are stimulated by cholinergic, $\alpha$-adrenergic, and $\beta$-adrenergic agonists; however, cholinergic stimulation provokes the largest response.[89] Spinal segments T-2 to T-4 supply sweat glands on the head and neck, T-2 to T-8 to glands of the upper limbs, T-6 to T-10 to the trunk, and T-11 to L-2 to the lower extremities.[89] Normell[90] provides an outline of the segmental arrangement of the thermoregulatory vasomotor innervation of the skin of the trunk and lower extremities. Autonomic dermatomes overlap several segments above and below the somatic level. Spinal lesions are associated with anhidrosis below the level of the lesion.[88,89] Normal evaporative cooling is still maintained in persons with spinal injury by increased compensatory sweating from sentient skin.[89,91]

Paraplegic men have been shown to have significant differences in skin blood flow response to hyperthermia when compared to intact control subjects.[86] When only insensate skin was heated (to 40°C) in paraplegic subjects, little or no increases in forearm blood flow (FBF) occurred, even with an elevation of oral temperature of 1° to 1.5°C over 59 to 71 minutes, though the subjects exhibited mild sweating on the upper body. In contrast, a normal subject exhibited vigorous vaso- and sudomotor responses to the same pattern of heating that was given to the paraplegic. In fact, the thermoregulatory responses of the normal subject were so effective it was impossible to push oral temperature above 37.5°C when lower body skin temperature heating was limited to 40°C. With whole-body heating of paraplegics, all but one exhibited sweating above the level of the spinal cord lesion, and FBF increased in all subjects. However, the increase in FBF in the paraplegic subjects was less than that reported for hyperthermic spinal cord–intact men. Freund and coworkers[86] suggested that one reason for the attenuated response of FBF to whole-body heating was diminished thermoregulatory effector outflow resulting from the diminished afferent input which, after SCI, could originate only from above the level of the lesion. Tam and colleagues[92] reached a similar conclusion. They reported that a person with T-6 paraplegia

had to achieve a higher core temperature threshold (37.2° to 37.9°C) to generate sweating and related vasodilatation responses, compared to the core temperature threshold (36.2° to 37.1°C) of a normal control subject. It can be concluded that paraplegic men appear to exhibit markedly attenuated skin blood flow in response to hyperthermia and thus are limited in their ability to dissipate excess heat.[86]

Another approach to the study of thermoregulation is to record the activity of vasoconstrictor and sudomotor impulses via microelectrodes in sympathetic skin nerves.[93] In quadriplegics, sympathetic skin nerve recordings from below the level of the lesion made while ambient temperature was varied demonstrated no changes in sympathetic outflow despite cooling that reduced tympanic temperature 2°C.[94] During this study, abdominal pressure over the bladder, as well as mechanical and electrical skin stimulation applied distal to the level of SCI, induced bursts of neural impulses recorded in the sympathetic skin nerve fascicles also below the level of SCI, indicating the presence of spinal vesicosympathetic and somatosympathetic reflexes. It has long been noted that increases in urinary bladder pressure elicit an increase in arterial blood pressure in quadriplegics.[95] Of note is that reflex vasoconstriction (below the level of SCI) induced by suprapubic pressure is prolonged during body cooling. The finding of increased vasoconstriction during cooling in persons with SCI may therefore not be a thermoregulatory response but simply an artifact induced by facilitation of vesicosympathetic reflexes.[94] This argues against the presence of physiologically significant spinal sympathetic thermoregulatory reflexes.

## Gastrointestinal Function

### Upper Gastrointestinal Tract

The stomach and intestinal wall contain intrinsic neurons that are part of the enteric nervous system, a system that has been referred to as the third division of the autonomic nervous system. It is noteworthy that there are as many neurons in the enteric nervous system ($10^8$) as there are in the spinal cord.[96] The enteric nervous system has two divisions: (1) the submucosal plexus (Meissner's plexus), which innervates the mucosa and regulates secretion, and (2) the myenteric plexus (Auerbach's plexus), which innervates the circular and longitudinal smooth muscle layers and regulates motility. The two plexuses communicate through interconnecting nerves. The enteric nervous system has three types of nerve cells: (1) motor neurons that innervate smooth muscle cells, (2) interneurons that connect different neurons, and (3) afferent neurons. Excitatory motor neurons of the enteric nervous system are cholinergic and so release the neurotransmitter acetylcholine. Inhibitory motor neurons are noncholinergic and nonadrenergic, and it is postulated that the putative neurotransmitters adenosine triphosphate and vasoactive intestinal peptide mediate the inhibition.[97]

Of the nerve fibers in the abdominal vagus, 80% or more are afferents with cell bodies in the nodose ganglia.[97] Mucosal afferent fibers arise from polymodal as well as selective receptors in the small intestine and stomach that respond to mechanical stimuli such as gentle stroking of the epithelium or chemical stimulation.[98] Thermoreceptors have also been identified in the cat duodenum and stomach.[99] Three types of chemoreceptors found in the small intestine are likely responsible for feedback control of gastric emptying by nutrients; they are osmoreceptors, lipid receptors, and receptors for amino acids.[98] Glucoreceptors and Ph receptors are also present in the small intestine. How stimulation of intestinal receptors mediates changes in gastric emptying has not been entirely resolved. In addition to mucosal afferent receptors there are also vagal afferents with receptors in the gastric, duodenal, and jejunal smooth muscle that respond to distension and contraction of the viscus.[99] The splanchnic nerves, which convey afferents from the gut to the spinal cord, are thought to mediate painful sensations, although vagus nerve afferents may also be involved in gut nociception.[99]

The sensation of hunger is reduced in vagotomized patients, but it is not eliminated, perhaps because the hypothalamus monitors the levels of circulating nutrients.[99] A detailed account of abdominal nociception, satiety, and appetite in high SCI patients would provide valuable information on the contribution of spinal afferents to these sensations.

The extrinsic innervation of the stomach and small intestine occurs through the parasympathetic and sympathetic divisions of the autonomic nervous system. In the abdomen, the parasympathetic preganglionic efferent fibers to the stomach are conveyed in the vagus nerve, which in turn gives rise to gastric branches that form synapses with neurons in the myenteric and the submucosal plexuses of the stomach.

Preganglionic sympathetic efferent fibers originate in the mediolateral gray matter of the spinal cord and course through the splanchnic nerves to the celiac and superior mesenteric plexuses. The stomach receives sympathetic postganglionic fibers principally from the celiac plexus but also from the left phrenic plexus, bilateral gastric and hepatic plexuses, and the sympathetic trunk. Postganglionic sympathetic efferent nerves emerge from the celiac and superior mesenteric prevertebral ganglia to run along mesenteric blood vessels and innervate the small intestine.

The vagus nerve is important for the motor activity of the stomach. The fundus of the stomach acts as a reservoir to accommodate the meal while the antrum is both a pump and a grinder. Vagal stimulation induces relaxation of the fundus and contraction of the antrum.[98] Mesenteric sympathetic nerve stimulation inhibits contraction in the small intestine.[98] The motor activity of the stomach and small intestine probably is modulated by reflexes with afferent and efferent components in the prevertebral ganglia without involving higher centers, as well as by reflexes with afferent and efferent components in the vagus nerve.

In the normal gastrointestinal tract of humans a cyclic wave begins in the stomach and duodenum and migrates to the terminal ileum. This activity, characterized by recurring periods of intense regular motor activity, is known as phase III of the interdigestive motor complex (IDMC).[100,101] The IDMC usually begins in the antrum and migrates to the proximal duodenum in a coordinated manner that is interrupted by feeding. Regulation of the IDMC is different for the antrum and small bowel. In the stomach, extrinsic nerves[102] and hormones[103] seem to be important influences, whereas the small bowel appears capable of generating its own IDMC as long as intrinsic neural elements are intact.[104,105]

In humans, gastric distension and ileus occur immediately after traumatic spinal cord transection, suggesting abnormal gastrointestinal motility.[106] In long-term quadriplegics an intact supraspinal sympathetic pathway is not an absolute requirement for initiation and propagation of antral phase III motor activity,[105] as there are no significant differences in the duration of phases of the IDMC, cycle length of the duodenal IDMC, or the propagation velocity of phase III of the IDMC from the duodenum to the jejunum[105] between subjects with quadriplegia (neurologic level above T-1), low paraplegia (neurologic level below T-10), or an intact spinal cord. In normal subjects 90% of phase IIIs originated in the antrum and migrated to the duodenum and jejunum, whereas in subjects with high SCI, fewer than 40% of their phase IIIs originated in the antrum. Some 80% of quadriplegic subjects had dissociation between antral and duodenal phase III motility manifested primarily as a pattern of persistent antral activity. In one subject with prominent recurrent autonomic hyperreflexia there was marked antral hypomotility. Antral quiescence was associated with the degree of reflex vascular hypertension resulting from spontaneous and suprapubic pressure-induced autonomic hyperreflexia, whereas duodenal motility was unaffected.[105] This suggests that motility in the antrum is modified by central sympathetic input and that excessive splanchnic sympathetic outflow may delay gastric emptying by inhibiting antral motility.[105] Sympathetic activity may influence gastric motility via a direct neural pathway to the gut wall or via indirect pathways that modulate the release of polypeptide gastrointestinal hormones.[105]

In dogs, a similar cyclic phenomenon characterizes the fasting pattern of myoelectric activity known as the migrating myoelectric complex (MMEC).[107] As each MMEC migrates distally, four distinct phases of activity are evident. One of these phases, phase III of the MMEC, is a period of intense spike activity usually lasting 5 minutes. During phase III of an MMEC in the stomach and duodenum, plasma levels of the endogenous hormone motilin reach peak concentration while infusion of motilin initiates phase III of the MMEC, suggesting that motilin is the hormone that controls initiation of phase III.[108] The so-called fed pattern

of myoelectric activity is characterized by an irregular pattern of spike activity. In dogs, after spinal cord transection the only long-term changes in the fed and fasted patterns of myoelectric activity in the stomach and small intestine is that the gastric component of the MMEC is shorter-lived.[108] In the early post–spinal cord transection period there were obvious disruptions of myoelectric activity in both the stomach and duodenum, but not in the jejunum and ileum. In the dog it took an average of 10 (range 1 to 36) days after spinal cord transection before normal MMECs returned to the duodenum, and 14 (range 40 to 50) days before MMEC-like myoelectric activity returned to the stomach. During the first 14 days after spinal cord transection gastric myoelectric activity resembled a fed pattern. There is evidence that the short-term changes seen in dogs persist longer in humans after SCI.[105]

Antral activity is limited in normal subjects fed a liquid meal, whereas two of five quadriplegics investigated had persistent antral motor activity after feeding.[105] The cumulative gastric emptying of all five quadriplegic subjects was reduced at 60 minutes postprandially, compared to subjects with paraplegia or with an intact spinal cord.[105] Paraplegics have been reported to have delayed gastric emptying, but this appears to be a nonspecific finding related to prolonged immobilization (see Chapter 17.)[109]

### Lower Gastrointestinal Tract

Vagal afferents supply the small intestine and the proximal two thirds of the colon coinciding with the vagal efferent innervation.[99] Vagal afferents respond to distension and contraction of the colon. It is probable that the colon has vagal mucosal mechanoreceptors and chemoreceptors as well, but further investigation is needed[99] before definitive statements can be made. Other afferent fibers from the colon travel with both sympathetic and parasympathetic axons and have cell bodies in the lumbar and sacral dorsal root ganglia; in addition, some afferents have cell bodies in the wall of the colon and project their axons centrally.[3]

The parasympathetic outflow to the colon and anorectum originates from brain stem nuclei and the sacral spinal cord. The ascending and transverse colon receives parasympathetic efferent fibers from the posterior vagus nerve, and the left half of the colon and rectum receives them from the pelvic nerve.[110] Preganglionic parasympathetic neurons project from the sacral segments S-2 to S-5 through the pelvic nerves and pass to the left colon and anorectum via the pelvic plexus.[3]

The sympathetic supply to the right colon arises from T-6 to T-12 and that to the left colon and upper rectum arises from L-1 to L-3.[110] Sympathetic preganglionic neurons to the colon and pelvic viscera send fibers through the lumbar splanchnic nerves to the superior and inferior mesenteric ganglion (IMG).[3] Postganglionic fibers from the superior mesenteric ganglion innervate the colon from the cecum to the distal transverse colon. Lumbar colonic nerves arise from the IMG and run along the inferior mesenteric artery to innervate the left side of the colon and the hypogastric nerves, which also arise from the IMG, join the pelvic plexus[3] (known as the *inferior hypogastric plexus*) to innervate the distal colon. Other sympathetic preganglionic axons enter paravertebral chain ganglia and form synapses with postganglionic neurons there (see Figure 4-11).[111]

Preganglionic sympathetic neurons projecting fibers into the lumbar splanchnic nerves are visceral vasoconstrictor neurons and motility-regulating (MR) neurons. Electrical stimulation of the sympathetic supply to the colon results in contraction of the internal anal sphincter and relaxation of the colon and rectum.[3] Transection of the low thoracic spinal cord in cats demonstrates that there is little spinal shock for the MR neurons, in comparison to the vasoconstrictor system.[3] The patterns of reflex discharge of MR neurons are determined within the lumbosacral spinal cord.[3]

Some postganglionic neurons directly innervate vascular or visceral smooth muscle. Other postganglionic neurons control the effector organs indirectly by influencing other peripheral neurons such as those in the submucosal ganglia (Meissner's plexus) or myenteric ganglia (Auerbach's plexus) of the enteric nervous system or in the prevertebral ganglia, via pre- or postsynaptic mechanisms.[110] The majority of lumbar sympathetic postganglionic neurons are noradrenergic, but many contain a peptide as well.[112] Sympathetic ganglia receive synaptic input from (1) preganglionic neurons with cell bodies in the spinal cord, (2) primary sensory neurons with cell bodies in the dorsal root ganglia, and (3) neurons arising in visceral intramural ganglia. The apparent convergence of multiple synaptic inputs onto individual principal ganglionic neurons suggests that the outflow from these neurons is the result of integration of synaptic information from several sources.[113] Therefore, it is reasonable to conclude that the peripheral autonomic nervous system may mediate complex reflex functions of the gastrointestinal system without the involvement of either supraspinal or spinal cord influences.

Research indicates that the lumbar sympathetic outflow exerts a tonic inhibitory influence on the motility of the colon. Studies in rats show that there is differential sympathetic inhibition of the proximal, transverse, and distal colon.[114] The distal colon receives a tonic inhibitory influence with a supraspinal organization, the transverse colon receives a tonic inhibitory influence with a spinal organization, and the proximal colon appears to be influenced by neither spinal nor supraspinal tonic inhibition.

The autonomic nervous system provides both the defecation reflex and the gastrocolic reflex. When food is ingested into the stomach there is an increase in colonic motor activity that is called the gastrocolic reflex.[115] The afferent limb of this reflex can be blocked by intragastric lidocaine, and the increase in distal colonic spike activity can be blocked by anticholinergics or naloxone, indicating participation of cholinergic and opiate receptors. The defecation reflex is the increase in rectal motor activity and the relaxation of the internal anal sphincter in response to rectal distension with an afferent and efferent component in the pelvic nerve.

Colonic cyclical organization in the rat, including enhancement of distal colonic cyclical activity as a secondary response to feeding (gastrocolic reflex), persists after ablation or section of the spinal cord.[114] This demonstrates that—at least for the distal colon—colonic cyclical organization is not initiated by lumbar spinal or supraspinal influences. The local enteric nervous system or the prevertebral ganglionic system, or both, are probably responsible for the cyclical organization of distal colonic motility in rats. However, the gastrocolic reflex in the transverse colon persists in rats after spinal cord transection but not after spinal cord ablation, suggesting that it was organized in the spinal cord.[114]

Analysis of colonic myoelectric spike activity of the rectal mucosa 6 to 15 cm from the anus revealed that in the fasting state persons with SCI above T-10 who were also more than three months post injury had significantly greater basal colonic myoelectric spike activity than control subjects.[116] Meal stimulation increased basal spike activity (gastrocolic reflex) in the control group compared to the fasting state. In the spinal cord–injured group there was no significant increase in myoelectric spike activity after the meal, compared to the fasting state. Because feeding did not significantly increase the already high basal spike activity of persons with SCI, the gastrocolic reflex could not be demonstrated. The loss of a tonic inhibitory supraspinal influence may cause the increase in basal colonic spike activity following SCI.[116] The absence of a gastrocolic reflex in this study is consistent with studies by Glick and colleagues,[117] who recorded at 12 to 18 cm from the anus, but the findings differ from those of the study of Connell and associates[118] who recorded intact gastrocolic reflexes at 15, 20, and 25 cm from the anus.[110]

After low thoracic spinal cord transection in cats, the defecation reflex remained intact and the resulting rectal motor activity was of greater amplitude than before spinal cord transection.[116] The defecation reflex in the cat was not present after transection of the pelvic nerves. Intact defecation reflexes are also identified in humans with or without SCI. Normal internal anal sphincter relaxation occurs after rectal distension in individuals with SCI above T-10 as well as in subjects without SCI.[116] Reflex contraction of the external anal sphincter is also mediated by a spinal reflex.[110]

The most obvious gastrointestinal consequence of SCI is the loss of voluntary control of the initiation of defecation. The most common problems complicating the neurogenic bowel are poorly localized abdominal pain (in 14% of cases studies by Stone's group), difficulty with bowel evacuation (20%), hemorrhoids (74%), abdominal distension (43%), and autonomic hyperreflexia arising from the gastrointestinal tract (43%).[119] As many as 27% of persons with SCI have significant chronic gastrointestinal problems, and those with more complete injuries are more likely to have symptoms (33%) than those with incomplete injuries (6%).[119] In persons with complete SCI above T-12 transit of contents is slowed throughout the large bowel, regardless of the level of the spinal cord lesion.[120] Delay of transit of contents was more marked in the descending colon, sigmoid, and rectum than in the cecum, ascending colon, and transverse colon.[120]

## Sexual Function

The penis receives innervation from both somatic and autonomic pathways.[121–124] Somatic afferent innervation to penile skin is carried in a terminal branch of the pudendal nerve called the dorsal nerve of the penis (DNP).[125] The penile and pelvic nerves also convey part of the sensory innervation to the urethra, rectum, and anus in male rats.[126]

In humans, sympathetic preganglionic fibers from T-11 to L-2 and parasympathetic preganglionic fibers from S-2 to S-4 are involved in erection and ejaculation.[127] Parasympathetic preganglionic fibers from the sacral spinal cord project in the pelvic nerve to the pelvic plexus.[123,125] One pathway for sympathetic preganglionic fibers to the penis is from the thoracolumbar spinal cord through the paravertebral chain ganglia to project via (1) the pelvic nerve and plexus into the penile nerve (also known as the cavernous nerve) or (2) the pudendal nerve to the penis.[121–123,125,128] The other pathway for sympathetic preganglionic fibers is through the lumbar splanchnic nerves to the IMG.[123,125] Postganglionic fibers from neurons in the IMG as well as preganglionic fibers project through the hypogastric nerves to the pelvic plexus.[129] Sympathetic and parasympathetic postganglionic efferent fibers project from the pelvic plexus to the penis via the penile nerves.

Physiologic activation of afferent pathways in the DNP elicits multiple sexual responses, including penile erection, seminal emission, and ejaculation.[130–133] In rats, stimulation of afferent fibers in the DNP or pelvic nerve has been shown to elicit reflexes in the penile nerve.[125] These reflexes on the penile nerve were mediated at the spinal cord level, since acute spinal cord transection failed to eliminate the responses.[125] The penile nerve contains a mixture of parasympathetic and sympathetic postganglionic axons that produce vas-odilatation of arteries supplying the corpus caver-nosum, resulting in penile tumescence.[125,128] This nerve also contains sympathetic vasoconstrictor axons that produce detumescence.[123,124,134] In the human male, the penile nerves travel just lateral to the vascular structures that are located poster-olateral to the prostate gland at about the 10–o'clock and 2–o'clock positions.[135] Erection involves parasympathetic cholinergic and sym-pathetic noncholinergic nonadrenergic mecha-nisms.[136] Vasoactive intestinal peptide has been implicated as a mediator of the noncholinergic nonadrenergic mechanism of erection.[136,137] It is known to relax smooth muscle from the human penis.[129,137] It has been shown that 92% of penile postganglionic neurons are positive for vasoactive intestinal peptide and 95% of penile postganglionic neurons have high levels of acetylcholinester-ase.[129] Acetylcholine may contribute to erection by inhibiting the effects of norepinephrine on pe-nile smooth muscle.[138] It may also relax smooth muscle via a direct action of muscarinic receptors on the smooth muscle, or by its action on vascular endothelium to release endothelium-derived relax-ing factor.[122]

The phenomenon of psychogenic erections in paraplegics with complete sacral lower motor neu-ron lesions and abolished reflexogenic erections indicates that a pathway for erection from the sym-pathetic outflow exists.[127] Reflex erections are me-diated via the sacral parasympathetics with afferent input from the pudendal nerve, and they are or-ganized in the sacral spinal cord.[127] More than two thirds of persons with complete SCI have some form of reflex penile erection.[139,140]

Emission of semen and seminal fluid is primar-ily under sympathetic control. Emission is fol-lowed by closure of the bladder neck and contrac-tion of the bulbourethral striated muscles, the latter being mediated by pudendal somatic efferents.[127] Some 5% to 10% of men with complete SCI ex-perience ejaculation or seminal emission.[127,139,140] For purposes of obtaining semen for artificial in-semination, an ejaculation reflex can be obtained by vibratory stimulation of the frenulum and lower surface of the glans penis.[141] The afferent pathway of this ejaculation reflex likely involves the pu-dendal nerves (DNP) and ascending tracts from the sacral spinal cord to the thoracolumbar T-12 to L-1 preganglionic sympathetic nerves.[139,142]

Testosterone levels have been shown to be nor-mal or slightly elevated in men with long-term SCI.[142,143] Levels of FSH and LH in young para-plegic subjects did not show evidence of primary testicular failure.[142,144]

Much less is known about sexual function in females with SCI than in males.[145] It is clear that a woman's libido and reproductive capability re-main intact following SCI.[146] There is transient anovulation in about 50% of women with SCI, but the preinjury menstrual pattern is reestablished in 3 to 6 months.[145–148] Mean menstrual cycle length and the duration of menses have been shown to fall within the normal range for fertile, able-bodied women, regardless of level or completeness of injury.[147] Menarche is not delayed if the SCI is preadolescent. Anovulation is thought to be a re-sult of the stress of the trauma and is not related to the level of injury or its degree of completeness.

The four components of the sexual response cycle—excitement, plateau, orgasm, and reso-lution[149]—are all present but may vary in degree in women with SCI.[145,146] The normal female sex-ual excitation phase consists of vaginal lubrication, swelling of the clitoral gland, and congestion of the labia.[145] With complete SCI there is absence of lubrication (reflex or psychogenic) when the injury is situated between T-10 and T-12 indicating that preganglionic neurons at this level of the spinal cord constitute the final efferent pathway for both reflex and centrally mediated lubrica-tion.[145] Reflex lubrication does occur with lesions above T-9 and psychogenic lubrication is present with injuries below T-12.[145]

The fertility rate and miscarriage rate are the same for women with SCI as for the general pop-ulation of sexually active women.[146] Pain in the first stage of labor is due to uterine contraction and cervical dilatation.[146] Since the afferent inner-vation of the uterus arises from T-10 to L-1, labor is painless for women with an SCI above T-10.[146] In the second stage, labor pain is from the peri-neum, innervated by the pudendal nerve and spinal cord segments S-2 to S-4. About 25% of pregnant spinal cord–injured women are unable to detect the onset of labor.[146]

Efferent uterine innervation arises from T-10 to T-12.[145] In women with SCI above the T-10 level, uterine contractions are effective and labor pro-gresses normally.[145] The uterus also contracts when its nerve supply is absent by using intermuscular communication.[146] The intensity of uterine contractions is not reduced,[148] and labor is of short duration, often with spasm of the abdominal muscles.[148] Most women with an SCI level above T-6 will develop autonomic hyperreflexia with uterine contractions.[146,150] Although an increase in the incidence of premature labor has been suggested,[151] a statistically significant increase in the incidence of premature delivery has not been documented.[146] Women with SCI may be expected to have a reasonably normal pregnancy outcome, provided that specific complications, particularly autonomic hyperreflexia, are anticipated and managed properly.[148]

## Micturition

Bladder mechanoreceptors are activated by bladder distension, mucosal deformation, and a shift in bladder position.[152] Pharmacologic experiments indicate that fluid-induced bladder distension results in the activation of capsaicin-sensitive mechanoreceptors, which provide the sensory input needed to facilitate the activation of both supraspinal- and spinal-mediated micturition reflexes.[153–155] Sensory inputs from the bladder[156] to the human lumbar spinal cord arise from T-11 to L-1, and perhaps as far proximal as T-9; sensory inputs from the bladder to the human sacral spinal cord arise from S-2 to S-4.

Preganglionic parasympathetic neurons in the IML of the sacral cord segments S-2 to S-4 project preganglionic fibers in the pelvic nerve to the pelvic plexus.[152] In the human bladder some pelvic plexus neurons are in the bladder wall.[152] Parasympathetic postganglionic nerves excite detrusor smooth muscle via release of acetylcholine, or possibly adenosine triphosphate.[157]

Sympathetic preganglionic neurons that project to the lower urinary tract are found in spinal cord segments T-10 to L-2 in humans.[152] Most preganglionic sympathetic fibers innervating the pelvic viscera form synapses in the IMG or the pelvic plexus.[3,152] Most preganglionic sympathetic fibers project through the lumbar splanchnic nerves to the IMG, and a smaller number of preganglionic sympathetic fibers project via the sacral paravertebral chain ganglia into the pelvic nerve to the pelvic plexus.[111] The hypogastric nerve (also

known as the presacral nerve) is composed of both preganglionic and postganglionic sympathetic fibers that pass from the IMG to the pelvic plexus.[3] β-Adrenergic receptors mediate inhibition of the detrusor smooth muscle, and α-adrenergic receptors mediate contraction of the smooth muscle of the bladder trigone as well as inhibition of parasympathetic ganglionic transmission.[157]

The urethral sphincter mechanism has two parts: the internal and external urethral sphincter (EUS).[158] The internal sphincter is the smooth muscle of the urethra that extends from the bladder outlet through the pelvic floor.[158] The striated muscle of the EUS also has two components, (1) the intrinsic EUS, which lies completely within the urethral wall, and (2) the extrinsic EUS, which is formed by the skeletal muscle fibers of the pelvic floor and urogenital diaphragm.[159] The intrinsic EUS is innervated by somatic pudendal nerve efferents but may have autonomic innervation as well.[158,160] The function of the cholinergic innervation of the EUS is not clear.[161] Adrenergic innervation of the EUS has been suggested, but adrenergic nerves have not been found in the human EUS except when the urinary bladder has been denervated.[161,162] The EUS is the most important active mechanism for maintenance of urinary continence.[158]

The activity of the urinary bladder detrusor muscle is regulated by parasympathetic and sympathetic reflex pathways that are organized in part within the lumbosacral spinal cord.[163] Activation of the parasympathetic pathways to the detrusor muscle and inhibition of somatic input to the intrinsic EUS are the essential neuronal events that initiate release of urine.

Reflex contractions of the urinary bladder and release of urine that occurs in response to bladder distension are mediated via a parasympathetic reflex pathway consisting of an afferent and a preganglionic parasympathetic efferent limb in the pelvic nerve.[163,164] The central component of the micturition reflex consists of a "spinobulbospinal" loop that includes a relay nucleus in the rostral pons known as the pontine micturition center.[165] The ascending and descending tracts from and to the urinary bladder and EUS are known from human and animal studies.[166–168] One ascending pathway travels in the paramedian superficial layer of the dorsal column and terminates in the medulla.[166] A second ascending pathway, travelling in the dorsolateral funiculus, projects from the sacral spinal cord to the nucleus juxtasolitarius ventral to the spinal trigeminal nucleus.[166,167] Animal studies indicate that the afferent information relayed to rostral structures by the dorsal columns is not essential for the production of bladder contraction and EUS relaxation.[169] The descending pathway of the micturition reflex is also in the dorsolateral funiculus, in close proximity to the ascending tracts.[168,169] The spinobulbospinal micturition reflex can be modulated at the spinal level by a variety of afferent inputs from the colon, vagina, penis, or perineum at various sites, including primary afferent terminals, interneurons, or bladder preganglionic neurons.[170]

Bilateral lesions in the rostral pons in the region of the locus ceruleus disrupt micturition and produce urine retention.[171,172] This area may represent the pontine micturition center. Electrical stimulation of the area of the locus ceruleus in cats induced bladder contractions and a simultaneous reduction in external urethral sphincter EMG activity, which was similar to what was seen in distension-induced reflex micturition contractions. Afferent feedback from bladder distension was necessary to maintain the micturition contractions elicited by electrical stimulation of the pons; however, afferent feedback was not required to inhibit the EUS, as stimulation of the brain stem elicited a bladder contraction and sphincter relaxation even when all afferent fibers from the bladder were severed. Whether EUS relaxation was mediated at a spinal cord– or supraspinal level is not clear.[172]

During continence, the spinal vesicosympathetic reflex pathways allow the urinary bladder to accommodate larger volumes by increasing the tone of the bladder neck, by depressing impulse transmission from the sacral spinal cord in pelvic vesical ganglia, and by direct inhibition of the detrusor muscle.[173,174] Vesicosympathetic reflexes are elicited by an intersegmental spinal pathway with afferents in the pelvic nerve and efferents in the hypogastric nerve.[157,175] The physiologic significance of the sympathetic innervation of the urinary bladder is unclear.

In addition to the spinobulbospinal pathway, which is thought to mediate normal micturition, a spinal micturition reflex pathway has been identified.[176] Research by de Groat and Ryall found that the spinal micturition reflex was present in some

intact cats and in all cats with chronic spinal cord transection.[164] It is thought that this spinal pathway mediates automatic micturition following chronic spinal cord transection.[163] Cutaneovesical reflexes have also been described. In rats, cutaneous stimulation resulted in a reflex bladder contraction both before and after spinal cord transection.[177] Neonatal cats exhibit a perineal-bladder reflex mediated in the spinal cord that disappears in adult life,[178,179] and this reflex reappears after spinal cord transection in adult cats.[173,178] Activation of spinal cutaneous somatovesical reflexes may be responsible for voiding elicited by suprapubic tapping or pulling pubic hair in persons with SCI above the sacral outflow.

Complete SCI proximal to the sacral spinal cord results in an upper motor neuron lesion characterized by a hyperreflexic detrusor, whereas injuries involving the sacral cord or cauda equina result in a lower motor neuron lesion characterized by an areflexic detrusor.[180] In a recent study of 489 persons with spinal cord lesions due to a variety of causes, all those who had suprasacral spinal cord lesions without evidence of additional sacral spinal cord or cauda equina involvement had either detrusor hyperreflexia (defined as involuntary bladder contractions with increased detrusor pressure of at least 6 cm $H_2O$) or detrusor–external urethral sphincter dyssynergia (DESD).[180] DESD has been defined as the presence of involuntary contractions of the external urethral sphincter during involuntary detrusor contractions.[181] DESD has been reported to occur during bladder contractions that are evoked either during urodynamic studies or by suprapubic tapping in as many as 86% of persons with SCI.[180,182] In such persons, abrupt discontinuation of suprapubic tapping resulted in brief relaxation of the EUS that was sufficient to result in some urine outflow in 68% of subjects.[182] The loss of reflex inhibition of the EUS during a micturition contraction of the urinary bladder, which occurs following SCI, is a major complicating factor in management of the neurogenic bladder.

## Summary

The function of the autonomic nervous system following injury or damage to the spinal cord cannot be considered only in terms of loss of descending supraspinal control. The neuronal components of the spinal cord, the peripheral autonomic ganglia, and the intrinsic enteric nervous system remain and are capable of complex integrative functions. Furthermore, researchers and clinicians must consider elements of neuronal plasticity and regeneration as contributing to the ultimate pattern of autonomic function following SCI. Plasticity may involve changes in synaptic contacts or physiology, changes in tonic or phasic firing patterns, and changes in neuromodulating peptides.[49]

# References

1. Felten SY, Carlson SL, Bellinger DL, et al. An overview of the efferent autonomic nervous system. In: Fredrickson RCA, Hendrie HC, Hingtgen JN, et al., eds. Neuroregulation of Autonomic, Endocrine and Immune Systems. Boston: Martinus Nijhoff, 1986;109–126.
2. Polinsky RJ. Clinical autonomic neuropharmacology, Clin Neuropharmacol 1990; 8:77–92.
3. Janig W, McLachlan EM. Organization of lumbar spinal outflow to distal colon and pelvic organs. Physiol Rev 1987; 67:1332–1404.
4. Langer SZ, Massingham R, Shepperson NB. $\alpha_1$- and $\alpha_2$-receptor subtypes: Relevance to antihypertensive therapy. In: Buckley JP, Ferrario CM, eds. Central Nervous Mechanisms in Hypertension: Perspectives in Cardiovascular Research, vol 6. New York: Raven Press. 1981;161–170.
5. Loewenstein W. Modulation of cutaneous mechanoreceptors by sympathetic stimulation. J Physiol 1956; 132:40–60.
6. Roberts WJ, Levitt GR. Histochemical evidence for sympathetic innervation of hair receptor afferents in cat skin. J Comp Neurol 1982; 210:204–209.
7. Himms-Hagen J. Thermogenesis in brown adipose tissue as an energy buffer. Implications for obesity. N Engl J Med 1984; 311:1549–1558.
8. Metz W, Forssmann WG. Innervation of the liver in the guinea pig and rat. Anat Embryol 1980; 160:239–252.
9. Simon OR, Schramm LP. The spinal and medullary termination of myelinated renal afferents in the rat. Brain Res 1984; 290:239–247.
10. Ciriello J, Caverson MM. Central organization of afferent renal nerve pathways. Clin Exper—Theory Pract 1987; A9(suppl 1):33–46.
11. DiBona GF. The functions of the renal nerves.

Rev Physiol Biochem Pharmacol 1982; 94:76–181.
12. Kooner JS, Frankel HL, Mirando N, et al. Haemodynamic, hormonal and urinary responses to postural change in tetraplegic and paraplegic man. Paraplegia 1988; 26:233–237.
13. Malliani A, Lombardi F, Pagani M. Sensory innervation of the heart. In: Cervero F, Morrison JFB, eds. Prog Brain Res 1986; 67:39–48.
14. Groomes TE, Huang C-T. Orthostatic hypotension after spinal cord injury: Treatment with fluocortisone and ergotamine. Arch Phys Med Rehabil 1991; 72:56–58.
15. Granata AR, Ruggiero AR, Park DA, et al. Brainstem area with C1 epinephrine neurons mediates baroreflex vasodepressor responses. Am J Physiol 1985; 248:H547–H567.
16. Yamada KA, McAllen RM, Loewy AD. GABA antagonists applied to the ventral surface of the medulla oblongata block the baroreceptor reflex. Brain Res 1984; 297:175–180.
17. McAllen RM. Identification and properties of subretrofacial bulbospinal neurones: A descending cardiovascular pathway in the cat. J Autonom Nerv Syst 1986; 17:151–164.
18. Coote JH, Macleod VH, Fleetwood-Walker SM, et al. Baroreceptor inhibition of sympathetic activity at a spinal site. Brain Res 1981; 220:81–93.
19. Gebber GL, Taylor DG, Weaver LC. Electrophysiological studies on organization of central vasopressor pathways. Am J Physiol 1973: 224:470–481.
20. Somers VK, Mark AL, Zavala DC, et al. Contrasting effects of hypoxia and hypercapnia on ventilation and sympathetic activity in humans. J Appl Physiol 1989; 67:2101–2106.
21. Somers VK, Mark AL, Zavala DC, et al. Influence of ventilation and hypocapnia on sympathetic nerve responses to hypoxia in normal humans. J Appl Physiol 1989; 67:2095–2100.
22. Reis DJ, Ruggiero DA, Morrison SF. The C1 area of the rostral ventrolateral medulla oblongata. A critical brainstem region for control of resting and reflex integration of arterial pressure. Am J Hypertens 1989; 2:363S–374S.
23. Kalia MP. Organization of central control of airways. Ann Rev Physiol 1987; 49:595–609.
24. Sato A, Schmidt RF. The modulation of visceral functions by somatic afferent activity. Jpn J Physiol 1987; 37:1–17.
25. Mitchell JH, Kaufman MP, Iwamoto GA. The exercise pressor reflex: Its cardiovascular effects afferent mechanisms and central pathways. Ann Rev Physiol 1983; 45:229–242.

26. Kumada M, Dampney RAL, Reis DJ. Profound hypotension and abolition of the vasomotor component of the cerebral ischemic response produced by restricted lesions of medulla oblongata: Relationship to the so-called tonic vasomotor center. Circ Res 1979; 45:63–70.

27. Doba N, Reis DJ. Localization within the lower brainstem of a receptive area mediating the pressor response to increased intracranial pressure (the Cushing response). Brain Res 1972; 47:487–491.

28. Schwaber JS. Neuroanatomical substrates of cardiovascular and emotional-autonomic regulation. In: Magro A, Osswald W, Reis O, et al., eds. Central and Peripheral Mechanisms of Cardiovascular Regulation. New York: Plenum Press, 1986;353–384.

29. Schramm LP. Spinal factors in sympathetic regulation. In: Magro A, Osswald W, Reis O, et al., eds. Central and Peripheral Mechanisms of Cardiovascular Regulation. New York: Plenum Press, 1986;303–352.

30. Banzett RB, Lansing RW, Reid MB, et al. 'Air hunger' arising from increased $Pco_2$ in mechanically ventilated quadriplegics. Respir Physiol 1989; 76:53–68.

31. Downey JA, Chiodi HP, Miller JM. The effect of inhalation of 5 per cent carbon dioxide in air on postural hypotension in quadriplegia. Arch Phys Med Rehabil 1966; 47:422–426.

32. Hilton S. The central nervous contribution to vasomotor tone. In: Magro A, Osswald W, Reis O, et al., eds. Central and Peripheral Mechanisms of Cardiovascular Regulation. New York: Plenum Press, 1986;465–486.

33. Yardley CP, Fitzsimons CL, Weaver LC. Cardiac and peripheral vascular contributions to hypotension in spinal cats. Am J Physiol 1989; 257:H1347–H1353.

34. Mathias CJ, Christensen NJ, Corbett JL, et al. Plasma catecholamines, plasma renin activity and plasma aldosterone in tetraplegic man, horizontal and tilted. Clin Sci Molec Med 1975; 49:291–299.

35. Guttman L, Munro AF, Robinson R et al. Effect of tilting on the cardiovascular responses and plasma catecholamine levels in spinal man. Paraplegia 1963; 1:4–18.

36. Krum H, Brown DJ, Rowe PR, et al. Steady state plasma [3H]-noradrenaline kinetics in quadriplegic chronic spinal cord injury patients. J Autonom Pharmacol 1990; 10:221–226.

37. Kooner JS, Birch R, Frankel HL, et al. Hemodynamic and neurohormonal effects of clonidine in patients with preganglionic and postganglionic sympathetic lesions. Circulation 1991; 84:75–83.

38. Gootman PM, Cohen MI. Sympathetic rhythms in spinal cats. J Autonom Nerv Syst 1981; 3:379–387.

39. Mannard A, Polosa C. Analysis of background firing of single sympathetic preganglionic neurons of cat cervical nerve. J Neurophysiol 1973; 36:398–408.

40. Meckler RL, Weaver LC. Splenic, renal, and cardiac nerves have unequal dependence upon tonic supraspinal inputs. Brain Res 1985; 338:123–135.

41. Qu L, Sherebrin R, Weaver LC. Blockade of spinal pathways decreases pre- and postganglionic discharge differentially. Am J Physiol 1988; 255:R946–R951.

42. Stein RD, Weaver LC. Multi- and single-fibre mesenteric and renal sympathetic responses to chemical stimulation of intestinal receptors in cats. J Physiol (Lond) 1988; 396:155–172.

43. Meckler RL, Weaver LC. Characteristics of ongoing and reflex discharge of single splenic and renal sympathetic postganglionic fibers in cats. J Physiol (Lond) 1988; 396:139–153.

44. Weaver LC, Meckler RL, Tobey JC, et al. Organization of differential sympathetic responses to activation of visceral receptors and arterial baroreceptors. In: Magro A, Osswald W, Reis O, et al. Central and Peripheral Mechanisms of Cardiovascular Regulation. New York: Plenum Press, 1986;269–301.

45. Weaver LC, Stein RD. Effects of spinal cord transection on sympathetic discharge in decerebrate-unanesthetized cats. Am J Physiol 1989; 257:R1506–R1511.

46. McCall RB, Gerber GL. Brain stem and spinal synchronization of sympathetic nervous discharge. Brain Res 1975; 89:139–143.

47. Stein RD, Weaver LC, Yardley CP. Ventrolateral medullary neurones: Effects on magnitude and rhythm of discharge of mesenteric and renal nerves in cats. J Physiol (Lond) 1989; 408:571–586.

48. Johnson RH, Park DM. Effect of change of posture on blood pressure and plasma renin concentration in men with spinal transections. Clin Sci 1973; 44:539–546.

49. Cole JD. The pathophysiology of the autonomic nervous system in spinal cord injury. In: Illis LS, ed. Spinal Cord Dyfunction Assessment. Oxford: Oxford Medical Publications, 1988; 201–235.

50. Osborn JW, Taylor RF, Schramm LP. Determinants of arterial pressure after chronic spinal transection in rats. Am J Physiol 1989; 256:R666–R673.

51. Davies IB, Mathias CJ, Sudera D, et al. Agonist regulation of alpha-adrenergic receptor responses

in man. J Cardiovasc Pharmacol 1982; 4:S139–S144.

52. Rodrigues GP, Clause-Walker J, Kent MC, et al. Adrenergic receptors in insensitive skin of spinal cord injured patients. Arch Phys Med Rehabil 1986; 67:177–180.

53. Mathias CJ, Frankel HL, Christensen NJ, et al. Enhanced pressor response to noradrenaline in patients with cervical spinal cord transection. Brain 1976; 99:757–770.

54. Mathias CJ, Christensen NJ, Frankel HL, et al. Renin release during head-up tilt occurs independently of sympathetic nervous activity in tetraplegic man. Clin Sci 1980; 59:251–256.

55. Mikami H, Bumpus FM, Ferrario CM. Hierarchy of blood pressure control mechanisms after spinal sympathectomy. J Hypertens 1983; 1(suppl 2):62–65.

56. Cardus D, McTaggart WG. Total body water and its distribution in men with spinal cord injury. Arch Phys Med Rehabil 1984; 65:509–512.

57. Osborn JW, Livingstone RH, Schramm LP. Elevated renal nerve activity after spinal transection: Effects on renal function. Am J Physiol 1987; 253:R619–R625.

58. Poole CJM, Williams TDM, Lightman SL, et al. Neuroendocrine control of vasopressin secretion and its effect on blood pressure in subjects with spinal cord transection. Brain 1987; 110:727–735.

59. Kooner JS, da Costa DF, Frankel HL, et al. Recumbency induces hypertension, diuresis and natriuresis in autonomic failure, but diuresis alone in tetraplegia. J Hypertens 1987; 5(suppl 5):S327–S329.

60. Kewalramani LS. Autonomic dysreflexia in traumatic myelopathy. Am J Phys Med Rehabil 1980; 59:1–21.

61. Braddom RL, Rocco JF. Autonomic dysreflexia. Am J Phys Med Rehabil 1991; 70:234–241.

62. Lindan R, Joiner E, Freehafer AA, et al. Incidence and clinical features of autonomic dysreflexia in patients with spinal cord injury. Paraplegia 1980; 18:285–292.

63. Stowe DF, Bernstein JS, Madsen KE, el al. Autonomic hyperrelexia in spinal cord injured patients during extracorporeal shock wave lithotripsy. Anesth Analg 1989; 68:788–791.

64. Lindan R, Leffler EJ, Kedia KR. A comparison of the efficacy of an alpha$_1$-adrenergic blocker and a slow calcium channel blocker in the control of autonomic dysreflexia. Paraplegia 1985; 23:34–38.

65. Giuliani S, Maggi CA, Meli A. Capsaicin-sensitive afferents in the rat urinary bladder activate a spinal sympathetic cardiovascular reflex. Naunyn-Schb Arch Pharmacol 1988; 338:411–416.

66. Holzer P. Local effector functions of capsaicin-sensitive sensory nerve endings: Involvement of tachykinins, calcitonin gene-related peptide and other neuropeptides. Neuroscience 1988; 24:739–768.

67. Mathias CJ, Frankel HI. Cardiovascular control in spinal man. Ann Rev Physiol 1988; 50:577–592.

68. Lehmann KG, Shandling AH, Yusi AU, et al. Altered ventricular repolarization in central sympathetic dysfunction associated with spinal cord injury. Am J Cardiol 1989; 63:1498–1504.

69. Coutts KD, Rhodes EC, McKenzie DC. Maximal exercise responses of tetraplegics and paraplegics. J Appl Physiol 1983; 55:479–482.

70. VanLoan MD, McCluer S, Loftin JM, et al. Comparison of physiological responses to maximal arm exercise among able-bodied, paraplegics and quadriplegics. Paraplegia 1987; 25:397–405.

71. Luce JM, Culver BH. Respiratory muscle function in health and disease. Chest 1982; 81:82–90.

72. McMichan JC, Michel L, Westbrook PR. Pulmonary dysfunction following traumatic quadriplegia. JAMA 1980; 243:528–531.

73. Axen K. Ventilatory responses to mechanical loads in cervical cord–injured humans. J Appl Physiol 1982; 52:748–756.

74. Banzett RB, Lansing RW, Brown R. High-level quadriplegics perceive lung volume change. J Appl Physiol 1987; 62:567–573.

75. Simon E. Temperature regulation: The spinal cord as a site of extrahypothalamic thermoregulatory functions. Rev Physiol Biochem Pharmacol 1974; 71:1–76.

76. Downey RJ, Downey JA, Newhouse E, et al. Hyperthermia in a quadriplegic: Evidence for a peripheral action of haloperidol in malignant neuroleptic syndrome. Chest 1992; 101:1728–1730.

77. Menard MR, Hahn G. Acute and chronic hypothermia in a man with spinal cord injury: Environmental and pharmacologic causes. Arch Phys Med Rehabil 1991; 72:421–424.

78. Downey JA, Chiodi HP, Darling RC. Central temperature regulation in the spinal man. J Appl Physiol 1967; 22:91–94.

79. Miller JM. Autonomic function in the isolated spinal cord. In: Downey JA, Darling RC, eds. Physiological Basis of Rehabilitation Medicine. Philadelphia: WB Saunders, 1971;265–281.

80. Cooper, KE, Ferres HM, Guttman L. Vasomotor responses in the foot to raising body temperature in the paraplegic patient. J Physiol (Lond) 1957; 136:547–555.

81. Appenzeller O, Schnieden H. Neurogenic pathways concerned in reflex vasodilatation in the hand with especial reference to stimuli affecting the afferent pathway. Clin Sci 1963; 25:413–421.

82. Benzinger TH. Heat regulation: Homeostasis of central temperature in man. Physiol Rev 1969; 49:671–759.

83. Tsai S-H, Shih C-J, Shyy T-T, et al. Recovery of vasomotor response in human spinal cord transection. J Neurosurg 1980; 52:808–811.

84. Corbett JL, Frankel HL, Harris PJ. Cardiovascular reflex responses to cutaneous and visceral stimuli in spinal man. J Physiol (Lond) 1971; 215:395–409.

85. Sahs AL, Fulton JF. Somatic and automatic reflexes in spinal monkeys. J Neurophysiol 1940; 3:258–268.

86. Freund PR, Brengelmann GL, Rowell LB, et al. Attenuated skin blood flow response to hyperthermia in paraplegic men. J Appl Physiol 1984; 56:1104–1109.

87. Johnson RH. Neurological studies in temperature regulation. Ann Ro Coll Surg Engl 1965; 36:339–352.

88. Downey JA, Huckaba CE, Kelley PS, et al. Sweating responses to central and peripheral heating in spinal man. J Appl Physiol 1976; 5:701–706.

89. Quinton PM. Sweating and its disorders. Annu Rev Med 1983; 34:429–452.

90. Normell LA. Distribution of impaired cutaneous vasomotor and sudomotor function in paraplegic man. Scand J Clin Lab Invest 1974; 33(suppl 138):25–41.

91. Huckaba CE, Frewin DB, Downey JA, et al. Sweating responses of normal, paraplegic and anhidrotic man. Arch Phys Med Rehabil 1976; 57:268–274.

92. Tam HS, Darling RC, Cheh HY, et al. The dead zone of thermoregulation in normal and paraplegic man. Can J Physiol Pharmacol 1978; 56:976–983.

93. Stjernberg L, Wallin BG. Sympathetic neural outflow in spinal man. A preliminary report. J Autonom Nerv Syst 1983; 7:313–318.

94. Wallin BG, Stjernberg L. Sympathetic activity in man after spinal cord injury. Brain 1984; 107:183–198.

95. Guttman L, Whitteridge D. Effects of bladder distension on autonomic mechanisms after spinal cord injuries. Brain 1947; 70:366–404.

96. Furness JB, Costa M. The Enteric Nervous System. Edinburgh:Churchill Livingstone, 1987.

97. Sarna SK, Otterson MF. Small intestinal physiology and pathophysiology. Gastroenterol Clin North Am 1989; 18:375–404.

98. Read NW, Houghton LA. Physiology of gastric emptying and pathophysiology of gastroparesis. Gastroenterol Clin North Am 1989; 18:359–372.

99. Andrews PLR. Vagal afferent innervation of the gastrointestinal tract. In: Cervero F, Morrison JFB, eds. Progress in Brain Research, vol 67, Visceral Sensation. Amsterdam: Elsevier, 1986;65–86.

100. Rees WDW, Malagelada JR, Miller LJ, et al. Human interdigestive and postprandial gastrointestinal motor and hormone patterns. Dig Dis Sci 1982; 27:321–329.

101. Stoddard CJ, Smallwood RH, Duthie HL. Migrating myoelectric complex in man. In: Duffy HL, ed. Proceedings of the Sixth International Motility Symposium. Baltimore: University Park Press, 1978;9–27.

102. Mroz CT, Kelly KA. The role of the extrinsic antral nerves in the regulation of gastric emptying. Surg Gynecol Obstet 1977; 145:369–377.

103. Vantrappen G, Janssens J, Peeters TL. Motilin and the interdigestive migrating motor complex in man. Dig Dis Sci 1979; 24:497–500.

104. Sarr MG, Kelly KA. Myoelectric activity of the autotransplanted canine jejunoileum. Gastroenterology 1981; 81:303–310.

105. Fealey RD, Szurszewski JH, Merritt JL, et al. Effect of traumatic spinal cord transection on human upper gastrointestinal motility and gastric emptying. Gastroenterology 1984; 87:69–75.

106. Guttman L. Spinal Cord Injuries (Comprehensive Management and Research), ed 2. Oxford: Blackwell Scientific, 1970; 237–473.

107. Szurszewski JH. A migrating electric complex of the canine small intestine. Am J Physiol 1969; 217:1757–1763.

108. Telford GL, Go VLW, Szurszewski JH. Effect of central sympathectomy on gastric and small intestinal myoelectric activity and plasma motilin concentrations in the dog. Gastroenterology 1985; 89:989–995.

109. Schuster M. Motor disorders of the stomach. Med Clin North Am 1981; 65:1269–1289.

110. Longo WE, Ballantyne GH, Modlin IM. The colon, anorectum, and spinal cord patient. A review of the functional alterations of the denervated hindgut. Dis Colon Rectum 1989; 32:261–267.

111. Kuo DC, Hisamitsu T, de Groat WC. A sympathetic projection from sacral paravertebral ganglia the pelvic nerve and to postganglionic nerves on the surface of the urinary bladder and large intestine of the cat. J Comp Neurol 1984; 226:76–86.

112. Lundberg JM, Hokfelt T, Anggard A, et al. Organizational principles in the peripheral sympathetic neurone system. Subdivision by co-existing peptides (somatostatin, avian pancreatic polypep-

tide, and vasoactive intestinal polypeptide–like immunoreactive materials.). Proc Natl Acad Sci USA 1982; 79:1303–1307.

113. Keef KD, Kreulen DL. Comparison of central versus peripheral nerve pathways to the guinea pig inferior mesenteric ganglion determined electrophysiologically after chronic nerve section. J Autonom Nerv Syst 1990; 29:95–112.

114. Du CH, Ferre JR, Ruckebusch Y. Spinal cord influences on the colonic myoelectrical activity of fed and fasted rats. J Physiol 1987; 383:395–404.

115. Hertz A, Newton A. The normal movement of the colon in man. J Physiol (Lond) 1913; 47:57–65.

116. Aaronson MJ, Freed MM, Burakoff R. Colonic myoelectric activity in persons with spinal cord injury. Dig Dis Sci 1985; 30:295–300.

117. Glick ME, Meshkinpour H, Haldeman S, et al. Colonic dysfunction in patients with thoracic spinal cord injury. Gastroenterology 1984; 86:287–294.

118. Connell AM, Frankel H, Guttman L. The motility of the pelvic colon following complete lesions of the spinal cord. Paraplegia 1963; 1:98–110.

119. Stone JM, Nino-Murcia M, Wolfe VA, et al. Chronic gastrointestinal problems in spinal cord injury patients: A prospective analysis. Am J Gastroenterol 1990; 85:1114–1119.

120. Menardo G, Bausano G, Corrazziari RE. Large bowel transit in paraplegic patients. Dis Colon Rectum 1987; 30:924–928.

121. de Groat WC, Booth AM. Physiology of male sexual function. Ann Intern Med 1980; 92:329–331.

122. de Groat WC, Steers WD. Neuroanatomy and neurophysiology of penile erection. In: Tanagho EA, Lue TF, McClure DD, eds. Contemporary Management of Impotence and Infertility. Baltimore: Williams & Wilkins, 1988;3–27.

123. Langley JM, Anderson HR. The innervation of the pelvic and adjoining viscera. Part II. The bladder. J Physiol (Lond) 1896; 19:71–84.

124. Semans JH, Langworthy OR. Observation on the neurophysiology of sexual function in the cat. J Urol 1938; 40:836–846.

125. Steers WD, Mallory B, de Groat WC. Electrophysiological study of neural activity in penile nerve of the rat. Am J Physiol 1988; 254:R989–R1000.

126. Peters LC, Kristal MB, Komisaruk BR. Sensory innervation of the external and internal genitalia of the female rat. Brain Res 1987; 408:197–204.

127. Yarkony GM. Enhancement of sexual function and fertility in spinal cord–injured males. Am J Phys Med Rehabil 1990; 69:81–87.

128. Lue TF, Zeineh SJ, Schmidt RA, et al. Neuroan-

atomy of penile erection: Its relevance to iatrogenic impotence. J Urol 1984; 131:273–280.

129. Dail WG, Minorsky N, Moll MA, et al. The hypogastric nerve pathway to penile erectile tissue: Histochemical evidence supporting a vasodilator role. J Autonom Nerv Syst 1986; 15:341–349.

130. Bors E, Comarr AE. Neurological disturbance of sexual function with special reference to 529 patients with spinal cord injury. Urol Surg 1960; 10:191–222.

131. Hart BL, Melese-D'Hospital PY. Penile mechanisms and the role of the striated penile muscle in penile reflexes. Physiol Behav 1983; 31:807–813.

132. Herbert J. The role of the dorsal nerves of the penis in the sexual behavior of the male rhesus monkey. Physiol Behav 1973; 10:292–300.

133. Sachs BD. Role of striated penile muscles in penile reflexes, copulation and induction of pregnancy in the rat. J Reprod Fertil 1982; 66:433–443.

134. de Tejada IS, Blanco R, Goldstein I, et al. Cholinergic neurotransmission in human penile corpus cavernosum smooth muscle. Fed Proc 1988; 256:454 (Abstr).

135. Lepor H, Gregerman M, Crosby R, et al. Precise localization of the autonomic nerves from the pelvic plexus to the corpora cavernosa: A detailed anatomical study of the adult male pelvis. J Urol 1985; 133:207–212.

136. Gu J, Polak M, Probert L, et al. Peptidergic innervation of the human male genital tract. J Urol 1983; 130:386–391.

137. Willis EA, Ottensen B, Wagner G, et al. Vasoactive intestinal polypeptide (VIP) as a putative neurotransmitter in penile erection. Life Sci 1983; 33:383–391.

138. Hedlund H, Andersson K-E, Mattiasson A. Pre- and post-junctional adreno- and muscarinic receptor functions in the isolated human corpus spongiosum urethrae. J Autonom Pharmacol 1984; 4:241–249.

139. Sarkarati M, Rossier AB, Fam BA. Experience in vibratory and electro-ejaculation techniques in spinal cord injury patients: A preliminary report. J Urol 1987; 138:59–62.

140. Brindley GS. The fertility of men with spinal injuries. Paraplegia 1984; 22:337–348.

141. Brindley GS. Reflex ejaculation under vibratory stimulation in paraplegic men. Paraplegia 1981; 19:299–302.

142. Chapelle PA, Roby-Rami A, Yakovleff A, et al. Neurologic correlations of ejaculation and testicular size in men with a complete spinal cord section. J Neurol Neurosurg Psychiatry 1988; 51:197–202.

143. Claus-Walker J, Scurry M, Carter M, et al. Steady-state hormonal secretion in traumatic quadriplegia. J Clin Endocrinol Metab 1977; 44:530–535.

144. Young RJ, Strachan RK, Seth J, et al. Is testicular endocrine function abnormal in young men with spinal cord injuries? J Clin Endocrinol Metab 1982; 17:303–306.

145. Berard EJJ. The sexuality of spinal cord injured women: Physiology and pathophysiology. A review. Paraplegia 1989; 27:99–112.

146. Nygaard I, Bartscht KD, Cole S. Sexuality and reproduction in spinal cord–injured women. Obstet Gynecol Surv 1992; 45:727–732.

147. Reame NE. A prospective study of the menstrual cycle and spinal cord injury. Am J Phys Med Rehabil 1992; 71:15–21.

148. Young BK, Katz M, Klein SA. Pregnancy after spinal cord injury: Altered maternal and fetal response to labor. Obstet Gynecol 1983; 62: 59–63.

149. Masters WH, Johnson VE. Human Sexual Response. Boston: Little, Brown, 1965; 65–130.

150. McGregor JA, Meeuwsen J. Autonomic hyperreflexia: A mortal danger for spinal cord–damaged women in labor. Am J Obstet Gynecol 1985; 151:330–333.

151. Seftel AD, Oates RD, Krane RJ. Disturbed sexual function in patients with spinal cord disease. Neurolol Clin 1991; 9:757–778.

152. Andersson KE, Sjogren C. Aspects on the physiology and pharmacology of the bladder and urethra. Prog Neurobiol 1982; 19:71–89.

153. Maggi CA, Santicioli P, Borsini F, et al. The role of the capsaicin-sensitive innervation of the rat urinary bladder in the activation of micturition reflex. Naunyn-Schmiedebergs Arch Pharmacol 1986; 332:276–283.

154. Santicioli P, Maggi CA, Meli A. Functional evidence for the existence of a capsaicin-sensitive innervation in the rat urinary bladder. J Pharm Pharmacol 1986; 38:446–451.

155. Maggi CA, Barbanti G, Santicioli P, et al. Cystometric evidence that capsaicin-sensitive nerves modulate the afferent branch of micturition reflex in humans. J Urol 1989; 142:150–154.

156. Janig W, McLachlan EM. Identification of distinct topographical distributions of lumbar sympathetic and sensory neurons projecting to end organs with different functions in the cat. J Comp Neurol 1986; 246:104–112.

157. de Groat WC, Booth AM. Physiology of the urinary bladder and urethra. Ann Intern Med 1980; 92:312–315.

158. McGuire F. The innervation and function of the lower urinary tract. J Neurosurg 1986; 65:278–285.

159. Elbadawi A. Neuromorphologic basis of vesicourethral function: Histochemistry, ultrastructure, and function of intrinsic nerves of the bladder and urethra. Neurourol Urodynam 1982; 1:3–50.

160. Elbadawi A. Ultrastructure of vesicourethral innervation. II. Postganglionic axoaxonal synapses in intrinsic innervation of the vesicourethral lissosphincter: A new structural and functional concept in micturition. J Urol 1984; 131:781–790.

161. Crowe R, Burnstock G. A histochemical and immunohistochemical study of the autonomic innervation of the lower urinary tract of the female pig. Is the pig a good model for the human bladder and urethra? J Urol 1989; 141:414–422.

162. Lincoln J, Crowe R, Bokor J, et al. Adrenergic and cholinergic innervation of smooth and striated muscle components of the urethra from patients with spinal cord injury. J Urol 1986; 135:402–408.

163. Mallory B, Steers WD, de Groat WC. Electrophysiological study of the micturition reflexes in rats. Am J Physiol 1989; 257:R410–R421.

164. de Groat WC, Ryall RW. Reflexes to sacral parasympathetic neurones concerned with micturition in the cat. J Physiol (Lond) 1969; 200:87–108.

165. Mallory B, Roppolo JR, de Groat WC. Pharmacologic modulation of the pontine micturition center. Brain Res 1991; Vol 546, 310-320.

166. Yamamoto S, Sugihara S, Kuru M. Microelectrode studies on sensory afferents in the posterior funiculus of cat. Jpn J Physiol 1956; 6:68–85.

167. Kuru M. The spino-bulbar tracts and the pelvic sensory vagus. Further contributions to the theory of the sensory dual innervation of the viscera. J Comp Neurol 1956; 104:207–231.

168. Kuru M. Nervous control of micturition. Physiol Rev 1965; 45:425–494.

169. Mallory B, Shefchyk SK. Effect of subtotal spinal cord lesions on brainstem evoked and peripheral reflex micturition in cats. Ann R Coll Phys Surg Can 1986.

170. Kruse MN, Mallory BS, Noto H, et al. Modulation of the spinobulbospinal micturition reflex pathway in cats. Am J Physiol 1992; 262:R478–R484.

171. Satoh K, Shimizu N, Tohyama M, et al. Localization of the micturition reflex center at dorsolateral pontine tegmentum of the rat. Neurosci Lett 1978; 8:27–33.

172. Kruse MN, Mallory BS, Noto H, et al. Properties of the descending limb of the spinobulbospinal micturition reflex pathway in the cat. Brain Res 1991; 556:6–12.

173. de Groat WC. Nervous control of the urinary bladder of the cat. Brain Res 1975; 87:201–211.

174. de Groat WC, Booth AM. Autonomic systems to

the urinary bladder and sexual organs. In: Dyck PJ, Thomas PK, Lambert EH, et al., eds. Peripheral Neuropathy, ed 2. Philadelphia: WB Saunders, 1984;285–299.

175. Schondorf R, Laskey W, Polosa C. Upper thoracic sympathetic neuron responses to input from urinary bladder afferents. Am J Physiol 1983; 245:R311–R320.

176. de Groat WC, Nadelhaft I, Milne RJ, et al. Organization of the sacral parasympathetic reflex pathways to the urinary bladder and large intestine. J Autonom Nerv Syst 1981; 3:135–160.

177. Sato A, Sato Y, Shimada F, et al. Changes in vesical function produced by cutaneous stimulation in rats. Brain Res 1975; 94:465–474.

178. Thor K, Kawatani M, de Groat WC. Plasticity in the reflex pathways to the lower urinary tract of the cat during postnatal development and following spinal cord injury. In: Goldberger M, Gorio A, Murray M, eds. Development and Plasticity of the Mammalian Spinal Cord. Padova: Liviana Press, 1985;105–121.

179. Thor KB, Blais DP, de Groat WC. Behavioral analysis of the postnatal development of micturition in kittens. Dev Brain Res 1989; 46:137–144.

180. Kaplan SA, Chancellor MB, Blaivas JG. Bladder and sphincter behavior in patients with spinal cord lesions. J Urol 1991; 146:113–117.

181. Blaivas JG, Sinha HP, Zayed AAH, et al. Detrusor–external sphincter dyssynergia. J Urol 1981; 125:542.

182. Wyndaele JJ. Urethral sphincter dyssynergia in spinal cord injury patients. Paraplegia 1987; 25:10–15.

# Chapter 21
# Peripheral Nerve Regeneration

MAZHER JAWEED

The peripheral nervous system was first described by Hippocrates (*ca*. 460 to 370 B.C.), but Galen (*ca*. 130 to 200 A.D.) probably was the first to study the effect of nerve transection on muscle size and power. Between the 16th and the 19th century, massive amounts of information were amassed on nerve excitability and muscle responses. With the invention of the microscope, new knowledge was obtained about the nature of peripheral nerves and myelin. After Galvani (1737 to 1798) demonstrated that electrical stimulation evoked responses in nerves and muscles, motor and sensory nerves were identified and associated with the ventral and dorsal roots in the spinal cord, respectively. In 1839, Schwann identified and characterized the nature of Schwann cell, and Purkinje discovered direct connections between the neuronal cell body and the axon.

In the mid-1800s, Waller reported that injury to the glossopharyngeal and hypoglossal nerves of the frog caused degenerative changes distal to the lesion. He also noted that regeneration was more rapid in younger frogs and was not enhanced by electrical stimulation. Waller concluded that the neuronal cell body functioned as a trophic center responsible for maintaining the nerve fiber and that an interruption due to injury resulted in death of the axon.[1]

In 1906, Golgi[2] and Ramon y Cajal[3] separately demonstrated that the nervous system is a network of individual nerve cells and functional connections. In the 20th century, Sunderland,[4] Sherring-ton, Seddon, Weiss, and Hoffmann, among others, contributed a great deal to the understanding of nerve-muscle interactions. As neurosciences advance, the roles of Schwann cells, the mechanisms of neural responses to injury, axonal growth and transport, and effect of the neural microenvironment continue to be elucidated.[5–8]

## Anatomy and Physiology of the Peripheral Nervous System

The peripheral nervous system (PNS) receives commands from the brain and relays information to target fibers or end organs such as muscle spindle or sympathetic neurons. The PNS comprises a complex composite structure of neuronal cell bodies in the spinal cord, their supportive connective tissue, and cellular elements. The neurons connect to the periphery, with the incoming or afferent nerve endings in the dorsal spinal roots and the outgoing (efferent) nerves originating in the ventral roots (Figure 21-1). Within the spinal cord, the neurons contact one another by their dendrites, but the connection with the periphery is via a single axon that terminates at the neuromuscular junction or sensory receptors. Myelinated efferent fibers innervate both the larger extrafusal fibers (alpha motor neurons) and the smaller intrafusal fibers (gamma motor neurons). Motor innervation to blood vessels and epidermal appendages is through the autonomic nervous system.[1,4,6]

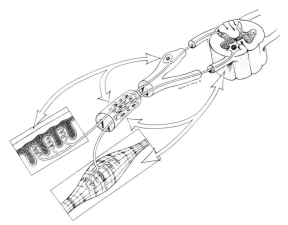

**Figure 21-1.** The PNS consists of afferent and efferent nerve endings in the dorsal and ventral roots, respectively. The afferent nerve axons originate from the periphery (e.g., spindle and the Golgi tendon) and terminate at the dorsal root ganglion (*upper arrows*). The efferent nerve axons (*lower arrows*) are the distal extensions of the alpha or gamma motor neurons, which synapse at the periphery (e.g., neuromuscular junction). (From Lundborg G, Dahlin LB. Structure and function of peripheral nerve. In: Gelberman RH, ed. Operative Nerve Repair and Reconstruction. Philadelphia: JB Lippincott, 1991.)

Both afferent and efferent nerve fibers are encased in bundles or fascicles bound by supportive connective tissue, which contributes approximately 25% to 85% of the bundle volume, depending on the type of nerve.[1] Sherrington[8] compared the composition of afferent and efferent nerves in fascicles of motor and sympathetic nerves, and observed that the larger afferent nerves predominated in the nerves innervating muscle. Eccles and Sherington[9] confirmed this observation and determined that fascicles consist of large and

small nerves, and include motor and sensory fibers. Several classifications for the peripheral nerves have been proposed, the most complete of which was advanced by Erlanger and Gasser[10] and later modified by Terzis and associates.[1] According to this classification, myelinated fibers can be grouped into A and B fibers, depending on their fiber diameter, conduction velocity, and function. Nonmyelinated fibers are identified as C fibers (Table 21-1); those of largest diameter are called group I, those of intermediate diameter groups II and III, and those of smaller diameter are identified as unmyelinated group IV fibers. The rates of both degeneration and regeneration of nerve fibers differ significantly in different nerves.

The peripheral nerves are associated with three separate and distinct supportive sheaths, the outer epineurium, the middle perineurium, and the inner endoneurium. These sheaths cover the nerve, the nerve fascicle, and the nerve axon, respectively (Figure 21-2). The perineurium, a mechanically strong membrane that can sustain intrafascicular pressure of as much as 300 to 750 mm Hg, acts as a barrier against mechanical trauma and diffusion from extracellular infiltrates. The perineurium blocks diffusion of proteins and ferritin[11,12] but is permeable to diphosphorus compounds, oxidative enzymes, and adenosine triphosphate.[13] The endoneurium protects the integrity of the axon and other endoneurial contents such as Schwann cells and axoplasm. Regeneration after injury to the peripheral nerves may depend on the extent of injury to these membranes. For example, if the endoneurial tube is intact after mild compression injury, the axon regenerates smoothly, the synapse is reestablished in the area of the degenerated endplate; by contrast, transection injury, in which a

**Table 21-1.** Nerve Fiber Classification

| Group | Myelin | Size | Conduction Presence | Fibers and Function |
|---|---|---|---|---|
| A | Myelinated | Largest | Fastest | Somatic afferents and efferents |
| A - α | Myelinated | 15–20 μ | Fast | Efferent |
| A - β | Myelinated | 8–15 μ | Fast | Afferent, touch |
| A - δ | Myelinated | 2–5 μ | Fast | Pricking, pain, temperature |
| B | Myelinated | 1–2 μ | Slow | Autonomic afferents and preganglionic |
| C | Unmyelinated | <1 μ | Slowest | Autonomic efferents and postganglionic Deep, burning pain |

Adapted from Erlanger J, Gasser H. Electrical Signs of Nervous Activity. Philadelphia: University of Pennsylvania Press, 1937.

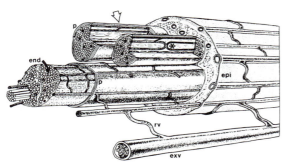

**Figure 21-2.** A peripheral nerve and ensheathing collagenous membranes. The outer epineurium (epi), the middle perineurium (p) and the inner endoneurium (end) encircle the nerve bundle, nerve fasicle, and the nerve axon, respectively. The asterisk represents a node. The nerve is richly vascular with radial vessels (rv) and external vessels (exv). The large arrow on the top shows the perineurium sheath surrounding the fasicle. From Lundborg and Dahlin (53a)

**Table 21-2.** Axonal Transport System and Major Components

| Transport System | Group | Velocity (mm/d) | Major Components |
|---|---|---|---|
| Anterograde | | | |
| Fast | I, II | 20–410 | Neurotransmitters and related enzymes and amino acids |
| Fast | III | 4–8 | Myosin-like actin-binding polypeptides |
| Slow | IV | 2–30 | Actin, clatrin |
| Slow | IV | 0.1–15 | Tubulin, neurofilaments |
| Retrograde | | | |
| Fast | – | ≤300 | Neurotropic factors, (NFG), lysosomes |
| Slow | – | 3–8 | Single protein |

Modified from Lundborg G, Dahlin LB. Structure and function of peripheral nerve. In: Gelberman RH, ed. Operative Nerve Repair and Reconstruction. Philadelphia: JB Lippincott, 1991.

guidance or navigation tube is absent, results in delayed reinnervation of the muscle. Thus, to examine or facilitate nerve regeneration and subsequent reinnervation, it is important to understand the behavior of factors that are linked to degeneration.[14,15]

One of the main factors that contributes to degeneration and regeneration of peripheral nerves is the transport of axoplasm, which carries a wide range of substances, including proteins, membranous vesicles, neurotransmitters, lipids, mitochondria, and RNA. Approximately 70% of these nutrients are lost during transport from the neuronal cell body to the peripheral target. The speed of axoplasmic transport contributes to the rate of regeneration of the nerves (Table 21-2). Lundborg and colleagues have identified five groups of anterograde transport.[16,17] The fast axonal transport system (20 to 410 mm per day, groups I and II) is used to pass membrane-bound materials and depends on the availability of energy; it can be blocked by metabolic and energy system inhibitors.[16,17] Inhibition of fast axonal transport thus interferes with synaptic transmission and, consequently, nerve regeneration of the axon. The slow transport system (0.1 to 30 mm per day), on the other hand, transports substances (mostly proteins) at speeds that vary from nerve to nerve. Retrograde transport from the periphery to the nerve cells in the spinal cord includes both fast (300 mm per day) and slow (4 to 8 mm per day) components. This system reportedly transports multivesicular and multilamellar organelles such as lysosomes, as well as growth factors and viruses. Retrograde chemotactic factors are also known to play an important role in stimulating or inhibiting peripheral nerve sprouting in partially denervated muscle.[18–20]

## Peripheral Nerve Degeneration

Peripheral nerve injury can be caused by a variety of lesions, by physical injury, or by environmental factors. The extent of an injury can be estimated by the level of degeneration of the neuron, the Schwann cell, the axon, and the target organ. Both Seddon[21] and Sunderland[22] developed schemes for classifying peripheral nerve injuries based on the damage to internal structures. The first, mildest degree of injury in this classification is neurapraxia, or nerve conduction block. In this type of injury, axonal continuity is maintained, and nerve conduction proximal and distal to the block is preserved. Recovery is relatively rapid (a few hours to several weeks),[23–25] and neither anterograde nor retrograde transport is interrupted. In this condition, the large fibers (A-alpha) are affected the most and are narrowed at the nodes of Ranvier. There is reason to believe that pressures as low as 30 mm Hg may impede fast conduction.

Pressures greater than 200 mm Hg may produce a block that can last 2 hours to 3 days, depending on the duration of compression.[1,4,24] Neurapraxic lesions are common in traumatic spinal cord injury. Prolonged pressure may lead to neural ischemia. Lundborg[24] observed ischemic changes in peripheral nerves with 4 to 6 hours of compression; compression for such periods resulted in increased intraneurial capillary permeability, leading to swelling and intraneurial pressure.[25]

Second-degree injury includes all the changes in first-degree lesions plus concomitant degeneration of the axon. Second-degree injuries are produced by crushing as well as by mild traction. The degenerative changes are visible within minutes, both proximally and distally. The pathologic changes depend on the degree and duration of ischemia, fiber size, proximity to cell body, and the age of the patient. In the initial phase of crush injury, organelles and metabolites accumulate in the proximal and distal stumps of the crushed nerve, leading to nerve swelling. The entire length of the distal segment then gradually begins to degenerate. The segment proximal to the lesion undergoes degeneration similar to that after cavitation of the spinal cord. Within 6 hours after injury, the neuronal cell bodies start to change, Nissl bodies disperse, neurofilaments disassemble, and ultimately the nucleus moves from the center of the cell to the periphery. Schwann cells, perhaps in response to these degenerative changes in the axon and myelin, are released from the nerve axons and

begin to multiply, increasing protein synthesis within the basal lamina tube.[27] This process, *wallerian degeneration*,[26] thus causes the axon to degenerate below the lesion. Figure 21-3 illustrates the degenerative changes observed in rat sciatic nerve 24 hours after L-4 spinal nerve sectioning. Although wallerian degeneration is visible in some axons, several myelinated and nonmyelinated axons are still intact, indicating that the degenerative process is both rapid and specific.

Third-degree peripheral nerve injury includes axonotmetic lesion(s), in which the continuity of the basal lamina is significantly disrupted. Damage to Schwann cells and their basement membranes is followed by hemorrhage, edema, and subsequent ischemia of the nerve axon. The accumulation of dead cells may complicate and limit the process of regeneration. The regenerated axon, without peripheral guidance, may not be able to form synapses with the appropriate end-organs, particularly in mixed sensory and motor nerves.[1,4,14,15]

Fourth-degree injury involves axonal, endoneurial, and perineurial injury, caused by severe crush or traction damage. The zone of injury is greater, the chance of fascicular organization negligible, and the loss of neurons frequent in this type of injury, leading to failure of regeneration.[1,4]

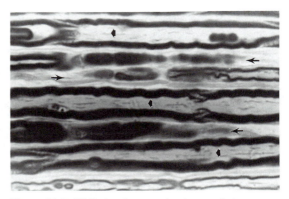

**Figure 21-3.** Wallerian degeneration in rat sciatic nerve 24 hours after partial nerve injury (L-5 spinal nerve sectioning). Note chromatolysis in denervated axons (*arrows*) while the intact axons show quite normal appearance (*arrowheads*). The dark material surrounding the axons is myelin sheath. The thin axon at the bottom is nonmyelinated.

The fifth and most severe degree of nerve damage is characterized by complete transection of the nerve trunk, and so carries minimal chance of spontaneous recovery. Transection injuries most often result from severe crushing or shearing. In this condition, abortive attempts at regeneration produce a tangled mass of axonal buds and neuromas.[1,4]

In summary, the effect of peripheral nerve injuries is quite variable; different degrees of injury can be associated with a single lesion. The first three degrees of injury can result in subsequent return of function, whereas fourth- and fifth-degree injuries may not. The degree of muscle reinnervation (or synapses with sympathetic neurons) thus depends on the type of injury to the axon.

## Mechanisms of Nerve Degeneration in Different Injuries

Nerve injuries can result from trauma, compression, stretch, ischemia, electrical shock, radiation, puncture, and laceration. Clinically, total and partial denervation can be caused by diseases such as Charcot-Marie-Tooth disease, diabetes, poliomyelitis, traumatic spinal cord injuries at the root level, Kugelberg-Welander disease, and several polyneuropathies. The extent of regeneration depends on the degree of injury. Brief discussions of some common injuries are presented below and in Table 21-3.

### Nerve Compression

Acute nerve compression can be produced by pressures as low as 30 mm Hg. At 60 mm Hg, nerve conduction block may be produced; pressures greater than 90 mm Hg may initiate damage to the internal structures.[28,29] Pressure on the nerve for 30 to 40 minutes leads to paresthesias, paralysis, and associated pathophysiologic changes in the nerve and muscle. More prolonged neurapraxic conditions lead to focal demyelination at the site of injury; the so-called Saturday night palsy results from local demyelination.[30]

Clinically, gunshot wounds and shrapnel cause similar acute nerve compression. Tissue damage is related to the velocity of the projectile; for example, when the kinetic energy of the shrapnel exceeds the speed of sound (335 m/sec) it becomes proportional to the third power of the velocity of the bullet.[1,30] Therefore, the compression produced by a bullet lodged in the muscle or connective tissue adjacent to the nerve may cause partial denervation leading to subsequently peripheral regeneration of the intact axons. This phenomenon is more common in proximal than the distal nerves. It has been proposed that compression-induced anoxia or ischemia could contribute to

**Table 21-3.** Peripheral Nerve Injury

| Nerve Injury | Symptoms | Tissue and Cellular Changes | Recovery Prognosis |
|---|---|---|---|
| Compressions | Neurapraxia, paresthesia, paralysis | Nerve conduction | Good |
| Stretch | Tingling, burning sensation, pain | Epineurial and perineurial sheath distention (tear) | Good |
| Ischemic injury (less than 6–8 hr) | Pain, paresthesia, hypersensitivity | Vascular damage | Good (>6-8 h is poor) |
| Electrical injury | Pain, burning | Nerve tissue coagulation; necrosis of nerve, vessels, skin, muscle | Unpredictable |
| Radiation injury | Pain | DNA damage, delayed mitosis, fibrosis | Questionable |
| Injection and laceration | Severe pain | Vascular damage, inflammatory changes | Fair |

Adapted from Terzis JK, Smith KL. The Peripheral Nerve. New York: Raven Press, 1990.

delayed conduction, loss of oxidative phosphorylation inside the nerve, and inhibition of sodium, potassium, and ATPase.[31–33] Electron microscopic studies of compressed nerves have revealed myofibroblast activation and proliferation in the epineurium and the appearance of small unmyelinated axons, indicating nerve regeneration.[34]

### Stretch Damage

Sudden overstretching of joints and muscles may damage superficial nerves. Nerve stretching is common in bone fractures, joint dislocations, obstetric trauma, and inadvertent traction during surgical repair of nerves. Of all stretch injuries, 95% are sustained in upper extremities; 16% in the peroneal nerves, and only 2% in the sciatic nerve.[35] The integrity of the three nerve-membrane sheaths is important. One of the common causes of traction injuries is the stretching of the epineurial and perineurial sheaths; however, when only the epineurium is distended, its elasticity protects the nerve. Nerve stretching also may cause proliferation of fibroblasts inside the nerve and hemorrhage in multiple areas, suggesting that stretch injuries may damage the collagen membranes as well as the capillaries and venules inside the nerve. Damaged vessels may form microemboli.[35,36]

### Ischemic Injury

Peripheral nerves are supplied with abundant oxygen through an elaborate vascular system to maintain cellular integrity, axoplasmic transport, and the generation, maintenance, and restoration of the membrane potential necessary for nerve conduction. Unlike the central nervous system, the PNS is fairly resistant to brief periods of ischemia. However, chronic hypoxia may cause weakness, referred pain, paresthesia, hypersensitivity, and sensory deficits.[1] Ischemia lasting more than 6 to 8 hours may cause necrosis and abnormal spontaneous potentials.[1,4,37,38] Ischemia can cause first- through fourth-degree nerve injury, as described above. Asphyxia for 10 minutes or more can result in severe damage in humans, including slowing of the resting potential, decrease in action potential, and ultimately failure of nerve excitability within 30 to 40 minutes. Reoxygenation can produce complete recovery within 10 minutes, indicating that ischemic changes in the nerve are metabolic rather than anatomic.[39,40]

### Electrical Injury

Injuries induced by electricity primarily involve motor nerves and produce immediate neurologic deficits associated with coagulation necrosis, heat production, and burn. This leads to abnormalities of nerve conduction (decrement of about 100 mA/mm of nerve diameter) in experimental animals.[41,42] Electrical injuries damage nerves, vessels, skin, or muscle tissue. Consequently, the associated fibrosis and scar formation is considerably greater than that of other injuries, and this impedes regeneration. The degree of recovery after electrical burns is quite unpredictable.

### Radiation Injury

The clinical effects of ionizing radiation on nerve and muscle are unknown. Radiation, either directly or indirectly, causes release of free radicals inside cell membranes, which contributes to neurolysis and delayed regeneration.[43] The target site for radiation damage is the DNA, causing genomic alterations followed by imprecise replication. In dividing cells, irradiation causes delayed mitosis, which limits cell division.[44,45] In humans, acute degenerative changes in peripheral nerves are aggravated by repeated or massive doses of radiation. Thus, secondary factors such as fibrosis and vascular impairment might become detrimental to the regeneration and elongation of individual axons.[43–46]

### Injection and Laceration Injuries

These types of injuries are associated with severe pain and inflammatory changes in the nerve, the degree of which is related to the degree of injury caused by the substance injected or the tearing produced by the laceration.[47,48]

In summary, a common factor among these different injuries appears to be vascular compromise and associated inflammatory changes. In addition, the collagen and fibroblast proliferation associated with tissue damage may form scar tissue, which significantly delays regeneration.

## Primary Growth Versus Nerve Regeneration

Although the developmental growth and regeneration of nerves may appear to be similar, the processes have some significant differences. Embryonic nerve cells are "cued" by neurotropic factors, which are used by the axons to initiate growth and attain their targets. The sources of neurotropic substances, which can stimulate or inhibit synapses with the appropriate targets, include the growth cone of the axon and the matrix of connective tissue or stromal cells, such as glial cells and fibroblasts.[1,4,49,50] The affinity of axons for inappropriate peripheral targets thus is limited during development and is governed by genetic templates to carry out the sequences of growth in a specific order.

Regeneration, on the other hand, is limited in its initiation of growth in unfavorable environments. Unlike the satellite cells in muscle, fibroblasts in skin, and regenerating hepatocytes in liver, nerves do not contain a reserve of regenerating cells. Degenerating Schwann cells at the periphery and other chemotactic factors signal destruction of the axon to the motor neurons via retrograde transport in the spinal cord. Several theories exist about the initiation of regeneration, the most prevalent being that nerve growth factor (NGF) and other chemotatic substances present at the peripheral targets and inside the sheaths surrounding the Schwann cells contribute in some way to the initiation and maintenance of nerve regeneration (see later).[51,52]

## Peripheral Nerve Regeneration

After injury to the peripheral nerve axon, the distal stump starts to undergo wallerian degeneration while the proximal stump begins to regenerate. The changes associated with regeneration begin within 24 hours after the injury (Figure 21-4). It has been reported that the dying axon somehow signals its condition to the neuronal cell body, which responds immediately to reestablish continuity with the periphery. The axonal growth rate and restoration of proper contact with the periphery is regulated by specific biochemical and biophysical factors.[53,54] For example, regeneration is significantly influenced by the integrity of the en-

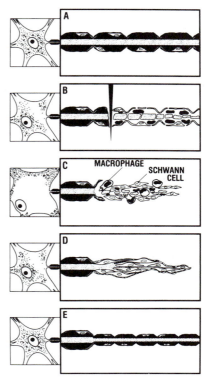

**Figure 21-4.** Diagram describing sequelae of reactions occurring in the distal segment of a peripheral nerve axon after injury to the axon. (*A*) Normal myelinated axon shown with intact axoplasm, nodes of Ranvier, and Schwann cells at the periphery. (*B*) Axonal injury, causing wallerian degeneration in the distal segment. Note the beginning of Nissl bodies rearrangement inside the neuronal cell body. (*C*) Total disintegration of the distal segment with microphagic infiltration and multiplication of Schwann cells. Note maximum rearrangement of Nissl bodies, migration of nucleus and overall hypertrophy in the cell body. (*D*) Growth cone formation and terminal regeneration of the proximal segment. The Schwann cells start to migrate towards the periphery. (*E*) Regenerated and elongated axon exhibits significant thinness. The regenerated axon does not attain the size of the original axon. Lundborg and Danielsen (53b)

doneurial tube; if the endoneurium is not damaged, the regeneration of axon is rather smooth, growing in the intact tube and ultimately finding the end target. In contrast, if the endoneurial wall is severed, the course of regeneration is delayed, possibly because of late neuronal recovery, passage of regenerated axons through the zone of injury or scarred area, elongation, and synapse with the end-organ. Therefore, functional recovery, defined as nerve conduction to the end-organ, is expected to be quicker in axon compression injuries than in traumatic or transection injuries.[1,4,14,15,51,52]

### Mechanism of Nerve Regeneration

Peripheral nerve regeneration involves complex interactions among the nerve cell body, the proximal and distal axon stumps, and neurotropic, neurite-promoting (NPF), and matrix factors. Soon after nerve injury, the neuronal cell body in the spinal cord becomes swollen, the Nissl bodies start to degenerate (chromatolysis), and the nucleus moves to the periphery in preparation for changing the metabolic priority from neurotransmitter synthesis to the production of materials required for axonal growth and elongation.[55] The cell must synthesize new messenger RNA, lipids, and proteins, especially cytoskeletal proteins such as tubulin and actin, neurofilaments, and gap-associated proteins (GAPs). GAPs, which are required to promote regeneration, are transported quickly to the distal end, at a rate of 400 mm per day. Synthesis of these proteins is 20 to 100 times higher during the early stages of regeneration than during normal growth. Cytoskeletal proteins, on the other hand, are moved much more slowly, at 5 to 6 mm per day.[56–58] Several investigators have suggested that during early regeneration the neuronal cell body behaves like an embryonic cell, with high growth-promoting activity and accumulation of growth factors.[59,60]

Cajal[61] was the first to demonstrate that viable nerve fibers grow out of the proximal stump of an injured neuron about 6 hours after injury, followed about 36 hours later by growth at the axon tip. Unlike the normal growth rate of 2 to 3 mm per day, regenerated axons grow through the scarred area very slowly (about 0.25 mm per day; see Table 21-5 for rates of regeneration in different nerves).[14] The growth of proximal axon is preceded by formation of a growth cone at the tip of the proximal stump. This is rich in smooth endoplasmic reticulum, microtubules, microfilaments, large mitochondria, lysosomes, and other vacuolar and vesicular structures of unknown function. It was suggested recently that before the regenerated axons emerge from the proximal stump the tip of the growth cone adheres to collagen surrounding

the degenerating distal stump, after which transmembrane events involving internal actin filaments lead to the release of a proteolytic substance that dissolves the matrix permitting elongation of the axon.[62–64]

Wallerian degeneration of the distal stump causes significant accumulation of collagenous material in and around the degenerating axon. By 28 to 35 days after injury, when robust regenerative activity is observed in the proximal axon, endoneurial collagen has accumulated in the distal segment, exerting pressure on the regenerated axons, decreasing their diameter and increasing the number of Schwann cells per unit of length of the regenerated axon. The newly regenerated axons also exhibit short internodal lengths and a vascular supply that is only 60% to 80% of its original cross-sectional area, even after remyelination.[65,66] This is interpreted to mean that the growth of regenerated axons is significantly influenced by the environment at the distal segment.

In addition to the interaction between the distal and proximal stumps, NGF and NPFs play significant roles in survival, neurite extension, and transmitter production in dorsal root ganglion and sympathetic neurons. NGF and other neurotropic factors are required to regulate cell division, cell death, axonal outgrowth, and synapses during fetal development and to facilitate regeneration after nerve injury.

NGF is synthesized in target tissue innervated by sympathetic and sensory neurons and is transported by retrograde transport to the neurons. NGF is a 26-kd polypeptide first isolated by Levi-Montalcini in 1987[67]; it influences neurite navigation, growth cone morphology, regeneration of proximal axons, and axonal elongation. Specific antibodies to NGF have been produced, and its genome has been located. Its concentration in the blood is very limited and it is measured primarily in target cells.[68–70] Binding studies with Iodine 125 have demonstrated the presence of specific and heterogeneous receptor sites in a variety of cells, including cells of neural crest origin, sympathetic and sensory neuronal cells, and the rat PC12 cell line. Low- and high-affinity receptors bind NGF at dissociation constants (Kd) of 8 nM and 0.2 nM, respectively.[71,72] The NGF receptor protein appears to be an acidic glycoprotein with an apparent molecular weight of 75 Kd existing as a disulfide dimer. The receptor is phosphorylated mainly at the serine sites. NGF-mediated modulation of PC12 cell line results in transport of tyrosine hydroxylase and amino acids.[73] The human NGF receptor gene contains about 25 kilobases and at least 3 axons. A better understanding of the biochemistry and physiology of NGF and similar growth factors in peripheral nerves may be necessary before we understand their roles in promoting growth and regeneration of sensory nerves.[73–75]

The role of NGF needs further definition with regard to regeneration in responsive cells. It has been understood that the genome encoding the NGF receptor is the same in the sympathetic and sensory cells[76] and that the signal for gene expression and functional alteration originates from internalization of NGF at the cell surface.[77,78] Therefore, to understand its mechanism of action it is necessary to determine the effects of NGF on membrane transport, membrane ruffling, and protein phosphorylation in regenerating nerves. Tanuichi[79] and Heumann and their coworkers[80] reported the largest amounts of NGF and its receptors to be at the terminal ends of the peripheral nerves. Expression of its response appears to be related to the Schwann cells in the neural sheaths surrounding both NGF-dependent and -independent axons, confirming the belief that the NGF is associated with repair mechanisms.

Similarly, NPFs are substrate-bound glycoproteins that bind to the polycationic substrata in nerve cultures and to the basal lamina of Schwann cells in vivo. Laminin, for example, a major component of the Schwann basal lamina, binds to collagen IV–type proteoglycan to facilitate target navigation.[81–83] Fibronectin, another NPF, promotes elongation of neurites in tissue culture by enhancing adhesion to the substrata or matrix. Other molecules presumed to enhance neurite growth are cell adhesion molecules (or N-CAM). N-CAMs are also membrane glycoproteins present in the developing nerve cells that promote adhesion.[84,85]

Finally, some matrix factors such as fibrin facilitate axonal regeneration by providing a medium for growth and elongation. During nerve repairs, for example, the proximal and distal ends of a cut nerve are passed through a silicone or semipermeable membrane guide laden with fibrin matrix to facilitate nerve regeneration. Fibrin, a product of

fibrinogen and fibronectin, interacts with many NPFs in ways that are not clearly understood.[86,87]

In summary, peripheral nerve regeneration is a complicated process regulated by interactions between intrinsic factors and the peripheral target. An absence of inputs from the periphery or a disturbance at the spinal cord level would significantly delay or impede the process of regeneration.

### *Factors Promoting Nerve Regeneration*

The extent and rate of nerve regeneration can be influenced much by extrinsic factors, including biologically active compounds, cerebral gangliosides, electrical or electromagnetic stimulation, and surgical procedures. The physiologic effects of these factors are described briefly below.

Estrogen, testosterone, insulin, and adrenal and thyroid hormones all reportedly affect nerve regeneration in varied and site-specific ways. For example, estrogen and insulin reportedly facilitate the growth of neurites in explants and tissue culture,[88–90] whereas testosterone and thyroid hormone stimulate regeneration of the sciatic nerve. Protease inhibitors such as glial-derived protease inhibitor[91] and leupeptin[92] inhibit the degeneration of the glial and distal axon, respectively, thus fostering nerve regeneration. Acidic fibroblast growth factor (FGF), a polypeptide present in brain tissue, appears to increase the number of myelinated fibers in the rat and to increase neurite growth in PC12 cell cultures. Beneficial effects of FGF in vivo are related to Schwann cell activation and blood supply enhancement. The action of FGF involves membrane-bound adenylcyclase, and cyclic AMP and is significantly affected by adding Forskolin, which in frog sciatic nerve increases sensory nerve regeneration by 40% or more. Similarly, inhibition of free radicals such as catalase[93,94] appears to enhance nerve regeneration by protecting the neurons from oxidative injury. The organic dye pyronin reportedly accelerates axonal sprouting at the nodes of Ranvier.[95] At present, FGF, Forskolin, and leupeptin are being tested for their ability to promote nerve regeneration.

Another group of compounds that have shown significant promise during the last decade are the cerebral gangliosides. These glycolipids are constituents of the neuronal plasma membrane, synthesized in the neural soma and transported to the periphery by fast axonal transport. In vitro preparations of gangliosides, especially GMI and GMIII, have been shown to promote neurite regeneration.[96–98] Gangliosides administered to intact animals enhance the formation of nerve sprouts and neuromuscular junctions and thus improve muscle reinnervation. The clinical utility of these compounds, however, is still controversial.

The use of physical modalities such as pulsed electromagnetic field and direct current stimulation to promote healing of neural tissue can be traced to the 18th century. During the last two decades, interest has been rekindled in the use of electrical stimulation (ES) and electromagnetic stimulation (EMS) to promote nerve regeneration. Despite differences in technique, such as whole-body or partial-body exposure, types of fields, and duration of treatment, most studies have demonstrated that pulsed EMS enhances nerve regeneration, particularly axon sprouting.[99–102] Cumulatively, ES and EMS reportedly increase the number of axons below the suture line or guide tube; the rate of axon regeneration, the number of motor axons forming synapses; the recovery of nerve conduction; and functional recovery.

In contrast, Murray and colleagues[103] and Cordiero and coworkers[104] have criticized these reports, noting that in most of them only one of many intrinsic factors was examined; the course of motor or sensory regeneration was not examined in relation to nerve conduction or other functional tests; pain tolerance was not documented; and the confounding role of ES and EMS in promoting collagen synthesis, which may enhance scar formation, was not evaluated.

Direct current electrical stimulation also has been reported to enhance sciatic nerve regeneration in adult rats. Weak cathode current (10 $\mu$amp/cm$^2$, field strength 100 mV/cm) or distal placement of cathode increased the reinnervation of hind limb muscles in the rat, as measured by electromyography. Interestingly, weak current was effective only after cut-and-suture techniques[105] and not after crush injuries, which appears to contradict the observation that axon regeneration is smoother when the endoneurium is intact.[106]

Similarly, low-voltage, pulsed ES of partially denervated muscle has been shown to improve the rate of neurotization and thereby improve muscle reinnervation in experimental animals.[106,107] Her-

bison, Jaweed, and Ditunno[108] stimulated partially sectioned sciatic nerves of rats using implanted electrodes and examined the isometric contractile properties of the plantar flexors. Electrical stimulation at 10 Hz for 2 to 4 hours, five times a week for 6 weeks produced increases in muscle mass and tetanic tension, whereas similar stimulation for 8 hours caused a significant decrease in muscle size and tension, suggesting that lengthy ES regimens may inhibit sprouting. Similar results were reported by Pestronk and Drachman,[18] who observed inhibition of axon sprouting after continuous electrical stimulation of muscle. It is also possible that stimulating muscle during axon sprouting may inhibit reinnervation. Jaweed and colleagues[109] observed inhibited muscle twitch force development in the partially denervated (L-5–sectioned) soleus muscles of adult male rats after whole-body EMS at 3 gauss per day for 4 weeks. Soleus mass was decreased and fatigue was increased, suggesting that ES and EMS procedures must be administered cautiously. The stimulation dosage and stage of nerve regeneration should be monitored carefully, and in treatment of humans compliance and pain tolerance must be considered.

After a nerve has been severed and the endoneurial tube disrupted regeneration is poor at best. Several surgical procedures, such as conditioning lesions, sectioning, and resuturing with nerve grafts, have been employed to facilitate nerve regeneration across the gap.[110–115] The rate of nerve regeneration is inversely proportional to the length of the gap produced by a nerve lesion. As shown in Table 21-4, the number of myelinated and nonmyelinated regenerated axons of the rat sciatic nerve declined as the length of the gap between the proximal and distal nerve segments increased from 4 to 8 mm.[112,113] Although axons have been regenerated across a 10-mm gap in the absence of endoneurial tubes,[113–115] Fields and Ellisman[116] found these new axons to be severely impaired. It appears that nerve regeneration and axon elongation are significantly slowed by disturbances in the endoneurial environment, including the presence of endoneurial fibroblasts and associated collagen accumulation plus many minifascicles in place of the original large fascicles. Isolating the regenerating axons from this milieu appears to allow normal elongation to be reestablished.

The concept of bridging the gap dates back to 1880, when Gluck[117] used decalcified bone as a

**Table 21-4.** Effect of the Length of Gap on Short-term (8 weeks) and Long-term (36 weeks) Reeneration of Rat Sciatic Nerve Axons

| Area of Injury (Gap) | Proximal Segment | | Gap | | Distal Segment | |
|---|---|---|---|---|---|---|
| | My | Un | My | Un | My | Un |
| Normal | 8,000 | 15,000 | —— | —— | —— | —— |
| 4 mm | | | | | | |
| 8 wk (N = 5) | —— | —— | 9,000 | 14,000 | 13,500 | 10,500 |
| 36 wk (N = 6) | —— | —— | 14,000 | 27,500 | 13,000 | 15,000 |
| 8 mm | | | | | | |
| 8 wk (N = 5) | —— | —— | 4,600 | 10,500 | 7,000 | 7,500 |
| 36 wk (N = 6) | —— | —— | 8,000 | 14,500 | 10,000 | 13,000 |

Key: My, myelinated axons; Un, unmyelinated axons.

Modified from Jenq C-B, Jenq LL, Bear HM, et al. Conditioning lesion of peripheral nerve changes regenerated axon numbers. Brain Res 1988; 457:63–69.

neural conduit. New procedures have been developed during the last decade to improve this model, with promising results.[115,116,118] The silicone nerve chambers first proposed by Lunborg and Hanson[17] and subsequently developed by Williams' group[86,87] are considered extremely useful in protecting nerve and fostering nerve regeneration.[15] These chambers offer several advantages. First, the surgical procedures during resuturing and placing the nerve in the nerve chambers probably cause far less trauma to the epineurium than other procedures. Second, the microenvironment is more conducive to regeneration because of the absence of minifascicles, scars, and distal nerve stump degeneration. Finally, growth-promoting and adhesion factors can be provided in these chambers. Williams and coworkers[87,114] have demonstrated phase-specific promotion of nerve regeneration in silicone nerve chambers (Table 21-5).

In summary, a number of new procedures have emerged in recent years that show promise for enhancing nerve regeneration. Though the mechanisms of action of these procedures are not understood completely, a combination of surgical procedures, physical modalities, and biochemical additives may improve nerve repair even after traumatic nerve injuries.

### Role of Schwann Cells in Regeneration

The Schwann and glial cells surrounding the axons of peripheral nerves are heavily laced with collagen fibers, which provide tensile strength to the nerve. Unlike motor neurons in the spinal cord, Schwann cells can reproduce freely and adapt to environmental demands during degeneration and regeneration of the axon. Schwann cells and pe-

**Table 21-5.** Nerve Regeneration Phases and Events in a Silicone Nerve Chamber

| Phases | Days | Events | Promoting Factors |
|---|---|---|---|
| Fluid phase | 1 | Accumulation of exudates from proximal and distal segments | Neurotropic factors |
| Matrix phase | 2–6 | Coalescence to fibrin matrix | Fibrin |
| Cellular phase | 7–14 | Migration of cells from distal and proximal segments | Perineurial, endothelial, Schwann cells |
| Axonal phase | 15–21 | Proximal segment growth (1–2 mm/d), myelination, distal segment entry | Capillaries, axons |

Data from Williams LR, et al.[87,114]

ripheral nerve neurons develop together from neural crest cells. The point at which the two cells separate from each other is unknown, though it is believed to be early, at the time of crest cell migration.[119] The number of Schwann cells increases with the number of motor and sensory fibers during development; reduction in nerve fibers due to damage or disease is associated with a decrease in Schwann-cell number.[120] The number of Schwann cells in the nerve is believed to be regulated by the neuronal cell body. Bunge[121] reviewed tissue culture techniques to isolate Schwann cells and examine their responses to axonal homogenates, mitogens, and spinal cord explants.[122–124] Biochemical, electron microscopic, and immunocytochemical analyses revealed that the Schwann cells in contact with axons can generate basal lamina (collagen type IV, laminin, and heparan sulfate proteoglycan). During early neural development and regeneration, each group of unmyelinated axons is harbored within the cytoplasm of a series of ensheathing Schwann cells; each myelinated fiber is provided with a series of Schwann cells over its length.[121] The significance of this phenomenon is not fully understood.

The roles of Schwann cells during axonal degeneration, however, have been known for some time. It appears from tissue-culture studies that the proliferation of Schwann cells after axonal injury results in release of a mitogenic substance that aids the degeneration of myelin.[125] During regeneration, the Schwann cells also contribute to the ensheathment of sensory axons smaller than 1 μ in diameter, and to the myelination of larger fibers. Axonal contacts may regulate the deposition of basal lamina by Schwann cells, which appear to be capable of forming basal lamina without the aid of fibroblasts. Finally, fibroblasts and Schwann cells both contribute to fibrous collagen present in the endoneurium; fibroblasts alone contribute to formation of the perineurium.

## Reinnervation of Muscle

The ultimate goal of nerve regeneration is to recreate a synapse with the end-organ. Motor nerve endings normally join the muscle at neuromuscular junctions, where they exert neurotropic effects. Denervation of muscle causes dramatic changes in the morphology, biochemistry, histochemistry, and physiology of the denervated muscle.[126–130] If the motor nerve is crushed, the axons regenerate smoothly and form another synapse, either in the original end-plate area or adjacent to it. Also, the latencies of nerve conduction to the muscle are delayed. Herbison, Jaweed, and others[128–130] demonstrated that crush-denervation of rat sciatic nerve produces degenerative changes in the gastrocnemius-soleus in accordance with the absence of nerve conduction and appearance of fibrillation potentials. Within 2 to 3 weeks after denervation, neuromuscular junctions are reestablished, after which nerve conduction is normalized and fibrillation disappears (Figure 21-5).

Muscle reinnervation after crush lesions results in 80% to 90% recovery of the muscle mass, protein content, cross-sectional area, and isometric tension in the slow-twitch and fast-twitch muscle fibers.[128–130] Regeneration of crushed or severed axons may be induced by yet unknown chemotactic factors residing in the muscle. Several investigators have reported that the formation of extrajunctional acetylcholine receptors at the periphery of denervated muscle is one of the stimuli for terminal regeneration of the axon.[18,20] Herbison and colleagues[128,131] demonstrated that overwork induced by synergistic tenotomy of the rat plantaris and gastrocnemius or 2 to 4 hours' daily swimming exercise during reinnervation (or synapsis) may delay the recovery of muscle contractile proteins in the soleus. These findings support the hypothesis that physical or electrical activity during neuromuscular synapsis may impair muscle recovery.[108]

After sectioning or trauma the regeneration of axons is quite slow compared to that after crush denervation. The rate of regeneration, navigation, and subsequent reinnervation are significantly delayed. Polyinnervation of muscle (i.e., multiple nerve endings making synapse with a single end-plate area) persists comparatively longer.

Partial injury to peripheral nerves causes degeneration of some axons while others are left intact. Regeneration of the intact axons causes reinnervation of the adjacent denervated muscle fibers. This process has been called peripheral reinnervation of the muscle.[18,20,132] After partial denervation in the rat, the intact axons regenerate within 3 to 5 days and neuromuscular synapsis is

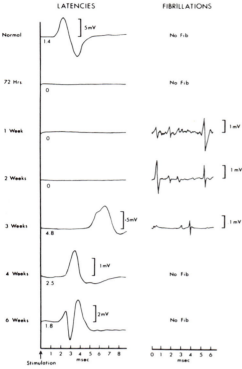

**Figure 21-5.** Changes in nerve conduction to the gastro-cnemius muscle and fibrillation potentials (FP) after crush denervation of rat sciatic nerve. Note disappearance of nerve conduction for up to 2 weeks and appearance of FPs within 72 hours after nerve injury. Nerve conduction to the muscle is reestablished with delayed latency between 2 and 3 weeks after nerve crush. This is accompanied by disappearance of FPs. By 6 weeks after nerve crush, the action potentials become polyphasic, indicating functional muscle reinnervation. (From Herbison GJ, Jaweed MM, Ditunno JF, et al. Effect of overwork during reinnervation of rat muscle. Exp Neurol 1973; 41:1–14.)

reestablished within 7 to 14 days. During this period, the neuromuscular junctions are polyinnervated. It normally takes 2 to 3 months for all synapses to become completely functional.[131–133] Reinnervation enlarges the innervation field of a motor unit to three to five times its original size.[134,135] Jaweed and colleagues[132] performed bilateral L-5 spinal nerve sectioning and simultaneous unilateral synergistic tenotomy of the rat plantaris and gastrocnemius to induce overwork in the soleus. After 7 days, neither damage from overwork nor decreased muscle mass was seen; however, the intact (10% to 12%) myelinated axons of the soleus nerve showed significant hypertrophy (22.5% vs control; Figure 21-6). This observation suggests that intact myelinated axons can adapt to overwork-induced stress. It is not clear, however, whether continued stress for prolonged periods might not produce deleterious effects. The significance of this phenomenon can be appreciated in diseases that include partial nerve injuries, such as diabetes, poliomyelitis, and amyotropic lateral sclerosis.

Rotshenker[136] outlined three mechanisms for the induction of sprouting and synapse formation during peripheral regeneration of the axon: trans-neuronal, central, and peripheral. The transneuronal mechanism involves inducing axon sprouting of intact motor neurons within the spinal cord (motor, sensory, or other). The central mechanism, which assumes that the site of regulation of axon growth is the neuronal cell body, proposes that muscle fibers may regulate sprouting and synapse formation by retrograde axoplasmic transport. The peripheral mechanism implicates neural growth-promoting factors present in the motor neuron extensions, including nerve endings or branches and target cells. Further investigations are necessary to characterize the interaction of these mechanisms in promoting peripheral regeneration.

## Conclusions

Peripheral nerve regeneration is a complex, well-coordinated process involving interactions between the neuron cell body in the spinal cord and its peripheral targets, the muscle or sympathetic neurons. Injury to the nerve induces wallerian degeneration of the axon below the site of the lesion, while the proximal stump undergoes immediate remodeling, terminal sprouting, and, ultimately, synapsing with the target organ or neuron. The signal for regeneration, believed to be transmitted from either the degenerating axon or the target cell, induces dramatic changes in the neuron within 24 hours. Depending on the degree and type of nerve injury, the nerve regeneration process begins within 36 to 48 hours after injury. The rate of elongation of the newly regenerated axon depends on the microenvironment surrounding it. Intrinsic factors influencing regeneration reside within and around the neuron—the neuronal cell

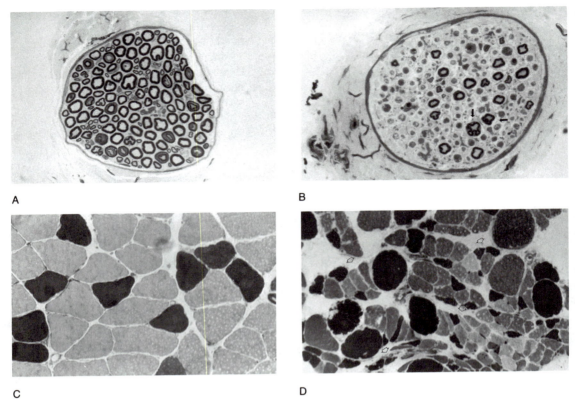

A

B

C

D

**Figure 21-6.** Effects of partial denervation in the rat. The soleus nerve and soleus muscle were examined 1 to 3 weeks after sectioning of the L-5 spinal nerve. (*A*) Normal rat soleus nerve showing cross-section of the whole nerve and the axons. All of the larger axons are myelinated; whereas the smaller axons consist of both the myelinated and unmyelinated fibers. (*B*) L-5 spinal nerve–sectioned rat soleus nerve, 1 week after partial denervation. Note a loss of approximately 90% of innervation due to spinal nerve sectioning. Some of the intact axons hypertrophy and show myelin abnormalities (*arrows*). (*C*) Normal rat soleus muscle showing slow-twitch (*light*) and fast-twitch (*dark*) muscle fibers. The differentiation of muscle fibers was based on the reactivity of myosin ATPase at pH 9.4. There is a normal distribution of the ST and FT fibers. (*D*) L-5 spinal nerve–sectioned rat soleus muscle, 3 weeks after partial denervation. Note significant hypertrophy of the intact ST and FT fibers (rounded fibers) due to overwork. The small triangulated fibers are denervated. The medium-sized fibers are presumed to be peripherally reinnervated fibers (*arrowheads*).

body, proximal and distal stumps, NGF, NPF, and matrix factors. Optimal interactions among these factors determine the success of regeneration.

Extrinsic factors that can promote nerve regeneration or elongation include biologically active compounds such as hormones, neuroactive peptides, and glycoproteins such as cerebral gangliosides, fibroblast growth factor, Forskolin, Isoxanine, and pyronin. Inhibitors of wallerian degeneration such as leupeptin may be useful in promoting axon elongation. Pulsed electrical or electromagnetic field stimulation of regenerating nerves or axons has been promising; however, ut-

most caution must be taken when the muscle rather than the nerve is being stimulated to enhance regeneration. ES and EMS procedures may also facilitate regeneration by decreasing fibrosis in the perineurial, epineurial, and endoneurial sheaths. Successful axon regeneration is manifested by synapse with muscle or sympathetic neurons and reestablishment of nerve conduction. Excessive physical or electrical activity imposed on muscle during axonal synapse (or muscle reinnervation) appears to have a negative influence. Although a suitable replacement for autogenous nerve grafts has not yet been identified, silicone nerve grafts laden with collagen and NGF and NPF are promising tools for protecting and enhancing nerve regeneration during surgery.

In summary, scientific advancements during the last decade have brought the field of nerve repair research to the threshold of a new era. It is hoped that improvements will make possible surgical manipulations that can aid peripheral nerve regeneration, and that this new knowledge can be expanded to promote and maintain nerve regeneration in the spinal cord.

## References

1. Terzis JK, Smith KL. The Peripheral Nerve. New York: Raven Press, 1990.
2. Golgi C. cited In: RK Daniel and JK Terzis, eds. Reconstructive Microsurgery. Boston: Little, Brown, 1977.
3. Cajal RS. Studien uber Nervenregenerationen. Leipzig, 1908. [cited in Weiss, 1941].
4. Sunderland S. The anatomy and physiology of nerve injury. Muscle Nerve 1990; 13:771–784.
5. Seddon HJ, Medawar PB, Smith H. Rate of regeneration of peripheral nerves in man. J Physiol (Lond) 1943; 102:191–215.
6. Hoffmann H. Local reinnervation in partially denervated muscle: A histopathological study. Aust J Exp Biol Med Sci 1950; 28:383–397.
7. Weiss P. The technology of nerve regeneration: A review. J Neurosurg 1944; 1:400–450.
8. Sherrington CS. On the anatomical constitution of nerves of skeletal muscles with remarks on recurrent fibers in the ventral spinal root. J Physiol (Lond) 1894; 17:211.
9. Eccles JC, Sherrington CS. Number and contraction values of individual motor units examined in some muscles of the limb. Proc R Soc London (Biol) 1930; 106:326.
10. Erlanger J, Gasser H. Electrical Signs of Nervous Activity. Philadelphia: University of Pennsylvania Press, 1937.
11. Thomas PK, Jones B. The cellular responses to nerve injury. J Anat 1967; 100:45–55.
12. Oldfors A. Permeability of perineurium of small nerve fascicles: An ultrastructural study using ferritin in rats. Neuropathol Appl Neurobiol 1981; 7:183–194.
13. Novikoff AB, Quintana N, Villaverde H, et al. Nucleoside phosphatase and choline esterase activities in dorsal root ganglion and peripheral nerve. J Cell Biol 1966; 29:525–545.
14. Miller RG. Injury to peripheral motor nerves. Muscle Nerve 1987; 10:698–710.
15. Seckel BR. Enhancement of peripheral nerve regeneration. Muscle Nerve 1990; 13:785–800.
16. Lundborg G, Dahlin LB. Structure and function of peripheral nerves. In: Gelberman RH Operative Nerve Repair and Reconstruction, vol I. Philadelphia: JB Lippincott, 1991;3–17.
17. Lundborg G, Hansson H. Regeneration of peripheral nerve through a preformed tissue space. Brain Res 1979; 178:573–576.
18. Pestronk A, Drachman DB. Motor nerve sprouting and acetylcholine receptors. Science 1978; 199:1223–1225.
19. Kuno M, Miyata Y, Munoz-Martinez EJ. Differential reaction of fast and slow alpha motoneurons to axotomy. J Physiol (Lond) 1974; 240:725–739.
20. Brown MC, Holland RC, Hopkins WG. Motor nerve sprouting. Ann Rev Neurosci 1981; 4:17–24.
21. Seddon HJ. Three types of nerve injury. Brain 1943; 66:237–261.
22. Sunderland S. Nerves and Nerve Injuries. Edinburgh: Churchill Livingstone, 1978;88–132.
23. Simpson JA. Nerve injuries, general aspects. In: Daniel RK, Terzis JK, eds. Reconstructive Microsurgery. Boston: Little, Brown, 1977;244–264.
24. Lundborg G. Structure and function of the intraneural microvessels as related to trauma, edema formation and nerve function. J Bone Joint Surg 1975; 57:725.
25. Costaldo JE, Ochoa JL. Mechanical injury of peripheral nerves, fine structure and dysfunction. Clin Plast Surg 1984; 11:9.
26. Waller A. Experiments on the section of glossopharyngeal nerves of frog and observations of the alterations produced thereby in the structure of their primitive fibers. Philos Trans R Soc Lond 1850; 140:423.
27. Bradley WG. Disorders of Peripheral Nerves. Oxford: Blackwell Scientific, 1974.
28. Orgel M, Terzis JK. Epineurial versus perineurial repair: An ultrastructural and electrophysiologic study of nerve regeneration. Plast Reconstr Surg 1977; 60:80–91.
29. Lundborg G, Gelberman RH, Minteer-Convery M, et al. Median nerve compression in the carpal-tunnel functional response to the experimentally induced controlled pressure. J Hand Surg 1982; 7:252–259.
30. Fowler TJ, Danta G, Gilliatt RW. Recovery of

The authors thank Christine Wogan and Michael Dean of the Baylor College of Medicine for their valuable assistance in preparation of this manuscript.

nerve conduction after a pneumatic tourniquet, observations on the hind limb of the baboon. J Neurol Neurosurg Psychiatry 1972; 35:638.

31. Swan KG, Swan RC. Gunshot Wound Pathophysiology and Management. Littleton, Mass: PSG, 1980.

32. Landon DN, Hall HS. The myelinated nerve fiber. In: Landon DN, ed. The Peripheral Nerve. London: Chapman and Hall, 1976.

33. Sunderland S. Nerve lesion in the carpal tunnel syndrome. J Neurol Neurosurg Psychiatry 1976; 39:615–626.

34. Mackinnon SE, Dellon AL. Experimental study of chronic nerve compression. Hand Clin 1986; 2:639–650.

35. Goodall RJ. Nerve injuries in fresh fractures. Texas State J Med 1956; 52:93.

36. Lundborg G, Rydevik B. Effects of stretching the tibial nerve of the rabbit. J Bone Joint Surg 1973; 55B:390–401.

37. Leone J, Ochs S. Anoxic block and recovery of axoplasmic transport and electrical excitability in nerve. J Neurobiol 1978; 9:229.

38. Gilliatt RW. Acute compression block. In: Sumner AJ, ed. The Physiology of Peripheral Nerve. W.B. Saunders Company, Philadelphia 1972;113.

39. Maruhashi J, Wright EB. Effect of oxygen lack in the single isolated mammalian (rat) nerve fiber. J Neurophysiol 1967; 30:434.

40. Yates SK, Hurst LM, Brown LF. The pathogenesis of pneumatic tourniquet paralysis in man. J Neurol Neurosurg Psychiatry 1981; 44:759–767.

41. Silverside J. The neurological sequelae of electrical injury. J Can Med Assoc 1964; 91:195–204.

42. Ponten B, Ericson U, Johansson S. New observations on tissue changes along the pathway of the current in electrical injury. Scand J Plastic Reconstr Surg 1970; 4:75–82.

43. Cavanaugh JB. Effects of x-irradiation on the proliferation of cells in peripheral nerve during wallerian degeneration in the rat. Br J Radiol 1968; 41:272–281.

44. Little JB. Cellular effects of ionizing radiation. N Engl J Med 1968; 278:308–315, 369–376.

45. Love S. An experimental study of nerve regeneration after x-irradiation. Brain 1983; 106:39–54.

46. Lundborg G, Schildt B. Microvascular permeability in irradiated rabbits. Acta Radiol 1971; 10(suppl):311–320.

47. Gentili F, Hudson AR, Hunter G. Peripheral nerve injection injury: An experimental study. Neurosurgery 1979; 4:244–253.

48. Hudson AR. Nerve injection injuries. In: Terzis JK, ed. Microconstruction of Nerve Injuries. Philadelphia: WB Saunders, 1987;173–179.

49. Katz B. Nerve Muscle and Synapse. New York: McGraw-Hill, 1966.

50. Peters A, Palay SL, Webster HdeF. The Fine Structure of the Nervous System. Philadelphia: WB Saunders, 1976.

51. Varon S, Skaper SD, Manthorpe M. Trophic activities for dorsal root and sympathetic ganglionic neurons in media conditioned by Schwann and other peripheral cells. Dev Brain Res 1981; 1:73–87.

52. Longo FM, Manthorpe M, Skaper SD, et al. Neurotrophic activities accumulate in vivo within silicone nerve regeneration chambers. Brain Res 1983; 261:109–117.

53a. Lundborg G, Dahlin LB. Structure and function of peripheral nerve. In: Gelberman RH, ed. Operative Nerve Repair and Reconstruction. Philadelphia: JB Lippincott, 1991.

53b. Lundborg G, Danielsen N. Injury degeneration and regeneration. In: RH Gelberman, ed. Operative Nerve Repair and Reconstruction. Philadelphia: JB Lippincott, 1991.

54. Smith J, Baroffio A, Dupin E, et al. Role of extrinsic factors in the development of the peripheral nervous system from the neural crest. In: Scarpini E, Fioro MG, Pleasure D, et al. Peripheral Nerve Development and Regeneration: Recent Advances and Clinical Applications. 1989;3–11.

55. Bray D. Isolated chick neurons for the study of axonal growth. In: Banker G, Goslin K, eds. Culturing Nerve Cells. Cambridge, Mass: MIT Press, 1991;137–154.

56. Lasek RJ, Hoffman PN. Neuronal cytoskeleton, axonal transport and axonal growth. In: Goldman, et al., eds. Microtubules and Related Proteins: Cell Proteins. New York: Cold Spring Harbor, 1976;1021–1049.

57. Bisby MA, Redshaw JD, Carlsen RC, et al. Growth-associated proteins (GAPS) and axonal regeneration. In: Gordon T, Stein RB and Smith PA eds. Neurology and Neurobiology: The Current Status of Peripheral Nerve Regeneration. New York: Alan R Liss, 1988;35–52.

58. Stoeckel K, Thoenen H. Retrograde axonal transport of nerve growth factor: Specificity and biological importance. Brain Res 1975; 85:337–341.

59. Richardson PM, Verge VM. The induction of a regenerative propensity in sensory neurons following peripheral axonal injury. J Neurocytol 1986; 15:585–594.

60. Smith PA, Shapiro J, Gurtu S, et al. The response of the ganglionic neurons to axotomy. In: Gordon, et al., eds. Neurology and Neurobiology: The Current Status of Peripheral Nerve Regeneration. New York: Alan R Liss, 1988;15–23.

61. Cajal RS. Degeneration and Regeneration of the Nervous System, vol I. London: Oxford University Press, 1928.

62. Crockett SA, Kiernan JA. Acceleration of peripheral nerve regeneration in vivo. Attraction of regrenerating axons by diffusable factors derived from cells in distal nerve stumps of transected peripheral nerves. Brain Res 1982; 253:1–12.

63. Sunderland S. The Future. In: Nerve Injuries and their Repair, 1991;519–525.

64. Letourneau PC. Cell to substratum adhesion and guidance of axonal elongation. Dev Biol 1975; 44:92.

65. Sunderland S, Bradley KC. Denervation atrophy of the distal stump of a severed nerve. J Comp Neurol 1950; 93:401–409.

66. Ducker TB, Kempe LG, Hatyes GJ. The metabolic background of peripheral nerve surgery. J Neurosurg 1969; 30:270–280.

67. Levi-Montalcini R. The nerve growth factor 35 years later. Science 1987; 237:1154–1162.

68. Herrup K, Shooter EM. Properties of the beta nerve growth factor receptor in development. Cell Biol 1975; 67:118–125.

69. Johnson EM, Tanuichi M, Clark HB, et al. Demonstration of retrograde transport of nerve growth factor receptor in the peripheral and central nervous system. J Neurosci 1987; 7:923–929.

70. Stephani A, Sutter A, Zimmerman A. Nerve growth factor in serum. J Neurosci Res 1987; 17:25–35.

71. Vale RD, Shooter EM. Assaying binding of nerve growth factor to cell surface receptors. Meth Enzymol 1985; 109:21–39.

72. Schechter AL, Bothwell MA. Nerve growth factor receptors on PC12 cells: Evidence for two receptor classes with differing cytoskeletal association. Cell 1981; 24:867–874.

73. Rowland EA, Muller TH, Goldstein M, et al. Cell-free detection and characterization of a novel nerve growth factor–activated protein kinase in PC12 cells. J Biol Chem 1987; 262:7504–7513.

74. Chandler CE, Parsons LM, Hosang M, et al. A monoclonal antibody modulates the interaction of nerve growth factor with PC12 cells. J Biol Chem 1984; 259:6882–6889.

75. Ross AH, Grob P, Bothwell M, et al. Characterization of nerve growth factor receptor in neural crest tumors using monoclonal antibodies. Proc Natl Acad Sci USA 1984; 81:6681–6685.

76. Green SH, Greene LA. A MW 103,000 $^{125}$I beta nerve growth factor-affinity labeled species represents both the low and high affinity nerve growth factor receptor. J Biol Chem 1986; 261:15316–15326.

77. Chao MV, Bothwell MA, Ross AH, et al. Gene transfer and molecular cloning of the human NGF receptor. Science 1986; 232:518–521.

78. Seeley PJ, Kieth CH, Shelanski ML, et al. Pressure microinjection of nerve growth factor into the nucleus and cytoplasm. J Neurosci 1983; 3:1488–1494.

79. Tanuichi M, Clark HB, Johnson EM. Induction of nerve growth factor receptor in Schwann cells after axotomy. Proc Natl Acad Sci USA 1986; 83:4094–4098.

80. Heumann R, Korsching S, Bandtlow C, et al. Changes in nerve growth factor synthesis in non-neuronal cells in response to sciatic nerve transection. J Cell Biol 1987; 104:1623–1631.

81. Baron-Van Evercooren A, Kleinman HK, Seppa HE, et al. Fibronectin promotes fast Schwann cell growth and motility. J Cell Biol 1982; 93:211–216.

82. Lander AD. Molecules that make axons grow. Mol Neurobiol 1987; 1:213–245.

83. Cornbrooks CJ, Carrey DJ, Timpl R, et al. Immunohistochemical visualization of fibronectin and laminin in adult rat peripheral nerve and peripheral nerve cells in culture. Soc Neurosci Abstr 1982; 8:240.

84. Dodd J, Jessell TM. Axon guidance and the pattern of neuronal projections in vertebrates. Science 1987; 242:692–699.

85. Dyck PJ, Karnes J, Lais A, et al. Pathological alterations of peripheral alterations of humans. In: Dyck PJ, Thomas PK, Lambert EH, et al. eds. Peripheral Neuropathy. Philadelphia: WB Saunders, 1984;760–870.

86. Williams LR, Danielsen N, Muller H, et al. Influence of the acellular fibrin on nerve regeneration success with the silicone chamber model. In: Gordon et al., eds. Neurology and Neurobiology: The Current Status of Peripheral Nerve Regeneration. New York: Alan R Liss, 1988;111–122.

87. Williams LR, Varon S. Modification of brain fibrin matrix formation in situ enhances nerve regeneration in silicone chambers. J Comp Neurol 1985; 231:209–220.

88. Vita G, Dattola R, Girlanda P, et al. Effects of steroid hormones on muscle reinnervation after nerve crush in rabbit. Exp Neurol 1983; 80:279–287.

89. Varon S, Bunge RP. Trophic mechanisms in the peripheral nervous system. Annu Rev Neurosci 1978; 1:327–361.

90. Bothwell M. Insulin and somatomedin MSA promote nerve growth factor–independent neurite formation by cultured chick dorsal root ganglion sensory neurons. J Neurosci Res 1982; 8:225–231.

91. Milesi H. Nerve grafting. Clin Plast Surg 1984; 11:105–113.

92. Hurst LC, Badalamente MA, Ellstein J, et al. Inhibition of neural and muscle degeneration after epineural neuropathy. J Hand Surg 1984; 9:564–572.

93. Longo FM, Hyman EG, Davis GE, et al. Neurite-promoting factors and extracellular matrix components accumulating in vivo within nerve regeneration chambers. Brain Res 1984; 309:105–117.

94. Muller H, Williams LR, Varon S. Nerve regeneration chamber: Evaluation of exogenous applied by multiple injections. Brain Res 1987; 413:320–326.

95. Keynes RJ. The effect of pyronin on sprouting and regeneration of mouse motor nerves. Brain Res 1982; 253:13–18.

96. Gorio A, Vitadello M. Ganglioside prevention of neuronal functional decay. In: Seil FJ, Herbert E, Carlson BM, eds. Progress in Brain Research, vol 71. Amsterdam: Elsevier, 1987;289–325.

97. Horowitz SH. Therapeutic strategies in promoting peripheral nerve regeneration. Muscle Nerve 1989; 12:314–322.

98. Gorio A, Marini P, Zanoni R. Muscle reinnervation. III. Motoneuron sprouting capacity, enhancement by gangliosides. Neuroscience 1983; 8:417–429.

99. Ito H, Bassett CAL. Effect of weak pulsing electromagnetic fields on neural regeneration in rat. Clin Orthop 1983; 181:283.

100. Ploitis MJ, Zanakis MF, Albala BJ. Facilitated regeneration in the rat peripheral nerve system using applied electrical fields. J Trauma 1988; 28:1375.

101. Raji ARM, Bowden REM. Effects of high peak electromagnetic fields on degeneration and regeneration of peroneal nerve in rats. J Bone Joint Surg 1983; 65:478–492.

102. Wilson DH, Jagadeesh P, Newman PP, et al. The effects of pulsed electromagnetic energy on peripheral nerve regeneration. Ann NY Acad Sci 1974; 238:575.

103. Murray HM, O'Brien WJ, Orgel MG. Pulsed electromagnetic fields and peripheral nerve regeneration in cat. J Bioelect 1984; 3:19.

104. Cordiero PG, Seckel BR, Miller CD, et al. Effects of high intensity magnetic field on sciatic nerve regeneration in the rat. Plast Reconstr Surg 1989; 83:207.

105. McDevitt L, Fortner P, Pomerantz B. Application of weak electrical field to the hind paw enhances sciatic motor nerve regeneration in the adult rat. Brain Res 1987; 416:308–314.

106. Borgens RB. Stimulation of neuronal regeneration and development by steady electrical fields. Adv Neurol 1988; 47:547–564.

107. Hoffman H. Acceleration and retardation of process of axon sprouting in partially denervated muscles. Aust J Exp Biol Med Sci 1952; 30:541–566.

108. Herbison GJ, Jaweed MM, Ditunno JF. Electrical stimulation of sciatic nerve of rats after partial denervation of soleus muscle. Arch Phys Med Rehabil 1986; 67:79–83.

109. Jaweed MM, Herbison GJ, Ditunno JF, et al. Effect of electromagnetic stimulation on terminal regeneration-caused peripheral reinnervation of the rat soleus. In: Proceedings of the International Symposium on Peripheral Nerve Regeneration. Washington, DC: American Association of Electromyography and Electrodiagnosis, August 1989.

110. Carlsen RC. Delayed induction of the cell body response and enhancement of regeneration following a condition/test lesion of frog peripheral nerve at 15 Co. Brain Res 1983; 279:9–18.

111. Bisby MA, Keen P. The effect of conditioning lesion on the regeneration rate of peripheral nerve axons containing substance P. Brain Res 1985; 336:201–206.

112. Jenq C-B, Jenq LL, Bear HM, et al. Conditioning lesion of peripheral nerve changes regenerated axon numbers. Brain Res 1988; 457:63–69.

113. Lundborg G, Dahlin LB, Danielsen N, et al. Nerve regeneration in silicone chambers: Influence of gap length and of distal stump components. Exp Neurol 1982; 76:361–375.

114. Williams LR, Longo FM, Powell HC, et al. Spatial temporal progress of peripheral nerve regeneration within a silicone chamber: Parameters for a bioassay. J Comp Neurol 1983; 218:460–470.

115. LeBeau JM, Ellisman MH, Powell HC. Ultrastructural and morphometric analysis of long term peripheral nerve regeneration through silicone tubes. J Neurocytology 1988; 17:161–172.

116. Fields RD, Ellisman MH. Axons regenerated through silicone tube splices. I. Conduction properties. Exp Neurol 1986; 92:48–60.

117. Gluck T. Uber Neuroplastik auf dem Wege der Transplantation. Arch Klin Chir 1880; 25:606–616.

118. Aebischer V, Guenard SR, Winn RF, et al. Blind-ended semipermeable guidance channel support peripheral nerve regeneration in the absence of a distal nerve stump. Brain Res 1988; 454:170–187.

119. LeDourian H. The Neural Crest. London: Oxford University Press, 1982.

120. Aguayo AJ, Epps J, Charron L, et al. Multipotentiality of Schwann cells in cross anastomized and

grafted myelinated and unmyelinated nerves. Quantitative microscopy and radioautography. Brain Res 1976; 104:1–20.

121. Bunge RP. Tissue culture observations relevant to the study of axon–Schwann cell interactions during peripheral nerve development and repair. J Exp Biol 1987; 132:21–34.

122. Slazer JL, Bunge RP, Glaser L. Studies of Schwann cell proliferation. III. Evidence for the surface localization of the neurite mitogen. J Cell Biol 1980; 84:767–778.

123. Cassel D, Wood PM, Bunge RP, et al. Mitogenicity of axolemma-enriched fractions for cultured Schwann cells. J Cell Biochem 1982; 18:433–446.

124. Sobue G, Kreider B, Asbury AK, et al. Specific and potent mitogenic effect of axolemmal fraction of Schwann cells from sciatic nerves in serum containing and defined media. Brain Res 1983; 28:263–275.

125. Spencer P. Reappraisal of the model for bulk axoplasmic flow. Nature 1972; 240:283–285.

126. Gutmann E, Malichna J, Syrovy I. Contractile properties and ATPase activities in fast and slow muscles of the rat during denervation. Exp Neurol 1972; 36:488.

127. Herbison GJ, Jaweed MM, Ditunno JF, et al. Effect of overwork during reinnervation of rat muscle. Exp Neurol 1973; 41:1–14.

128. Jaweed MM, Herbison GJ, Ditunno JF. Denervation and reinnervation of fast and slow muscles: A histochemical study in rats. J Histochem Cytochem 1975; 23:808–827.

129. Jaweed MM, Herbison GJ, Ditunno JF. Direct

130. Lai KS, Jaweed MM, Herbison GJ, et al. Changes in nerve conduction and phosphorus magnetic resonance ($^{31}$P-NMR) spectra of the gastrocnemius-soleus muscles of rats during denervation and reinnervation. Arch Phys Med Rehabil 1992; 73:1155–1159.

131. Herbison GJ, Jaweed MM, Ditunno JF. Effect of swimming on reinnervation of rat skeletal muscle. J Neurol Neurosurg Psychiatry 1974; 37:1247–1251.

132. Jaweed MM, Herbison GJ, Ditunno JF. Overwork-induced axonal hypertrophy in the soleus nerve of the rat. Arch Phys Med Rehabil 1989; 68:706–709.

133. Coers C, Tellerman-Toppett N, Gerard J-M. Terminal innervation ratio in neuromuscular disease. I. Methods and controls. Arch Neurol 1973; 29:210–214.

134. Thompson W, Jansen JKS. Extent of sprouting of remaining motor units in partly denervated immature and adult rat soleus. Neuroscience 1977; 5:523–535.

135. Hopkins WG, Brown MC. Distribution of nodal sprouts in paralyzed or partially denervated mouse muscle. Neuroscience 1982; 7:37–44.

136. Rotshenker S. Transneural, peripheral and central mechanisms for the induction of sprouting. In: Gordon T, Stein R, and Smith P, eds. The Current Status of Peripheral Nerve Regeneration. New York: Alan R Liss, 1988;63–75.

electrical stimulation of rat soleus during denervation and reinnervation. Exp Neurol 1982; 75:589–599.

# Chapter 22
# Biofeedback

STEVEN L. WOLF

Since its first conceptualization in 1969, biofeedback has been viewed as both a clinical revelation and a misplaced enigma. This disparity is best attributed to the variability in biofeedback's reputed effectiveness when applied to different clinical problems. In the field of rehabilitation, however, the literature is replete with studies demonstrating biofeedback's clinical efficacy for a host of neuromuscular and musculoskeletal disorders. In fact, the accumulated evidence of the benefits of feedback in reducing spasms and hyperactive muscle responses has been convincing to most third-party payers of medical costs. This chapter reviews historical and contemporary perspectives on biofeedback, discusses clinical findings, explores the notion of kinesiologic electromyography, and discusses mechanisms to account for changes in movement control subsequent to electromyographic (EMG) biofeedback interventions.

## Examining the Concept of Feedback

Traditionally, I have used the term *biofeedback* to describe the use of instrumentation to make a covert physiologic process obvious to the user by providing timely and specific visual and/or auditory representations of that process.[1] For rehabilitation, electromyographic (EMG), position, or force feedback is most commonly provided. The visual and auditory cues are supplied virtually instantaneously, and the information is specified by the proximity of the signal transducers (e.g., surface electrodes, potentiometers, strain gauges, force plates) to the signal source.

The behavior of the user (patient) appears stereotypic. At first, most patients are intently attuned to both visual and auditory feedback cues. With time and practice, patients direct their visual attention toward the limb segment while still being mindful of auditory signals. Eventually, patients may abandon both auditory and visual cues, but still demand that they be available as a reference.[2] An integral aspect of this typical scenario is the need for the clinician periodically to withdraw all feedback cues from the patient. Then, the patient is asked to produce an output that approaches a known threshold or target level. Once this attempt has been made the patient may then view the stored response to determine how accurately the target level was reproduced. Inevitably, success at these tasks must be linked to a relearned appreciation of internal cues, perhaps even representative of a recalibrated proprioceptive system.[3]

The foregoing perspective is provided in contrast to the interest in motor control theory appropriately manifested by clinicians specializing in the rehabilitation of patients with neurologic lesions. Winstein[4] has provided an excellent account of feedback in the context of *knowledge and results* (KR). Most clinical applications of feedback are extrinsic, and, in most settings, the feedback would be verbal and not instrumented. In fact, most feedback is more attuned to performance than to discrete selection of individual muscles or muscle groups.[5] Motor learning theorists have divided the learning of a movement into acquisition and transfer phases.[6] Recent data have shown that for *normal persons,* providing periodic KR rather than continuous KR enhances learning and retention.[7,8] Explanations for these results include (1) a *guidance hypothesis,* which suggests that too much reliance on guidance properties might retard response-produced feedback, thereby preventing improvement in error detection capability, and (2) a *consistency hypothesis* predicated on the belief that too much feedback leads to maladaptive corrections and heightened response variability (see, for example reference 9). The validity of these explanations to account for performance changes in patients has been questioned.[4,10]

Table 22-1 is designed to contrast the notion of feedback in motor learning and biofeedback contexts (apologies are offered to any proponent of either context who feels unduly insulted by this perspective). Contrary to the perception of many clinicians and motor theorists, while verbal feedback is continuous (and helpful), it is delayed. In the context of *motor relearning,* any delay impedes the relearning process. Additionally, verbal feedback inevitably lacks informational specificity. For example, how much "harder" is contextually conveyed in the command, That's good, now try harder? As noted earlier, clinical experience dictates that patients with disrupted control

of the peripheral nervous system voraciously "consume" specificity of feedback in the early relearning phase. Removal of feedback must be continuously graded, in the confines of the unique sensory or motor deficits of each patient. Undoubtedly, controlled research paradigms, such as those expressed by Mulder,[11] will have to be tested to validate this point. In the interim, clinicians must remember an inherent distinction when interpreting data from most motor control studies and from clinical muscle biofeedback investigations; namely that in the first case the studies are undertaken among subjects with intact sensorium and movement control as patterns of movement are measured, and in the second the investigations are made among patients with disrupted systems and measure specific muscle activity rather than patterns of movement. Within the past few years, however, biofeedback practitioners have been encouraged to quantify more functional and limb-specific activities.[12]

### Other Feedback Options

KR need not be limited to information derived from muscle. Figure 22-1 shows an electrogoniometer applied to an interphalangeal joint. The leads are attached to a potentiometer through which a small current is passed. The parallelogram arrangement moves as the finger is extended, causing the potentiometer to rotate about its axis. As

**Table 22-1.** Comparing the Notion "of Feedback"

| Component | Motor Learning Therapy | Clinical Biofeedback |
| --- | --- | --- |
| Type | Extrinsic | Extrinsic |
| Source | Usually verbal | Instrumental |
| Timing | Delayed when verbal | Instantaneous |
| Specificity | Nonspecific | Specific, defined by transducer and its placement |
| Best frequency of feedback | Occasional (50%) | 100% |
| Application | Nonpatient | Patient |
| Task | Movement pattern | Joint or muscle specific |

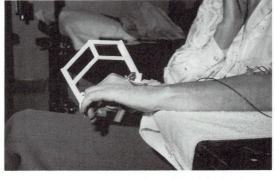

**Figure 22-1.** Electrogoniometric positional feedback device placed about metacarpal-phalangeal joint of left index finger. Note potentiometer at base of modified goniometer.

this rotation occurs, a small amount of current is passed through a strip of linearly placed resistors, each having progressively greater resistance. In keeping with Ohm's law,

$$I = V/R$$

the current remains constant but the resistance values (R) change, and the voltage (V) varies linearly with the resistance. This voltage change is reflected on the lead-emitting diode display in Figure 22-1, which has been arranged to correspond to joint angles. By incorporating a level detector or threshold, the clinician can add an audio tone that changes in quality when the ''threshold'' or desired joint angle is achieved.

Another form of feedback, force or pressure feedback, is represented in Figure 22-2. Force transducers, housed within the shoe inserts, produce a linear voltage change proportional to the force exerted through the foot. Once again, a tone may be emitted through an audio amplifier (Figure 22-2, background). This application is relevant to training amputees to transfer weight onto a prosthesis,[13] training older patients for postural stability,[14] or assessing gait characteristics.[15] The construction and application of these devices is presented in great detail elsewhere.[16,17]

## Applications of Muscle Biofeedback

To date, more than 300 clinical studies addressing feedback applications in physical rehabilitation

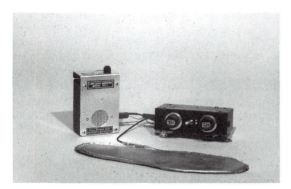

**Figure 22-2.** Shoe insert housing force plate to convey voltage signal proportional to force exerted through plate placed in a properly fitted shoe.

have been published. This survey does not include publications that address feedback or behavior modification approaches to patients whose primary symptom is pain, for the number of articles on that one problem exceeds the total number of biofeedback articles for all other problems involving limitation of movement. Here I focus on the most recent information on common musculoskeletal and neuromuscular disorders. For more historical perspectives, the reader is referred to several classic texts.[18–23]

### *Musculoskeletal Disorders*

In 1987 we noted that most patients with musculoskeletal disorders need to restore strength and mobility without being excessively concerned about proprioceptive and cutaneous loss or cognitive dysfunction precipitated by central nervous system trauma or demyelinating disease.[24] To this group one might add sensorimotor return from peripheral nerve injury, though impaired kinesthesia cannot be discarded as a contributor to reduced motor drive, even with the provision of muscle feedback. In retrospect, the paucity of clinical research using feedback interfaces for musculoskeletal injury patients could probably be attributed to a collective belief in the obvious benefits of immediate quantification of muscle signals during strengthening programs. One of the first documented studies to support this contention was reported by Lucca and Recchiuti,[25] who showed that women who performed isometric contractions that produced visual EMG feedback gained more peak torque than an exercise group or a no-treatment group. A similar study by Croce[26] showed that integrated EMG levels from the quadriceps muscle showed significantly greater increases over a 5-week training period under conditions of isokinetic exercise (at a speed of 30 degrees per second) for male subjects who received feedback compared to groups that received deceptive (false) feedback or none.

Another variation on a similar theme addressed whether normal subjects could differentially activate vastus medialis and lateralis, two muscles of the quadriceps mass innervated by the femoral nerve.[27] Under precise and specified training controls, subjects were able to "downtrain" the vastus lateralis and "uptrain" the vastus medialis. Because it has now been proven that patients with patellofemoral pain have abnormal vastus medialis–vastus lateralis EMG ratios during specific functional tasks[28] it is time to ascertain (1) whether targeted biofeedback training to these two muscles can properly alter this ratio and (2) whether the change affects patellofemoral pain and knee function.

Following the suggestion by Fernie and coworkers[29] that above-knee amputees might gain better knee control if given force feedback, controlled clinical trials have been completed. The results have demonstrated that feedback can augment control in both upper[30] and lower[31] extremity amputees. In the former study, subjects who used a prosthetic limb performed most accurately when audio-augmented feedback was concurrent with the elbow joint movement response as compared to no feedback or postural feedback. In the second study, lower-extremity amputees showed equal improvements in sway reduction whether with mirror feedback and feedback through pressure exerted on a force plate in the prosthetic foot; however, force feedback provided better quantification and control of weight bearing.

The prospects for utilizing force feedback are limited only by the imagination of the user. As an example of exceptional inventiveness, Clarkson and coworkers[32] demonstrated that force feedback from a transducer placed on the instep reduced excessive foot pronation more than control or sham conditions. Force feedback can also be derived from assistive devices such as a feedback cane. Strain gauges can be placed along the shaft of the cane, producing a tone when the torque generated through the shaft exceeds a preset threshold.[33] In essence, the patient is obliged to bear more weight through the limbs and less through the cane as the audio threshold is lowered and the patient is instructed to prevent the sound from occurring.

The future holds promise for applying biofeedback principles to a host of orthopedic problems far beyond the management of chronic back pain. For example, Draper[34] applied muscle feedback to the quadriceps of 11 anterior cruciate ligament (ACL) repair patients within 1 week of reconstructive surgery. Compared to a matched group of 11 ACL patients who served as feedback controls, the group that received feedback showed a significant improvement in peak torque at 45, 60, and 90-degree joint angles over the 12-week rehabilitation period. In a different study, Lee and colleagues[35] were able to show that feedback of force through the hands of students learning spinal mobilization techniques yielded more "ideal" forces at training and at 1-week follow-up than those seen in a control group of students given no feedback on the manual forces used in their applications. These data support the use of feedback as a teaching tool and as a technique to train musculoskeletal injury patients.

Pressure feedback is now incorporated into many devices designed to resolve center of mass and provide visual feedback in the form of a cursor displayed on a monitor. The resolution is the result of as many as eight voltages, derived from individual transducers, that are computed into one final output. Slight postural sway causes the cursor (center of mass) to move. If the clinician marks targets on the monitor, patients can practice weight shifting in multiple directions. When the clinician adds to this technology the capability of actually moving the floor or surrounding surfaces on which the subject is standing, an exceptionally dynamic environment is created. Under these circumstances, it is possible, for example, to train elderly persons who have a history of falls to gain enhanced postural stability under conditions of postural perturbations; that is, when the platform or environment is moved. This unique integration of force feedback and mechanical dynamics offers great promise as a training vehicle to reduce falls or other postural abnormalities.

In 1978, Keef and Surwit[36] issued an admonition that was judiciously recalled 10 years later by John Basmajian.[37] In essence, a note of optimism was sounded over the myriad applications of biofeedback for the rehabilitation community. The major proviso was that the outcome studies be undertaken that were rigorously designed and used appropriate control groups. In the area of many musculoskeletal disorders, this concern has been addressed since Basmajian's 1988 comment. The underlying optimism is well-founded when the interface between biofeedback and diseases of neuromuscular origin is considered.

### Neuromuscular Disorders

Perhaps no single biofeedback application in rehabilitation has been researched as much as the relationship between EMG feedback and motor improvement among stroke patients.[38] While there are numerous examples of treatment strategies and controlled clinical trials of biofeedback treatments for other neuromuscular disorders such as spinal cord injury, multiple sclerosis, and cerebral palsy (see reference 24 for an overview), in this chapter I concentrate on the feedback–stroke patient interface.

The pioneering work of Basmajian[39] and Brudny[40] drew particular attention to the prospects for chronic stroke patients learning to walk with few or no assistive devices. Presumably, by training such patients to recruit anterior leg compartment muscles while inhibiting the triceps surae with the use of muscle biofeedback, control of ankle movement during the swing phase of gait would be improved more than it would by a conventional exercise program. While it is encouraging, this early work did not account for ankle inversion and eversion control in particular; nor were other factors that contribute to successful ambulation, including cutaneous or proprioceptive integrity or degree of cognitive impairment, evaluated. Through systematic study of lower extremity performance among chronic stroke patients receiving muscle feedback training we learned that proprioception and cognitive integrity were essential to maximizing ambulatory independence.[41,42] Subsequent controlled clinical trials[43–45] revealed that muscle feedback training was superior to no treatment or relaxation training alternatives. More recent data corroborate the value of feedback to enhance ambulatory control in normal subjects[46] and in stroke patients given positional feedback.[47]

The value of muscle feedback to improve upper extremity movement control has also been studied vigorously. Initial results, however, were more equivocal (see, for example, references 41, 48, 49). This fact was probably attributable to variations in method and discrepancies in what constituted upper extremity improvement, especially in light of limitations in manual skills. These problems have been thoughtfully reviewed by Ince and coworkers,[50] but as noted by Basmajian[51] in his more recent review, the provision of controlled studies has changed this perspective dramatically.

One paper by Basmajian's group[52] demonstrated that biofeedback applications to stroke patients classified as "early mild" resulted in major upper extremity improvement while those to patients labelled as "late severe" did not. Among many measures of function, patients who received EMG biofeedback along with physical therapy showed greater quantitative improvement than those who received only a standard exercise program. Wolf and Binder-Macleod[53] examined all neuromuscular, range-of-motion, and quantified-timed functional tasks among groups of chronic stroke patients who received either exclusive EMG feedback training or no treatment at all. Blind evaluations revealed that most patients' assistive capacity to use the involved upper extremity improved. Among the subgroup that regained independent use of the hemiparetic hand, all subjects had the pretreatment ability to initiate some voluntary extensor activity in the wrist or fingers. This factor was the single best predictor of total upper limb return with biofeedback training. Control patients showed no improvement; but once placed into a treatment group, the two subjects who had isolated finger or wrist extension activity subsequently gained independent manual use.

We took these criteria to suggest that chronic stroke or head-injured patients could improve their upper extremity and hand use. In a subsequent study[54] we demonstrated that these new patients were able to improve to the same extent as the former group,[53] whether they received conventional targeted feedback training or a new technique called *motor copy*. In the latter treatment, homologous muscles of the upper extremities were used to produce matched outputs from the intact and involved limb, using only differences in amplifier gain to shape responses. Since that time, similar approaches[55] have been applied.

## On Treatment Strategy

The task of treating musculoskeletal injuries or reinnervating peripheral nerve injuries is relatively straightforward—to increase EMG output and shape responses by reducing the amplifier gain and elevating the threshold at any one sensitivity setting. In treating patients with central nervous system involvement, the training strategy is much more complex. Table 22-2 summarizes the general approach, sometimes referred to as "conventional" or "targeted" biofeedback training.

The progression stems from assumptions derived from the teachings of Bobath[56]; specifically, that muscles should be treated in a proximal-to-distal manner and that hyperactive muscles should be relaxed (inhibited) before weak antagonists are recruited. As a result, the typical muscles or muscle groups shown in Table 22-2 are trained by presuming that the upper extremity possesses predominantly flexor synergy and the lower extremity extensor synergy.

The notion that hyperactive muscles should be inhibited and weak muscles recruited has met with some opposition. Recently several clinicians[57–59] suggested that treatment orientation should be geared toward function. This thought suggests

some unique possibilities that can be systematically explored through clinical research efforts. For example, might better results with EMG feedback be obtained through direct training of the weaker muscle group without first downtraining spastic muscles? Is there a need to select muscles by synergy groupings or joint specifications as opposed to simple choice of muscle monitoring based upon requirements to accomplish a specific task?

## The Concept of Kinesiologic Electromyography

Several years ago we suggested that in addition to training patients with EMG biofeedback the information could be processed and quantified on line, so that direct evidence of treatment effectiveness could be obtained or an immediate change could be made in treatment plan or patient handling. The

**Table 22-2.** Typical "Conventional" Electromyographic Training Strategies in the Treatment of Stroke Patients

| Location | Movement | Inhibit | Recruit |
|---|---|---|---|
| **Upper Extremity** | | | |
| Scapula | Adduction | | Serratus anterior |
| Shoulder | Elevation | Upper trapezius | |
| | Internal rotation | Pectoralis major | |
| | External rotation | | Infraspinatus |
| | Flexion | | Anterior deltoid |
| | Abduction | | Middle deltoid |
| Elbow | Flexion | Biceps | |
| | Extension | | Triceps |
| Wrist | Flexion | Flexor mass | |
| | Extension | | Extensor mass |
| Fingers | Flexion | Finger flexors | |
| | Extension | | Finger extensors |
| Thumb | Abduction | Thenar eminence | |
| | Extension | | Wrist-dorsum |
| **Lower Extremity** | | | |
| Hip | Abductor | | Gluteus medias |
| | Extension | | Gluteus maximus |
| | Flexion | | Sartorius |
| | Adduction | Adductor mass | |
| Knee | Extension | Quadriceps | |
| | Flexion | | Biceps femoris |
| Ankle | Plantar flexion | Triceps surae | |
| | Dorsiflexion | | Anterior leg compartment |
| | Eversion | | Extensor digitorum brevis |

issue no longer was one of proving or disproving the usefulness of a treatment approach but rather of altering any aspect of that intervention *via feedback to the clinician and the patient simultaneously.* No longer would the clinician be dependent only on vision and palpation. We coined the acronym CAMA, for concurrent assessment of muscle activity.[60]

An example of this approach can be seen in Figures 22-3 and 22-4. A stroke patient is being asked to recruit the weaker left hamstring muscles during a sit-to-stand task. Not only does the patient observe the response, but the clinician, by keying on the feedback signal, can offer guidance or suggestions to the patient to help activate this muscle group. The interval of the training and the response are defined by a remote foot switch engaged by the clinician. On activating the switch a second

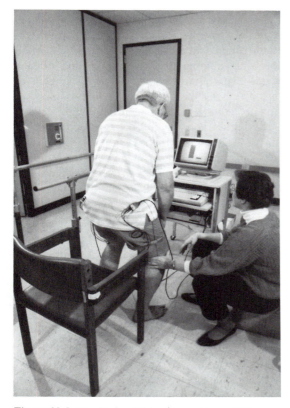

```
TRIAL#:04          00;15
CHANNEL 1
  AVERAGE:      .300    UV*SEC
  MAXIMA:       .410    UV*SEC
  MINIMA:       .136    UV*SEC
CHANNEL 2
  AVERAGE:      .148    UV*SEC
  MAXIMA:       .238    UV*SEC
  MINIMA:       .050    UV*SEC


***PRESS ANY KEY TO CONTINUE***
```

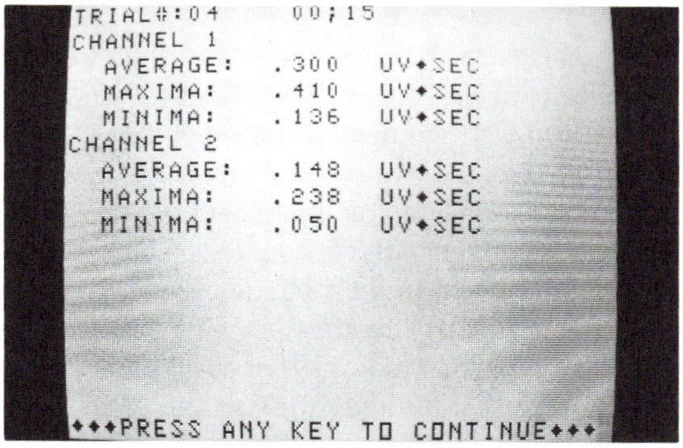

**Figure 22-4.** Representative output of EMG effort from each hamstring muscle group in task shown in Figure 22-3.

time, the duration of the task and the quantification of the response are recorded for the patient's record (Figure 22-4). Within the past year, other investigators have used this approach or variations thereof (see reference 61 for a review).

Integrating quantified EMG values into the treatment assessment or recording procedure is beneficial, as these data offer one more piece of evidence to support the value of a clinical intervention. This validation factor is becoming progressively more important as third-party payers seek proof of rehabilitation treatment benefits before reimbursement is rendered. In addition, while EMG values in and of themselves may not be conclusive in confirming the efficacy of treatment, combined with other measures (e.g., range of motion, torque, time to complete tasks), they help to complete the picture. In this regard, EMG biofeedback instrumentation is of particular interest because such equipment combines treatment capability with evaluation through quantification.

**Figure 22-3.** Monitoring bilateral hamstring activity as stroke patient practices sit-to-stand activity with effort designed to provide feedback of EMG in weaker muscle group while quantifying muscle activity for the duration of the task.

## How Might Muscle Feedback Work?

One major benefit of EMG feedback, particularly if it is adopted after more traditional therapy has been offered, is that it promotes expanded discussions about the possibilities for patients to improve, especially those with long-standing limitations. We pondered this question previously.[62] Based on the stereotypic nature of patient responses, clearly the *speed* with which information is provided to the patient and the *specificity* of that information, defined by the locus of electrode placements, constitute the unique attributes of the modality.

The neurophysiologic factors that allow processing of a visual or auditory representation of a biofeedback signal are complex and poorly understood.[51,63] Undoubtedly, for patients whose central nervous system is intact the timing of feedback serves to create a "feedforward" mechanism designed to augment motor drive. This situation is most prevalent in training for strength or mobility after disturbances that cause muscle weakness and limit joint range of motion.

With diseases that have affected the central nervous system so that the continuity of sensory inflow and motor output has been disrupted, our understanding of the relationship of instrumented feedback signals to enhanced movement performance is exceptionally vague. If one observes patient interaction with feedback devices, however, there appears to be an effort at recalibrating sensorimotor timing. At first patients tend to focus compulsively on both forms of feedback; only later do they observe the limb segment under training while attending to auditory cues. Over time, it appears that patients no longer attend to either cue but insist they be available. This consistently reproducible behavior suggests that with practice and training patients grow to rely more on proprioceptive and interoceptive cues and less on the original exteroceptive cues, which, in reality, were only representations of self-generated muscle activity. In short, the patient may have regained an appreciation or sensitivity to length changes caused by eccentric or concentric muscle efforts.

Many neurologic disease patients are aware of the tasks they should accomplish but fail to execute them. This implies that the specific sensory engram is intact and the disorder must lie in the motor system or between the sensory cortex and the motor command system; that is, in the sensory association cortex. Ostensibly then, the feedback loops in the brain would be incapable of successfully modifying the temporal-spatial requirements for appropriate motor behavior. Successful use of the feedback signals probably rests on the capacity for employing these inputs to activate subsidiary functional sets of motor cells through either direct or reflex loops. Such mechanisms should not be construed to demonstrate true neuroplasticity;

rather, central synapses previously unused in the execution of specific motor commands are now accessed in a way that conventional rehabilitation could not achieve. This phenomenon has been referred to as *unmasking* by Bach-y-Rita and colleagues.[64]

As biofeedback retraining progresses, available and responsive motor cells are called into play. With continued training, patients are able to improve performance. It is interesting to speculate that the sensory engram has established an increasingly reliable linkage with functional transmitting cells, thus making the patient more reliant on proprioceptive feedback and less dependent on an artificial form of information (i.e., biofeedback).

Our understanding of how the feedback signal is processed into meaningful movement is still fragmentary, and we do not yet fully comprehend the circumstances that permit this instrumented effort at relearning to be successfully completed by some patients and not by others, even when all ostensibly have the same diagnosis and lesion site. Furthermore, we have yet to determine whether feedback training that is totally goal-oriented yields better function than single movement–directed training or individual muscle training, especially among patients with neurologic deficits. Should clinicians favor one approach over another? Is there merit in viewing muscles as having subcompartments, each of which possesses unique retraining requirements? Answers to these and other questions await investigation, which, unquestionably, will be easier to conduct with future generations of more sophisticated instruments.

## References

1. Wolf SL. Electromyographic biofeedback: An overview. In: Nelson RM, Currier DP, eds. Clinical Electromyography, ed 2. Norwalk, Conn: Appleton & Lange, 1991;361–384.
2. Wolf SL, Binder-Macleod SA. Electromyographic biofeedback in the physical therapy clinic. In: Basmajian JV, ed. Biofeedback: Principles and Practice for Clinicians, ed 3. Baltimore: Williams & Wilkins, 1989;91–103.
3. Wolf SL. EMG biofeedback applications in rehabilitation. Physiother Can 1979; 31:65–72.
4. Winstein CJ. Motor learning consideration in stroke rehabilitation. In: Duncan PW, Badke MB, eds.

Stroke Rehabilitation: The Recovery of Motor Function. Chicago: Year Book, 1987;109–134.

5. Gentile AM. A working model of skill acquisition with application to teaching. Quest 1972; 17:3–23.

6. Adams JA, Reynolds B. Effect of shift on distribution of practice conditions following an interpolated rest. J Exp Psychol 1954; 47:32–36.

7. Schmidt RA, Young DE, Swinnen S. Summary knowledge of results for skill acquisition: Support for the guidance hypothesis. J Exp Psychol [Learn Mem Cogn] 1989; 15:352–359.

8. Winstein CJ, Schmidt RA. Reduced frequency of knowledge of results enhances motor skill learning. J Exp Psychol [Learn Mem Cogn] 1990; 10:677–691.

9. Lee TD, White MA, Carnahan H. On the role of knowledge of results in motor learning: Exploring the guidance hypothesis. J Motor Behav 1990; 22:191–208.

10. Winstein CJ. Knowledge of results and motor learning—implications for physical therapy. Phys Ther 1991; 71:140–149.

11. Mulder T. The Learning of Motor Control Following Brain Damage: Experimental and Clinical Studies. Berwyn, Pa: Swets North America; 1985.

12. LeCraw DE, Wolf SL. Contemporary perspectives on electromyographic feedback for rehabilitation clinicians. In: Gersh MR, ed. Electrotherapy. Philadelphia: FA Davis, 1991.

13. Wannstedt GT, Herman RM. Use of augmented sensory feedback to achieve symmetrical standing. Phys Ther 1978; 58:553–559.

14. Woollacott MH. Gait and postural control in the aging adult. In: Bles W, Brandt T, eds. Disorders of Posture and Gait. New York: Elsevier, 1986;325–336.

15. Wolf SL, Binder-Macleod SA. Use of the Krusen limb load monitor to quantify temporal and loading measurements of gait. Phys Ther 1982; 62:976–984.

16. Wolf SL. Biofeedback applications in rehabilitation medicine: Implications for performance in sports. In: Sandweiss JH, Wolf SL, eds. Biofeedback and Sports Science. New York: Plenum, 1985;159–180.

17. Brown DM, Nahai F. Biofeedback strategies of the occupational therapist in total hand rehabilitation. In: Basmajian JV, ed. Biofeedback: Principles and Practice for Clinicians, ed 3. Baltimore: Williams & Wilkins, 1989;123–135.

18. Brown BB. Stress and the Art of Biofeedback. New York: Harper and Row, 1977.

19. Yates AJ. Biofeedback and the Modification of Behavior. New York, Plenum, 1980.

20. Olton DS, Noonberg AR. Biofeedback: Clinical Applications in Behavioral Medicine. Englewood Cliffs, NJ: Prentice Hall, 1980.

21. Ince LP. Behavioral Psychology in Rehabilitation Medicine: Clinical Applications. Baltimore: Williams & Wilkins, 1980.

22. Sandweiss JH, Wolf SL. Biofeedback and Sports Science. New York: Plenum, 1985.

23. Marcer D. Biofeedback and Related Therapies in Clinical Practice. Rockville, Md: Aspen, 1986.

24. Wolf SL, Fischer-Williams M. The use of biofeedback in disorders of motor function. In: Hatch JP, Fisher JG, Rugh JD, eds. Biofeedback: Studies in Clinical Efficacy. New York: Plenum, 1987;153–177.

25. Lucca JA, Recchiuti SJ. Effect of electromyographic biofeedback on an isometric strengthening program. Phys Ther 1983; 63:200–203.

26. Croce RV. The effects of EMG biofeedback on strength acquisition. Biofeedback Self Regul 1986; 11:299–310.

27. LeVeau BF, Rogers C. Selective training of the vastus medialis muscle using EMG biofeedback. Phys Ther 1980; 60:1410–1415.

28. Souza DR, Gross MT. Comparison of vastus medialis obliques: vastus lateralis muscle integrated electromyographic ratios between healthy subjects and patients with patellofemoral pain. Phys Ther 1991; 71:310–319.

29. Fernie G, Holden J, Soto M. Biofeedback training of knee control in the above-knee amputee. Am J Phys Med 1978; 57:161–166.

30. Patterson P, Shea CH. Augmented auditory information in the control of upper-limb prostheses. Arch Phys Med Rehabil 1985; 66:243–245.

31. Gauthier-Gagnon C, St. Pierre D, Drouin G, et al. Augmented sensory feedback in the early training of standing balance of below-knee amputees. Physiother Can 1986; 38:137–142.

32. Clarkson PM, James R, Watkins A, et al. The effect of augmented feedback on foot pronation during barre exercise in dance. Res Q 1986; 57:33–40.

33. Baker M, Hudson J, Wolf SL. A "feedback" cane to improve the hemiplegic patient's gait. Phys Ther 1979; 59:170–171.

34. Draper V. Electromyographic biofeedback and recovery of quadriceps femoris muscle function following anterior cruciate ligament reconstruction. Phys Ther 1990; 70:11–17.

35. Lee M, Moseley A, Refshauge K. Effect of feedback on learning a vertebral joint mobilization skill. Phys Ther 1990; 70:97–104.

36. Keef FJ, Surwit RS. Electromyographic biofeedback: Behavioral treatment of neuromuscular disorders. J Behavioral Med 1978; 1:13–24.

37. Basmajian JV. Research foundations of EMG biofeedback in rehabilitation. Biofeedback Self Regul 1988; 13:275–298.

38. Wolf SL. Electromyographic biofeedback applications to stroke patients: A critical review. Phys Ther 1983; 63:1448–1455.

39. Basmajian JV, Kukulka CG, Narayan MG. Biofeedback treatment of foot-drop after stroke compared with standard rehabilitation technique: Effects on voluntary control and strength. Arch Phys Med Rehabil 1975; 56:231–236.

40. Brudny J, Korein J, Grynbaum B, et al. Sensory feedback therapy as a modality of treatment in central nervous system disorders of voluntary movement. Neurology 1974; 24:925–932.

41. Wolf SL, Baker MP, Kelly JL. EMG biofeedback in stroke: Effect of patient characteristics. Arch Phys Med Rehabil 1979; 60:96–102.

42. Wolf, SL, Baker MP, Kelly JL. EMG biofeedback in stroke: A 1-year follow-up on the effect of patient characteristics. Arch Phys Med Rehabil 1980; 61:351–355.

43. Middaugh SJ, Miller MC. Electromyographic feedback: Effects on voluntary contractions in paretic patients. Arch Phys Med Rehabil 1980; 61:24–29.

44. Wolf SL, Binder-Macleod SA. Electromyographic biofeedback applications to the hemiplegic patient: Changes in lower extremity neuromuscular and functional status. Phys Ther 1983; 63:1404–1413.

45. Binder SA, Moll CB, Wolf SL. Evaluation of electromyographic biofeedback as an adjunct to therapeutic exercise in treating the lower extremities of hemiplegic patients. Phys Ther 1981; 61:886–893.

46. Colborne CR, Olney SJ. Feedback of joint angle and EMG in gait of able-bodied subjects. Arch Phys Med Rehabil 1990; 71:478–483.

47. Mandel AR, Nymark JR, Balmer SJ, et al. Electromyographic versus rhythmic positional biofeedback in computerized gait training with stroke patients. Arch Phys Med Rehabil 1990; 71:649–654.

48. Brudny J, Korein J, Grynbaum BB, et al. Helping hemiparetics to help themselves. Sensory feedback therapy. JAMA 1979; 241:814–818.

49. Prevo AJH, Visser SL, Vogelaar TW. Effect of EMG feedback on paretic muscles and abnormal co-contraction in the hemiplegic arm, compared with conventional physical therapy. Scand J Rehabil Med 1982; 14:121–131.

50. Ince LP, Leon MS, Christidis D. EMG biofeedback for improvement of upper extremity function: A critical review of the literature. Physiother Can 1985; 37:12–17.

51. Basmajian JV. Biofeedback for neuromuscular rehabilitation. Crit Rev Phys Med Rehabil 1989; 1:37–58.

52. Basmajian JV, Gowland C, Brandstater ME, et al. EMG feedback treatment of upper limb in hemiplegic stroke patients: Pilot study. Arch Phys Med Rehabil 1982; 63:613–616.

53. Wolf SL, Binder-Macleod SA. EMG biofeedback applications to the hemiplegic patient: Changes in upper extremity neuromuscular and functional status. Phys Ther 1983; 63:1403–1413.

54. Wolf SL, LeCraw DE, Barton LA, et al. A comparison of motor copy and targeted feedback training techniques for restitution of upper extremity function among neurologic patients. Phys Ther 1989; 69:719–735.

55. Wissel J, Ebersbach G, Gutjahr L, et al. Treating chronic hemiparesis with modified biofeedback. Arch Phys Med Rehabil 1989; 70:612–617.

56. Bobath B. Adult Hemiplegia: Evaluation and Treatment, ed 2. London: Heinemann, 1978.

57. Lord JP, Hall K. Neuromuscular reeducation versus traditional programs for stroke rehabilitation. Arch Phys Med Rehabil 1986; 67:88–91.

58. Sivenius J, Pyorala K, Heininen OP, et al. The significance of intensity of rehabilitation of stroke—controlled trial. Stroke 1985; 16:928–931.

59. Ballantyne B. Factors contributing to voluntary movement deficit and spasticity following cerebral vascular accidents. Neurol Rep 1991; 15:15–18.

60. Wolf SL, Edwards DI, Shutter LA. Concurrent assessment of muscle activity (CAMA): A procedural approach to assess treatment goals. Phys Ther 1986; 66:218–224.

61. Anderson PA, Hobart DJ, Danoff JV, eds. Electromyographical Kinesiology. New York: Excerpta Medica, 1991.

62. Wolf SL. Electromyographic biofeedback: An overview. In: Nelson RM, Currier DP, eds. Clinical Electrotherapy, ed 2. Norwalk, Conn: Appelton & Lange, 1991;361–384.

63. Wolf SL, Binder-Macleod SA. Neurophysiological factors in electromyographic feedback for neuromotor disturbances. In: Basmajian JV, ed. Biofeedback: Principles and Practice for Clinicians, ed 3. Baltimore: Williams & Wilkins, 1989;17–36.

64. Bach-y-Rita P, Balliet R. Recovery from stroke. In: Duncan PW, Badke M, eds. Stroke Rehabilitation. New York: Year Book, 1987;79–108.

# Chapter 23

# The Physiologic Aspects and Clinical Application of Functional Electrical Stimulation in Rehabilitation

KRISTJAN T. RAGNARSSON

Functional electrical stimulation (FES) may be defined as the application of electrical currents to neural tissue for the purpose of restoring a degree of control over abnormal or absent body functions. Electricity has been applied either experimentally or clinically for many purposes—to improve hearing and sight, to prevent bladder and bowel incontinence and to control evacuation, to regulate heart rhythm, to reduce spasticity, to allow ventilator-free breathing, to correct scoliosis, and to usefully move paralyzed limbs. In this chapter I address one specific form of FES, usually referred to by scientists as *functional neuromuscular stimulation* (FNS), which restricts the electrical stimulation to the neuromuscular system for the purpose of controlling skeletal muscle contractions. Though FNS may be applied successfully for different forms of paralytic conditions caused by upper motor neuron lesions (e.g., stroke, traumatic brain injury, cerebral palsy) in this chapter its application after spinal cord injury is principally discussed.

## History

Electricity has been used therapeutically for different human ailments, including treatment of paralysis, for hundreds of years.[1] Gilbert is usually credited with having laid the scientific foundations of electrotherapy with his studies and publications in the 16th century on magnetism and electricity,[2] though Krueger, in 1744, may have been the first to use electricity in a scientific fashion for therapeutic purposes. Development of electrostatic generators during the 18th century made electricity widely available for experimental and clinical application. During that age, the work of Galvani and Volta[2] led to the clinical use of interrupted direct currents to produce muscle contractions. In the early 19th century, Faraday introduced the alternating current generator, which a number of clinicians, most prominently Duchenne, were soon using for therapeutic purposes. Scientific developments in the fields of electrophysiology and electrical engineering during the second half of the 19th century and during the entire 20th century led to vastly increased knowledge, which, for instance, was useful in promoting the clinical field of electrodiagnosis. The ability to detect and amplify small amounts of electricity in the body was of particular clinical importance, as was the recognition that certain forms of electricity are better suited than others for electrostimulation of neuromuscular structures. A body of work also helped to clarify the limits of the therapeutic use of electricity. For example, it became clear that stimulation of a denervated muscle is very difficult and that electrostimulation does not significantly change the course of recovery after neurologic injury. On the other hand, stimulation of an innervated muscle was found to be easy and facilitated by the presence of upper motor neuron damage and the resulting hypertonicity.

The first attempts to restore useful movement of limbs by electrostimulation of muscles paralyzed by upper motor neuron lesions are generally credited to Liberson,[3] who reported in 1961 on his work to produce dorsiflexion of the ankle in hemiplegic patients during the swing phase of gait. At the same time, in a little noted report Kantrowitz described a paraplegic patient who was enabled to stand by electrical stimulation of the quadriceps muscles.[4] Shortly thereafter, Long and Masciarelli reported on their attempts to restore wrist and hand movement for functional grasp and release by using a hybrid system of electrical stimulation and wrist-hand orthosis.[5] These early clinical investigators were hampered in their work by the limitations of the available technology, but during the 1970s improved electronic technology and increased understanding of neuromuscular physiology intensified interest in this field. Kinesiologic electromyography was used to clearly identify all the muscles responsible for completing a given motor task. Researchers thought that computer-controlled multichannel stimulators using this information would be able to replicate any particular motion accurately by circumducting the lesion in the central nervous system and thus bypassing the injured upper motor neuron by directly stimulating the peripheral nerve or the motor point of the muscle at the desired preprogrammed times and intensity. Numerous investigators in different countries have since contributed to FNS technology and its clinical application; some focused primarily on the lower limbs for ambulation[6-10] while others worked on hand function[1-14] or respiration for ventilator-free breathing.[15-17] While a number of technical and physiologic problems have been overcome, many others remain unsolved.

## Motor System Anatomy and Physiology

Although the physiology and anatomy of motion are addressed in other chapters in this book, it is important to review the basic structure of the motor system to understand all the events related to its electrical excitation. In the simplest terms, the initial motion signal is normally generated by the upper motor neuron in the motor cortex of the brain. This signal travels down the spinal cord, connects with the lower motor neuron at the anterior horn of the cord and is transmitted through the peripheral nerve to the muscle fibers, which shorten and cause a movement of the body part. Sensory feedback to the spinal cord and brain occurs continuously, in order to control and modify the motions and to accomplish the motor task in a safe and effective manner. The continuous sensory feedback results in constant changes in the number of fibers that are stimulated to contract within each muscle, and in the number of protagonist, antagonist, and synergist muscles that participate in the desired motor task. These constant alterations in fiber contractions occur at a subconscious level, perhaps even at the level of the spinal cord, through a complicated learning process that depends on different parts of the central nervous system and reciprocal inhibition and facilitation. A voluntary motion is thus considered voluntary only in its purpose, not in the means by which it is accomplished.

Voluntary movements are impaired not only by damage to the efferent neural pathways, which results in paralytic conditions, but whenever there is an interruption of the afferent channels to the brain from the different sensory organs. The countless normal physiologic events that continuously occur with even the simplest motor task are clearly far more complex than what can currently be accomplished by artificially stimulating the neuromuscular system, even with the most sophisticated technology with computer-controlled multichannel stimulators and closed-loop sensory feedback.

Completion of a motor task, whether by voluntary effort, by reflex action, or by FNS, is accomplished by activation of the intact lower motor unit, which consists of the alpha motor neuron, located in the anterior horn of the spinal cord, its axonal nerve fiber, the myoneural junction, and the group of muscle fibers that it innervates. The number of muscle fibers innervated by a single but branching axonal nerve fiber varies inversely with the precision of the movement performed by the muscle (e.g., a motor unit may contain hundreds of muscle fibers in the limb muscles, but in the eye muscles it may contain less than five). A single muscle thus consists of many motor units, the exact number of which depends on the size of the muscle and its specific function. Within the muscle the fibers from different motor units lie intermingled with each other. All the efferent nerve fibers to a striated skeletal muscle are excitatory (i.e., they always produce contraction of the muscle, but never relaxation by inhibition), in contrast to efferent nerve supply to smooth and cardiac muscle, which also may cause relaxation upon stimulation. Upon excitation, all the muscle fibers of a single motor unit are activated to contract. An electrical stimulus of threshold strength theoretically may activate only one motor nerve fiber and all the muscle fibers it innervates, whereas a maximal stimulus strength may activate all the nerve fibers with consequent contraction of all the muscle fibers. The activation of an increasing number of motor units within a muscle upon contraction is referred to as *recruitment*. A succession of maximal stimuli will produce different results depending on the firing rate (i.e., rate of activation). A second maximal stimulus given during the latent period (the first milliseconds of the first stimulus), produces no additional contraction, as the muscle is in its refractory state, whereas if the stimulus is given slightly later, the muscle tension generated is greater than that generated by the first stimulus. A series of maximal stimuli applied at progressively shorter intervals, at low rates (10 to 20 stimuli per second), produces a subcutaneous tremulous response, whereas at higher rates (60 per second), full tetanus results, with greater tension of the muscle fibers and a steadier pull. The increased firing rate of active motor units is referred to as *temporal summation*. Recruitment and temporal summation are the two main mechanisms that regulate the strength of muscle contraction during voluntary activation, and usually these mechanisms act simultaneously. Synchronized activation of a different number of motor units results in a smooth, voluntary contraction of a muscle. While modern FNS systems strive toward achieving precise control that results in smooth muscle contraction, this has not been possible because of the limitations of current technology.

Not all alpha motor neurons are identical, and neither are the muscle fibers. The alpha motor neurons differ in both size and function. Small alpha motor neurons usually innervate slow muscle fibers, and the large neurons innervate fast fibers. The small motor neurons physiologically have the lowest activation threshold. All the muscle fibers within a single motor unit are usually thought to be histologically identical, whereas within a whole muscle they are not. Muscle fibers are usually considered to be of two different types, referred to as *type I* (red, slow, aerobic) and *type II* (white, fast, anaerobic). Histologically, the *type I muscle fibers* are of relatively small diameter, as they have relatively small amounts of contractile proteins. Their smaller diameter facilitates oxygen diffusion from the surrounding capillaries into the fiber. These fibers are rich in glycolytic and oxidative enzymes, substances that give them their dark or red appearance, and metabolically provide them with aerobic capacity for different endurance tasks (e.g., maintenance of posture, walking, distance running, bicycling). Physiologically, type I fibers have a slow twitch speed upon stimulation and are activated at low electrical frequencies for tonic contraction. They are recruited first upon physiologic stimulation and can continue to contract for prolonged periods. *Type II muscle fibers,* in contrast, are larger, have less glycolytic and oxidative enzymes, appear pale or white, have low aerobic capacity and slow speed of twitch, and are activated at higher electrical frequency levels for phasic but relatively strong contractions of short duration.

Clearly, type I and type II muscle fibers are metabolically suited to perform different tasks. Normally, type I and type II muscle fibers are recruited selectively by the central nervous system in order to perform different tasks, but with recruitment by electrical stimulation such differentiation is not possible. Upon sustained or repeated contractions, muscle fatigue occurs, apparently because of changes in the muscle fiber induced by anoxia and accumulation of metabolites, regardless of the type of fiber. Fatigue may be offset or delayed by exclusive activation of type I fibers and maintenance of adequate blood supply. The blood flow and oxygenation of the muscle fiber, however, are reduced during a sustained contraction of the muscle, and in the presence of impaired physiologic response of the cardiovascular and respiratory systems.

There is ample evidence for the transformation of type I muscle fibers into type II fibers with inactivity and paralysis and for the reversibility of this process with appropriate external stimulus, (e.g., endurance exercise or regular prolonged electrical stimulation of the paralyzed muscle.)[18–22] Similarly, endurance training may improve the physiologic responses and work capacity of the healthy but deconditioned cardiovascular system, a process that is necessary to sustain the desired work of the muscles.

The function of a skeletal muscle is to generate force with or without movement. The muscles' ability to generate force and movement depends on two different relationships: the length-tension relationship and the force-velocity relationship.[23] The *length-tension relationship* means that isometric muscle force (the force developed at constant muscle length), varies as a function of muscle length. The length-tension force may be assessed by measuring the force generated by maximal stimulation at different muscle lengths. The *force-velocity relationship* means that isotonic velocity (contraction velocity against a constant force) varies as a function of muscle force. Assessment of the force-velocity relationship may be done by subjecting the muscle to a constant force, stimulating maximally and measuring the initial contraction velocity at each force level. The length-tension, as well as the force-velocity relationship, are related to the histochemical properties of the muscle fibers (i.e., type I or type II), which in turn are affected by and may be altered by appropriate external stimuli.[19,20,25] While electrical stimulation of the isolated muscle under experimental circumstances can produce different and predictable length-tension and force-velocity relationships, this is much more difficult during clinical application of FNS in the human body.

## Components of Functional Neuromuscular Stimulation Systems

The FNS systems that are currently used are fundamentally quite similar. They are designed to deliver pulses of electrical currents at predetermined frequencies and amplitudes to nerves, myoneural junctions, or muscles. The main components of such systems include a portable power source for the electrical stimulation device, control mechanism, lead wires, electrodes, and, in the more sophisticated systems, peripherally placed

sensors and microprocessor (computer) for preprogrammed or automatic control (Figure 23-1). Most FNS systems are completely external to the body. Certain systems, however, utilize implanted electrodes with percutaneous lead wires. Currently, experiments are being conducted on completely implantable systems.

### *The Electrical Stimulation Device*

Muscle contraction may be obtained by electrical excitation of the muscle itself or, more commonly, of a peripheral motor nerve, either well before or near the point where the nerve connects with the muscle (at the motor point). A muscle that is paralyzed by damage to the lower motor neuron has no motor point. The motor point of a muscle is a relatively small area where the motor nerve ending connects with the muscle and where sensitivity to stimulation is high. A denervated muscle (one without a motor point), responds only to very high levels of electrical current (i.e., duration of at least 100 msec), compared to less than 1 msec for an innervated muscle. The current must pass through all the denervated muscle fibers in order to gen-

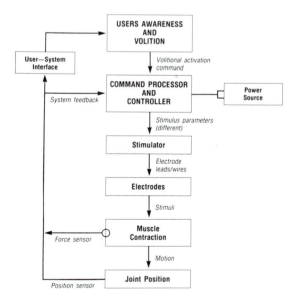

**FNS SYSTEM: MAIN COMPONENTS AND ACTION SEQUENCE**

**Figure 23-1.** Schematic drawing of an FNS system's main components and sequence of action.

erate an effective contraction. Such high current levels may be both dangerous and very painful for a subject with preserved sensation. For these reasons, a muscle denervated by a lower motor neuron lesion cannot be subjected to FNS, given the current state of technology and knowledge.

The electrical stimulus used most frequently for FNS to generate depolarization and action potential (figure 23-2) is usually a pulsed direct current waveform. There is a predictable relationship between the stimulus pulse amplitude and the pulse width that is necessary to reach the threshold required for nerve excitation and muscle contraction (Figure 23-3). When the pulse is long, the excitation thresholds for muscle and nerve are nearly equal, but for short pulses, which are usually used for FNS, the nerve has much lower threshold than the muscle. Therefore, upon stimulation of the nerve or of the motor point, when using short electrical pulse widths, there is little direct activation of the muscle fibers and contraction occurs mostly by nerve excitation. For clinical purposes, series of short-duration (i.e., 10 to 100 μsec) charge-balanced biphasic stimuli are used[26,27] with pulse widths (amplitude), no greater than 50 mA, though stimuli of longer duration and amplitude have been used experimentally with both surface and implanted electrodes.[28,29]

Greater pulse duration and amplitude is required for stimulation by surface electrodes (i.e., 300 μsec and 60 mA, respectively).[28] A biphasic

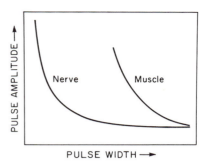

**Figure 23-3.** The relationship between the electrical stimulus pulse amplitude and the pulse width necessary to reach the threshold required for nerve excitation and muscle contraction. When the pulse width is long, the thresholds are almost equal, but for the more commonly used short pulse widths the nerve has a much lower threshold than the muscle.

pulse form is preferable to a monophasic form (see Figure 23-2), as it may provide better control of recruitment and thus muscle contraction force.[30] Control may be further improved by decreasing pulse amplitude and width.[30,31] Nerve cuff electrodes require the least electrical charge to elicit contraction. It is clear that some tissue damage may result from long-term electrical stimulation of implanted electrodes. Such damage is felt to be related to the charge intensity of the stimulus, as well as to current intensity. By maintaining equal charge in both the negative and positive phases of the waveform, a greater charge may be used without causing tissue damage.[32,33]

Researchers have observed that a muscle fatigues more rapidly when stimulated by artificial means than when stimulated by voluntary action, the cause apparently being due to the different order in which motor units are recruited.[34,35] By voluntary contraction, the slow and aerobic type I muscle fibers are recruited first and the rapidly fatiguing type II fibers last. This order of recruitment may be reversed during FNS, since excitation current threshold varies inversely with the diameter of the nerve fiber. The small-diameter nerve fibers within a bundle of fibers have the lowest threshold to electrical stimulation, and these tend to stimulate the fast, type II fibers. Special stimulation techniques have been tested in animals to recruit first the slow, type I muscle fibers by employing high currents and additional electrodes,

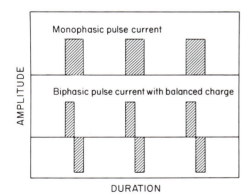

**Figure 23-2.** Pulsed direct current waveforms with either monophasic (*above*) or biphasic (*below*) action potentials are used for neuromuscular electrical stimulation. To minimize tissue damage, a biphasic pulsed current with equal positive and negative charge is preferred.

but they have not been tried in humans.[36] Muscle endurance can be increased to a certain extent by restricting the electrical stimulation frequency, which is usually in the range of 15 to 50 Hz.[29,37,38] This frequency range roughly equals the ranges found during weak to strong voluntary isometric contractions, respectively. In general, low-frequency stimulation is clearly preferred. Muscle endurance can also be increased experimentally by sequentially stimulating different groups of motor units within each muscle by means of multipolar nerve electrode designs.[39] Additionally, endurance may be increased by altering the contractile properties of the muscle fibers by regular electrical stimulation and consequent alteration of muscle fibers from type II to type I.[38]

The electrical stimulation device usually has high-output impedance for generation of a "constant current," which is desirable in order to minimize the effect of changing tissue impedance, a situation that might alter the stimulus delivered to the tissues.[32] The electrical stimulation device must be electrically safe and must operate reliably. Good insulation and battery power prevent dangerous electrical shocks, and mechanical failure may best be prevented by use of solid-state electronics, reverse circuits, and warning signals.

### Electrodes

The selection of electrode design for FNS systems depends on the specific purpose of application, and on availability of equipment, clinical experience, and other variables. Four main electrode designs are currently available: skin surface, epimysial (muscle surface), intramuscular with percutaneous leads, and surgically implanted nerve cuff electrodes (Figure 23-4). No electrode meets all the ideal criteria for safety, reliability, efficiency, specificity, durability, low cost, ease of application, and minimal maintenance. Though *surface electrodes* clearly are the safest, least invasive, easiest, and simplest to apply, they do not always provide adequate selectivity of excitation, particularly not for excitation of deep muscles, nor can they provide accurate repeatability in muscle responses. Minor displacement of such electrodes on the skin surface may result in a major alteration in the muscle response. Surface electrodes may be adequate for therapeutic purposes or for a short-term trial of FNS, which employs a system with relatively few stimulation channels, usually eight or fewer, but for long-term application of FNS systems with greater number of channels, researchers generally prefer implanted electrodes.[11] Despite their inherent shortcomings, skin surface electrodes have improved in quality and now may provide excellent skin contact and can be left in place for days without causing irritation. In the clinical setting, single electrodes are usually used, but for long-term FNS participation the electrodes may be sewn into skin-tight garments for the subject to wear when stimulation is desired.[40]

*Intramuscular electrodes with percutaneous leads* are usually fabricated from a fine multifila-

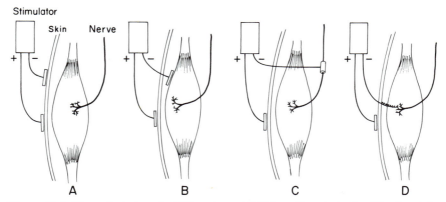

**Figure 23-4.** Electrode designs for FNS systems: (*A*) Skin surface electrode, (*B*) epimysial (muscle surface) electrode, (*C*) nerve cuff electrode, (*D*) intramuscular electrode with percutaneous lead.

ment stainless steel wire with Teflon insulation in a coiled configuration with an exposed tip. These electrodes may be inserted easily through the skin using a large-gauge hypodermic needle (i.e., gauge 19 to 26), and placed subcutaneously, epimysially on the surface of the muscle, or into the muscle itself.[11,41] A barb at the end of the coil secures the electrode in place until it becomes encapsulated by fibrous tissue. Whatever the exact form of the percutaneous placement, the electrode is placed at the motor point of the muscle and thus stimulation elicits muscle contraction through nerve stimulation rather than by direct muscle fiber excitation. These electrodes may be left in place for months or even years.[11] They provide excellent selectivity of muscle contraction. Infection and electrode burns reportedly are rare, and the mechanical failure rate is relatively low, approximately 1% to 2% per month.[9,42] In general, percutaneous electrodes are preferable to surface electrodes when more than eight-channel stimulation is performed, for upper limb application in order to obtain fine control of small muscles, and for stimulation of poorly accessible muscle.

### Implanted Electrodes

Electrodes may also be inserted surgically and then placed either epimysially[13,43] or directly over or around the nerve by a cuff. A special FNS system design that uses a surgically implanted nerve cuff electrode is the Neuromuscular Assist device (Medtronics, Inc). Here, radio-frequency signals are transmitted through the skin transcutaneously from an external antenna and a small stimulator to stimulate the peroneal nerve and correct foot drop in hemiplegic patients.[7] While such surgically implanted cuff electrodes under radio frequency control have been used for limb muscles,[13,44] their clinical use currently appears to be more restricted to diaphragmatic pacing by stimulation of the phrenic nerve[15] or to bladder evacuation by stimulation of the sacral anterior nerve roots.[44] Materials for implanted electrodes and the leads must be carefully selected. There must be minimal biologic reaction to the material, which should be strong, flexible, resistant to fatigue and corrosion, and of low impedance. Metals such as stainless steel or platinum or alloys of platinum and iridium or of nickel, cobalt, chromium and molybdenum have been used in the fabrication of such electrodes and leads.[32] Though implanted cuff electrodes provide good muscle specificity and allow stimulation with relatively low current, the implantation is quite invasive and surgical reinsertion is difficult without damaging the nerve. Though the experience of some clinicians has shown that properly implanted electrodes using correct stimulation parameters do not appear to damage the nerve functionally,[6] other clinicians have expressed concern that the nerve may be damaged either by the electrical stimulation itself or mechanically by the electrodes' attachment to the stimulated tissue.[42,45] Continuous stimulation at frequencies of 50 Hz or greater for constant periods of 8 to 16 hours daily may damage the nerve irreversibly.[45]

### Sensors

Sensors are essential parts of all sophisticated FNS systems and are necessary for proper interaction with the user and the environment. Normally, the five senses provide the brain and the spinal cord with information about the external and internal environment of the body through innumerable sensory nerve end-organs, in order to make motor activity accurate and effective. Without such sensory feedback, motor activity becomes grossly uncoordinated and essentially useless. Coordinated motor activity requires accurate sensory information on the positions and motions of individual joints, as well as of whole limbs, in addition to sensory feedback on impact force, pressure, and tendon tension. Tiny signals from the sensory nerve end-organs can be detected by percutaneous intraneural electrodes, but utilization of this information for FNS systems would require a large number of implantable microelectrodes and a highly intelligent microprocessor.[46] Neither is currently available.[47] The types of sensors required for FNS systems are similar to the transducers used in industry for measurements and controls of manufactured devices. These sensors, however, must meet the additional criteria of reliability, ease of use, small size, low mass, easy mounting, flexibility, cosmesis, and they should not interfere with normal joint function.[47] Currently, sensory feedback signals from the limbs are obtained primarily from externally mounted goniometers or potentiometers on ankles and knees that measure joint position and allow, from the absolute sense of position, velocity and acceleration of movement to be calculated by the systems microprocessor, which in turn controls the stimulator.[48] At present, no sensors exist that can monitor from their placement on the body surface the tension developed by a contracting skeletal muscle, though such capability would be ideal for sensory feedback.

### Control of Functional Neuromuscular Stimulation Systems

FNS systems are frequently described as user-interactive devices, where the user is able to control the electrical stimulation to the muscles by different means, including a joystick, push-button switches, voice recognition, breath force, myoelectric signals, or motion sensors. A visual display (e.g., by liquid crystal or an audible sound), may inform the user of the system's status. A computer may provide additional automatic control either by an open-loop or closed-loop mechanism. In an *open-loop control* system, preprogrammed patterns of electrical stimulation are generated for a specific function and for a specific individual but there is no automatic correction for changes in the external environment, in the mechanical function of the system, or in muscle contraction. In a *closed loop control* system, the computer receives feedback information from sensors about a particular motion and institutes a remedial action or gives a warning if motion is not possible or should be altered.

## Alterations in Exercise Capacity Following Spinal Cord Injury

Spinal cord injury (SCI) results in numerous degenerative physiologic changes that to some extent affect most, if not all, organ systems of the body. Many of these physiologic changes result in diminished work capacity and physical fitness, which may not only impair the patient's ability to use FNS systems but may also negatively affect their general health and well-being. Though some

of these changes are unalterable and directly related to the loss of supraspinal control over voluntary and autonomic motor functions, the enforced sedentary lifestyle and lack of exercise programs for the pursuit of physical fitness further compound the problem. The following paragraphs briefly address some of the major degenerative physiologic changes that can diminish work performance after SCI.

### Skeletal Muscles

During the initial areflexic state of SCI, rapid and progressive atrophy of the paralyzed muscles occurs, which appears to continue for several months. When reflex activity and tone return to muscles that are paralyzed by an upper motor neuron lesion, further atrophy may not develop, but even in the presence of significant spasticity, muscle bulk usually is not restored to normal. On excitation of the muscle, maximum contraction strength and endurance are diminished. Morphologic studies have shown that after SCI, as with other causes of paralysis and immobilization, many muscle fibers change from type I (slow, aerobic) to type II (fast, anaerobic).[22,49,50] This change is accompanied by reduction in mitochondria concentration, glycolytic and oxidative enzyme level, and the number of capillaries in the muscle. As type II fibers become preponderant, the contractile properties of the muscle change dramatically. There is increased speed of muscle contraction and relaxation, and the muscle becomes unable to generate prolonged contractions (i.e., the type of contractions that are normally required of most "antigravity" muscles in the lower limbs during standing and locomotion). Strength of individual muscle fibers, as measured by maximum tetanic tension, may not decrease,[50] though it appears clinically that on electrical stimulation of an entire muscle the strength is significantly diminished compared to that of a muscle contracting voluntarily. Muscle endurance (the ability of the muscle to contract repeatedly against little or no resistance) is clinically reduced, as fatigue is usually observed after relatively few contractions that are elicited by electrical stimulation. Skeletal muscle has remarkable adaptability, and many of the changes associated with disuse are reversible, though perhaps not completely.

### Cardiovascular System

Numerous studies have shown that cardiovascular fitness, expressed as physical work capacity and maximum oxygen consumption ($VO_2$ max), is diminished in most individuals with SCI, particularly those with high cord lesions.[51-60] Two major factors are considered to be responsible for this reduction: the muscle mass available for voluntary exercise is diminished, and responses of the autonomic nervous system are altered. Both are the result of lost supraspinal control. Secondarily, there is loss of cardiovascular fitness as a result of the sedentary lifestyle.

$VO_2$ max is customarily used as a measure of cardiovascular fitness (i.e., endurance or aerobic capacity). In able-bodied persons obtainable $VO_2$ max is influenced by many factors, including sex, age, genetics, endurance training, type of exercise, organ health, and environment. SCI typically results in extensive muscle paralysis, and consequently the muscle mass that remains under voluntary control is significantly decreased. It is thus clear than a person with high-level quadriplegia is not capable of significantly increasing $VO_2$ max through exercise of the few residual functional muscles, whereas a paraplegic person may be able to increase $VO_2$ max considerably through upper extremity endurance exercise. Numerous investigators have shown that the physical work and aerobic exercise capacity after SCI are reduced proportionally with the muscle mass available for voluntary exercise.[61-67] It is not clear if involuntary FNS exercise can significantly increase $VO_2$ max, but it appears that such a potential increase may depend to a certain degree on the level of the lesion and autonomic control of the cardiovascular system.

The extent of autonomic dysfunction following SCI depends on the level of the cord lesion. Quadriplegics lose all supraspinal control of the sympathetic nervous system and of the sacral parasympathetic efferent flow while retaining essentially normal and uninhibited vagal parasympathetic function. Individuals with high-level paraplegia (i.e., T-5 or above) similarly experience severe loss of supraspinal sympathetic control, primarily control over the splanchnic nerve supply rather than that for cardiopulmonary functions. Paraplegia with a cord lesion lower than T-5 seems to affect autonomic dysfunction less. It has been reasonably argued that loss of supraspinal sympathetic control limits maximum heart rate, contractility of the heart muscle, stroke volume, and cardiac output during strenuous physical exercise.[68] Further, loss of supraspinal sympathetic control predictably may impair effective dilatation of arterioles supplying working muscles and compensatory vasoconstriction to resting organs such as intestines, kidneys, and skin. As a consequence, maximum work capacity may be limited for both voluntary upper limb exercise and electrically stimulated lower limb endurance activities. Several studies have shown that the cardiac output of persons with SCI, both at rest and during maximum arm exercise, is lower than that of able-bodied persons, that the arteriovenous oxygen gradient is high, and that serum lactate levels are elevated.[51,52,54] Oxygen pulse (milliliters of oxygen consumed per heart beat), a parameter frequently used as a noninvasive measure of stroke volume, has been shown to be decreased to a greater extent in persons with high cord lesions than in those with lower levels of paraplegia,[64,69-72] It is obvious that if neurologic recovery does not occur the individual with high-level cord injury will not regain supraspinal sympathetic control and exercise performance will be limited. There is evidence, however, that, in response to a different form of physical stress, (i.e., head-up tilt), a limited reflex sympathetic activity occurs, as evidenced by a rise in serum dopamine-β-hydroxylase and plasma renin.[73] Additionally, there may be increased vascular reactivity to normal levels of norepinephrine and other vasoconstricting agents.[74] Both the reflex sympathetic activity and increased sensitivity to the neurotransmitters may have some beneficial effect during physical exercise for persons with quadriplegia.

Thermoregulation during rest and exercise is to a large extent a sympathetically mediated process that consists of vasoconstriction or vasodilatation, as well as sweating, shivering, and so on. Concern has been expressed that persons with high spinal cord lesions subjected to strenuous exercise may experience an excessive rise of body temperature, but no such increase has been reported.

SCI may impair both venous and arterial circulation in the peripheral areas of the paralyzed parts. It is well-recognized that paralysis of muscles in the lower limbs and abdominal wall, along with decreased venomotor tone, may contribute to peripheral pooling of venous blood and consequently cause reduced venous return to the heart. The reduced return of venous blood to the heart may further contribute to reduction in stroke volume and cardiac output during physical exercise, especially during exercise performed in an upright position, as during ambulation by means of FNS or orthoses or crutches, arm cranking, and FNS cycle ergometry.

Arteries in the chronically paralyzed lower limbs have been shown to become small and atrophic, perhaps owing to lack of muscle activity and chronically reduced blood flow. While this condition has not been noted clinically to lead to frank ischemia, except in the presence of other risk factors, such as cigarette smoking and diabetes, it is possible that atrophic arteries may limit oxygen supply to muscles subjected to endurance exercise by FNS following years of inactivity, which would contribute to early development of muscle fatigue. Narrowed lower limb arteries, however, may prevent excessive shunting of blood to these body parts, a condition that may be helpful during upper limb voluntary exercise.

### Respiratory Function

Paralysis of the intercostal and abdominal muscles impairs the respiratory capacity of persons with SCI. Several studies have shown that with each ascending level of the spinal cord lesion there is a progressive reduction of vital capacity.[61,75–77] This impairment, however, does not appear to significantly affect exercise capacity, which is primarily limited by the available muscle mass. Thus, respiration and oxygenation of blood seem to be sufficient for most endurance exercises[61] that persons with SCI are capable of performing with the residual voluntary muscles. Reduced respiratory capacity may only limit exercise capacity in some highly

trained paraplegic athletes during high-level endurance activities.

### Endocrine Function

Normally, several hormones are secreted in response to strenuous exercise. These are primarily hormones that increase the rate of lipolysis, glycolysis, and gluconeogenesis, (i.e., epinephrine, norepinephrine, growth hormone, adrenocorticotropin, cortisol, glucagon, thyroid-stimulating hormone, thyroid hormone), and hormones that are important for regulation of body fluids and electrolytes (aldosterone, antidiuretic hormone). In contrast, there is decreased secretion of hormones that increase synthesis of fat and glycogen. Insulin is the most important of these. The first and most significant hormonal response to sudden exercise is sympathetically mediated secretion of catecholamines (epinephrine and norepinephrine), both from nerve endings and the adrenal medulla, in amounts that are proportional to the increase in work load and the duration of the exercise.[78] It is probable that secretion of catecholamines during such exercise may be impaired with high cord lesions and a dysfunctional sympathetic nervous system. In general, however, secretion of different hormones in response to sudden vigorous exercise or prolonged exercise training program after SCI has not yet been adequately studied. Currently, it does not appear that endocrine imbalance significantly affects exercise response in this condition.

## Clinical Applications

Clinicians have long practiced the application of controlled currents of electricity to nerves or to motor points of muscles in order to generate a contraction for therapeutic purposes. Earlier in this chapter, reference was made to the use of relatively simple systems of FNS for correction of scoliosis and for generating ankle dorsiflexion during the swing phase of gait in subjects with stroke, usually with a single stimulation channel. The discussion here addresses the clinical application of computer-controlled multichannel FNS systems for the purposes of restoring prehension to the hand or achieving ventilator-free breathing or the ability to stand, walk and leg pedal.

### Upper Limb Control

Injury to the cervical spinal cord usually causes paralysis of the upper and lower limbs. The paralysis of the upper limbs most consistently involves the hands and thus reduces the person's self-care skills and vocational potential. Depending upon the extent and distribution of the cord damage, the paralysis is caused in varying proportions by both upper and lower motor neuron destruction. Rehabilitation interventions to improve upper limb function after such paralysis have traditionally consisted of maintaining joints range of motion, strengthening residual muscles, teaching new skills, providing orthoses and adaptive equipment, and surgically reconstructing the hand. Recently, FNS systems have been successfully developed for quadriplegic persons with lesions at C-5 and C-6, but whose the lower motor neuron is preserved for the C-7 and C-8 segments.[11,13,79,80]

Restoration of upper limb function by FNS aims at reestablishing the ability of the person to position the arm in space and to grasp or to release objects from the hand. Either one or both of these key components of upper limb function may be impaired or lost after cervical SCI, and traditional rehabilitation methods may not provide adequate functional restoration. Because persons with quadriplegia at C-5 and C-6 have voluntary control of shoulder muscles and elbow flexors, they are generally capable of positioning their arms and hands over a working surface in front of them, however, they do not have functional prehension of the hands, owing to paralysis of the more distal muscles. Consequently, functional restoration by means of FNS for these persons has focused on achieving opening and closing of the hand by means of stimulating flexors and extensors of the fingers and thumb. Systems have been developed[14] for simultaneous FNS control of both the hand muscles and the more proximal upper limb muscles paralyzed by cord lesions at C-4 or above. The task is very complicated, and extensive research and development are needed before clinical application can be attempted.

Long first described a hybrid upper limb FNS system,[5] in which an orthosis provided stability of the wrist, thumb, and the interphalangeal joints of the fingers, an electrical stimulation device generated finger extension, and a spring across the metacarpophalangeal joints generated flexion torque. Most users rejected this crude device because of its unsightly appearance and the rapid muscle fatigue they experienced when using it. Subsequent work by Peckham and associates has led to the development of a portable FNS hand neuroprosthesis[11,13,79] for persons with C-5 and C-6 quadriplegia. In a retrospective study, this device was shown to have measurably increased the function of the users, though the relative improvement was greater for C-5 than for C-6 quadriplegics.[80] This neuroprosthesis has eight stimulation channels that provide palmar prehension (three jaw chuck pinch) and lateral prehension (key grip) for closing the hand, and an extension movement for opening. A single channel of cutaneous stimulation provides sensory feedback from the anesthetic hand of persons with C-5 quadriplegia. Control of the muscle force upon contraction is regulated by recruitment modulation, which in turn is controlled by the duration/width of the primary stimulus pulse. The hand muscles are thus activated in a synergistic or an antagonistic pattern, to move the fingers through the desired range. While it is possible to use different voluntary commands sources—voice recognition, breath power, myoelectric signals—to control the whole FNS-generated motion of the fingers, the hand neuroprosthesis uses voluntary movement of the opposite shoulder to generate a single continuously variable command and control signal. The voluntary shoulder motions, which are rapid, precise, and easily repeatable in C-5 and C-6 quadriplegics, are transduced to a position sensor mounted on the anterior chest, which in turn converts these motions to logical and proportional signals.[12] The neuroprosthesis operates as an open-loop system that employs visual feedback to ensure adequate grasp of the object. Intramuscular electrodes with percutaneous leads primarily have been used, with all the leads and the electronic controller and stimulator placed externally on the body. A neuroprosthesis with completely implantable electrodes, leads, receiver and stimulator, powered by radio frequency and controlled by an external portable computer has been developed (Figure 23-5) and clinically tested,[13,81,82] but it is not yet available to clinicians.

In certain cases of quadriplegia, upper limb surgical reconstruction with tendon transfers and anastomoses and fusions of certain finger joints has long been shown clinically to increase hand function.[83,84] Such reconstruction has also been used in combination with FNS, particularly when FNS of the usual muscles cannot elicit suitable finger motion and no adjacent voluntary muscles can be used for transfer. Under these circumstances, spastic hand muscles, which are paralyzed by upper motor neuron lesions and lie close to flaccid paralyzed muscles or their tendons, may be used for transfers in a fashion identical to the traditional transfers of tendons from voluntarily contracting muscles.[13] Thumb and finger joints to be fused, as well as the tendons to be transferred,

are selected individually based upon availability of excitable muscles and the biomechanics of the hand. The transferred spastic muscles are subsequently stimulated for functional purposes in a manner similar to that of the other spastic muscles.

Functional evaluation done retrospectively on 22 quadriplegic patients who used a hand neuroprosthesis has shown that performance of 10 different functional hand tasks was 89% successful with the use of the FNS neuroprosthesis, but only 49% successful without it. The improvement in performance with the neuroprosthesis was significantly greater with the C-5–injuries than with C-6 quadriplegia.[80] This FNS system, which employs percutaneous electrodes, is presently being clinically tested in several centers.[85]

### Stimulation of the Diaphragm

Quadriplegic persons with cord lesions at C-3 or higher lose the phrenic nerve control of the diaphragm, become unable to breath on their own, and for survival usually require mechanical ventilation by negative or positive pressure. When the lesion in the spinal cord is at C-1 or C-2 and spares the lower motor neurons for the phrenic nerve at the third, fourth, and fifth cervical segments, it is possible to stimulate the nerve anywhere between the neck and its motor points in the diaphragm, and thus reduce or eliminate the need for mechanical ventilation.[15,16] *Electrophrenic respiration* (EPR), as this technique is often called, was initially used at night for persons with sleep apnea who were otherwise healthy, but it has since proved to be a reliable mode of ventilation for quadriplegic persons. It is an attractive alternative to mechanical ventilation, since the tracheostomy can be plugged, the transmitter box can be inconspicuously attached to the wheelchair, and the ventilator tubing can be eliminated.[86] Candidates for electrostimulation of the diaphragm must be chosen very carefully. The cervical cord injury must have happened at least 6 months earlier to allow spontaneous improvement to have occurred, and all respiratory complications must have been effectively treated. There should be no evidence of atelectasis, pneumonitis, bronchiectasis, chronic obstructive pulmonary disease, or significant stenosis of the trachea. The patient must have ade-

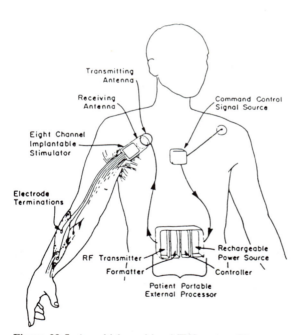

**Figure 23-5.** A multichannel hand FNS system ("neuroprosthesis") with completely implantable motor and sensory electrodes, lead wires and receiver-stimulator, powered and controlled by radio frequency and an external portable computer. (From Keith MW, Peckham PH, Thrope GB, et al. Functional neuromuscular stimulation neuroprosthesis for the tetraplegic hand. Clin Orthop 1988; 233:25–33, permission.)

quate sitting tolerance and be able to tolerate room air without supplemental oxygen. Children younger than 6 years of age generally are not considered good candidates. Family members must be not only emotionally supportive but able to learn how to use and maintain the equipment. Careful evaluation of the viability of the phrenic nerve is most important. This usually involves fluoroscopic assessment of diaphragm motions, both during voluntary effort and during electrical stimulation of the phrenic nerve in the neck with a recording electrode attached to the chest wall just below the insertion of the diaphragm (Figure 23-6). The diaphragmatic excursions on fluoroscopy should measure 4 to 6 cm, and the latency of the phrenic nerve on stimulation should average 6 to 9 msec.[86]

Ordinarily, stimulating cuff electrodes are surgically implanted around the phrenic nerve, either at the base of the neck or more commonly along the route of the phrenic nerve in the chest (Figure 23-7) in a subcutaneous pocket, either on the lower anterior chest wall or at a point where it is easier to locate. The receiver and stimulator is surgically implanted in the abdominal wall below the costal border. Subcutaneous lead wires connect the device with the stimulating electrodes. An external transmitter with a circular antenna controls the stimulation parameters. Postoperatively, a careful and gradually incremental program of electrostimulation is initiated, to recondition the diaphragm while minimizing muscle fatigue. Since stimula-

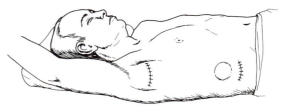

A

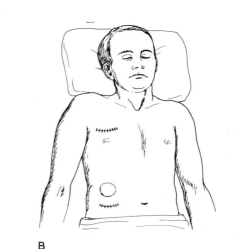

B

**Figure 23-7.** Surgical approaches for insertion of intrathoracic phrenic nerve stimulation electrodes (A) through the axilla at the third intercostal space or (B) through the anterior chest wall at the second intercostal space. The receiver is placed subcutaneously, either (A) anteriorly on the lower chest wall or (B) in the abdominal wall below the costal border.

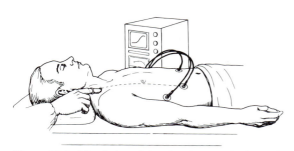

**Figure 23-6.** Stimulation of the phrenic nerve in the neck by an external electrode with recording electrodes attached to the chest wall at approximately the eighth intercostal space, close to where the diaphragm inserts on the chest wall (Adapted from Shaw RK, Glenn WWL, Hogan JF, et al. Electrophysiological evaluation of phrenic nerve function in candidates for diaphragm pacing. J Neurosurg 1980; 53:345–354.)

tion of half of the diaphragm is usually adequate for ventilation while resting in the supine position, alternate stimulation of each half of the diaphragm may be desirable to avoid muscle fatigue, but unfortunately such stimulation is not adequate while the patient is sitting. Blood gases are carefully monitored during the reconditioning phase, which may last 2 to 4 months or until the user is able to breathe without any other ventilatory support except as a safety backup.

Almost 20 years of clinical experience have demonstrated the efficacy and safety of EPR for appropriate candidates.[15,86] It is clear that continuous stimulation of the phrenic nerve bilaterally can be safely applied if the stimulation frequencies are low (8 to 12 Hz).[15] Excessive stimulation, may damage the nerve, as can physical contact between the nerve and the electrode, localized infection, or fibrosis. It has therefore been suggested that electrodes that are implanted intramuscularly into the diaphragm may prove safer and require a less invasive implantation procedure,[87] but apparently, clinical implementation of this system has not reached realization.

### Lower Limb Control

Restoration of lower limb function by FNS has received much attention in recent years. Research projects have demonstrated that with FNS paraplegic persons can stand and walk short distances, negotiate stairs, curbs and inclines, and pedal exercise cycles for physical fitness training. Despite promising results in the laboratory and improved technology, clinical application of FNS for ambulation has been slow. Only one commercially available system has been introduced in the United States, and no paraplegic persons have reported using this technology as their primary means for mobility. In contrast to the limited clinical application of FNS ambulation systems, an FNS ergometer has been available commercially for several years, and many with quadriplegia or paraplegia have used it regularly to exercise paralyzed limbs for physical fitness and potential health benefits.

### Standing and Ambulation

The early clinical attempts to use FNS involved electrical stimulation of the ankle dorsiflexors in a hemiplegic limb in order to obtain foot clearance during the swing phase of gait[3,88] and stimulation of the quadriceps muscles in paraplegic limbs to maintain a standing position.[4] For the last 20 years extensive research and development efforts in different countries have been directed toward enabling paraplegic individuals to functionally stand and ambulate by means of FNS. Additionally, it has been suggested that FNS systems can be used to restore gait after stroke or traumatic brain injury.[9] Despite the extensive work, currently no FNS system for ambulation adequately meets all the requirements; this partly accounts for their limited clinical application and commercial availability.

In concept, FNS systems for ambulation and standing may differ in several ways with respect to their purposes and to the components used. The simplest systems have a single channel for muscle stimulation. One such system, which stimulates the peroneal nerve to correct the foot drop of hemiplegia, has been rejected clinically because similar correction may be obtained by wearing a regular ankle-foot orthosis.[88,89] A simple two-channel device for bilateral stimulation of the quadriceps muscles with the hips positioned in hyperextension has been shown to be adequate for standing, and it might be useful for more SCI patients than the more complex systems used for ambulation.[90,91] The Parastep,[92] the first FNS ambulation system to be commercially available in the United States, uses a four-channel stimulator for surface stimulation of the knee extensors and hip flexors bilaterally. The more complex systems (Figure 23-8) have multiple stimulation channels, implanted electrodes, closed-loop control, and multiple sensors.

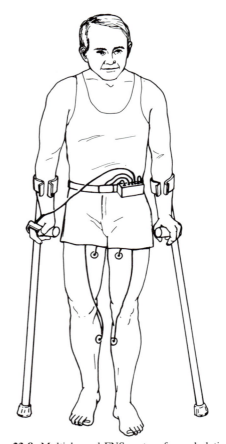

**Figure 23-8.** Multichannel FNS system for ambulation.

## Electrodes

For practical clinical reasons, FNS systems using skin surface electrodes should have no more than four stimulation channels. Intramuscular electrodes with percutaneous leads or surgically implanted electrodes are generally preferred for multiple channel systems, owing to their greater accuracy in stimulating deep or small muscles, greater effectiveness in producing repeated muscle responses, and less irritation to the skin. These electrodes, however, have a considerable failure rate[9] and occasionally even cause a burn or an infection.

## Control

FNS systems that are designed for accomplishing a relatively simple task, such as stimulation of one or two groups of muscles for ankle dorsiflexion or knee extension, are best preprogrammed with an open-loop control, whereas the more complicated multichannel systems are designed with peripherally placed sensors and a closed-loop control. The stimulation patterns for different lower limb tasks are evaluated individually for each subject and are properly adjusted before the patterns are programmed and transferred into the portable computer-stimulator's memory. The number of such preprogrammed activities may vary much, but sophisticated systems for capable users may at present have as many as 24 different tasks patterned. The user operates a manual switch to select the desired programmed activity (e.g., standing up from sitting, sitting down, prolonged standing, walking on a level surface, negotiating stairs, performing different exercises). A visual display on the computer-stimulator provides the user information on the activated function. In an open-loop control system, sensory feedback is obtained simply by using residual sensory functions (visual, auditory, vestibular), but in systems with closed-loop controls, artificial sensors are placed in the paralyzed limbs and these can provide the computer-stimulator with information on joint position and pressure on the limb, which in turn may institute a remedial action or give a warning signal.

Ideally, an FNS system for ambulation should allow the paralyzed person to walk without any other assistive devices, but currently this is not possible, since standing and ambulation balance cannot be provided even with the most sophisticated FNS systems, which are equipped with multiple sensors and closed-loop control. All users of such systems require arm support from gait aids—canes, crutches, or walker. Additionally, lower limb orthoses of different designs are used by many, if not most, FNS systems to provide joint stability, prevent joint injuries, reduce oxygen consumption, provide mounting for sensors, increase limb control, and reduce the number of electrodes and stimulation channels required. These orthoses may vary in design from a simple ankle-foot orthosis to a knee-ankle-foot orthosis with trunk extensions (i.e., a reciprocating gait orthosis).[93]

Despite advances in biomechanical technology and better understanding of the pathophysiology of SCI, numerous obstacles must be overcome before FNS systems for ambulation become widely used. Electrodes must be made that are reliable for long-term stimulation, perfectly safe, and easily implantable. Currently used surface and percutaneous electrodes may occasionally produce skin burns, and implanted nerve cuff electrodes may cause nerve damage. The failure rate of percutaneous electrodes is reportedly high (45% after 3 months of use and 60% after 6 months),[9] apparently owing to suboptimal placement, movement of the electrode away from the motor point, or mechanical failure. A totally implantable microelectronic computer-stimulator-receiver package for multichannel stimulation must be engineered and designed. Such a package must be adapted and easily connected not only to implanted leads and electrodes but to peripherally placed sensors. Current FNS systems demand a high level of attentiveness on the part of the user, whereas optimally the sensory feedback should result in automatic correction of limb movement to control posture and gait. Preliminary work on FNS control has relied on computer simulation models, which consist of nonlinear muscle-tendon dynamics, nonlinear body segment dynamics, and linear output-feedback control law.[94] The physiology of muscle contraction and aerobic metabolism during chronic electrical stimulation needs to be better understood, and methods must be developed effectively to restore adequate strength and endurance to muscles atrophied by disuse. Undesirable spinal reflexes and spasticity elicited or aggravated by the electrical stimulation and consequent sensory neuron discharge must be suppressed or better utilized for functional purposes. Interventions must be identified to restore optimal cardiovascular function during prolonged ambulation, especially for persons with high-level SCI who have limited supraspinal control, if any, over the sympathetic nervous system. In order to ambulate functionally, the user has to be able to obtain an acceptable speed of gait and be able to travel significant distances and negotiate different surfaces (e.g., stairs and inclines). FNS ambulation speed has been reported to be very slow—between 12 and 18 m per minute,[8] maximum in the best subjects 50 to 60 m per minute. The usual distance traveled on level surfaces is 100 to 200 m; the maximum distance approximately 400 m.[9] Most FNS systems are preprogrammed for ambulation on level surfaces only, though the more sophisticated systems allow the patient to ascend and descend stairs and inclines. Energy cost of FNS ambulation has been found to be similar to that measured for paraplegics using bilateral knee-ankle-foot orthoses and crutches for ambulation, which is two or three times higher than oxygen consumption per minute during walking for persons without disabilities.[95] There are indications, however, that as the speed of FNS ambulation increases with training and improved skills there is no significant rise in oxygen consumption.[95] Another study showed a smaller energy cost during ambulation with a hybrid reciprocating gait orthosis–FNS system than with the orthosis alone.[93] Thus, FNS ambulation eventually may compare favorably with the more traditional paraplegic ambulation with knee-ankle-foot orthoses and crutches.

From the user's perspective, an FNS system must be easy to use. Intensive training for at least 4 to 6 weeks is required before the system can be used safely. Application of the system takes an average of 15 minutes, and daily care of the percutaneous electrodes may take as much as 30 minutes. The external stimulator, leads, and electrodes are quite conspicuous and are generally found to be cosmetically inadequate.

The safety of FNS systems for ambulation has not yet been adequately documented. It has been reported that skin burns and infections associated with use of electrodes with percutaneous leads are relatively rare,[9] but it may easily be anticipated that extensive clinical use may cause injuries to anesthetic joints, resulting in the development of neuropathic joint disease (Charcot joints), and that with minor trauma or as a result of falls osteoporotic bones in the paralyzed limbs may fracture.

Clearly, not all SCI patients are candidates for even the most ideal yet-to-be-designed FNS ambulation. Those with T-4 to T-12 cord lesions are the ideal users, but they represent only about 25% of all SCI patients. In addition, different health problems may reduce this number significantly. Quadriplegics and paraplegics with lower motor neuron paralysis in general would not qualify. One study refers to 500 persons who recently sustained SCI who over a 9-year period were admitted and evaluated for FNS system use. The system was prescribed and implemented when the application criteria were met,[8] but only 76 persons, 15% of the entire group, met the criteria. Fifty of them had complete cord lesions, and all were followed and evaluated regularly. Only 25% of the 50 subjects with complete cord lesions were able to ambulate effectively with the FNS system, and for various reasons nine subjects soon stopped using the system. Thus, only 16 subjects remained ambulatory by this means, a small percentage of the 500 patients originally evaluated. Given the current state of technology and training, it appears that for the near future only the exceptional SCI person will be able to use FNS systems for community ambulation.

### Lower Limb Exercise

FNS systems have been designed and commercially marketed to provide strengthening and endurance exercise for lower limb muscles that have been paralyzed by upper motor neuron lesions in the spinal cord (Figure 23-9). Hundreds of such devices have been sold, and it is probable that thousands of persons with SCI have used this clinical intervention. The systems were first developed as a byproduct of research and development on FNS systems for ambulation. During the early clinical experiments with FNS systems for ambulation it was recognized that considerable training of the paralyzed muscles was necessary if functional ambulation was to be obtained with synchronized electrical stimulation by subjects who

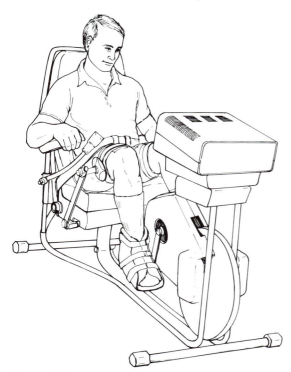

**Figure 23-9.** Multichannel FNS system for lower limb cycle ergometry.

were significantly deconditioned owing to disuse and immobilization. Preparation for ambulation thus required strengthening exercises by regular stimulation of the key lower limb muscles (quadriceps and gluteus), either by isometric (or preferably by isotonic) muscle contraction by which the knee was raised against gravity and some degree of resistance. To further improve the oxidative capacity of the muscles, the subjects trained by pedaling an exercise cycle against different degrees of resistance. While only a few of the subjects involved in such training programs eventually progressed to experimental FNS system ambulation, most indicated that subjectively their physical and mental condition had improved during this preparatory therapy. While such subjective observations do not have a ready scientific explanation, speculative and hypothetical explanations abound. It has long been recognized that immobilization for any reason, including the sedentary lifestyle forced by SCI, results in many adverse physiologic changes[96] and that many of these changes may be

reversed by regular and sustained physical exercise. Additionally, numerous scientific studies[57,97,98] have demonstrated various beneficial effects of regular physical exercise on health and longevity in able-bodied persons.

Earlier in this chapter I described some of the degenerative physiologic changes secondary to SCI, including those due primarily to disuse and a sedentary lifestyle. Clinicians have speculated that many of the clinical symptoms and signs noted during long-term follow-up evaluation of SCI patients may be related to, or aggravated by, the lack of physical exercise, both for nonparalyzed upper limb muscles and in particular for the large muscle mass of the paralyzed lower limbs.[99] Clinicians speculate further that these symptoms and signs, often refractory to customary interventions, may be reduced through fitness training of upper and lower limb muscles.[100] Sedentary lifestyle and the consequent reduced cardiovascular fitness after SCI[63,101] have been linked hypothetically[100] to the high reported mortality rate from cardiovascular conditions after SCI,[102] a rate that may be exceeded only by that of pulmonary complications. While numerous forms of wheelchair sports, activities, and upper limb exercise programs exist for upper body fitness training, FNS provides the optimal means of actively exercising the large mass of paralyzed muscles in the lower limbs. In recent years a large number of persons with SCI have participated in FNS ergometry training programs. As a result, a considerable body of clinical and research data has been gathered on its effects. Description of the FNS ergometer and some of the reported results from this application are summarized below.

The most commonly used FNS exercise ergometer is the ERGYS Clinical Rehabilitation System (Therapeutic Technologies, Inc.); (Figure 23-9). This consists of a remote-control keyboard for the computer, a stimulus control unit, six channels for sequential muscle stimulation through skin surface electrodes, position and resistance sensors, and the patient's chair. By proper programming and by closed-loop control through feedback from the sensors, the exact stimulus amplitude is provided to generate a constant pedaling speed of 35 to 50 revolutions per minute against a precise prescribed resistance. The amount of resistance provided by this ergometer is much lower than that of a conventional exercise cycle—0 to 7/8 kp (1 kp = 9.80665 Newton units of force) compared to 0 to 10 kp for conventional exercise cycles.[103] Judging from the relative dearth of reports on adverse effects, this treatment appears to be relatively safe; nonetheless all users must meet defined clinical criteria (Table 23-1), in order to further ensure safety, comfort, and suitability for this form of exercise. The therapeutic effects of FNS ergometry, hypothetically, are many, though only relatively few have been confirmed scientifically. Some of these are discussed in the following paragraphs.

*Muscles*

FNS has repeatedly been shown to reverse to a certain extent the reduced bulk, strength, and endurance of muscles paralyzed by SCI.[18,103–105] As noted above, chronic low-frequency electrical stimulation and other forms of increased muscle use have been shown to reverse the biochemical, morphologic, and functional changes that occur during muscle disuse (i.e., to change a muscle from a predominantly type II [fast, anaerobic] to type I [slow, aerobic] fiber type.[18,19,24,25] To examine whether such alteration in muscle fibers does occur during FNS ergometry, comparison of muscle biopsy specimens taken before and after training would be needed. No such studies on SCI subjects have been completed and reported. An alternative method of measuring the relative contributions of type I and type II fibers during muscle contraction may be done by comparing quadriceps twitch time before and after FNS strengthening and endurance training. Such evaluation has shown a significant decrease in the initial slope of quadriceps twitch time with training, which suggests increased contributions from type I fibers to muscle contraction.[106]

*Cardiovascular System*

Though no amount of FNS-induced exercise can alter the SCI patient's reduced exercise capacity, which results from lost supraspinal control over the sympathetic nervous system, both voluntary exercise of the nonparalyzed muscles and FNS exercise of paralyzed muscles may significantly increase $Vo_2$ max. Many studies have shown that with upper limb exercise alone even patients who have a high-level spinal lesion can increase $Vo2$ max and other corresponding measured parameters by as much as 50%.[64,72] Similarly, people with cervical and high thoracic cord lesions who participated in FNS ergometry programs have become able to pedal the ergometer for increasingly longer periods and against progressively greater resistance[106] while demonstrating improved peak work performance and aerobic capacity (i.e., increased $Vo_2$, $Vco_2$, minute ventilation, etc.). The aerobic capacity appeared to increase rapidly during the early phase of training, but after a point, a number of relevant exercise stress test parameters remained relatively constant, though pedaling time continued to improve. This suggests that the maximum effect on the cardiovascular system may have been obtained early and that peripheral muscle strength and oxidative capacity continued to increase. It is probable that the exercise quickly becomes anaerobic and that the serum lactate level increases owing to poor return of venous blood to the heart, which in turn is caused by inadequate vasoconstriction to nonworking muscles and organs, weak venomotor tone, ineffective muscle pump, and lower intraabdominal pressure. This in turn results in insufficient stroke volume, cardiac output, and delivery of oxygen to the exercising muscles.[107] This exercise response in persons with high cord lesions is not restricted to FNS exercise; similar results are noted during performance of maximum upper limb exercises.[61] While this modest exercise response may prevent persons with high cord lesions from performing work that requires sustained high output, it is possible that such exercise may be adequate to secure certain cardiovascular health benefits.[107]

No reports exist on quantitative assessment of peripheral arterial and venous circulation during FNS training. Single-channel electrical stimulation of the gastrocnemius muscle during the early phases of SCI, especially when combined with administration of subcutaneous low-dose heparin, has been reported to reduce the incidence of deep venous thrombosis and pulmonary embolism,[108] and it may be speculated that FNS exercise in the chronic phase of SCI may help to increase both venous and arterial circulation of the exercising lower limbs with similar preventive effect. Anecdotal reports describe clinically reduced acrocy-

**Table 23.1.** Selection Criteria for FNS Ergometry[107]

| |
|---|
| Upper motor neuron lesion |
| Impaired sensation in order to tolerate stimulus |
| Minimal to moderate spasticity |
| Joint range of motion in lower extremities is within functional limits |
| Roentgenographic exam of lower extremities is unremarkable |
| Health generally good |
| Emotionally stable, reliable, and realistic |

anosis of the lower limbs with FNS exercise and reduction of pedal edema.[109]

Clinicians speculate that FNS exercise may have another—indirect—beneficial effect on the cardiovascular system, especially the coronary arteries, by raising the serum levels of high-density lipoproteins (HDL).[107,110] It is well-documented that serum HDL levels are significantly lower in SCI patients than in the nondisabled population, which may in part be due to their sedentary lifestyle. It has also been shown that although wheelchair athletes have relatively low serum HDL, their levels are higher than those of inactive SCI patients.[58] No studies, however, exist that show any change in serum HDL with FNS exercise.

Though the incidence of obesity during the chronic phase of SCI is not well-documented, body composition studies have shown that even in the absence of clinical obesity there is decreased lean body mass and increased total body fat, especially with higher cord lesions.[111] This change in body composition is attributed to physical inactivity and oversupply of energy relative to energy expenditure. Although obesity is known to be a major risk factor for coronary heart disease and development of adult onset diabetes mellitus, it is not known whether the reduced lean body mass after SCI is clinically harmful or, if so, whether regular FNS or voluntary muscle exercise and modifications of diet would have a beneficial effect on this condition.

*Respiratory System*

As noted previously in this chapter, respiratory capacity, although diminished by SCI, has been found to be sufficient for whatever voluntary exercise a person with an SCI is capable of performing. Similarly, no reports demonstrate that respiratory capacity may be inadequate for FNS exercise, even during simultaneous voluntary upper limb exercise by arm cranking.

*Endocrine Function*

The sedentary lifestyle after SCI may affect secretion of insulin as well as the sensitivity to the hormone itself of insulin receptor sites in the muscles. It has been well-documented in able-bodied people that insulin sensitivity at its receptor sites increases as physical fitness improves,[112] with consequent reduction in insulin secretion, and that the reverse process may occur with inactivity and physical deconditioning. Research also confirms that persons with chronic SCI have an increased prevalence of abnormal carbohydrate metabolism (i.e., abnormal glucose tolerance test, hyperinsulinemia, insulin resistance).[113-115] Although it may be hypothesized that increased physical fitness through both upper limb voluntary exercise and lower limb FNS ergometry may improve carbohydrate metabolism after SCI and insulin sensitivity, no studies exist to support this hypothesis.

While patients' altered self-image and depression in both the acute and chronic phases of SCI are primarily an emotional reaction to the disability, the depression may be aggravated by neuroendocrine dysfunction (i.e., excessive secretion of cortisol and inadequate secretion of β-endorphin (BEP). BEP is a peptide with opium-like properties that is normally secreted in the brain and other body tissues and appears to influence a number of physiologic and psychological functions.[116-118] Plasma levels of BEP and its precursor β-lipotropin have been shown to be increased by physical exercise, and fitness training reportedly augments the effects of these natural chemicals.[117,119] The majority of SCI patients who participated in a clinical FNS ergometry program reported improved self-image and perceived that their appearance was better after participation in this program.[120] It has since been shown that SCI is associated with a decreased level of BEP and flattened circadian rhythm, as well as dysregulated cortisol serum level.[121] The same study showed that regular FNS exercise caused a significant and sustained increase in BEP, along with regulation of the cortisol level and improved depression scores. The efficacy of upper limb endurance exercise in stimulating BEP secretion after SCI has not been reported.

*Skeletal System*

SCI is followed by immediate and significant loss of bone minerals and bone mass in the paralyzed body parts. This bone loss continues many months and may not come to a halt until 2 to 3 years after the injury.[122,123] The evidence is increased excretion of calcium and hydroxyproline in the urine.[124] The mechanisms for this pathogenic bone loss are generally believed to be immobilization and inadequate bone stress, which is normally generated by active muscle contraction and longitudinal weight bearing. Endocrine dysfunction does not seem to play a major role in the bone loss, as the nonparalyzed limbs are not affected, but dysfunction of the sympathetic nervous system resulting in inadequate trophic support and blood flow regulation has been thought to have some effect.[125,126] Although bone loss eventually halts, no known interventions increase the rate of bone formation. In contrast, able-bodied persons can reverse immobilization osteoporosis if they resume physical activity following a period of disuse.[127–129] The persistent osteoporosis increases the risk of long bone fractures, which can occur with minor injury.[130] Concern has been expressed that FNS of the paralyzed and osteoporotic lower limbs, either during ambulation or ergometry exercise, may cause fractures of the bones, and, indeed, anecdotal reports of such injuries exist. In general, however, the degree of osteoporosis found in most SCI patients does not appear to present a significant clinical risk during FNS.

The osteoporosis observed in paralyzed body parts is felt to be unalterable by any known clinical means—chemical treatment, daily standing with orthoses—or the development of spasticity.[122] Lower limb FNS for ambulation or ergometry exercise has frequently been mentioned hypothetically as an effective therapy for osteoporosis after SCI,[131] but investigators who have evaluated the impact of this technology on bone mineral density have failed to show any increase in bone density.[100,132]

## Conclusion

The clinical use of electricity allows physiatrists and other rehabilitation specialists to effectively diagnose neuromuscular disorders, to prevent and manage disease, and to enhance function. In recent years, a better understanding of the physiology of the neuromuscular system and of physical exercise, along with rapid progress in electronic technology, has enhanced the use of electricity for functional restoration in persons with disease or disability. At times it is difficult to distinguish between the use of electricity for therapeutic purposes and its application for functional restoration. Indications and contraindications for prescribing different forms of FNS have been described in the literature and in this chapter. Promising results of this intervention have raised hopes that in the near future FNS technology may dramatically change the lives of many persons with physical disability, but caution is advised. Compared to performance of the intact human body, that produced by the current technology, which is used to restore lost neuromuscular function, is crude and cannot be described as well-coordinated movement. The maximum success of FNS as a clinical intervention depends on the solution of innumerable technological problems, better understanding of neuromuscular physiology, and improved training methods. Such developments may then afford more accurate control over paralyzed but otherwise essentially intact body parts by methods that effectively bypass the damaged motor and sensory pathways in the central nervous system.

While the application of FNS systems for the purposes of improving upper limb function, allowing respirator-free ventilation, and inducing lower limb exercise may all at present have greater clinical potential than FNS systems for ambulation, FNS has received far more public attention. If everyday ambulation in the community by FNS is to become a practical reality, the stimulation of individual muscles must be highly selective, contraction must be uniform throughout the muscle,

The writing of this chapter was supported in part by the Mount Sinai Spinal Cord Injury System of Care grant #H133N00009 from the National Institute of Disability and Rehabilitation Research, United States Department of Education, Washington, D.C.

incremental activation of muscle must be reproducible, complete reconditioning of the muscle must occur with training, metabolic requirements must be fully met, muscle fatigue upon repeated artificial stimulation must be reduced, spasticity must be controllable, balance with canes and crutches must be good, and full miniaturization of more accurate devices for total body implantation must be developed. Eventually, FNS systems for different purposes may produce valuable clinical alternatives to wheelchairs, orthoses, and other forms of assistive devices now prescribed to improve the health, mobility, and self-care skills of many paralyzed persons.

## References

1. Licht S. Therapeutic electricity and ultraviolet radiation, ed 2. New Haven, Conn: Elizabeth Licht, 1967;1–70.
2. Krusen FH. Physical medicine, the employment of physical agents for diagnosis and therapy. In: History of Physical Therapy. Philadelphia: WB Saunders, 1941;9–41.
3. Liberson WT, Holmquest HJ, Scot D, et al. Functional electrotherapy: Stimulation of the peroneal nerve synchronized with the swing phase of gait of hemiplegic patients. Arch Phys Med Rehabil 1961; 42:101–105.
4. Kantrowitz A. Electronic Physiologic Aids. Brooklyn: Maimonides Hospital, 1960;4–5.
5. Long C, Masciarelli VD. An electrophysiologic splint for the hand. Arch Phys Med Rehabil 1963; 44:499–503.
6. Waters RL, McNeal D, Tasto J. Peroneal nerve conduction velocity after chronic electrical stimulation. Arch Phys Med Rehabil 1975; 56:240–243.
7. Waters RL, McNeal DR, Perry J. Experimental correcting of foot drop by electrical stimulation of peroneal nerve. Bone Joint Surg 1975; 57A:1047.
8. Kralj A, Bajd R, Turk R. Enhancement of gait restoration in spinal-injured patients by functional electrical stimulation. Clin Orthop 1988; 233:34–43.
9. Marsolais EB, Kobetic R. Development of a practical electrical stimulation system for restoring gait in a paralyzed patient. Clin Orthop 1988; 233:64–74.
10. Petrofsky JS, Phillips CA. Computer controlled walking in the paralyzed individual. Neurol Orthop Surg 1983; 4:153–164.
11. Peckham PH. Functional electrical stimulation: Current status and future prospects of applications to the neuromuscular system in spinal cord injury. Paraplegia 1987; 25:279–288.
12. Keith MW, Peckham PH, Thrope GB, et al. Functional neuromuscular stimulation, neuroprosthesis for the tetraplegic hand. Clin Orthop 1988; 233:25–33.
13. Keith MW, Peckham PH, Thrope GB, et al. Implantable functional neuromuscular stimulation in the tetraplegic hand. J Hand Surg 1989; 3:524–530.
14. Nathan RH. Generation of functional arm movements in C4 quadriplegics by neuromuscular stimulation. In: Rose FC, Jones T, Urbova, eds. Comprehensive Neurologic Rehabilitation vol 3, Neuromuscular Stimulation: Basics, Concepts and Clinical Implications. New York: Demos, 1989; 273–284.
15. Glenn WWL, Hogan JF, Loke JS, et al. Ventilatory support by pacing of the conditioned diaphragm in quadriplegics. N Engl J Med 1984; 310:1150–1155.
16. Glenn WWL. The treatment of respiratory paralysis by diaphragmatic pacing. Ann Thorac Surg 1980; 30:106–109.
17. Nochomowitz ML, Hopkins M, Brodkey J, et al. Conditioning of the diaphragm with phrenic nerve stimulation following prolonged disuse. Am Rev Respir Dis 1984; 130:686–688.
18. Lieber RL. Comparison between animal and human studies of skeletal muscle adaptation to chronic stimulation. Clin Orthop 1988; 233:19–24.
19. Salmons S, Henriksson J. The adaptive response of skeletal muscle to increased used. Muscle Nerve 1981; 4:94–105.
20. Munsat TL, McNeal D, Waters R. Effects of nerve stimulation on human muscle. Arch Neuro 1975; 33:176–182.
21. Grimby G, Nordwall A, Hulten B, et al. Changes in histochemical profile of muscle after long-term electrical stimulation in patients with idiopathic scoliosis. Scand J Rehabil Med 1985; 17:191–196.
22. Peckham PH, Mortimer JT, Marsolais EB. Alterations in the force and fatiguability of skeletal muscle in quadriplegic humans following exercise induced by chronic electrical stimulation. Clin Orthop 1976; 114:326–334.
23. Lieber RL. Skeletal muscle adaptability I: Review of basic properties. Dev Med Child Neurol 1986; 28:390–397.
24. Pette D, Vrbova G. Neural control of phenotypic expression in mammalian muscle fibers. Muscle Nerve 1985; 8:676–689.
25. Jolesz F, Sreter FA. Development, innervation and

activity pattern–induced changes in skeletal muscle. Annu Rev Physiol 1981; 43:531–552.

26. Van den Honert C, Mortimer JT. The response of the myelinated nerve fiber to short duration biphasic stimulating currents. Ann Biomed Eng 1979; 7:117–125.

27. Van den Honert C, Mortimer JT. A technique for collision block of peripheral nerve: Single stimulus analysis. IEEE Trans Biomed Eng 1981; 28:373–378.

28. McNeil DR, Baker LL. Stimulating the quadriceps and hamstrings with surface electrodes. In: Proceedings of the 8th Annual Conference of Rehabilitation Eng. Soc. N. America, 1101 Connecticut Ave NW Wash. D.C. 20036 1985;651–653.

29. Thrope GB, Peckham PH, Crago BE. A computer controlled multichannel stimulation system for laboratory use in functional neuromuscular stimulation. IEEE Trans Biomed Eng 1985; 32:363–370.

30. Gorman PH, Mortimer JT. The effect of stimulus parameters on the recruitment characteristics of direct nerve stimulation. IEEE Trans Biomed Eng 1983; 30:407–414.

31. McNeil DR, Baker LL, Symons J. Recruitment data for nerve cuff and epimysial electrodes. In: Proceedings of RESNA -Rehabilitation Engineering Society of North America (tel: 202-857-1199) 10th Annual Conf. of Rehabilitation Eng. Soc. N. America, 1101 Connecticut Ave NW Wash. D.C. 20036 1987;651–653.

32. Peckham PH. Functional neuromuscular stimulation. Phys Technol 1981; 12:114–121.

33. Mortimer JT. Motor prosthesis. In: Handbook of Physiology, The Nervous System II. Bethesda, Md: American Physiological Society, 1981;155–187.

34. Peckham PH. Electrical excitation of skeletal muscle: Alterations in force, fatigue and metabolic properties. Doctoral thesis. Case Western Reserve University, Cleveland Oh; 1972.

35. Campbell J. Efficacy of volitional versus electrically evoked knee extension exercise. In: Proceedings RESNA 10th Amer. Conf. San Jose, Calif, June 19–23. 1987;648–650.

36. Fang ZP. Presentation at the Engineering Foundation Conference on Neuroprosthesis: Motor System. Potosi, Missouri, July 17–22, 1988.

37. Petrofsky JS, Phillips CA. Microprocessor-controlled simulation in paralyzed muscle. IEEE NAECON Rec 1979; 79:198–210, 1979a.

38. Kralj AR, Bajd T. Functional electrical stimulation: Standing and walking after spinal cord injury. Boca Raton, Fl: CRC, 1989.

39. Petrofsky JS. Sequential motor unit stimulation through peripheral motor nerves in a cat. Med Biol Eng Comput V 1979; 17:87–93.

40. Patterson RP, Lockwood JS, Dykstra DD. A functional electric stimulation using an electrode garment. Arch Phys Med Rehabil 1990; 71:340–342.

41. Marsolais EB, Kobetic R. Functional electrical stimulation for walking in paraplegia. Bone Joint Surg 1987; 69A:728–733.

42. Mortimer JT, Kaufman D, Roessmann U. Intramuscular electrical stimulation: Tissue damage. Biomed Eng 1980; 8:235–244.

43. Waters RL, Campbell JM, Nakai R. Therapeutic electrical stimulation of the lower limb by epimysial electrodes. Clin Orthop 1988; 233:44–52.

44. Brindley GS, Rushton DN: Long-term follow-up of patients with sacral anterior root stimulators. Paraplegia 1990; 28:469–475.

45. Agnew WF, McCreery DB, Yuen TG, et al. Histologic and physiologic evaluation of electrically stimulated peripheral nerve: Considerations for the selection of parameters. Ann Biomed Eng 1989; 17:39–60.

46. Loeb GE, Walmsley B, Duysens J. Obtaining proprioceptive information from natural limbs: Implantable transducers versus somatosensory neuron recordings. In: Neuman MR, et al. ed. Solid State Physical Sensors for Biomedical Applications. Boca Raton, Fla: CRC, 1980.

47. Crago PE, Chizeck HJ, Neuman MR, et al. Sensors for use with functional neuromuscular stimulation. IEEE Trans Biomed Eng 1986; 33:256–268.

48. Petrofsky JS, Phillips CA, Stafford DE. Closed-loop control for restoration of movement in paralyzed muscle. Orthopaedics 1984; 7:1289–1302.

49. Grimby G, Broberg C, Krotkiewska I, et al. Muscle fiber composition in patients with traumatic cord lesions. Scand J Rehabil Med 1976; 8:37–42.

50. Lieber RL: Skeletal muscle adaptability II: Muscle properties following SCI. Dev Med Child Neurol 1986; 28:533–542.

51. Heigenhauscher GF, Ruff GL, Miller B, et al. Cardiovascular response of paraplegics during graded arm ergometry. Med Sci Sports Exer 1976; 8:68.

52. Hjeltnes N. Oxygen uptake and cardiac output in graded arm exercise in paraplegics with low-level spinal lesions. Scand J Rehabil Med 1977; 9:107–113.

53. Hjeltnes N. Cardiorespiratory capacity in tetra- and paraplegia shortly after injury. Scand J Rehabil Med 1986; 18:65–70.

54. VanLoan M, McCluer S, Loftin JM, et al. Com-

parison of maximal physiological responses to arm exercise among able-bodied paraplegics and quadriplegics. Med Sci Sports Exer 1985;17:250.

55. Glaser RM, Sawka MN, Brune MF, et al. Physical responses to maximal effort wheelchair and arm crank ergometry. J Appl Physiol 1980; 48:1060–1064.

56. Knutsson E, Lewenhaupt-Olsson E, Thorsen M. Physical work capacity and physical conditioning in paraplegic patients. Paraplegia 1973; 11:205–216.

57. Blair SN, Kohl HW, Pattenbarger RS, et al. Physical fitness and all-cause mortality. A prospective study of healthy men and women. JAMA 1989; 262:2395–2401.

58. Brenes G, Dearwater S, Shapera R, et al. High density lipoprotein cholesterol concentrations in physically active and sedentary spinal cord injured patients. Arch Phys Med Rehabil 1986; 67:445–450.

59. Ferrara MS, Davis RW. Injuries to the elite wheelchair athletes. Paraplegia 1990; 28:335–341.

60. DeBoer LB, Kallal JE, Longo MR. Upper extremity prone position exercise as aerobic capacity indicator. Arch Phys Med Rehabil 1982; 63:467–471.

61. Coutts DK, Rhodes EC, McKenzie DC. Maximal exercise responses of tetraplegics and paraplegics. J Appl Physiol 1983; 55:479–482.

62. Davis GM, Kofsky PR, Kelsey JC, et al. Cardiorespiratory fitness and muscular strength of wheelchair uses. Can Med Assoc J 1981; 125:1317–1323.

63. Figoni SF. Spinal cord injury and maximal aerobic power. Am Correct Ther J 1984; 38:44–50.

64. Gass GC, Watson J, Camp EM, et al. Effects of physical training on high-level spinal lesion patients. Scand J Rehabil Med 1980; 12:61–65.

65. Hass F, Axen K, Pineda H. Aerobic capacity in spinal cord injured people. Cent Nerv Syst Trauma 1986; 3:77–91.

66. Wicks JR, Oldridge NB, Cameron BJ, et al. Arm cranking and wheelchair ergometry in elite spinal cord injured athletes. Med Sci Sports Exerc 1983; 15:224–231.

67. Drory Y, Ohry A, Brooks ME, et al. Arm crank ergometry in chronic spinal cord injured patients. Arch Phys Med Rehabil 1990; 71:389–392.

68. Freyschuss U, Knuttson E. Cardiovascular control in man with transverse cervical cord lesions. Life Sci 1969; 8:421–424.

69. Coutts KD. Prediction of oxygen uptake from power output in tetraplegics and paraplegics during wheelchair ergometry. Med Sci Sports Exerc 1983; 15:181.

70. Gass GC, Camp EM. The maximum physiological responses during incremental wheelchair and arm cranking exercise in male paraplegics. Med Sci Sports Exerc 1984; 16:355–359.

71. Sawka MM, Glaser RM, Laubach LL, et al. Wheelchair exercise performance of the young, middle-aged and elderly. J Appl Physiol 1981; 50:824–828.

72. Whiting RB, Dreisinger TE, Dalton RB, et al. Improved physical fitness and work capacity in quadriplegics by wheelchair exercise. J Cardiac Rehabil 1983; 3:251–255.

73. Kamelhar DL, Steele JM, Schact RG, et al. Plasma renin and serum dopamine-beta-hydroxylase during orthostatic hypotension in quadriplegic man. Arch Phys Med Rehabil 1978; 59:212–216.

74. Naftchi NE, Ragnarsson KJ, Sell GH, et al. Increased digital vascular reactivity to L-norepinephrine in quadriplegics. Arch Phys Med Rehabil 1975; 56:554.

75. Fugl-Meyer AR. Effects of respiratory muscle paralysis in tetraplegia and paraplegia patients. Scand J Rehabil Med 1971; 3:141–150.

76. Kokkola K, Moller K, Lehtonen T. Pulmonary function in tetraplegia and paraplegia patients. Ann Clin Res 1975; 7:76–80.

77. Rhodes EC, McKenzie DC, Coutts KD, et al. A field test for the prediction of aerobic capacity in male paraplegics and quadriplegics. Can J Appl Sports Sci 1981; 6:182–186.

78. Bunt JC. Hormonal alterations due to exercise. Sports Med 1986; 3:331–345.

79. Peckham PH, Keith MW, Freehafer AA. Restoration of functional control by electrical stimulation in the upper extremity of the quadriplegic patient. J Bone Joint Surg 1988; 70A:144–148.

80. Wijman CAC, Stroh KC, Van Doren CL, et al. Functional evaluation of quadriplegic patients using a hand neuroprosthesis. Arch Phys Med Rehabil 1990; 71:1053–1057.

81. Smith B, Peckham PH, Roscoe DD, et al. An externally powered multichannel implantable stimulator for versatile control of paralyzed muscles. IEEE Trans Biomed Eng 1987; 34:499–508.

82. Brindley GS, Donaldson N, Perkins TA, et al. Two-stage key grip by joy stick from an eleven-channel upper limb FES implant in C6 tetraplegia. Proceedings Biology Engineering Society, Hexham, England, 41 1989.

83. Moberg E. The Upper Limb and Tetraplegia: A New Approach to Surgical Rehabilitation, Stuttgart: George Thieme, 1978.

84. House JH, Shannon MA. Restoration of strong grasp and lateral pinch in tetraplegia: A compari-

son of two methods of thumb control in each patient. J Hand Surg 1985; 10:22–29.

85. Peckham PH. Personal communication. 1991.

86. Carter RE: Available respiratory options. In: Whiteneck G., et al. eds. The Management of High Quadriplegia. New York: Demos, 1989.

87. Nochomovitz ML, DiMarco AF, Mortimer JT, et al. Diaphragm activation with intramuscular stimulation. Am Rev Respir Dis 1983; 127:325–329.

88. Waters R, McNeal D, Perry J. Experimental correction of foot drop by electrical stimulation of the peroneal nerve. J Bone Joint Surg 1975; 57A:1047–1054.

89. Merletti R, Andina A, Galante N, et al. Clinical experience of electrical peroneal stimulators in fifty hemiparetic patients. Scand J Rehabil Med 1979; 11:111–121.

90. Jaeger RJ, Yarkony GM, Roth EJ, et al. Estimating the user population of a simple electrical system for standing. Paraplegia 1990; 28:505–511.

91. Yarkony GM, Jaeger RJ, Roth EJ, et al. Functional neuromuscular stimulation for standing after spinal cord injury. Arch Phys Med Rehabil 1990; 71:201–206.

92. Technological Advancements in Rehabilitation: Independent Standing & Short Distance Walking for the Spinal Cord Injured. An Overview of the Parastep ® System Sigmedics Inc. One Northfield Plaza, Suite 410, Northfield, Illinois 60093, 1991

93. Nene AB, Patrick JH. Energy cost of paraplegic locomotion using the Parawalker/electrical stimulation hybrid orthosis. Arch Phys Med Rehabil 1990; 71:116–120.

94. Khang G, Zajac FE. Paraplegic standing controlled by functional neuromuscular stimulation: Part I and Part II: Computer model and control system design; computer stimulation studies. IEEE Trans Biomech Eng 1989; 36:873–894.

95. Marsolais EB, Edwards BG. Energy cost of walking and standing with functional neuromuscular stimulation and long leg braces. Arch Phys Med Rehabil 1988; 69:243–249.

96. Dietrich JE, Whedon GD, Shorr E. Effects of immobilization upon various metabolic and physiological functions of normal man. Am J Med 1948; 4:3–36.

97. Rippe JM, Ward A, Porcari JP, et al. Walking for health and fitness. JAMA 1988; 259:2720–2724.

98. Harris SS, Caspersen CJ, DeFriese GH, et al. Physical activity counseling for healthy adults as primary preventive intervention in a clinical setting: Report for the US Preventive Service Task Force. JAMA 1989; 261:3590–3598.

99. Ragnarsson KT. Spinal cord injury: Old problems, new approaches. Bull NY Acad Med 1986; 62: 174–181.

100. Ragnarsson KT. Physiologic effects of functional electrical stimulation–induced exercises in spinal cord injured individuals. Clin Orthop 1988; 233:53–63.

101. Figoni SF. Perspectives on cardiovascular fitness and SCI. J Am Parapleg Soc 1990; 13:63–71.

102. Stover SL, Fine PR. Spinal Cord Injury: Facts and Figures. Birmingham, Ala: The University of Alabama at Birmingham, 1986.

103. Ragnarsson KT, Pollack S, O'Daniel W, et al. Clinical evaluation of computerized functional electrical stimulation after spinal cord injury: A multicenter pilot study. Arch Phys Med Rehabil 1988; 69:672–677.

104. Gruner JA, Glaser RM, Feinberg SD, et al. A system for evaluation and exercise conditioning of paralyzed muscles. J Rehabil Res Dev 1983; 20:21–30.

105. Faghri PD, Glaser RM, Figoni SF, et al. Feasibility of using two FNS exercise modes for spinal cord injured patients. Clin Kinesiol 1989; 43:62–68.

106. Pollack SF, Axen K, Spielholtz N, et al. Aerobic training effects of electrically induced lower extremity exercises in spinal cord injured people. Arch Phys Med Rehabil 1989; 70:214–219.

107. Ragnarsson KT, Pollack SF, Twist D. Lower limb endurance exercise after spinal cord injury: Implications for health and functional ambulation. J Neurol Rehabil 1991, 5:37–48

108. Merli GJ, Herbison GJ, Ditunno JF, et al. Deep vein thrombosis: Prophylaxis in acute spinal cord injured patients. Arch Phys Med Rehabil 1988; 69:661–664.

109. Twist DF. Acrocyanosis in spinal cord injured patients: Effects of computer-controlled neuromuscular electrical stimulation: A case report. Phys Ther 1990; 70:45–49.

110. Brenes G, McDermott AL, Sikora JM. The effect of computerized functional electrical stimulation on lipoprotein cholesterol in the spinal cord injured. In: Proceedings of the Fifteenth Annual Scientific Meeting, American Spinal Injury Association, Las Vegas, Nevada, 1989. : , ; 78. Publishers: Am Spinal Injury Assoc., Atlanta Georgia, 1989.

111. Nuhlicek DNR, Spurr GB, Barboriak JJ, et al. Body composition of patients with spinal cord injury. Eur J Clin Nutr 1988; 42:765–773.

112. Mondon CE, Dolkas CB, Reaven GM. Site of enhanced insulin sensitivity in exercise trained rats at rest. Am J Physiol 1980; 239:E169.

113. Duckworth WC, Solomon SS, Jallpalli P, et al. Glucose intolerance due to insulin resistance in patients with spinal cord injuries. Diabetes 1980; 29:906–910.

114. Duckworth WC, Jappalli P, Solomon SS. Glucose intolerance in spinal cord injury. Arch Phys Med Rehabil 1983; 64:107–110.

115. Bauman WA, Yalow RS, Zhang RL, et al. Glucose intolerance in diabetes mellitus in paraplegic veterans. J Am Parapleg Soc 1991; 14:195.

116. Byck R. Peptide transmitters: A unifying hypothesis for euphoria, respiration, sleep and the action of lithium. Lancet 1976; 2:72–73.

117. Carr DB, Bullen BA, Skrinar GS, et al. Physical conditioning facilitates the exercise induced secretion of beta-endorphine and beta-alipotropin in women. N Eng J Med 1981; 305:560–563.

118. Pasternak GW. Multiple morphine and encephalon receptors and the relief of pain. JAMA 1988; 259:1362–1367.

119. Harber VJ, Sutton JR. Endorphines and exercise. Sports Med 1984; 1:154–171.

120. Sipski ML, DeLisa JA, Schweer S. Functional electrical stimulation by cycle ergometry: Patient perceptions. Am J Phys Med Rehabil 1989; 68:147–149.

121. Twist DJ, Culpepper-Morgan JA, Ragnarsson KT, et al. Neuroendocrine parameters in spinal cord injured involved in a computerized functional electrical stimulation exercise program. Am J Phys Med Rehabil 1992; 71:156–163.

122. Biering-Sorensen F, Bohr H, Schaadt O. Bone mineral content of the lumbar spine and lower extremities years after spinal cord lesion. Paraplegia 1988; 26:293–301.

123. Naftchi NE, Viau AT, Sell GH, et al. Mineral metabolism in spinal cord injury. Arch Phys Med Rehabil 1980; 61:139–142.

124. Claus-Walker J, Comporse RJ, Carter RE, et al. Calcium excretion in quadriplegia. Arch Phys Med Rehabil 1972; 53:14–20.

125. Dietz FR. Effect of peripheral nerve on limb development. J Orthop Res 1986; 5:576–585.

126. Gillis BJA. The nature of the bone changes associated with nerve injuries and disuse. J Bone Joint Surg 1954; 36B:464–473.

127. Donaldson CL, Hulley SB, Vogel JM, et al. Effect of prolonged bedrest on bone mineral. Metabolism 1970; 19:1071–1084.

128. Uhtoff HK, Jaworski ZFG. Bone loss and response to long term immobilization. J Bone Joint Surg 1978; 60B:420–429.

129. Ruben CT, Lanyon LE. Regulation of bone formation by applied dynamic loads. J Bone Joint Surg 1984; 66A:397–402.

130. Ragnarsson KT, Sell GH. Lower extremity fractures after SCI: A retrospective study. Arch Phys Med Rehabil 1981; 62:418–422.

131. Phillips CA, Petrofsky JS, Hendershot DM, et al. Functional electrical exercise: A comprehensive approach for physical conditioning of the spinal cord injured patient. Orthopaedics 1984; 7:1112–1123.

132. Leeds EM, Klose KJ, Ganz W, et al. Bone mineral density after bicycle ergometry training. Arch Phys Med Rehabil 1990; 71:207–219.

# Chapter 24

# Central Nervous System Plasticity and Cognitive Remediation

YASOMA B. CHALLENOR
RICHARD B. BORKOW

The processes of rehabilitation therapy follow the trend of much of modern medical therapeutics: strategies for intervention that are observed to be effective may await clarification of the underlying mechanisms that account for the efficacy.

In this chapter we explore central nervous system (CNS) plasticity, mechanisms of recovery that may suggest therapeutic strategies, especially in pediatric rehabilitation and particularly in the growing area of cognitive remediation. The latter area has direct implications for addressing the needs of children and adults with traumatic brain injury, cerebral palsy, learning disabilities, attention deficit disorders, and a host of other disorders that impair function in mature and growing brains.

> Learning . . . disposeth the constitution of the mind not to be fixed or settled in the defects thereof, but still to be capable and susceptible of growth and reformation.
> *Sir Francis Bacon*
> *The Advancement of Learning*
> *Book I*

## Central Nervous System Plasticity

### Central Nervous System Regeneration

In the mammalian peripheral nervous system nerve injury is followed by some degree of regeneration of the nerve axon from the point of injury toward the peripheral structure to be innervated. In contrast, in the CNS regeneration is severely limited.

This limitation apparently is greater for the mature mammals than for immature ones.

Several reasons have been proposed for the restriction of CNS regenerative capability. Glial scarring may block the pathway for sprouting of axons; though, even without demonstrable scarring, regrowth is limited. Axon maturity may mean that the axon is no longer capable of renewing its embryonic growth potential. Why this should be the case in axons of the CNS and not of the peripheral nervous system is not clear. Target cell trophic factors or growth factors may give a specific feedback to promote nerve regrowth; these factors may be lacking in the CNS.[1] Alternatively, substances such as nerve growth factor may be time- and concentration-dependent in order to stimulate growth across a lesion site.[2,3] The concentration of nerve growth factor in the CNS, if any at all is present, may be insufficient or too slow to accumulate to produce nerve regeneration.

The blood-brain barrier normally prevents antibody-producing cells from entering the CNS. Physical or chemical injury may weaken or remove this barrier and may afford antibody-producing cells access to nerve tissue, so autoimmune factors may be implicated in the limited capacity for CNS regeneration.[4,5] The CNS of young rodents is capable of regrowth of nerve across lesioned areas if immunologic competence has not yet developed; with immune system maturity, autoimmunity to nerve tissue may prevent regeneration. Synaptic receptor sites may become nonreceptive to new innervation once they have been for a time free of the influence of the innervating axon. On the other hand, when limited CNS sprouting does occur, it may fail to reach the synapse, reach an inappropriate or aberrant synapse, or reach a synapse that cannot be reinnervated.

Whatever the capacity for CNS regrowth after lesions, and whatever the reasons for the severe restriction of regrowth, some functional recovery can occur. We will consider animal experimental models of CNS plasticity, correlate them to clinical models of human plasticity, and then attempt to understand the mechanisms of recovery and the therapeutic strategies these observations may suggest.

### Animal Models of Plasticity

The capacity for nerve regrowth in the mammalian CNS may be specific to certain CNS loci or certain types of nerve cells. Dendritic and axonal sprouting phenomena have been extensively observed in several animal models. Liu and Chambers[6] noted increased fiber terminal density following section of dorsal roots in cat spinal cord. This suggested that intact intraspinous processes of spinal sensory neurons of the cat could react to partial denervation by forming new processes. Glees and Cole[7] have observed recovery of limb function in monkeys after localized lesions in the sensorimotor cortex. Subsequent excision of cortex immediately surrounding the original area of damage again produced a motor deficit, suggesting that sprouting to the area surrounding the first lesion had occurred.

Sprouting of intact dendrites or axons may promote synaptic rearrangement. Hypothalamic fibers and others traveling along the medial forebrain bundle sprout to replace synaptic endings transiently eliminated by transection of the fornix.[8-10] Other areas in the CNS in which electron or light microscopic evidence of sprouting has been observed include the ventral cochlear nucleus,[11] visual thalamus,[12,13] and spinal trigeminal nucleus.[14] Histochemical studies have shown sprouting of acetylcholinesterase-containing fibers triggered by lesions of the entorhinal cortex. The new fibers originated in the septal region of the brain, and subsequent lesioning of the septum caused immediate loss of acetylcholinesterase staining of the dentate gyrus. However, Nerve sprouting does not occur in all loci after injury. Goodman and Horel[12] found that the optic tract sprouted into only two of 13 potential, deafferented visual system sites of rat brain after damage to one occipital cortex.

Heterotopic sprouting in the CNS may occur,[2] and some loci appear to have specific patterns of axonal sprouting. Goodman and coworkers[16] showed that when lesions were carefully limited to the optic tracts, only visual system axons successfully filled vacated synaptic sites. However, Sotelo and colleagues[17] viewed the process of neuronal sprouting as a natural rather than a regenerative phenomenon, because they observed that healthy adult rats show a process of axonal degeneration and hypertrophy with constantly changing synaptic contacts, despite the absence of neural lesions. Similarly, Matthews and colleagues[18] demonstrated that a continuous process of new sprouts taking over existing synapses, as well as formation of new synapses, is a natural occurrence in the adult CNS; this process may be accentuated by pathologic processes.

A major question is whether collateral sprouting is merely associated with recovery after brain damage or is directly responsible for it. Evidence for the association can be derived from observations of the effects on recovery after CNS injury of age, environment, rate of lesion growth, and specific training.

Visual system lesions in kittens elicit substantially less deficit if they are produced during a certain early critical period. Enucleation of one eye of a kitten produced significant translaminar sprouting in the visual cortex; such sprouting was not seen after enucleation at a later age.[19-21] The ability to induce and reverse amblyopia or blindness following monocular occlusion has reinforced the observation of a critical period in the early life of kittens and monkeys, which corresponds to a critical period of reversibility in humans.[22,23] Tsang[24] noted that infant rats required removal of up to 50% of their visual cortex to produce the same amount of impairment in maze-solving tasks that adult rats exhibited after removal of only 7.4% of their cortex. Similarly, when somatosensory cortical ablation was performed on the sixth day of life kittens learned to perform well on tasks of smooth-rough texture determination, whereas adult cats with lesions of corresponding size and location could not learn even the simplest such task.[25] Comparable observations have been made in rats and monkeys.[26–28]

Several investigators have exposed animals to an enriched environment before inducing brain lesions, in order to observe a possible "sparing" effect, but results have been disappointing.[29] On the other hand, "postlesion" enrichment does appear to reduce the behavioral deficit in several experimental situations, particularly if the exposure to the enriched environment takes place just after the experimental animal is weaned.[30] Greenough observed a histologic correlate to the behavioral observations: upper visual cortical neurons of rats reared from weaning in an enriched environment had about 20% larger dendritic fields than the control rats reared in individual cages, without environmental complexity (presence of litter mates and toys, shapes for visual and motor exploration).[31,32] He also observed that rats trained to reach into a tube for food using the nondominant forepaw showed, in the motor cortex region governing that forepaw, an increase in the dendritic field size of the neurons that project to the spinal cord region innervating the forelimb, as compared to the opposite hemisphere. (Rats show a "handedness" preference, without a population bias, and in untrained rats the dendritic fields associated with the preferred paw are usually larger).[33] Greenough suggests that the brain is amenable to modification by experience and training. The corollary would be that therapeutic procedures may be able to alter functional neural organization. An additional tantalizing observation[34] is that animals that may perform very poorly on a behavioral task immediately after a brain lesion may be trained to perform nearly normally if they are advanced through easy, staged tasks. This has been observed with and without serial lesions.

Pharmacologic therapy to promote recovery from brain damage has been explored using pyrogens, thyroid hormone, adrenocorticotropin (ACTH) and cortisone, proteolytic enzymes, and anticholinesterases. Except for steroids used early after injury, the results of most pharmacologic agents have been equivocal at best.[35–37] Locus-specific neurotransmitters, denervation supersensitivity, collateral sprouting, and axon proliferation may all mediate altered sensitivity to pharmacologic agents.[38] Bach-y-Rita adds to the list of factors that modify drug effects: molecular size and configuration, degree of ionization, lipid solubility and the subject's hormone status, genetic substrate, and nutritional status.[39]

### Human Central Nervous System Plasticity

Surgical removal of the complete left hemisphere of children because of intractable seizures and hemiparesis after brain injury had little deleterious effect on language function *when the original damage occurred early in life*. This observation suggests that linguistic function has shifted from its usual locus in the left hemisphere to the right. The critical period of transferability appears to be the first 5 years of life.[40] Milner[41] suggested that early in life both hemispheres can subserve language functions, to different extents. With maturation, the left hemisphere "inhibits" the language mechanisms of the right; but if a lesion is acquired early in life, the right hemisphere language functions are "disinhibited" so that the right hemisphere takes charge. This transfer of language function seems to have a cost: decreased verbal and nonverbal IQ scores are thought by Milner to be due to "crowding" too many functions into the remaining intact brain.

Supportive evidence for these hypotheses comes from studies in which the right hemisphere is suppressed by intracarotid injection of amytal. In left hemisphere–damaged children, this procedure produces reversible aphasia. Similarly, damage to the right side of the brain in children may cause temporary aphasia; this does not occur in adults with similar damage.[42] It is interesting to note that Sigmund Freud was one of the first to observe, in 1897, that temporary aphasia in children could occur after either right or left hemisphere insults. Recently developed evoked potential techniques have suggested that intrahemispheric, rather than interhemispheric, reorganization may sometimes account for the relatively good return of language following left hemisphere lesions in young children.[43]

Lenneburg reported that language recovery after perinatal lesions can be rapid and complete if the damage occurs before age 2 years, but if aphasia develops after age 10 years, recovery is slower and less complete.[44]

Zihl[45] has reported that scotomas in patients with damage to the visual cortex improved following progressive visual discrimination training. Blakemore[46] has described recovery in patients with left temporal lobectomy with verbal function deficits, and in patients with right temporal lobectomy with subsequent nonverbal functional decrements. These patients' verbal test scores returned to their preoperative levels by the end of 1 year. The group with left temporal lobectomy showed improvement in paired associate learning: by the fifth postoperative year scores matched those on preoperative tests. It is possible that the immature, or less mature, brain may have other equipotential areas, though it is difficult to find additional examples of this in humans.

Large numbers of people sustained brain injuries in World War II and in the Korean Conflict. Many experienced an initial period of functional recovery followed by slower continued recovery, which could go on 5 years or longer. Patients who received immediate physical and occupational therapy performed significantly better than those whose therapy was delayed 6 to 12 months,[47] and the younger the victim, the better was the functional recovery.[48]

***Theoretical Mechanism for Plasticity***

*Mechanisms Underlying Short-Term Improvement*

Clinical recovery of function after CNS injury may begin within hours or days, or may begin and continue after months. Patterns of recovery vary, and the reasons for this are not all known.

Resolution of cerebral edema and arterial spasm are tempting and logical explanations for *early* recovery (within days after injury). The concept of *diaschisis,* which implies a suspension of function or a state of neural shock without anatomic disruption of the corresponding brain tissue, has been invoked to explain recovery beginning weeks after brain insult. Diaschisis has a peripheral corollary in the state of neurapraxia, or the state of transient physiologic peripheral nerve block without structural disorder. Luria[49] and Meyer[50] have suggested that this state of physiologic block to function can be improved, or lifting of the block

can be hastened by CNS stimulants such as anticholinesterase agents or *d*-amphetamine.

The unmasking of silent synapses, which begin to function only after the primary functional synapses are disrupted, has been postulated to contribute to recovery after brain injury, and in animal studies unmasking may occur within hours after injury.[51] Unmasking of function may also be invoked in conjunction with the theory of equipotentiality in certain brain areas, in that a lesion in one area may unmask latent function inherent in an equipotential area. Initially, the newly functioning area of the brain may not have the speed and efficiency of the primary area, but with repeated training over time it may improve. The unmasked pathway may, in fact, have had a comparable but subservient role to that of the primary path or area. Alternatively, the unmasking may cause facilitation of synaptic access of fibers to cells that have lost their primary input.[51a] In the same hypothetical context, unmasking may involve facilitation of uncrossed pyramidal or extrapyramidal pathways.[51a]

*Hemispheric transfer* was described earlier in the case of hemispherectomy and language function. Whether or not other functions are amenable to such transfer is not known. Bach-y-Rita cites three cases that appear to show hemispheric transfer of sensorimotor ability, albeit partial, after hemispherectomy for intractable seizures.[52] Even more difficult to document with human clinical examples is the possibility of locus transfer within one hemisphere.[53] One step farther out on the theoretical limb is the concept of reorganization of functional systems proposed by Luria and others. While hemispheric transfer of function involved its restoration in nearly original form, *functional reorganization* of systems takes longer, and functional restoration is not complete. An example of functional restoration of cortical interpretation and control is seen in patients who, because of peripheral nerve injury, have lost sensation in the prehensile digits. One treatment for such deficits is an island pedicle flap taken from an area with intact sensation and outside the area critical to prehension. For example, the skin of the ulnar border of the ring finger, together with its nerve and vascular supply, is transferred to the insensitive digit. On initial testing with vision occluded, the patient reports and interprets tactile input to the transferred island as a touch on the ring finger. With a few weeks' training the patient begins to perceive the island as belonging to the previously insensitive digit and as no longer belonging to its original site. Clearly, a reorganization of cortical perception or interpretation, or both, has occurred.

Luria uses as an example of functional reorganization of systems the case of retraining a patient to read in the presence of visual agnosia. He observes that patients taught to trace large, rough letters while phonating the appropriate sound are making use of alternate motor and sensory pathways to supplement the deficient visual system. Again, with time and training, the supplements are used less and less.[49] In the motor system, Luria advocates analyzing the component sections of each complex movement, working to retrain the isolated components, then sequencing them into a continuous program. With time, the expanded program is performed more smoothly, in a shorter time, and it becomes a "contracted" program.[49] Further consideration of Luria's approach to learning, memory, and executive functioning, as well as other mental capacities, is covered in the section on Visual and Auditory Perceptual Learning.

Bach-y-Rita has reviewed the possibility that the cerebellum plays an important role in motor reorganization by modifying input-output relationships, thus compensating for changes in information processing resulting from CNS lesions.[54] The cerebral motor cortex is the common receptor of inputs from cerebellar pathways and from thalamocortical pathways from the basal ganglia. Hore[55] has shown that the severe disruption of motor function that follows globus pallidus cooling can be ameliorated by providing visual feedback for control of motion. The comparison is made to patients with parkinsonism, who perform motor activities better with visual guidance than with kinesthetic guidance alone. This, too, may fall into the category of functional reorganization of systems, though some observers view it as a simple substitution. Reorganization might be the case if, with training, the substitute system could be withdrawn without causing deterioration in function.

Table 24-1 summarizes some of the proposed processes that may represent CNS plasticity. Much research is needed to clarify these processes. Even more important may be the use of newer anatomic imaging techniques (computed tomography and magnetic resonance imaging), combined with physiologic imaging techniques (evoked potentials, brain electrical activity mapping, and positron emission tomography) to supplement clinical neurologic and neuropsychological observations of the processes of recovery of function.

To what extent CNS plasticity underlies recovery of function remains as a mystery. Fortunately, researchers have many clues to follow. As the editor of *The Lancet* commented, "Surprisingly little in the nervous system is final—except autolysis."[56]

## Learning and Cognitive Remediation

What neurophysiologic processes enable human beings to learn vast quantities of factual information and to master complex procedures and skills? According to current understanding, these learning capacities imply an enormous potential for plastic alteration at synaptic, and perhaps other, neuronal sites. Important synaptic mechanisms supporting plasticity appear to include N-methyl-D-aspartate (NMDA) receptor activity, second messenger processes, and associated dendritic transformations, all discussed in more detail later. The synaptic and macromolecular components that permit these

**Table 24-1.** Theoretical Mechanisms Underlying Plasticity

| Time Course | Quality of Return | Theoretical Mechanism |
|---|---|---|
| Days | Return of exact function | Resolution of cerebral edema, resolution of arterial spasm |
| Weeks | Return of exact function | Diaschisis, deinhibition, unmasking of synapses |
| Months | Return of nearly the same functional quality | Sensory substitution, learning of alternate strategies, hemispheral transfer, sprouting of intact neurons, modulation of existing synapses, denervation hypersensitivity |
| Months to years | Return of distorted function | Reorganization of functional systems, unmasking of silent pathways, unmasking of equipotential cells, sprouting of intact axons |

events may be viewed as the organic hardware of the learning process. The past two decades have witnessed explosive growth in our knowledge of these hardware components. Some of the milestones are reviewed in the section on memory.

A theoretical understanding of the *software* of the learning system, however, has been more elusive. We lack a general-purpose set of laws and relationships to account for all the cognitive programs, routines, procedures, and strategies, which, in sum, would comprise an all-embracing learning theory. We necessarily lack as well grand theories of cognitive instruction and remediation.[57,58] Nevertheless, many principles of learning and of remediation have emerged empirically and have generally proven useful for purposes of cognitive instruction. (Included in the general category of "cognitive instruction" are training techniques explicitly intended to improve memory functions, attentional processes, and reasoning, problem-solving, and other executive functions). Many approaches have been taken in the development of cognitive remediation curricula. One approach was to borrow and modify psychological and neuropsychological tests such as those used in the laboratory for investigational purposes and to convert them into therapeutic tools. Thus, the continuous processing test, originally developed to *assess* attentional capacity, was recently adopted for the *treatment* of patients with attention deficits. A second approach has been to teach patients the cognitive strategies that (it is believed) unimpaired persons utilize naturally and without special instruction. For example, patients with frontal lobe injury are trained to use explicit goal-setting and self-monitoring procedures and are taught to balance divergent and convergent thinking when faced with novel tasks and problems. The underlying assumption is that the sequential components that, covertly, comprise executive functioning in neurologically intact persons can be identified and made explicit and overt for purposes of remediation. A third avenue of curriculum development has been to borrow techniques used in the training of exceptional cognitive skills, again in unimpaired persons, and to adapt this training for remediational programs. Teaching specialized mnemonic strategies is an example of this last approach. In short, theories of cognition and of learning, as incomplete and open-ended as they may be at present, have contributed in important

ways to the theory and practice of cognitive remediation. Some of the most significant of these contributions are discussed below.

## Behavioristic and Cognitive Frames of Reference

Historically, behavioristic and cognitive formulations of learning theory have represented opposite conceptual poles. The relevant questions in the behaviorist framework are the environmental antecedents to behavior, the overt behavior itself, and the consequences, or reinforcement characteristics, of that behavior. For purposes of instruction or remediation, the behaviorist approach suggests that the message or task to be learned be broken down into clear, concrete steps and that the results (success or failure in learning) be immediately and accurately conveyed to the patient. Through a sequence of small steps and successive approximations (*shaping*) the patient eventually attains the learning objective or other target behavior. In its most radical form behaviorism contends that learning processes can be understood without recourse to internal or cognitive explanations. This viewpoint dominated American psychology in the first half of this century.

Since midcentury, however, with advances in cybernetics and with the parallel development of theories on information processing, interest in human cognition has grown enormously. The cognitive frame of reference concerns the flow of information in the central nervous system. Attentional and memory capacities are examined as minutely as possible. Treatment emphasizes training of planning, conceptualizing, and attentiveness skills and instruction in the application of internal mediators such as private speech, inner dialogues, and visual imagery.

Also clustered at the cognitive pole are other nonbehavioristic approaches, most notably the Piagetian school of structuralist psychology. Piaget and his followers argue that intellectual development in childhood has distinct stages; each stage is characterized by constraints on learning capability that are dependent on the degree of CNS maturity; these constraints are biologically based and are not breachable by any environmental manipulation. The central issues in the structuralist approach to cognition revolve around these constraints. Instruction and remediation therapy must be adjusted to accommodate them.

Despite the historical conflict between behavioristic and cognitive schools of thought, clinical experience confirms that both contribute to construction of effective models of remediation.[57] In recent decades the accumulating clinical evidence tends to justify the inclusion of principles from both explanatory spheres when treating persons with attention deficits or memory and executive function disorder. Cognitive behavioral therapy is an excellent example of an eclectic approach of this sort.[59] Developed by Meichenbaum, Kendall and Braswell, and others primarily for the management of attention deficit disorder and impulsiveness in children, cognitive behavioral therapy simply draws from both behaviorist and cognitive models.[60,61] In this form of therapy self-regulatory speech is targeted for treatment. Impulsive children are taught to utilize internal dialogue, that is, covert private speech, in order to modify their outward behavior.[61p.1]

## Visual and Auditory Aspects of Learning

To a large extent, learning is modally specific. Thus, some neuronal structures serve exclusively as visual analyzers, others respond exclusively to auditory input, and others register only somesthetic signals. In this section we deal with visual and auditory perceptual learning and with the cerebral basis for modal exclusivity. In what ways can visual registration and retention of information, for example, be distinguished from auditory registration and retention of information; and to what extent can we identify the regions of the brain responsible for each? In investigating these questions, the influential writings of Soviet neuropsychologist Aleksandr Luria will be a superb guide. In *The Working Brain,* Luria outlined a hierarchical approach to the understanding of human learning, memory, executive function, and other mental capacities.[62] Comprehended most broadly, human mental processes are divided by Luria into three major functional units: ''a unit for regulating tone or waking (corresponding anatomically to the ascending reticular activating system); a unit for obtaining, processing, and storing information arriving from the outside world (corresponding

anatomically to the occipital, temporal, and parietal cortices); and a unit for programming, regulating, and verifying mental activity (corresponding anatomically to the prefrontal cortex).'' Luria emphasizes that these units function together, not independently. In conscious mental activity especially, ''Man's mental processes . . . always take place with the participation of all three units, each of which has its role to play.''[62p.43] These three functional units are dealt with more fully when executive functions, attentional processes, and memory are addressed as distinct cognitive operations. For discussion of modality-specific aspects of learning, however, Luria's second functional unit (responsible for ''obtaining, processing, and storing information arriving from the outside world'') is of primary importance.

Luria writes that all of the basic units are themselves ''hierarchical in structure and (consist) of at least three cortical zones, built one above the other: the primary (projection) area, which receives impulses from or sends impulses to the periphery, the secondary (projection-association), where incoming information is processed or programs are prepared, and finally, the tertiary (zones of overlapping), the latest systems of the cerebral hemispheres to develop and responsible in man for the most complex forms of mental activity requiring the concerted participation of many cortical areas.''[62p.43]

### Feature Analyzers of the Visual Pathway

Portions of the primary (projection) visual cortex have been mapped in detail by Hubel and Wiesel, who in 1981 were awarded the Nobel Prize for their work. Their studies were based on earlier investigations by Kuffler,[63] whose pioneering microelectrode studies demonstrated that the nervous system is predisposed to register even the simplest visual sensations with a high degree of bias. It was his work that identified a sound physiologic basis for brightness contrast bias in the visual system.

Utilizing microelectrodes to record the firing patterns of single ganglion cells in the cat's retina, Kuffler noted the existence of tiny retinal fields, each consisting of several retinal ganglion cells. Typically, each retinal field was divided into two zones, a central circular area and a surrounding ringlike (annular) area. A bias to register only contrasts in brightness comes about because the two zones are antagonistic to each other. Where central zones are excitatory, annular zones are inhibitory, and vice versa. Thus, diffuse light is ineffective as a stimulus: though it causes the excitatory zone cells to discharge, inhibitory cells discharge at the same time. The excitatory effect is canceled by the inhibitory cells; there is no *net* discharge from the retinal field. Compare this result with the effect of a contrast in brightness. If a spot of light with a brightness boundary exactly fills the excitatory zone and does not encroach on the inhibitory zone, net firing from the retinal field is maximal. A net excitatory effect of intermediate degree can be expected when there is modest encroachment on the inhibitory zone and substantial filling of the excitatory zone. In summary, the retinal system declines to register external stimuli impartially and accepts (and in fact enhances) only contrasts in brightness.

Bringing the study of the visual perceptual system to structures deep within the brain, Hubel and Wiesel found this same tendency toward feature enhancement in cells of the lateral geniculate bodies and cells of the striate (visual) cortex (Brodmann's area 17). Using microelectrode techniques and recording the activity of individual neurons of the lateral geniculate bodies, and of cortical layer IV (the first cortical relay station for the visual system) Hubel and Wiesel noted that these neurons were supplied by retinal fields almost indistinguishable from the retinal fields serving retinal ganglion cells. Cortical cells outside of layer IV, and farther along the pathway of visual analysis, behaved differently, however, and could be divided into three types: *simple, complex,* and *hypercomplex.*

Simple cortical cells responded most energetically to *bars* of light located at specific positions in the retinal field. Complex cells appeared to be subject to the converging influences of several simple cells. Complex cells therefore surveyed more broadly than simple cells and responded to *all* bars of light, regardless of their position within the retinal field. Hypercomplex cells, in turn, combined the information supplied to them by several complex cells, and appeared to be able to read more narrowly specified patterns than complex cells could—corners, for example, and bars of specific length and width.[64–66]

The cells of the primary visual receptive cortex,

Brodmann's area 17, thus respond selectively to elementary visual forms and patterns, albeit with varying degrees of complexity. Electrical stimulation of area 17 produces elementary visual hallucinations—"flashes of light, tongues of flame and colored spots."[62p.114] Representations of complete visual images, on the other hand, apparently depend on the immediately adjacent peristriate cortex, Brodmann's areas 18 and 19.[62p.115] Electrical stimulation there produces hallucinations of complete images (flowers, animals, familiar faces), and lesions of these zones produce visual agnosia wherein the patient perceives the elementary patterns but cannot make sense of them.[62p.116]

The anatomic basis for this arrangement can partly be understood by application of Flechsig's rule,[67] which states that the primary sensory cortical areas (including the primary visual cortex) make *no distant connections whatsoever* but rather send all of their intercortical efferents to the immediately contiguous perisensory regions. Thus, the primary visual cortex has no direct communication with cortical areas subserving other modalities (e.g., audition, somatic sensation) and has no interhemispheric connections. The perisensory cortex, on the other hand, has *extensive connections with distant cortical regions,* including an abundance of callosal connections with the opposite hemisphere. These far-ranging connections excite the tertiary cortical zones, with their integrating, generalizing, and symbol-forming functions. The tertiary zones permit intermodal and abstract analysis of perceptual information and establish as well the anatomic basis for a degree of lateralization of that analysis.[62p.78] Two major organizing principles of the human cerebral cortex thus emerge: the principle of increasing abstraction as analysis proceeds and the principle of increasing lateralization of function.[68] The learning of visual shape discrimination, for example, appears to be dependent on tertiary zone TE, comprising the middle and inferior temporal gyri.[62p.76] Spatial vision, including the ability to know and remember an object's location relative to other locations and the general ability to form mental maps, depends on another tertiary region, the posterior parietal cortex.[69] The perceptual analysis of facial features, particularly the emotional connotations of those features, is overwhelmingly a right hemispheric function.[62p.149]

In principle, we can try to account for all of

visual perception on the basis of serial processing of this sort, with progressive integration of information as the data are channeled from station to station.[70] Thus, we can imagine a hierarchical information flow, from the hypercomplex cells of the primary visual cortex, to cells within secondary cortex, and thence to definitive analysis in the tertiary cortical areas, where hypothetical cells are capable of surveying, registering, and combining the enormous data array of a single visual percept. Such a hypothetical construct, however, must be rejected as extraordinarily unlikely. It would require us to assume that there are separate cells capable of responding selectively to each and every pattern of the myriad patterns that are part of our visual universe. There are not enough neurons in the visual network for such an arrangement to be possible. It is far more reasonable to postulate that each visual percept requires a vast amount of *parallel processing* simultaneous with the serial or convergence processing already outlined. And there is evidence that such elementary features as color, movement, depth, and other aspects of the visual scene are processed in parallel, utilizing separate information channels.[70]

### Feature Analyzers of the Auditory Pathway

The neurons of the primary auditory cortex (Brodmann's area 41), located on the supratemporal plane, deep within the sylvian fissure[71] are excited only by particular acoustic signals such as tone bursts of specific frequency. There is evidence that neurons of the medial sectors of area 41 register high tones and that lateral neurons respond to low-frequency tones.[62pp.131–132] With this limited range of response, individual cells of the primary auditory cortex resemble counterpart cells of the primary visual cortex. As we follow the auditory signals centrally, we find additional similarities between the two systems. There is a hierarchical arrangement between auditory zones: the secondary auditory cortex, located on the temporal convexity (and thus inferior to the primary cortex), synthesizes the raw and segregated acoustic information arriving from area 41 into sound combinations of various sorts. There is increasing lateralization of brain function as signals are processed more and more centrally, particularly at the point where signals pass from the primary to the sec-

ondary zones.[62pp.77,132–137] Functional distinctions cannot be made between right and left *primary* cortices, but there is separation of function for the *secondary* auditory cortices; only one of the secondary cortices is specialized for the analysis of speech sounds (usually the left).[62pp.132–137] When the specialized cortex of children younger than 8 to 10 years is damaged, they are able to develop excellent speech-analyzing capability in the undamaged contralateral hemisphere. If the damage occurs in the adult years, however, the potential to train the spared hemisphere to carry out speech analysis has been lost.[72]

The tertiary auditory cortex, posterior to the left secondary auditory cortex near the boundary between temporal and occipital lobes, can be divided into frontotemporal, posterior temporal, and other overlapping regions.[62p.73] "The cardinal symptoms of . . . lesions (of the posterior left temporal zone) is disturbance both of the nominative function of speech (the naming of objects) and of the ability to evoke visual images in response to a given word. This is manifested not only by great difficulty in finding the meaning of a given word (which this time is based not so much on a disturbance of phonemic hearing as on a disturbance of the link between the cortical zones of the auditory and visual analyzers), but also as gross inability to draw a picture of an object named although the patient is still perfectly capable of copying."[62p.145] The tertiary auditory cortex is concerned with a more abstract level of analysis than is the secondary auditory cortex. The left posterior temporal zone is concerned with semantics, with the symbolic connotations of words (i.e., of phonemic combinations), whereas the left secondary cortex focuses on acoustic content, on the differentiation of one phoneme from another, without regard to semantic associations.

There is substantial crossing of fibers along the course of the auditory pathways at relay ganglia in the brain stem (the cochlear and olivary nuclei) and in the midbrain (inferior colliculi), so that each temporal region receives input from both ears.[71p.59] In both right and left temporal cortices, however, the contralateral ear is more strongly represented than the ipsilateral one. It is thus possible, by means of dichotic listening experiments, to find one hemisphere or the other to be dominant for selected types of acoustic input. A right ear advantage has been demonstrated for many kinds of verbal material, such as consonant-vowel combinations and single words and phrases; left ear advantages have been reported for recall of melody, for environmental sounds, and, intriguingly, also for interpretation of emotional tone in speech.[73]

## A Sampling of Treatment Methods for Remediation of Perceptual Disorders

There are two general methods of managing disorders of visual and auditory perception: (1) approaches that are fundamentally compensatory and seek to bypass the perceptual impairment and (2) approaches that are remediational and attempt to treat the perceptual disorder directly. In the following illustrative example a school-aged child discussed by Gaddes[71p.170] was managed with compensatory techniques in the classroom, but only after his cognitive profile and his aptitudes had been clarified:

Sam developed meningitis at age 6 weeks and had onset of a seizure disorder with the focus in the left cerebral hemisphere. At age 12 years, when first seen for neuropsychological evaluation, he had poor academic performance, deficient verbal abilities, and had been placed in a slow learner's class since starting school. On the Wechsler Intelligence Scale for Children (WISC) assessment Sam's verbal abilities were below average (verbal IQ score 87), but he did quite well on the performance part of the WISC (performance IQ 110) and his score on the block design subtest was very superior. Gaddes concluded, "Sam was a classic example of left hemisphere dysfunction, with his poor verbal skills and his strong right-hemisphere (spatial-constructional) abilities." The neuropsychological report emphasized Sam's superior spatial abilities and predicted a high level of achievement in subjects such as geometry, map reading in geography, and interpretation of mechanical drawings and blueprints, and urged that he be placed in a regular class. It was recommended that he receive daily remedial drill in reading and spelling. He was transferred to a regular class. As the phonemic analyzers of the left temporal cortex were most likely damaged, efforts to teach him reading and spelling by phonics were discontinued. Instead, because of his aptitude for visuospatial analysis, a largely compensatory approach was attempted, emphasizing visual and motor techniques. With this change of classroom and instructional method Sam made astonishing progress. The following year psychometric testing reported his performance IQ on the WISC to be 132 (99th percentile), and his feelings of inferiority had started to abate. With

a compensatory approach for the remainder of his school years, Sam himself was able to choose an "occupational program" (drafting, mechanics and industrial arts), from the ninth grade on, and after graduation he took an automechanics apprenticeship.

Sam's progress was primarily in those areas where he had already shown superior ability on neuropsychological assessment; his language skills remained extremely delayed on all follow-up evaluations. As Gaddes observes, children with left hemisphere dysfunction are likely to be treated unfairly in contemporary educational systems, where special emphasis is placed on verbal skills and right hemispheric talents such as drawing, construction, and map design and blueprint comprehension are largely ignored.

Evidence from laboratory studies of perceptual learning support the need for a "multisensory" or "intersensory" training model for remediation of perceptual deficits, such as that advocated by Ayres and utilized by many occupational therapists. Two landmark studies will be cited here:

(1) Normal humans have an extraordinary capacity to adapt to distorting perceptual input and reinterpret it to cancel out the distortion. Almost a century ago, Stratton[73] reported that when he wore lenses that prevented inversion of the retinal image he found visually guided behavior of all sorts to be extremely difficult at first. Yet after several days he had accommodated and was able to walk about, reach and grasp, and engage in other types of visually directed activity. This implied that the mature intact CNS was capable of a high degree of perceptual learning involving multisensory integration. That is, input from kinesthetic, proprioceptive, vestibular, and perhaps other channels must have participated in crucial ways to permit the visual perceptual learning that occurred.[71p.131]

In 1960, Held and Hein demonstrated that visual perceptual learning does not occur unless the learning experience includes at the same time both visual input and self-produced movement. In one experiment they raised kittens in a dark room for 21 hours of each 24-hour period. For the remaining 3 hours of the day, half the kittens had an opportunity to see and walk at the same time in a well-lit cylindrical room on the walls of which vertical stripes were clearly demarcated. The other kittens also spent those 3 hours in the bright cylindrical room, but they were kept in snug boxes, conveyable, and tethered to the active kittens. As the active kittens walked and viewed the striped wall, they dragged along the passive kittens, who thus had no opportunity to walk in the lighted room but who were exposed to almost identical visual input. The active kittens developed good eye-paw coordination and good paw-protective responses, but the passive kittens, deprived of self-produced movement, did not. The protective responses of the passive kittens were poor, and they would often fail to avoid visual cliffs.[74]

Ayres and Kephart interpreted these findings to support their contention that visual-perceptual learning benefits much from a multimodal and sensory integrative approach (including motor training). The effectiveness of multisensorimotor treatment programs for purposes of remediation of perceptual deficits remains a subject of considerable controversy.[75–77]

Some years ago, Weinberg and colleagues in a controlled trial demonstrated the effectiveness of a perceptual retraining program for patients with right hemispheric damage due to cerebrovascular accident.[78] The objectives of remediation were to improve visual scanning and reading skills and to increase sensory awareness and spatial organization in 30 right brain–damaged persons, who, characteristically, showed some degree of neglect of left visual space. Patients in both the experimental and control groups were continued on conventional therapy programs, but the experimental group received 20 hours' special perceptual training in addition. Perceptual training included target tracking, size estimation, and searching for lights over the visual field. The method used to train sensory awareness is of special interest: "A mannequin was designed to replicate the upper back portion of a human torso. . . . It was studded with 12 lights . . . placed 5 cm to 10 cm apart on three distinct horizontal levels with four lights on each level. The activation of these lights was controlled by the examiner using a separate (set of) switches." The patient faced the mannequin during training and wore a jacket, with locations on the back of the jacket that corresponded to the locations of the studded lights on the mannequin. There was a highly systematic training protocol with operant conditioning components. The patient was asked to indicate on the mannequin when the

corresponding spot on his back was touched by the examiner. *Immediate and accurate reinforcement* (knowledge of success or failure) was provided: if the response was correct, the appropriate light flickered on and off; if the response was incorrect, the light remained on. The training was divided into eight *sequential stages,* starting with relatively easy-to-identify locations and proceeding to more randomized and difficult locations. At each stage, the identification task began on the unimpaired side and proceeded to the impaired side. Thus, correct responses were highly likely at the beginning of the program and at the beginning of each stage. Step by step, the patient developed sensory awareness for successively more difficult locations. With this specialized training there was significant improvement in the experimental group, as compared with the controls, for several visual and nonvisual perceptual parameters.

## The Executive Functions

Cognition, in the broadest sense, refers to our general capacity for knowledge, but understood more concretely, it comprises the set of mental functions that permit registration, channeling, storage, and retrieval of information (Luria's second functional unit). As such, cognition should be viewed as a fundamentally *subordinate* activity, always under the control of the executive functions (Luria's highest functional unit), which set goals and directions. Thus, in intact persons cognitive processes never act without purpose or plan, but at all times are under the governance of executive processes.[62p.83] According to this hierarchical concept, the executive functions, through their planning, regulating, monitoring, and verifying aspects, always participate in conscious mental activities in concert with cognition, making their particular organizing and governing contributions.

The prefrontal cortex, together with its extensive intercortical and subcortical connections, appears to provide the neuronal substrate essential for these superordinate executive activities. The executive processes cannot be precisely anatomic,[79] but some very general conclusions appear reasonable.[79p.221] With destruction of the frontal lobes behavior is disinhibited. Luria observes, "The normal animal always aims at a certain goal, inhibiting its response to irrelevant, unimportant stimuli; the dog with destroyed frontal lobes, on the other hand, responds to all irrelevant stimuli . . . distractions by these unimportant elements of the environment disturb the plans and programs of its behavior, making it fragmentary and uncontrolled.[62p.89]

While removal of the frontal lobes thus leads to a profound disturbance of attention, it would be erroneous to conclude that all aspects of attention are equally disrupted. Attentional processes can be subdivided into voluntary (or effortful) forms and involuntary (or effortless, passive) forms.[80] Patients with frontal lobe damage have *only the voluntary type of attention impaired,* especially the attentional forms that are activated with the aid of language. Involuntary attentional processes "not only remain intact, but may actually be enhanced" in the presence of irrelevant stimuli.[62p.197]

"Involuntary" attentional processes include those that control the multitude of automatic and nearly automatic activities we engage in from moment to moment, the routine programs that trigger specific overlearned actions or skills "such as drinking from a container, doing long division, making breakfast, or finding one's way home from work.[81] These more or less automatic activities do not require continuous monitoring or overtly conscious attention. We attend to them, but peripherally and almost effortlessly. Because many such automatic programs exist, however, and because they can be activated by totally independent triggering mechanisms, there must be a selection process to prevent overloading of our limited cognitive and effector resources.

Norman and Shallice have proposed that two selective attention systems exist.[81] One, conscious and supervisory, is reserved for activities that are not routine and require a high level of mental efforts (e.g. reasoning, concentration, weighing of evidence). This is the *supervisory attentional system* (SAS). The second selection system, called *contention scheduling,* and operative when not overruled by the SAS, allocates attentional resources between the competing routine programs in a "crude but fast" manner. Automatic perceptual, emotional, or cognitive triggers determine which routines are put into operation at any one time, and these are played out until their goals are reached (if the SAS does not intervene).

With specific disruption of the SAS, this model predicts that routine tasks would still be performed in a satisfactory manner but that novel tasks that require initiative and planning would suffer. In particular, the ability to inhibit the effects of the contention-scheduling system and its automatic triggering function would be impaired. Thus, many of the characteristics of frontal lobe dysfunction, including adynamia, disorders of planning, and disinhibition, can be seen and explained in the context of this two-tiered theory of selective attention.

Disinhibition, the most striking of these impairments, appears to be localized in the prefrontal cortex, specifically the lateral, dorsolateral, and lateral-orbital surfaces of the frontal lobes. Patients with *lateral* frontal lobe lesions are described as "restless, hyperkinetic, explosive and impulsive" whereas patients with *medial* frontal lobe damage are "slow, lethargic, and apathetic," lacking initiative and spontaneity.[79p.224] Deficits of the latter type can be subsumed under the broader categories of impairment of drive, motivation, and will, and the adynamia often seen after traumatic brain injury is attributed primarily to medial prefrontal damage. The lateral frontal syndrome includes disinhibition, as suggested above, but also appears to encompass related dysfunctions, including impaired ability to integrate behavior in a planned and sequential manner.

## Procedural and Declarative Knowledge

Contemporary learning theory distinguishes between procedural and declarative forms of knowledge.[82,83] The acquisition of procedural knowledge—learning of skills and conditioned habits—is largely unconscious. The knowledge gained is accessible only through performance.[82] Declarative knowledge, on the other hand, is "explicit and accessible to conscious awareness."[83] Its acquisition results in the storage of all the factual and conceptual (or *semantic*) knowledge and all the autobiographical (or *episodic*) knowledge gained through experience and study. Nonverbal mental contents (e.g., visual images), if retrievable from memory and accessible to consciousness, are also included within declarative knowledge. As declarative knowledge includes all retrievable autobiographic information, it "permits the storage of information as single events that happened in particular times and places, . . . (affording) a sense of familiarity about previous events."[84p.162]

The learning processes utilized for declarative knowledge and for procedural knowledge are distinct but are dynamically linked.[58] Declarative knowledge, explicit and conscious, rapidly connects with vast stores of related information, including well-established and automatic procedural programs. When faced with the task of learning a new skill (for example, learning to drive a standard shift automobile), the novice first acquires information about the skill in a declarative form. Thus, he or she gains factual knowledge about the relationship of clutch and gearshift before beginning to acquire "knowledge-how" procedures for clutch and gearshift control. In this early stage, "the learner acquires an initial, often verbal, characterization of the skill, which is sufficient to generate the desired behavior to at least some crude approximation. In this stage it is common to observe verbal mediation, in which the learner (consciously) rehearses the information required to execute the skill."[58] It is possible to bypass the declarative stage and train automatic procedures directly, for example through operant conditioning techniques, but this is a relatively slow process. Learning is greatly speeded by starting with the declarative stage. Declarative knowledge permits analogous reasoning, cause-and-effect thinking, and similarity-difference analysis. Through these processes the learner gains rapid access to potentially useful procedures, retained by virtue of previous experience. Sometimes new tasks have very familiar elements, and our declarative knowledge network helps us recognize the areas of familiarity. In such cases, as we try to master the new task, we may be able to call upon rather specific procedures already stored in memory that are appropriate to the familiar components. Even when the task at hand is unfamiliar, we are likely to proceed first with conscious declarative learning. Through our declarative knowledge base we are able to categorize and analyze, at least to some degree, even the most novel tasks, and we may choose to summon and employ stored procedures useful for general problem-solving purposes.

As our procedural and declarative knowledge bases increase, at least two patterns of learning

seem to be operative. Trial-and-error learning (operant conditioning) is primarily involved with the fine tuning and progressive automatization of skills; thus, while trial-and-error techniques may affect the growth of declarative knowledge, this learning mode is more readily associated with the elaboration of unconscious procedures. As described in traditional operant conditioning theory, skilled procedures are learned because correct responses are rewarded and incorrect responses are not. Learning occurs in a stepwise fashion, and the optimal skill level is attained through a series of successive approximations. A second major mode of learning, however, does not occur in a step-by-step process but seems rather to involve leaps of insight and reconceptualization of the task.[85] Reconceptualization appears to involve a sudden change in the structure of our knowledge base. Conscious declarative knowledge, both the verbal propositional type and the imagery-based perceptual type, is critically affected and advanced by insightful learning. Typically, the moment of reconceptualization is preceded by a stage of confusion, a period in which there has been no improvement, or even a decrement, in performance. When a task or problem can be effectively reconceptualized, a discontinuity in the learning curve will be the likely result, and an abrupt advance to a new and higher level of performance can be expected. Although sudden reconceptualizations are infrequent during knowledge acquisition, they must nevertheless be considered fundamental (if inadequately understood) characteristics of human learning.

## Procedural Knowledge, Declarative Knowledge and Remediation of the Executive Functions

When the CNS is intact, knowledge bases grow by virtue of a balance between declarative learning and procedural learning. In remediation of the patient with a damaged CNS it is desirable to establish a similar balance, wherever possible. In certain clinical circumstances, such as dense amnesia, a balanced approach is extremely difficult to achieve; nevertheless, it often is possible to give substantial remedial attention to both declarative and procedural learning. The cognitive cycle model of Gross and Schutz[114] is an example. These authors propose a cognitive cycle consisting of a set of five specific cognitive operations, considered to comprise the basic components of executive mental functioning: (1) goal setting; (2) prediction of the conditions under which goal satisfaction might occur; (3) preparation of a plan of action; (4) initiation of the planned action, and, (5) feedback, which can be viewed as the observation of: (*i*) the consequences of the action, and (*ii*) the degree of match of consequences to both goals and predictions. In goal setting, the first-operation goals are accessible to consciousness and retrievable from declarative knowledge stores; in the other four operations, an interplay between declarative and procedural knowledge is essential. Operations 2 and 3 utilize declarative memory of causal relationships (if *x* happens, *y* will result) so that alternative action procedures that might realize the goal can be summoned and prepared. When the situation is judged to be appropriate, operation 4, the planned action, automatic and part of the procedural knowledge base, is put into effect. Operation 5, feedback, allows reconceptualization of goals and modification or correction, as necessary, of the if-then assumptions utilized in operation 2. Thus, with operation 5 we are cycled back to operations 1 and 2, albeit in modified forms.

For the patient with traumatic diffuse or anterior brain injury, one or several of these five cognitive operations are likely to be impaired. The Gross-Schutz model, as well as other similar conceptualizations (see, for example, the formulation suggested by Ben-Yishai and colleagues),[87] allows the therapist to separate out fundamental subcomponents of the executive functions and focus attention selectively and systematically on the individual segments of the cycle. As this model is employed in rehabilitation practice, a large part of the therapeutic effort is directed toward increasing patients' *metacognition*—that is, toward increasing their awareness of their own cognitive processes. Thus, they are taught the five operations of the cycle and are encouraged to refer to them and review each in turn when dealing with novel or problematic situations. The chief virtue of a metacognitive approach is its generalizability. Patients who understand their cognitive processes and strengths and weaknesses can, if they are sufficiently practiced, apply general cognitive strategies to a wide variety of situations. Metacognition, and methods for teaching the elements of problem solving and organizational skills, are described further in the section on management of attention disorders.

## Attentional Processes: The Principal Brain Loci

*Attention* refers to a broad spectrum of processes that affect cognition and executive functioning at all levels. The term refers both to a *general* state of arousal and to the process of focusing on *specific* stimuli. When applied to specific stimuli, attention denotes integration of sensory features into a coherent percept, the focusing of an attentional spotlight. The term also implies *selectivity,* the ability to ignore irrelevant information and to shift processing resources rapidly from one object to another. Another dimension is *endurance,* or the capacity to sustain attention toward a single task over time.

The mesencephalic reticular formation (MRF) is associated with *nonselective* aspects of attention, especially wakefulness and general arousal, such as that seen in the orientation response.[62pp.54–56] It has been shown that stimulation of the MRF leads to generalized and pronounced facilitation of all sensory cortical evoked potentials, confirming the nonselective nature of MRF arousal.[62p.46] The neuroanatomic basis of *selective* attention has not been clearly established, but speculation has recently centered on the reticular nucleus of the thalamus, a thin but extensive sheet of neurons that lies between the cortex and the thalamus proper.[88,89] Stimulation of this nucleus selectively and profoundly attenuates cortical evoked responses and localized thalamic transmission of afferent signals. The prefrontal cortex (see earlier section on the executive functions) exercises highly selective regulation over the thalamic reticular nucleus, and it is suggested that this sheet of neurons, under prefrontal control, might serve as a thalamic gatekeeper or filter.[88,89]

Alternating attention, or the capability to shift attention rapidly from one point of focus to another, a function of the right parietal cortex, is often impaired in patients with traumatic brain injury. Patients with severe right parietal cortical damage, with signs of left visual field neglect, ordinarily fail to respond to visual stimuli presented in the left visual field. Yet these patients are reportedly able to attend to left visual stimuli if there has been no right visual field input in the moments immediately prior to the left visual field stimulation. The interesting possibility is that left visual field neglect in patients with right parietal damage may in large part be due to the inability to shift spatial attention.[90]

## The Management of Attentional Disorders: A Sampling of Remediational Approaches

In their process-specific approach to attentional remediation Sohlberg and Mateer pay due regard to this very broad and multidimensional spectrum.[91] Their treatment model deals with attentiveness and attention disturbances under five headings: (1) *focused* attention, "the ability to respond discretely to specific visual, auditory, or tactile stimuli"; (2) *sustained* attention, "the ability to maintain a consistent behavioral response during continuous and repetitive activity"; (3) *selective* attention, "the ability to maintain a behavioral or cognitive set in the face of distracting or competing stimuli", (4) *alternating* attention, "the capacity for mental flexibility that allows individuals to shift their focus of attention and move between tasks having different cognitive requirements, thus controlling which information will be selectively attended to"; and (5) *divided* attention, "the ability to respond simultaneously to multiple tasks or multiple task demands."

Many of the specific treatment techniques for the remediation of these five forms of attention disturbance can be viewed as *forced usage,* that is, the *direct practice* of identified neuropsychological deficits: "Forced usage of an impaired behavior is the most straightforward way to approach cognitive rehabilitation. One simply collects baseline neuropsychological data, identifies the major cognitive deficits to be addressed, and asks the patient to practice the lost skill."[90p.255] In the process-specific approach, a large set of forced usage attentional training tasks has been developed and grouped by attention category. Sustained auditory attention is trained through a series of exercises that require the patient to listen for target items (letters or numbers or words) presented by audiotape. The targets are mixed with nontarget items. When patients hear the targets they are required to respond consistently (by pressing a buzzer). At the simplest level, a patient might be told to press a buzzer every time he or she hears the number 4 in a series such as 6, 4, 1, 4, 4, 2, 7. Another exercise, the Big-Little task, has been developed for the training of alternating visual attention: when presented with a written series such as BIG, little, LITTLE, big, BIG, LITTLE, big, little, big . . . the patient might first be asked to read the series as words (ignoring the size of the letters) and then asked to switch attention set and state the size of the letters in each word (now ignoring the meaning of the written words).[91pp. 122,125;92]

The Orientation Remediation Module (ORM), developed by Ben-Yishai and colleagues, also involves a forced usage approach to the remediation of attention deficits. Patients with severe head injury and consequent disturbances of basic arousal are taken through a series of exercises of steadily increasing attention demand. The five component tasks of the ORM are primarily targeted on arousal and vigilance aspects of attentional dysfunction. Several of the tasks require the patient to practice vigilance and concentration skills such as environmental scanning (for particular visual signals), time estimation, and the speeding of reaction time. The most demanding ORM task requires the patient to synchronize the pressing of a telegraph key with a complex auditory signal (a variety of Morse code–like rhythms). The authors have found that ORM training results in (1) stable, persisting improvement in the specific ORM tasks themselves, and (2) higher scores on those psychometric tests that have important attentional components; in addition, improvements in daily functioning are often seen. A highly disoriented 27-year-old patient who sustained severe traumatic brain injury 21 months before systematic training on the ORM provides a good example. At the outset of the training the patient had very severe attention disorders. He was taken through the ORM program 2 hours a day over a period of 3 months. Posttraining assessment showed significantly improved orientation to his environment and high levels of alertness and reflectiveness generally, which enabled him to "become a pupil again," able to assimilate new information relevant to his rehabilitation needs.[93,94]

Instruction in the use of verbal mediators and private speech is a different approach to attentional remediation and serves, in essence, as a method to train control of the SAS (see page 610). Much recent work in the treatment of impulsive, nonreflective behavior patterns in children with attention deficit disorder has involved teaching the conscious use of internal dialogue (*private speech*). The children are trained to cue themselves, monitor their own behavior, and reinforce positive (more reflective) behavior by means of internal, covert verbal mediators. Initially, they are taught to voice the verbal mediators aloud. Once overt expression is learned, the children are instructed to "fade" to a barely audible level, and then, finally, to engage in the same self-talk subvocally and covertly. Impulsive children are viewed as having "metacognitive deficits" (i.e., insufficiently developed strategies for dealing with novel problems or new learning) and are thought to need verbal mediation training to supply them with metacognitive strategies that develop naturally in normal (i.e., reflective) children.[59]

Training in the use of verbal mediation and private speech is essentially a method for teaching control of the SAS, so this approach has application in the remediation of disinhibition subtypes of frontal lobe impairment. Verbal mediation training can be directly linked, for example, to the cognitive cycle model,[86] and it is discussed in the section on remediation of executive function disorders. Let us assume that the task before the patient is the preparation of a breakfast of pancakes. Verbal mediators that refer to problem-solving strategy in a general way (metacognitive strategy) can be taught, and also verbal mediators that pertain very specifically to the task at hand. If using the cognitive cycle model, the patient will be instructed to ask himself several questions in sequence, of the following sort: What is my goal? What methods are available to achieve the goal? Am I monitoring the results? Are the results turning out as anticipated? Am I remembering to consult memory retrieval aids (such as lists—prepared earlier—of the steps that need to be taken)? Am I complimenting myself on successful completion of each step? Am I using errors to self-correct? Am I complimenting myself for monitoring errors successfully and for self-correcting? Task-specific private dialogue would include questions that relate to the actual implements needed for pancake preparation and the separate egg-beating, batter-mixing, and cooking protocol. There is really nothing artificial about any of these questions; they are used by anyone who attempts to solve a problem. For the person with frontal lobe impairment, however, effective organization of tasks may depend on a training procedure in which the questions are made explicit.

Verbal mediation is most effectively taught in a highly systematic manner. The five-stage protocol described by Meichenbaum and Goodman[95] presents a carefully guided, step-by-step approach: (1) modeling by the instructor: the instructor verbalizes aloud, using the target verbal mediators, while performing the task; (2) transition to patient verbalization: the instructor verbalizes aloud while the patient performs the task; (3) patient self-instruction aloud: the patient verbalizes aloud while performing the task; (4) "fading" to internalized self-instruction: the patient verbalizes in a whisper while performing the task; and (5) private speech: the patient verbalizes self-instruction covertly while performing the task.

## Memory and Learning

Research into the nature of human memory has lent strong support to the view that memory is fundamentally *dichotomous* and consists of (1) *a nonconsolidated and labile short-term form of memory (STM),* associated with consciousness and attentiveness, and capable of holding approximately seven entries or "chunks" of information, and (2) *a relatively consolidated and robust long-term form of memory (LTM),* readily accessible to consciousness but not part of it, persisting despite long periods of inattention, and capable of holding vast stores of information. LTM appears to contain several subcompartments, some distinguished by ease of consolidation. Procedural memories, for example, are consolidated with much less difficulty than factual information, a distinction that can be exploited in the management of memory disorders, as we shall see presently. (Memory theory recognizes, as well, as third quasi-memory compartment, an extremely brief *sensory buffer* that momentarily holds rapidly fading visual and auditory impressions. These *iconic* and *echoic* traces disappear almost entirely within 1 or 2 seconds.)

STM, or "working memory," is the locus for consciously keeping track of all present items of interest, for employing strategies of learning, reasoning, and also strategies of retrieval from LTM.[96] STM can be illustrated by considering what happens when we look up an unfamiliar telephone number in a directory some distance from the telephone. We find the listing, and for a fraction of a second an iconic trace of much of the column of numbers occupies the sensory buffer. This trace quickly fades, but what is the fate of the seven numerical entries of primary interest? If these numbers have some unexpected significance, and can be readily associated with concepts already consolidated in LTM, they may join the older entries and themselves become consolidated as items in LTM. It is far more likely, though, that the fresh items will be placed in the labile short-term stores. As we approach the telephone, the seven numbers will not remain in the proper sequence for long unless we keep attending to them by rehearsing them or possibly by using more elaborate strategies. Attention can stray for a moment, and the numbers may be retained but if we are distracted by something pressing, even if only for several seconds, the seven entries will begin to decay.

What is the fate of the items in STM when rehearsal is prevented? A 1959 study by Peterson and Peterson convincingly established this boundary condition for STM, and since that time it has served as a major point of reference for memory theory.[97] The investigators showed subjects three consonants (a consonant trigram) and instructed them to retain it as long as possible. Rehearsal was prevented by requiring the subjects to attend to a distractor (counting) task immediately after seeing the trigram. Under these conditions decay of information was rapid. Recall was roughly 80% correct at 3 seconds, 40% correct at 6 seconds and 10% correct at 18 seconds. Thus, in the absence of attention, STM traces have become quite unreliable by 6 seconds and have all but disappeared by 20 seconds.

There appear to be separate neuronal systems for nonconsolidated memory and consolidated memory. In one study of memory consolidation, rats were trained to stay on a wooden platform to avoid a shock to the feet if they stepped down to an electrified metal floor beneath. Trained rats, when placed on the wooden platform the following day, avoid stepping down onto the metal floor. If the foot shock experience during training is followed within 1 or 2 seconds by electroconvulsive shock, rats do not avoid the metal floor on subsequent trials and will step down as quickly as untrained rats. But if the interval between training foot shock and electroconvulsive shock is longer, the training effect is retained and avoidance learning is successful—increasingly so with increasingly prolonged delays. These results suggest that two quite different neuronal systems support memory in these animals, a nonconsolidated neuronal network, vulnerable to total disruption by electroconvulsive shock, and a consolidated system, presumably relying on far more robust neuronal alterations, and relatively unsusceptible to electroconvulsive shock disruption.[98]

Clinical observations in humans point to the same division of memory. Retrograde amnesia, the loss of memory for events just preceding major head injury, appears to be at least partially based on disruption of a nonconsolidated memory (STM) system. After head injury, retrograde amnesia may extend back to events that occurred many years before the trauma. Often improvement occurs, and eventually the amnesia encompasses only events that occurred a few seconds to minutes before the injury. This ultimate and irreducible amnesia may reflect complete disappearance of memory traces from the preconsolidated system.

Evidence supportive of the dichotomous concept of memory was found in the clinical course of patient H.M., who, in 1953, aged 27, underwent bilateral medial temporal lobe resection for intractable and frequent grand mal seizures.[99] Resection included the uncus, amygdala, hippocampus, and hippocampal gyrus. After surgery, seizure frequency was very significantly reduced and many intellectual functions seemed to be preserved. I.Q. on the Wechsler Adult Intelligence Scale was above average before and after surgery. His STM was only slightly impaired. There was some retrograde amnesia for events in the 2-year period before surgery, but he demonstrated excellent ability to retrieve items from LTM stores. He did have severely disabling amnesia that took the form of nearly complete inability to register new information in LTM. He was unable to learn any new facts; there was almost no transformation of verbal or of visual information to a consolidated state. He would read a magazine article with interest but would be unable to report anything about the article after reading it. After carrying on a conversation, he would have no recollection of the experience. He was unable to recognize close family friends or neighbors if he did not know them before surgery. H.M. was able to learn certain motor tasks, even complex ones (such as mirror writing) and also showed some perceptual learning ability (improved recognition of incomplete pictures after practice), though he had no recollection of the practice sessions themselves.[100] Because of his intact STM and normal access to preoperatively encoded LTM stores, language comprehension was unimpaired. He was sociable and at ease in conversation and able to get the point of conversational subtleties and jokes.[99]

Some forms of conscious learning, including much of verbal and visual learning, seem to require an initial period of rumination in the labile or nonconsolidated store before the information can be transferred to LTM. H.M.'s amnesia, and the memory characteristics of patients with similar histories, point to the hippocampus and related structures (including the amygdala and medial diencephalon) as being essential for this information transfer. Some learning, however, appears to proceed without conscious effort and without a need for transfer from STM to LTM. Most types of motor learning seem to bypass STM and enter LTM directly, presumably without the need for hippocampal involvement. Likewise, the two principal modes of conditioning, classical (pavlovian) and instrumental (or operant), seem to enter LTM directly.

## Kandel Synapses and Conditioning

Conditioning is a familiar concept, but review of the components of this phenomenon and of its basic terminology may be helpful. Eric Kandel and his associates studied the cellular and biochemical mechanisms responsible for the conditioning of an avoidance response, mantle withdrawal, in the marine snail, *Aplysia*.[101] The mantle shelf of this invertebrate is a covering that protects the animal's gill and respiratory chamber (the mantle cavity). Noxious stimuli cause the mantle shelf, the gill, and adjacent structures to contract and withdraw into the mantle cavity. This forceful withdrawal is an unconditioned (native) response (UR), and the noxious sensation that triggers it is the unconditioned stimulus (UCS). In their conditioning experiments Carew and coworkers[102] delivered a strong shock (the UCS) to the snail's tail, simultaneously giving a gentle stimulus to the siphon of the animal (the CS). (The siphon is a snoutlike structure at the tip of the mantle shelf.) Siphon contact, by itself, and in the absence of such a pairing history, does not lead to a withdrawal response. However, with conditioning the *Aplysia* responds to gentle siphon stimulation with a vigorous conditioned withdrawal reflex (the CR). It is essential in classical conditioning that the CS and the UCS be delivered at almost the same time, the CS *just* preceding the UCS. In these experiments with *Aplysia* the CS typically preceded the UCS by about 0.5 second. Initially, the CS produced only a weak withdrawal response, but after repeated pairings "the CS . . . becomes much more effective and elicits a powerful gill and siphon withdrawal reflex."[102] Further experiments established that the conditioning was quite specific to the site of stimulation. After siphon conditioning, stimulation of the mantle shelf proper failed to produce the same highly enhanced withdrawal response. Similarly, mantle shelf contact could serve as a specific CS, and under those circumstances, stimulation of the nearby siphon would fail to lead to an effective CR.

Earlier work by the Kandel group had generated enormous excitement because, through their efforts, many of the synaptic and biochemical mechanisms underlying extremely simple forms of learning—habituation and sensitization—had been identified for the first time. However, neither habituation nor sensitization involves learning new associations. Both of these nonassociative learning nodes are characterized by very general changes in the responsiveness of an animal to a single stimulus. Doubts, therefore, could still be raised concerning the relevance of their findings to more complex associative forms of learning. Thus, their subsequent success in identifying important components of the synaptic and biochemical mechanisms for associative learning (conditioning) in

*Aplysia* marked a second important milestone. Furthermore, of special interest was their report that the mechanisms and sites of synaptic modification for nonassociative learning (sensitization) and for avoidance response conditioning were, in fact, quite similar.

*Presynaptic facilitation* was found to be the basis for both forms of learning in the *Aplysia,*[103] the facilitation synapse being the one that links the siphon skin sensory neuron with the motor neuron that effects the withdrawal response. The key to the mechanism is a facilitator interneuron that is activated by the shock stimulus to the tail and that modifies the sensory neuron presynaptically, at a site close to the synapse, initiating a cascade of intracellular reactions (including increased production of cyclic AMP and activation of a second enzyme, cyclic AMP–dependent protein kinase). The $K^+$ channel and the $Ca^{2+}$ channel effects that result from these intracellular biochemical events permit a large $Ca^{2+}$ influx into the terminal region of the axon. It is the high intraterminal $Ca^{2+}$ levels that bring about substantial increases in transmitter release and, consequently, in synaptic efficiency. This sequence of steps forms the basis both for sensitization and for conditioning, but conditioning appears to involve an additional feature: some form of augmentation of this chemical cascade through effects of the spike potential, as yet unidentified.[104]

The neuronal circuitry that subserves conditioning in higher animals is far more intricate. The circuitry that allows conditioning of a defensive eye blink, for example, includes the nucleus interpositus of the cerebellum and complex pathways in the cerebellar cortex.[105] The hippocampus is not a necessary structure, in general, for conditioning or for other forms of automatic learning, but it is, nevertheless, likely to be active during conditioning,[106] and may serve to enhance the learning process.

## Hebb Synapses and Long-Term Potentiation

In 1949, on the basis of what was then hypothesized about learning in animals and man, Donald Hebb, a Canadian psychologist, in effect "invented a nervous system."[107] Hebb tried to conceptualize the types of neuronal circuits that would

be needed to support the prevailing models of learning and memory. His concepts have stood up well and have proven to be roughly compatible with current neurobiologic information. The simplest Hebb circuits are the cell assemblies and the phase sequences. The cell assembly provides for recurrent cycling of a discharge after a stimulus has served as a trigger and has then been withdrawn. Because of the looping character of the cell assembly, a reverbatory circuit is established. Hebb's phase sequence represents the functional connection of two or more cell assemblies. In the circuit design (Figure 24-1), cell assembly A has established connections with cell assembly B, and, consequently, a new and larger functional unit has resulted.

Complex phase assemblies representing new visual associations, perhaps, or new auditory associations, and also new intermodal connections between visual and auditory inputs could be designed. Hebb further proposed that repeated discharge of cell assemblies and phase sequences might lead to *synaptic alterations,* rendering these

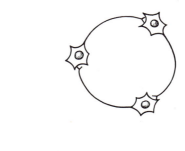

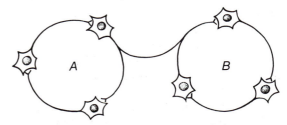

**Figure 24-1.** Cell assembly (*top*) and phase sequence (*bottom*). Both types of designs allow reverberatory circuits to be established, which persist even after the triggering stimulus has been withdrawn (see text). (After Bugelski BR. Principles of Learning and Memory. New York: Praeger, 1979;156.)

neuronal clusters more and more likely to fire as a unit.[107p.60] Associationist learning and LTM, according to Hebb, were based on the consolidation of strong connections between cell assemblies through *increased synaptic efficiency.* Temporal contiguity was another important concept in the Hebbian model. Learning depended on it, for the initial linkage between two or more cell assemblies depended on their simultaneous or nearly simultaneous firing.

Neurobiologists have had some success in identifying these Hebbian components. The discovery of long-term potentiation (LTP) in the hippocampus by Bliss and Lomo in 1983 stands as a landmark in this regard.[108] These investigators found that a single, extremely brief, high-frequency tetanic electrical stimulation of a major afferent pathway to the hippocampus (namely the perforant pathway to the dentate gyrus) results in markedly increased synaptic efficiency for the connections made to the dentate, persisting for weeks. The possibility was raised at once that LTP might be a mechanism for learning and for memory consolidation. It is established with great rapidity, and its effects are tenacious. The discovery of LTP in the hippocampus was also very suggestive. At first, in fact, it was thought to be a phenomenon unique to the hippocampus, but it has more recently been observed in the cerebral cortex also.

Investigations since this first report have tended to strengthen the case for LTP as a likely LTM mechanism. Barnes found that the speed of maze learning in rats corresponded to the recorded magnitude of LTP.[109] Administration of the drug AP5 (aminophosphonovaleric acid) blocks induction of LTP and markedly interferes with place learning in rats, even though the drug has no detectable effect on ordinary synaptic transmission in the rat hippocampus. This AP5-blocking effect seems to be selective for hippocampus-based learning.[110] Visual discrimination learning, which is not vulnerable to hippocampal damage, was not impaired by AP5 infusion.

AP5 can selectively block the induction of LTP in hippocampal neurons yet leave ordinary synaptic transmission in these cells unaffected, because of the presence of multiple kinds of neurotransmitter receptors on the postsynaptic membrane. Three principal subclasses of neurotransmitter receptor (all responsive to the neurotransmitter L-glutamate) have been identified: two of these, the kainate receptors and the quisqualate receptors, are not antagonized by AP5. The third subclass, the NMDA receptors, is subject to AP5 block.[111] It would appear, then, that NMDA receptors are the chemical mediators of LTP in the hippocampus, whereas the other postsynaptic receptor subtypes are presumed to mediate ordinary forms of transmission at the same hippocampal synapses. Additionally, it is known that LTP is established by virtue of $Ca^{2+}$ influx into the postsynaptic cell, and NMDA receptors are thought to be the sole $Ca^{2+}$ channel gatekeepers on the postsynaptic membrane. These $Ca^{2+}$ channels are voltage dependent and are blocked during ordinary synaptic transmission (most probably by magnesium ions). The tetanizing bursts that initiate LTP are presumed to open these channels by extruding the magnesium ions, thereby exposing the intradendritic environment to influx of $Ca^{2+}$.[111]

Memory consolidation requires the building of linkages between previously unassociated impressions. The temporal coincidence of the impression is what links them initially. If LTP, as mediated by NMDA receptors and $Ca^{2+}$ influx, underlies memory consolidation, one must postulate that LTP responds to finely timed convergence of inputs. These timing conditions would be met if we assumed that the first stage of the LTP process involves the priming of a target postsynaptic cell by means of an initial pulse of excitation. The next stage in the process would depend on the nearly coincident arrival of a second pulse (and probably additional pulses) of excitation, and consequently sufficient permeation of $Ca^{2+}$ into the postsynaptic cell to bring about LTP.[112] Experimental evidence of temporal linkage of this type has been reported.[113] LTP priming effects appear to develop in about 50 msec and do not persist beyond 2 seconds. The long-term potentiation process is associated with significant postsynaptic morphologic changes, including the rounding of target dendritic spines. These morphologic changes appear to be the result of breakdown and restructuring of the submembranous cytoskeleton of the dendritic spine due to the action of calcium-dependent proteases (calpains).[114]

Where in the brain are the long-term memory repositories? It is unlikely that long-term memories are stored in the hippocampus or in related subcortical structures such as amygdala or diencephalon, because long-term memories are retained despite total excision of the hippocampus and adjacent structures bilaterally. It has been suggested that the very cortical structures and cells responsible for our initial and unconsolidated perceptions and conceptualizations serve also, after synaptic alteration occurs, as the loci of our memories.[69] It is a parsimonious arrangement. Through a form of intimate feedback to the cortex, the hippocampus and other related subcortical stations would play a critical role of the consolidation of novel cortical associations. Once memory is established via enhanced synaptic efficiency, the same circuits that receive impressions would also serve to recall them.[115] NMDA receptors function at a cortical level, and they may be crucial to the process. Additionally, cholinergic and noradrenergic neurons appear to play a modulatory role and probably affect the efficiency of the consolidation mechanism.[116] This modulating role has important therapeutic implications, and they have been exploited in recent years. Encouraging but controversial are the reports of memory improvement in patients with early Alzheimer's disease who are treated with 1,2,3,4,-tetrahydro-9-aminoacridine (THA), a relatively long-acting anticholinesterase.[117,118]

## The Remediation of Memory Deficits: A Sampling of Treatment Methods

Patients with amnesia can acquire some types of new information rather effectively. This clinical and experimental observation has clear implications for treatment. How can we anticipate and distinguish which materials and skills amnesic patients are likely to be able to retain? The distinction between procedural and declarative knowledge appears to be critical in this regard. Severely amnesic patients usually have far greater difficulty with declarative than with procedural learning, and attempts to treat memory disorders in these patients have on occasion led to dramatic demonstrations of the distinction between the two forms of learning. In one study that involved teaching computer operation skills and procedures to head-injured patients with memory impairment of varying severity,[119] it was found at the conclusion of the training

program that the most severely amnesic of these patients had no memory of the many computer training sessions (more than 100). He denied that he had ever worked on a computer. Yet he had become adept at all of the basic computer procedures that were taught. These results, and corroborative findings with normal subjects, suggest that the distinction between procedural and declarative memory is a fundamental one: procedural learning processes are considered much older phylogenetically than declarative ones, and the two systems are thought to be based on substantially different neuronal pathways and mechanisms.

A verbal proposition (e.g., *Maryland is one of the fifty states*) is most efficiently acquired through declarative learning techniques (e.g., conscious study, conscious linkage with associated propositions, familiarization through the establishment of personally meaningful connections), yet most amnesic patients retain information best through procedural learning and, so, must be taught by procedural learning methods. In the computer training program mentioned above the investigators capitalized on an important procedural learning process known as *priming,* a special type of cueing effect that facilitates verbal learning. When amnesic patients are primed (that is, exposed either to concepts or to word fragments that resemble the target words or propositions, in this case, computer-relevant vocabulary and computer commands), they show enhanced ability to produce the target material. What is striking about priming is that amnesics seem to benefit as much from its effects as do normal subjects. Priming is not based on conscious familiarity or conscious memories of previously presented materials but seems more closely akin to automatic conditioned behavior. In this study, priming cues were gradually reduced as patients became more skillful at remembering computer terminology and computer procedures ("method of vanishing cues").

Additional principles relevant to memory remediation have been summarized by Baddeley[120]:

1. Learning and consolidation of memory cannot be effective when attention is poor. Seen in this light, attention is not merely one additional cognitive area for remediation; it may be the first and most fundamental treatment concern in cases of memory impairment.

2. New information is most successfully incorporated into long-term memory stores when it can be related to schemas, conceptual networks, and organized systems that are already well-established in memory. "... An expert chess player can acquire in a single glimpse of a game more information than a novice player can acquire in four or five glimpses. A football enthusiast can hear the results and recall them much more effectively than someone who has merely a passing interest in football...."[120p.22] This principle leads directly to the twin concepts that elaborative rehearsal and "deep" encoding of new material enhance the learning of new material. "Efficient deep processing (is characterized) by the following features:

Elaboration: Working on the detail of material and relating it to what one already knows appears to enhance learning.

Compatibility: Material that is consistent with existing knowledge is easier to learn than inconsistent material, and neutral material is best learned by attempting to relate it to what is already known.

Self-reference: Learners who are asked to judge how material relates to themselves seem to remember it better than if they are required to judge its relevance to other people."[113]

3. In general terms, rehearsal is necessary both to maintain information in STM and to transfer information from STM to LTM. Rehearsal, however, can take several forms; simple repetition of the material is one. While repetition may hold material in STM for a while, it is a relatively poor way to consolidate information. Elaborative processing, the attempt to graft the new material onto what already exists (see principle 2, above) is far more effective.[120p.21] The principle of elaborative rehearsal need not call upon existing LTM stores, however. Malek and Questad, for example, applied the principle to memory remediation by instructing a patient to weave the new information into a simple but coherent narrative (a simple story) and then to make a mental picture of the story, using as much visual detail as possible. They found this training technique to be both effective and practical.[162]

External aids, such as alarm watches, timers, calendars, and memory notebooks, can be extremely helpful to patients with memory deficits, but some patients forget to use them! As the regular use of external aids depends on procedural learning, with enough practice, many patients can develop the necessary habits of use. Most memory remediation programs use external aids, but *staff should include the requisite practice activities,* often extensive and prolonged, as part of the remediation effort.

When forced usage methods and repetitive practice of cognitive capacities are attempted, what degree of generalization of these capacities can be expected? To what extent does direct training of attentiveness, for example, or direct training of memory, lead to the kind of general strengthening of these cognitive skills that can transfer over into daily life? The evidence thus far indicates that desktop computer and computer console training procedures for remediation of attention deficits, improve attentiveness generally and that for many patients benefits carry over into everyday life.[91,93] It is important to note, however, that memory, unlike attention, does not appear to be trainable as a general capacity. "The notion that a damaged memory can be restored or improved in some general sense through practice or repetitive drills continues to persist among many workers in rehabilitation settings, despite the complete lack of empirical evidence that such general improvements ever occur. . . . Although there is evidence that memory-impaired patients can learn some specific pieces of information through repeated practice, there is no evidence that such practice improves memory for any other materials; that is, training does not appear to generalize to other situations, tasks, or stimuli. Even with concentrated practice sessions over long periods of time, significant benefits of drilling on overall memory performance have not been found."[119] Certainly, amnesic patients can be helped to remember through learning and application of memory strategies, through use of external aids, and through utilization of special techniques such as priming (described above). Memory remediation efforts should be focused on techniques such as these and not squandered on memory drills if such drills demand the retention of material that is irrelevant to daily life.

# References

1. Scott D Jr, Liu CN. Factors promoting regeneration of spinal neurons: Positive influence of nerve growth factor. Progr Brain Res 1964; 13:127–150.
2. Bjorklund A, Steneve U. Growth of central catecholamine neurons into smooth muscle grafts in the rat mesencephalon. Brain Res 1971; 31:1–20.
3. Bjorklund A, Bjerre B, Stenevi U. Has nerve growth factor a role in the regeneration of central and peripheral catecholamine neurones? In: Fuxe L, et al., eds. Dynamics of Degeneration and Growth in Neurons. New York: Pergamon, 389–409.
4. Feringa ER, Gurden GG, Strodel W, et al. Descending spinal motor tract regeneration after spinal cord transection. Neurology 1973; 23:599–608.
5. Berry M, Riches AC. An immunological approach to regeneration in the central nervous system. Br Med Bull 1974; 30:135–140.
6. Liu CN, Chambers WW. Intraspinal sprouting of dorsal root axons. Arch Neurol 1958; 79:46–61.
7. Glees P, Cole J. Recovery of skilled motor functions after small repeated lesions of motor cortex in macaque. J Neurophysiol 1950; 13:137–148.
8. Raisman G. Neuronal plasticity in the septal nucleii of the adult rat. Brain Res 1969; 14:25–48.
9. Moore RY, Bjorklund R. Stenevi U. Plastic changes in the adrenergic innervation of the rat septal area in response to denervation. Brain Res 1971; 33:13–35.
10. Raisman G, Field PM. A quantitative investigation of the development of collateral reinnervation after partial deafferentation of the septal nucleii. Brain Res 1973; 50:241–264.
11. Gentshcev T, Sotelo C. Degenerative patterns in the ventral cochlear nucleus of the rat after primary deafferentation. Brain Res 1973; 62:37–60.
12. Goodman DC, Horel JR. Sprouting of optic projections in the brainstem of the rat. J Compar Neurol 1966; 127:71–88.
13. Ralston HJ, Chow HL. Synaptic reorganization in the degenerating lateral geniculate nucleus of the rabbit. J Compar Neurol 1973; 147:321–350.
14. Westrum LE, Black RG. Fine structural aspects of the synaptic organization of the spinal trigeminal nucleus of the cat. Brain Res 1971; 25:265–287.
15. Lynch G, Matthews D, Mosko S, et al. Induced acetylcholinesterase-rich layer in rat dentate gyrus. Brain Res 1972; 42:311–318.
16. Goodman DC, Bogdasarian RS, Horel JR. Axonal sprouting of ipsilateral optic tract following opposite eye removal. Brain, Behav Evol 1973; 8:27–50.
17. Sotelo C, Palay SL. Altered axons and axon terminals in the lateral vestibular nucleus of the rat. Lab Invest 1971; 25:633–672.
18. Matthews Do, Cotman CW, Lynch G. An electron microscopic study of lesion-induced synaptogenesis of the dentate gyrus of the adult rat. Brain Res 1978; 115:1–21.
19. Guillery RW. Experiments to determine whether retinogeniculate axons can form translaminar collateral sprouts in the dorsal lateral geniculate nucleus of the cat. J Compar Neurol 1972; 146:407–420.
20. Halil RE. Formation of new retinogeniculate connections in kittens: Effects of age and visual experience. Anat Rec 1973; 175:353–356.
21. Hickey TL. Translaminar growth of axons in the kitten dorsal lateral geniculate nucleus following removal of one eye. J Compar Neurol 1975; 161:359–382.
22. Dews PB, Wiesel TN. Consequences of monocular deprivation on visual behaviour in kittens. J Physiol (Lond) 1970; 206:437–455.
23. von Noorden GH. Experimental amblyopia in monkeys. Invest Ophthalmol 1973; 12:721–726.
24. Tsang YC. Maze learning in rats dehemicorticated in infancy. J Compar Psychol 1937; 24:221–254.
25. Benjamin RM, Thompson RF. Differential effects of cortical lesions in infant and adult cats on roughness discrimination. 1959; 1:305–321.
26. Wetzel RB, Thonpson VE, Horel JR, et al. Some consequences of perinatal lesions of the visual cortex of the cat. Psychonom Sci 1965; 3:381–382.
27. Harlow HF, Blumquist RJ, Thompson CI, et al. Effects of induction age and size of frontal lobe lesions in learning rhesus monkeys. In: Isaacson RL, ed. The Neuropsychology of Development. New York: John Wiley, 1968;79–120.
28. Chow HL, Steward DL. Reversal of structural and functional effects of long term visual deprivation in cats. Exp Neurol 1972; 34:409–433.
29. Finger S. Environmental attenuation of brain-lesion symptoms. In: Finger S, ed. Recovery from Brain Damage—Research and Theory. New York: Plenum, 1978;297–309.
30. Frommer GP. Subtotal lesions: Implications for coding and recovery of function. In Ibid. 1978;176–178.
31. Greenough WT. Experimental modification of the developing brain. Am Sci 1975; 63:37–46.
32. Greenough WT, Fass B, DeVoogd TJ. The influence of experience on recovery following brain

damage in rodents. In: Walsh RN, Greenough WT, eds. Environments as Therapy for Brain Dysfunction. New York: Plenum, 1976;10–50.

33. Greenough WT. Presentattion at the Annual Meeting of the American Academy of Physical Medicine and Rehabilitation. Boston, Mass, October 25, 1984.

34. Finger S. Environmental and experiential determinants of recovery of function. In: Finger S, Stein DG, eds. Brain Damage and Recovery. New York: Academic Press, 1982;195.

35. Finger S. Drugs and recovery: Pyrogens and hormones. In: Ibid.

36. Luria AR, Naydin VL, Tretkova LS, et al. Restoration and higher cortical functions following local brain damage. In: Vinken PJ, Bruyn GW, eds. Handbook of Clinical Neurology. Amsterdam: North Holland, 1969;368–433.

37. Stricker E, Zigmond M. Recovery of function after damage to central catecholamine-containing neurons. In: Sprague JM, Epstein AN, eds. Progress in Psychobiology and Physiological Psychology, vol 6. New York: Academic Press, 1976;121–172.

38. Glick SD, Zimmerberg B. Pharmacological modification and brain lesion syndromes. In: Finger S, ed. Recovery of Function from Brain Damage. New York: Plenum, 1978;281–293.

39. Brailowsky S. Neuropharmacological aspects of brain plasticity. In: Bach-y-Rita P, ed. Recovery of Function: Theoretical Considerations for Brain Injury Rehabilitation. Baltimore: University Park Press, 1980;191–192.

40. Illis LS, Sedgwick EM, Glanville HJ. Rehabilitation of the Neurological Patient. Oxford: Blackwell, 1980;282.

41. Milner B. Sparing of language functions after early unilateral brain damage. In: Eidelberg E, Stein DG, eds. Functional Recovery After Lesions of the Nervous System. Neuroscience Research Program Bulletin. 1974; 12:213–216.

42. Hecaen H. Albert ML. Human Neuropsychology. New York: John Wiley, 1978.

43. Freud S. Die infantile Cerebralahmung. In: Nothnagel, Specielle Pathologie und Therapie IV. Vienna: Holder, 1897.

44. Lenneberg EH. Biological Foundations of Language. New York: John Wiley, 1967.

45. Zihl J. Shrinkage of visual field defects associated with specific training after brain damage. Paper presented at the European Brain and Behavior Society Workshop, "Recovery from Brain Damage", Rotterdam April 1981. In: Hof van MW, Mohn G, eds. Functional Recovery From Brain Damage. Amsterdam: Elsevier, 1981;189–202.

46. Blakemore, Falconer MA. Long-term effects of anterior temporal lobectomy on certain cognitive functions. J Neurol Neurosurg Psychiatry 1967; 30:364–367.

47. Finger S. Stein DG. Recovery and the human patient. In Finger S, Stein DG, eds. Brain Damage and Recovery. New York: Academic Press, 1982;330.

48. Teuber HL. Recovery of function after brain injury in man. In: Outcome of Severe Damage to the Central Nervous System. Ciba Foundation Symposium 34. Amsterdam: Elsevier, 1975;160–180.

49. Luria AR, Naydin VL, Tsvetkova LS, et al. Restoration of higher cortical function following brain damage. In: Vinken PJ, Bruyn GW, eds. Handbook of Clinical Neurology III. Amsterdam: North Holland, 1969;368–433.

50. Meyer PM, Horel JA, Meyer DR. Effects of d-amphetamine upon placing responses in neodecorticate cats. J Compar Physiologic Psychol 1963; 56:402–404.

51. Wall PD. The presence of ineffective synapses and the circumstances which unmask them. Philo Trans R Soc Lond (ser B) 1977; 278:361–372.

51a. Bach-y-Rita P. Central nervous system lesions: Sprouting and unmasking in rehabilitation. Arch Phys Med Rehabil 1981; 62:413–417.

52. Glees P. Functional reorganization following hemispherectomy in man and after small experimental lesions in primates. In: Bach-y-Rita R, ed. Recovery of Function: Theoretical Considerations for Brain Injury Rehabilitation. Baltimore: University Park Press, 1980;106–113.

53. Finger S, Stein DG. Vicariation theory and radical reorganization and function. In: Finger S, Stein DG, eds. Brain Damage and Recovery. New York, Academic Press: 1982;293–295.

54. Evarts E. Brain control of movement: Possible mechanisms of functional reorganization. In: Bach-y-Rita P, ed. Recovery of Function: Theoretical Considerations for Brain Injury Rehabilitation. Baltimore: University Park Press, 1980;184–185.

55. Hore J, Meyer-Lohmann J, Brooks VB. Basal ganglia cooling disables learned arm movements of monkeys in the absence of visual guidance. Science 1977; 195:584–586.

56. When do neurons stop changing? [Editorial]. Lancet 1978; 2:667–668.

57. Rosenthal TL. Some organizing hints for communicating applied information. In: Gholson B, Rosenthal TL, eds. Applications of Cognitive-Developmental Theory. Orlando, Fla: Academic Press, 1984.

58. Anderson JR. The Architecture of Cognition.

Cambridge, Mass: Harvard University Press, 1983;2.

59. Ryan EB, Short EJ, Weed KA. The role of cognitive strategy training in improving the academic performance of learning-disabled children. J Learn Disabil 1986;19:521.

60. Meichenbaum D. Cognitive-Behavior Modification. New York: Plenum Press, 1977.

61. Kendall PC, Braswell L. Cognitive-Behavioral Therapy for Impulsive Children. New York: Guilford, 1985.

62. Luria AR. The Working Brain. New York: Basic Books, 1973.

63. Kuffler SW. Discharge patterns and functional organization of mammalian retina. J Neurophysiol 1953; 16:37–68.

64. Kandel ER. Processing of form and movement in the visual system. In: Kandel ER, Schwartz JH, eds. Principles of Neural Science, ed 2. New York: Elsevier North Holland, 1985.

65. Hubel DH, Wiesel TN. Receptive fields, binocular interaction and functional architecture in the cat's visual cortex. J Physiol (Lond) 1962; 160:106–154.

66. Hubel DH, Wiesel TN. Brain mechanisms of vision. Sci Am 1979; 241:150–162.

67. Geschwind N. Disconnection syndromes in animals and man. Brain 1965; 88:237–294.

68. Luria AR. Restoration of function after brain injury. New York: Macmillan, 1963.

69. Mishkin M, Appenzeller T. The anatomy of memory. Sci Am 1987; 256:80–89.

70. Kandel ER. Processing of form and movement in the visual system. In: Kandel ER, Schwartz JH, eds. Principles of Neural Science, ed 2. New York: Elsevier North Holland, 1985.

71. Gaddes WH. Learning Disabilities and Brain Dysfunction, ed 2. New York: Springer-Verlag, 1985.

72. Rapin I. Children with Brain Dysfunction: Neurology, Cognition, Language and Behavior. New York: Raven Press, 1982.

73. Hiscock M. Behavioral asymmetries in normal children. In: Molfrese DL, Segalowitz SJ, eds. Brain Lateralization in Children. New York: Guilford, 1988.

74. Held R, Hein A. Movement produced stimulation in the development of visually guided behavior. J Compar Physiol Psychol 1963; 56:872–876.

75. Ayres AJ. Sensory Integration and Learning Disorders. Los Angeles: Western Psychological Services, 1972.

76. Kephart N. The Slow Learner in the Classroom, ed 2. Columbus, Oh: Merrill, 1971.

77. Critchley M, Critchley EA. Dyslexia Defined. Chichester: Thomas, 1978.

78. Weinberg J, Diller L, Gordon WA, et al. Training sensory awareness and spatial organization in people with right brain damage. Arch Phys Med Rehabil 1979; 60:491–496.

79. Stuss DT, Benson DF. The Frontal Lobes. New York: Raven Press, 1986.

80. James W. Attention and will. In: Roth JK, ed. The Moral Philosophy of William James. New York: Thomas Y Crowell, 1969.

81. Shallice T. Specific impairments of planning. Philos Trans R Soc Lond [Biol] 1982; 298:199–209.

82. Squire LR. Memory and Brain. New York: Oxford University Press, 1987;151.

83. Squire LR. Science 1986; 232:1612–1619.

85. Norman DA. Learning and Memory. New York: WH Freeman, 1982;83.

86. Gross Y, Schutz LE. Intervention models in neuropsychology. In: Uzzell BP, Gross Y, eds. Clinical Neuropsychology of Intervention. Boston: Martinus Nijhoff, 1986.

87. Ben-Yishai Y, Lakin P, Ross B, et al. A modular approach to training (verbal) abstract reasoning in traumatic head-injured patients. In: Working Approaches to Remediation of Cognitive Deficits in Brain Damaged Persons, Institute of Rehabilitation Medicine, New York University Medical Center, Department of Behavioral Sciences, New York: 1980.

88. Yingling CD, Skinner JE. Selective regulation of thalamic sensory relay nuclei by nucleus reticularis thalami. Electroencephalogr Clin Neurophysiol 1976; 41:476–482.

89. Crick F. Function of the thalamic reticular complex: The searchlight hypothesis. Proc Natl Acad Sci USA 1984; 82:4586–4590.

90. Gummow L, Miller P, Dustman RE. Attention and brain injury: A case for cognitive rehabilitation of attentional deficits. Clin Psychol Rev 1983; 3:255–274.

91. Sohlberg MM, Mateer CA. Introduction to Cognitive Rehabilitation. New York: Guilford Press, 1989.

92. Sohlberg N, Mateer C. Effectiveness of an attention-training program. J Clin Exp Neuropsychol 1987; 9:117–130.

93. Ben-Yishai Y, Piasetsky EB, Rattok J. A systematic method for ameliorating disorders in basic attention. In: Meier MJ, Benton AL, Diller L, eds. Neuropsychological Rehabilitation. New York: Guilford, 1987.

94. Piasetsky EB, Rattok J, Ben-Yishai Y, et al. Computerized ORM: A manual for clinical research use. In: Working Approaches to Remediation of Cognitive Deficits in Brain Damaged Persons.

New York: Institute of Rehabilitation Medicine, New York University Medical Center, Department of Behavioral Sciences, New York: 1983.

95. Meichenbaum D, Goodman J. Training impulsive children to talk to themselves: A means of developing self-control. J Abnorm Psychol 1971; 77:115–126.

96. Baddeley A. Working Memory. Oxford: Clarendon Press, 1986.

97. Peterson LR, Peterson MJ. Short-term retention of individual verbal items. J Exp Psychol 1959; 58:193–198.

98. Kalat JW. Biological Psychology. Belmont, Calif: Wadsworth, 1980;383.

99. Milner B, Corkin S, Teuber H-L. Further analysis of the hippocampic amnesic syndrome: 14-year follow-up study of H.M. Neuropsychologia 1968; 6:215–234.

100. Wickelgren WA. Sparing of short-term memory in an amnesic patient: Implications for strength theory of memory. Neuropsychologia 1968; 6:235–244.

101. Kandel ER. Small systems of neurons. Sci Am 1979:66–76.

102. Carew TJ, Hawkins RD, Kandel ER. Differential classical conditioning of a defensive withdrawal reflex in *Aplysia californica*. Science 1983; 219:397–400.

103. Kandel ER, Castellucci VF, Goelet P, et al. Cell-biological interrelationships between short-term and long-term memory. In: Kandel ER, ed. Molecular Neurobiology in Neurology and Psychiatry. New York: Raven, 1987.

104. Hawkins RD, Kandel ER. Steps toward a cell-biological alphabet for elementary forms of learning. In: Lynch G, McGaugh JL, Weinberger NM, eds. Neurobiology of Learning and Memory. New York: Guilford, 1984.

105. Thompson RF. The neurobiology of learning and memory. Science 1986; 233:941–947.

106. Berger TW, Laham RI, Thompson RF. Hippocampal unit–behavior correlations during classical conditioning. Brain Res 1980; 193:229–248.

107. Bugelski BR. Principles of Learning and Memory. New York: Praeger, 1979;156.

108. Bliss TVP, Lomo T. Long lasting potentiation of synaptic transmission in the dentate area of the anaesthetized rabbit following stimulation of the perforant path. J Physiol (Lond) 1973; 232:331–356.

109. Barnes CA. Memory deficits associated with senescence: A neurophysiological and behavioral study in the rat. J Comp Physiol Psychol 1979; 93:74–104.

110. Morris RGM, Anderson E, Lynch GS, et al. Selective impairment of learning and blockade of long-term potentiation by an N-methyl-D-aspartate receptor antagonist, AP5. Nature 1986; 319:774–776.

111. Collingridge GL. Long term potentiation in the hipocampus: Mechanisms of initiation and modulation by neurotransmitters. Trends Pharmacol Sci 1985;407.

112. Larson J, Lynch G. Induction of synaptic potentiation in hippocampus by patterned stimulation involves two events. Science 1986; 232:985–988.

113. McNaughton BL, Douglas RM, Goddard GV. Synaptic enhancement in fascia dentata: Cooperativity among coactive afferents. Brain Res 1978; 157:277–293.

114. Lynch G, Baudry M. The biochemistry of memory: A new and specific hypothesis. Science 1984; 224:1057.

115. Squire LR. Mechanisms of memory. Science 1986; 232:1612–1619.

116. Mayes AM. Human Organic Memory Disorders. Cambridge: Cambridge University Press, 1988;214.

117. Summers WK, Majovski LV, Marsh GM, et al. Oral tetrahydroaminoacridine in long-term treatment of senile dementia, Alzheimer type. N Engl J Med 1986; 315:1241–1245.

118. Mayeux R. Therapeutic strategies in Alzheimer's disease. Neurology 1990; 40:175–180.

119. Glisky E, Schacter D. Remediation of organic memory disorders. J Head Trauma Rehabil 1986; 1:54–63.

120. Baddeley AD. Memory theory and memory therapy. In: Wilson, BA, Moffat N, eds. Clinical Management of Memory Problems. Rockville, Md: Aspen, 1984.

121. Malek J, Questad K. Rehabilitation of memory after craniocerebral trauma: Case report. Arch Phys Med Rehabil 1983; 64:436–438.

# Chapter 25

# Aging of the Reproductive System in Women: Menopause

FREDI KRONENBERG
JOHN A. DOWNEY

Aging of the reproductive system in women is integrally interwoven with the inexorable aging process. As a result, it is difficult to separate the consequences of aging from those of menopause. The passage of time causes changes in skin, bone, muscle, blood vessels, and other tissues, and these changes can be modulated by hormones such as estrogen.

Menopause has been the focus of some controversy in medicine. At one extreme are physicians who view menopause as a natural process that requires minimal intervention, if any. At the other extreme are those who view menopause as an estrogen deficiency disease or an endocrinopathy that requires aggressive treatment.

In this chapter we focus on the biology of menopause—the changes in biologic structure and function that occur in the years during and subsequent to the transition from reproductive cyclicity to nonreproductive acyclicity. The rate and magnitude of these changes vary considerably, as do individual responses to them. Many women have a relatively smooth transition; others, a more difficult one. Thus, physiologic change does not necessarily imply major clinical problems.

## Definitions

The word *menopause* is derived from the Greek *mene* (month) and *pausis* (stop). Strictly speaking, menopause is the occurrence of the last menstrual period, but in popular usage it is the period of years during which menstrual cycles become increasingly irregular, culminating in the cessation of menses, and followed by a variable number of years during which the body continues to adjust to its new, noncycling state. To facilitate comparisons among research studies we have attempted to standardize definitions and to distinguish discrete stages of reproductive function within what is really a continuum. Definitions are based principally on the degree of regularity of the menstrual cycle. *Perimenopause* generally refers to the transition period prior to menopause and shortly after the last menstrual period. It typically lasts several years and is characterized by changes in menstrual cycle length or bleeding pattern interspersed with periods of amenorrhea, presumably reflecting hormone fluctuations. *Menopause* is the permanent cessation of menstruation, marking the decrease of ovarian activity. *Natural menopause*, which usually occurs as part of the normal maturation process, is most commonly defined as the absence of menses for 12 consecutive months. Menopause can also occur prematurely, because of surgical removal of both ovaries (*surgical menopause*), or following radiation, chemotherapy, or other drugs that suppress ovarian function (*artificial menopause*). Postmenopause is generally considered to be the period beginning at, or 12 months after, the cessation of menses and continuing indefinitely thereafter. The term *menopause*, or *the menopausal period*, is commonly used to mean the time from menopause onward, or even more broadly, to encompass the perimenopausal period as well. Here, the latter, broader, sense of the word is used.

## Age at Natural Menopause

Estimates of the median age at menopause are fairly consistent, ranging from age 49 to 51 years[1-8] using different population samples, and despite inconsistent definitions of menopause and various methods of analysis. The distribution of ages at menopause (Figure 25-1) illustrates the wide range of ages at which cessation of menses occurs.[8]

A variety of physiologic, environmental, and sociodemographic factors have been examined to determine their influence on age at menopause. The data are sparse and contradictory. The most compelling data are for cigarette smoking, which is associated with 1 to 2 years earlier onset of menopause in most studies,[9-13] though not in all.[13] A woman's reproductive history may influence her age at menopause. Menstrual irregularity before age 25 seems to predict earlier menopause.[13] Data on parity are conflicting. Some investigators have reported that nulliparous women experience earlier menopause than parous women,[7,13] but others found no association.[1,12,14] There is also lack of agreement in reports of relationships between age at natural menopause and age at menarche, age at first birth, number of live births, oral contraceptive use, race, income, and education.[3,7,13]

## The Transition to Menopause

The transition from regular menstrual cyclicity to menopausal acyclicity is usually a gradual process that lasts several years. Women's level of circulating estradiol reaches a peak in the fourth decade of life and then decreases gradually. Although the end result is the same (i.e., cessation of menses), the time course, pattern, and magnitude of physical and endocrine changes vary between women, and within women from month to month.

### The Menstrual Cycle

During the reproductive years, cyclic production of sex steroids and gonadotropins characterizes the menstrual cycle. The ovary is responsible for the cyclic synthesis and secretion of steroid hormones and the release of oocytes. Ovary, hypothalamus, and anterior pituitary act in concert to regulate the endocrine and gametogenic events of the menstrual cycle. The principal ovarian steroids are estradiol produced primarily by the granulosa cells, androstenedione produced primarily by the stroma and thecal cells and progesterone, produced by the corpus luteum. Ovarian function is regulated by the gonadotropins follicle-stimulating hormone (FSH) and luteinizing hormone (LH), which are peptides secreted by the anterior pituitary in response to stimulation by gonadotropin-releasing hormone (GnRH) from hypothalamic neurons. The ovarian steroids feed back to the hypothalamus and pituitary and modulate secretion of gonadotropin. GnRH is secreted in pulses, and this episodic secretion is critical to stimulating the pulsatile secretion of LH and FSH. LH pulses vary in frequency and amplitude across the menstrual cycle, being more frequent but lower in amplitude in the follicular than in the luteal phase. These changes in pulsatility are modulated by feedback of steroid

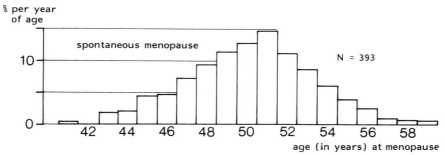

**Figure 25-1.** Age at menopause. (From Treloar AE. Menstrual cyclicity and the premenopause. Maturitas 1981; 3:255, with permission.)

hormones, especially progesterone, on the hypothalamus and pituitary.[15]

Endogenous opioid peptides also play a role in the steroid-gonadotropin interrelationships. Endogenous opiates are modulated by ovarian steroids. From a nadir in the early follicular phase, circulating β-endorphin levels rise to peak at midcycle.[16] β-Endorphin exerts inhibitory control on gonadotropin secretion.[17,18]

At the start of a menstrual cycle, when estrogen and progesterone levels are low, the FSH level begins to rise, stimulating follicular growth. Inhibin, a peptide produced by granulosa cells in response to FSH, facilitates the development of one primary follicle through suppression of FSH.[19] The LH also rises (negative feedback). Soon, one follicle dominates and others become atretic. The maturing dominant follicle produces an increasing amount of estradiol, which by negative feedback leads to a decline in FSH level and by positive feedback culminates in a peak of estradiol. The high level of estrogen exerts a stimulatory (positive feedback) effect on LH release, whereas LH release is suppressed at low estrogen levels.[20] This high estrogen level just prior to midcycle triggers the pituitary to release a burst of LH and a concomitant surge of FSH. The follicle ruptures and ovulation occurs. The high midcycle LH peak is closely followed by a decrease in the estradiol level.

The ovulatory follicle undergoes changes, including vascularization and incorporation of lipids and lutein, a yellow pigment. This luteinization begins prior to ovulation, resulting in an increase in progesterone. The progesterone facilitates the surge of LH and FSH.[21] After ovulation, the ruptured follicle is converted into a corpus luteum (yellow body), which secretes large amounts of progesterone and some estrogen. These hormone levels increase, reach a peak in the midluteal phase, and via negative feedback inhibit secretion by the pituitary of LH and FSH and thus reduce the stimulus for follicular development. If the oocyte is not fertilized, the corpus luteum deteriorates as lipid levels decline and vascularity decreases. Progesterone and estradiol levels return to the lower follicular phase levels. This decline in the levels of these steroids results in spasm of the spiral arteries of the endometrium, and menses occurs. LH and FSH levels rise owing to release of negative feedback inhibition, permitting the de-

velopment of a new cohort of follicles and the start of a new menstrual cycle.

This repetitive menstrual cycle pattern becomes irregular during the transition into menopause, principally owing to changes in the structure and function of the ovary.

### Changes in the Ovary

The ovaries of older women differ structurally and functionally from those of younger women. With aging, the ovaries become smaller, stromal tissue increases and fewer oocytes are present.[22] The decline in the number of oocytes begins before birth. The number of oocytes is greatest (about 7 million) in the ovaries of a fetus of about 20 weeks. By birth, the number has fallen to about 2 million, and by puberty, to less than 300,000.[23] The oocytes are largely lost to atresia, plus a small number to ovulation. Some primordial follicles and corpora lutea have been found in ovaries several years after menopause,[24,25] with some follicular growth and hormone secretion, but fewer and fewer follicles reach maturity, ovulation, and luteinization.[25]

### Changes in Menstrual Cyclicity

About age 40 years, while regular menstrual bleeding may continue, hormone patterns may become increasingly variable, apparently owing to aging of the ovary. During this perimenopausal period, changes in menstrual cycle length begin. The patterns of these changes have been documented in two major longitudinal, prospective studies—Treloar's in the United States[26] and Vollman's in Switzerland.[27] Records of women's menstrual histories from menarche to menopause establish that the years just preceding menopause are characterized by menstrual cycle irregularity reminiscent of that in the years just after menarche (Figure 25-2). The mean duration of this perimenopausal menstrual cycle irregularity was 5.0 years (Figure 25-3).[8]

Vollman's subjects recorded their daily basal body temperature (BBT) and reported no midcycle increase in BBT. This suggested that perimenopausal menstrual cycle irregularity was characterized by an increasing number of anovulatory

HUMAN MENSTRUAL CYCLE VARIATION

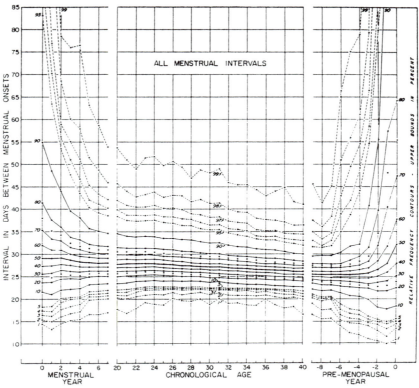

**Figure 25-2.** Menstrual cycle lengths: puberty to menopause. (From Treloar AE, Boynton RE, Behn BG, et al. Variation of the human menstrual cycle through reproductive life. Int J Fertil 1967; 12:93, with permission.)

cycles and that shorter cycles resulted from a shorter follicular phase.[27] The menstrual irregularity may be manifested clinically as oligomenorrhea, polymenorrhea, or amenorrhea, but changes in the menstrual pattern do not predict when the final menses will occur.[28]

### Endocrine Changes

During the perimenopause, the general trend is one of increasing levels of circulating FSH, while changes in the LH pattern lag somewhat, usually just prior to menopause, when marked increases in LH are noted (Figure 25-4).[29–31] Estrogen level generally is not markedly decreased in this period.[32] Within these general trends, individual patterns of gonadotropins vary, not only between

women, but in one woman over time. The range of hormone levels during this period is from normal premenopausal levels to levels characteristic of postmenopausal women. While menstrual cycles continue, there may be increases in circulating FSH and decreases in peak levels of estradiol at midcycle and during the luteal phase; LH concentrations remain relatively unchanged. Other observed endocrine patterns include (1) high levels of estrogen, FSH, and LH and (2) high LH but low FSH.[33] The various patterns of FSH and LH may reflect decreased sensitivity to estrogen or altered regulation by the hypothalamus or pituitary, or they may be the result of decreasing levels if inhibin, an ovarian hormone that contributes to the regulation of FSH.[19,20,29,34,35] Circulating FSH and LH levels may continue to rise for 2 to 3 years after menopause. Thereafter, FSH and LH concen-

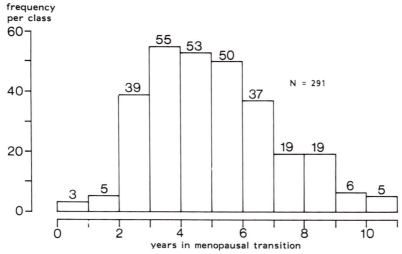

Figure 25-3. Duration of the menopausal transition. (From Treloar AE. Menstrual cyclicity and the premenopause. Maturitas 1981; 3:260, with permission.)

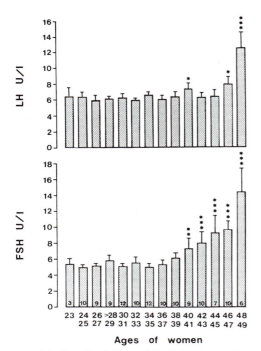

**Figure 25-4.** Age distribution of geometric mean (± error of the mean) of LH and FSH plasma concentrations in 127 women aged 23 to 49 years. The number of women in each age group is given at the base of each column. (*P<.05; **P<.01; ***P<.001.) (From Lenton EA, Sexton L, Lee S, et al. Progressive changes in LH and FSH and LH:FSH ratio in women throughout reproductive life. Maturitas 1988; 10:39, with permission.)

trations begin to fall (Figure 25-5).[36–38] Postmenopausally, a pulsatile pattern of release still characterizes both LH and FSH secretion.[39]

During reproductive life the principal ovarian steroid is 17β-estradiol, produced by developing follicles. The ovary also secretes estrone, progesterone, androstenedione, and testosterone.[40] Smaller amounts of estrone, a biologically weaker estrogen than estradiol, are produced by peripheral conversion of androstenedione.[41–43]

During the menopausal period, with the continuing reduction in the number of follicles, cyclical ovarian production of estradiol and progesterone eventually stops, though for several years postmenopausally the ovary is capable of some small degree of estrogen production.[44–47] In postmenopausal women, estrone, produced largely by conversion of adrenal androstenedione, becomes the primary circulating estrogen.[48] This conversion to estrone takes place largely in adipose tissue[45,49] but also in bone, muscle, and other tissue.[50] With age, conversion of androstenedione to estrone becomes more efficient.[51] Estrogen level in postmenopausal women is correlated with body weight, and is particularly high in obese women.[43,45,46,49,52] Circulating estradiol is derived primarily from peripheral conversion of estrone.[53] The progesterone level does not change substantially with age.[52]

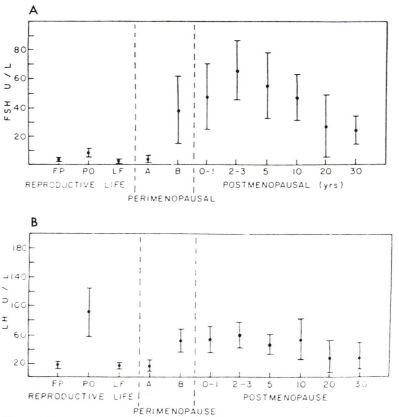

**Figure 25-5.** Plasma FSH (*A*) and LH (*B*) values (mean ± S.D.) at different ages. The normal values in the reproductive phase are given as follicular phase, peak ovulatory phase, and luteal phase. Groups A and B refer to women who are still menstruating who attended the menopausal clinic with apparent climacteric symptoms. Group A had no hot flushes. Group B represents the patients who complained of hot flushes symptoms. FSH and LH values at various years after the menopause are also shown. (From Studd J, Chakravarti S, Oran D. The climacteric. Clin Obstet Gynaecol 1977; 4:6, with permission.)

Most of the androgen circulating postmenopausally is produced by the adrenal gland. The level of circulating androstenedione is about half what it was before menopause: the postmenopausal ovary produces about 20% of the circulating androstenedione.[32,39,45,47,52,54] Ovarian testosterone secretion drops only slightly, if at all, and the total circulating testosterone level is only slightly lower postmenopausally than it was premenopausally.[32,39,54,55] The drop in ovarian estrogen production relative to the amount of ovarian testosterone being produced may account for the

increased hirsutism some women experience after menopause.[55] Thus, the postmenopausal endocrine environment is quite different from the premenopausal (Figure 25-6).

### Fertility in the Perimenopause

Between age 40 and 50 years, when menstrual cycles may become increasingly irregular with long periods of amenorrhea interspersed between occasional menses, women may not know whether

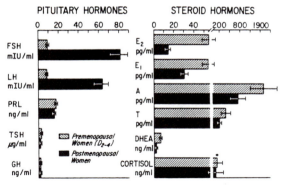

PITUITARY HORMONES          STEROID HORMONES

**Figure 25-6.** Circulating levels of pituitary and steroid hormone in postmenopausal women as contrasted with premenopausal women (days 2 to 4 of menstrual cycle). (From Yen SSC. The biology of menopause. J Reprod Med 1977; 18:290, with permission.)

they are still ovulating, and thus fertile. Ovulation has been documented in women throughout the menopausal transition, even when menstrual cycles are irregular and gonadotropin levels are elevated, and as long as 3 years after the last menstrual period.[24,29,56] The incidence of pregnancy is low after age 45, and rare after age 50.[24] Although there is histologic evidence of corpus luteum formation in women after age 50,[24] biochemically, the corpus luteum may be incapable of supporting a pregnancy and the ova may be inadequate for fertilization or implantation.[24,57]

### Signs, Symptoms, and Sequelae of Menopause

The nature and severity of symptoms women experience during the menopausal years vary much.

Some women cease to menstruate and have no associated symptoms; others experience many problems. When symptoms do appear, they may begin in the perimenopausal period and continue long after menstrual cycles stop, or they may first be manifested after cessation of menses. (Figure 25-7).

Hot flashes (hot flushes) are most clearly associated with menopause and a low estrogen level (described later); atrophic vaginitis is also consistently associated with a decline in estrogen level. Many other symptoms have been attributed to menopause, though inconsistently. These include fatigue, headache, memory loss, irritability, poor concentration, crying spells, and dizziness. There is no consensus among physicians, social scientists, and women themselves about which symptoms are attributable to physiologic changes underlying menopause, which are due to general physiologic aging, and which are the result of simultaneous psychological or social factors that may beset women at midlife.

To resolve these issues, it must be kept in mind that menopause is a biological process and a sociocultural phenomenon. Women in different cultures have different experiences of menopause and different expectations of symptoms. Both depend in part on their culture's attitudes toward and stereotypes of menopausal women. Whether a woman reports any symptoms, or which symptoms a woman relates to menopause, is influenced by her culture's definition of menopause.[58–60] In Western societies, hot flashes are the concomitant of menopause most widely accepted as having a biologic basis. In Japan and Indonesia, the reported frequency of hot flashes is far less than in the United States.[61,62] Mayan women in Yucatan, Mexico, do

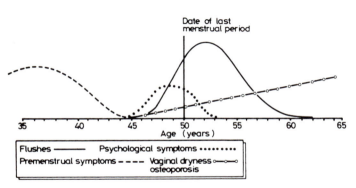

**Figure 25-7.** Occurrence of common problems with respect to the date of the last menstrual period. (From Coope J. Menopause: Diagnosis and treatment. Br Med J 1984; 289:888–890, with permission.)

not report any symptoms at menopause other than menstrual cycle irregularity.[63] In cultures in which hot flashes are not frequently reported, it is not known whether the physiological changes such as increased heart rate, sweating, and skin temperature, measured in association with hot flashes, are absent, or are present but not attributed to menopause. In Africa, the sweating of hot flashes is sometimes misdiagnosed as malaria.[64] Physiological processes may be affected by factors such as diet, exercise, climate, and the reproductive practices of a culture. It is, therefore, not surprising that the reported prevalence of hot flashes varies widely from culture to culture.

## Multiple Effects of Decreased Estrogen Level

Estrogen has multiple effects on the body, especially on the reproductive and urinary systems. Estrogen receptors are present in the ovaries, vagina, cervix, fallopian tubes, distal urethra, and bladder.[65] The rate and magnitude of the change in circulating estrogen level varies among women, as does the rate and extent of the resultant target tissue changes. For some women, physical and physiological changes occur slowly and are barely noticeable; for others, changes are marked and occur rather rapidly. This may be due to the rate of fall of hormones, since sudden changes are particularly evident in women whose ovaries have been surgically removed or rendered nonfunctional by radiation or chemotherapy. Drugs or diseases that alter the estrogen level may also affect the extent of the estrogen-related changes. Whether clinical problems are caused by the decline in estrogen level depends on a complex interplay of factors. A synergistic interaction between aging and estrogen depletion causes urogenital atrophy, but the relative contributions of the two components have not been determined.

### Vulva

The external genitalia, which are highly vascular during reproductive years,[66] become less vascular as estrogen levels decline.[66] The labia become less sensitive, and less responsive to sexual stimulation.[67] The lower estrogen level leads to a decrease in vulvar skin elasticity and other atrophic changes. Skin conditions such as lichen sclerosis become more prevalent.[68,69] Pubic hair thins and the labia majora, which previously contained much subcutaneous fat, become smaller and more wrinkled as this fat layer is reduced.[68]

### Vagina

With a decline in ovarian estrogen production, the vaginal epithelium becomes thin and more susceptible to irritation (atrophic vaginitis). The vagina becomes shorter, narrower, and less flexible and distensible. Vaginal blood flow decreases and vaginal secretions diminish, reducing the protective layer of moisture on the cells lining the vagina and decreasing sexually stimulated fluid production.[70,71] Inadequate lubrication and dryness of the vagina, in conjunction with the structural changes, can result in discomfort during intercourse (dyspareunia), and even bleeding.[68] Women who are sexually active tend to have less vaginal atrophy than women of similar age and estrogen level who are not.[72] These atrophic changes are responsive to estrogen treatment (topical or oral), which increases the thickness of the vaginal mucosa, increases vaginal perfusion, restores vaginal fluid production, and results in lowered pH.[73,74]

The population of microorganisms in the vagina is also affected by estrogen. Doderlein's lactobacilli and other acidophilic bacteria normally present in the vagina, metabolize glycogen, which is plentiful in well-estrogenized cells. The organic acids produced by this metabolism help keep the vaginal pH acidic, thus favoring the lactobacilli over pathogenic bacteria and minimizing vaginal infections.[74] As estrogen levels decline, there are fewer layers of epithelial cells lining the vagina, and cell glycogen content is reduced. There is a reduction in the number of lactobacilli, and a resulting change in pH from acidic to alkaline. This alkaline environment increases the risk of vaginal infection by bacteria such as staphylococci and streptococci.[70,74] Estrogen treatment helps reduce vaginal pH and restore a more favorable balance to the bacterial population.

The range and severity of these problems is

great. Some women have minor discomfort, which is remedied by short-term, local estrogen treatment. Others experience significant pain and vaginal dryness so extreme as to make even walking uncomfortable.[75] Few statistics are available on the incidence of these symptoms.

### Cervix and Uterus

As estrogen levels decline, atrophic changes occur in the epithelium of the cervix and less mucus is produced by the endocervical glands. The cervix, which once protruded into the vagina, may retract and become flush with the wall of the vagina.[67,76] The uterus decreases in size, the endometrial lining becomes thin, and there is decreased vascularization. Epithelial cells flatten and the glands become inactive. Myometrial fibers change in structure and become atrophic. If fibroids are present, they tend to shrink.[65,68]

Relaxation of the pelvic muscles and other structures supporting the uterus and urinary tract organs may result in a descensus of these organs, and consequent discomfort,[67,77] though pelvic relaxation may also be related to parity, birth trauma, and obesity.[50]

### Breasts

The breast is also a target organ for estrogen. In the postmenopausal years as a result of a decrease in glandular and subcutaneous fatty tissue the breasts tend to shrink and become less elastic.[68] Some women's breasts retain their normal appearance, even at an advanced age, and a small number of women report increased breast size, though the explanation for this is not clear.[78]

### Skin and Hair

Skin changes with age. It becomes less elastic and more pigmented; sweat and sebaceous gland activity is reduced,[79] and the skin becomes drier. The epidermis thins and subcutaneous fat is reduced, resulting in wrinkling of the skin. Skin contains estrogen receptors and is thus a target tissue for

estrogen,[80,81] and it has been demonstrated that estrogen therapy increases epidermal thickness in surgically menopausal women.[82] Hair loss may be noted at sites that are influenced by loss of estrogen (e.g., pubic, axillary, scalp), whereas hair growth may increase on sites presumably affected by the greater relative amount of androgen (e.g., chin, upper lip).

### Urinary System

The lower portion of the urinary tract and the lower reproductive tract tissues have a common embryonic origin. Thus, urinary tract tissues are also estrogen sensitive and undergo atrophic changes similar to those in the vaginal epithelium. As estrogen levels decline, the urethral mucosa becomes thin and friable, and vascularity diminishes.[83] These changes may manifest as reduced ability to control urine. Urethral closure pressure, important in the maintenance of continence, may diminish in the years after menopause.[67] Cystitis, urinary frequency, urgency, suprapubic pain, and dysuria may increase after menopause (atrophic urethritis).[50,67,77,78,84] Some of these symptoms respond favorably to estrogen treatment.[78,85] Estrogen loss may also be one cause of a reduction in the support of pelvic organs provided by pelvic muscles, ligaments, and fascia. This may facilitate the occurrence of cystocele, cystourethrocele, and rectocele.[50,67,86] Reduction in the support of the bladder and urethra contributes to diminished urinary control, since periurethral muscles contract less effectively.

Although urinary problems are a troubling complaint of menopausal women, the incidence or seriousness of these problems in the general population is not known. Hagstad and Janson[87] found no significant differences in the percentage of urinary incontinence between menstruating (8.1%) and postmenopausal (11.1%) women; others have observed a significantly higher rate of incontinence in older women.[88,89] Notelovitz[78] reported that 30% of women aged 45 to 65 years reported nocturia. And Rekers[90] reported that among a random sample of postmenopausal women in Holland, the frequency of urinary symptoms were approximately these: incontinence 26%, urgency 15%, frequency 20%, nocturia 18%, and dysuria 11%.

### Lipoproteins and Coronary Heart Disease

Between puberty and menopause women have a much lower incidence of coronary heart disease (CHD) than men.[91] After menopause, CHD becomes a leading cause of death in women.[92,95] Menopause, not age per se, is the critical factor, as postmenopausal women have a higher risk of CHD than age-matched, menstruating women.[92,96] Clinical and epidemiologic studies have demonstrated that a low level of low-density lipoprotein (LDL) cholesterol and an elevated level of high-density lipoprotein (HDL) cholesterol are predictors of reduced risk of CHD in both men and women.[97,98] Throughout adult life, HDL cholesterol levels in women exceed those of men, whereas LDL cholesterol levels in women are lower than those of men until age 50, when they increase and surpass those of men.[99]

There is substantial evidence that sex steroids play a significant role in the regulation of these serum lipids and lipoproteins. The increase in the female to male ratio of deaths from CHD that occurs at menopause, and the fact that CHD is rare in younger women but high in men younger than 50 years, suggests that estrogen is a critical factor in women's favorable lipoprotein profile and lower risk of CHD prior to menopause. Studies of the effects of estrogens on lipoproteins, including exogenous estrogen administration to postmenopausal women, have consistently, over many years, demonstrated that estrogens increase HDL cholesterol and decrease LDL cholesterol.[100–103]

Thus, estrogen's role in producing a lipid profile that is correlated with reduced CHD is compelling, despite continued controversy about the effect of postmenopausal estrogen treatment on CHD. Though some studies show no statistically significant effect of estrogen on CHD[93,104] or elevated risk,[105] most demonstrate a beneficial effect.[94,95,100,106–108]

### Skeletal System

Estrogen's role in bone metabolism becomes extremely significant in postmenopausal women. Chapter 27 Skeletal Physiology and Osteoporosis is devoted to osteoporosis, and to bone metabolism.

### Hot Flashes

Hot flashes, which affect many women in the menopausal years, are recurrent, transient periods of heat sensation, flushing, sweating, palpitations, and a sense of anxiety, often followed by chills. The terms *hot flash, hot flush, night sweat,* and *vasomotor instability* are used interchangeably. More women seek medical treatment for hot flashes than any other menopausal complaint; yet the specific cause and physiology of hot flashes, the most characteristic manifestation of the menopausal period, are still unknown.

### Epidemiology

Information on the prevalence of hot flashes is based principally on studies of menopausal symptoms conducted in several Western countries (Great Britain, the Netherlands, Scotland, Sweden, the United States). The prevalence of hot flashes ranges from 24% to 92%, being highest in the first 2 years after menopause and gradually declining after that.[109–116] Hot flash prevalence rates tend to be higher with surgical menopause than with natural menopause, at least for the first year after ovariectomy.[115–119] Hot flashes have been reported in many different cultures and ethnic groups, including Japanese, Indian, African, American Indian, Mexican American, and Mayan.[61,63,120–124] Findings of studies to identify characteristics that might predispose women to hot flashes have been contradictory.

Pre- and perimenopausal women also report hot flashes; reported prevalences range from 6% to 61%.[5,87,109–112,116,121] In a study of women who reported hot flashes, 50% of participants reported onset of hot flashes prior to menopause (sometimes 5, 10, or 15 years before), when menstrual cycles were still regular or were becoming irregular (Figure 25-8).[116] Some women do not begin having hot flashes until a number of years after menstruation has stopped. Hot flashes typically subside within 6 months to 2 years, though they can continue many years, even as long as 40 years after cessation of menstrual cycles (Figures 25-9).[116]

Within and among individuals, the frequency, intensity, and duration of hot flashes vary. For the

## Age and Menstrual Cycle Status at Onset of Hot Flashes

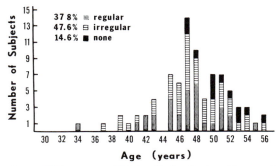

**Figure 25-8.** Age at which hot flashes begin with respect to menstrual cycle status at that time.

majority of women experiencing them, frequency and severity peak during the first 2 to 5 years following menopause. Hot flashes may occur monthly, weekly, or hourly. For about 15% of affected women, hot flashes occur many times a day. In the perimenopausal period hot flashes may come and go as menstrual cycles stop and start again. The intensity of hot flashes can vary from mild to severe, and the duration of each episode, while typically lasting 3 to 5 minutes, occasionally can last 30 minutes or more (Figure 25-10).[125]

Many women experience an aura when a hot flash is about to begin. It is described as a sense of anxiety, a change in heart rate, or a sense of "dis-ease." The hot flash itself, in addition to the sweating, sensation of heat, and flushing, may include a feeling of panic, suffocation, or frustration.[116]

Hot flashes occur spontaneously; however, some women report specific triggers for their hot flashes, including a warm or confined environment, coffee, alcohol, sex, or stress.[116] Hot flashes are particularly distressing at night, when a woman's sleep often is disrupted several times because she awakens drenched in sweat and must change her nightclothes and sheets. This pattern of sleep, punctuated by awakenings associated with hot flashes, is illustrated in Figure 25-11. The concomitant decreases in chest skin temperature reflect evaporative cooling with each sudden, transient outpouring of sweat. Rapid, marked increases in heart rate accompany the hot flashes. The disrupted sleep leads to fatigue and irritability and can adversely affect spousal and other family and work relationships.

### Thermoregulatory Physiology

Hot flashes appear to be the result of a perturbation of the brain's thermoregulatory center, activating heat loss (vasodilation and sweating at hot flash onset) and heat conservation (vasoconstriction and shivering at termination of the hot flash) mechanisms. Hot flashes are marked by a characteristic

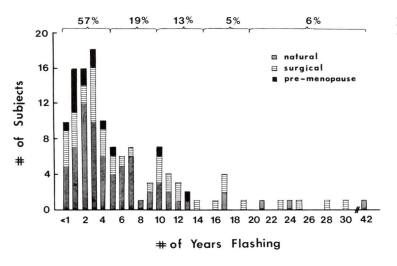

**Figure 25-9.** Number of years women experience hot flashes.

A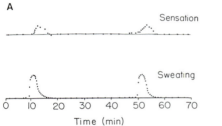

B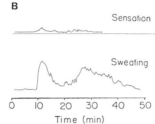

**Figure 25-10.** Subjective sensation and sweating patterns in discrete and prolonged hot flashes. (From Kronenberg F, Downey JA. Thermoregulatory physiology of menopausal hot flashes: A review. Can J Physiol Pharmacol 1987; 65:1315, with permission.

pattern of thermoregulatory responses and hormone changes that are well-documented (Figure 25-12).[116,125–132]

Immediately before the onset of the hot flash, women often report a brief aura that alerts them to an impending hot flash. Increases in heart rate (up to 38%)[116,133,134] and blood flow (four to 30 times)[116,133] occur during this aura, slightly before the hot flash is sensed. Most women report that their sensation of heat and sweating is predominantly in and on the upper body, and in particular, the chest, neck, face, and scalp. The wave of heat typically is described as spreading upward. Sweat on the chest and forehead evaporates, resulting in cooling of the skin; it can be measured indirectly as a decrease in skin temperature (Figure 25-11). The rapid rise in finger temperature (1° to 7°C)

that follows the vasodilatation,[116,135,136] in combination with sweating and the resulting evaporative cooling (thermoregulatory heat loss responses), results in a decrease in internal body temperature (0.1° to 0.9°C).[116,126,128,131]

Hot flashes appear to be the body's response to sudden, transient downward resetting of the body's thermostat (temperature set-point), which is located in the hypothalamus.[116,128] This set-point resetting would cause the sensation of intense heat and activation of heat loss responses, including behavioral adjustments, cutaneous vasodilatation and sweating, and a drop in core temperature. When subsequently the temperature set-point returns to normal, the sensation becomes one of chilliness, as body temperature has fallen below normal, and heat conservation (vasoconstriction),

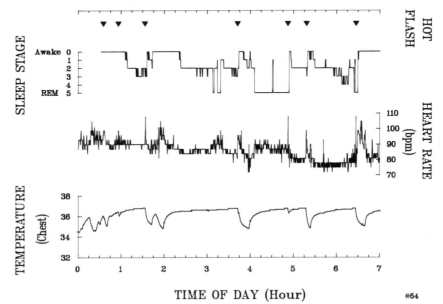

**Figure 25-11.** Association of nocturnal awakenings with hot flashes in a postmenopausal woman (temperatures in Celsius scale).

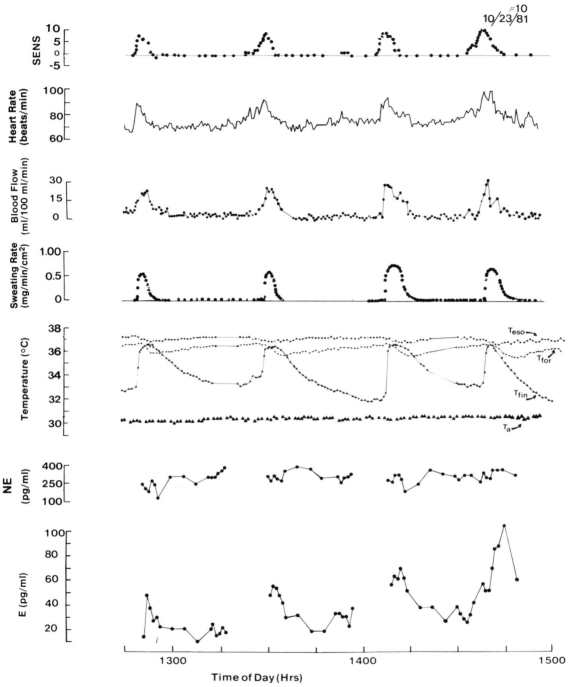

**Figure 25-12.** Pattern of cardiovascular, thermoregulatory, and endocrine changes for four consecutive hot flashes over a 2-hour period. Changes in sensation (SENS), heart rate, blood flow (finger), sweating rate, temperatures (esophageal, forehead, finger, ambient), norepinephrine (NE), and epinephrine (E) are depicted. (From Kronenberg F, Downey JA. Thermoregulatory physiology of menopausal hot flashes: A review. Can J Physiol Pharmacol 1987; 65:1314, with permission.)

heat production (shivering), and behavioral adjustments are activated to bring body temperature back to normal.[135] This constellation of physiologic and behavioral changes that characterize a hot flash suggests an integrated thermoregulatory event whose pattern is the inverse of that during a fever.[132]

### Endocrinology

Observation of an abrupt onset of hot flashes following bilateral ovariectomy and the relief of hot flashes with estrogen therapy suggested a relationship between low plasma estrogen levels and hot flashes.[119,137] Reports that levels of circulating estrone and estradiol are lower in women with hot flashes than in women with no hot flashes provide further support for this relationship[138–140]; however, a low estrogen level is not the complete explanation for hot flashes. All postmenopausal women have a low estrogen level, but some never have hot flashes and others have them only sporadically or only for a short while.

Hot flashes are not triggered by the high or pulsatile gonadotropin patterns characteristic of menopause, as, despite continued high gonadotropin levels, hot flashes often decline or stop after menopause. Although LH pulses may be temporally correlated with hot flashes,[116,135,136,141] hot flashes occur in women who have no episodic LH release, such as those who have undergone hypophysectomy,[142] in pre- or postmenopausal women whose pulsatile LH release has been suppressed by treatment with a GnRH analogue[143–145] and in women with pituitary insufficiency and hypoestrogenism.[146]

A variety of substances have been found to increase in the peripheral blood in association with hot flashes, including epinephrine,[125,147] neurotensin,[131] β-endorphin, β-lipotropin, adrenocorticotropin,[130] cortisol, androstenedione, dehydroepiandrosterone,[130,141] and growth hormone.[129] Norepinephrine (NE) decreases during hot flash episodes[125]; levels of estradiol, estrone,[141] FSH,[135,148] prolactin,[129,136,148] dopamine,[136] and TSH remain the same.[129] Thus, though there is some relationship between low estrogen level and hot flashes, other factors clearly are involved in triggering individual hot flash episodes.

### Modulating Factors

Environmental temperature influences the frequency and intensity of hot flashes: cool ambient temperatures reduce the frequency and intensity of hot flashes, warmer temperatures increase them.[149] Thus, sleeping in a cool room generally may be expected to decrease the prevalence of hot flashes and resultant awakenings.

## Sleep Patterns

Several survey studies of menopausal symptoms have reported increased complaints of insomnia after menopause as compared with menstruating women.[4,5,110,112] Nighttime awakenings in menopausal women are often associated with hot flashes.[150] Sometimes women awaken 30 to 60 seconds before feeling the hot flash; at other times they awaken already drenched in sweat. Figure 25-12 illustrates the abrupt change in sleep state associated with the reported hot flashes. If the hot flash is mild, the woman may quickly fall asleep again. If the sweating is profuse she may have to further disrupt her sleep by getting up to change clothes and bedding. Sometimes, the changes in heart rate, sweating, and skin temperature characteristic of hot flashes continue throughout the night and are associated with transient electroencephalogram-documented arousals that do not cause conscious awakening (Kronenberg, unpublished observations). These brief arousals may also contribute to poorer quality sleep and diminished functioning the next day.[151] Treatment with estrogen has been shown to decrease nocturnal hot flashes, reduce the frequency of awakenings,[150,152] and decrease the amount of wake time.[153]

Many other complaints of menopausal women —depression, poor concentration, irritability, anxiety—can negatively affect sleep.[154] Ravnikar[155] suggested that these problems, and the insomnia and hot flashes, may all be interrelated, and related to the hormone changes at menopause. Schiff and colleagues[153] reported that estrogen administration improved clinically rated psychological adjustment and reduced hot flashes and improved the quality of sleep. In a survey of women aged 40 to 55 years, Ballinger[156] found the highest incidence of psychiatric problems in women 45 to 49 years old, but observed no clear relationship between psychiatric problems and hot flashes. Ballinger[157] found no correlation between sleep disturbance and menopausal status and reported that sleep disturbances occurred in women both with and without psychiatric disorders. She concluded that while it seems that relationships may exist between hormone levels and hot flashes and hormone levels and psychological function, they may not be the same relationships.

Estrogen's influence on sleep and mood has yet to be clearly defined. Estrogen does affect enzymes that control biogenic amines involved in regulating both sleep and mood state,[155] but further research is needed to understand more fully the interrelationships between the many central and peripheral actions of estrogen.

## Sexual Functioning

Most research in human sexuality has focused on sexual functioning as it relates to intercourse and orgasm. Now, a broader perspective of the meaning of a satisfying sexual and sensual life for people of all ages is becoming widely accepted.[158,159] Sexuality, sensuality, love, and affection are important to healthy living for people of all ages. Recent information on the sex lives of middle-aged and older people,[160] supporting earlier reports,[161,162] indicates that healthy women can retain interest in and enjoyment of sex throughout life. This information is calling into question stereotyped notions of menopausal women as uninterested in or incapable of enjoying sex. Certainly, postmenopausal changes in anatomy and physiology consequent to a decline in estrogen level can affect sexual functioning, but existing research suggests that though hormone changes may impinge on optimal sexual functioning, the degree to which the hormone-induced changes actually disrupt this functioning depends on social, psychological, and health factors.

### Anatomic and Physiologic Changes

Most of what is known about changes in sexual functioning associated with menopause involves changes in sexual anatomy and physiology that are principally due to diminished estrogen level and the resultant decrease in blood flow to the genitourinary area. Change in sexual responsiveness is manifested in a slightly slower time to arousal, lubrication, and clitoral response; in less lubrication, less vasocongestion, and a shorter-lived and less intense orgasm.[66,163] The breast continues to respond to sexual arousal, but with diminished vasocongestive response. Painful uterine contractions may occur with orgasm.[66,162] The reduction in vaginal lubrication and the dryness and irritation of the vaginal wall predispose to vaginitis. This, in combination with a narrower, less flexible vagina, can lead to discomfort, or even pain, during intercourse.

Maintaining sexual activity reduces vaginal atrophy and helps preserve the functional capacity for lubrication.[50,72,86,162,164] Self-stimulation also helps maintain sexual responsiveness and contributes to reducing atrophic changes.[164] Administration of oral or local estrogen can help increase vaginal blood flow, mucosal wall thickness, and vaginal lubrication.[73]

### *Modification of Function*

Despite the age-related reduction in estrogen level and physiological changes in the urogenital system, women can remain sexually interested and responsive throughout life. A *change* in function does not imply *dys*function. The majority of women experience no change in libido; some report an increase of sexual desire that possibly is due in part to the relative increase in circulating androgens,[165–167] but also to feeling relief from the fear of pregnancy and the annoyance of birth control. Yet physical discomfort, such as dyspareunia and hot flashes, may cause anxiety and tension, which can negatively affect the desire for sex, and therefore, sexual responsiveness.[72]

Little research has been done on the physiology of the sexual response in postmenopausal women. Masters and Johnson[162] documented that the capacity for orgasm remains intact, though the intensity and duration of the orgasm may be reduced and the overall sexual response is decreased and requires more stimulation. Morrell and coworkers[163] reported that postmenopausal women demonstrate lower estrogen levels and less sexual responsiveness to erotic films than younger (mean age 31) normally cycling women, and older (mean age 51) cycling women, as measured by vaginal pulse amplitude. Thus, it seems that menopausal status, not age per se, is the critical factor.

Many women are concerned about maintaining a satisfying sexual relationship as they enter their postmenopausal years. An individual's sexual behavior after menopause depends to a great extent on her satisfaction with her sex life before menopause, and on the responsiveness and sensitivity of her partner.[161] Genital tract changes do not necessarily affect a woman's capacity as a lover. The problems a woman faces also can be due to physical changes in her partner, to a partner ignorant of the changes that both may be experiencing, or, more likely, to the lack of a partner.[168] Demographics indicate that there are far more older women than available men. Masturbation and homosexuality are not practiced by many older women today; thus, many have no sexual outlet. If they do have a partner of the same age or older, his sexual responsiveness is likely to have declined, a phenomenon manifested as increased time to achieve erection and decreased ability to maintain it. Surgery or medication may also affect men's sexual functioning.

But a changing body does not have to mean a reduction in the quality of sexual interaction. Sex is, of course, more than just intercourse, orgasm, and the anatomy and physiology of sex organs. Sensual and sexual arousal can involve the whole body. The slower arousal time that both men and women experience as they grow older can provide an opportunity to explore new ways to heighten sexual enjoyment.

## Conclusions

In the last 10 years, menopause has emerged as a significant area of clinical and basic research. In this chapter we have presented current information about menopause, including an indication of the range of symptom patterns that may be seen in clinical practice. Though we have focused on symptoms that have been described extensively in Western populations, physicians in North America may see patients from a variety of cultural and ethnic backgrounds. It is helpful, therefore, to be aware that women of different cultures may have different perceptions and definitions of whether or how their problems, both psychological and physiological, relate to menopause.

Currently, about a third of American women are 45 years of age or older.[169] Health issues of concern to them, such as osteoporosis and cardiovascular disease, and the relationship of these diseases to the hormone changes of menopause, have made their way into the media. Today, physicians are treating women who have more medical information than ever before, who ask many questions, and who deserve informed and considered responses.

In concentrating on the physiology of menopause, one risks giving the impression that the changes described are due solely to menopause, and that all women experience them as problems. While the biological changes that occur with menopause can cause serious problems for some women, for many others they pose few, if any. Changes associated with menopause are complexly interrelated with concomitant aging processes. The ability and capacity to adapt to these changes varies with each person. We do well to keep in mind Margaret Mead, who spoke of her menopausal years as an energetic and creative time and reported that women in most societies exhibit a *postmenopausal zest*.[170]

## References

1. Jaszmann L, Van Lith ND, Zaat JCA. The age at menopause in the Netherlands: The statistical analysis of a survey. Med Gynaecol Androl Sociol 1969; 4:256–262.
2. Frere G. Mean age at menopause and menarche in South Africa. S Afr J Med Sci 1971; 36:21–24.
3. McKinlay S, Jefferys M, Thompson B. An investigation of the age at menopause. J Biosoc Sci 1972; 4:161–173.
4. Jaszmann L. Epidemiology of climacteric and post climacteric complaints. Front Horm Res 1973; 2:22–34.
5. Thompson B, Hart SA, Durno D. Menopausal age and symptomatology in a general practice. J Biosoc Sci 1973; 5:71–82.
6. Treloar AE. Menarche, menopause, and intervening fecundability. Hum Biol 1974; 46(1):89–107.

7. van Keep PA, Brand PC, Lehert P. Factors affecting the age at menopause. J Biosoc Sci 1979; 6(suppl):37–55.

8. Treloar AE. Menstrual cyclicity and the premenopause. Maturitas 1981; 3:249–264.

9. Jick H, Porter J, Morrison AS. Relation between smoking and natural menopause. Lancet 1977; 1:1354–1355.

10. Kaufman DW, Slone D, Rosenburg L, et al. Cigarette smoking and age at natural menopause. Am J Public Health 1980; 70:420–422.

11. Willett W, Stampfer MJ, Bain C, et al. Cigarette smoking, relative weight, and menopause. Am J Epidemiol 1983; 117:651–658.

12. McKinlay SM, Bifano N, McKinlay JB. Smoking and age at menopause in women. Ann Intern Med 1985; 103:350–356.

13. Stanford JL, Hartge P, Brinton LA, et al. Factors influencing the age at natural menopause. J Chron Dis 1987; 40:995–1002.

14. Brand PC, Lehert PH. A new way of looking at environmental variables that may affect the age at menopause. Maturitas 1978; 1:121–132.

15. Veldhuis JD, Christiansen E, Evans WS, et al. Physiological profiles of episodic progesterone release during the midluteal phase of the human menstrual cycle: Analysis of circadian and ultradian rhythms, discrete pulse properties, and correlations with simultaneous luteinizing hormone release. J Clin Endocrinol Metab 1988; 66:414–421.

16. Wehrenberg WB, Wardlaw SL, Frantz AG, et al. β-Endorphin in hypophyseal portal blood: Variations throughout the menstrual cycle. Endocrinology 1982; 111:879–881.

17. Reid RL, Hoff JD, Yen SSC, et al. Effect of exogenous β-endorphin on pituitary hormone secretion and its disappearance rate in normal human subjects. J Clin Endocrinol Metab 1981; 52:1179–1183.

18. Ferin M, Van Vugt D, Wardlaw S. The hypothalamic control of the menstrual cycle and the role of endogenous opioid peptides. Recent Prog Horm Res 1984; 40:441–485.

19. McLachlan RI, Robertson DM, Healy DL, et al. Circulating immunoreactive inhibin levels during the normal human menstrual cycle. J Clin Endocrinol Metab 1987; 65:954.

20. Speroff L, Glass RH, Kase NG. Clinical Gynecologic Endocrinology & Infertility. Baltimore: Williams & Wilkins, 1989.

21. March CM, Marrs RP, Goebelsmann U, et al. Feedback effects of estradiol and progesterone upon gonadotropin and prolactin release. Obstet Gynecol 1981; 58:10–16.

22. Nicosia SV. The aging ovary. Med Clin North Am 1987; 71:1–10.

23. Baker TG. A quantitative and cytological study of germ cells in human ovaries. Proc R Soc Lond [Biol] 1963; 158:417–433.

24. Novak ER. Ovulation after fifty. Obstet Gynecol 1970; 36:903–910.

25. Costoff A, Mahesh VB. Primordial follicles with normal oocytes in the ovaries of postmenopausal women. J Am Geriatr Soc 1975; 23:193–195.

26. Treloar AE, Boynton RE, Behn BG, et al. Variation of the human menstrual cycle through reproductive life. Int J Fertil 1967; 12:77–126.

27. Vollman RF. The Menstrual Cycle. Philadelphia: WB Saunders, 1977.

28. Kaufert PA, Gilbert P, Tate R. Defining menopausal status: The impact of longitudinal data. Maturitas 1987; 9:217–226.

29. Sherman BM, West JH, Korenman SG. The menopausal transition: Analysis of LH, FSH, estradiol, and progesterone concentrations during menstrual cycles of older women. J Clin Endocrinol Metab 1976; 42:629–636.

30. Reyes FI, Winter JSD, Faiman C. Pituitary-ovarian relationships preceding the menopause. Am J Obstet Gynecol 1977; 129:557–563.

31. Lenton EA, Sexton L, Lee S, et al. Progressive changes in LH and FSH and LH:FSH ratio in women throughout reproductive life. Maturitas 1988; 10:35–43.

32. Chang RJ, Judd HL. The ovary after menopause. Clin Obstet Gynecol 1981; 24:181–191.

33. Metcalf MG, Donald RA, Livesey JH. Pituitary-ovarian function in normal women during the menopausal transition. Clin Endocrinol 1981; 14:245–255.

34. Marrs RP, Lobo R, Campeau JD, et al. Correlation of human follicular fluid inhibin activity with spontaneous induced follicular maturation. J Clin Endocrinol Metab 1984; 58:704–709.

35. Sherman BM. Endocrinologic and menstrual alterations. In: Mishell DR Jr, ed. Menopause: Physiology and Pharmacology. Chicago: Year Book, 1987;41–51.

36. Wide L, Nillius SJ, Gensell C, et al. Radioimmunosorbent assay of follicle-stimulating hormone and luteinizing hormone in serum and urine from men and women. Acta Endocrinol (Copenh) 1973; 174:1–58.

37. Chakravarti S, Collins WP, Forecast JD, et al. Hormonal profiles after the menopause. Br Med J 1976; 2:784–786.

38. Studd J, Chakravarti S, Oram D. The climacteric. Clin Obstet Gynaecol 1977; 4:3–29.

39. Judd HL. Reproductive hormone metabolism in

postmenopausal women. In: Eskin BA, ed. The Menopause. Comprehensive Management. New York: Masson, 1980;55–71.

40. Somma M, Sandor T, Lanthier A. Site of origin of androgenic and estrogenic steriods in the normal human ovary. J Clin Endocrinol 1969; 29:457–466.

41. Baird DT, Horton R, Longcope C. Steriod dynamics under steady-state conditions. Recent Prog Horm Res 1969; 25:611–664.

42. Baird DT, Fraser IS. Blood production and ovarian secretion rates of estradiol-17β and estrone in women throughout the menstrual cycle. J Clin Endocrinol Metab 1974; 38:1009–1017.

43. Casey ML, MacDonald PC. Origin of estrogen and regulation of its formation in postmenopausal women. In: Buschman HJ, ed. The Menopause. New York: Springer-Verlag, 1983;1–8.

44. Poliak A, Jones GES, Goldberg B, et al. Effect of human chorionic gonadotropin on postmenopausal women. Am J Obstet Gynecol 1968; 101:731–739.

45. Vermeulen A, Verdonck L. Factors affecting sex hormone levels in postmenopausal women. J Steroid Biochem 1979; 11:899–904.

46. Vermeulen A. Sex hormone status of the postmenopausal woman. Maturitas 1980; 2:81–89.

47. Longcope C, Hunter R, Franz C. Steroid secretion by the postmenopausal ovary. Am J Obstet Gynecol 1980; 138:564–568.

48. Grodin JM, Siiteri PK, MacDonald PC. Source of estrogen production in post-menopausal women. J Clin Endocrinol Metab 1973; 36:207–214.

49. MacDonald PC, Edman CD, Hemsell DL, et al. Effect of obesity on conversion of plasma androstenedione to estrone in postmenopausal women with and without endometrial cancer. Am J Obstet Gynecol 1978; 130:448–455.

50. Edman CD. The climacteric. In: Buchsbaum HJ, ed. The Menopause. New York: Springer-Verlag, 1983;23–33.

51. Hemsell DL, Grodin JM, Brenner PF, et al. Plasma precursors of estrogen. II. Correlation of the extent of conversion of plasma androstenedione to estrone with age. J Clin Endocrinol Metab 1974; 38:476–479.

52. Meldrum DR, Davidson BJ, Tataryn IV, et al. Changes in circulating steroids with aging in postmenopausal women. Obstet Gynecol 1981; 57:624–628.

53. Judd HL, Shamonki IM, Frumar AM, et al. Origin of serum estradiol in postmenopausal women. Obstet Gynecol 1982; 59:680–686.

54. Vermeulen A. The hormonal activity of the postmenopausal ovary. J Clin Endocrinol Metab 1976; 42:247–253.

55. Judd HL, Judd GE, Lucas WE, et al. Endocrine function of the postmenopausal ovary: Concentration of androgens and estrogens in ovarian and peripheral blood. J Clin Endocrinol Metab 1974; 39:1020–1024.

56. Sherman BM, Korenman SG. Hormonal characteristics of the human menstrual cycle throughout reproductive life. J Clin Invest 1975; 55:699–706.

57. Kaufman SA. The menopause. In: McElin TW, Sciarra JJ, eds. Gynecology and Obstetrics. New York: Harper and Row, 1981;1–11.

58. Flint M. The menopause: Reward or punishment. Psychosomatics 1975; 16:161–163.

59. Kaufert P, Syrotuik J. Symptom reporting at the menopause. Soc Sci Med 1981; 15E:173–184.

60. Kaufert PA, Gilbert P, Hassard T. Researching the symptoms of menopause: An exercise in methodology. Maturitas 1988; 10:117–131.

61. Lock M, Kaufert P, Gilbert P. Cultural construction of the menopausal syndrome: the Japanese case. Maturitas 1988; 10:317–332.

62. Agoestina T, van Keep PA. The climacteric in Bandung, West Java province, Indonesia; A survey of 1025 women between 40–55 years of age. Maturitas 1984; 6:327–333.

63. Beyene Y. Cultural significance and physiological manifestations of menopause: A biocultural analysis. Cult Med Psychiatry 1986; 10:47–71.

64. Thornton JG. Menopausal hot flushes: Personal experience in Africa. Trop Doct 1984; 140:135.

65. Brown KH, Hammond CB. Urogenital atrophy. Obstet Gynecol Clin North Am 1987; 15:13–32.

66. Sarrel PM. Sexuality in the middle years. Obstet Gynecol Clin North Am 1987; 4:49–62.

67. Bergman A, Brenner PF. Alterations in the urogenital system. In: Mishell DR Jr., ed. Menopause: Physiology and Pharmacology. Chicago: Year Book, 1987;67–75.

68. Voet RL. End organ response to estrogen deprivation. In: Buchsbaum HJ, ed. The Menopause. New York: Springer-Verlag, 1983;9–22.

69. Barber HRK. Perimenopausal and Geriatric Gynecology. New York: Macmillan, 1988.

70. Semmens JP, Wagner G. Estrogen deprivation and vaginal function in postmenopausal women. JAMA 1982; 248:445–448.

71. Tsai CC, Semmens JP, Semmens EC, et al. Vaginal physiology in postmenopausal women: pH value, transvaginal electropotential difference, and estimated blood flow. South Med J 1987; 80:987–990.

72. Bachmann GA, Lieblum SR, Kemmann E, et al. Sexual expression and its determinants in the postmenopausal woman. Maturitas 1984; 6:19–29.

73. Semmens JP, Tsai CC, Semmens EC, et al. Effects

of estrogen therapy on vaginal physiology during menopause. Obstet Gynecol 1985; 66:15–18.

74. Bergh PA. Vaginal changes with aging. In: Breen JL, ed. The Gynecologist and the Older Patient. Rockville: Aspen, 1988;299–311.

75. Cobb JO. Understanding Menopause. Toronto: Key Porter Books, 1988.

76. Singer A. The uterine cervix from adolescence to the menopause. Br J Obstet Gynaecol 1975; 82:81–99.

77. Karafin LJ, Coll ME. Lower urinary tract disorders in the postmenopausal woman. Med Clin North Am 1987; 71:111–122.

78. Notelovitz M. Gynecologic problems of menopausal women: Part 3. Changes in extragenital tissues and sexuality. Geriatrics 1978; 33:51–58.

79. Kligman AM, Grove GL, Balin AK. Aging of human skin. In: Finch CE, Schneider EL, eds. The Biology of Aging. New York: Van Nostrand Reinhold, 1985;820–841.

80. Stumpf WE, Sar M, Joshi SG. Estrogen target cells in the skin. Experientia 1974; 30:196–198.

81. Hasslequist MB, Goldberg N, Schroeter A, et al. Isolation and characterization of the estrogen receptor in human skin. J Clin Endocrinol Metab 1980; 50:76–82.

82. Brincat M, Studd J. Skin and menopause. In: Mishell DR Jr, ed. Menopause: Physiology and Pharmacology. Chicago: Year Book, 1987;103–114.

83. Corlett RC. Urinary tract disorders. In: Buchsbaum HJ, ed. The Menopause. New York: Springer Verlag, 1983;131–138.

84. Smith P. Age changes in the female urethra. Br J Urol 1972; 44:667–676.

85. Brown ADG. Postmenopausal urinary problems. Clin Obstet Gynecol 1977; 4:181–206.

86. Notelovitz M. Gynecologic problems of menopausal women: Part 1. Changes in genital tissues. Geriatrics 1978; 33:24–30.

87. Hagstad A, Janson PO. The epidemiology of climacteric symptoms. Acta Obstet Gynecol Scand Suppl 1986; 134:59–65.

88. Thomas TM, Plymat KR, Blannin J, et al. Prevalence of urinary incontinence. Br Med J 1980; 281:1243–1245.

89. Brocklehurst JC, Fry J, Griffiths LL, et al. Urinary infection and symptoms of dysuria in women aged 45–64 years, their relevance to similar findings in the elderly. Age Ageing 1972; 1:41–47.

90. Rekers H. Urogenital problems. In:Zichella L, Whitehead M, van Keep PA, eds. The Climacteric and Beyond. New Jersey: Parthenon, 1988;145–146.

91. Tsang R, Gleuck CJ. Atherosclerosis, a pediatric perspective. Curr Probl Pediatr 1979; 9:3–37.

92. Gordon T, Kannel WB, Hjortland MC, et al. Menopause and coronary heart disease: The Framingham Study. Ann Intern Med 1978; 89:157–161.

93. Pfeffer RI, Whipple GA, Kurosak TT, Chapman JM. Coronary risk and estrogen use in postmenopausal women. Am J Epidemiol 1978; 107:479–487.

94. Ross RK, Paganini-Hill A, Mack TM, et al. Menopausal oestrogen therapy and protection from death from ischaemic heart disease. Lancet 1981; 1:858–860.

95. Bush TL, Miller VT. EFfects of pharmacologic agents used during menopause: Impact on lipids and lipoproteins. In: Mishell DR Jr, ed. Menopause: Physiology and Pharmacology. Chicago: Year Book, 1987;187–208.

96. Kannel WB, Hjortland MC, McNamara PM, et al. Menopause and risk of cardiovascular disease. The Framingham Study. Ann Intern Med 1976; 85:447–452.

97. Castelli WB, Doyle JT, Gordon T, et al. HDL cholesterol and other lipids in coronary heart disease. The Cooperative Lipoprotein Phenotyping study. Circulation 1977; 55:767–772.

98. Gordon T, Castelli WP, Hjortland MP, et al. The Framingham Study. High lipoprotein as a protective factor against coronary heart disease. Am J Med 1977; 62:707–714.

99. Heiss G, Tamir I, Davis CE, et al. Lipoprotein-cholesterol distributions in selected North American populations: The Lipid Research Program prevalence study. Circulation 1980; 61:302–315.

100. Bush TL, Barrett-Connor E. Noncontraceptive estrogen use and cardiovascular disease. Epidemiol Rev 1985; 7:80–104.

101. Wallace RB, Hoover J, Barrett-Connor E, et al. Altered plasma lipid and lipoprotein levels associated with oral contraceptive and oestrogen use. Lancet 1979; 2:111–115.

102. Cauley JA, LaPorte RE, Kuller LH, et al. Menopausal estrogen use, high density lipoprotein cholesterol subfractions and liver function. Arteriosclerosis 1983; 49:31–39.

103. Wahl P, Walden C, Knopp R, et al. Effect of estrogen/progestin potency on lipid/lipoprotein cholesterol. N Engl J Med 1983; 308:862–867.

104. Rosenberg L, Armstrong B, Jick H. Myocardial infarction and estrogen therapy in post-menopausal women. N Engl J Med 1976; 294:1256–1259.

105. Wilson PWF, Garrison RJ, Castelli WP. Postmenopausal estrogen use, cigarette smoking, and cardiovascular morbidity in women over 50. N Engl J Med 1985; 313:1038–1043.

106. Bain C, Willett W, Hennekens CH, et al. Use of

postmenopausal hormones and risk of myocardial infarction. Circulation 1981; 64:42–46.

107. Stampfer MJ, Colditz GA, Willett WC, et al. Postmenopausal estrogen therapy and cardiovascular disease. N Engl J Med 1991; 325:756–762.

108. Kennedy DL, Baum C, Forbes MB. Noncontraceptive estrogens and progestins: Use patterns over time. Obstet Gynecol 1985; 65:441–446.

109. Goodman MJ, Stewart CJ, Gilbert F Jr. Patterns of menopause. A study of certain medical and physiological variables among Caucasian and Japanese women living in Hawaii. J Gerontol 1977; 32:291–298.

110. McKinlay SM, Jefferys M. The menopausal syndrome. Br J Prev Soc Med 1974; 28:108–115.

111. Jaszmann L, Van Lith ND, Zaat JAC. The perimenopausal symptoms: The statistical analysis of a survey. Part A & B. Med Gynaecol Androl Sociol 1969; 4:268–277.

112. Neugarten BL, Kraines RJ. "Menopausal symptoms" in women of various ages. Psychosomat Med 1965; 27:266–273.

113. Smith G, Waters WE. An epidemiological study of factors associated with perimenopausal hot flushes. Publ Hlth 1983; 97:347–351.

114. James CE, Breeson AJ, Kovacs G, et al. The symptomatology of the climacteric in relation to hormonal and cytological factors. Br J Obstet Gynaecol 1984; 91:56–62.

115. Feldman BM, Voda AM, Gronseth E. The prevalence of hot flash and associated variables among perimenopausal women. Res Nurs Health 1985; 8:261–268.

116. Kronenberg F. Hot flashes: Epidemiology and physiology. Ann NY Acad Sci 1990; 592:52–86.

117. Sherman BM, Wallace RB, Bean JA, et al. The relationship of menopausal hot flushes to medical and reproductive experience. J Gerontol 1981; 36:306–309.

118. Chakravarti S, Collins WP, Newton JR, et al. Endocrine changes and symptomatology after oophorectomy in premenopausal women. Br J Obstet Gynaecol 1977; 84:769–775.

119. Utian WH. The true clinical features of postmenopause and oophorectomy, and their response to oestrogen therapy. S Afr Med J 1972; 46:732–737.

120. Lock M. Ambiguities of aging: Japanese experience and perceptions of menopause. Cult Med Psychiatry 1986; 10:23–46.

121. Sharma VK, Saxena MSL. Climacteric symptoms: A study in the Indian context. Maturitas 1981; 3:11–20.

122. Moore B. Climacteric symptoms in an African community. Maturitas 1981; 3:25–29.

123. Wright AL. On the calculation of climacteric symptoms. Maturitas 1981; 3:55–63.

124. Kay M, Voda AM, Olivas G, et al. Ethnography of the menopause-related hot flash. Maturitas 1982; 4:217–227.

125. Kronenberg F, Cote LJ, Linkie DM, et al. Menopausal hot flashes: Thermoregulatory, cardiovascular, and circulating catecholamine and LH changes. Maturitas 1984; 6:31–43.

126. Molnar GW. Body temperatures during menopausal hot flashes. J Appl Physiol 1975; 38:499–503.

127. Sturdee DW, Wilson KA, Pipili E, et al. Physiological aspects of menopausal hot flash. Br Med J 1978; 2:79–80.

128. Tataryn IV, Lomax P, Bajorek JG, et al. Postmenopausal hot flushes: A disorder of thermoregulation. Maturitas 1980; 2:101–107.

129. Meldrum DR, DeFazio JD, Erlik Y, et al. Pituitary hormones during the menopausal hot flash. Obstet Gynecol 1984; 64:752–756.

130. Genazzani AR, Petraglia F, Facchinetti F, et al. Increase of proopiomelanocortin-related peptides during subjective menopausal flushes. Am J Obstet Gynecol 1984; 149:775–779.

131. Kronenberg F, Carraway RE. Changes in neurotensin-like immunoreactivity during menopausal hot flashes. J Clin Endocrinol Metab 1985; 60:1081–1086.

132. Kronenberg F, Downey JA. Thermoregulatory physiology of menopausal hot flashes: A review. Can J Physiol Pharmacol 1987; 65:1312–1324.

133. Ginsberg J, Swinhoe J, O'Reilly B. Cardiovascular responses during the menopausal hot flush. Br J Obstet Gynaecol 1981; 88:925–930.

134. Nesheim BI, Saetre T. Changes in skin blood flow and body temperatures during climacteric hot flashes. Maturitas 1982; 4:49–55.

135. Tataryn IV, Meldrum DR, Lu KH, et al. FSH and skin temperature during menopausal hot flush. J Clin Endocrinol Metab 1979; 49:152–154.

136. Casper RF, Yen SSC, Wilkes MM. Menopausal flushes: A neuroendocrine link with pulsatile luteinizing hormone secretion. Science 1979; 205:823–825.

137. Aksel S, Schomberg DW, Iyrey L, et al. Vasomotor symptoms, serum estrogens and gonadotropin levels in surgical menopause. Am J Obstet Gynecol 1976; 12:165–169.

138. Erlik Y, Meldrum DR, Judd HL. Estrogen levels in postmenopausal women with hot flashes. Obstet Gynecol 1982; 59:403–407.

139. Abe T, Furvhashi N, Yamaya Y, et al. Correlation between climacteric symptoms and serum levels of estradiol, progesterone, follicle-stimulating

hormone, and luteinizing hormone. Am J Obstet Gynecol 1977; 129:65–67.

140. Chakravarti S, Collins WP, Thom MH, et al. Relation between plasma hormone profiles, symptoms, and responses to oestrogen treatment in women approaching the menopause. Br Med J 1979; 1:983–985.

141. Meldrum DR, Tataryn IV, Frumar AM, et al. Gonadotropins, estrogens, and adrenal steroids during the menopausal hot flash. J Clin Endocrinol Metab 1980; 50:685–689.

142. Mulley G, Mitchell JRA, Tattersall RB. Hot flushes after hypophysectomy. Br Med J 1977; 2:1062.

143. Casper RF, Yen SSC. Menopausal flushes: Effect of pituitary gonadotropin desensitization by a potent luteinizing hormone releasing factor agonist. J Clin Endocrinol Metab 1981; 53:1056–1058.

144. Lightman SL, Jacobs SJ, Maguire AK. Downregulation of gonadotropin secretion in postmenopausal women by superactive LHRH analogue: Lack of effect on menopausal flushing. Br J Obstet Gynaecol 1982; 89:977–980.

145. DeFazio J, Meldrum DR, Laufer L, et al. Induction of hot flashes in premenopausal women treated with a long-acting GnRH agonist. J Clin Endocrinol Metab 1983; 56:445–448.

146. Meldrum DR, Erlik Y, Lu JKH, et al. Objectively recorded hot flushes in patients with pituitary insufficiency. J Clin Endocrinol Metab 1981; 52:684–687.

147. Mashchak CA, Kletzky OA, Artal R, et al. The relation of physiological changes to subjective symptoms in postmenopausal women with and without hot flushes. Maturitas 1984; 6:301–308.

148. Lightman SL, Jacobs HS, Maguire AK, et al. Climacteric flushing: Clinical and endocrine response to infusion of naloxone. Br J Obstet Gynaecol 1981; 88:919–924.

149. Kronenberg F, Barnard RM. Modulation of menopausal hot flashes by ambient temperature. J Therm Biol 1992; 17:43–49.

150. Erlik Y, Tataryn IV, Meldrum DR, et al. Association of waking episodes with menopausal hot flushes. JAMA 1981; 245:1741–1744.

151. Carskadon MA, Dement WC. Nocturnal determinants of daytime sleepiness. Sleep 1982; 5:573–581.

152. Thomson J, Oswald I. Effects of oestrogen on the sleep, mood, and anxiety of menopausal women. Br Med J 1977;2:1317–1319.

153. Schiff I, Regestein Q, Tulchinsky D, et al. Effects of estrogens on sleep and psychological states of hypogonadal women. JAMA 1979; 242:2405–2407.

154. Fry JM. Sleep disorders. Med Clin North Am 1987; 71:95–111.

155. Ravnikar VA, Schiff I, Regestein QR. Menopause and sleep. In: Buchsbaum HJ, ed. The Menopause. New York: Springer-Verlag, 1983;161–171.

156. Ballinger CB. Psychiatric morbidity and the menopause: Screening of general population sample. Br Med J 1975; 3:344–346.

157. Ballinger CB. Subjective sleep disturbance at the menopause. J Psychosomat Res 1976; 20:509–513.

158. Davidson JM. The psychobiology of sexual experience. In: Davidson JM, Davidson RJ, eds. The Psychobiology of Consciousness. New York: Plenum, 1980;271–332.

159. Weg RB. Sexuality in the menopause. In: Mishell DR Jr, ed. Menopause: Physiology and Pharmacology. Chicago: Year Book, 1987;127–138.

160. Brecher EM. Love, sex, and aging: A summary. In: Brecher EM, ed. Love, Sex, and Aging. A Consumers Union Report. Boston: Little, Brown, 1984;403–408.

161. Kinsey A, Pomeroy W, Clyde M. Sexual Behavior in the Human Female. Philadelphia: WB Saunders, 1953.

162. Masters WH, Johnson VE. Human Sexual Responses. Boston: Little, Brown, 1966.

163. Morrell MJ, Dixen JM, Carter CS, et al. The influence of age and cycling status on sexual arousability in women. Am J Obstet Gynecol 1984; 148:66–71.

164. Leiblum S, Bachmann G, Kemmann E, et al. Vaginal atrophy in the postmenopausal woman. JAMA 1983; 249:2195–2198.

165. Persky H, Dreisbach L, Miller W, et al. The relation of plasma androgen levels to sexual behaviors and attitudes of women. Psychosomat Med 1982; 44:305–319.

166. Sherwin BB, Gelfand MM, Brender W. Androgen enhances sexual motivation in females: A prospective, crossover study of sex steroid administration in the surgical menopause. Psychosomat Med 1985; 47:339–351.

167. Bachmann GA, Leilblum SR, Sandler B, et al. Correlates of sexual desire in postmenopausal women. Maturitas 1985; 7:211–216.

168. Weg RB. The physiological perspective. In: Weg RB, ed. Sexuality in The Later Years. New York: Academic Press, 1983;39–80.

169. U.S.Department of Commerce Bureau of Census. Current Population Reports. Series P-25,Nos 512,917,1022. Washington, D.C.: US Bureau of the Census, 1980.

170. Mead M. PMZ at work. Behav Today 1975;498.

# Chapter 26

# Aphasia, Apraxia, and Agnosia

JOHN C. M. BRUST

## Handedness and Cerebral Dominance

Approximately 90% of people are "right handed"; they have better motor dexterity with their right limbs and prefer to use them in complex motor tasks such as throwing a ball or writing.[1,2] More than 90% of right-handers process language in the left cerebral hemisphere (left cerebral dominance), damage to which causes aphasia. Ten per cent of people are left handed, though among them the degree of left preference varies considerably and some are left-handed as a result of cerebral disease. Approximately half of left-handers also have left cerebral dominance for language, and the other half have right dominance. Overall, the hemispheric specialization of left-handers appears to be less pronounced, which may account for the observation that when they develop aphasia it is more likely than in right-handers to be mild or to resolve.

## Aphasia: Definition and Historical Background

*Aphasia* is a disturbance of language unexplained by articulatory impairment or sensory loss. Abnormal speech (dysarthria) secondary to paresis, spasticity, incoordination, abnormal movements, or dysphonia is not aphasia, and reading difficulty secondary to poor vision is not alexia. Aphasia is a disturbance of higher cortical function resulting from cerebral damage. Though it can occur in isolation, especially after head injury or stroke, aphasia is often a feature of a dementing illness such as Alzheimer's disease, and most severe aphasics have additional cognitive impairment not related to language.

The modern study of aphasia began in the 1860s with Broca's description of left hemispheric lesions in patients with language disturbance.[3,4] Although details of the neurologic examinations were sparse and the lesions were large (including temporal and frontal lobes and insula), Broca's reports led not only to the recognition that language was usually processed in the left hemisphere but to the notion that the left frontal pars opercularis ("Broca's area") was the "center" for speech, destruction of which caused *expressive aphasia*.

A decade later, Wernicke described infarction of the posterior superior temporal gyrus in patients with impaired speech comprehension.[5] Analogous to Broca's area, this posterior opercular region ("Wernicke's area") became regarded as the "center" for speech comprehension. Wernicke also attributed difficulty in naming and repetition to lesions in the deep white matter tract connecting Wernicke's and Broca's area (the arcuate fasciculus) and called the resulting disorder *conduction aphasia*.

These reports were followed by a spate of clinical-anatomic correlations that attempted to define "centers" not only for particular language skills such as reading and writing but for nonlanguage cognitive activities as well.[6] (For example, as late as the 1920s, Henschen claimed there were centers for musical expression and reception, with a separate center for violin playing.[7]) Early skepticism for such compartmentalization was expressed by Hughlings Jackson, who stressed that loss of function following a focal lesion does not necessarily mean that the damaged region is a "center" for that function.[8] This controversy—between those who sought to understand language by focusing on anatomic localization and those whose emphasis was psychological or linguistic—persists today, and a consequence has been a bewildering diversity of aphasia classifications.[9–19] In the United States, a classification that has found its way into many current medical and neurologic texts is that of Geschwind.[20,21] Oriented to the concept of centers and disconnections between them, it is as controversial as its historical predecessors. The advantage for clinicians of Geschwind's system, however, is that while it may seem pathophysiologically and linguistically simplistic, it depends on easily assessible symptoms and signs and a relatively unambiguous definition of aphasia subtypes. Geschwind's approach, which lends itself either to brief bedside screening or more formal testing such as the Boston Diagnostic Aphasia Examination,[22] can be said to *work* practically, even if its ultimate neuropsychological or linguistic validity remains uncertain.

## Examination of the Patient

Language assessment consists of six parts: spontaneous speech, speech comprehension, naming, repetition, writing, and reading. Abnormalities in one sphere obviously influence strategies employed to test others. Equally obvious is that nonlanguage mental abnormalities (e.g., obtundation, delirium, schizophrenia, dementia) can make language assessment difficult or impossible. Conversely, assessment of memory or cognition can be impossible when aphasia is present. The following outline is based on the assumption that the patient is cooperative and that language is impaired out of proportion to any coexisting mental abnormalities.

One assesses spontaneous speech by posing questions or remarks designed to elicit full-sentence replies. *Fluency* refers to the amount of speech produced over time (normally more than 50 words per minute.)[23] Word-finding difficulty can produce nonfluent hesitations, but except with very severe anomia the patient is usually able to produce several consecutive words or syllables at a normal rate. By contrast, the speech of so-called Broca's aphasia (defined later) is severely and consistently nonfluent independently of word-finding per se and often marked by long delays in initiation and hesitations between words and syllables.

*Prosody* refers to the musical qualities of speech, including rhythm, accent, and pitch.[24–26] It gives languages and dialects their special oral character. There are different kinds of prosody. That which characterizes the emotional quality of speech ("sad, glad, mad") is believed to depend on right hemisphere processing. Prosody also provides propositional information, for example the pitch inflections that characterize a sentence as interrogative or imperative, or, in languages such as Chinese or Thai, that convey the semantic meaning of words. Propositionally linked prosody is processed in the language hemisphere and can be impaired in some kinds of aphasia.

The term *paraphasia* describes incorrect words unintentionally substituted for correct ones. There are two types of paraphasic errors. In *literal* or *phonemic* paraphasia, words produced phonetically resemble the intended word but contain one or more substituted syllables (e.g., "hosicle" for "hospital"). When such alterations have the character of real words, they are called *neologisms;* sometimes ingeniously concocted (e.g., "nork" for a combination of knife and fork), they are not specific to aphasia, occurring also in psychotic speech. In *verbal* or *semantic* paraphasia, real but unintended words are produced (e.g., "hotel" for "hospital"); the substituted word is often semantically close to the intended word. In some patients, paraphasic errors are occasional contaminants of speech. In others, they almost entirely replace it; such speech is called *jargon.*

Even in the absence of paraphasia, the content of aphasic speech may be difficult to grasp. Severely restricted vocabulary may cause logorrheic but empty speech rather than word-finding hesitations. For example, an answer to the question, "Why are you in the hospital?" went, "Well, it was when I did that, that they said I should and so I did here." The term *paragrammatism* refers to the seemingly preserved syntax amidst such profoundly restricted semantic content. By contrast, syntactic or relational words (e.g., prepositions, conjunctions, possessives, verb tenses) are sometimes conspicuously abnormal or absent in aphasic speech, especially with Broca's aphasia; such speech, practically reduced to nouns and verbs, is called *agrammatic* or *telegrammatic*.

Some patients, again especially those with Broca's aphasia, have markedly restricted and nonfluent propositional speech yet produce outbursts of relatively fluent emotional or "inferior" speech. Such dissociation led Jackson to postulate that nonpropositional speech (e.g., amenities or invective cursing) is processed in the nondominant hemisphere. Sometimes aphasic speech is limited largely to a single sentence, cliche, or even syllable, so-called recurrent utterance.

Having assessed spontaneous speech, the examiner proceeds to the patient's own speech comprehension, for if that is impaired, the rest of the examination must be restructured. Strikingly abnormal speech comprehension may become apparent only on shifting from open-ended conversation to specific testing. Moreover, abnormalities of speech comprehension (like any neurologic sign) may be mild or severe, or may become more severe as the examination progresses.

Assessment of speech comprehension should be as independent as possible of the patient's own verbal output: a wrong answer to a question could signify a paraphasic error rather than failure to understand the question. Asking the patient to follow spoken commands carries similar potential ambiguities. If a command, simple or complex, is followed, and if the examiner has remembered to avoid nonverbal cues, it can be presumed that it was understood. Failure to follow a command, however, could have different possible explanations, for example paralysis, apraxia, pain, or negativism.

A more reliable method of testing speech comprehension is to ask yes-no questions. Even patients whose own speech is so severely restricted that they cannot say the words *yes* or *no* can usually indicate affirmative or negative. The correct answers must of course be known to both the patient and the examiner. Failure to identify a public figure, for example, could signify loss of memory or lack of interest rather than impaired speech comprehension. Appropriate questions might include, "Is your name Mrs. Jones?" or (if the patient can see), "Am I wearing a hat?" The informational content of questions can be steadily increased (e.g., "Am I wearing a red striped necktie?").

Alternatively, the patient can be asked to point to objects or body parts; motor disability such as apraxia is less likely to interfere with such tasks than with command following. Again, questions can be made increasingly complex (e.g., from "Where is the ceiling?" to "Where is the source of artificial illumination in this room?" to "Where did we enter this room?" A variant of the formal Token Test[27] relies on similar identification of increasingly information-laden images; shown an array of drawings the patient might be asked to point first to a circle (not a square), then to a large (not a small) circle, then to a large red (not a large blue) circle.

These strategies detect disorders of semantic comprehension. As with abnormal speech output, semantic and syntactic or relational comprehension can dissociate.[28] Syntactic or relational comprehension can be assessed (in patients with adequate motor ability) by object manipulation. First identifying, say, a comb, a pen, and a key, the patient is asked to put the key *on top of* the comb, or the comb *between* the key and the pen. Alternatively, the patient could be given a statement such as, "Tom's aunt's husband has blue eyes," and then be asked, "Is the person with blue eyes a man or a women?"

Naming ability is tested in patients with adequate vision by showing them objects, body parts, colors, or pictures of actions ("confrontation naming"). Patients with impaired vision can be asked to name body parts being touched or to name from description (e.g., "What do you shave with?" "What is the color of grass?"). Patients with impaired speech comprehension may not grasp the nature of the task. A variety of abnormal responses indicate anomia. Some patients produce literal or verbal paraphasias, which may or may not then be self-corrected. Some hesitate and effortfully grope for the correct word (tip-of-the-tongue phenomenon); such patients, though unable to come up with the word on their own, may correctly select it from a spoken list or say it correctly after being given its first letter or phoneme or an incomplete sentence that the word would appropriately complete (contextual prompting).[29] Other patients describe rather than name the object (e.g., "It's what you wear around your neck," [instead of "necktie"]). Infrequently, anomic patients say simply, "I don't know," or "I've forgotten."

In some aphasics confrontation naming may be unexpectedly good compared to the apparent degree of word-finding difficulty in spontaneous speech. Seeing an object may facilitate lexical entry, and so such patients may have much greater difficulty listing names within a category (e.g., articles of clothing, animals, objects of furniture). Not infrequently, only three or four items can be named.

Repetition is tested by having the patient repeat several sentences (e.g., "Today is a sunny day"; "In the winter the President lives in Washington"). Syntactically loaded sentences may be especially difficult (e.g., "If he were to come, I would go out"). (The phrase, "No *ifs, ands,* or *buts*" has been considered particularly suitable for identifying difficulty with syntax;[21] such an assertion is dubious, because, though the words are all prepositions or conjunctions, they are not being used in a syntactical sense. Moreover, if a sentence is unfamiliar or makes no sense to a patient, difficulty repeating it might have nothing to do with aphasia.) Repetition errors most often consist of paraphasic substitutions.

Testing of writing can begin by having the patient sign his or her name. If that cannot be accomplished, more elaborate tests will almost surely fail. The examiner must be aware, however, that writing one's name does not necessarily rely on language processing per se; in many people it is an "overlearned motor act" more akin to a golf swing than true graphia. One should therefore proceed to dictated sentences, words, or letters, or to spontaneous writing such as describing what one sees in the room. Right hemiparesis need not deter such testing; most people can write, however awkwardly, with their left hand, and the test here is one of language, not penmanship. Left-handed writing would not explain gross spelling errors or paragraphic substitutions. If writing is abnormal, the patient can be asked to spell aloud, type, or use block or other anagram letters. Abnormalities on such tests signify a disorder affecting more than the mechanism of writing; in other words not only letter production but letter choice.[30] Some patients with severe agraphia on spontaneous or dictated writing are able to *copy* writing in a slavish fashion.

A number of abnormal writing patterns have been described. For example, in *lexical agraphia* there is impaired spelling of orthographcially irregular words with preserved spelling of phonologically regular words or nonwords.[31] In *phonologic agraphia* the reverse occurs.[32] Pure agraphia without other language disturbances can occur with metabolic encephalopathy and with focal lesions affecting the frontal, parietal, or temporal lobes. Agraphia is present in most aphasics, and it may be a prominent residual following recovery of speech.

Reading is tested both orally and for comprehension. Using large print (patients often blame reading difficulty on impaired vision), the patient reads aloud simple sentences, words, or letters. Reading comprehension testing can parallel speech comprehension testing. Written commands often involve actions that were successfully executed in response to oral commands and yes-no questions or object identification requests can be posed in writing.

Dissociations between oral reading and reading comprehension can be striking.[33] Some patients understand quite well what they read, yet oral reading quickly disintegrates into incomprehensible paralexia. Others can read aloud with astonishing accuracy and yet comprehend little or nothing of what they read. The term *deep dyslexia* refers to loss of the ability to read aloud phonetically with relative preservation of semantic comprehension.[34] Such patients make frequent verbal paralexic substitutions when reading aloud and may appear not to comprehend what they have read, yet they correctly match the seemingly uncomprehended word with an appropriate picture. By contrast, patients with *surface dyslexia* can read phonetically both real words and nonwords but can no longer attach semantic meaning to what they read.[35]

## Aphasic Syndromes

Assessing spontaneous speech, speech comprehension, naming, repetition, writing, and reading enables one to determine not only the presence of aphasia but its subtype, the approximate location of the lesion, and the patient's particular functional limitations. Regarding aphasia subtypes, one should keep two concepts in mind. First, the variables that define these subtypes are difficult to quantify beyond such terms as mild, moderate, or severe, and labels chosen for particular patients really represent points along a continuum. (Some investigators have asserted that as many as 60% of aphasias cannot be subclassified at all into so-called classical syndromes.[36–38]) Second, though the following classification differs from others in terminology and pathophysiologic interpretation, the clinical phenomena described are similar for different authors.[39,40]

Broca's aphasia is characterized by such extremely nonfluent and nonprosodic speech that the abnormality is easily recognized, even when the patient speaks only a foreign language. There is often dysarthric slurring as well, and the effortful delivery and incompletely executed words and sentences may be incomprehensible because of combined articulatory distortion and paraphasic substitution. Speech, so far as it is understandable, may be agrammatic, with relatively preserved emotional outbursts or recurrent utterances. The patient appears quite aware of his difficulty and is often visibly depressed.

Writing is usually at least as affected as speech and it may not be executed at all: the patient may grasp the pen but not attempt to use it. Speech comprehension and reading are relatively preserved but not normal; errors can usually be demonstrated with specific testing. Ability to name or repeat varies. Some patients name unexpectedly well to confrontation. When repetition is relatively intact compared to spontaneous speech the aphasia is sometimes called *transcortical motor aphasia;* responsible lesions have been observed either superior or anterior to the pars opercularis.[41] Independently of repetition, Broca's aphasics sometimes have remarkably preserved singing ability, with or without words.[42]

Broca's aphasia implies involvement (though not exclusively) of frontal lobe structures. What features of the syndrome are related to the pars opercularis (Broca's area) is still, after more than a century, uncertain.[43] One report correlated nonfluency with computed tomographic lesions affecting the subcallosal fasciculus and periventricular white matter beneath the area of sensorimotor cortex that represents the mouth.[44] In any case, frontal lobe involvement accounts for the observation that the great majority of patients with Broca's aphasia have moderate to severe right hemi-

paresis. They also frequently have buccolingual apraxia (see below).

If pre-, peri-, or subrolandic lesions account for the nonfluency and loss of prosody in Broca's aphasia, then sparing of these regions should predict preserved fluency and prosody. This is the common denominator of several aphasia subtypes caused by lesions restricted to the parietal or temporal lobes. Classification of those subtypes is based on speech comprehension and repetition.

Aphasia characterized by fluent, prosodic speech and moderate or severe impairment of both comprehension and repetition is called *Wernicke's aphasia*. The lesion most often lies in the area originally described by Wernicke, namely the posterior superior temporal gyrus. Speech usually, but not always, is contaminated by paraphasic verbalizations, especially the literal kind; when they are abundant incomprehensible jargon is produced. The preserved fluency and prosody, however, give the speech a normal sound, so that if the patient speaks only a foreign language, aphasia may be unrecognized. Moreover, patients with severe Wernicke's aphasia often fail to recognize that they have any disability (anosognosia) and, preserving paralinguistic aspects of speech (e.g., pausing appropriately for the examiner to speak), participate in a lengthy "conversation," apparently unaware that they do not understand what is being said to them or that they make no sense to others. When testable, naming, writing, and reading are usually, but not always, severely impaired in Wernicke's aphasia; the types of impairment vary much.

When speech is fluent and prosodic and repetition is much more affected than speech comprehension, the patient has *conduction aphasia*. Wernicke, and later Geschwind, placed the responsible lesion in the arcuate fasciculus, allegedly disconnecting Wernicke's and Broca's areas. Others have found greater correlation of symptoms with lesions in the inferior parietal lobule (supramarginal and angular gyri). Patients with conduction aphasia usually have impaired naming and writing. Reading ability varies; frequently observed is nearly normal reading comprehension with paralexic oral reading.

*Anomic aphasia* consists of fluent prosodic speech with normal or nearly normal speech comprehension and repetition. The major difficulty is word finding, usually apparent on spontaneous speech (sometimes so severe that hesitations compromise fluency), confrontation and list naming, and writing. Restricted vocabulary leads to substitution of phrases for missing words and lengthy, "empty" or "circumlocutory" speech. Manifestations of semantic paraphasia occur; those of literal paraphasia and neologisms are usually infrequent.[39] Reading ability varies. When the anomia is of the tip-of-the-tongue type, the term *amnestic aphasia* has been used. That term is misleading, however, as it implies a true memory dysfunction. In fact, memory is usually normal in patients with this type of aphasia, and conversely, patients with severe amnestic disorders (e.g., Korsakoff's syndrome) have normal naming ability. Anomic aphasia is the least localizable of aphasia subtypes; it is a frequent aftermath of more severe aphasic subtypes (e.g., Wernicke's), and it frequently accompanies diffuse dementing illness (e.g., Alzheimer's disease). When it acutely follows a focal lesion such as stroke or trauma, the inferior parietal lobule is often affected; such patients often have agraphia, alexia, or Gerstmann's syndrome (see later). Anomic aphasia can follow damage to any part of the language areas, or even to the nonlanguage hemisphere.

Persons with *transcortical sensory aphasia* produce fluent prosodic speech; repetition is preserved relative to speech comprehension. Responsible lesions have been parietal-occipital, sparing periopercular parietotemporal language areas.[45] Transcortical sensory aphasia has also followed lesions of the posterior thalamus.[46] (A frequent, though nonspecific feature of "subcortical" aphasia is a tendency for even a severe language disturbance to improve rapidly. The role of thalamic or basal ganglia damage per se in such aphasias remains controversial.[39])

As might be predicted anatomically, posterior aphasia syndromes characterized by fluent prosodic speech are usually accompanied by little or no hemiparesis, if any. Homonymous hemianopia and sensory loss are variable. Ideomotor apraxia, when testable, is not unusual (see later).

The term *expressive aphasia* is usually equated with Broca's aphasia, and *receptive aphasia* with Wernicke's aphasia. The terms are misleading: expression is as compromised in severe Wernicke's aphasia as in Broca's aphasia.

Muteness is common in aphasia of sudden onset and has little localizing value (i.e., it does not

signify ultimate nonfluency). Whether aphasia is severe or mild, it is unusual for complete muteness to last more than several days.

The aphasia subtypes discussed so far follow damage to particular periopercular areas while others are spared; they are frequently the result of middle cerebral artery branch occlusions. When damage extends to the entire periopercular, the resulting aphasia can have mixed features (e.g., speech of Broca's type plus loss of speech comprehension). When severe, such mixed aphasias are called *global*. Naming, repetition, writing, and reading are also severely affected. Usually the result of extensive cerebral convexity lesions (e.g., infarction in the entire middle cerebral artery territory, massive head injury, cerebral neoplasm), global aphasia is usually accompanied by hemiplegia, sensory loss, and homonymous hemianopia. (Global aphasia with little or no hemiplegia can follow separate lesions of Broca's and Wernicke's areas, as from embolic strokes.[47]) Global aphasia with preserved repetition is called *mixed transcortical aphasia*. Such patients sometimes repeat what they hear in a compulsive fashion (echolalia), and sometimes, even when they have no speech comprehension, they make correct grammatical transpositions (e.g., on hearing the examiner inquire, "How are you today?" the patient might reply, "How am I today?") Other patients can complete cliches or familiar proverbs or, after getting started with cues, successfully recite "serial speech," such as days of the week. Some demonstrate strikingly preserved singing, with or without words.

In an autopsy case of mixed transcortical aphasia, there was infarction of cerebral cortex surrounding the periopercular language areas, which were themselves intact.[48] A proposed formulation for the transcortical aphasias is that they disconnect the periopercular language areas from the rest of the brain, impairing speech output, speech comprehension, or both, yet allowing repetition through the preserved Wernicke's area, arcuate fasciculus, and Broca's area. Accepting such a formulation, Geschwind referred to mixed transcortical aphasia as *isolation aphasia*.[46] Needless to say, not everyone agrees.

As noted, aphasia subtypes represent artificial compartmentalizations. Moreover, it is not unusual during recovery for Wernicke's aphasia to evolve into conduction and then anomic aphasia, or for global aphasia to evolve into Broca's aphasia.[49,50] Recognizing the oversimplification involved, the clinician can usefully employ aphasia subtypes as guideposts.

A number of other language disturbances do not easily fit into the above spectrum. *Aphemia,* or *anarthria,* refers to speech of Broca's type but without the other language abnormalities often seen with Broca's aphasia, including agraphia.[51] It is a disturbance more of speech than of language. The lesion is believed to be frontal, but whether it involves the pars opercularis, the deep white matter, or other structures remains controversial.

Analogously, *pure word deafness* refers to loss of speech comprehension without the other language abnormalities that usually accompany Wernicke's aphasia, including loss of reading comprehension and paraphasic speech. Nonverbal sounds (e.g., a trumpet sounding, a telephone ringing, or a dog barking) are normally identified. The syndrome is rare. Unilateral or bilateral lesions have involved fibers connecting both auditory cortices (Heschl's gyrus) with the language-dominant auditory association cortex (Wernicke's area). What is heard is thus disconnected from periopercular language areas, which themselves are intact and connected to visual pathways.[52]

*Pure alexia,* or *alexia without agraphia,* describes loss of the ability to read in the absence of any other aphasic features. The patient can write spontaneously or to dictation but is then unable to read what he has written.[53,54] Most often the result of left posterior cerebral artery occlusion, the syndrome usually (but not always) includes right homonymous hemianopia; alexia is attributed to posterior corpus callosum damage with disconnection of what is seen (by the right occipital lobe) from the left hemisphere. (When homonymous hemianopia is absent, the lesion is presumed to disconnect both visual cortices from left hemispheric language areas.) Patients with pure alexia can sometimes slowly read individual letters. Color anomia is frequently present.

Unilateral or bilateral damage to the medial frontal lobe (supplementary motor cortex and cingulate gyrus) can cause difficulty initiating and sustaining speech and writing. Whether such language disturbance should be called aphasic is questionable; paraphasias generally do not occur, and the patient is often abulic (*bradyphrenic,* without initiative).[55,56]

Gerstmann's syndrome consists of agraphia, acalculia, left-right confusion, and finger agnosia (failure to recognize, not simply to name). Considerable unresolved speculation has addressed why these features should occasionally be so linked.[57,58] The responsible lesion usually affects the language-dominant inferior parietal lobule.

## Apraxia

The term *apraxia* is problematic, for, over the years, it has been used to describe very disparate phenomena. In its broadest sense, *apraxia* refers to impaired motor activity not explained by weakness, incoordination, abnormal tone, bradykinesia, movement disorder, dementia, aphasia, or poor cooperation. Failure to perform an act at all is not apractic; it should be performed incorrectly. Parts of the act might be omitted, abnormally sequenced, or incorrectly orientated in space. Or, any or all components of the act may be performed imprecisely. Heilman[59] suggests four types of testing: (1) gesture ("Show me how you would. . . ."), (2) imitation ("Watch how I . . . , then you do it"), (3) use of an actual object ("Here is a. . . . Show me how you would use it"), and (4) imitation of examiner using the object. Tests include limb gestures (e.g., waving goodbye, hitchhiking), limb manipulation (e.g., opening a door with a key, flipping a coin), buccofacial gesture (e.g., sticking out tongue), buccofacial manipulation (e.g., blowing out a match), and serial acts (e.g., folding a letter, putting it in envelope, sealing envelope, and place stamp on it).

Liepmann classified apraxia as ideational, ideomotor, and limb-kinetic.[60] *Ideomotor apraxia* consisted of inability to perform learned or complex motor acts though primary executive skills are preserved, as is the "idea" of the act (its *engram,* or physiologic memory trace). Affected patients accurately describe what they are supposed to do and correctly perform individual components of the act. Moreover, when the mode of input is switched (e.g., from a spoken command to a visual stimulus), they can sometimes perform the act in its entirety. (Liepmann saw ideomotor apraxia as a functional—if not anatomic—disconnection between the idea of a motor act and its execution.

Ideomotor apraxia can be demonstrated by asking the patient to *pretend* to perform a learned act such as striking a match and blowing it out. The act is attempted but done incorrectly. The patient is able to describe the act and to perform the individual motor movements that subserve it. When handed the real objects (match and matchbook) or, less often, after watching the examiner perform the act, the patient correctly executes it.

By contrast, in *ideational apraxia* the patient cannot accurately describe the act, and presentation of the real object produces no improvement; the patient might tear the match in half and chew one end. Here the lesion appears to affect the engram itself. In *limb-kinetic* apraxia the idea is understood but neither the act itself nor its individual components can be performed, with or without the objects. Presumably, the lesion affects the executive apparatus—not enough to cause frank weakness or ataxia, but enough to prevent accurate motor performance.

It is questionable whether the term *apraxia* is appropriate for the ideational and limb-kinetic types. Ideational apraxia is usually the result of bihemispheric disease and is often associated with obvious dementia. Limb-kinetic apraxia is part of a spectrum of cerebral motor disturbances that include altered tone, power, and coordination. One apractic subtype, so-called gait apraxia, is loosely applied to any impaired gait when strength and coordination of both legs are preserved. The term *constructional apraxia* is even less appropriate.

*Ideomotor apraxia* is what most neurologists mean when they describe a disturbance as *apractic* It most often affects the limbs bilaterally following lesions of the language-dominant parietal or temporal lobe. Such location means that apraxia is often missed, for accompanying aphasia and impaired speech comprehension make testing difficult. Ideomotor apraxia can also affect the *left* limbs of patients with left anterior cerebral artery occlusion and right leg weakness (*sympathetic apraxia*); the responsible lesion is presumed to involve the anterior corpus callosum and to disconnect the right motor cortex from left hemispheric language areas or from the motor engram itself.[61] (Such patients, for similar reasons, often

have left-handed agraphia and tactile anomia.) A subtype of ideomotor apraxia, buccolingual apraxia, affects lip and tongue movements and is a frequent accompaniment of Broca's aphasia. Probably related, *apraxia of speech* refers to the abnormalities of phonologic selection and sequencing that often accompany aphasia (especially Broca's, though Broca's aphasia and oral apraxia can dissociate).[62,63]

### Agnosias and Disorders of Spatial Perception and Manipulation

*Agnosia* is a failure of recognition that is not explained by impaired primary sensation (tactile, visual, auditory) or cognitive impairment. It has been described as "perception stripped of its meaning."[64] Agnosia differs from anomia in that the patient cannot name the confronted object nor select it from a group nor match it to a likeness. In *tactile agnosia (astereognosis)*, touch threshold is normal, yet the object cannot be tactilely identified. Some patients with tactile agnosia cannot even describe fundamental features of the object such as roundness or smoothness (*aperceptive agnosia*); others can identify the primary features but are unable to synthesize them into full object recognition (*associative agnosia*). Although astereognosis can be the predominant symptom of peripheral lesions (e.g., diabetic sensory neuropathy), when it occurs ipsilaterally, either alone or with other discriminative sensory loss (e.g., proprioception or two-point discrimination), the lesion is likely to affect the contralateral parietal sensory cortex or association areas.

Comparable agnosias exist in the visual and auditory spheres. Responsible lesions are likely to be bilateral, and so visual and auditory agnosias are rare. *Simultanagnosia* is inability to recognize the meaning of a whole scene or object, even though its individual components are correctly perceived and recognized. It is sometimes a feature of so-called Balint's syndrome, defined as an inability to look voluntarily into the peripheral visual field, plus optic ataxia (erroneous pointing to objects in space) and decreased visual attention for extrafoveal space. Such patients usually have biparietal lesions.[65,66]

*Prosopagnosia* is selective inability to recognize familiar faces. The problem seems to be one of fine tuning; affected patients can recognize a face as a face (or a dog as a dog) but are unable to identify *which one*. To date, all patients examined at autopsy have shown bilateral occipitotemporal lesions; whether unilateral lesions can cause prosopagnosia remains controversial.[67,68]

Posterior cerebral lesions can also cause agnosia for colors or so-called central achromatopsia, either hemianopic or throughout the visual fields.[69] Unilateral or bilateral lesions usually affect the inferior medial occipital lobe.

Just as the left hemisphere is usually the major processor of language (and related analytic skills), so the right hemisphere processes spatial information. Right hemisphere lesions (especially parietal) cause impairment of spatial perception and manipulation. There may be difficulty reading maps or finding one's way about (*topographagnosia*), copying simple pictures or shapes, or drawing simple objects such as a flower or a clock face (so-called constructional apraxia or apractagnosia). Clothing may be put on backward or upside down (so-called dressing apraxia).

Even more striking is the tendency of a patient with a right hemispheric lesion to ignore the left half of his own body or of meaningful or novel objects in left extracorporeal space (*hemineglect*). The patient may fail to recognize severe hemiplegia (*anosognosia*) or even to acknowledge left body parts as his own (*asomatognosia*), insisting, for example, that a paralyzed limb belongs to someone else or complaining that his own left limbs are missing. Objects or voices in contralateral space are ignored, and grooming or dressing may be restricted to the right half of the body. Asked to bisect a line, the patient indicates a point to the right of midline. Picture copying may omit the left half, and a drawn clock face may have all the numbers neatly arranged on the right side. As with aphasia, when this syndrome is severe there is usually additional cognitive impairment, but not enough to explain the spatial disturbance. Neither is hemineglect the result of homonymous hemianopia.

Constructional apraxia can also follow damage to the language-dominant hemisphere. So can contralateral hemineglect, though the syndrome is usually less obvious in an aphasic patient. Even

when aphasia is accounted for, however, hemineglect is more frequently associated with lesions contralateral to the language-dominant hemisphere.[70] As with aphasia, hemineglect also occurs with thalamic and diencephalic lesions.[71]

## Calculation and Music

Disorders of calculation (*acalculia*) are of several types, including alexia or agraphia for numbers, spatial disorganization of numbers, and true anarithmetria.[72] Consequently, acalculia has followed lesions of either hemisphere. (The fundamental process of calculation appears to be in the domain of the left hemisphere.[73]) Similarly, music involves the processing skills of both hemispheres, and so-called amusia, affecting either productive or receptive aspects of music, has been associated with both left and right brain lesions.[74]

## Aphasia Treatment

The treatment of aphasia—speech therapy—is controversial.[75–78] As to whether it helps patients, most agree that it does. Less clear is whether the perceived benefit is the result of the specific strategies employed or of general psychological support and whether the benefit consists of restored neuropsychological function, of adaptation and compensatory use of preserved function, or simply of improved attention and mood. The fact that aphasia (like other neurologic impairment) can improve without treatment for months or even years makes speech therapy (like physiotherapy) difficult to assess, and controlled studies have been understandably infrequent. In one study, where patients were randomly assigned to treatment or no treatment, there was no significant difference in outcome at 24 weeks.[79] In another study, one group of patients began treatment at entry to the study and continued it for 12 weeks; another group began a similar course of treatment 12 weeks after entry. At 12 weeks, the early treated group was significantly more improved than the deferred treatment group, which, however, caught up at 24 weeks.[80] As with psychotherapy the variables involved make comparison of such studies difficult. What one can reasonably expect from speech therapy was summarized as follows: "Clinical aphasiologists are not naive enough to believe that they fix damaged brains. Rather, they provide alternative compensatory mechanisms or strategies for approximating adequate (if imperfect) means for meeting daily needs."[81]

# References

1. Subirana A. Handedness and cerebral dominance. In: Vinken PJ, Bruyn GW, eds. Handbook of Clinical Neurology, vol 4, Disorders of Speech, Perception, and Symbolic Behavior. Amsterdam: North Holland, 1969;248–272.
2. Springer SP, Deutsch G. Left Brain, Right Brain. San Francisco: WH Freeman, 1981;103–120.
3. Broca P. Perte de la parole. Ramollissement chronique et destruction partielle du lobe antérieur gauche du cerveau. Bu Soc Anthropol Paris 1861; 2:235–238.
4. Broca P. Sur la faculté du language articulé. Bull Soc Anthropol Paris 1865; 6:337–393.
5. Wernicke C. Der Aphasiche Symptomencomplex. Breslau: Cohn & Weigart, 1874.
6. Lichtheim L. On aphasia. Brain 1885; 7:433–484.
7. Henschen SE. On the function of the right hemisphere of the brain in relation to the left in speech, music, and calculation. Brain 1926; 49:110–123.
8. Jackson JH. On the physiology of language. Med Times Gaz 1868; 2:275. [Reprinted in Brain 1915; 38:59–64.]
9. Marie P. Revision de la question de l'aphasie. Semin Med 1906; 26:241–247, 493–500, 565–571.
10. Pick A. Die Agrammatischen Sprachstörungen. Berlin: Springer, 1913.
11. Head H. Aphasia and Kindred Disorders of Speech. New York: MacMillan, 1926.
12. Weisenberg T, McBride KE. Aphasia. A Clinical and Psychological Study. New York: The Commonwealth Fund, 1935.
13. Nielsen JM. Agnosia, Apraxia, Aphasia. Their Value in Cerebral Localization. New York: Hoeber, 1946.
14. Goldstein K. Language and Language Disturbances. New York: Grune & Stratton, 1948.
15. Schuell H, Jenkins JJ, Jiminez-Pabon E. Aphasia in Adults. New York: Hoeber, 1964.
16. Bay E. Principles of classification and their influence on our concepts of aphasia. In: De Reuk AVS, O'Connor M, eds. Disorders of Language. Boston: Little, Brown, 1964.
17. Brain WR. Speech Disorders. Aphasia, Apraxia and Agnosia. London: Buttersworth, 1965.
18. Hecaen H, Albert M. Human Neuropsychology, New York: Wiley, 1978.
19. Luria AR. Higher Cortical Functions in Man, ed 2. New York: 1980.
20. Geschwind N. Disconnection syndromes in animals and man. Brain 1965; 88:237–294, 585–644.
21. Benson DF, Geschwind N. Aphasia and related disorders: A clinical approach. In: Mesulam M-M, ed. Principles of Behavioral Neurology. Philadelphia: FA Davis, 1985;193–238.
22. Goodglass H, Kaplan E. The Assessment of Aphasia and Related Disorders. Philadelphia: Lea & Febiger, 1972.
23. Wagenaar E, Snow C, Prins R. Spontaneous speech of aphasic patients: A psycholinguistic analysis. Brain Lang 1975; 3:281–303.
24. Monrad-Krohn GH. Dysprosody or altered melody of language. Brain 1947; 70:405–415.
25. Ross ED. The aprosodias: Functional-anatomic organization of the affective components of language in the right hemisphere. Arch Neurol 1981; 38:561–569.
26. Fromkin VA. The state of brain/language research. In: Plum F, ed. Language, Communication, and the Brain. New York: Raven, 1988;1–8.
27. DeRenzi E, Vignolo LA. The token test: A sensitive test to detect receptive disturbances in aphasics. Brain 1962; 85:665–678.
28. Caramazza A, Berndt RS. Semantic and syntactic processes in aphasia: A review of the literature. Psychol Bull 1978; 85:898–918.
29. Barton M, Maruszeqski M, Urrea D. Variation of stimulus context and its effect on word-finding ability in aphasics. Cortex 1969; 5:351–365.
30. Roeltgen D. Agraphia. In: Heilman KM, Valenstein E, eds. Clinical Neuropsychology, ed 2. New York: Oxford University Press, 1985;75–96.
31. Roeltgen D. Lexical agraphia. Further support for the two-system hypothesis of linguistic agraphia. Brain 1984; 107:811–827.
32. Roeltgen D, Sevush S, Heilman KM. Phonological agraphia: Writing by the lexical-semantic route. Neurology 1983; 33:755–765.
33. Lytton WW, Brust JCM. Direct dyslexia. Preserved oral reading of real words in Wernicke's aphasia. Brain 1989; 112:583–594.
34. Marshall JC, Newcombe F. The conceptual status of deep dyslexia: An historical perspective. In: Coltheart M, Patterson K, Marshall JC, eds. Deep Dyslexia, ed 2. London: Routledge & Kegan Paul, 1987;1–21.
35. Newcombe F, Marshall JC. Reading and writing by

letter sounds. In: Patterson KE, Marshall JC, Coltheart M, eds. Surface Dyslexia: Neuropsychological and Cognitive Studies of Phonological Reading. London: Lawrence Erlbaum, 1985;35–51.

36. Alexander MP, Fischette MR, Fischer RS. Crossed aphasias can be mirror images or anomalous. Case reports, review and hypothesis. Brain 1989;953–974.

37. Albert ML, Goodglass H, Helm-Estabrooks N, et al. Clinical Aspects of Dysphasia. New York: Springer-Verlag, 1981;219–223.

38. Basso A, Lecours AR, Moraschini S, et al. Anatomoclinical correlations of the aphasias as defined through computerized tomography: Exceptions. Brain Lang 1985; 26:201–229.

39. Benson DF. Aphasia. In: Heilman KM, Valenstein E. Clinical Neuropsychology, ed 2. New York: Oxford University Press, 1985;17–47.

40. Brust JCM, Shafer SQ, Richter RW, et al. Aphasia in acute stroke. 1976; 7:167–174.

41. Freedman M, Alexander MP, Naeser MA. Anatomic basis of transcranial motor aphasia. Neurology 1984; 34:409–417.

42. Yamadori A, Osumi Y, Masuhara S, et al. Preservation of singing in Broca's aphasia. J Neurol Neurosurg Psychiatry 1977; 40:221–224.

43. Mohr JP, Pessin MS, Finkelstein S, et al. Broca aphasia: Pathologic and clinical aspects. Neurology 1978; 28:311–324.

44. Naeser MA, Palumbo CL, Helm-Estabrooks N, et al. Severe non-fluency in aphasia. Role of the medial subcallosal fasciculus and other white matter pathways in recovery of spontaneous speech. Brain 1989; 112:1–38.

45. Kertesz A, Sheppard A, MacKenzie R. Localization in transcortical sensory aphasia. Arch Neurol 1982; 39:475–478.

46. Alexander MP, LoVerme SR. Aphasia after left hemispheric intracerebral hemorrhage. Neurology 1980; 30:1193–1202.

47. Legatt AD, Rubin MJ, Kaplan LR, et al. Global aphasia without hemiparesis: Multiple etiologies. Neurology 1987; 37:201–205.

48. Geschwind N, Quadfasel FA, Segarra J. Isolation of the speech area. Neurolopsychologia 1968; 6:327–340.

49. Kertesz A, McCabe P. Recovery patterns and prognosis in aphasia. Brain 1977; 100:1–18.

50. Vignolo L. Evolution of aphasia and language rehabilitation. A retrospective exploratory study. Cortex 1964; 1:344–367.

51. Schiff HB, Alexander MP, Naeser MA, et al. Aphemia. Arch Neurol 1983; 40:720–727.

52. Auerbach SH, Alland T, Naeser M, et al. Pure word deafness: Analysis of a case with bilateral lesions and a defect at the prephonemic level. Brain 1982; 105:271–300.

53. Dejerine J. Contribution a l'étude anatomo-pathologiques et clinique des differentes variétés de cecite verbale. Mem Soc Biol 1892; 4:61–90.

54. Damasio AR, Damasio H. The anatomic basis of pure alexia. Neurology 1983; 33:1573–1583.

55. Masdeu JC, Schoene WC, Funkenstein H. Aphasia following infarction of the left supplementary motor area. Neurology 1978; 28:1220–1223.

56. Brust JCM, Plank C, Burke A, et al. Language disorder in a right-hander after occlusion of the right anterior cerebral artery. Neurology 1982; 32:492–497.

57. Benton AL. Reflection on the Gerstmann syndrome. Brain Lang 1977; 4:45–62.

58. Roeltgen DP, Sevush S, Heilman KM. Pure Gerstmann's syndrome from a focal lesion. Arch Neurol 1983; 40:46–47.

59. Heilman KM, Rothi LJG: Apraxia. In: Heilman KM, Valenstein E, eds. Clinical Neuropsychology, ed 2. New York: Oxford University Press, 1985; 131–150.

60. Liepmann H. Apraxia. Erbgn Ges Med 1920; 1:516–543.

61. Liepmann H, Maas O. Fall von linksseitiger Agraphie und Apraxie bei rechtsseitiger Lähmung. Z L Psychol Neurol 1907; 10:214–227.

62. Darley Fl, Aronson AE, Brown JR. Motor Speech Disorders. Philadelphia: W B Saunders, 1975; 250–269.

63. Heilman KM, Gonyea EF, Geschwind N. Apraxia and agraphia in a right-hander. Brain 1974; 96:21–28.

64. Bauer RM, Rubens AB. Agnosia. In: Heilman KM, Valenstein E. Clinical Neuropsychology, ed 2. New York: Oxford University Press, 1985;187–241.

65. Hecaen H, de Arjuriaguerra J. Balint's syndrome (psychic paralysis of visual fixation) and its minor forms. Brain 1954; 77:373–400.

66. Levine DN, Calvanio R. A study of the visual defect in verbal alexia simultanagnosia. Brain 1978; 101:65–81.

67. Damasio AR, Damasio H, Van Hoesen GW. Prosopagnosia: Anatomic basis and behavioral mechanisms. Neurology 1982; 32:331–341.

68. Sergent J, Villemure J-G. Prosopagnosia in a right hemispherectomized patient. Brain 1989; 112:975–996.

69. Green GL, Lessell S. Acquired cerebral dyschromatopsia. Arch Ophthalmol 1977; 95:121–128.

70. Heilman KM, Van den Abell T. Right hemisphere

dominance for attention: The mechanism underlying hemispheric asymmetries of inattention (neglect). Neurology 1980; 30:327–330.

71. Healton EB, Navarro C, Bressman S, et al. Subcortical neglect. Neurology 1982; 32:776–778.

72. Levin HS, Spiers PA. Acalculia. In: Heilman KM, Valenstein E, eds. Clinical Neuropsychology, ed 2. New York: Oxford University Press, 1985;97–114.

73. Warrington EK. The fractionation of arithmetical skills: Single case study. Q J Exp Psychol 1982; 34A:31–51.

74. Brust JCM. Music and language. Musical alexia and agraphia. Brain 1980; 103:367–392.

75. Darley FL. Aphasia. Philadelphia: WB Saunders, 1982;144–185.

76. Vignolo LA. Evolution of aphasia and language rehabilitation: A retrospective exploratory study. Cortex 1964; 1:344–367.

77. Sarno MT, Silverman M, Sands E. Speech therapy and language recovery in severe aphasia. J Speech Hearing Res 1970; 13:607–623.

78. Brust JCM. Neurology. In: Haller RM, Sheldon N, eds. Speech Pathology and Audiology in Medical Settings. New York: Stratton Intercontinental Medical Book Corporation, 1976;49–57.

79. Lincoln DB, Mully GP, Jones AL, et al. Effectiveness of speech therapy for aphasic stroke patients. Lancet 1984; 1:1197–1200.

80. Wertz RT, Weiss DG, Aten JL, et al. Comparison of clinic, home, and deferred language treatment for aphasia. A Veterans Administration Cooperative study. Arch Neurol 1986; 43:653–658.

81. Holland AL, Wertz RT. Measuring aphasia treatment effects: Large-group, small-group, and single-subject studies. In: Plum F, ed. Language, Communication, and the Brain. New York: Raven Press, 1988;267–273.

# Chapter 27
# Skeletal Physiology and Osteoporosis

FELICIA COSMAN
ROBERT LINDSAY

## Physiology of Bone Metabolism

### Functions of the Skeletal System

The skeleton has critical mechanical functions, including protecting vital organs, acting as a framework for the body, and anchoring muscles. The skull and vertebral column protect brain and spinal cord, sternum and ribs protect thoracic and upper abdominal viscera, and the pelvis protects genitourinary structures. Additionally, bones surround and protect hematopoietic marrow, creating a physically secure, compartmentalized microenvironment in which blood cells are made and subsequently released into the circulation. In infants, this hematopoietic activity occurs in all bones; in adults it occurs primarily in the flat bones (sternum, ribs, skull, vertebrae, and innominate bones) and in only the proximal ends of long bones such as the humerus and femur. In addition to its protective mechanical functions, the skeleton serves to maintain erect posture, acts as a focus of locomotion, and provides a system of levers to which muscles attach for all movement. Muscles attach through the collagenous fibers of tendons, interweaving through the periosteum, the fibrous outer sheath surrounding bone surfaces.

Bone also acts as the storage site for calcium and phosphate. In order to serve this function, a readily accessible part of bone is always available for dissolution when the supply of electrolytes diminishes. Likewise, minerals can be redeposited into bone when the ion supply is plentiful. Finally, toxins, again usually minerals such as lead or aluminum, are stored in bone until they can be excreted.

The skeletal system's function in maintaining a normal extracellular calcium level takes precedence over its mechanical functions. In times of calcium deficiency, for example, in order to maintain serum calcium, mineral can be rapidly resorbed from the skeleton, causing it to weaken, fracture easily, and lose the ability to protect and to support posture and locomotion.

### Gross Structure and Growth of the Skeleton

The skeleton is comprised of bones that differ markedly in their gross structures, so that no two bones are identical. Microscopically, however, there is much less variability. Generally, long bones are laid down on a cartilaginous *Anlage,* whereas flat bones are ossified in a membranous matrix. Flat bones comprise the axial skeleton whereas tubular bones generally form the appendicular skeleton. Linear growth of bones is a phenomenon that occurs only at the specialized cartilaginous growth plates (epiphyseal plates) that separate bone into shaft (diaphysis) and end (metaphysis). The regulation of bone length involves different genetic, endocrine, and environmental controls than those that regulate bone shape, thickness, or diameter. Although genetic endowment probably defines the basic structure of each bone, environmental influences modify the structure significantly. Genetic endowment also controls (at least in part) environmental factors such as body mass and muscle mass. Figure 27-1 provides a model of how genetic and environmental factors may operate and interact to determine ultimate bone size and structure.[1]

Bone modeling—the sculpting of size (diameter) and gross architecture (macrogeometry)—occurs during growth of the skeleton in all known bony vertebrates and continues into adulthood. Modeling of bone shape and thickness should be distinguished from cartilaginous phenomena such as linear growth. Modeling must also be distinguished from remodeling, which is a preventive maintenance process of coupled resorption and formation that occurs throughout life as old bone is replaced with new to maintain structural integrity. Remodeling does not affect the external shape of bone or move bone through space relative to a defined body axis, as bone modeling does.[2]

Wolff hypothesized more than a century ago that altered mechanical loads could induce appropriate architectural changes in bone. In general, mechanical use increases cortical (compact) bone mass and lack of it has the opposite effect. The difference in bone mass between congenitally paralyzed and normally mobile growing limbs suggests that mechanical use during growth is responsible for 20% to 50% of the ultimate dimensions of the normal young adult skeleton.[3] Figure 27-2 exemplifies the difference in thickness and structure of an animal bone after a period of disuse.[4]

Frost's flexural strain theory extends Wolff's law. In essence, he states that, in growing mammals (or in adults during fracture repair), under repetitive, uniformly oriented, nontrivial, dynamic flexural strains (causing slight bending or angular deformation of bone), bone growth proceeds in the direction of the concavity, with bone formation on the concave surface and resorption on the convex surface.[1] It is generally well-accepted that compression strain stimulates bone growth and tension strain stimulates bone resorption.[5] The resultant drift or movement of the bone in space ultimately

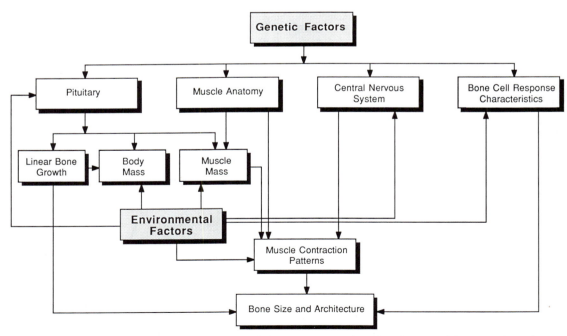

**Figure 27-1.** A schematic representation of the association between genetic and environmental factors as determinants of bone size and structure. (Adapted from Frost HM. Mechanical determinants of bone remodeling. Metab Bone Dis Rel Res 1982; 4:217–229, with permission.)

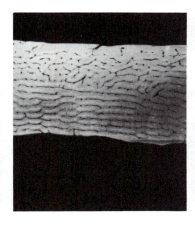
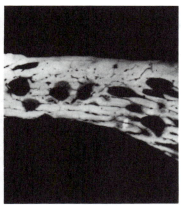

**Figure 27-2.** (*A*) Microradiograph of a 100-μ thick transverse section from the midshaft of a normal male turkey ulna. (*B*) Similar microradiograph from a bone following 8-week loss of functional load bearing. Bone is thinned and porous from endosteal resorption. (From Lanyon LE. Functional strain as a determinant of bone remodeling. Calcif Tiss Int 1984; 36:556–561, with permission.)

reduces compression stress and strain in the concave cortex and tension stress and strain in the convex cortex. This general principle explains to some extent the final macrogeometry of ribs, clavicles, and vertebrae and predicts the eventual correction of fracture malunions. Figure 27-3 is a schematic representation of the events that normally follow a femoral fracture that healed with angulated malunion and ultimately corrected through the modeling process.[1] Tension forces probably contribute in a different way (non-resorbing stimulus) to a few highly specialized macroscopic cortical thickenings or outpouchings, such as those that occur at the insertions of powerful tendons from the iliopsoas and gastrocnemius muscles.[5]

Exactly how mechanical factors (such as compression strain) translate into the cellular processes of bone modeling is unknown. Mechanisms that may be involved include the strain itself (directly stimulating or inhibiting bone cells), release of local matrix factors or cellular growth factors, changes in intrabone pressure, fluid flow, pH, oxygen tension, and streaming electrical potentials.[4]

### Macroscopic Bone Structure

Just as genetic codes specify some aspects of general skeletal size and shape, they encode some differences in the internal structure of bone. One variable is the relative amounts of cancellous (spongy or trabecular) and cortical (compact)

bone. Overall, the skeleton contains 80% cortical and 20% trabecular bone by mass.[6] Nearly every bone in the skeleton contains some cancellous and some compact bone, though the proportions of each are highly variable. The calcaneus contains almost solely cancellous bone, whereas the mid-

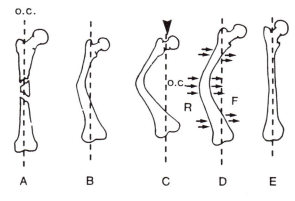

▼ LOAD

**Figure 27-3.** (*A*) Fractured femur of a young child (O.C., original centroid of bone). (*B*) Healing with angulation of the diaphysis. (*C*) With each vertical load, angulation increases slightly. (*D*) Modeling occurs with bone formation on the side of the concavity (*right*) owing to increased stress and strain components (F). Bone resorption (R) occurs with increased tension in the lateral cortex (*left*). This causes the diaphysis to move back toward the original centroid. (*E*) Modeling has resulted in a return of the original configuration of the bone. (Adapted from Frost HM. Mechanical determinants of bone remodeling. Metab Bone Dis Rel Res 1982; 4:217–229, with permission.)

shaft regions of the femur and radius are almost entirely compact bone. Vertebrae contain 45% to 80% cancellous bone, and the femoral neck contains 75% cortical bone. Various proportions occur in other parts of the skeleton.[7,8]

Compact and trabecular bone contain all the same elements, though they are organized differently. In cancellous bone, each small bone fragment (trabeculum) is surrounded by marrow rather than by other packets of bone. Compact bone contains bone units that are densely packed, and only the few that form the corticoendosteal (inner cortical) surface are contiguous with bone marrow (Figure 27-4). Cancellous bone, therefore, has a much higher surface-to-bone volume ratio, providing a large diffusion surface or bone–blood vessel interface for mineral exchange from bone to blood.

Cortical bone contains longitudinally oriented, parallel, cylindrically shaped packets called haversian systems or osteons. Each haversian system consists of a central blood vessel, nerve, and lymphatic channel surrounded concentrically by rings of osteocytes (mature osteoblasts) embedded in calcified bone matrix. Each osteocyte is interconnected to other osteocytes and to a central blood vessel by filamentous cell processes that course through tiny canals (canaliculi) in the mineralized matrix. The haversian system has an average cross-sectional diameter of 250 microns; thus, no cell is farther than that from a blood vessel.[2] The fluid that bathes the bone cells is a specialized derivative of extracellular fluid maintained by both the capillary endothelial cells and the membranous osteocyte cell processes.

Cancellous bone is composed of a series of interconnected plates, often arranged in parallel. Just as mechanical factors help determine the shape and thickness of cortical bone during modeling, they also influence the structure of trabecular bone during skeletal remodeling. This trajectorial theory of trabecular bone architecture was first put forth by Culmann and von Meyer and expounded by Wolff and Roux.[5] In addition to affecting the overall trabecular bone mass, mechanical vectors affect the orientation of the trabeculae, the degree of connectedness, the thickness, and the separation between trabeculae. The long axis of trabecular orientation is parallel to the deformational forces of weight bearing and muscle contraction.[9] Figure 27-5 shows the predominant trabeculae and their orientation parallel to the major compressive forces in the femoral head and tibial plateau.[5] The relative stiffness or strength of trabecular bone depends, as does that of cortical bone, on its overall mineral density.[10] Trabecular contiguity, the frequency of perpendicular trabecular interconnections and thus reinforcement of strength (Figure 27-6), however, is also important.[11] Moreover, the age of bone tissue is a critically important factor in determining strength and ability to resist fatigue damage.[2]

Because cancellous bone has a greater surface and is more richly vascular, it contributes much more toward the function of mineral exchange than compact bone even though it comprises only a small proportion of the overall skeletal mass. Though its relative stiffness or strength is an order of magnitude smaller than that of cortical bone,[10–12] it is lighter than cortical bone. It is therefore structurally economical, preventing bone from being unnecessarily heavy while still contributing significantly to compressive strength, for example in the vertebrae, where estimates suggest that cancellous bone is responsible for 25% to 90% of the total compressive strength.[10,12,13] Although cancellous bone is not as stiff as cortical bone, it is more resistant to deformation (strain or bending forces); resistance to fracture is associated with a greater proportionate length change than of cortical bone. Cancellous bone is thus more compliant, allowing better protection of joint surfaces and transmission of forces from joints to bone shafts.[12]

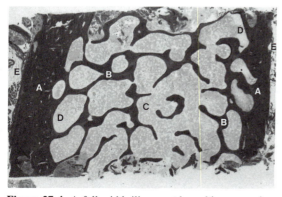

**Figure 27-4.** A full-width iliac crest bone biopsy specimen showing cortices (A), cancellous bone (B), marrow cavity (C), corticoendosteal surfaces (D), and periosteal surfaces (E). (Courtesy of Dr. David Dempster.)

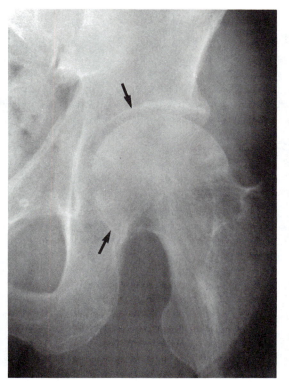
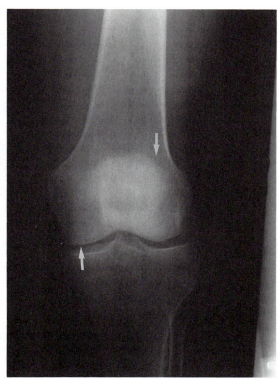

A                                                    B

**Figure 27-5.** (*A*) Note that two major trabecular orientations are seen in the femoral head. The major vertical orientation (*top arrow*) is parallel to the major weight-bearing forces on the bone. The arched, transversely oriented trabeculae (*lower arrow*) correspond to deformational forces produced by compression against the lower acetabulum. (*B*) In the femoral condyles, note that almost all trabeculae are vertically oriented, since almost all compressive forces are exerted vertically and there is little transverse or lateral pressure.

## Microscopic Bone Structure

Like all connective tissue, bone is composed of cells, matrix, and organic fibers. Its compressive strength is due principally to hydroxyapatite mineral and its tensile strength to type I collagen fibers. The extracellular matrix of bone is 35% organic by weight (50% organic by volume).

### Organic Phase

The organic component of bone matrix is 90% collagen, a triple polypeptide helix that associates into fibrillar networks, giving bone its tensile strength and serving as a framework for the deposition of bone mineral and bone cell attachment.[19] A large number of noncollagen proteins (NCPs)

have also been found in the bone matrix (Table 27-1).[14–19] The major NCPs, at least in terms of quantity, are bone gla protein (BGP or osteocalcin) and osteonectin. The functions of these proteins are unknown. In addition to collagen and NCP, the organic phase of bone contains a small amount of lipid.[14]

BGP, a major noncollagen protein, accounts for 15% to 20% of NCP or 1% to 2% of total bone protein. This 49–amino acid protein has three glutamic acid (gla) residues, which become γ-carboxylated in a posttranslational modification. The protein is highly conserved among mammals, birds, and fish.[20] It is also highly specific, being found in only dentin and plasma besides bone matrix. BGP is secreted by osteoblasts during bone formation and has an affinity for hydroxyapatite (see

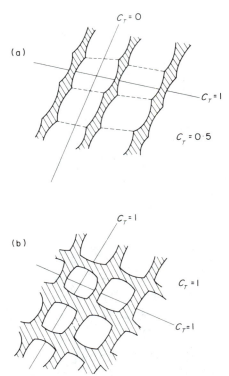

**Figure 27-6.** Idealized trabecular bone structure. (*Top*) Since trabecular contiguity ($^CT$) is O in vertical direction and 1 in horizontal direction, overall $^CT = 0.5$. (*Bottom*) Overall $^CT$ is 1, with much greater strength. (From Pugh JW, Rose RM, Radin EL. Elastic and viscoelastic properties of trabecular bone: Dependence on structure. J Biomech 1973; 6:475–485.)

later) when fully γ-carboxylated, and thus is incorporated into bone matrix. The protein is chemotactic for monocytes and may induce formation of osteoclast precursors and initiate bone resorption.[21] It has also been reported to inhibit the precipitation of hydroxyapatite, and thus prevents excess mineralization. During coumadin treatment, gla residues cannot be added to BGP. Whether this affects bone formation or not has yet to be determined.[22] Matrix gla protein (MGP), with 79 amino acids and five gla residues, has significant sequence homology with BGP, suggesting common derivation. It is also secreted by some osteoblast-like cells in addition to cartilaginous cells.[23] MGP is often found in association with bone morphogenetic protein[20] and may reflect an earlier stage in bone formation than BGP.[23]

Osteonectin is as abundant as BGP (15% of NCP) and is both glycosylated and phosphorylated. It binds both hydroxyapatite and collagen through different regions of the molecule. In vitro, this protein promotes mineral deposition onto collagen. It is possible that in vivo, after binding to collagen, it nucleates hydroxyapatite crystal deposition. Osteonectin, which is immunologically and electrophoretically identical to bone osteonectin, is also found in platelets. During clotting, osteonectin is released into the circulation so that the majority of serum osteonectin is derived from platelets, not bone. Osteonectin may also be made by megakaryocytes.[24] In general the amount of osteonectin in bone correlates with the amount of lamellar bone. Osteonectin is distinct from both fibronectin and thrombospondin, larger proteins that also bind collagen and probably contribute to cell attachment capability.[17,18]

BMP was originally described by Urist as an extract of bone that had the ability to induce endochondral bone formation from extraskeletal mesenchymal tissue in rats.[25] Recently, BMP was recognized as a family of proteins, each independently having similar potential bone induction activity. The three polypeptides have been fully sequenced, and complementary DNA has been isolated. Two of these polypeptides are closely related to other growth factors (although none of the related growth factors has bone induction potential) and the third appears to be a completely novel regulatory protein.[15] The cellular origin of BMP is unknown.

*Mineral Phase*

The mineral phase of bone matrix accounts for 50% of its volume and 65% of its weight. The mineral phase contains both well-formed hydroxyapatite (calcium and phosphate) crystals and amorphous calcium phosphates. The amorphous form has a lower calcium-phosphate ratio than hydroxyapatite, but the two forms are rapidly interchangeable. Mineral deposition occurs in close relation to collagen fibrils (within spaces between triple helices) and within 2 to 10 microns from the osteoblast cell surface. Mineralization normally begins within 5 to 10 days after newly synthesized osteoid is laid down.[14]

**Table 27-1.** Bone Matrix Proteins

| Protein | Mol. Wt. (kd) | Comments |
|---|---|---|
| Type I collagen | 285 | 90% of bone protein; three polypeptides (α chains) in triple helix, high proline and hydroxyproline content; glycosylated |
| Osteocalcin (BGP) | 5.8 | 15–20% of NCP; highly specific to bone dentin; contains three gla residues |
| Osteonectin | 32 | 15% of NCP, abundant in both bone and platelets; phosphorylated glycoprotein |
| Other phosphoproteins | 24–75 | Possibly three different proteins |
| Matrix gla protein | 10 | Contains five gla residues, has homology with BGP, associated with BMP |
| Bone morphogenic protein | 16–30 | Family of three polypeptides, induces cartilage and bone growth in vivo |
| Serum proteins: Albumin, α₂-glycoprotein, transferrin | | Made in liver, secreted into circulation, concentrated in bone matrix, together probably comprise approximately 25% of NCP |
| Proteoglycans I and II | 85–120 | Contain long chondroitin sulfate chains, 10% of NCP |
| Sialoproteins: osteopontin, others | 44 | May be involved in cell attachment, together probably 7.5% NCP |
| Thrombospondin | 450 | Trimeric molecule; like osteonectin is made in bone and platelets, but also wide variety of other tissues; may be involved in cell attachment |
| Fibronectin | 450 | Dimeric molecule; also involved in cell attachment; binds collagen, fibrin, heparin; involved in differentiation of osteoprogenitor cells |

### Bone Cells

Bone cells account for only 3% of bone volume. They include osteoblasts, osteoclasts, and osteocytes (mature osteoblasts or bone lining cells) as well as bone cell precursors. Osteoblasts derive from stromal tissue in the bone marrow, which also gives rise to fibroblasts, adipocytes, and reticular cells in addition to preosteoblasts.[26] Osteoblasts are the cells primarily responsible for bone formation, and they have an important role in activating bone resorption. Osteoblasts elaborate a variety of organic matrix components, including collagen, BGP, osteonectin, thrombospondin, osteopontin, MGP, in addition to various growth factors (possibly BMP) and osteoclast-stimulating factors, some of which are prostaglandins that stimulate resorption and activate bone remodeling. Differences in the ability to secrete these products occur among different osteoblast-like cell lines and at different stages in cell differentiation.[6,16,17] Osteoblasts also secrete alkaline phosphatase, which is expressed on the cell membrane. This enzyme degrades inorganic pyrophosphates (inhibitors of bone mineralization) and may promote mineralization. Osteoblasts probably also synthesize 1,25-dihydroxyvitamin D from 25-hydroxyvitamin D.[27] When active, osteoblasts are cuboidal in shape and contain intracellular organelles characteristic of cells engaged in active protein synthesis.[6]

Osteoblast function is mediated by numerous hormones and local factors, many of which are listed in Table 27-2.[6,28–30] Parathyroid hormone (PTH) probably signals osteoblasts to activate osteoclasts, which then begin resorption, and exerts a direct trophic effect on osteoblasts.[6] There is also accumulating evidence that PTH may stimulate the formation of some osteoblast products, such as BGP[31] and alkaline phosphatase under certain conditions.

Calcitriol regulates some aspects of osteoblast function, such as increasing production of BGP (in vivo and in vitro), MGP, and alkaline phosphatase and modulating osteoblast proliferation.[21,23,33] Calcitriol probably also stimulates

**Table 27-2.** Mediators of Osteoblast Function

Parathyroid hormone
1,25-Dihydroxyvitamin D
(?) Other vitamin D metabolites, including 25-hydroxyvitamin D or 24, 25-dihydroxyvitamin D
Glucocorticoids
Estrogens
Prostaglandins
Insulin
Retinoids
Interleukins (especially IL 1)
Thyroxine
Tumor necrosis factors
Growth factors: somatomedins (IGF-I, II); epidermal, fibroblast, platelet, and bone-derived growth factors; transforming growth factors
Fluoride
Others

rapid bone resorption through osteoblastic activation of osteoclasts.[33]

Glucocorticoids inhibit osteoblast function with respect to BGP formation both in vivo and in vitro[34,35] and reduce bone formation rates as determined by analysis of bone biopsy specimens, probably through a direct inhibitory effect on osteoblast function.[36] They also diminish the stimulatory effect of calcitriol on BGP formation in vivo.[35] On the other hand, glucocorticoids may serve a permissive role in the differentiation of osteoblasts.[29]

Estrogens may exert at least some of their skeletal effects directly on osteoblasts. Estrogen receptors were recently identified on osteoblasts and osteoblast-like cells,[37,38] but the responses of these cells in vivo are unknown. In vitro, estradiol stimulates osteoblast proliferation and collagen synthesis,[39] and it has been shown to increase the secretion of various products of osteoblast-like cells, including alkaline phosphatase, other cellular enzymes, and type 1 insulin-like growth factor (IGF-1).[40–42] Estrogen may also affect the skeleton indirectly through reducing monocytic interleukin 1 (IL-1) synthesis.[43] IL 1, a potent bone-resorbing factor, exerts some of its effects directly through the osteoblast.[6]

Insulin probably increases bone formation directly and acts indirectly by modulating levels of IGF-1.[29] Thyroid hormones stimulate osteoblastic function directly and nonspecifically.[30] Certain

prostaglandins may stimulate bone resorption indirectly through osteoblasts, whereas others are capable of increasing bone formation.[6] Tumor necrosis factors stimulate bone resorption through osteoblastic regulation.[6] Fluoride directly stimulates osteoblastic activity, particularly in the trabecular part of the skeleton.[44]

Osteoclasts derive from mononuclear cells (most likely of the monocyte-macrophage series) in hematopoietic tissue. Precursors undergo first differentiation and then fusion to become multinucleate giant-cells with many mitochondria and lysosomes. Once activated (a process that appears to be under osteoblastic control), osteoclasts demonstrate a ruffled, membranous border with numerous projections and a large surface area where bone resorption occurs. The ruffled border is surrounded by a clear zone delineated by relatively smooth plasma membrane in direct apposition to underlying bone. This clear or sealing zone has no organelles but contains bundles of actin that attach the osteoclast tightly to the underlying bone surface, separating the bone and cell compartment from the surrounding extracellular space to create and maintain a favorable microenvironment for bone resorption. It is generally well-accepted now that osteoclasts are responsible for resorption of both the mineral and the organic phase of bone matrix. Osteoclastic carbonic anhydrase and ruffled-border proton pump enable osteoclasts to secrete acid into the subosteoclastic resorption zone to dissolve hydroxyapatite and create the acidic environment optimal for the function of lysosomal enzymes, including acid phosphatase and cysteine proteases, which solubilize and remove the organic matrix.[45,46,176] The role of collagenase, secreted by osteoblasts, not osteoclasts, in bone resorption remains unclear. It may be required to digest the nonmineralized osteoid lining the mineralized surface to allow optimal osteoclastic activation and action.[45]

Calcitonin is the only known hormone that acts directly on osteoclasts; it is a potent inhibitor of bone resorption, causing rapid obliteration of the active ruffled border and loss of osteoclastic motility.[47,177] Certain prostaglandins may also transiently inhibit osteoclastic function directly. Estrogen and diphosphonates probably inhibit function indirectly. Osteoclast function is stimulated by parathyroid hormone (PTH), calcitriol, prostaglandins $E_2$ and $I_2$, thyroxine, and many cytokines including IL 1, tumor necrosis factors, tissue growth factors, transforming growth factors, and osteoclast-activating factors, all probably acting indirectly through osteoblasts.[6,45] Glucocorticoids stimulate osteoclastic activity, possibly by hypersecretion of PTH.[36]

## Bone Remodeling

Bone remodeling is a process of cyclic resorption and formation that begins in childhood and continues throughout life, at varying rates. It maintains the strength and integrity of bone, prevents mechanical failure, and repairs microfractures. Remodeling also maintains a dynamic state that allows mineral release into extracellular fluid when needed and subsequent redeposition into bone. Remodeling activity is proportionately much greater in the trabecular part of the skeleton: at any one time, approximately 20% of the trabecular surface is actively undergoing remodeling but only 5% of the intracortical bone surface. Consequently, 25% of the total trabecular bone mass, but only 5% to 10% of the cortical bone mass, is renewed each year.[2]

There are several important distinctions between remodeling and modeling of bone. Remodeling is a coupled process of erosion and repair on the same bone surface with long quiescent periods between remodeling cycles. Modeling may involve formation and resorption, each on separate bone surfaces, and these processes may continue long without interruption. Remodeling does not result in grossly perceptible changes in bone shape, whereas the *purpose* of modeling is to alter the macrostructure of the bone. Finally, the net effect of remodeling in adults is bone loss and the net effect of modeling is bone accrual.[2]

Bone remodeling occurs in anatomically discrete packets of bone where the bone and cells involved are called bone remodeling units (BRUs). The process involves a characteristic sequence of events: activation, resorption, reversal, formation, and quiescence (Figure 27-7).[46,48] Remodeling occurs on all bone surfaces, including those deep within cortical bone, where the surface is adjacent

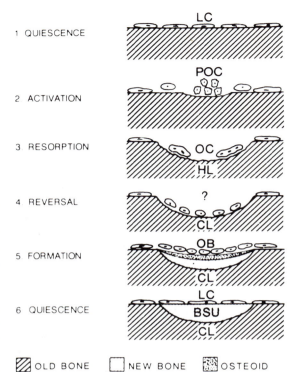

Figure 27-7. Normal adult bone remodeling sequence. Key: LC, lining cell; POC, preosteoclast (mononuclear cell); OC, osteoclast; HC, Howship's lacuna; CL, cement line; OB, osteoblast; BSC, bone structural unit. (From Parfitt AM, The cellular basis of bone remodeling: The quantum concept reexamined in light of recent advances in the cell biology of bone. Calcif Tiss Int 1984; 36:537–545, with permission.)

to a haversian canal. Rates of remodeling vary, not only in different regions of the skeleton but also in different areas of any bone, areas commonly divided into periosteal, intracortical, corticoendosteal, and trabecular bone envelopes (see Figure 27-4). How a systemic hormone such as PTH, probably the most important activator of skeletal remodeling, can activate the remodeling sequence in some quiescent bone regions without affecting others is unknown.

Osteocyte lining cells (the terminal cells of the osteoblast lineage) probably play a role in local remodeling activation. These cells retract their cell processes, removing the non-mineralized lining material and exposing the mineralized bone surface, which is probably chemotactic for osteoclast precursors.[2] Activated multinucleated osteoclasts then resorb bone, creating cavities of a characteristic shape and depth over a 1- to 3-week period. Resorption cavities are called *Howship's lacunae* in trabecular bone and *cutting cones* in cortical bone. Though the initial cavity is formed by osteoclasts alone, the final resorption stage, which is much slower, includes mononuclear cells.

The reversal stage, which follows resorption, lasts 1 to 2 weeks and appears to be responsible for the coupling of formation to resorption, though the precise mechanisms are unknown. Some of the reversal (mononuclear) cells deposit a thin layer of cement substance, smoothing and preparing the surface for bone formation. Osteoblast precursors from connective tissue or marrow stroma are recruited to the resorption cavity and mature into osteoblasts.

Osteoblasts commence formation by secreting the organic components of bone matrix. Mineral deposition begins through basically unknown mechanisms approximately 5 to 10 days after the first osteoid has been secreted but generally before the organic phase of formation is completed. As the resorption cavity is filled, osteoblasts make a gradual morphologic and functional transformation from highly active cells to the quiescent bone lining cells, called *osteocytes* at this stage. Maturation and increasing density of bone mineral continue to occur, extending the total formation phase to about 3 months and the total remodeling sequence to an average of 4 months (range 3 to 24 months).[49]

The duration of the remodeling sequence, extent of resorption cavities, extent of repair with newly formed bone, and rate of remodeling site activation are some of the variable parts of this process that are under complicated regulatory control, including genetic, endocrine, nutritional, mechanical, and age-related factors. In general, though formation is coupled to resorption, the exact balance of these processes is such that at any one surface there may be a net loss or gain of bone. Characteristically, in adulthood, there is a small net gain of bone on the periosteal surface and a net decrease of bone on endosteal and trabecular surfaces. The latter overwhelms the periosteal increases and results in net loss of bone from the skeleton over time. This is a universal age-related phenomenon, though it occurs in varying degrees depending on the factors already mentioned.

## Mineral Homeostasis

### Calcium

Nearly all of the body's calcium (99%) is stored in bone, and only 1% is spread throughout other tissues, extracellular fluid, and blood. Approximately half the circulating calcium is bound to protein and half is in ionized form with a small amount complexed to bicarbonate, citrate, or phosphate.[50] It is critical to maintain the extracellular calcium within tight limits because small increases or decreases can cause severe neurologic, neuromuscular, or renal disturbances that can lead to death. Calcium intake is highly variable, usually correlating with total calorie, protein, and phosphorous intake. Calcium absorption occurs primarily in the upper intestine through both an active mechanism dependent on the presence of active vitamin D (1,25[OH]$_2$D) and passive diffusion. We normally absorb only about 25% of the calcium we consume. Although the total amount of calcium absorbed increases with increased intake, the proportion of dietary calcium absorbed, particularly the active fraction, declines with increased intake.[51] Excess dietary calcium, together with calcium secreted into the gastrointestinal tract, is eliminated in the feces. The majority of absorbed calcium is normally excreted by the kidney. While 98% of the filtered calcium normally is reabsorbed, this can be increased to almost 100% when strict calcium conservation is required. During states of calcium deprivation, increased PTH causes increased renal tubular reabsorption of calcium and increased bone resorption. It also increases the level of 1,25(OH)$_2$D, which in turn increases the efficiency of intestinal calcium absorption. These three mechanisms maintain a normal serum calcium level despite great fluctuations in intake.

### Phosphorous

A large proportion of the body's phosphorous is also in the skeleton, both in association with calcium in the hydroxyapatite crystal and in the organic bone matrix with organophosphorous compounds such as phospholipids, phosphoproteins, and nucleic acids. In the blood, only 13% of phosphorous is protein bound, and of the rest approximately equal amounts are present as ions and complexes. We normally absorb about 90% of the phosphate that we consume. Absorption is mostly passive and less dependent on vitamin D than is calcium absorption. Dietary phosphorous deficiency and malabsorption are, therefore, rare. The kidney is the major site of phosphorous regulation; renal tubular reabsorption rates depend on the PTH level.[50]

### Endocrine Control of Mineral Homeostasis

PTH and calcitriol are the major hormonal controls on mineral levels; calcitonin has a less important role. Other regulators such as thyroid hormone, gonadal steroids, glucocorticoids, and catecholamines, among others, may also affect mineral homeostasis, especially when they are frankly low or high.

PTH is synthesized initially as preproparathyroid hormone, which then undergoes two intracellular cleavages, ultimately being secreted as the intact PTH molecule with 84 amino acids. It undergoes rapid peripheral metabolism to amino (N)-terminal fragments, most containing 34 amino acids, and carboxy (C)-terminal fragments. Bioactivity seems to reside in the N-terminal portion of the molecule, as the N-terminal fragments and intact molecule are active while the C-terminal fragments are biologically inert.[50] PTH causes an increase in bone resorption, calcitriol production, and renal reabsorption of calcium. It also decreases the renal threshold for phosphate reabsorption, causing phosphaturia. PTH secretion is increased by low serum calcium or high serum phosphate. The hormone acts by increasing both cyclic adenosine monophosphate[48] and intracellular calcium in its target tissues, bone and kidney.[52,53]

Intake of vitamin D is very variable. It is present primarily in enriched foods and foods that contain small bones such as fish. Despite tremendous dietary variability, vitamin D deficiency is rare because the body is able to synthesize the vitamin from a precursor in the skin (7-dehydrocholesterol) when the skin is exposed to sunlight. People who avoid the sun or who live in areas of the world where penetration of sunlight is limited are still vulnerable to vitamin D deficiency.[54] Absorption of dietary vitamin D, a fat-soluble vitamin, depends on normal hepatobiliary, pancreatic, and probably gastric function to digest fat, and on a normal intestinal surface to absorb it. Figure 27-8 gives an overview of this and subsequent steps in vitamin D metabolism.[55]

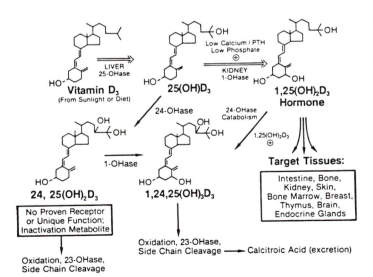

**Figure 27-8.** The vitamin D endocrine system. (From Meunier P, et al. Physiological senile involution and pathological rarefaction of bone. Clin Endocrinol Metab 1973; 2:239–256, with permission.)

Once in the blood, choleciferol associates with D-binding protein, an α-globulin, and is transported to the liver, where it is converted to 25(OH)D. This conversion is not strictly regulated and correlates well with dietary intake and cutaneous formation. 25(OH)D is the principal circulating metabolite and occupies the majority of D-binding protein. It is converted to 1,25(OH)$_2$D by the renal 1 alpha-hydroxylase enzyme. This enzyme is regulated principally by PTH, which increases its activity, and by phosphorous, which decreases its activity. Because of tight regulation of this enzyme, calcitriol levels are constant over a large range of 25(OH)D levels. In states of suppressed PTH secretion, as when calcium supply is abundant, 25(OH)D is preferentially converted to 24,25-dihydroxyvitamin D, a metabolite presumed, but not proven, to be essentially inactive.[33] That the most active form of vitamin D is 1,25(OH)$_2$D is relatively indisputable, but possible contributions from other metabolites to the regulation of bone and mineral homeostasis cannot be fully excluded.

1,25(OH)$_2$D increases fractional calcium absorption from the intestine, its major target organ. Through this indirect effect on calcium supply, it exerts its major influence on bone formation. 1,25(OH)$_2$D has been shown to modulate several aspects of osteoblast function directly (see later), but the physiologic relevance of these effects is unknown. The better-characterized effect on the skeleton is its ability to resorb bone and mobilize calcium. This activity occurs both rapidly (within hours) and slowly (over days). The latter effect is probably mediated by an increased number of osteoclast cells resulting from increased precursor differentiation. Like other steroid hormones, 1,23(OH)$_2$D complexes with an intracellular receptor and enters the target cell nucleus, where it exerts its effects by modulating mRNA production. Some cellular effects are felt to be too rapid to have occurred through this mechanism and consequently other non-genomic pathways of 1,25(OH)$_2$D action have been proposed. The plasma half-life of 1,25(OH)$_2$D is on the order of minutes; its biologic half-life is hours. 1,25(OH)$_2$D is excreted mostly in bile and reabsorbed through the enterohepatic circulation.[33]

Calcitonin is a small peptide hormone (32 amino acids) synthesized by parafollicular or C cells in the thyroid gland. THe physiologic function of this hormone is unknown. In pharmacologic doses, it inhibits osteoclast activity, resulting in decreased bone resorption and increased renal calcium clearance. These two effects can cause a moderate decrease in serum calcium. Unlike deficiencies of PTH and 1,25(OH)$_2$D, which cause well-described diseases, no definite disease state has been described as a result of calcitonin deficiency or excess. It is likely, therefore, that calcitonin plays a less important physiologic role in mineral metabolism than PTH or calcitriol.[56,57]

Numerous other hormones and factors affect mineral metabolism, particularly frank excesses or deficiencies, but they only rarely produce changes in serum levels of calcium because of dominant regulation by PTH and calcitriol. For example, deficiency of estrogen is well-known to cause increased skeletal turnover, but it does not produce frank hypercalcemia because PTH release may be suppressed. Likewise, excessive adrenal or exogenous glucocorticoid causes osteoblastic dysfunction and calcium malabsorption, resulting in osteoporosis but not hypocalcemia, because excess PTH is secreted. In contrast, thyrotoxicosis (excess thyroid hormone), particularly when severe, may occasionally cause mild hypercalcemia, despite complete suppression of PTH and calcitriol, suggesting that certain disease states can overwhelm the physiologic adaptations of the calciotropic hormones.

## Metabolic Bone Disease

Metabolic bone disease is generally defined as a disorder of the skeleton secondary to alteration in bone cell function. In most cases these are diffuse diseases that result from abnormalities in the hormones, minerals, or other regulators of function. Though the abnormal cell processes usually occur throughout the skeleton, they may cause more marked changes or symptoms in characteristic localized areas. Generally, although the mechanisms underlying these diseases are very different, the common end-point is most often loss of skeletal integrity and strength and a predisposition to fracture with minimal trauma or none. The major metabolic bone diseases are osteoporosis, Paget's disease, hyperparathyroidism, osteomalacia, renal osteodystrophy, and congenital diseases such as osteogenesis imperfecta and osteopetrosis. As osteoporosis is by far the most common of these disorders for the rehabilitation physician, in the remainder of this chapter I will discuss that disease. Recent reviews of the other disorders have been published.[179–184]

## Osteoporosis

### Definition

Osteoporosis, characterized by a generalized loss of skeletal tissue mass and disruption of skeletal microarchitecture, is most common in aged persons, particularly women. There is a proportionate loss of both hydroxyapatite mineral and organic bone constituents, but it is principally the loss of bone mineral that decreases bone strength and increases the risk of fracture. The clinical hallmark of the disease is fracture, which most characteristically occurs in the spine, femoral neck, or distal radius, though it may occur in the pelvis, humerus, or any other bone.

Bone loss is universally associated with aging (Figure 27-9)[7,64–66]: everyone who lives long enough will develop osteoporosis. Acceleration of the bone loss process, especially when accompanied by low peak bone mass, increases the likelihood of osteoporotic fracture.

A precise, consistent, and universally accepted definition of osteoporosis does not exist. Patients of all ages who present with fractures sustained from minimal trauma who have no evidence of other underlying bone disorders probably have osteoporosis. We also consider patients osteoporotic

if their bone mass value is more than 2 standard deviations below the average bone mass values for *young normal* persons (Figure 27-10). This definition includes 50% or more of the population older than 70 years (i.e., even those with average or above average bone mass for that age are considered osteoporotic). This definition makes no distinction between a natural aging process and a more extreme or exaggerated process that probably occurs in only a small percentage of the population and is perhaps more consistent with the usual definition of a disease process. This difficulty in separating natural aging from disease is common to other aging phenomena, such as memory loss, systolic hypertension, glucose intolerance, and aortic atherosclerosis. A different commonly used definition includes all patients with bone mass values more than 2 standard deviations below the mean for normal individuals of the *same age and sex* (Figure 27-10). Though this definition does make a distinction between the majority of people and a small outlying fraction (the lowest 2.5%), the former definition is probably more important physiologically, in that it is the absolute amount of bone, rather than the relationship of bone mass to others of that age, that predicts the risk of fracture. Not surprisingly, then, bone mass values of patients who fracture do overlap bone mass measurements of those who are "normal for age" and who have not had a fracture.[67]

### Epidemiology

As bone mass declines with menopause and age, fracture frequency also increases with age (Figure 27-11).[68,69] Osteoporosis is therefore most common in postmenopausal women and in elderly per-

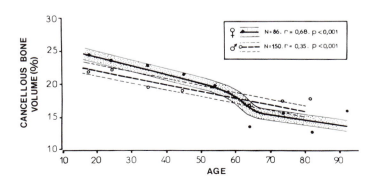

**Figure 27-9.** Changes in iliac trabecular bone volume with age and sex in 236 controls (curves statistically smoothed). (From Meunier P, et al. Physiological senile involution and pathological rarefaction of bone. Clin Endocrinol Metab 1973; 2:239–256, with permission.)

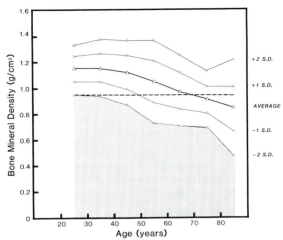

**Figure 27-10.** Defining osteoporosis. BMD (measured by dual-photon absorptiometry) as a function of age in the lumbar spine. Middle bold line is mean at every age; other curves represent 1 and 2 standard deviations above and below the mean. By definition 1 (see text), all patients below the dotted line have osteoporosis. By definition 2 (see text), all patients in shaded area have osteoporosis.

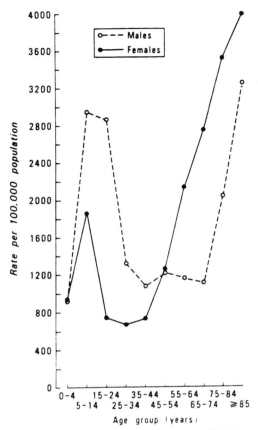

**Figure 27-11.** Age- and sex-specific rates for limb fractures. (From with permission.)

sons of both sexes; in younger patients it is usually secondary to an underlying condition such as alcoholism or endocrine disease. The most common fractures are compressions of the vertebrae of which an estimated 500,000 cases occur annually in the United States, approximately 90% in women. The female-male ratio is somewhere between 6:1 and 10:1.[7] Accurate incidence and prevalence rates of these fractures are difficult to obtain, since the fractures are often asymptomatic and are not recorded in epidemiologic data. Approximately 50% of 80-year-old women have evidence of vertebral fractures.[70-71] Fractures of the distal radius, proximal humerus, and pelvis are four to eight times more common in women than in men.[72,73] Hip fracture is the most serious complication of osteoporosis; about 300,000 of these occur each year in the United States, more than 90% in those older than 70 years. Although the female-male ratio is only about 2:1, 80% of hip fractures occur in women because more women live to an older age.[72-75] The number of hip fractures is increasing as the percentage of aged persons in the population increases,[72-76] and it may also be increasing independently of this factor, for reasons that are not yet clear.[73,74,76]

*Pathophysiology*

**Bone Mass.**    Bone mass is the major determinant of fracture risk, with bone strength being 80% to 90% dependent on bone mass.[64] Although bone mass measurements in patients with fractures overlap those without fractures, the prevalence of vertebral fracture and incidence of hip and radius fracture are inversely proportional to bone mass values at the respective sites.[68,69] Bone mass at any adult age is determined by peak bone mass and the amount of bone subsequently lost, a product of both rate and duration of loss. Peak mass is usually achieved in the fourth decade of life, at which point slow, continuous bone loss begins that continues throughout life (see Figure 27-10). In women, the rate of bone loss accelerates for several years prior to actual menopause (during partial ovarian failure), and for as long as 10 years after complete cessation of ovarian function.[64-66,68,77-79]

The majority of evidence supports the importance of estrogen deficiency at menopause as the major factor in rapid bone loss and subsequent osteoporotic fractures.[79-82]

**Estrogen Deficiency.** The loss of estrogen at menopause increases the activation rate of new bone remodeling sites. Because resorption slightly exceeds formation in remodeling units (after peak bone mass is achieved), this elevated activation rate causes a net increase in skeletal resorption. In addition, estrogen withdrawal may result in actual eradication of some trabecular units, this being caused by increased size or depth of resorption cavities.[83] This results in decreased trabecular connectivity or contiguity (see Figure 27-6), causing loss of reinforcing strength. These additional architectural changes cause more loss of bone strength than would be expected by the loss of mass alone.[83-87]

The increased skeletal remodeling associated with estrogen withdrawal is consistent with the biochemical and calcium kinetic changes observed across menopause. Levels of calcium and phosphate in the serum and urine increase but remain within the normal range.[79] Increases in serum alkaline phosphatase, BGP, and urine hydroxyproline are also consistent with increased skeletal turnover.[21,79] In a series of studies, Heaney showed that at menopause there is increased transit of calcium into and out of the skeleton, decreased intestinal calcium absorption, and decreased renal tubular calcium reabsorption.[88-90] These latter effects are probably secondary to the increased skeletal liberation of calcium, which in turn suppresses PTH and calcitriol.

Because estrogen receptors were not identified in bone until recently, several theories put forth previously depict indirect action of estrogen on the skeleton. One of the most appealing was that estrogen stimulated calcitonin release, thus suppressing bone resorption. Calcitonin levels are lower in women than men at all ages, and levels decrease with age.[91,92] One study reported that basal calcitonin levels correlated strongly with circulating

estrone levels and were significantly lower in postmenopausal than in menopausal women.[93] Moreover, calcitonin production rates were significantly lower in postmenopausal osteoporotics than in premenopausal or normal postmenopausal women, suggesting that an independent calcitonin deficiency in osteoporotics might be superimposed on menopause and age-related changes. There is little other evidence to support this theory, however; several investigators find higher calcitonin levels in postmenopausal osteoporotic women than in normal ones.[94,95]

Another possible mechanism of estrogen's effect on skeletal turnover is modulation of IL-1 secretion. IL 1 has been shown to be a powerful bone-resorbing agent, and it has been suggested that monocytic IL-1 production increases at menopause and can be suppressed by treatment with estrogen, although not all studies agree.[43,96] Osteoporotic women, especially those with a high bone turnover rate, may produce more IL 1 than nonosteoporotic women.[97] Recent evidence showing estrogen receptors on osteoblast cells[37,38] supports the theory that estrogen acts, at least in part, directly on bone tissue. Direct effects of estrogen on bone cells have been demonstrated in vitro, including stimulation of osteoblast proliferation and collagen synthesis, and IGF-1 production.[39-42]

**Age.** The mechanism of the slower, continuous bone loss associated with age alone is also ill-understood. From the fourth decade onward, there is a remodeling imbalance at individual foci such that less bone is formed than is resorbed in most modeling units. This may be caused by impaired regulation of the osteoblast population rather than by intrinsic cellular osteoblast dysfunction.[68] Intestinal calcium absorption efficiency decreases with age and is concomitant with decreased $1,25(OH)_2D$ level.[51] In contrast to the perimenopausal state, however, PTH usually increases with advancing age. This suggests that the primary defect may be in $1,25(OH)_2D$ production or increased resistance to $1,25(OH)_2D$ with regard to at least the gastrointestinal tract, associated with a compensatory and secondary increase in PTH to maintain calcium homeostasis,[51,98] which would result in a net increase in bone resorption. Other age-related factors, such as decreased mechanical stress from decreased activity, muscle mass, or weight loss, may also be involved.

To compare the relative importance of bone loss associated with estrogen deficiency to that associated with age alone, Richelson assessed bone mineral density (BMD) in women whose mean ages differed by 20 years but who had undergone either natural or surgical menopause the same number of years before they entered the study. He found that BMD was not significantly different between these groups at any site, despite the 20-year age disparity. This suggests that the interval after cessation of ovarian function is a stronger determinant of BMD than age.[81]

**Other Causes of Bone Loss.** Other factors besides age and menopause that are thought to affect the degree of bone loss are listed in Table 27-3.[99] Early age at menopause or any significant periods of hypogonadism in both women and men (from anorexia nervosa, hyperprolactinemia, extreme exercise, or other cause) are likely to result in more bone loss than unaffected persons exhibit.[84–95,100–113] Endocrine diseases such as thyrotoxicosis, Cushing's syndrome, insulin-dependent diabetes mellitus, and primary hyperparathyroidism may accelerate bone loss.[36,72,114–117] Smoking increases bone loss because of its association with a thin body habitus, its ability to induce early menopause, and perhaps through the stimulation of estrogen degradation/metabolism and consequent lowering of serum estrogen levels.[111,118–120] Excessive alcohol ingestion increases skeletal loss by inducing a defect in bone formation resulting in greater net resorption of bone.[119,121,122] Immobilization is well-known to accelerate bone loss,[123] and increased physical activity may help prevent bone loss. Medicines, including glucocorticoids, excess thyroid hormone, antiepileptics, heparin, and some chemotherapy drugs (methotrexate) all adversely affect the skeleton.[36,96,114,124–128]

The influence of dietary calcium intake on bone density and bone loss in postmenopausal adults remains controversial. Some studies suggest a definite relationship between low dietary calcium intake in adults and bone loss, some show a very modest effect on cortical bone only, and others have been unable to show that a large amount of dietary calcium has any effect at all on decreasing bone loss.[129–133] Other dietary factors, including

**Table 27-3.** Causes of Increased Bone Loss

Premature hypogonadism
  Early menopause, 84,106
  Oligomenorrhea/amenorrhea
    Exercise-induced 85,86
    Anorexia nervosa 87,88
    Hyperprolactinemia 89,90
  Low testosterone in males
  Hyperprolactinemia 91,92
  Idiopathic 92,94,95
  Anorexia nervosa 93,127
Other endocrine disorders
  Cushing's syndrome 36,96
  Thyrotoxicosis 62,97
  Insulin-dependent diabetes mellitus 62,98
  Primary hyperparathyroidism 62,97
  Addison's disease 99
Lifestyle
  Smoking 62,95,100,101
  Alcohol consumption 95,101,102,115
  Thin body habitus 62,95,100
  Immobilization/inactivity 103
  Insufficient dietary calcium
  Too much protein, caffeine, phosphorus, sodium 62,104,105
Drugs
  Glucocorticoids 36,96
  Excessive thyroid hormone 107,108
  Antiepileptics 109
  Chemotherapy 110,112
  Heparin 112
Systemic disease 83,110
  Gastrectomy
  Malabsorption
  Chronic obstructive pulmonary disease
  Some hematopoietic/neoplastic disorders (lymphoma/leukemia)
  Radiotherapy (localized)

excessive protein, phosphorous, caffeine, or sodium intake, may also increase bone loss to some extent by increasing calciuria.[129,130] Underlying systemic diseases such as postgastrectomy states, malabsorption, certain liver diseases, and chronic obstructive lung disease have all been associated with low bone mass.[118,127]

*Peak Bone Mass*

Factors thought to affect peak bone mass are listed in Table 27-4. The major determinants are probably genetic, including race, gender, and body build. Men have about 5% to 10% higher bone density than women throughout youth and early

**Table 27-4.** Factors That Affect Peak Bone Mass

Genetics: race, sex, body build, skin type
Genetic diseases: Turner's syndrome, osteogenesis imperfecta, homocysteinuria, Ehler-Danlos syndrome
Calcium intake
Level of physical activity
Late menarche
Periods of hypogonadism (exercise, anorexia nervosa, hyperprolactinemia, idiopathic)

adulthood, and the difference increases as ovarian failure approaches.[7,64,67,72] Blacks have bone densities about 5% to 10% higher than whites from an early age.[134,135] Thin, small, pale-skinned women are at greater risk than large, obese, or dark-skinned women.[62,72,134] Studies have shown a high level of concordance of bone mass measurements between monozygotic twins as compared to dizygotic pairs.[136–139] Daughters of osteoporotic mothers have exhibited reduced bone mass in the lumbar spine, and possibly, the femoral neck, in some,[140] but not all, studies.[141] Both male and female children and siblings of osteoporotics have been found to have lower spinal bone mass than control subjects.[142] Certain genetic diseases such as Turner's syndrome and osteogenesis imperfecta are associated with low peak bone mass.[62,143,144]

The total duration of the skeleton's exposure to estrogen levels that are compatible with menstrual function is a major determinant of bone mass, affecting peak mass as well as the rate of bone loss. Thus, those who have late menarche (after age 16) are more likely to have diminished peak bone mass compared than those whose menarche occurred at the average age.[112] Women who experience periods of amenorrhea in youth (induced by the same factors mentioned above) suffer lower peak BMD.[101–106] Estrogen deficiency is at least one of the causes of low bone mass in Turner's syndrome.[144] Furthermore, all of the factors listed in Table 27-3 that increase bone loss, might reduce peak bone mass if they occurred during the period of skeletal accrual.

In addition to genetic influences and gonadal insufficiency in youth, peak bone mass is affected by dietary calcium intake during childhood, adolescence, and young adulthood.[145] That calcium intake is a determinant of peak bone mass is less controversial than the importance of calcium intake as a factor in bone loss. A study of two Yugoslavian populations that differed primarily in their lifelong calcium intake showed higher peak bone density to be associated with higher calcium intake.[146] Studies of postmenopausal women showed that those who reported consuming much milk during childhood and adolescence had higher bone density than age-matched women whose milk intake during youth was lower.[147,148] In a study of young normal premenopausal women, bone density was significantly correlated with total calcium intake once effects of different activity levels were eliminated.[149]

Several studies in young adults show a correlation between BMD and physical activity level, suggesting that exercise might increase peak bone mass.[149–151] Physical activity level, measured as daily energy expenditure in walking (using a pedometer) and nonwalking leisure activity, was found to correlate significantly with vertebral BMD in young premenopausal females.[149] In another study of premenopausal women, activity level measured by a motion sensor correlated with both spinal BMD and total body calcium.[150] In young men, spinal BMD was significantly greater in those who engaged in regular, vigorous exercise than in relatively sedentary persons.[151] Lifelong cross-country runners (longer than 25 years in sport) had greater bone mineral mass in seven sites in their skeletons than sedentary age-matched controls.[152] A study comparing male athletes and nonathletes showed higher femur densities in the athletic group. Of the nonathletes, the exercisers had greater bone density than the nonexercisers.[153] Weight lifters and ballet dancers who began training early in life had higher forearm and leg densities and bone widths than healthy age-matched controls.[154] All of these studies suggest that the amount of various types of physical activity in youth is an important determinant of peak skeletal mass. Along the same lines, immobilization or reduction in weight-bearing physical activity is well-known to reduce bone mass, as demonstrated in paraplegia, poliomyelitis, space flight, and bed rest for unrelated conditions.[123]

*Qualitative Factors*

In addition to bone mass or quantity, several qualitative factors increase the probability of fracture. One is the phenomenon of complete elimination of trabecular plates that occurs during bone loss after ovarian failure. Highly active remodeling with deep resorption cavities results in trabecular perforation followed by resorption of the remaining free ends of trabeculae (Figure 27-12). The actual eradication of trabecular units causes loss of structural reinforcement, which, as described earlier, is a major determinant of the strength of trabecular bone. This architectural abnormality causes a greater predisposition to fracture than the loss of bone mass alone.[83,86,87] The age of bone is also important in determining its ability to resist fracture. Bone that is not remodeled effectively can accumulate fatigue damage that weakens it and makes it more liable to fracture.[85] Other changes in the chemical composition of bone may occur, such as a reduction in the calcium content per unit volume of bone. Age-related changes such as increased diameter of the medullary canal of bones and increased cortical bone diameter are adaptations that maximize strength in the face of an overall reduction in mass. This is accomplished to some extent through local remodeling imbalances that favor endosteal bone resorption and periosteal bone formation.[155,156]

*Falls*

Though vertebral fractures may occur spontaneously, almost all other fractures occur only after a traumatic event, usually a fall. Falling is especially common in elderly persons; poor sight, balance problems, postural hypotension, dementia, and drugs such as hypnotics, antidepressants, antipsychotics, antihypertensives, diuretics, and hypoglycemics all probably play a role. Alcohol ingestion, with its effects on vision, coordination, and concentration, is also potentially very dangerous and likely to cause falls in elders.[157] Certain acute and chronic diseases, including those that cause nocturia, may precipitate falls. Environmental hazards in the home such as slippery surfaces, especially in the shower and bath, poor room lighting, floor wires, throw rugs, and poorly placed furniture also contribute to the risk of falling. Ill-fitting shoes or excessively long trousers or skirts are additional risks for tripping and falling. Moreover, elders may not tolerate falls as well as younger persons because of their reduced soft tissue padding, weaker muscles, and slowed reflexes with consequent greater force transmission to bones.[71]

*Clinical Presentation*

Osteoporosis may present with symptoms of an acute fracture, chronic back pain, painless kyphosis, or height reduction. Acute vertebral crush fracture often causes sudden severe localized back

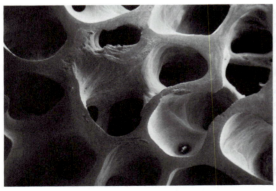
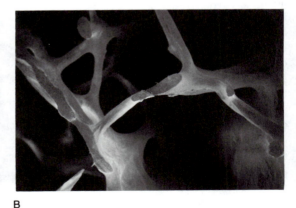

A                                    B

**Figure 27-12.** Low-power electron micrographs of iliac crest biopsies. (*A*) Normal 44-year-old male. (*B*) 47-year-old osteoporotic woman. Notice substantial loss of bone volume with complete eradication of many trabecular plates. (From Dempster DW, Shane E, Holbert W, et al. A simple method for correlative light and scanning electron microscopy of human iliac crest biopsies. J Bone Miner Res 1986; 1:15–21, with permission.)

pain precipitated by movements such as lifting, reaching, flexing, or rotating. Paraspinal muscle spasms and pain radiating in the dermatomal distribution of the proximal nerve root may occur. The patient may be unable to recline and may need to sleep in a sitting position. There may be tenderness and palpable muscle spasm at the site, but physical examination findings are generally otherwise negative. The diagnosis is usually clear on plain radiography, where a crush or wedge compression fracture is seen (Figure 27-13), though it may take several days for the radiographic changes to develop. Acute fractures of other sites present with localized pain after minor trauma. Rib fractures may be precipitated by a cough, sneeze, or hug. Groin pain may signify a pelvic fracture. Hip and wrist fractures cause pain, swelling, deformity, and loss of motion at their respective sites, and are easily diagnosed.

Multiple thoracic vertebral fractures produce a characteristic spinal deformity of exaggerated kyphosis (dowager's hump), because generally, vertebral height loss is more marked anteriorly than posteriorly, thrusting the spine forward (Figure 27-13). This spinal configuration causes stretching of ligaments, tendons, and paraspinal muscles that may result in chronic generalized back pain.[158] Because the center of gravity is farther anterior with marked kyphosis, a patient may acquire exaggerated lumbar lordosis as a compensatory measure to neutralize this altered center of gravity. This may also cause ligament and muscle strain with resultant lower back pain. Alternatively, if the lumbar vertebrae themselves are fractured, there may be loss of the natural lumbar lordosis. Loss of spinal range of motion is an accompaniment of these spinal deformities. Patients with multiple fractures and chronic back pain may have low sitting or standing tolerance and may require frequent periods of rest in a reclining position.

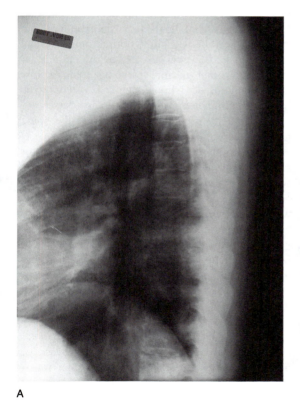
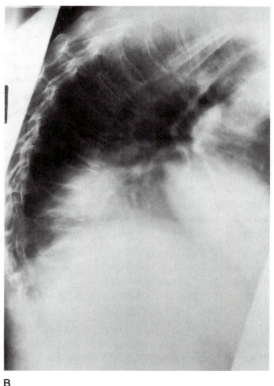

A                                    B

**Figure 27-13.** (*A*) Thoracic spine of normal 60-year-old woman with preservation of vertebral height in all vertebrae. (*B*) Severely kyphotic thoracic spine with compression fractures of essentially all vertebrae.

Patients who have lost enough height for the lower rib cage to rest on the iliac crests may have chronic lower rib and flank pain.[158] Why some patients suffer severe pain syndromes and others have deformity without pain is not known. Some researchers have suggested that elderly osteoporotics who present with hip fracture more often have asymptomatic vertebral wedging whereas younger postmenopausal patients develop painful crush fractures. This may relate to different rates or amounts of cancellous and cortical bone loss and to different underlying pathophysiologic mechanisms in these possibly distinct forms of the disease.

### Diagnosis and Evaluation

When back pain is not associated with vertebral fractures, height loss, or kyphosis, osteoporosis is unlikely to be the underlying disease. Other common causes of back pain must be considered, including muscle or ligament sprain, degenerative joint or disc disease, enthesopathy, spondyloarthropathy, malignancy with vertebral metastases, and vertebral osteomyelitis. A complete history and physical, basic laboratory evaluation, plain radiographs, and special imaging studies when indicated (technetium bone scan, computed tomography, magnetic resonance imaging) should make the diagnosis. Patients with vertebral fractures, with or without back pain, should also have a full evaluation to exclude any concomitant diagnoses. Laboratory evaluation should include serum levels of calcium, phosphorous, other nutritional parameters such as protein and cholesterol, alkaline phosphatase, hepatic and renal function profiles, blood counts, and erythrocyte sedimentation rate. Secondary causes of osteoporosis—multiple myeloma, thyrotoxicosis or excessive thyroid replacement, and Cushing's syndrome—should be excluded by appropriate diagnostic tests. In men, symptoms of hypogonadism should be solicited and serum testosterone levels obtained. In suggestive cases, in addition to the serum evaluation, urinary calcium, phosphorus, and hydroxyproline, and serum PTH and vitamin D levels should be measured, to rule out other metabolic bone diseases such as osteomalacia, hyperparathyroidism, and Paget's disease.

### Bone Mass Measurements

Bone mass measurements are used clinically to establish the severity of the skeletal deterioration, to evaluate asymptomatic persons for their risk of developing the disease, and at times to monitor the skeletal response to treatment. Various techniques have developed, including single-photon absorptiometry (SPA), dual-photon absorptiometry (DPA), dual energy x-ray (DEXA), and quantitative computed tomography (QCT).[159,160] SPA is used solely to measure the radius; the other techniques can measure hip, spine, and other areas. Each technique is quite precise and reliable, with DEXA offering an overall advantage.[160] The major difference between QCT and the other two methods is that radiation exposure is substantially higher for QCT, so it is less than optimal for use in asymptomatic individuals and for serial follow-up over long periods.[159]

Although a low BMD measurement (DPA, DEXA; expressed in grams per square centimeter) in a patient with fractures induced by minimal trauma suggests a diagnosis of osteoporosis, bone mass may well be within the normal range for age and sex. It is, however, usually below the normal range for young normal persons. Even a low BMD, though, does not distinguish osteoporosis from certain other metabolic bone disorders.

Artifactually high measurements of the spine may be due to degenerative calcifications, for example osteophytes and vascular calcifications, or to measurement over sites of vertebral compression. Old traumatic fractures that were not previously diagnosed might be evident later in an otherwise asymptomatic person. If none of these artifacts is present, a high BMD value in a patient with atraumatic fractures is unusual. It is particularly important in such cases to rule out other underlying bone diseases, such as osteomalacia or Paget's disease. A radionuclide bone scan can help distinguish old healed fractures from active disease, but increased tracer uptake can be secondary to recent fractures of any cause or to other metabolic bone diseases such as Paget's disease or osteomalacia. Where concern about other metabolic bone diseases exists and diagnosis can not be confirmed by serum or urine measurements or radionuclide scan, a transiliac crest bone biopsy may be required. Bone histomorphometry is also useful in defining qualitative abnormalities that might predispose an osteoporotic patient to fracture.[83,86,87] It also allows assessment of the level of skeletal turnover and may help direct therapy accordingly, though the advantages of basing osteoporosis treatment on skeletal turnover rates have yet to be validated.[161]

Bone mass measurements to screen asymptomatic persons at risk are being requested more often. It is in this asymptomatic stage, particularly at menopause, that therapeutic intervention aimed at preventing further skeletal deterioration is most likely to be efficacious.

## Treatment

### Asymptomatic Low Bone Mass

The aim of therapy in a patient with asymptomatic low bone mass is prevention of further bone loss and fracture. Medicines known to accelerate bone loss should be discontinued or decreased in dosage if possible (e.g., steroids, excess thyroxine). Lifestyle factors known to contribute to decreased bone mass, such as smoking and consuming excessive amounts of alcohol and caffeine, should be discontinued. Optimal calcium intake is still not known, but the generally accepted guidelines are 1000 mg per day in adult women, increasing to 1500 mg in women who are at particular risk of osteoporosis. These guidelines are based on Heaney's kinetic data documenting what amount of calcium intake is required to prevent net loss of body calcium at various ages.[88] A patient who cannot modify diet to increase calcium intake appropriately should take a calcium supplement.

The best exercise regimen for this patient population has not been determined. Weight-bearing activity is thought to be critical to skeletal integrity, but the optimal level is unknown. Generally, aerobic exercises such as rapid walking, running, or upright calisthenics or aerobics are recommended. Several studies suggest that these weight-bearing aerobic exercises may increase or maintain BMD. Aloia and colleagues studied postmenopausal women. Those who exercised 3 hours per week for 1 year, increased their total body calcium while the calcium level of controls decreased significantly, although forearm BMD did not change significantly in either group.[162] After both 9 and 22 months Dalsky and coworkers found a significant increase in lumbar BMD above baseline, and above the values for bone-losing controls in postmenopausal women who exercised 3 hours per week.[163] Chow's group randomized postmenopausal women to participate in aerobic, aerobics plus strengthening, or no exercise three times per week for 1 year and found significantly increased bone mass in the exercising groups, as compared to those who did no exercise.[164] Smith and associates found various indices of bone mass in the forearm to be increased in middle-aged women who performed approximately 3 hours of aerobic exercise per week over a 4-year period.[165] Not all studies are supportive, however. In a 3-year randomized trial of the effects of walking on postmenopausal women, forearm bone density decreased in both groups though in a subset of patients (those with high grip strength), radius cross-sectional area increased in the exercisers but not in the controls.[166] Additionally, another study of brisk walking in postmenopausal women showed equivalent decrements in bone mass of the spine in both walkers and nonwalkers after 1 year.[167]

Whether or not exercising specific muscle groups adds density or prevents loss of mass in the underlying skeletal site has yet to be determined. BMD of the lumbar vertebrae was found to correlate significantly with the strength of back extensor muscles.[168] Spinal extension exercises have been shown to increase spinal muscle strength[169] but have not yet been shown to increase bone mass. It is possible that strengthening back extensors may help protect against vertebral bone loss and subsequent fracture. In tennis players, BMD values are well-known to be significantly higher in the dominant arm than in the other one.[170] Clinical trials are required to investigate whether building muscle strength in the spine, hip, wrist, or intercostal region in the postmenopausal age group increases BMD and decreases fracture rates in the respective sites. Patients with average or below-average bone mass may be candidates for pharmacologic intervention. Estrogen, in the form of Premarin, 0.625 mg orally per day (or its equivalent), is the best-tested regimen in terms of efficacy and toxicity.[171–174] Replacing estrogen in postmenopausal women prevents further bone loss and decreases the risk of fracture.[174–177] The route of estrogen administration (oral or transdermal) is probably not important as long as estrogen is absorbed and serum levels are measurable. There is some evidence that supplementing calcium intake to total 1500 mg per day may allow reduction of the estrogen dose to 0.3 mg and still afford the same protective effect on the skeleton.[178] Parenteral (subcutaneous) calcitonin therapy has also been shown to be effective in stopping bone loss.[161,179,180] New routes of administration, such as intranasal calcitonin spray, may make this a more widely used agent should it prove to be equally effective.[181]

### Patients with Established Disease

Patients who have low bone mass and have already sustained a fracture represent a more challenging problem than those with only asymptomatic low bone mass. Appropriate medicine for pain relief—anti-inflammatory agents, muscle relaxants, if necessary narcotic analgesics—is critical. Physical modalities should be tried, including hydrotherapy, hot packs, ultrasound massage, and transcutaneous nerve stimulation. Although bed rest right after a fracture is usually recommended, patients should be mobilized as soon as pain is tolerable, as more prolonged immobilization could aggravate osteoporosis. Occasionally, a thoracic brace, usually made of soft elastic material, helps patients feel better and become ambulatory faster. Stiff metal and plastic braces are not recommended because they are extremely uncomfortable, they facilitate awkward and potentially imbalanced movements, and they often encourage patients to spend more time in bed than they would otherwise. Proper body mechanics should be taught, including avoidance of unnecessary spinal compression forces like those associated with spinal flexion, twisting, rapid jarring, and forward-reaching movements.[182]

When the patient is ready, a program of both weight-bearing aerobic exercise (low impact) and spinal extension exercise should be prescribed. These recommendations are based on a few preliminary studies of the effects of exercise in osteo-porotic women. Krolner and coworkers studied middle-aged osteoporotic women (all had had a wrist fracture), half of whom participated in a supervised and varied exercise program 2 hours per week for 8 months. BMD of the lumbar spine increased in exercisers while it decreased significantly in controls, though forearm BMD decreased slightly in both groups.[183] Sinaki and colleagues studied the effects of spinal exercises on postmenopausal osteoporotics. Those who performed regular spine extension exercises had a lower fracture recurrence rate than those who performed flexion exercises or had no exercise regimen.[184] Over 5 months, various dynamic loading exercises of the forearm increased radius BMD in postmenopausal osteoporotics, as compared with decreased BMD in controls.[185] More studies are obviously required to confirm and extend these results so that specific exercise programs can be prescribed for osteoporotic women.

Adequate calcium intake must be ensured, either through dietary modification or calcium supplementation such that deficient calcium intake does not exacerbate the problem. In many cases, an antiresorptive agent such as estrogen or calcitonin should be prescribed to prevent further bone loss. Preliminary data suggest that some diphosphonates may also be effective in preventing bone loss,[186–189] but antifracture efficacy has yet to be shown. In selected cases, a trial of fluoride, the only agent in the current therapeutic armamentarium that directly stimulates bone formation, may be warranted. Unfortunately this agent frequently causes intolerable gastrointestinal toxicity, including pain, nausea, and bleeding, as well as arthralgias. The bone that is formed is not normal: fluoride is incorporated into the hydroxyapatite crystals. Though it has been suggested that fluoride decreases vertebral fractures in those who can tolerate it, it does not prevent hip fracture and may actually increase that risk.[190] The exact role of fluoride in osteoporosis remains controversial at present. Two rather large double-blind, placebo-controlled trials were recently completed. Findings showed positive effects on bone mass in both the spine and hip but no decrease in fracture frequency in the treated groups.[191,192]

Pharmacologic regimens that take into account the remodeling cycle—activate, depress, free, repeat (ADFR)—have been and are actively under investigation.[193,194] These regimens use various agents known to activate skeletal remodeling such as phosphorus, calcitriol, or PTH, followed by agents that depress bone resorption such as calcitonin or diphosphonate, in a sequential fashion. This is then followed by a drug-free period during which formation proceeds unimpeded. The sequence is then repeated with hopes that remodeling imbalance will favor formation and result in increased bone density. Results so far have been variable, and conclusions await further investigation. Intermittent therapy is similar to ADFR, except that only antiresorptive agents are used, and remodeling activation occurs naturally. Other clinical trials investigating the efficacy of continuous parathyroid hormone and IGF-1 therapies are also under way. These offer new hope for more effective ways to halt and reverse this disabling disorder.

# References

1. Frost HM. Review article. Mechanical determinants of bone modeling. Metab Bone Dis Rel Res 1982; 4:217–229.
2. Parfitt AM. Bone remodeling: Relationship to the amount and structure of bone, and the pathogenesis and prevention of fractures. In: Riggs BL, Melton LJ III, (eds). Osteporosis: Etiology, Diagnosis and Management. New York: Raven Press, 1988;45–93.
3. Frost HM. Vital biomechanics: Proposed general concepts for skeletal adaptations to mechanical usage. Calcif Tissue Int 1988; 42:145–156.
4. Lanyon LE. Functional strain as a determinant for bone remodeling. Calcif Tissue Int 1984; 36:S56–S61.
5. Trueta J. Mechanical forces and bone shape. In: Studies of the Development and Decay of the Human Frame. Philadelphia: WB Saunders, 1968;37–41.
6. Martin TJ, Ng KW, Nicholson GC. Cell biology of bone. In: Martin TJ, ed. Bailliere's Clinical Endocrinology and Metabolism, vol 2. Metabolic Bone Disease. London: Bailliere Tindall, 1988;1–29.
7. Riggs BL, Wahner HW, Seeman E, et al. Changes in bone mineral density of the proximal femur and spine with aging. J Clin Invest 1982; 70:716–723.
8. Wasnich RD, Ross PD, Vogel JM. Letter to the editor. N Engl J Med 1985; 313:325–326.
9. Cowin SC. Wolff's law of trabecular architecture at remodeling equilibrium. J Biomech Eng 1986; 108:83–88.
10. Hayes WC, Gerhart TN. Biomechanics of bone: Applications for assessment of bone strength. In: Peck WA, ed. Bone and Mineral Research, vol 3. Amsterdam: Elsevier, 1985;259–294.
11. Pugh JW, Rose RM, Radin EL. Elastic and viscoelastic properties of trabecular bone: Dependence on structure. J Biomech 1973; 6:475–485.
12. Melton LJ III, Chao EYS, Lane J. Biomechanical aspects of fractures. In: Riggs BL, Melton LJ III, eds. Osteoporosis: Etiology, Diagnosis, and Management. New York: Raven Press, 1988;111–131.
13. Rockoff SD, Sweet E, Bleustein J. The relative contribution of trabecular and cortical bone to the strength of human lumbar vertebrae. Calcif Tissue Res 1969; 3:163–175.
14. Robey PG, Fisher LW, Young MF, et al. The biochemistry of bone. In: Riggs BL, Melton LJ III, eds. Osteoporosis: Etiology, Diagnosis, and Management. New York: Raven Press, 1988;95–109.
15. Wozney JM, Rosen V, Celeste AJ, et al. Novel regulators of bone formation: Molecular clones and activities. Science 1988; 242:1528–1534.
16. Noda M, Rodan GA. Transcriptional regulation of osteopontin production in rat osteoblast-like cells by parathyroid hormone. J Cell Biol 1989; 108:713–718.
17. Robey PG, Young MF, Fisher LW, et al. Thrombospondin is an osteoblast-derived component of mineralized extracellular matrix. J Cell Biol 1989; 108:719–727.
18. Yamada KM, Olden K. Review article. Fibronectins—adhesive glycoproteins of cell surface and blood. Nature 1978; 275:179–184.
19. Kleinman HK, Klebe RJ, Martin GR. Role of collagenous matrices in the adhesion and growth of cells. J Cell Biol 1981; 88:473–485.
20. Price P. Osteocalcin. In: Peck WA, ed. Bone and Mineral Research, vol 1. Amsterdam: Excerpta Medica, 1983;157–190.
21. Lian JB, Gundberg CM. Basic science and pathology. Osteocalcin biochemical considerations and clinical applications. Clin Orthop 1988; 226:267–291.
22. Menon RK, Gill DS, Thomas M, et al. Impaired carboxylation of osteocain in Warfarin-treated patients. J Clin Endocrinol Metab 1987; 64:59–61.
23. Fraser JD, Otawara Y, Price PA. 1,25-Dihydroxy-vitamin $D_3$ stimulates the synthesis of matrix

gamma-carboxyglutamic acid protein by osteosarcoma cells. Mutually exclusive expression of vitamin K–dependent bone proteins by clonal osteoblastic cell lines. J Biol Chem 1988; 263:911–916.

24. Tracy RP, Shull S, Riggs BL, et al. Minireview. The osteonectin family of proteins. Int J Biochem 1988; 20:653–660.

25. Urist MR, Nillsson OS, Hudak R, et al. Immunologic evidence of a bone morphogenetic protein in the milieu interieur. Ann Biol Clin 1985; 43:755–766.

26. Owen M. Lineage of osteogenic cells and their relationship to the stromal system. In: Peck WA, ed. Bone and Mineral Research, vol 3. Amsterdam: Elsevier, 1985;1–25.

27. Turner RT, Howard GA, Puzas JE, et al. Calvarial cells synthesize 1,25-dihydroxyvitamin $D_3$ from 25-hydroxyvitamin $D_3$. Biochemistry 1983; 22:1073–1076.

28. Raisz LG, Kream BE. Regulation of bone formation. First of 2 parts. N Engl J Med 1983; 309:29–35.

29. Raisz LG, Kream BE. Regulation of bone formation. Second of 2 parts. N Engl J Med 1983; 309:83–89.

30. Rizzoli R, Poser J, Burgi U. Nuclear thyroid hormone receptors in cultured bone cells. Metabolism 1986; 35:71–74.

31. Noda M, Yoon K, Rodan GA. Parathyroid hormone (PTH) enhances osteocalcin mRNA expression in rat osteosarcoma cells (Abstr). J Bone Miner Res 1988; 3(suppl 1):s144.

32. McPartlin J, Skrabanek D, Powell D. Bone alkaline phosphatase: Quantitative cytochemical characterization and response to parathyrin in vitro. Biochem Soc Trans 1984; 123:894–898.

33. Reichel H, Koeffler HP, Norman AW. The role of the vitamin D endocrine system in health and disease. N Engl J Med 1989; 320:980–991.

34. Ekenstam E, Stalenheim G, Hallgren R. The acute effect of high dose corticosteroid treatment on serum osteocalcin. Metabolism 1988; 37:141–144.

35. Beresford JN, Gallagher JA, Poser JW, et al. Production of osteocalcin by human bone cells in vitro: Effects of $1,25(OH)_2D_3$, $24,25(OH)_2D_3$, parathyroid hormone and glucocorticoids. Metab Bone Dis Rel Res 1984; 5:229–234.

36. Dempster DW. Perspectives. Bone histomorphometry in glucocorticoid-induced osteoporosis. J Bone Miner Res 1989; 4:137–141.

37. Komm BS, Terpening CM, Benz DJ, et al. Estrogen binding, receptor mRNA, and biologic response in osteoblast-like osteosarcoma cells. Science 1988; 241:81–84.

38. Eriksen EF, Colvard DS, Berg NJ, et al. Evidence of estrogen receptors in normal human osteoblast-like cells. Science 1988; 241:84–86.

39. Ernst M, Schmid C, Froesch ER. Enhanced osteoblast proliferation and collagen gene expression by estradiol. Proc Nat Acad Sci USA 1988; 85:2307–2310.

40. Gray TK, Flynn TC, Gray KM, et al. 17-Beta-estradiol acts directly on the clonal osteoblastic cell line UMR106. Proc Nat Acad Sci USA 1987; 84:6267–6271.

41. Bankson DD, Rifai N, Williams ME, et al. Biochemical effects of 1-beta-estradiol on UMR106 cells. Bone Miner 1989; 6:55–63.

42. Gray TK, Mohan S, Linkhart TA, et al. Estradiol stimulates in vitro the secretion of insulin-like growth factors by the clonal osteoblastic cell line, UMR106. Biochem Biophys Res Comm 1989; 158:407–412.

43. Pacifici R, Rifas L, McCracken R, et al. Ovarian steroid treatment blocks a postmenopausal increase in blood monocyte interleukin-1 release. Proc Nat Acad Sci USA 1989; 86:2398–2402.

44. Peck WA, Woods WL. The cells of bone. In: Riggs BL, Melton LJ III, eds. Osteoporosis: Etiology, Diagnosis, and Management. New York; Raven Press, 1988;1–44.

45. Vaes G. Cellular biology and biochemical mechanism of bone resorption. A review of recent developments on the formation, activation, and mode of action of osteoclasts. Clin Orthop 1988; 231:239–271.

46. Arnett TR, Dempster DW. Effect of pH on bone resorption by rat osteoclasts in vitro. Endocrinology 1986; 119:119–124.

47. Murrills RJ, Shane E, Lindsay R, et al. Bone resorption by isolated human osteoclasts in vitro: Effects of calcitonin. J Bone Miner Res 1989; 4:259–268.

48. Parfitt AM. The cellular basis of bone remodeling: The quantum concept reexamined in light of recent advances in the cell biology of bone. Calcif Tiss Int 1984; 36:S37–S45.

49. Recker RR, Kimmel DB, Parfitt AM, et al. Static and tetracycline-based bone histomorphometric data from 34 normal postmenopausal females. J Bone Miner Res 1988; 3:133–144.

50. Auerbach GD, Marx SJ, Spiegel AM. Parathyroid hormone, calcitonin, and the calciferols. In: Wilson JD, Foster DW, eds. Williams' Textbook of Endocrinology, ed. Philadelphia: WB Saunders, 1985;1137–1217.

51. Heaney RP, Gallagher JC, Johnston CC, et al. Calcium nutrition and bone health in the elderly. Am J Clin Nutr 1982; 36:986–1013.

52. Reid IR, Civitelli R, Halstead LR, et al. Parathyroid hormone acutely elevates intracellular calcium in osteoblastlike cells. Am J Physiol 1987; 252:E45–E51.

53. Hruska KA, Goligorsky M, Scoble J, et al. Effects of parathyroid hormone on cytosolic calcium in renal proximal tubular primary cultures. Am J Physiol 1986; 251:F188–F198.

54. Audran M, Kumar R. The physiology and pathophysiology of vitamin D. Mayo Clin Proc 1985; 60:851–866.

55. Haussler MR, Mangelsdorf DJ, Komm BS, et al. Molecular biology of the vitamin D hormone. Recent Prog Horm Res 1988; 44:263–305.

56. Talmage RV, Cooper CW, Toverud SU. The physiological significance of calcitonin. In: Peck WA, ed. Bone and Mineral Research, vol 1. Amsterdam: Excerpta Medica, 1983;74–143.

57. Hurley DL, Tiegs RD, Wahner HW, et al. Axial and appendicular bone mineral density in patients with long-term deficiency or excess of calcitonin. N Engl J Med 1987; 317:537–541.

58. Bijvojet OLM, Vellenga CJLR, Harinck HIJ. Paget's disease of bones: Assessment, therapy, and secondary prevention. In: Kleerekoper M, Krane SM, eds. Clinical Disorders of Bone and Mineral Metabolism. New York: Mary Ann Liebert, 1989;525–542.

59. Bilezikian JP. Clinical disorders of the parathyroid glands. In: Raisz LG, Martin TJ, eds. Clinical Endocrinology of Calcium Metabolism. New York: Marcel Dekker, 1987;53–97.

60. Labat M, Milhaud G. Osteopetrosis and the immune deficiency syndrome. In: Peck WA, ed. Bone and Mineral Research, vol 4. Amsterdam: Elsevier, 1986;131–212.

61. Ritz E, Drueke T, Merke J, et al. Genesis of bone disease in uremia. In: Peck WA ed. Bone and Mineral Research, vol 5. Amsterdam: Elsevier, 1987;309–374.

62. Sillence D. Osteogenesis imperfecta: An expanding panorama of variants. Clin Orthop 1981; 159:11–25.

63. Marel GM, McKenna MJ, Frame B. Osteomalacia. In: Peck WA, ed. Bone and Mineral Research, vol 4. Amsterdam: Elsevier, 1986;335–412.

64. Mazess RB. On aging bone loss. Clin Orthop 1982; 165:239–252.

65. Krolner B, Nielsen SP. Bone mineral content of the lumbar spine in normal and osteoporotic women: Cross-sectional and longitudinal studies. Clin Sci 1982; 62:329–336.

66. Meunier P, Courpron P, Edouard C, et al. Physiological senile involution and pathological rarefaction of bone. Quantitative and comparative histological data. Clin Endocrinol Metab 1973; 2:239–256.

67. Riggs BL, Wahner HW, Dunn WL, et al. Differential changes in bone mineral density of the appendicular and axial skeleton with aging. Relationship to spinal osteoporosis. J Clin Invest 1981; 67:328–335.

68. Riggs BL, Melton LJ III. Involutional osteoporosis. N Engl J Med 1986; 314:1676–1686.

69. Hui SL, Slemenda CW, Johnston CC Jr. Age and bone mass as predictors of fracture in a prospective study. J Clin Invest 1988; 81:1804–1809.

70. Kanis JA, McCloskey EV. Epidemiology of vertebral osteoporosis. Bone 1992; 13:S1–S10.

71. Resnick NM, Greenspan SL. Senile osteoporosis reconsidered. JAMA 1989; 261:1025–1029.

72. Cummings SR, Kelsey JL, Nevitt MC, et al. Epidemiology of osteoporosis and osteoporotic fractures. Epidemiol Rev 1985; 7:178–208.

73. Melton LJ III. Epidemiology of fractures. In: Riggs BL, Melton LJ III, eds. Osteoporosis: Etiology, Diagnosis and Management. New York: Raven Press 1988;133–154.

74. Melton LJ III, O'Fallon WM, Riggs BL. Secular trends in the incidence of hip fractures. Calcif Tiss Int 1987; 41:57–64.

75. Lindsay R, Dempster DW, Clemens T, et al. Incidence, cost, and risk factors of fracture of the proximal femur in the USA. In: Christiansen C, Arnaud CD, et al, eds. Osteoporosis I, Copenhagen International Symposium, Aalborg Srifts bogtrykkeri Copenhagen, Denmark, 1984;311–315.

76. O'Brant KJ, Bengner U, Johnell O, et al. Increasing age-adjusted risk of fragility fractures: A sign of increasing osteoporosis in successive generations? Calcif Tiss Int 1989; 44:157–167.

77. Genant HK, Cann CE, Ettinger B, et al. Quantitative computed tomography of vertebral spongiosa: A sensitive method for detecting early bone loss after oophorectomy. Ann Intern Med 1982; 97:699–705.

78. Johnston CC, Hui SL, Witt RM, et al. Early menopausal changes in bone mass and sex steroids. J Clin Endocrinol Metab 1985; 61:905–911.

79. Lindsay R. Sex steroids in the pathogenesis and prevention of osteoporosis. In: Riggs BL, Melton LJ III, eds. Osteoporosis: Etiology, Diagnosis and Management. New York: Raven Press, 1988;333–358.

80. Aitken JM, Hart DM, Anderson JB, et al. Osteoporosis after oophorectomy for non-malignant disease in premenopausal women. Br Med J 1973; i:325–328.

81. Richelson LS, Wahner HW, Melton LJ III, et al. Relative contributions of aging and estrogen de-

ficiency to postmenopausal bone loss. N Engl J Med 1984; 311:1273–1275.

82. Nilas L, Christiansen C. Bone mass and its relationship to age and the menopause. J Clin Endocrinol Metab 1987; 65:697–702.

83. Parfitt AM. Trabecular bone architecture in the pathogenesis and prevention of fracture. Am J Med 1987; 82 (supp1B):68–72.

84. Eriksen EF, Mosekilde L, Melsen F. Trabecular bone resorption depth decreases with age: Differences between normal males and females. Bone 1985; 6:141–146.

85. Heaney RP. Osteoporotic fracture space: An hypothesis. Bone Miner 1989; 6:1–13.

86. Kleerekoper M, Villanueva AR, Stanciu J, et al. The role of three-dimensional trabecular microstructure in the pathogenesis of vertebral compression fractures. Calcif Tiss Int 1985; 37:594–597.

87. Dempster DW, Shane E, Horbert W, et al. A simple method for correlative light and scanning electron microscopy of human iliac crest bone biopsies: Qualitative observations in normal and osteoporotic subjects. J Bone Miner Res 1986; 1:15–21.

88. Heaney RP, Recker RR, Saville PD. Calcium balance and calcium requirements in middle-aged women. Am J Clin Nutr 1977; 30:1603–1611.

89. Heaney RP, Recker RR, Saville PD. Menopausal changes in calcium balance performance. J Lab Clin Med 1978; 92:953–963.

90. Heaney RP, Recker RR, Saville PD. Menopausal changes in bone remodeling. J Lab Clin Med 1978; 92:964–970.

91. Heath H III, Sizemore GW. Plasma calcitonin in normal man. J Clin Invest 1977; 60:1135–1140.

92. Deftos LJ, Weisman MH, Williams GW, et al. Influence of age and sex on plasma calcitonin in human beings. N Engl J Med 1980; 302:1351–1353.

93. Reginster JY, Deroisy R, Albert A, et al. Relationship between whole plasma calcitonin levels, calcitonin secretory capacity, and plasma levels of estrone in healthy women and postmenopausal osteoporotics. J Clin Invest 1989; 83:1073–1077.

94. Tiegs RD, Body JJ, Wahner HW, et al. Calcitonin secretion in postmenopausal osteoporosis. N Engl J Med 1985; 312:1097–1100.

95. Prince RL, Dick IM, Price RI. Plasma calcitonin levels are not lower than normal in osteoporotic women. J Clin Endocrinol Metab 1989; 68:684–687.

96. Stock JL, Coderre JA, McDonald B, et al. Effects of estrogen in vivo and in vitro on spontaneous interleukin-1 release by monocytes from postmenopausal women. J Clin Endocrinol Metab 1989; 68:364–368.

97. Pacifici R, Rifas L, Teitelbaum S, et al. Spontaneous release of interleukin-1 from human blood monocytes reflects bone formation in idiopathic osteoporosis. Proc Natl Acad Sci USA 1987; 84:4616–4620.

98. Gallagher JC, Riggs BL, Jerpbak CM, et al. The effect of age on serum immunoreactive parathyroid hormone in normal and osteoporotic women. J Lab Clin Med 1980; 95:373–385.

99. Eastell R, Riggs BL. Diagnostic evaluation of osteoporosis. Endocrinol Metab Clin North Am 1988; 17:547–571.

100. Aloia JF, Cohn SH, Vaswani A, et al. Risk factors for postmenopausal osteoporosis. Am J Med 1985; 78:95–100.

101. Drinkwater BL, Nilson K, Chesnut CH, et al. Bone mineral content of amenorrheic and eumenorrhic athletes. N Engl J Med 1984; 311:277–281.

102. Marcus R, Cann C, Madvig P, et al. Menstrual function and bone mass in elite women distance runners. Ann Intern Med 1985; 102:158–163.

103. Rigotti NA, Nussbaum SR, Herzog DB, et al. Osteoporosis in women with anorexia nervosa. N Engl J Med 1984; 311:1601–1606.

104. Biller BMK, Saxe V, Herzog DB, et al. Mechanisms of osteoporosis in adult and adolescent women with anorexia nervosa. J Clin Endocrinol Metab 1989; 68:548–554.

105. Klibanski A, Greenspan SL. Increase in bone mass after treatment of hyperprolactinemic amenorrhea. N Engl J Med 1986; 315:542–546.

106. Schlechte J, El-khoury G, Kathol M, et al. Forearm and vertebral bone mineral in treated and untreated hyperprolactinemic amenorrhea. J Clin Endocrinol Metab 1987; 64:1021–1026.

107. Greenspan SL, Neer RM, Ridgway EC, et al. Osteoporosis in men with hyperprolactinemic hypogonadism. Ann Intern Med 1986; 104:777–782.

108. Jackson JA, Kleerekoper M, Parfitt AM, et al. Bone histomorphometry in hypogonadal and eugonadal men with spinal osteoporosis. J Clin Endocrinol Metab 1987; 65:53–58.

109. Rigotti NA, Neer RM, Jameson L. Osteopenia and bone fractures in a man with anorexia nervosa and hypogonadism. JAMA 1986; 256:385–388.

110. Finkelstein JS, Klibanski A, Neer RM, et al. Osteoporosis in men with idiopathic hypogonadotropic hypogonadism. Ann Intern Med 1987; 106:354–361.

111. Seeman E, Melton LJ III, O'Fallon WM, et al. Risk factors for spinal osteoporosis in men. Am J Med 1983; 75:977–983.

112. Johnell O, Nilsson BE. Lifestyle and bone mineral mass in perimenopausal women. Calcif Tiss Int 1984; 36:354–356.

113. Fonseca VA, D'Sousa V, Houlder S, et al. Vitamin D deficiency and low osteocalcin concentrations in anorexia nervosa. J Clin Pathol 1988; 41:195–197.

114. Reid IR. Pathogenesis and treatment of steroid osteoporosis. Clin Endocrinol 1989; 30:83–103.

115. Seeman E, Wahner HW, Offord KP, et al. Differential effects of endocrine dysfunction on the axial and the appendicular skeleton. J Clin Invest 1982; 69:1302–1309.

116. Hui SL, Epstein S, Johnston CC Jr. A prospective study of bone mass in patients with type I diabetes. J Clin Endocrinol Metab 1985; 60:74–80.

117. Devogelaer JP, Crabbe J, De Deuxchaisnes CN. Bone mineral density in Addison's disease: Evidence for an effect of adrenal androgens on bone mass. Br Med J 1987; 294:798–800.

118. Daniell HW. Osteoporosis of the slender smoker: Vertebral compression fractures and loss of metacarpal cortex in relation to postmenopausal cigarette smoking and lack of obesity. Arch Intern Med 1976; 136:298–304.

119. De Vernejoul MC, Bielakoff J, Herve M, et al. Evidence for defective osteoblastic function: A role for alcohol and tobacco consumption in osteoporosis in middle-aged men. Clin Orthop 1983; 179:107–115.

120. Jensen J, Christiansen C, Rodbro P. Cigarette smoking, serum estrogens, and bone loss during hormone-replacement therapy early after menopause. N Engl J Med 1985; 313:973–975.

121. Crilly RG, Anderson C, Hogan D, et al. Bone histomorphometry, bone mass, and related parameters in alcoholic males. Calcif Tiss Int 1988; 43:269–276.

122. Diamond T, Stiel D, Lunzer M, et al. Ethanol reduces bone formation and may cause osteoporosis. Am J Med 1989; 86:282–288.

123. Steinberg FU. The effects of immobilization on bone. In: The Immobilized Patient: Functional Pathology and Management. New York: Plenum 1980;33–64.

124. Ettinger B, Winger J. Thyroid supplements: Effect on bone mass. West J Med 1982; 136:472–476.

125. Fallon MD, Perry HM, Bergfeld M, et al. Exogenous hyperthyroidism with osteoporosis. Arch Intern Med 1983; 143:442–444.

126. Hahn TJ. Drug–induced disorders of vitamin D and mineral metabolism. Clin Endocrinol Metab 1980; 9:107–129.

127. Melton LJ III, Riggs BL. Clinical spectrum. In: Riggs BL, Melton LJ III, eds. Osteoporosis: Etiology, Diagnosis, and Management. New York: Raven Press, 1988;155–260.

128. Mazanec DJ, Grisanti JM. Drug-induced osteoporosis. Cleve Clin J Med 1989; 56:297–303.

129. Heaney RP, Recker RR. Effects of nitrogen, phosphorus, and caffeine on calcium balance in women. J Lab Clin Med 1982; 99:46–55.

130. Parfitt AM. Dietary risk factors for age-related bone loss and fractures. Lancet 1983; 2:1181–1185.

131. Riggs BL, Wahner HW, Melton LJ III, et al. Dietary calcium intake and rates of bone loss in women. J Clin Invest 1987; 80:979–982.

132. Kanis JA, Passmore R. Calcium supplementation of the diet - II. Br Med J 1989; 298:205–208.

133. Riis B, Thomsen K, Christiansen C. Does calcium supplementation prevent postmenopausal bone loss? A double-blind, controlled clinical study. N Engl J Med 1987; 316:173–177.

134. Liel Y, Edwards J, Shary J, et al. The effects of race and body habitus on bone mineral density of the radius, hip, and spine in premenopausal women. J Clin Endocrinol Metab 1988; 66:1247–1250.

135. Weinstein RS, Bell NH. Diminished rates of bone formation in normal black adults. N Engl J Med 1988; 319:1698–1701.

136. Moller M, Horsman A, Harvald B, et al. Metacarpal morphometry in monozygotic and dizygotic elderly twins. Calcif Tiss Res 1978; 25:197–201.

137. Pocock NA, Eisman JA, Hopper JL, et al. Genetic determinants of bone mass in adults. A twin study. J Clin Invest 1987; 80:706–710.

138. Dequeker J, Nijs J, Verstraeten A, et al. Genetic determinants of bone mineral content at the spine and radius: A twin study. Bone 1987; 8:207–209.

139. Christian JC, Pao-Lo Y, Slemenda CW, et al. Heritability of bone mass: A longitudinal study in aging male twins. Am J Hum Genet 1989; 44:429–433.

140. Seeman E, Hopper JL, Bach LA, et al. Reduced bone mass in daughters of women with osteoporosis. N Engl J Med 1989; 320:554–558.

141. Gardsell P, Lindberg H, Obrant KJ. Osteoporosis and heredity. Clin Orthop 1989; 240:164–167.

142. Evans RA, Marel GM, Lancaster EK, et al. Bone mass is low in relatives of osteoporotic patients. Ann Intern Med 1988; 109:870–873.

143. Beals RK. Orthopedic aspects of the XO (Turner's) syndrome. Clin Orthop 1973; 97:19–39.

144. Stepan JJ, Musilova J, Pacovsky V. Bone demineralization, biochemical indices of bone remodeling, and estrogen replacement therapy in adults with Turner's syndrome. J Bone Miner Res 1989; 4:193–198.

145. Kleerekoper M, Tolia K, Parfitt AM. Nutritional, endocrine, and demographic aspects of osteoporosis. Orthop Clin North Am 1981; 12:547–559.

146. Matkovic V, Kostial K, Simonovic I, et al. Bone status and fracture rates in two regions of Yugoslavia. Am J Clin Nutr 1979; 32:540–549.

147. Sandler RB, Slemenda CW, LaPorte RE, et al. Postmenopausal bone density and milk consumption in childhood and adolescence. Am J Clin Nutr 1985; 42:270–274.

148. Cauley JA, Gutai JP, Kuller LH, et al. Endogenous estrogen levels and calcium intakes in postmenopausal women. Relationships with cortical bone measures. JAMA 1988; 260:3150–3155.

149. Kanders B, Dempster DW, Lindsay R. Interaction of calcium nutrition and physical activity on bone mass in young women. J Bone Miner Res 1988; 3:145–149.

150. Aloia JF, Vaswani AN, Yeh JK, et al. Premenopausal bone mass is related to physical activity. Arch Intern Med 1988; 148:121–123.

151. Block JE, Genant HK, Black D. Greater vertebral bone mineral mass in exercising young men. West J Med 1986; 145:39–42.

152. Dalen N, Olsson KE. Bone mineral content and physical activity. Acta Orthop Scand 1974; 45:170–174.

153. Nilsson BE, Westlin NE. Bone density in athletes. Clin Orthop 1971; 77:179–182.

154. Nilsson BE, Andersson SM, Havdrup T, et al. Ballet dancing and weight lifting—effects on BMC (abstr). AJR 1978; 131:541–542.

155. Ruff CB, Hayes WC. Subperiosteal expansion and cortical remodeling of the human femur and tibia with aging. Science 1982; 217:945–948.

156. Zagba-Mongalima G, Goret-Nicaise M, Dhem A. Age changes in human bone: A microradiographic and histological study of subperiosteal and periosteal calcifications. Gerontology 1988; 34:264–276.

157. Tinetti ME, Speechley M. Prevention of falls among the elderly. N Engl J Med 1989; 320:1055–1059.

158. Sinaki M. Postmenopausal spinal osteoporosis. Mayo Clin Proc 1982; 57:699–703.

159. Cummings SR. Bone mineral densitometry. Ann Intern Med 1987; 107:932–936.

160. Wahner HW, Dunn WL, Brown ML, et al. Comparison of dual energy x-ray absorptiometry and dual photon absorptiometry for bone mineral measurements of the lumbar spine. Mayo Clin Proc 1988; 63:1075–1084.

161. Civitelli R, Gonnelli S, Zacchei F, et al. Bone turnover in postmenopausal osteoporosis. Effect of calcitonin treatment. J Clin Invest 1988; 82:1268–1274.

162. Aloia JF, Cohn SH, Ostuni JA, et al. Prevention of involutional bone loss by exercise. Ann Intern Med 1978; 89:356–358.

163. Dalsky GP, Stocke KS, Ehsani AA, et al. Weight-bearing exercise training and lumbar bone mineral content in postmenopausal women. Ann Intern Med 1988; 108:824–828.

164. Chow R, Harrison JE, Notarius C. Effect of two randomized exercise programmes on bone mass of healthy postmenopausal women. Br Med J 1987; 295:1441–1444.

165. Smith EL, Gilligan C, McAdam M, et al. Deterring bone loss by exercise intervention in premenopausal and postmenopausal women. Calcif Tiss Int 1989; 44:312–321.

166. Black-Sandler R, Cauley JA, Hom DL, et al. The effects of walking on the cross-sectional dimensions of the radius in postmenopausal women. Calcif Tiss Int 1987; 41:65–69.

167. Cavanaugh DJ, Cann CE. Brisk walking does not stop bone loss in postmenopausal women. Bone 1988; 9:201–204.

168. Sinaki M, McPhee MC, Hodgson SF, et al. Relationship between bone mineral density of spine and strength of back extensors in healthy postmenopausal women. Mayo Clin Proc 1986; 61:116–122.

169. Sinaki M, Grubbs NC. Back-strengthening exercises: Quantitative evaluation of their efficacy for women aged 40 to 65 years. Arch Phys Med Rehabil 1989; 70:16–20.

170. Huddleston AL, Rockwell D, Kulund DN. Bone mass in lifetime tennis athletes. JAMA 1980; 244:1107–1109.

171. Lindsay R, Aitken JM, Andersen JB, et al. Long-term prevention of postmenopausal osteoporosis by estrogen. Lancet 1976; 1:1038–1040.

172. Aitken JM, Lindsay R, Hart DM. Long-term estrogens for the prevention of postmenopausal osteoporosis. Postgrad Med J 1976; 52 (suppl 6):18–25.

173. Lindsay R, Hart DM, Forrest C, et al. Prevention of spinal osteoporosis in oophorectomised women. Lancet 1980; ii:1151–1154.

174. Lindsay R, Hart DM, Clark DM. The minimum effective dose of estrogen for prevention of postmenopausal bone loss. Obstet Gynecol 1984; 63:759–763.

175. Ettinger B, Genant HK, Cann CE. Long-term estrogen replacement therapy prevents bone loss and fractures. Ann Intern Med 1985; 102:319–324.

176. Kiel DP, Felson DT, Anderson JJ, et al. Hip frac-

ture and the use of estrogens in postmenopausal women. The Framingham Study. N Engl J Med 1987; 317:1169–1174.

177. Barzel US. Estrogens in the prevention and treatment of postmenopausal osteoporosis: A review. Am J Med 1988; 85:847–850.

178. Ettinger B, Genant HK, Cann CE. Postmenopausal bone loss is prevented by treatment with low-dosage estrogen with calcium. Ann Intern Med 1987; 106:40–45.

179. Macintyre I, Whitehead MI, Banks LM, et al. Calcitonin for prevention of postmenopausal bone loss. Lancet 1988;900–902.

180. Fatourechi V, Heath H III. Salmon calcitonin in the treatment of postmenopausal osteoporosis. Ann Intern Med 1987; 107:923–925.

181. Reginster JY, Albert A, Lecart MP, et al. One-year randomised trial of prevention of early postmenopausal bone loss by intranasal calcitonin. Lancet 1987; ii1481–1483.

182. MacKinnon JL: Osteoporosis. A review. Phys Ther 1988; 68:1533–1540.

183. Krolner B, Toft B, Nielsen SP, et al. Physical exercise as prophylaxis against involutional vertebral bone loss: A controlled trial. Clin Sci 1983; 64:541–546.

184. Sinaki M, Mikkelsen BA. Postmenopausal spinal osteoporosis: Flexion versus extension exercises. Arch Phys Med Rehabil 1984; 65:593–596.

185. Simkin A, Ayalon J, Leichter I. Increased trabecular bone density due to bone-loading exercises in postmenopausal osteoporotic women. Calcif Tiss Int 1987; 40:59–63.

186. Smith ML, Fogelman I, Hart DM, et al. Effect of etidronate disodium on bone turnover following surgical menopause. Calcif Tiss Int 1989; 44:74–79.

187. Storm T, Thamsborg G, Steiniche T, et al. Effects of intermittent cyclical etidronate therapy on bone mass and fracture rate in women with postmenopausal osteoporosis. N Engl J Med 1990; 322:1265–1271.

188. Watts NB, Harris ST, Genant HK, et al. Intermittent cyclical etidronate treatment of postmenopausal osteoporosis. N Engl J Med 1990; 323:73–79.

189. Chestnut CH III. Optimizing bone mass in the perimenopause: Calcitonin and diphosphonates. In: Kleerekoper M, Krane SM, eds. Clinical Disorders of Bone and Mineral Metabolism. New York: Mary Ann Liebert, 1989;199–201.

190. Hedlund LR, Gallagher JC. Increased incidence of hip fracture in osteoporotic women treated with sodium fluoride. J Bone Miner Res 1989; 4:223–225.

191. Riggs BL, Hodgson SF, O'Fallon WM, et al. Effects of fluoride treatment on the fracture rate in postmenopausal women with osteoporosis. N Engl J Med 1990; 322:802–809.

192. Kleerekoper M, Peterson EL, Nelson DA, et al. A randomized trial of sodium fluoride as a treatment for postmenopausal osteoporosis. Osteoporosis International 1991; 1:155–161.

193. Pedrazzoni M, Palummeri E, Pioli G, et al. Involutional osteoporosis and ADFR treatment: A controlled pilot study. Curr Ther Res 1989; 45:188–197.

194. Hesch R, Busch U, Prokop M, et al. Increase of vertebral density by combination therapy with pulsatile 1-38hPTH and sequential addition of calcitonin nasal spray in osteoporotic patients. Calcif Tiss Int 1989; 44:176–180.

# Chapter 28

# Biology of Aging in Humans

JOSE A. ALONSO
LUCIEN J. COTE

In the past few decades the aging of the American population has greatly increased the need for a better understanding of the normal physiology of aging in humans and of the pathologic states associated with it.

In 1900, the mean life expectancy at birth in America was 49 years; in 1985, it was 72 years for men and 79 years for women, and it continues to rise.[1] The maximum human life span is estimated to be 110 to 120 years. Needless to say, with rapidly advancing medical knowledge, new and more effective drugs, and greater emphasis on proper diet and exercise programs, we are certain to have a greater number of centenarians in the future. Today, in fact, people 65 years of age and older are the most rapidly increasing segment of the population. The marked rise in the population of elders brings with it an increased number of medical problems, among them osteoporosis, stroke, emphysema, and Alzheimer's disease, which are now reaching epidemic incidence. To deal effectively with these problems is one of the most challenging tasks we face as we approach the 21st century. If we are to make inroads in these aged-related disorders, we must broaden our knowledge of normal aging.

To the best of our knowledge, normal aging is a series of events that, like development, are genetically programmed. Because the events are also affected by environmental factors, life stresses, disease states, and other variables, it is difficult to isolate the normal aging changes. Nonetheless, even in the time of Aristotle, it was recognized that each species had its own maximum life span. Most gerontologists (research scientists interested in normal aging) believe that we have genes that guide us through life, playing a role in the normal physiologic changes of aging and eventually death. The primary goal of a geriatrician should be to maintain the quality of life by preventing age-related diseases or by treating them effectively. To prolong any life without respect for the quality of life is a dubious achievement.

## Systemic Changes Associated with Aging

### Cardiovascular System

The age-related changes of the cardiovascular system at rest and during exercise have been reviewed.[2] A major difficulty in studying these changes lies in distinguishing pathologic processes that increase with age from those that are due solely to biologic aging.

Histologic and cellular changes of the aging heart include accumulation of lipofuscin in the nuclei of cardiac muscle cells[3] and diminution in the number of pacemaker cells in the sinoatrial node.[4] Wei[5] reviewed the age-related changes in blood vessels; the intima shows irregularity in shape and size of endothelial cells with an increased number of giant multinucleated cells; the subendothelial layer shows increased amounts of connective tissue and lipid deposits, as well as increased calcification; the media, likewise, shows increased calcification as well as increasing fragmentation of elastic laminae; changes in the adventitia have not been clearly established.

Macroscopic changes in the aging heart include an increase in heart weight,[2] and an increase in the thickness of the left ventricular wall, which is thought to be due to cellular hypertrophy rather than hyperplasia.[6]

At rest, overall cardiac function can be measured by determining the cardiac output (the product of heart rate and stroke volume). Whether cardiac output at rest decreases or remains unchanged with aging is a matter of controversy. Brandfonbrener and coworkers[7] noted an age-related decrement in stroke volume and an average diminution of cardiac output of 1% per year, but Rodeheffer and colleagues[8] reported no change in resting cardiac output or stroke volume with increasing age. The difference in the findings may be due to the fact that a significant number of elderly people with latent coronary artery disease participated in the former study but such subjects were carefully excluded from the latter one. Thus, pathologic changes, rather than changes due to true biologic aging, may be responsible for the decrement in cardiac output and stroke volume seen in some elders.

Stroke volume, in turn, depends on preload, myocardial contractility, and afterload. Rodeheffer's group[8] noted no age-related change in preload; however, Miyatake and associates[9] recorded among older subjects, using intracardiac Doppler flowmetry, augmentation of atrial contribution to left ventricular flow. This increase possibly serves to compensate for the age-associated decreased compliance of the left ventricle. It is also thought that myocardial contractility is not significantly affected by aging, though prolongation of isometric relaxation has been noted. Fleg[2] reviewed the possible causes of the increase in afterload associated with greater age. They include structural and functional changes in the aorta and other large arteries (e.g., alterations in pulse contour, increase in pulse wave velocity, and increase in the static circumferential modulus). Humoral and autonomic factors, including the association of increased levels of plasma norepinephrine with advancing age,

also contribute to the increase in afterload. The increase in afterload with aging is clinically manifested by an increase in systolic blood pressure and compensatory left ventricular hypertrophy occurs to permit normal wall tension and stroke volume.

Overall cardiovascular fitness can be estimated by measuring the maximal oxygen consumption ($Vo_2$max) during exercise. Several investigators[10,11] have noted diminution of $Vo_2$ max with increasing age. $Vo_2$ max is proportional to the arteriovenous oxygen difference ($a - \overline{V}o_2$), as well as cardiac output. Seals and coworkers[12] noted reduction in the maximal arteriovenous oxygen difference with aging, suggesting increased difficulty of muscles in extracting and utilizing oxygen or problems with redistribution of blood flow to skeletal muscle during exercise, or both.

Whether with increasing age maximal cardiac output with exercise decreases or remains unchanged is a matter of controversy. Julius and coworkers[13] note an age-related decrement in maximal cardiac output that is thought to be due primarily to a decline in maximal heart rate and, to a lesser extent, to a decline in stroke volume. In contrast, Rodeheffer and colleagues[8] found no change in maximal cardiac output with increasing age; though maximal heart rate decreased with age, this was counteracted by an increase in maximal stroke volume. The difference in the results may be due to inclusion of a significant number of elderly people with latent coronary disease in the former case but not in the latter.

Stroke volume during exercise, as at rest, is dependent on preload, myocardial contractility, and afterload. Rodeheffer's group[8] found an age-related increase in end-diastolic volume and cardiac dilatation during exercise; the increase in venous return (preload) promotes diastolic filling, and thus enhances stroke volume, in keeping with the Frank-Starling mechanism. The same authors found no change in age-related myocardial contractility or afterload during exercise. This is in contrast to results noted by Borer and coworkers,[14] who observed a decline in myocardial contractility (as measured by the ejection fraction) and Julius and associates,[13] who reported increased afterload during maximal exercise. The contrast between the findings of Rodeheffer's group and other researchers, as previously noted, may be due to inclusion of patients with coronary artery disease in the other studies. However, in the study mentioned here, Rodeheffer's group do note a decrement in the absolute ejection fraction at maximal effort in their elderly subjects, and this is attributed to decreased sensitivity of the aging heart to catecholamines.

With increasing age, the cardiovascular response to orthostasis also changes, so that an increase in heart rate is blunted during orthostatic changes.[5] A postprandial hypotensive response has also been noted in elders.[15]

## Pulmonary System

The age-related changes of the pulmonary system have been reviewed previously.[16,17] Chest wall compliance decreases owing to stiffening and calcification at the costovertebral joints, decreased elasticity of costal cartilage, decreased thoracic disc height, and increased thoracic kyphosis. The decrease in the elastic recoil of the lung is thought to be due to increased collagen fiber cross-linkages and to a reduction in the thickness and number of elastic fibers.[18,19] The combination of diminished chest wall compliance and elastic recoil of the lung are thought to contribute to the increase in functional residual capacity (FRC), and residual volume (RV), and the decrease in vital capacity (VC) associated with aging.

Reddan[20] reports age-related changes in the bronchial tree, including thickening of the mucus layer, and increase in the number of bronchial mucous glands, and a decrease in the elastic properties of bronchial cartilage. These changes result in increased airway resistance and contribute to the decrement in forced expiratory volume ($FEV_1L/sec$) and peak expiratory flow rate associated with aging.

The decreased compliance and increased airway resistance add to the work of breathing for the respiratory muscles, which, like other skeletal muscles, are rendered less capable of meeting the increasing work demands by age-related changes. This is especially true during periods of stress such as exercise. The maximal minute ventilation ($V_E$) during exercise is decreased in older persons, who, in contrast to younger ones, depend more on an increase in respiratory rate than on an increase in tidal volume ($V_T$) to attain a given $V_E$; the result is increased work of breathing, which increases the likelihood of respiratory muscle fatigue.[21]

An age-related decrement also occurs in gas diffusion from the alveoli into the capillaries. This results from a decrease in alveolar surface area and a decrement in diffusing capacity.[22] Owing to changes in ventilation/perfusion ratios, the anatomic and the physiologic dead space are increased in older persons.[23] Arterial oxygenation ($Pao_2$) and oxygen saturation ($So_2$) decrease with aging, but arterial carbon dioxide ($Paco_2$) remains unchanged.[24]

## Muscular System

The functional, morphologic, and biochemical age-related changes of muscle were reviewed by Cress and coworkers.[25] Functional changes of aging include loss of lean muscle mass, muscle atrophy, and decline in absolute muscle strength. Muscle endurance relative to maximal strength does not appear to diminish with age.

Tzankoff[26] noted a 40% decline in lean muscle mass with increasing age when comparing 80-year-old and 30-year-old men, and Borkan and colleagues[27] reported an 11.7% loss in lean muscle mass when comparing middle-aged men to older ones.

An age-related decrement in muscle strength has been noted in several studies. Aniansson and colleagues[28] in a longitudinal study of muscle strength in healthy elderly subjects, followed 19 men and 21 women from age 70 until age 75 years. This study found that over the 5-year period, isometric and isokinetic knee extensor strength of both men and women declined. The researchers also reported a decline in strength of the elbow flexors and extensors but noted no change in hand grip strength—especially in the key grip, which is used very frequently in activities of daily living. A positive correlation between isokinetic muscle strength in the knee flexors and extensors and a higher level of physical activity in men was also observed. This positive correlation, as well as the maintenance of hand-grip strength with aging, led the authors to hypothesize that the age-related decline in muscle strength may be based on a changed activity pattern and may be reversible if elderly people remain physically active. Pearson and colleagues,[29] in a cross-sectional study, found a decrement in isometric strength and muscle area of the triceps surae and biceps brachii when they compared 100 women and 84 men between ages 65 and 90 years to younger subjects. In a study of 114 boys and men aged 11 to 70 years, Larsson and associates[30] noted increasing dynamic and isometric quadriceps strength until 35 years of age, and no significant further change until age 50; after age 50 men's strength and velocity of contraction declined. Davies and colleagues[31] studied the electrically evoked mechanical properties of the triceps surae in 69-year-old and 22-year-old men and women and found an increased time to peak tension of the twitch, a lower force–cross-sectional area, and easier fatiguability in the muscles of the elderly subjects. In reviewing the literature, Brown[32] found that though there is a range in the magnitude of decline in isometric muscle strength with aging, a trend of declining strength with increasing age is evident, while when subjects in their 60s and 70s were compared to those in their 30s, the isometric strength of the older group was 20% to 50% less than that of the younger group. The age-related decline in muscle strength appears to be greater in back and lower extremity muscles than in upper extremity muscles, and greater in proximal lower extremity muscles than in distal ones.[33–37]

Two factors have often been cited to explain loss of muscle strength with age. One is the reduction of the number of functional motor units with age[38]; the other is the decrease in some customary activities of elders that may lead to relative disuse of certain muscles.[39,40] As Knortz' review[37] shows, several factors have been proposed to explain the decrease in the number of functional motor units with age: changes in neuromuscular transmission, reduced number of neurons, decreased number of muscle fibers. In a cross-sectional study of 56 men and 66 women older than 65 years who were living independently, Bassey and coworkers[40] measured both maximal voluntary strength of the triceps surae and the amount and speed of walking, a customary activity. They found that triceps surae strength in men had a

positive correlation with walking speed and total walking distance, but it declined with age. Muscle strength in women was significantly associated with walking speed and leisure pursuits, but it also declined with age. Though total walking distance was the same for women and men, the amount of walking was not significantly related to muscle strength for women, though it was for men. The authors theorize that this difference may be due to different patterns of walking among men and women. Women in the group tended to walk more inside the house, men more outdoors. The authors note that the women's short distance walking around the house would not load the plantar flexors as much as several periods of continuous outdoor walking. Even after adjustment for body weight, men were significantly stronger and walked significantly faster than women. Given these findings, the authors raise the possibility that the loss of muscle strength with aging may be partly reversed by increasing certain types of daily physical activities.

Relative muscle endurance does not appear to decrease with age. Brown[32] notes that as long as older people work at the same relative intensity (same percentage of their maximum strength) as younger ones, the older ones are able to continue a particular activity as long as the younger ones. No change in quadriceps femoris[41] or hand grip endurance[42] has been associated with increasing age when work intensity has been maintained at equivalent percentages of maximum strength for older and younger subjects.

Researchers note that some of the morphologic changes observed with aging are closely related to the reduction in muscle mass. Before discussing the morphologic age-related changes of muscle, a review of the metabolic and mechanical properties of the different types of skeletal muscle fibers may prove helpful. Kidd and colleagues[43] discuss the different properties of type I (slow-twitch, oxidative), type IIa (fast-twitch, oxidative-glycolytic), and type IIb (fast-twitch, glycolytic) muscle fibers. Type I fibers, characterized by small muscle fiber diameter, contract slowly and fatigue slowly; their major source of adenosine triphosphate (ATP) is oxidative phosphorylation, so they have numerous mitochondria, high myoglobin content, dense capillarity, but low glycogen content, glycolytic enzyme activity, and myosin APTase activity. Type IIb fibers have a large muscle fiber diameter and have fast speed of contraction and rate of fatigue. Their major source of ATP is glycolysis; thus, they have few mitochondria, low myoglobin content, sparse capillarity, but high glycogen content, glycolytic enzyme activity, and myosin ATPase activity. Type IIa fibers have a fast speed of contraction and an intermediate rate of fatigue compared to type I and IIb fibers. The major source of ATP for type IIa fibers is oxidative phosphorylation, but they also use glycolysis and thus have intermediate aerobic capacity; they have numerous mitochondria, high myoglobin content, dense capillarity, high myosin ATPase activity, and intermediate glycogen content and glycolytic enzyme activity as compared to type I and type IIb fibers. Thus, type II fibers are well-suited for generating large forces quickly (weight-lifting–type activities), whereas type I fibers are better suited for endurance-type activities that require less intense effort over a longer time.

The decline in muscle mass with aging has been related to a reduction in the total number of muscle fibers or a reduction in size of type II fibers. Though most investigators agree that there is relative stability of type I fibers with age, the mechanism of loss of lean muscle mass secondary to changes in the type II fiber population has not been as clearly defined.[25] Grimby and colleagues[44] attribute the loss to a declining number of type II fibers; Larsson[45] attributes the decline to a reduction in fiber size. Grimby and colleagues[35] also note that the reduction in the cross-sectional area of type II fibers is not equal for all muscle groups. Large weight-bearing muscle groups show greater loss of cross-sectional area than non–weight-bearing muscles of the upper extremities. Cress and colleagues[25] speculate that the unequal changes in fiber types observed in weight-bearing and non–weight-bearing muscles may be due to decreased weight-bearing activity by elders as compared to relative continuation of more sedentary activities that require use of non–weight-bearing muscles of the arms.

Other morphologic changes in older muscle include changes in the size or number of mitochondria[46] and fine structural changes detected by electron microscopy. The electron mi-

croscopic age-related changes were summarized by Cress and coworkers[25] and include changes in the sarcolemma and sarcoplasmic reticulum, Z lines, T system, and mitochondria.

The biochemical age-related changes of skeletal muscle were previously reviewed.[25] The data on anaerobic enzymes are conflicting. While levels of creatine phosphokinase and lactate dehydrogenase have been reported by some investigators to increase with age,[47] others found no change in lactate dehydrogenase level and a decline in phosphofructokinase level.[48] Aerobic enzyme concentrations seem to be relatively unchanged with increasing age, as evidenced by maintenance of lactate dehydrogenase-H levels.[45]

## Skeletal System

Tonna observed involutional changes of the skeletal system with aging.[49] Using the BNL mouse model, Tonna identified a decline in the proliferative capacity of cartilage and bone cells from birth to age 8 weeks; following this, the proliferative activity remained low. Of note is that the median life span of BNL mice is 1 year, even though some mice survive as long as 2 years. Electron micrographs of osteoblasts from the femoral periosteum of 5-week-old mice revealed well-developed Golgi apparatus and rough endoplasmic reticulum. By 26 weeks of age there is little rough endoplasmic reticulum, Golgi apparatus, or mitochondria, and the nuclei become hyperchromatic. By 1 and 2 years of age degenerative changes are marked; granules of lipofuscin appear inside the osteoblasts and severe loss of cell contact and cell death are noted. With aging, as more bone is deposited by apposition at the periosteal surface, osteocytes become situated farther from the surface, and thus disposal of cellular waste and acquisition of necessary nutrients become more difficult. This, in turn, is thought to contribute to the accelerated degenerative changes that ensue, including deposition of lipofuscin granules and subsequent cell lysis. Though involutional skeletal changes are evident with aging, it has not been determined whether they represent normal skeletal biologic aging or disease activity. Whether degenerative joint disease or osteoporosis is dependent or independent of normal skeletal biologic aging remains to be determined. Garn[50] has reported the changing pattern of bone deposition and resorption with increasing age in humans. He notes that during adolescence both bone deposition and resorption are rapid, but subsequently they slow down markedly until the fourth decade; after the fourth decade, the rate of resorption tends to be greater than the rate of apposition. The age of onset and rate of bone loss differ for men and women. In women, bone loss begins about age 30 to 35 years and the rate of loss is approximately 1% per year before menopause and 2% to 3% per year after menopause. In contrast, bone loss in men begins at approximately age 50 at a rate of about 0.4% per year.[51,52]

Tissue flexibility has been noted to decrease 20% to 30% in elders.[53] Most of this loss in flexibility, according to Johns and associates,[54] is due to changes in the connective tissue in tendons, joint capsules, muscles, and ligaments. Changes in the structure of collagen and an increase in the cross-linkages of elastic fibers are among the changes noted in these structures, and these can lead to loss of flexibility.[55,56]

## *Integument*

Aging causes many changes in the skin; most make it more vulnerable to damage and disease. The skin's moisture content decreases, rendering it more brittle and more likely to tear. The rate of epidermal renewal and repair slows. The dermis becomes thinner and adheres less well to the epidermis. Skin elasticity, sebum secretion, vascular supply, hair and nail growth, and sensitivity to touch, pain, and temperature all decrease. These numerous changes render aging skin very vulnerable to breakdown, but proper preventive skin care, started early in life, can help minimize the consequences of age-related alterations and prevent many pathologic changes in the skin of elders.

## *Gastrointestinal Tract*

Though the gastrointestinal tract maintains physiologic functions relatively well even in advanced age, changes do occur. The pharyngeal muscles

tend to weaken, leading to excessive relaxation of the cricopharyngeal region and the pooling of fluids and food, posing a potential danger for aspiration. Esophageal mobility appears to be well preserved with age, though very old persons may have reflux from the stomach. Acid production in the stomach decreases with age, and in very old persons emptying time may be delayed. The small intestine shows relatively little change with age, but there is evidence that absorption of calcium, vitamin D, and iron decreases. The colon shows mucosal atrophy but hypertrophy of the muscular layer. Transit in the colon is delayed with age, but constipation in elders has been linked more to decreased water content in the feces than to slower transit. Diverticulosis is seen in about one third of the healthy 65-year-old population and two thirds of 80-year-olds.[57] With aging the liver shrinks some and is less capable of metabolizing certain drugs, such as benzodiazepines.[58]

## *Kidneys*

The kidneys shrink by about 20% with aging, and blood flow and filtration rate decrease. Vascular changes are seen, and interstitial fibrosis is common. These age-related changes per se do not cause difficulty, but if the kidneys become diseased elders may be more vulnerable to renal failure.

The prostate gland commonly causes problems for elderly men—benign prostatic hyperplasia (BPH) and carcinoma. The incidence of BPH increases to about 90% by age 80 years. The probability that a 50-year-old man will require prostatectomy sometime during his life is about 25%.[59] Carcinoma of the prostate is rare before age 50, but nearly every man has neoplastic cells in the prostate by age 80 years.[60]

## *Female Reproductive System*

Menopause is an important transitional period in a woman's life. The average age at menopause is about 50 years, so women can expect to be postmenopausal for at least 30 years. Many physiologic and psychologic changes take place during the menopausal period, and women often have difficulty dealing with them. For instance, hot flashes, which can occur many times any day or night, are extremely uncomfortable and stressful (see Chapter 25).

## Hematopoietic System

Research findings suggest that aging causes no significant changes in basal hematopoiesis, but reserve capacity decreases.[61] In normal elders hematopoiesis is difficult to evaluate, because many extraneous factors can alter the normal hematologic profile. Lipshitz and colleagues reported that serum iron is slightly lower in elders whereas the ferritin level is increased by about 75%.[62]

Anemia is relatively common in elders, but in several control studies with healthy aged humans researchers noted no significant reduction in hemoglobin.[63] Anemia in elders appears to be related to exogenous factors, among them diet, infections, medications, and chronic disease.

## Endocrine System

Age-related changes in the endocrine system occur at several levels, including in the hypothalamus, pituitary gland, and end-organs. Aminergic and neuropeptidergic neurons show reduced activity with age.[64] With aging, the hypothalamus-pituitary-adrenal axis shows decreased feedback inhibition of corticotropin-releasing hormone and of adrenocorticotropic hormone by glucocorticoids.[65] This delays return to baseline of glucocorticoid levels following stress. Growth hormone in the circulation shows a decline with aging, and growth hormone surges are reduced.

In men normal aging is associated with a moderate degree of testicular failure. The testes shrink and Leydig cells which make testosterone and Sertoli cells which produce are lost.[66]

## Nervous System

The brain decreases in weight by 15% to 20% by age 80 years, and protein content is reduced by 25% to 30%.[67] Nerve cells do not divide and thus are not replaced when they die. On the other hand,

glia cells, supporting cells that interact intimately with nerve cells, can proliferate. Age brings loss of neurons, by as much as 60% in areas of the brain such as the substantia nigra, locus ceruleus, neocortex, cerebellum, and hippocampus. Other areas of the brain, such as the nucleus basalis of Meynert and the cranial nerve nuclei, do not show any significant loss of nerve cells with normal aging. Furthermore, dendritic processes increase with age in areas of the brain such as in the hippocampus and cerebral cortex. Thus, changes in the aging brain vary much from area to area. With age, intraneuronal organelles such as neurofibrillary tangles (i.e., bundles of abnormal filaments), lipofuscin, and granulovacuoles accumulate. Senile plaques form. These roughly spherical lesions range in size from ten to several hundred microns. They contain amyloid deposits, degenerating hypertrophic neuritic processes, and intracellular organelles (microsomes, mitochondria, etc.) and are surrounded by glia cells. The changes, including plaques and neurofibrillary tangles, are seen in normal aged persons, but when they are more pronounced than normal, and especially when they are localized to certain areas of the brain (hippocampus, amygdala) dementia of the Alzheimer's type occurs. Our present knowledge does not provide a clear dividing line between normal aging changes in the brain and Alzheimer's disease.

Many non–life-threatening neurobehavioral changes occur with age that do not seriously compromise the quality of life, such as alterations in motor, sleep, and mental functions.[83] Elders have a slower gait with shorter stride length and fewer associative movements; posture is less erect than that of young adults. Postural reflexes are often sluggish, making elders more susceptible to falling. The motor changes are caused by many factors, involving both central nervous system mechanisms and peripheral changes such as reduced position sense, muscle weakness, and skeletal changes.

Elders' sleep is different—marked by more awake periods after falling asleep and decreased sleep time. Stage 1 of non–rapid eye movement sleep increases in elders, while stages 3 and 4 are reduced, as is rapid eye movement sleep. These changes, which are consistently observed with aging, can be troublesome and can result in chronic sleep deprivation.

Age-related mental changes occur, but they vary much among individuals. There is a decline in the ability to retain a large body of new information over a long period; however, performance on the vocabulary subtest of the Wechsler Adult Intelligence Scale is well-maintained into the 80s. Semantic knowledge, such as rapidly naming objects shown or naming as many words as possible that start with a given letter, declines with age. Visuospatial ability, such as arranging blocks into a design or drawing a three-dimensional figure such as a cube, is impaired in many elders. Starting in the 60s, general intelligence shows a mild decline that continues with advancing age. Thus, several aspects of cognition change with age, but they do not significantly impair the quality of life. That our grandparents sometimes forget things (benign forgetfulness) is not a sin or a reason to underrate their wisdom.

## The Role of Exercise in Aging

Exercise programs for elders should be carefully evaluated before being prescribed, as they offer both benefits and complications for the various organ systems. An appropriate exercise program helps maximize elders' ability to function while minimizing untoward effects.

The possible positive effects of endurance training on the cardiovascular system for elders are reviewed in the literature,[17,68] and changes in resting blood pressure and heart rate have been reported. Larsson and colleagues[69] in a cross-sectional study, compared 18 athletic men of mean age of 65 years to 648 nonathletic men at age 67. The study reported significantly lower resting heart rates and systolic blood pressures among the athletes but no significant difference in diastolic blood pressure. (The authors acknowledge the possibility that atypical subjects were selected for this study.) In a longitudinal study, DeVries[70] notes a decrement in both systolic and diastolic blood pressure at rest in a group of older subjects, after a 6-week endurance training program. Researchers have also observed reductions in heart rate for a given submaximal workload after training.[71,72] Seals and colleagues,[12] in a longitudinal study of older subjects who participated for a year in an endurance training program, noted not only a lower heart rate

at a given submaximal workload, but they also reported an increment in submaximal stroke volume, maximal stroke volume, maximal arteriovenous oxygen difference, and maximal oxygen consumption ($VO_2$max). However, this study reported no changes in submaximal cardiac output, maximal cardiac output, submaximal arteriovenous oxygen difference, or maximal heart rate. Other investigators[73,74] have also reported increase in $VO_2$ max after training. Sidney and colleagues[75] reported a significant decrement in ST depression after endurance training.

Frontera's group reviewed the possible positive effects of endurance training on the pulmonary system of elders.[17] In their study, Seals and coworkers[12] report a decrease in $V_E$ at a given submaximal workload, as well as an increase in maximal $V_E$ after endurance training. In a cross-sectional study, Verg and associates[73] compare older athletes to sedentary control subjects. A similar increase in maximal $V_E$ and decrease in $V_E$ at a given submaximal workload were observed in the athletes.

The possible benefits for elders of an exercise program for the neuromuscular system were reviewed earlier.[76,77] The number of terminal sprouts of neurons in the soleus muscles of older rats that had undergone a five-month treadmill exercise program increased over those of a control group.[78] In studies involving human subjects, reaction time has been found to increase with increasing age, though less for physically active persons than for sedentary ones.[79,80] Aniansson[81,82] reported increases in isokinetic and isometric strength in subjects older than 70 years who have undergone a strengthening program as compared to younger persons; the postulated mechanisms for this increase in strength include increased recruitment and increased size of motor units supplying type IIA (fast-twitch) fibers. Moritani and associates[83] compared the effects of a strengthening program on the elbow flexors of men in their 60s and 70s to that of men in their teens and 20s. They noted that, after training, the older group showed increased recruitment of motor units by electromyography and no change in muscle hypertrophy. Though strength acquisition was similar in the younger and the older groups, in the younger group increasing strength correlated with muscle hypertrophy and increased neural activity.

In elders increases in strength may be due partly to nervous system adaptations, but muscle changes may also contribute. Larsson[84] reported reversal of type I and type II fiber atrophy in men in their 50s and 60s who participated in a quadriceps strengthening program. Animal studies report similar reduction in the fiber atrophy associated with aging. Brown[85] has noted that soleus muscle of older rats subjected for 1 year to a running program had a larger area of type I fibers and their extensor digitorum longus a greater area of type II fibers than a nonexercised control group. Similarly, Stebbins and coworkers[86] reported fewer atrophic muscle fibers in the gastrocnemius of older female rats subjected for 5 months to treadmill endurance training, as compared to nonexercised controls.

Endurance training has also been noted to increase aerobic enzyme activity in elders. Sanchez and colleagues[87] found increased levels of the aerobic enzyme citrate synthetase in the soleus and extensor digitorum longus of older rats subjected to a 3-month running program. Suominen's group[88] reported increased levels of malate dehydrogenase and succinate dehydrogenase in sedentary men in the fifth through the seventh decade who participated in an 8-week bicycle training program. Kiessling and colleagues[89] found that sedentary middle-aged men who followed a 13-week endurance training program had increased levels of cytox, an aerobic enzyme, though their increment in aerobic enzyme activity was still only half that of trained athletes.

The positive effects of physical activity on the skeletal system were also reviewed earlier.[90,91] Though some negative results have been reported, in general most cross-sectional studies suggest that a higher level of physical activity is associated with greater bone mass. In a study involving 14- to 50-year-old professional tennis players, Jones and coworkers[92] noted a greater cortical thickness in the dominant humerus when compared to the nondominant (control) arm. A similar pattern has been found in tennis players aged 70 to 84 years.[93] Jacobson and colleagues[94] reported lower bone mineral content and ratio of bone mineral to width in the distal radius and midradius of physically inactive women in the teens through the 30s and in the 40s through the 60s, as compared to physically active controls. This same study noted a different distribution of bone mineral content in swimmers and tennis players than in age-matched controls. The swimmers also had greater mineral content in the radius and metatarsals, but no change in mineral content in the lumbar spine. The tennis players had greater mineral content at all three sites than the control group, and more lumbar and metatarsal bone mineral content than the swimmers. This suggests that bone hypertrophy in specific areas depends on individual activity patterns. Swimming, a non–weight-bearing activity, does not load the lumbar spine and metatarsals as much as tennis, a weight-bearing activity, does.

Cross-sectional studies suggest that physical activity increases bone mass in elders, but researchers must remain aware of the possible errors introduced by selection in these studies. Do elderly professional athletes and physically active elders have greater bone density than controls only because they exercise more, or did their genes code for heavier bones that made them stronger and less liable to injuries so that they tend to choose a more active lifestyle? This factor can be overcome by performing longitudinal studies, but, even in longitudinal studies, difficulties with randomization, with intercorrelations of bone density in different skeletal regions, and limitations of measurement techniques make fully accurate interpretation of studies problematic.[91] As with cross-sectional studies, although some negative results have been reported, in general, most longitudinal studies suggest that a higher level of physical activity is associated with greater bone mass.

In a longitudinal study involving women aged 69 years and older, Smith and colleagues[95] found an increase in bone mineral content and bone mineral–width ratio in the radius of the women involved in a 3-year aerobic exercise program, as compared to a loss of bone mass in the women in the control group. Krolner and associates[96] noted an increase in lumbar bone mineral content after an 8-month exercise program in postmenopausal osteoporotic women who had sustained a Colles' fracture within the past 2 years. Alovia and coworkers[97] reported a higher level of total body calcium in postmenopausal women who had undergone a 1-year aerobic exercise program than in controls.

One difficulty of study design is measuring bone changes after a general exercise program that is not designed specifically to load the bone from which measurements are taken. Simkin and colleagues[98] designed an exercise program that would specifically load the distal radius, from which bone density measurements were taken after using a Compton scattering technique. After a 5-month program, the osteoporotic postmenopausal women showed greater distal radius bone density than the control group; in fact, these same women experienced significant loss of bone density elsewhere, similar to that of the control group, for the year before the beginning of the exercise program. There is evidence that a regular exercise program can increase bone mass in elders, but no known studies have shown that such activity reduces the risk of fracture, though one mnight expect this to be true.[91]

Aerobic exercise training has been shown to improve the neuropsychological function of older persons. Dustman and coworkers[99] reported that a group of 55- to 70-year-old sedentary persons who engaged in a 4-month supervised aerobic exercise program demonstrated significantly greater improvement on a neuropsychological test battery than the control group. Because depression scores, visual acuity, and sensory thresholds did not change, the aerobic training program appears to have central rather than peripheral effects. Peri and Templer[100] also report a significantly greater perceived internal locus of control and increase in self-concept in elders after they participated in a 14-week aerobic training program.

A properly designed and carefully managed aerobic exercise training program should also provide these benefits for elders: increased lean body mass and decreased body fat, increased levels of high-density lipoproteins, lower lipid concentrations, improved glucose tolerance, greater flexibility, better digestion, less constipation, lower serum catecholamine levels, and better quality of life.[101,102]

Though exercise benefits elders in many ways, health professionals need to be aware of possible complications. Elkowitz[103] notes several possible adverse consequences. Patients with a history of ischemic heart disease may develop exercise-induced myocardial ischemia, infarction, or arrhythmias; those with osteoporosis may develop fractures while jogging, skiing, or skating. Persons with arthritis may find their symptoms worsen after activities such as jogging that overload already damaged structures or activities that involve excessive repetitive movements. Elders are more susceptible to heat stress, heat exhaustion, and heat stroke owing to age-related changes in thermoregulation. With increasing age, thirst is not an adequate measure of fluid needs, and fluid replacement often lags 2 to 3 days behind actual needs, especially in a hot climate. The delayed onset of sweating, as well as the increased percentage of body fat of elders, make heat dissipation more difficult. Likewise, the diminished ability of the kidneys to concentrate urine and the age-related decrease in total body water, predispose to dehydration.

In a longitudinal study, Steinhagen-Thiessen and colleagues[104] reported possible detrimental effects of a short-term endurance program on the skeletal and cardiac muscles of mice. They were forced to run in electrically-driven running wheels and eight to 10 mice from each running group, and their controls, were sacrificed at age 9, 14, 18, 21, 22, and 27 months. The researchers measured hind leg weight and assessed samples of skeletal and cardiac muscles for creatine kinase, adolase, and superoxide dismutase activity. Young mice that underwent a short-term training program adapted easily. In contrast, intermediate mice (21 months) showed loss of adaptation capacity, and old mice (25 and 27 months) showed no training effect or even a negative training effect. On the other hand, old mice subjected throughout life to a long-term training program—*provided that it started no later than 15 months of age*—maintained a positive adaptation similar to that seen in the younger mice.

To maximize the benefits and minimize the untoward effects of exercise for elders, any program should be medically evaluated and carefully prescribed. Lampman[101] and Elkowitz[103] discuss a practical approach to this. Before beginning an exercise program, even apparently healthy elders should receive a thorough history and physical examination to check for underlying disorders that could predispose them to exercise-induced complications. Disorders that require caution include coronary and peripheral vascular disease, hypertension, orthostatic hypotension, arrhythmias, pulmonary disease, degenerative bone and joint disease, neurologic disease, nutritional deficiencies, anemia, and hypokalemia. Most of these disorders do not preclude an exercise program, but they do require caution: an elderly person's blood pressure control should be maximized and electrolyte imbalances corrected before starting an exercise program. The physician should review the patient's medication regimen, giving special attention to drugs that interact with physical training. For example, diuretics may lead to hypokalemia, which may result in exercise-induced arrhythmias. The effects of insulin and oral hypoglycemic agents may be potentiated by a vigorous exercise program and result in symptomatic hypoglycemia; the dose, type, and time of administration may need to be changed to prevent hypoglycemia. Nitroglycerin taken too close to the exercise period may cause hypotension, yet it could also be taken prophylactically to prevent exercise-induced angina. Neuroleptics, tricyclic antidepressants, and other drugs known to cause orthostatic hypotension could cause symptomatic orthostasis during exercise. A regular exercise program may lower blood pressure, so it may be necessary to reduce the dose of antihypertensive medication. For patients with bronchospastic lung disease, addition of low-flow (2 L/min) oxygen via nasal cannula or prophylactic $B_2$ agonists via nebulizer given 15-20 minutes before exercise may increase exercise tolerance.

An appropriate exercise prescription must be individualized for each patient, taking into account the risk-benefit ratio of the program. A prescription needs to address issues such as intensity, duration, frequency, and type of exercise—and precautions. Environmental factors—including access to exercise equipment, patient motivation, ability to comply—must be considered.

The optimum intensity of aerobic exercise is most safely determined from the results of a graded exercise tolerance test, especially for patients with risk factors for atherosclerotic heart disease. Detailed discussion of exercise-stress testing is beyond the scope of this chapter; it is discussed in greater detail in the cardiopulmonary system chapter. It is enough to say that the training heart rate should range between 65% and 75% of the maximum heart rate attained during exercise stress testing. Exercise stress testing may not be readily available, especially for patients with physical impairments secondary to amputation or stroke who require specially modified exercise testing equip-

ment. If exercise stress testing or Persantine thallium stress testing is not available, caution suggests starting elderly persons initially at 60% to 70% of age-predicted maximum heart rate, though recommended training heart rates range between 70% and 85% of the age-predicted maximum for younger persons. The physician should observe closely for untoward effects.

The duration of aerobic training should be 15 to 60 minutes per session, and initially periods of vigorous aerobic training should be interspersed with periods of less vigorous activity. More intense activity should be increased gradually over several months, until a maintenance program of 30 to 60 minutes of more vigorous aerobic exercise can be performed continuously.

The frequency of aerobic exercise should be at least three to five times per week, though flexibility training can be performed daily. Daily aerobic training is also possible, but initially days of higher-intensity exercise should alternate with days of milder-intensity exercise. Only after several months of vigorous training three to five times per week should more vigorous training be performed daily. Even then, the rate of orthopedic complications rises with daily exercise.

Although the type of exercise needs to be individualized for a given patient, general guidelines for an exercise program for elders include: (1) involvement of as many joints and large muscle groups as possible; (2) taking all joints through their full range of motion; (3) an aerobic component.

Beginning an exercise program with low-intensity warm-up activities such as flexibility and range-of-motion exercises can prevent contractures, and stretching the areas of the body that will be used during the aerobic portion of the program may help avoid injury. Also warm-up and cooldown activities such as walking or bicycling prior to more vigorous aerobic training may help prevent exercise-induced arrhythmias and musculoskeletal injuries. A warm-up period may allow a sufficient gradual rise in deep muscle temperature to encourage vasodilatation, so that hypertension does not occur during exercise.

Walking is a simple means of exercising for elders; it improves aerobic capacity but does not require much equipment. Swimming, if easily accessible, is another excellent form of exercise, as it provides the benefits of aerobic training and uses most of the body's muscle groups. The buoyancy of the water helps support weak muscles and joints while the water's resistance strengthens muscles. Increasing the water temperature may provide relief for patients with arthritis and myofascial pain, though possible untoward effects of hydrotherapy must be considered. Increasing the water temperature may easily increase the body core temperature beyond that required by the exercise, given age-related changes in thermoregulation. An abnormal increase in core temperature may increase myocardial demand, which may predispose to development of myocardial ischemia, infarction, or arrhythmias. Patients should be cautioned about diving, which may increase the risk of retinal detachment.

Both swimming and walking offer the elderly psychological benefits, as they provide an opportunity for leaving the home and socializing with others. Bicycling and dancing also offer this advantage, and they too can improve aerobic capacity. Older persons should use sliding dancing steps, to prevent excessive loading on symptomatic joints.

Elders should embark on weight-lifting activities with caution, using light weights (5% to 20% of body weight) after an adequate warm-up consisting of rhythmic exercise involving the arms and legs. Isometric exercises, especially those associated with Valsalva's maneuver, should be avoided, as they can increase myocardial demand and result in hernias or detached retinas.

Patients whose physical impairments prevent them from undertaking such activities may benefit from specially adapted exercise equipment. For example, a stroke patient may be able to participate in a stationary bicycling program by modifying a bicycle ergometer to allow use of the uninvolved upper and lower extremity to attain an acceptable training heart rate, which may not be attainable using only one lower or upper extremity.

The physician prescribing an exercise program for an elder must consider environmental issues as well as safety. The propensity for heat-related complications has been noted, especially in very hot or humid weather. Safety tips suggested by Eisenman[105] include: (1) wearing loose clothing that "breathes"; (2) exercising during the cooler periods of the day or in an air-conditioned facility;

(3) realizing that thirst is not a guide to the need for fluid replacement; (4) drinking fluids often during vigorous physical activity (as much as 6 to 8 ounces of water every 15 minutes to replace sweat-mediated losses); (5) keeping a record of body weight and drinking 1 pint of fluid for each pound lost, and ensuring that body weight is within 2% of normal before the next exercise session; (6) pouring water over the head, legs, and arms to help promote evaporative heat loss; (7) drinking an additional 16 to 32 ounces of fluid a half hour before vigorous exercise; (8) avoiding alcoholic beverages, which impair sweating; and (9) observing closely for signs of heat stress such as light-headedness, weakness, confusion, headaches or nausea, and stopping the activity if any of these occurs.

Cold weather may be just as problematic as hot weather for the elderly person undergoing an exercise program. Cold leads to vasoconstriction, and often higher blood pressure, during exercise, which may result in greater myocardial demand, increasing the likelihood of exercise-induced myocardial ischemia or infarction. Cold can also induce bronchospasm and coronary ischemia. Decreased sensory feedback from the feet, hands, and ears could result in frostbite. Elders who wish to perform outdoor activities in cold weather should do so for only short periods, after a slow, gradual start, and while wearing proper winter clothing.

Physicians prescribing exercise programs and elderly people undertaking them should give attention to proper visibility outdoors and to provision of adequate lighting and environmental cues indoors to help compensate for the decreased visual acuity and depth perception common in the elderly. The exercise route should be planned to avoid uneven terrain or slippery surfaces. Good quality shoes are essential to ensure maximal stability and provide shock-absorbing relief of joints at heel strike.

Even a properly prescribed exercise program is worthless unless a patient is motivated to exercise regularly. To promote compliance, an exercise program should minimize complications and take into account the patient's wishes and lifestyle. Education in the benefits of exercise, as well as the danger signals, is crucial. Compliance may be better if a variety of activities are prescribed in a group setting that permits socialization rather than a single activity to be performed in isolation. A structured program is often helpful for the elderly patient with memory impairment, and music often can make activities more enjoyable. The accessibility and cost of an exercise program also needs to be considered.

The relationship between age-related impairment, disability in activities of daily living, and the role of exercise in elders requires comment. Young[106] mentions the concept of threshold values of physical ability: the age-related decline in $Vo_2$max results in the significant reduction of the safety margin between the absolute level of energy expenditure and the amount of energy required to accomplish certain activities of daily living. A minor intercurrent illness is all that is needed to lower the $Vo_2$ max slightly, and render the patient incapable of performing certain activities of daily living that require aerobic metabolism. Likewise, it appears that a healthy elderly person is very close to the threshold value of quadriceps strength below which he or she would be unable to arise unassisted from a low armless chair or toilet seat. An exercise program for the healthy elderly can result in improvement in aerobic power and strength and can reverse the effects of immobilization after an illness. A very small gain in strength or aerobic power, if it slightly exceeds the threshold value, may result in significant functional improvement. What is not always clear is to what extend the aging process can be influenced by exercise. Also, there is a paucity of studies that attempt to correlate measurements of muscle strength and aerobic power with performance of activities of daily living. Both areas are critically important for the advancement of exercise physiology in geriatric practice.

## Conclusion

In conclusion, aging affects all organ systems to some degree, but these changes per se are not fatal. No one dies of old age. The increased vulnerability of the elderly to serious illnesses—cancer, heart and lung diseases, stroke, Alzheimer's disease along them—superimposed on the biologic changes associated with aging, become overwhelming and incompatible with life.

## References

1. National Center for Health Statistics. Vital Statistics of the United States, 1985, vol II, sec 6, Life Tables. DHHS (PHS) 88–104. Washington, DC: US Government Printing Office, 1988.
2. Fleg JL. Alterations in cardiovascular structure and function with advancing age. Am J Cardiol 1986; 57:33C–44C.
3. Pomerance A. Pathology of the myocardium and valves. In: Caird, FI, Dalle JLC, Kennedy RD, eds. Cardiology in Old Age. New York, Plenum Press, 1976, pp. 11–53.
4. Wei JY. Heart Disease in the elderly. Cardiovasc Med 1984; 9:971–982.
5. Wei JY. Cardiovascular anatomic and physiologic changes with age. Topics in Geriatric Rehabilitation 1986; 2:10–16.
6. Unverferth DV, Fetter JK, Unverferth BJ, et al. Human myocardial histologic characteristics in congestive heart failure. Circulation 1983; 68:1194–1200.
7. Brandfonbrener M, Landowne M, Shock NW. Changes in cardiac output with age. Circulation 1955; 12:557–566.
8. Rodeheffer RJ, Gerstenblith G, Becker LC, et al. Exercise cardiac output in maintained or advancing age in healthy human subjects: Cardiac dilation and increased stroke volume compensate for a diminished heart rate. Circulation 1984; 69:203–213.
9. Miyatake K, Okamoto J, Kimoshita N, et al. Augmentation of atrial contribution to left ventricular flow with aging as assessed by intracardial Doppler flowmetry. Am J Cardiol 1984; 53:586–589.
10. Bruce RA. Exercise, functional aerobic capacity, and aging—another viewpoint. Med Sci Sports Exerc 1984; 16:8–13.
11. Dehn, MN, Bruce RA. Longitudinal variations in maximal oxygen intake with age and activity. J Appl Physiol 1972; 33:805–807.
12. Seals DR, Hagberg JM, Hurley BF, et al. Endurance training in older men and women. Cardiovascular responses to exercise. J Appl Physiol 1984; 57:1024–1029.
13. Julius S, Avery A, Whitlock LS, et al. Influence of age on the hemodynamic response to exercise. Circulation 1976; 36:222–230.
14. Borer J, Bachrach S, Green M, et al. Real time radionuclide cineangiography in the non-invasive evaluation of global and regional left ventricular function at rest and at exercise in patients with coronary artery disease. N Engl J Med 1977; 296:839–845.

15. Lipsitz LA, Nyquist RP, Wei JY, et al. Postprandial reduction in blood pressure in the elderly. N Engl J Med 1983; 309:81–83.

16. Zadai CC. Pulmonary physiology of aging: The role of rehabilitation. Topics in Geriatric Rehabilitation 1985; 1:49–57.

17. Frontera W, Evans W. Exercise performance and endurance training in the elderly. Topics in Geriatric Rehabilitation 1986; 2:17–32.

18. Kenney RA. Physiology of Aging. Chicago: Year Book, 1982.

19. Wright RR. Elastic tissue of normal and emphysematous lungs. Am J Pathol 1961; 39:355–367.

20. Reddan WG. Respiratory system and aging. In: Smith E, Serfass R, eds. Exercise and Aging: The Scientific Basis. Hillside, New Jersey, Enslow Publishers, 1981.

21. Bye PTB, Farkos GA, Rousso CH. Respiratory factors limiting exercise. Annu Rev Physiol 1983; 45:439–451.

22. Campbell EJ, Lefrak SS. How aging affects the structure and function of the respiratory system. Geriatrics 1978; 33:68–78.

23. Chebotarev DF, Korlsushko CV, Ivanov LA. Mechanisms of hypoxia in the elderly. J Gerontol 1974; 29:393–400.

24. Morris, JF, Koski A, Johnson LC. Spirometric standards for healthy non-smoking adults. Am Rev Respir Dis 1971; 103:57–67.

25. Cress, ME, Schultz E. Aging muscle: Functional, morphologic, biochemical and regenerative capacity. Topics in Geriatric Rehabilitation 1985; 1:11–19.

26. Tzankoff, SP, Morris AH. Effect of muscle mass decrease on age-related BMR changes. J Appl Physiol 1977; 43:1001–1006.

27. Borkan GA, Hults DE, Gerzof SG, et al. Age changes in body composition revealed by computed tomography. J Gerontol 1983; 38:673–677.

28. Aniansson A, Sperling L, Rundgren A, et al. Muscle function in 75-year-old men and women. A longitudinal study. Scand J Rehabil Med 1983; 9(suppl):92–102.

29. Pearson MB, Bassey EJ, Bendall MJ. Muscle strength and anthropometric indices in elderly men and women. Age Ageing 1985; 14:49–54.

30. Larsson L, Grimby G, Karlsson J. Muscle strength and speed of movement in relation to age and muscle morphology. J Appl Physiol 1979; 46:451–456.

31. Davies CTM, Thomas DO, White MJ. Mechanical properties of young and elderly human muscle. Acta Med Scand Suppl 1986; 711:219–226.

32. Brown M. Selected physical performance changes with aging. Topics Geriatr Rehabil 1987; 2:68–76.

33. Sperling L. Evaluation of upper extremity function in 70-year-old males and females. Scand J Rehabil Med 1980; 12:139–144.

34. Tomonaga M. Histochemical and ultrastructural changes in senile human skeletal muscle. J Am Geriatr Soc 1977; 3:125–131.

35. Larsson L, Sjodin B, Karlsson J. Histochemical and biochemical changes in human skeletal muscle with age in sedentary males, age 22–65 years. Acta Physiol Scand 1978; 103:31–39.

36. Grimby G, Danneskiold-Samsoe B, Huid K, et al. Morphology and enzymatic capacity in arm and leg muscles in 78- to 81-year-old men and women. Acta Physiol Scand 1982; 115:123–134.

37. Knortz KA. Muscle physiology applied to geriatric rehabilitation. Topics Geriatr Rehabil 1987; 2:1–12.

38. Campbell M, McComas A, Petito F. Physiological changes in ageing muscle. J Neurol Neurosurg Psychiatry 1973; 36:174–182.

39. Patrick JM, Bassey EJ, Fentem PH. Changes in body fat and muscle in manual workers at and after retirement. Eur J Appl Physiol 1982; 49:187–196.

40. Bassey EJ, Bendell MJ, Pearson M. Muscle strength in the triceps surae and objectively measured customary walking activity in men and women over 65 years of age. Clin Sci 1988; 74:85–89.

41. Larsson L, Karlsson J. Isometric and dynamic endurance as a function of age and skeletal muscle characteristics. Acta Physiol Scand 1978; 104:129–136.

42. Aniansson A, Grimby G, Krotkiewski I, et al. Muscle strength and endurance in elderly people with special reference to muscle morphology. In: Asmussen E, Jorgensen K, eds. Biomechanics VI-A. Baltimore, University Park Press, 1978.

43. Kidd G, Broline P. The motor unit. Physiotherapy 1980; 66:146–152.

44. Grimby G, Saltin B. The aging muscle. Clin Physiol 1983; 3:209–218.

45. Larsson L. Morphological and functional characteristics of ageing skeletal muscle in man. Acta Physiol Scand 1978:457.

46. Kiesseling KH, Pilareom L, Karlsson J, et al. Mitochondrial volume in skeletal muscle from young physically untrained and trained healthy men and from alcoholics. Clin Sci 1973; 44:547–554.

47. Suominen E, Keikkinen E, Parkatti T. Effect of eight weeks of physical training on muscle and

connective tissue on the m. vastus lateralis in 69-year-old men and women. J Gerontol 1977; 32:33–37.

48. Orlander J, Kiessling KH, Karlsson J, et al. Low intensity training, inactivity and resumed training in sedentary men. Acta Physiol Scand 1977; 101:351–362.

49. Tonna EA. Aging in the skeletal system normal versus disease. In: Johnson HA, ed. Normal Aging and Disease. New York, Raven Press, 1985.

50. Garn SM. The Earlier Gain and the Later Loss of Cortical Bone. Springfield, Ill: Charles C Thomas, 1970.

51. Barry HC. Exercise prescriptions for the elderly. American Family Physician 1986; 34(3):155–162.

52. Smith EL. Exercise for the prevention of osteoporosis, a review. Physiol Sports Med 1982; 10:72–83.

53. Benison B, Hogstel MO. Aging and movement therapy: Essential interventions for the immobile elderly. J Gerontol Nurs 1986; 12(2):8–16.

54. Johns RJ, Wright V. Relative importance of various tissues in joint stiffness. J Appl Physiol 1962; 117:824–828.

55. Wright V, Johns RJ. Physical factors concerned with the stiffness of normal and diseased joints. Bull Johns Hopkins Hosp 1960; 106:215–231.

56. LaBelle FS, Paul G. Structure of collagen from human tendons as influenced by age and sex. J Gerontol 1963; 20:54–57.

57. Whiteway J, Morson BC. Pathology of aging—diverticular disease. Clin Gastroenterol 1985; 14:829.

58. Jori A, et al. Rate of aminopyrine disappearance in young and aged humans. Pharmacology 1972; 8:273.

59. Birkhoff JD. Natural history of benign prostatic hypertrophy. In: Hinman F, ed. Benign Prostatic Hypertrophy. New York: Springer-Verlag.

60. Catalona WF, Scott WW. Carcinoma of the prostate. In: Walsh PC, et al., eds. Campbell's Urology, ed 5. Philadelphia: WB Saunders.

61. Everitt AV, Webb C. The blood picture of the aging male rat. J Gerontol 1958; 13:255.

62. Lipschitz DA, Udupa KB, Milton KY, et al. Effect of age on hematopoiesis in man. Blood 1984; 63:502.

63. Garry PJ, Goodwin JS, Hunt WC. Iron status and anemia in the elderly. J Am Geriatr Soc 1983; 31:389.

64. Simpkins JW, Millard WJ. Influence of age on neurotransmitter function. Endocrinol Metab Clin North Am 1987; 16:893.

65. Sapolsy R, et al. The neuroendocrinology of stress and aging: The glucocorticoid cascade hypothesis. Endocrine Rev 1986; 7:284.

66. Neaves W, et al. Leydig cell numbers, daily sperm production and serum gonadotrophin levels in aging men. J Clin Endocrinol Metab 1984; 59:756.

67. Goldman J, Cote LJ. Aging of the brain: Dementia of the Alzheimer's Type. In: Kandel E, Schwartz J, Jessell TM, eds. Principles of Neural Science ed 3. 1991; 974–983.

68. Posner JD, Gorman KM, Klein HS, et al. Exercise capacity in the elderly. Am J Cardiol 1986; 57:52C–58C.

69. Larsson B, Renstrom P, Svardsudd K, et al. Health and aging characteristics of highly physically active 65-year-old men. Eur Heart J 1984; 5(suppl E):31–35.

70. DeVries HA. Physiological effects of an exercise training regimen upon men aged 52 to 88. J Gerontol 1970; 25:325–336.

71. Haber P, Honiger B, Kliepera M, et al. Effects in elderly people 67-76 years of age of three-month endurance training on a bicycle ergometer. Eur Heart J 1984; 5(suppl E):37–39.

72. Nunimaa V, Shephard RJ. Training and oxygen conductance in the elderly. II. The cardiovascular system. J Gerontol 1978; 33:362–367.

73. Verg JE, Seals DR, Hagberg JM, et al. Effect of endurance training on ventilatory function in older individuals. J Appl Physiol 1985; 58:791–794.

74. Ekblom B. Effect of physical training on oxygen transport system in man. Acta Physiol Scand 1969; 328(suppl):9–45.

75. Sidney KH, Shephard RJ. Training and electrocardiographic abnormalities in the elderly. Br Heart J 1977; 39:1114–1120.

76. Brown M, Rose SJ. The effects of aging and exercise on skeletal muscle: Clinical considerations. Topics in Geriatric Rehabilitation 1985; 1:20–30.

77. Grimby G. Physical activity and muscle training in the elderly. Acta Med Scand; 711:233–237.

78. Stebbins CL, Schultz E, Smith RT, et al. Effects of chronic exercise during aging on muscle and endplate morphology in rats. J Appl Physiol 1985; 58:45–51.

79. Sherwood DE, Selder DJ. Cardiorespiratory health, reaction time and aging. Med Sci Sports 1979; 11:186–189.

80. Kroll W, Clarkson PM. Age, isometric knee extension strength, and fractionated resisted response time. Exp Aging Res 1978; 4:389–409.

81. Aniansson A, Gustafsson E. Physical training in old men with special reference to quadriceps mus-

cle strength and morphology. Clin Physiol 1981; 1:87–98.

82. Aniansson A, Ljungberg P, Rundgren A, et al. Effects of a training programme for pensioners on condition and muscular strength. Arch Gerontol Geriatr 1984; 3:229–241.

83. Moritani T, DeVries H. Potential for gross muscle hypertrophy in older men. J Gerontol 1980; 35:672–682.

84. Larsson L. Physical training effects on muscle morphology in sedentary males at different ages. Med Sci Sports Exerc 1982; 14:203–206.

85. Brown M. Long-term endurance exercise effects on skeletal muscle in aging rats. Med Sci Sports Exerc 1985; 27:245.

86. Stebbins CL, Schultz E, Smith RT, et al. Effects of chronic exercise during aging on muscle and endplate morphology in rats. J Appl Physiol 1985; 58:45–51.

87. Sanchez J, Bastien C, Monod H. Enzymatic adaptations to treadmill training in skeletal muscle of young and old rats. Eur J Appl Physiol 1983; 52:69–74.

88. Suominen H, Heikkinen E, Liesen H, et al. Effects of 8 weeks' endurance training on skeletal muscle metabolism in 56- to 70-year-old sedentary men. Eur J Appl Physiol 1977; 37:173–180.

89. Kiessling KH, Pelstrom L, Bylund A, et al. Enzyme activities and morphometry in skeletal muscle of middle-aged men after training. Scand J Clin Lab Invest 1974; 33:63–69.

90. Raab DM, Smith EL. Exercise and aging effects on bone. Topics in Geriatric Rehabilitation 1985; 1:31–39.

91. Martin AD, Brown E. The effects of physical activity on the human skeleton. Topics Geriatr Rehabil 1989; 4:25–35.

92. Jones HH, Priest JD, Hayes WC. Humeral hypertrophy in response to exercise. J Bone Joint Surg 1977; 59:204–208.

93. Huddleston AL, Rockwell D, Kulund DN, et al. Bone mass in lifetime tennis athletes. JAMA 1980; 244:1107–1109.

94. Jacobson P, Beaver W, Grubb S, et al. Bone density in women: College athletes and older athletic women. J Orthop Res 1984; 2:328–332.

95. Smith EL, Reddan W, Smith PE. Physical activity and calcium modalities for bone mineral increase in aged women. Med Sci Sports Exerc 1981; 13:60–64.

96. Krolner B, Toft B, Nielsen SP, et al. Physical exercise as prophylaxis against involutional vertebral bone loss: A controlled trial. Clin Sci 1983; 64:541–546.

97. Alovia JF, Cohn SH, Ostuni JA, et al. Prevention of involutional bone loss by exercise. Ann Intern Med 1978; 89:356–358.

98. Simkin A, Ayalon J, Leichter I. Increased trabecular bone density due to bone-loading exercises in postmenopausal osteoporotic women. Calcif Tissue Int 1987; 40:59–63.

99. Dustman RE, Ruhling RO, Russel EM, et al. Aerobic exercise training and improved neuropsychological function in older individuals. Aging 1984; 5:35–42.

100. Perri S, Templer DI. The effects of an aerobic exercise program on psychological variables in older adults. Int J Aging Human Dev 1984-85; 20:167–172.

101. Lampman RM. Evaluating and prescribing exercise for elderly patients. Geriatrics 1987; 42:63–76.

102. Council on Scientific Affairs of the American Medical Association. Physician-supervised exercise programs in rehabilitation patients with coronary heart disease. JAMA Assoc 1981; 1463.

103. Elkowitz EB, Elkowitz D. Adding life to later years through exercise. Postgrad Med 1986; 80:91–103.

104. Steinhagen-Thiessen E, Reznick AZ, Ringe JD. Age-dependent variations in cardiac and skeletal muscle during short and long term treadmill-running mice. Eur Heart J 1984; 4(suppl E):27–30.

105. Eisenman PA. Hot weather, exercise, old age, and the kidneys. Geriatrics 1986; 4:108–114.

106. Young A. Exercise physiology in geriatric practice. Acta Med Scand 1986; 711(suppl):227–232.

# Chapter 29
# Pain and Suffering

W. CRAWFORD CLARK

My purpose in this chapter is to review all aspects of our current knowledge of the mechanisms and treatment of acute and chronic pain. The title, Pain and Suffering, emphasizes the view taken throughout this chapter that the emotional aspect of pain may be as important, or even more important, than the sensory component. The chapter begins with an introduction to the evaluation of the sensory and psychological determinants of clinical and experimentally induced pain and suffering. Next the neuroanatomic and neurophysiologic mechanisms of pain and its modulation are described. The influence of ethnic and cultural differences and personality on the patient's report of pain and suffering are then outlined. This is followed by a description of pharmacologic, surgical, and behavioral treatments for pain and suffering. The chapter concludes with a discussion of the relation between the patient's beliefs and the effectiveness of more controversial treatment approaches, including acupuncture, transcutaneous electrical stimulation, and hypnosis.

## Introduction to Clinical Pain

Pain is an unpleasant subjective experience familiar to all of us. Most of the time, it signals that something is wrong: some tissue has been injured or has become inflamed, or our bodies are being assaulted by extremes of heat, cold, pressure, or other noxious stimuli. We can infer its presence in

others by their vocalizations and behavior. When an injured or inflamed part is touched, the patient winces or writhes and withdraws from the stimulus. In addition, autonomic symptoms such as pallor, flushing, or perspiration may be apparent, and the general pattern of activity may be altered; the patient becomes restless or, alternatively, relatively immobile and passive. Most important, the patient's behavior appears to center on pain, as if the experience had preempted consciousness and altered motivation. The emotional (anxiety, depression) and psychosocial (job loss, marital difficulties, social isolation) effects of pain not only are inseparable from the pain sensations themselves but may be more devastating. For these reasons the term *pain and suffering* is appropriate, particularly when the patient is experiencing persistent pain.[1,2]

The practitioner bases the initial assessment of pain on observable behavior and a physical examination of the patient. The patient's subjective report may be very useful, because different pain qualities are associated with specific disorders. For example, a report of chronic burning pain could support a diagnosis of causalgia, whereas paroxysmal facial pain touched off by pressure could support a diagnosis of trigeminal neuralgia. Variations in intensity, locus, and persistence are also important here. Pain may be dull or sharp, diffuse or localized, deep or superficial, continuous or intermittent. Migraine headaches throb; tension headaches typically do not. Cutaneous pain tends to be sharp and well-localized, whereas internal pain originating in muscles and viscera tends to be diffuse, aching, and poorly localized. The patient's report can also aid diagnosis by indicating what circumstances initiate, ease, or exacerbate the pain or change its quality. As with other symptoms, observation and inquiry are essential aspects of the diagnostic work-up. In addition, the patient must be viewed as a whole person.

Cassel[3] contends that the distinction between suffering and physical distress has received scant attention in the medical literature. Suffering may include physical symptoms, but it is not limited to them. Cassel maintains that the patient may be in pain, uncomfortable, and distressed but that these complaints do not constitute suffering. The separate expressions *pain* and *suffering* simply continue the Cartesian body and mind dualism; the expression *pain and suffering* is used in this chapter in an attempt to overcome this dichotomy. Suffering has its source in the threat to the intactness of the *persona* as a psychosocial entity. Even though a specific treatment relieves the pain itself, a physician's failure to comprehend the emotional focus of the patient's suffering can increase the total suffering. Cassel emphasizes three points: (1) Suffering is experienced by persons, not minds or bodies; it is the person that must be treated. (2) Suffering occurs when the impending disintegration of the person is perceived. Suffering may occur in the presence of pain and other physical symptoms, but it does not necessarily; the meaning of the symptom to the patient is all-important. (3) Suffering can occur with respect to altered social and career roles, loss of loved ones, loss of a perceived future, or changed spiritual values. Recovering from suffering is always enhanced by help from family, friends, and health care professionals. To accomplish this, it is often more important that the patient be seen as a total person than that the immediate physical distress be treated.

### Attempts to Define Pain

A complete classification of chronic pain syndromes has been prepared by the International Association for the Study of Pain.[4] Pain has been defined by the Subcommittee on Taxonomy as "an

unpleasant sensory or emotional experience associated with actual or potential tissue damage, or described in terms of such damage." This definition is oversimplified and presents immediate difficulties. Not only can damage occur without pain, as it does within some malignancies, mild sunburn, or tooth decay, but pain also can continue long after the initial injury has healed, as in phantom limb pain or sympathetic dystrophy. Psychological intervention may ameliorate pain, though the tissue damage remains the same. Further, the same amount of tissue damage, insofar as this can be determined, may produce quite different intensities of pain in different persons or in one person at different times. Objective and detectable tissue damage, though it usually produces pain, represents only a part of the total complex of conditions that produce the experience of pain. In many instances of chronic pain, the pain and suffering persists long after healing is complete.

Alternative approaches are to give up on a definition of pain and agree that pain is anything the patient says it is, or to agree with Popper[5] and avoid definitions entirely. He notes that attempts to define a term lead to an infinite regress that can only be halted by agreeing that some terms cannot be defined, which might as well be conceded at the outset. He also notes that the physical sciences advanced when scientists stopped asking questions such as, What is matter? and formulated questions that would lead to an experiment: How does this piece of material behave under these particular physical conditions? The same approach should bear fruit in the study of pain and suffering. One asks, How does this patient behave (behavior includes verbal report) following this particular treatment regimen?

*Pain* describes a broad spectrum of unpleasant sensory and emotional experiences and pain behaviors. At one end are the brief, localized, protective sensations such as those produced by noxious heat, cold, pinch, prick, and chemical stimuli. Without this type of warning sensation, survival would be difficult. At the other end of the spectrum are the nonprotective, pathologic, persistent pains associated with chronic disease states. Such pain and suffering experiences provoke emotional disturbances including anxiety, fear, and depression.

Thus, pain and suffering can be considered a *construct;* that is, a label for categorizing a constellation of observations or symptoms. As one of the senses, then, pain is paradoxical in the extent to which the presumed intensity of the noxious stimulus (amount of apparent damage) is dissociated from the subjective or behavioral reactions to it. The report of pain, particularly chronic pain, is less veridical than reports about hearing, vision, or touch, in which the response can be predicted quite exactly in most instances once the intensity of the stimulus is known. In contrast, the intensity of our pain experience is influenced substantially by psychological variables, by redirection of attention, by expectations of relief or of exacerbation, by a physician or dentist convincing us that nothing is wrong or predicting catastrophic illness, or, in little children, by a mother's kiss to "make it stop hurting."

## Evaluating the Complaint of Pain

Considering the complexity of pain and suffering, it is not surprising that patients have much difficulty communicating their experiences. The information they provide is further distorted by psychological and psychosocial factors. Kolb[6] has drawn attention to the complaint of chronic pain as an expression of attachment behavior that becomes organized into an individual's total pattern of personality adaptation. He points out that the experience of pain has multiple functions. When communicated to the physician (or friends and relatives) as a complaint, the implication is that there is something wrong with the patient's body, that there is something that must be done to relieve the discomfort. While the experience of pain appears to be an innate response to injury, the associated verbal complaint may be modified by learning, which is specific to the family and the culture. Thus, the complaint of some tissue damage may also convey a message of social importance—a bid for help or attention, an attempt to gain emotional support from other persons or to dominate them, for example. Psychic factors thus influence the intensity of the complaint, independently of the severity of the organic injury, accounting for intense complaints in persons with little or no discernible injury or faint complaints in those who wish to deny their pain and illness.

Evaluating a patient's pain is difficult. There is

no "thermometer" for pain, as there is for temperature. The practitioner cannot share the patient's urgent experience of pain; it must be inferred. The initial assessment of pain is most frequently based on the history, in combination with objective findings and an evaluation of the patient's psychological status. We ask ourselves, "How valid is the report of pain? Is the patient expressing mental anguish rather than physical pain? Is he or she by nature stoic or not?" The primary problem here is not the patient's veracity, but the manifold meanings that people attach to the word *pain*. Patients have enough difficulty interpreting and conveying their experiences, but clinicians are faced with an even more arduous task: they must attempt to unravel the sensory, psychological, and other components of the patient's message. This is particularly true where the physical findings provided by x-rays, computerized tomography (CT), and other objective medical tests do not support the patient's complaints.

Three books that deal with the problems and approaches (one hesitates to say solutions) to the measurement of pain and suffering have appeared in recent years.[7-9] A number of questionnaires have been developed, and in some cases standardized, in attempts to measure the multitudinous facets of chronic pain. Responses to these questionnaires have been used in attempts to aid diagnosis, to assess the effect of medication, to measure improvement, and to determine "organicity." Though they have their drawbacks, certainly these questionnaires provide a more objective assessment than a clinical judgment of *worse, same, better*. Such tests are essential in any research protocol. A thorough review of many of these measurement approaches is available.[10]

### Dimensions of Pain and Suffering

If we are to understand and relieve pain and suffering we must be able to measure it, but, quantitation is difficult because pain is a multidimensional experience that varies over a wide range of intensities and possesses an almost infinite number of qualities. While thousands of words have been used to describe pain and suffering, our ability to understand and treat pain would be much enhanced if these words could be reduced to a dozen or so "dimensions." Because the number and the characteristics of the dimensions are currently in dispute, the first step toward the quantitation of pain is a better understanding of its dimensions.[11]

The history of speculation concerning the dimensions of pain and suffering was reviewed by Melzack.[12] He notes that while Aristotle thought of pain as an emotion, not a sensation, 19th-century physiologists thought of pain as a sensory modality devoid of emotion. Sherrington combined these views and held that pain had two dimensions: sensory and affective. Melzack and Casey[13] argue for three dimensions. The *sensory-discriminative* dimension is the sensory aspect of pain, including intensive, temporal, and spatial properties and somatosensory qualities. The *affective-motivational* dimension reflects the emotional and aversive aspects of pain and suffering. The *cognitive-evaluative* dimension reflects the patient's evaluation of the meaning and possible consequences of the pain, including the quality of life and death itself. This three-dimensional model is widely accepted, because it succeeds in integrating much of what is known about the physiology and psychology of pain and suffering.

A view that expands upon Melzack and Casey's by placing even greater emphasis on the emotional and behavioral dimensions has been presented by Loeser[1] and Fordyce.[2] They describe four aspects of pain and suffering: *nociception,* the activation of A-delta and C fibers by tissue-damaging stimuli; *pain,* the sensation that usually, but not always, follows nociceptive stimulation; *suffering,* which includes the affective or emotional response of the central nervous system and includes anxiety, depression, and fear; and *pain behaviors,* the observable muscular and autonomic activities of patients experiencing pain or suffering. The Melzack-Casey and Loeser-Fordyce views, which are compatible, are now widely accepted, but recent multidimensional scaling research suggests there may be many more dimensions.

Multidimensional scaling represents an objective approach to discovering the number and kinds of dimensions of pain and suffering.[11] To date, evidence has been found for the following dimensions: pure sensory pain, somatosensory qualities, emotional qualities, aversiveness, and pain behaviors. A major advantage of this model is that it indexes the dimensions that are most salient to each subject. The view that pain and suffering may be represented by specific dimensions and that individual patients are located at different points along these dimensions represents an important advance toward understanding and being able to treat pain and suffering. This work is discussed in more detail later.

## Pain Puzzles

The amount of pain experienced in certain syndromes, such as reflex sympathetic dystrophy, postherpetic neuralgia, phantom limb, or central thalamic pain, is paradoxical in being out of all proportion to the apparent quantity or quality of sensory input. This disproportion poses problems for any approach that views pain as a simple sensory modality. It also poses problems for those who suffer from these disabilities, and for those who attempt to treat them. Later in this chapter some of the neural mechanisms responsible for these paradoxical pains are discussed.

Reflex sympathetic dystrophy is characterized by intense, continuous burning pain, sympathetically mediated increases in vasomotor tone, profuse sweating, and physical changes in the skin of the affected limb. It follows trauma that is often mild and is not associated with noticeable nerve injury. Pain may arise spontaneously or in response to peripheral touch (*hyperpathia* and *allodynia*), or even as a result of emotional stress. Hyperpathia is a painful syndrome characterized by amplification of strong stimuli and decreased sensitivity to weak stimuli, whereas allodynia refers to pain produced by what is normally an innocuous stimulus intensity. These symptoms of *dysesthesia* (an unpleasant, but not necessarily painful, abnormal sensation—spontaneous or evoked) are particularly interesting. The neural mechanisms responsible for "sympathetic" pain are beginning to be understood.

Postherpetic neuralgia may occur subsequent to herpes zoster, an infectious disease characterized by inflammation of dorsal root or cranial nerve ganglia and the distal portion (axon) of the primary afferent nerves. The spontaneously occurring pain is intense and may be accompanied by unbearable itching. Though the affected area becomes less sensitive to nonnoxious touch or temperature stimulation, repeated mild stimulation of the area (a trigger zone) can provoke an excruciating attack of pain after a brief delay. The condition may last years and resist all forms of therapy, including procaine block, resection of peripheral nerve, dorsal root, or ganglion, and excision of sensory cortex. Recent work by Dworkin and colleagues[14] suggests an added complexity, namely that patients who are depressed during the early stages of the infection (and hence may have a compromised immune system) appear to be more apt to develop postherpetic neuralgia.

Phantom limb pain is another puzzle. Most recent amputees experience a complex of sensations patterned in a way that makes them feel as if they still had a limb of normal size, shape, and mobility. Usually, this phantom limb gradually shrinks and eventually disappears, but in a small proportion of cases, particularly when the limb was painful before the amputation, severe pain continues to be felt in the phantom limb. Some causes are understandable. Neuromas may develop at the severed nerve endings at the amputation site, and these can be stimulated accidentally. Neurosurgery or local anesthetic injected at the site eliminates this peripheral source of pain, though often only temporarily. Patients whose pain is not improved by surgery pose a problem. What is the source of the spontaneously recurring pain? Even dorsal root resections that remove all pain sensibility from the stump itself may not eliminate phantom limb pain.

Centrally mediated pain, which is recurring, excruciating, and typically possesses a burning quality, may be caused by vascular, traumatic, or degenerative lesions at any level of the neuraxis, but it occurs more frequently with thalamic and mesencephalic lesions than with lesions at lower or higher levels.

Fibromyalgia—characterized by complaints of chronic diffuse musculoskeletal aching and stiffness and by tender points at specific anatomic sites (myalgia), fatigue, and unrefreshing sleep—has baffled physicians for a long time. Other terms for the illness include fibrositis, neurasthenia, masked depression, chronic fatigue syndrome, and somatoform pain disorder. Theories of causation include psychological disturbance, pathologic immune system response, and inflammation following viral infection. In the absence of any specific cause, doubts have been raised about the diagnostic legitimacy of this syndrome; however, Moldofsky[15] argues that the illness is characterized by an alpha-frequency electroencephalographic (EEG), non–rapid eye movement sleep anomaly that is absent in healthy controls and in insomniacs. Although the EEG sleep anomaly is frequently correlated with the fibromyalgia syndrome, it has relatively low specificity, being found in some 15% of asymptomatic patients. Moldofsky postulates a close relation between the immune system, immunologically active peptides, and the brain, particularly the serotoninergic pain-inhibitory system. Obviously, much more remains to be learned about the cause of this controversial syndrome.

In sum, paradoxical pain is characterized not only by pain that is out of all proportion to the discernible stimulus, but also by these features: (1) Gentle touch may produce extreme pain, yet additional stimulation sometimes relieves it. (2) The pain response may be delayed or may persist long after stimulation has ceased. (3) Superficial touch at sites far removed from the pathologic tissue may trigger an attack (thus the name *trigger zones*). (4) Surgical lesions of the pain pathways frequently fail to produce relief.

## Experimentally Induced Pain

Clinical pain and suffering is an almost hopelessly complex subject. Accordingly, a number of investigators take the view that progress can best be made by first understanding simpler types of pain, such as that induced in the laboratory by precisely calibrated noxious stimuli of varying intensities. Experimental or laboratory pain procedures have been used to study the effects of culture, personality, age, sex, drugs, hypnosis, and acupuncture on the response to noxious stimuli. Much has been learned from the responses of volunteers and patients to precisely calibrated noxious stimulation that could not be learned from the study of clinical pain, where the intensity of the noxious stimulus cannot be determined with any degree of precision and emotional factors distort the response.

Most experimental approaches to sensation, including vision, audition, and pain, emphasize the application of graded intensities of the physical stimulus and require the subject (the observer) to make some judgment about the presence, absence, or intensity of the stimulus. For pain, the major methodologic approaches include pain detection and pain tolerance (withdrawal) thresholds obtained by the method of serial exploration or "limits," by magnitude estimation, by sensory decision theory, and by multidimensional scaling. Procedural and statistical controls, designed to minimize error in these reports, are usually elaborate and include careful control of stimulus and test conditions, placebo controls, and the use of single- or double-blind controls. (In the latter, neither subject nor treatment deliverer knows which treatment has been given.)

Experimental pain stimuli must produce short-term and reversible effects. Electrical stimulation of tooth pulp or skin, immersion of a limb in ice water, stimulation of the skin with radiant heat, pressure over superficial bony structures, pinch, and tourniquet procedures that produce ischemic pain by obstructing circulation are options. Internal stimuli include esophageal, lower bowel, and rectal distension by pressurized balloons and infusion of dilute acids into the lower esophagus.[16]

Many different response modes to noxious stimulation have been investigated. Some investigators have sought pain indicators that would be more objective than verbal report, which is easily influenced by attitude, expectations, and the social demand characteristics of the experimental situation. Orne[17] originated the term *social demand characteristics* to refer to the compelling influence on subjects of what is expected of them by an audience or of the social norms implicit in the situation. "Objective" tests have employed a variety of physiologic responses not ordinarily considered to be under voluntary control: pulse rate, blood pressure, shift of blood flow from viscera to striated muscles, inhibition of salivary and gastric secretions, pupil dilation, blood glucose, corticosteroid and epinephrine levels, palmar skin potential, altered EEG, together with reflexive wincing and withdrawal. Unfortunately, none of these measures is more useful than verbal report, as none is truly specific to pain, as opposed to, say, surprise, stress, or fear. For example, the palmar skin potential may show a greater increase in response to an unexpected soft sound than to an expected noxious electrical pulse. Furthermore, like verbal report, these so-called objective indicators also are influenced by psychological varia-

bles, including fear, surprise, stress, and social demand characteristics. The physiologic measures may, however, provide useful information to supplement verbal report.

### Method of Limits

In the method of limits or serial exploration, the observer responds to each of a series of brief, physically calibrated thermal, pressure, pinch, or electrical stimuli, which are gradually increased in intensity. The pain *sensitivity* threshold is the intensity at which the subject first reports pain; the pain *tolerance* threshold is the intensity at which the subject withdraws from the stimulus. Although the threshold was once thought to be a pure measure of sensory function, it is now clear that it is heavily influenced by nonsensory factors, especially the subject's expectations and attitudes. Nevertheless, it remains a useful way of approximating the threshold and determining intensities to be used in the more sophisticated procedures described below.

### Sensory Decision Theory Measures

A major problem in understanding pain and suffering is the seemingly inseparable mixture of sensory and psychological variables. This is as true for experimental pain as for the clinical entity. Recent developments in psychophysical measurement, particularly what is variously called *medical decision making theory, signal detection,* or *sensory decision theory* procedures, offer considerable promise, at least for measurement of experimental pain. These procedures separate the sensory component of the traditional method of limits threshold from its otherwise hidden psychological or attitudinal component. The method can be used with untrained subjects and has been applied not only to verbal report but also to physiological and motor indicators of pain. The *discriminability index, d'* or *P(A)*, is related to the functioning of the neurosensory system. High values suggest that neurosensory functioning is normal; low values, either that the signal-related neurosensory activity has been attenuated, as it might be by an analgesic, or that spontaneous neural noise has increased, as it might after an extended period of chronic pain. Discriminability has been shown to be decreased by analgesics such as morphine and by nerve blocks, which attenuate neural activity and, so, the amount of information that reaches higher centers.[18] Unlike the pain threshold, $d'$ or $P(A)$ has been shown to be essentially independent of changes in the subject's expectation, mood, and motivation. The other measure of perceptual performance is the report criterion, $Lx$ or $B$; it measures response bias, which is the willingness or reluctance of a subject to use a particular response. The criterion is related to the subject's attitude (which in turn often depends on emotional factors such as anxiety and depression) toward reporting painful experiences. A high criterion reflects stoicism, while a low criterion indicates that the subject readily reports pain even to innocuous stimulus intensities. In terms of the pain and suffering dimensions discussed earlier, discriminability is related to sensory dimensions and criterion to emotional dimensions. Fernandez and Turk[19] present an extensive review of the experimental literature on this question.

Many studies (reviewed by Clark and Yang[18]) have used sensory decision theory to demonstrate the effect of attitudinal and emotional variables on the pain report criterion. For example, a placebo described and accepted by the subjects as a powerful analgesic, raised the threshold; that is, it apparently decreased pain sensitivity according to the traditional method of limits. Analysis by sensory decision theory, however, demonstrated that only the pain report criterion had been raised (fewer pain reports); discriminability, $d'$, did not change. Thus, the placebo-induced reduction in pain report was due, not to an analgesic effect of the placebo on neurosensory function, but to a criterion shift made in response to the social demand characteristics of the situation.

## Magnitude Estimation

In the magnitude estimation or ratio scaling procedure, the subject is assigned a simple number, such as 10, to describe a calibrated stimulus of an intensity (the modulus) in the mildly painful range. The subject then assigns numbers to subsequently presented variable stimulus intensities that range above and below the modulus value. These numbers reflect the ratios between the sensations produced by the modulus and the variable intensity stimuli. Gracely and coworkers[20] report an interesting study that demonstrated that subjects could separately rate electrocutaneous stimuli with respect to sensory (pain) and affect (unpleasantness) dimensions. An anxiety-reducing drug (diazepam) reduced intensity ratings on the affect, but not on the sensory dimension. In another study, Gracely, McGrath, and Dubner[21] found that a narcotic reduced sensory pain intensity ratings but not, surprisingly, the affect intensity ratings. The results of these studies are in accord with the known tranquilizing and analgesic effects of these drugs and support the concept of separate sensory and emotional components of pain and suffering. In spite of the results of these well-designed experiments, other studies have raised questions about the reliability of the affect dimension[19] and of the subjective assignment of words to the various dimensions.[11]

## Multidimensional Scaling

The pain and suffering dimensions associated with laboratory pain induced by electrical and thermal stimulation have been investigated by a new technique, *multidimensional scaling*. Studies in this area were summarized recently.[11] An important advantage of this method is that, unlike the laboratory procedures just described, it is equally at home with verbal descriptors of pain and suffering and with physical stimuli. Thus, it can be used to uncover the dimensions of acute and chronic clinical pain.

The multidimensional scaling procedure yields a geometric configuration of points in the pain and suffering space, as on a map, where each point corresponds to one of the stimuli. This map allows inferences to be made about the structure or dimensions of the pain and suffering universe. Unlike the dimensions described earlier, which were based on ad hoc opinions, these dimensions are obtained in an objective manner, because the subject, not the experimenter, determines the type and number of the dimensions. In addition to defining the group stimulus space, the method also generates a subject weight space, which represents the relative importance or salience of each dimension for a particular subject or patient and which may be said to provide an "address" for each individual in the multidimensional pain and suffering space.

Clark and colleagues[22] used multidimensional scaling to study a group of patients suffering cancer-related pain and a matched group of healthy volunteers. The subjects made pairwise similarity judgments between all possible pairings of the following cancer-related pain words: *burning, cramping, shooting, annoying, miserable, sickening, mild pain, intense pain, unbearable pain.* Three dimensions emerged in the group stimulus space, namely, Pain Intensity, Emotional Quality, and Somatosensory Quality. The subject weight space revealed that, although there were individual differences, on average the Pain Intensity dimension was most important for the patients, while the Emotional Quality dimension was most important for the healthy volunteers. If the multidimensional scaling approaches fulfill their promise, we should soon be nearing a better understanding of the variables that affect clinical pain and suffering.

## Modulation of Pain and Suffering

We turn now to studies in which pain and suffering is attenuated by arousal, stress, counterirritant stimulation, and various psychological factors. It is common knowledge that injuries sustained during strenuous physical activity may go unnoticed at the time or be perceived as not especially painful. The power of counterirritant stimuli to relieve pain seems firmly implanted in folk medicine (it appears, for example, in the human tendency to grasp firmly or rub vigorously an area adjacent to a limb injury) and has received some experimental validation.

### Central Processes

Generally, investigators concerned with pain as a clinical problem recognize that the severity of the pain is based not only on sensory input but also on one or more kinds of central processing. The details of such processing are still obscure, but anxiety and motivation are believed to influence the perceived significance of the pain. Feedback mechanisms, both physiologic and psychophysiologic, also complicate the picture. For example, a pain-induced muscle spasm may augment the original pain, or attention to a mild headache may cause fear, which increases blood pressure and, in turn, increases the headache. Goals, purposes, and general activity levels also appear to modulate the pain experience. In some circumstances reactions to ordinarily painful tissue damage may be surprisingly slight, as in "painless childbirth" or in primitive puberty rites (e.g., penile incision among Polynesians). A football player who cracks an ankle bone in an active scrimmage may not feel a great deal of pain until later, when the excitement has subsided and he is physically inactive. Here, sensory inputs that might ordinarily be perceived as painful signify the achievement of valued goals. Activity and excitement are at a high pitch. The physiologic and cognitive responses to this acute stress combine to limit sharply the perception of pain.

Central pain-inhibitory mechanisms must be invoked to account for some of the complex responses to injury. For example, Beecher[23] described how men wounded at the Anzio beachhead complained little of pain from their wounds but bitterly about inept venipuncture. Thus, the general excitement of the situation and the relief of leaving battle with a "good" wound did not make them generally hypoalgesic; rather, the perception of pain was highly selective. Learned pain inhibition is selective also with respect to locus. Pavlov[24] showed that dogs that repeatedly received food (unconditioned stimulus) immediately after shock or burn (conditioned stimulus) soon stopped reacting in the usual way to these noxious stimuli and ignored them when they occurred. Very small changes in the locus and character of the noxious stimulation, however, produced the usual vocalizations, arousal, and attempts to escape. The site specificity of these analgesic effects prove that higher centers in the brain, in addition to general arousal and endocrine effects, must be involved in pain suppression. These are the "central control mechanisms" described by Melzack and Wall[25] and discussed later.

Variability in the response strength of central control mechanisms could account for the poor correlation often observed between the amount of tissue damage and the severity of the reported pain. Central processing variables—experience, selective attention, arousal, activity, and emotion—could alter the pain experience. The effectiveness of these psychological factors nevertheless depends in part on the sensory input. If the intensity of pain increases very rapidly (as in colic or cardiac pain), central inhibition might not occur rapidly enough to block the pain experience. Gradually rising pain inputs may be easier to manage by mild counterstimulation and conscious psychological maneuvers.

### Stress-Induced Changes in Response to Pain

The effect of stress on pain and pain-suppressing mechanisms has recently become the object of intensive investigation.[26] Arousal and stress can influence pain perception in many ways. Increased neurohumoral secretions, increased distribution of blood to heart and skeletal muscle, and redirected attention all can play a role in reducing pain. Stress mobilizes a defense system that involves the nervous system, endogenous analgesics, and the hypothalamic-pituitary-adrenal (HPA) axis. Atkinson and associates[27] found that chronic pain patients had higher levels of plasma β-endorphin (a naturally occurring opioid) than a group of psychiatric patients, who in turn had higher levels than healthy controls. It should be borne in mind, however, that although plasma levels of β-endorphin rise in response to stress of any type, brain and spinal levels of β-endorphin (where the analgesic effect is most likely to occur) are not necessarily correlated with plasma levels. Other endocrine secretions also can modulate pain sensitivity; Goolkasian,[28] using sensory decision methods, demonstrated reduced discriminability of calibrated noxious thermal stimulation during the ovulatory phase of the menstrual cycle.

Janal and coworkers[29] studied a group of marathon runners before and after a 10-km run and observed analgesic effects following the run, namely, decreased discriminability to noxious thermal stimulation and decreased sensitivity to tourniquet ischemic pain. In addition, the runners were in a euphoric mood. Both the analgesia and the euphoria suggest increased endogenous opioid activity. This hypothesis was further confirmed

when these effects did not appear on a second occasion when the runners were administered naloxone, which blocks the central effects of opioids. This finding suggests that the stress decreased pain by increasing brain levels of endogenous opioids. The run also elevated plasma levels of β-endorphin, adrenocorticotropic hormone, prolactin, and growth hormone, demonstrating the effect of exercise stress on HPA axis activity.

Neuroendocrine changes may explain the results obtained by Yang and associates,[30] who used the sensory decision theory approach to study the responses of chronic back pain patients to brief, calibrated thermal stimuli. Compared to healthy volunteers, the patients were less able to discriminate among the stimuli (lower $d'$) and reported less pain (set a high criterion, $L_x$). These findings, similar to those produced by analgesics, suggest stress-induced activation of some endogenous analgesic. Apparently the endogenous analgesic mechanism triggered by the stress was sufficient to blunt the response to the relatively low-intensity thermal stimuli but was insufficient to ameliorate the more intense endogenous stimulation responsible for the back pain. The stoical criterion suggests that, in comparison to their clinical pain, the pain induced by the brief thermal stimuli appeared relatively innocuous.

Arousal by pleasurable stimulation can also inhibit pain responses. Whipple and Komisaruk[31] demonstrated in a group of college students that vaginal self-stimulation increased the threshold of noxious finger compression. No change was found in the ability to detect innocuous touch stimuli, demonstrating that the decreased sensitivity to pain was not caused by distraction.

## Neuroanatomic Basis of Pain: 1965

A thorough understanding of the neuroanatomic and neurophysiologic characteristics of the intact and injured systems underlying pain perception is essential for the treatment of the pain patient. A historical overview of the pain system as it was conceived more than 20 years ago[32] is presented first, for two reasons: a simple scheme structures the complexities of recent discoveries that are presented in the next section, and a historical perspective emphasizes how much has been learned.

Abundant experimental and clinical evidence indicates that, up to a point, the pain system is organized and responds in much the same way as other sensory systems. At moderate levels of stimulation, where the emotional component is minimal, responses can be obtained that relate subjects' judgments of pain to intensity of physical stimulation as precisely as those obtained with the other senses. That is, an invariant relation exists between noxious stimulus intensity and magnitude of sensation. To this limited degree, a "specificity theory" of pain can be entertained, namely, a relatively direct pathway conducts stimulus-related neural activity from the periphery to "higher" pain centers in the brain.

*Two Major Nociceptive Systems*

Primary or first-order nociceptive neurons extend from the axon tip in the periphery (skin, muscle, viscera) to the dorsal horn in the spinal column. Second-order neurons extend from the dorsal horn to the thalamus, and third-order neurons from thalamus to cortex. It will soon become clear that this is a gross oversimplification, though it is true in some instances. The receptors for pain are fine, unmyelinated nerve endings, the axon tips of the first-order neurons. These endings are present in a variety of tissues that are sensitive to pain—skin, viscera, joints, muscles, teeth, bones, and blood vessels, particularly arteries. The once popular view that these fine nerve endings subserve only pain has been discarded. Tissues such as the cornea, which contain only free nerve endings, are sensitive to touch, warmth, and cold, as well as to noxious stimuli.

Transmission of pain after the impulses from the primary neurons arrive at the dorsal horn has been attributed to two major systems (Figure 29-1). The *spinothalamic system,* which is phylogenetically recent, is a relatively direct, rapidly conducting system that involves few neurons and mediates accurately localized, sharp pain that is precisely discriminated with respect to intensity and duration. This classic sensory-discriminative pain system resembles other sensory systems, such as touch. Its function is to warn of impending tissue damage, to mediate reflex withdrawal, and to transmit the pain of minor trauma. Second-order

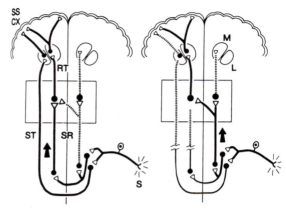

**Figure 29-1.** Redundancy and plasticity of central pain pathways. (*Left*) Under normal circumstances, noxious stimuli (S) activate the contralateral spinothalamic (ST) and the spinoreticulothalamic (SR) pathways (*solid lines, arrow*). ST projects directly to the lateral thalamus (L), which projects to the somatosensory cortex (SSCX). SR projects to the reticular system of the medulla, pons, and midbrain, indicated within the rectangle. The reticulothalamic (RT) projection terminates in the medial thalamus (M), which projects to wide areas of cortex, including SSCX. Noxious stimuli also activate the ipsilateral spinoreticulothalamic pathway (*dashed line*); however, the profound analgesic effect that initially follows contralateral cordotomy indicates that ipsilateral SR pathways normally contribute little to nociception. A possible mechanism for the progressive recovery of nociceptive function after cordotomy appears on the right. Because the ipsilateral SR pathway projects bilaterally to RT neurons, it can provide a "bypass" (*arrow*) for the pain message to the contralateral thalamus and cortex. (From Fields, Ref 35, 1987; 159, with permission.)

neurons ascend contralaterally to the lateral thalamus and somatosensory cortex in a somatotopic manner; that is, the geography of the body is preserved, or mapped, in the nervous system.

The *spinoreticulothalamic system* is a phylogenetically older, multisynaptic system that mediates diffuse, poorly localized pain that has a long latency and persists after the noxious stimulus has been removed. After receiving input from the first-order neurons, the long fibers of the spinoreticular and spinotectal tracts project through ipsilateral and contralateral tracts to the reticular system of the medulla, pons, and midbrain before ending on the nonspecific nuclei of the medial thalamus. This system is not well-organized somatotopically but instead forms a diffuse projection system. Fibers from it ascend to the limbic system, including the hippocampus, amygdala, and other rhinencephalic structures, as well as to the hypothalamus and, through it, to the pituitary gland. Thus, the spinoreticular system is involved in arousal, avoidance, and emotional and defensive reactions.

The major effect of hemisection of the spinal tract is contralateral analgesia. Because the neurons of the spinothalamic system travel to the opposite side, surgical hemisection for intractable pain usually fails to last, presumably because activity increases in the second pain system. A possible explanation of the transient effects of surgery, which involves these two pain systems, appears in Figure 29-1.

## Melzack-Wall Gate Control Theory: 1965

The gate control theory holds that nonpainful sensory inputs can inhibit nociceptive activity; thus it successfully integrated diverse clinical and physical observations. According to Melzack and Wall,[25] large-fiber activity initiated by touch or vibration inhibits small-fiber activity, which mediates pain at the level of the first synapse in the spinal dorsal horn. The ratio of small-fiber to large-fiber activity determines the activity in the pain transmission or T cells (second-order neurons). A reduction in large-fiber input, while small-fiber input is maintained, opens the gate, creating hyperalgesia, as in causalgia, diabetic neuropathy, and phantom limb pain. On the other hand, if the small-fiber system is relatively intact, increasing large-fiber sensory input closes the gate and relieves pain. Thus, gentle tapping of the stump sometimes relieves phantom limb pain, and mild electrical stimulation or damp warm or cold towels may alleviate causalgia. In some patients, electrical stimulation of large-diameter sensory fibers relieves chronic pain resulting from peripheral nerve damage even after termination of the stimulating current.[33] The model also allows for descending nerve impulses from the brain to close the gate; this mechanism would account for the influence of cognitive-behavioral therapy as a means of controlling pain. This theory has been greatly refined in the past 25 years, but its essential concepts remain.

## Neuroanatomical Basis for Pain: 1991

The aforementioned general observations of the nociceptive system may now be updated and viewed in greater detail. Price[34] and Fields[35,36] have presented excellent outlines of the neuroanatomy and physiology of pain. Berkley[37] cogently argues that there are many pains, and accordingly, that different neural mechanisms probably underlie pain sensations arising from different loci such as skin, muscle, and various viscera. Each of these distinct sensory experiences can be subclassified further on the basis of their duration. Different neural mechanisms must underlie pain that lasts for milliseconds, for minutes, for days, for weeks, and for months. Furthermore, the interaction between non-nociceptive and nociceptive systems requires much more investigation. Other recent findings on pain mechanisms may be found in the *Proceedings of the International Association for the Study of Pain*. These sources should be consulted for further details and very informative illustrations.

An overview of primary and secondary neurons appears in Figures 29-2 and 29-3. As portrayed in Figure 29-2, it is widely accepted that the primary afferent neurons for touch end in the dorsal column nuclei, whereas those for pain and temperature end in the spinal gray matter. However, this simplistic view is yielding to the much more complex mapping portrayed in Figure 29-3. Recent animal studies have led to hypotheses that the ventral posterolateral nucleus of the thalamus may be involved in tactile sensibility, acute cutaneous pain, or chronic musculoskeletal pain, depending on circumstances and on the history of the animal.[37]

### *Primary Afferent Neurons*

The axon tip of the first neuron innervates skin, muscle, tendons, viscera, bone, and teeth; the cell body and dendrites terminate in the dorsal horn of the spinal cord (see Figure 29-3). Pain sensibility on the body's surface is not uniformly acute. Each sensory area, which may be smaller than 1 cm in diameter, transmits a unique pattern of excitation to higher centers, permitting localization and two-point discrimination. Individual receptive fields are innervated by several nerve fibers, which en-

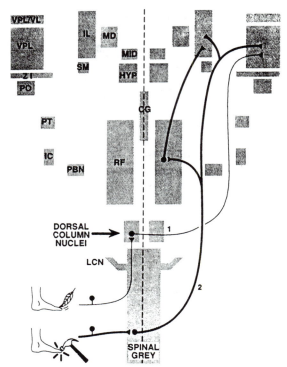

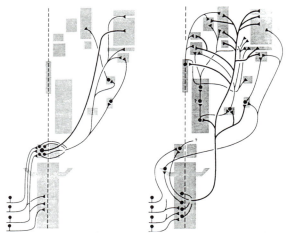

**Figure 29-2.** A simple, but out-of-date, current conceptualization of somatovisceral sensory pathways is found in many modern textbooks. Pathway 1, in which the primary neuron forms synapses in the dorsal column nuclei (thin lines) and hence directly to ventral posterolateral nuclei of the thalamus mediates the sensation of touch, whereas pathway 2 from the spinal cord (thick lines) mediates pain and temperature sensations (see text for details). Key: CG, central gray; HYP, hypothalamus; IC, intercollicular area; IL, intralaminar nuclei; LCN, lateral cervical nuclei; MD, medial dorsal nuclei; MID, midline nuclei of thalamus; PBN, parabrachial nuclei which mediate somatovisceral and cardiovascular functions; PO, posterior group complex; PT, pretectum; RF, reticular formation; SM, submedius nuclei; VPL, ventral posterolateral nuclei of the thalamus (which project to the somatosensory cortex); VPL/VL, border of VPL with the ventral lateral nuclei; ZI, zona incerta. (From Berkley KJ. Suspension of neural pathways for pain and nociception. J Cardiovasc Electrophysiol 1991; 2(suppl):S13–S17, with permission.)

**Figure 29-3.** A current conceptualization of somatovisceral sensory pathways incorporating evidence obtained during the past 25 years. Connections that mediate touch, originating from the dorsal column nuclei, are illustrated on the left side of the figure. Connections originating from neurons in the spinal gray matter are illustrated on the right. The blocks representing neural regions are the same as those identified in Figure 29-2. For clarity, a considerable amount of information has been omitted from this figure, including output from thalamus to cortex, cerebellar and related connections, ipsilateral connections (except those from the central gray), internal variations within all nuclei, and, perhaps most important, descending connections. (From Berkley KJ. Suspension of neural pathways for pain and nociception. J Cardiovasc Electrophysiol 1991; 2(suppl):S13–S17, with permission.)

sures multiple projections to the neuraxis. The various fibers that serve temperature, touch, and pain sensibility in a given region come together as a peripheral nerve on their way to the spinal cord. The sensory territory of any peripheral nerve widely overlaps that of adjoining nerves. Thus, several peripheral nerve trunks or dorsal roots usually must be cut to eliminate pain in a particular area. The amount of overlap varies much from region to region in the body, but every locus on the skin appears to be supplied by at least two dorsal roots.

Pain sensibility in deeper tissues is less well-understood, but it is known that a deep branch of a spinal nerve may supply areas in fascia, skeletal muscle, and bone that are remote from the superficial areas supplied by other branches of the same nerve. The viscera have pain sensibility, particularly when the whole organ is involved and a sufficient number of the sparsely distributed stretch receptors are stimulated. Adequate stimuli include rapid distension or contraction of hollow organs, distension of the capsule of solid organs such as the liver, damage to blood vessels, and ischemia. Intense pain from deep somatic structures and viscera often produces such autonomic symptoms as nausea, decreased blood pressure, and syncope. Pain fibers from deep tissues, such as viscera, muscles, and periosteum are more sparsely distributed than somatic pain fibers. These visceral afferents are anatomically associated with sympathetic efferent fibers to smooth muscles and glands, but they do not differ from other somatic afferents and are not part of the sympathetic system.

The three principal types of primary afferent neurons, A-beta, A-delta, and C, are classified by their diameters and by the presence or absence of a myelin sheath, both attributes that determine speed of conduction. The A-beta fibers are heavily myelinated, fast conducting, and respond to low intensity, nonpainful, proprioceptive and light mechanical stimuli. The A-delta nociceptive fibers are thinly myelinated, fast conducting, tend to be modality specific, and produce a well-localized, sharp, "bright" pain. They are well-designed to mediate rapid withdrawal from a noxious stimulus. The C nociceptive afferents are smaller-diameter, unmyelinated, and slowly conducting and produce a delayed, poorly localized, dull pain. They tend to be polymodal; that is, they respond to a variety of stimuli.

Depending on the type of stimulus to which they are most sensitive, the high-threshold primary nociceptive cutaneous afferents are classified as thermal (heat and cold), mechanical, or chemical. In healthy tissue they show no spontaneous activity and do not respond to innocuous stimulation; thus, they are often referred to as *nociceptive specific fibers*. The C fibers constitute the great majority of nociceptive afferents; they are termed *polymodal nociceptors* because they respond maximally to noxious thermal, cold, mechanical, and chemical stimuli. Some thermal, mechanical, and mechanothermal nociceptive afferents, however, are high-threshold A-delta fibers. Though we are concerned with nociception, it should be borne in mind that innocuous stimuli also have their afferents. Touch and vibration stimulate large A-beta and low-threshold C fibers; cold, low-threshold A-delta fibers; warmth, A-delta and C fibers. The response rate of the A-beta fibers reflects the in-

tensity of innocuous mechanical stimulation but shows no further change to, and therefore does not signal, noxious intensity.

### Second-Order Neurons

Fibers from the primary afferents project to spinal cord gray matter, which is organized into anatomically distinct layers (Rexed laminae) of the dorsal horn (see Figures 29-3, 29-4.) Here, facilitation and inhibition cause the peripheral input to be radically transformed. In addition, inputs from autonomic and somatomotor systems, as well as from descending brain stem centers, are integrated. Lamina I neurons respond maximally to noxious stimulation. A single lamina I neuron may receive input from both C and A-delta fibers; such cells are called *nociceptive specific* or high-threshold neurons. Lamina I also receives *wide dynamic range* neurons, which respond to both innocuous and noxious stimuli and so must have inputs from both A-delta and C nociceptive and A-beta nonnociceptive primary afferents. Nociceptive specific neurons also terminate in laminae II, and to a lesser extent, often via interneurons, in lamina V, where many cells are of the wide dynamic range type. Lamina II neurons (originally known as the substantia gelatinosa) receive the primary nociceptive C fibers. Although some lamina II neurons project to brain stem and thalamus, most appear to be interneurons that synapse within lamina II and modulate the activity of other projection neurons.

Interneurons in laminae I and III appear to play an inhibitory role. Nonnociceptive (low-threshold) afferents terminate in laminae III and IV. The majority of cells in laminae III and IV also receive collaterals from large, myelinated primary afferents (A-beta), which mediate light touch and pressure and ascend in the dorsal column; they do not respond to changes in the intensity of noxious stimulation but may exert an inhibitory effect on the nociceptive system. When this inhibitory input is reduced (for example, by nerve injury), sensitivity to weak stimuli is decreased, but, paradoxically, stronger innocuous stimuli cause a poorly localized burning pain (causalgia). While laminae I to IV principally process cutaneous input, lami-

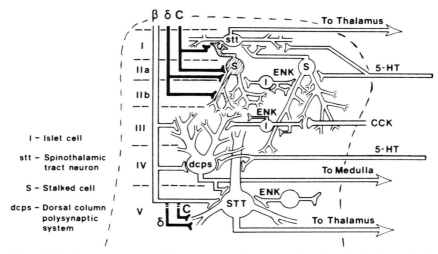

**Figure 29-4.** Schematic diagram illustrates the major morphologic-functional characteristics of neurons and neural interconnections in dorsal horn layers I to V (dorsal is at top of figure, ventral at bottom). The primary afferent C fibers enter laminae I, IIa, and V; the A-delta fibers, laminae II, and IIb; and the nonnociceptive A-beta fibers, laminae III, IV, and V. Sensory projection neurons to thalamus and medulla are indicated in layers I, IV, and V. These include nociceptive-specific (NS) and wide dynamic range (WDR) spinothalamic tracts as well as dorsal column postsynaptic neurons (DCPS). Layer I neurons receive mainly excitatory, and perhaps some inhibitory, connections from stalked cells in layer II. Stalked cells are either NS or WDR, depending on the ventral extent of their dendrites. Those that extend into only II are NS; those that extend more ventrally (where mechanoreceptive afferents synapse) are WDR. Layer V projection neurons may receive connections from layer IV neurons as well as direct primary afferent nociceptive input from A-delta and C fibers. Several types of inhibitory neurons, some of which are enkephalinergic or dynorphinergic, are indicated. The lamina II NS islet cell receives input exclusively from nociceptive afferents, and it inhibits output of stalked cells via various types of inhibitory synaptic connections. The more ventral islet cells receive input from sensitive mechanoreceptive afferents from laminae III and IV. Other types of low-threshold mechanoreceptive inhibitory neurons exist in the dorsal horn. Descending inhibitory fibers contain serotonin and cholecystokinin. (From Price DD. Psychological and Neural Mechanisms of Pain. New York: Raven Press, 1988;131, with permission.)

nae V and VI give rise to wide dynamic range neurons, which receive proprioceptive and nociceptive inputs from joints, muscle, and viscera. Laminae VII and VIII receive nociceptive inputs from very large receptive fields covering as much as half the body, including muscle and viscera. Lamina X cells are predominantly nociceptive, and some project to the brain stem reticular formation, suggesting that they have a role in the alerting and motivational dimensions of pain.

Given the complexity of transmission described above, it is obvious that coding of intensity by changes in impulse frequency alone could not possibly transmit all the information that is present. Complex temporal and spatial patterns of neural impulses are necessary and they have been demonstrated.

### Vagal Inhibition and Facilitation

The convergence of cutaneous, muscle, and visceral afferent inputs onto the wide dynamic range and nociceptive-specific neurons suggests the basis of referred pain localized to these deeper tissues. Diagnosing the cause of visceral pain on the basis of symptom report is extremely difficult. For example, pain resulting from myocardial ischemia or from gastric acid reflux in the esophagus can cause referred pain to the chest, arm, shoulder, face, or teeth. Moreover, the warning signs do not always work. Silent myocardia ischemia is a coronary artery disease syndrome in which cardiac ischemia fails to provoke angina; that is, the warning signs of oxygen insufficiency are absent. Whether the absence of pain report is due to a sensory deficit or to a stoic pain report criterion is being studied currently with the sensory decision theory model described earlier. Apparently, sensory loss, rather than a stoical criterion, is responsible for these patients' failure to report pain.

Vagal afferents have long been known to play a role in cardiopulmonary and gastrointestinal function. Gebhart and Randich[38] discuss recent work in which vagal afferent and spinopetal (descending) systems modulate pain. Vagal afferent stimulation inhibits responses in spinothalamic and spinoreticular neurons in the spinal cord to cutaneous stimuli, cardiac sympathetic afferent stimulation, or urinary bladder distension. Whether inhibition or facilitation occurs depends on the intensity of stimulation. Low-intensity vagal efferent stimulation generally facilitates nociceptive responses, probably in A-delta afferents, whereas higher intensities inhibit nociceptive responses, probably in C fibers. The changes observed in nociception are accompanied by cardiovascular and respiratory responses. For example, inhibitory effects are accompanied by a cardiac depressor response and brief apnea. Although the responses are correlated, studies suggest that different vagal afferents mediate nociception and cardiopulmonary reflexes. Inhibitory and facilitory vagal afferents project to the nucleus of the solitary tract, which connects with other brain stem nuclei, and are sources of the descending noradrenergic and serotonergic nociceptive inhibitory systems.

The axons of the second-order neurons travel from the dorsal horn to the thalamus and other structures at higher levels (see Figures 29-1 through 29-4). Axons that mediate touch travel in the dorsal columns of the spinal cord, while those that mediate pain and temperature form the anterolateral columns of the spinal cord. Surgical interruption of the latter path eliminates pain for contralateral cutaneous and (less completely) for deep structures in regions below the lesion, but over a period of months most patients experience partial return of pain sensation, owing to functional changes in other (e.g., spinoreticulothal-

amic) pathways. The fact that pain and touch fibers travel in separate tracts has led to a controversial treatment for lower body pain. The procedure involves long-term implantation of electrodes over the dorsal columns. Mild electrical stimulation of the dorsal column elicits neural impulses that travel to the dorsal column nuclei as well as antidromically to the dorsal horn. According to the Melzack-Wall gate hypothesis, this should have an inhibitory effect on the pain transmission neurons. A large proportion of patients do report pain relief initially, but the long-term results are disappointing.

The second-order nociceptive and non-nociceptive systems form synapses in various thalamic nuclei (see Figures 29-2, 29-3). The input to the thalamus is arranged somatotopically and also projects somatotopically to the somatosensory cortex. Lesions of the ventral posterior lateral and medial thalamic nuclei, made electively in humans to control intractable pain, have reduced acute pain, while electrical stimulation of these sites provoked burning sensations. Thus, these nuclei, as well as those that receive projections originating in the contralateral laminae I and IV through VII, are clearly related to the Melzack-Casey sensory-discriminative dimension. Lesions within the medial dorsal thalamic nuclei, which project to prefrontal cortex (a region deprived of input by the prefrontal lobotomies of an earlier are) reduce the aversive, emotional component of pain. The centre median and parafascicularis nuclei of the thalamus may be involved in arousal and motor reactions associated with pain. These nuclei appear to be related to the Melzack-Casey motivation-affective dimension.

### Third-Order Neurons and the Cerebral Cortex

Third-order neurons project from the thalamus to somatosensory areas I and II and other regions of cortex. Until recently, there was little evidence that the cortex was involved in pain perception. For example, electrical stimulation over most of the somatosensory cortex and all of the association cortex (a necessary precaution routinely performed during certain surgical procedures to avoid excision of critical "speech center" tissue) failed to elicit pain sensation. Initially, this was puzzling, because the ventral posterior lateral nucleus projects in a somatotopic fashion to somatosensory areas I and II. Recently, however, Talbot and associates[39] demonstrated with modern brain-imaging techniques that noxious thermal stimuli applied to the forearm do indeed produce neural activity in contralateral primary and secondary somatosensory cortex. In addition, they found activity in the anterior cingulate gyrus, a party of the limbic system known to regulate emotional responses. This study confirms that the Melzack-Casey sensory-discriminative and affective-motivational dimensions are represented in the cortex.

Removal (lobotomy) or isolation (leukotomy) of the anterior and orbital portions of the frontal lobes markedly reduces pain behavior, even though these areas are not ordinarily regarded as sensory. Following the operation, which at one time was performed for intractable cancer pain, patients reported that they felt the pain but that it did not hurt, nor did they request analgesics. Presumably, their rather strange description means that they felt the intensity of the sensory input but that it lacked the aversive quality of pain. Because nonspecific dorsal thalamic nuclei project to and receive fibers from this area as well as the limbic system (which mediates emotions), it would appear that the operation produces changes in the functioning of the diffuse spinoreticulothalamic system and its cortical projections, and thus attenuates the affective component of pain.

In contrast to prefrontal lobotomy, which often produced drastic personality changes, contemporary brain surgery destroys small, selected areas of brain tissue. Corkin and colleagues[40] found that bilateral anterior cingulotomy relieves persistent, non-neoplastic pain, as well as depression (but not schizophrenia or obsessive-compulsive disorder). In meticulous, well-designed studies of cognitive function, these investigators found no evidence of lasting neurologic or behavioral deficit; in fact, there were significant gains on tests of general intelligence. At the time, the mechanisms responsible for these effects were not clear, though it was noted that serotonin and endorphin pathways terminated in the region of the cingulotomy. The recent work of Talbot and associates[39] described above, serves, at last, to provide a rationale for the beneficial effects of the surgery. The involvement of these higher centers suggests ways in which experience, attention, input from other senses, and, perhaps, even hypnotic suggestion, could modify the pain experience through central processing mechanisms. Thus, evidence that supports the Melzack-Casey cognitive-evaluative dimension of pain and suffering is beginning to emerge.

## Neurotransmitter and Modulatory Substances

Clinical pain lasts far longer than that produced by brief noxious stimuli, and it may be accompanied by inflammation, tenderness, and hyperalgesia. Sources of such persistent pain include the various chemical substances released following tissue injury, such as potassium ions, bradykinin, histamine, serotonin, prostaglandins, and substance P. Norepinephrine is involved in sympathetically maintained pain states (e.g., reflex sympathetic dystrophy). The cellular mechanisms by which these substances sensitize nociceptors remain largely unknown; however, the action of substance P, a polypeptide released by the peripheral terminals of some primary afferent C fibers following noxious stimulation, is becoming understood. Substance P is found in many tissues, including blood vessels, where (along with histamine, which it releases) it is involved in the hyperalgesia, vasodilatation (often accompanied by warmth and erythrema), and edema that follow injury or infection.

Price[34] presents an excellent discussion of the neurochemical and neuroanatomic mechanisms responsible for the complex interactions among ascending, descending, and interneurons of the various systems that mediate pain. Figure 29-4 portrays the distribution of the afferent A-beta, A-delta, and C fibers in the various Rexed laminae, and their direct (via spinothalamic tract neurons) and indirect (via stalked cells, islet cells, and dorsal column cells to the medulla) routes to higher centers. Descending inhibitory 5-hydroxytryptamine (5-HT) and cholecystokinin (CCK) fibers, which release enkephalins and similarly acting endogenous opioids at the spinal level, are also portrayed.

A variety of substances that may act as neurotransmitters have been demonstrated in primary and secondary neurons. Neuropeptides such as vasoactive intestinal peptide, somatostatin, cholecystokinin and substance P are believed to mediate the slow component of pain, whereas fast excitatory neurotransmitter candidates include amino acids such as glutamate or aspartate and nucleotides such as adenosine triphosphate (ATP). Fast and slow transmitters are found in primary afferent neurons and in their synaptic terminals in laminae I and II.

## Endogenous Opioids

One of the most exciting advances in understanding pain has been the discovery of a large family of endogenous opiate-like peptides, the endorphins, enkephalins, and dynorphins. These naturally occurring peptides act at the same receptor sites in the brain and spinal cord as opiates such as morphine, to produce profound analgesia. In the spinal cord, pain is inhibited by local interneurons in laminae I, II, III, and V which contain the endogenous opioid peptides. The action of both endogenous opioids and morphine is blocked by naloxone, a synthetic substance that preferentially occupies the receptor site. Thus, a person taking morphine who has become tolerant to narcotics is thrown into withdrawal by administration of naloxone because, as far as the body is concerned, the narcotic has vanished. Physical exercise in humans increases plasma levels of β-endorphin and produces "stress-induced analgesia," which is partially blocked by naloxone,[29] suggesting that brain levels of endogenous opioids have also been increased. The fact that the analgesic effect is only partially blocked strongly suggests that non-opioid endogenous analgesics also play a role in analgesia.

The opioids do much more than produce analgesia. The opioid system has also been shown to be involved in food consumption, temperature regulation, pituitary hormone release, respiration, and cardiovascular regulation. Opioid peptides and opioid receptors have been found in the brain, spinal cord, blood vessels, heart, kidneys and adrenal medulla.

The suppression of pain by exogenous or endogenous opioids depends on the binding of these substances to several classes of opiate receptors.

There are at least four classes of opiate receptors, including *mu* (morphine), *delta* (enkephalin), *kappa* (ketocyclazocine), and *epsilon* (β-endorphin). Drug tolerance following repeated administration of narcotics for chronic pain causes a decrease in the number of receptor sites or a reduction in their binding affinity (down-regulation). Thus, tolerant subjects require larger doses of opiates to activate the few remaining or down-regulated receptors. Stevens and coworkers[41] have demonstrated in rats that the inflammatory pain of experimentally induced arthritis down-regulates spinal opioid receptors, and, presumably, increases the pain. Why such a maladaptive response should occur is unclear, but it could account in part for chronic arthritis pain in humans and for the observation that administration of naloxone to chronic pain patients fails to have the expected effect of increasing the pain.

Activation of endogenous pain inhibitory circuits requires noxious stimuli or cues to signal such events. This response is adaptive, because an injured but analgesic animal is better able to cope with an emergency situation. Once the emergency has passed, however, the animal must become aware of, and immediately attend to its injuries if it is to survive. Wiertelak and coworkers[42] have demonstrated an endogenous analgesia inhibitory system in rats that is activated by environmental safety signals. They found that a safety signal reversed morphine analgesia by initiating processes that act at the spinal cord. Moreover, the administration of a cholecystokinin (CCK) antagonist prevented the safety signal from abolishing the morphine analgesia; that is, the antianalgesia system was inhibited. Their work suggests that in nature a safety signal at the level of the cerebral cortex releases CCK in the spinal cord. The authors conclude that pain depends on the interplay of pain-inhibitory and anti–pain-inhibitory processes. Note in Figure 29-4 that descending CCK fibers are portrayed as forming synapses on enkephalinergic islet cells.

## Serotonin and Norepinephrine

There is now overwhelming evidence for inhibition of dorsal horn neurons, particularly in laminae I, II, and V, by a serotonergic (5-HT) pathway that descends from the midbrain periaqueductal gray via the raphe magnus. (These are the 5-HT neurons portrayed in Figure 29-4.) These brain sites produce analgesia when activated by microinjection of opioids. Electrical stimulation of these midbrain regions activates the descending inhibitory pathway, which in turn releases enkephalin. This "stimulation-produced analgesia," which does not differ from morphine-induced analgesia, has been demonstrated in humans. Pain-inhibitory effects are also mediated by an independent noradrenergic system that descends from the brain stem. It is worth noting here that clinical depression is associated with a deficiency of catecholamines (e.g., norepinephrine and dopamine) and indolamines (e.g., serotonin), and furthermore, that tricyclic antidepressants, which increase the concentration of these neurotransmitters by blocking their re-uptake at the synapse, have sometimes proved successful in the treatment of intractable pain, including cancer pain. Though such a mechanism is plausible, the effectiveness of antidepressants in the treatment of pain remains controversial.

## Neural Plasticity

Persistent pain and other sensory abnormalities are often reported after nerve injury.[43] These abnormalities include paresthesias, dysesthesias, allodynia, and hyperalgesia. A partial explanation of symptoms that follow nerve injury lies in the fact that the C (and probably A-delta) nociceptive afferents have a greater capacity to regrow into the denervated region than do the larger axons that mediate touch (thus, the dysesthesia). This imbalance would cause loss of large-fiber inhibition of the nociceptive neurons; that is, it would open the Melzack-Wall gate. The problems just described usually disappear after some months, when the larger, A-beta nerves have regrown and can once again act to close the gate.

In some cases pain persists after complete regrowth of the large fibers. Dubner[44] reviewed the latest findings on the causes of long-term allodynia and hyperalgesia following tissue damage, inflammation, edema, and erythema. Neuropathic hyperalgesia (frequently with burning (causalgic) pain) may appear after nerve injury by trauma

(sympathetic dystrophy), infection (postherpetic neuralgia), or metabolic disease (diabetic neuropathy). The pathophysiologic mechanisms underlying these hyperalgesic states are becoming better understood. They involve long-term alterations in central nervous system functioning. For example, following injury to the skin, previously innocuous stimuli provoke activity in myelinated and unmyelinated mechanical, thermal, and polymodal nociceptive afferent fibers. Or, following nerve trauma, axons may sprout and form a neuroma that emits spontaneous discharges and is sensitive to thermal, mechanical, and chemical stimulation. Surprisingly, both inflammatory and neuropathic allodynia appear to be mediated by input from large myelinated afferents, which never signal pain when the tissue is healthy. Both inflammatory and neuropathic hyperalgesias are associated with prolonged hyperexcitability of the spinal dorsal horn wide dynamic range and nociceptive-specific neurons, and are maintained by both peripheral input and local circuit activity. The hyperexcitability probably involves both increased activity in excitatory fibers and reduced activity of inhibitory neurons, including descending inputs from supraspinal sites. A different mechanism may operate in the viscera, where, according to Handwerker and Reeh,[45] small afferents in the bladder and colon (some studies implicate the skin as well) that under healthy conditions are not activated by noxious stimulation, become activated when tissues are inflamed.

Dubner[44] postulates the following series of events to explain continued pain after healing is apparently complete. Continuous noxious stimulation following the initial injury produces massive discharge from primary axons in the periphery. This discharge leads to increased depolarization of neurons with N-methyl-D-aspartate (NMDA) receptor sites. The depolarization is facilitated by the release of neuropeptides such as substance P and calcitonin gene–related peptide (GRP), as well as by the endogenous opioid dynorphin. In brief, the neural hyperexcitability leads to excitatory amino acid toxicity. The result is cell dysfunction and loss of inhibitory mechanisms, which causes an increase in the size of receptive fields, hyperexcitability, and an increase in pain. If the noxious stimulation is very prolonged, these changes could become irreversible and progress to cell death; the pain then could be centrally maintained without further peripheral input.

The long-term changes in neural function involve changes in gene expression. Exciting research on this topic is now under way.[46] The *c-fos* proto-oncogene (*oncogene* indicates that it is involved in cell growth, as in cancer) is rapidly induced by various normal and pathologic stimuli. The *c-fos* protein (FOS) binds to DNA, where it acts as a transcription regulator; it is thought to mediate long-term changes in neural responsivity. Noxious stimulation has been shown to increase, and morphine to reduce, neuronal levels of *c-fos* in laminae I, II, V. The action of *c-fos* is to increase the intracellular calcium ion flow induced by substance P and glutamate. Such a mechanism could mediate the long-term (months and years) central pain that persists in the absence of afferent nociceptive input. The blocking action of morphine on *c-fos* synthesis emphasizes the importance of using this drug during surgery to control postoperative pain.

A different type of structural change in the nervous system appears to be responsible for the pain associated with reflex sympathetic dystrophy or causalgia. In some cases, nerve injury is apparent, in others it is only suspected. These patients suffer persistent, intense burning pain that is out of proportion to the initial injury, for example, a fracture that months ago healed and was forgotten. These patients' pain often depends on sympathetic activity in the affected area; thus, the term *sympathetically maintained pain*. Campbell, Meyer, and Srinivasa[47] suggest that following a barrage of activity in nociceptive fibers produced by the initial injury, alpha$_1$-adrenoreceptors become expressed on primary afferent nociceptors and are activated by the release of norepinephrine from postganglionic sympathetic terminals. (The normal function of the alpha$_1$-receptor is to mediate vasoconstriction induced by norepinephrine release.) One line of evidence for the presence of these receptors is that the pain is eliminated by an anesthetic or surgical block of the relevant sympathetic ganglia or by regional infusion of guanethidine, which is thought to act by depleting norepinephrine. Injection of norepinephrine produces no hyperalgesia in a healthy subject; this further suggests that sympathetically maintained pain is a receptor disease.

The devastating effect of hyperactivity within neural systems that mediate pain forces a complete shift in the way we think about pain. Pain is not only a manifestation of an underlying disease; pain can be a disease itself, one that can profoundly alter the functioning of the nervous system and delay healing and recovery, and that, at its worst, can kill. With this realization, there is now considerable discussion about premedication with local anesthetics at the surgical site to prevent intense nociceptive stimulation.

## The Gate Control Theory: 1991

In light of the considerable neurophysiologic research done since 1971, the gate theory was recently updated.[48] The original concept that impulses in low-threshold touch fibers inhibit nociceptive fibers has been supported. In addition, it has now been demonstrated that direct stimulation of nociceptive afferents also results in inhibition of spinothalamic neurons; this provides a physiologic rationale for the pain relief sometimes induced by noxious counterirritant stimulation, including acupuncture and transcutaneous electrical nerve stimulation (TENS). It is also now known that some of the second-order pain transmission cells do not receive input from low-threshold warmth and touch afferents, and thus cannot be inhibited by the gate mechanism. The original hypothesis that input at the level of the dorsal horn might be inhibited by descending impulses from higher centers has been amply confirmed. The interactions governing sensory transmission in the dorsal horn, midbrain, and thalamus are far more complex than was originally envisioned. Wide dynamic range and nociceptive-specific fibers are controlled by local circuit neurons as well as by descending systems to the dorsal horn.

Though it is now recognized that pain may arise from activity at any level in the nervous system, this was not always understood. Nineteenth century specificity theory held that the intensity of the pain experience was directly related to the intensity of the noxious stimulus and the resulting afferent input in primary neurons. The early gate theory attempted to explain how the afferent input could be modulated by secondary neurons at the spinal level, but not above. Now, Melzack[48] describes a case of phantom pain that persisted when there was no neural activity at either of these levels. After an accident that rendered him paraplegic, the patient underwent cordectomy (complete removal of a section of the spinal cord) for the intractable pain that radiated from his legs and body below the lesion. The operation gave complete relief for 11 years, until he again reported daily shooting pains in both legs and the back. This striking case of central pain without any peripheral input poses a problem for theories of peripheral pain modulation. To explain this case of phantom pain, Melzack postulates a widespread network of positive and negative feedback, in third-order neurons and above, with loops between thalamus, cortex, and limbic (emotional) systems. He postulates further that this neural network is normally activated and modulated by afferent inputs but that such afferent activity is not essential. The brain can drive itself. It is possible that centrally mediated pain may play a role in other types of chronic pain; for example, about three quarters of patients with low back pain continue to suffer in spite of a variety of therapies, including disc surgery, trigger-point injection of analgesics or steroids, physical therapy, and behavior therapy. These treatments may fail because the pain is maintained at least in part by independent central mechanisms.

The neurophysiologic evidence for pain inhibition is overwhelming; now, other studies at the neurophysiologic level suggest the presence of a central modulatory system that enhances pain.[49] Thus, it is possible that afferent sensory input and its modulation by the inhibitory system is not the only source of pain sensation. Such a central excitatory system could drive nociceptive transmission neurons without afferent nociceptive input. Thus, cognitive activities such as attention and suggestion could contribute to the perceived intensity of pain. Much more work is needed, but it now seems likely that cognitive control of pain, postulated by Melzack and Wall,[25] will be demonstrated at the neural level.

## Physical Treatment for Pain and Suffering

Drug therapy is the mainstay of the management of pain and suffering, but pain is frequently un-

dermedicated because practitioners fail to recognize its presence and patients frequently tolerate pain without complaint unless they are specifically questioned about it. Groups who may fail to communicate include children, patients from different language or ethnocultural groups, and mentally retarded or emotionally disturbed persons. Another source of confusion is that physical signs associated with acute pain–tachycardia, sweating, hypertension, pallor–are frequently absent in the instance of chronic pain.[50]

### Opiates

Two classes of analgesic drugs are the opioids and the nonsteroidal antiinflammatory drugs (NSAIDS), which include salicylates. These are discussed here with respect to what is known about their mechanisms of action, rather than rules for their therapeutic use. Other drugs that are used to ameliorate pain and suffering include sedatives, psychotropics, anticonvulsants, and antihistamines, and adjuvants such as caffeine. Injection of local anesthetics produces temporary local nerve block; alcohol and phenol injections have more permanent effects. Local injection of steroids reduces inflammation, and, so, pain.

Drugs of the opioid family are the most effective substances available for the management of severe pain such as postsurgical or cancer pain. The mechanisms of analgesia of the centrally acting substances are now relatively well-understood. Morphine and morphinelike drugs produce analgesia by acting on the *mu* receptor, the receptor that responds to endogenous opioid peptides. Morphine activates pain-modulating serotonergic neurons in the brain stem that project to the dorsal horn and inhibit primary afferent input. In addition, a separate opioid system at the spinal level contributes to morphine analgesia. Although morphine is an excellent analgesic, in larger doses it produces vomiting, respiratory depression, sedation, constipation, and mood changes, and prolonged use produces tolerance (the drug becomes less effective) and dependence (withdrawal syndrome characterized by nausea, fever, abdominal pain, hypertension, insomnia). Only a small percentage of patients who receive opioids in a hospital for acute pain become addicted, but hard data are difficult to obtain. A thorough discussion of concerns about drug abuse potential of patients who receive narcotics and other substances over an extended period may be found in a book by Fields.[35]

## Nonsteroidal Antiinflammatory Drugs

Salicylates such as aspirin and other NSAIDs are useful for the treatment of moderate pain from a number of causes, including surgery, inflammation (e.g., arthritis), and cancer at an early stage. They are less effective for intense, sharp pains, which respond only to narcotics. NSAIDS now are known to act centrally as well as peripherally. In the periphery, pain is caused by prostaglandins, which induce inflammation and directly facilitate C fiber activity. Prostaglandins are produced by the action of the enzyme cyclooxygenase on arachidonic acid. NSAIDS reduce prostaglandin levels by inhibiting the action of cyclooxygenase. Recently, Malmberg and Yaksh[51] demonstrated that NSAIDS also act centrally at the spinal level. Activation of C-fiber afferents by noxious stimulation causes spinal release of the excitatory amino acids glutamate and aspartate, as well as substance P. These substances activate pharmacologically distinct receptor sites to produce hyperalgesia and, in some way still unknown, to increase spinal levels of arachidonic acid, which augments the hyperalgesia. NSAIDs also act centrally to produce analgesia, in the same manner as in the periphery—via cyclooxygenase inhibition. NSAIDs such as ibuprofen and ketoprofen are generally more efficacious than aspirin; however, all NSAIDs inhibit platelet aggregation, by inhibiting prostaglandin synthetase, and can have adverse gastrointestinal, renal, and hepatic effects.

## Antidepressants

Tricyclic antidepressants (e.g., amitriptyline and imipramine), although not classified as analgesics, are used to treat neuropathic pain such as diabetic neuropathy, postherpetic neuralgia, tension and migraine headaches, rheumatoid arthritis, low back pain, and malignant nerve infiltration. In many instances the antidepressant probably is act-

ing on the emotional component of pain and suffering, but, at least in the instance of neuropathy and postherpetic neuralgia, pain relief occurs regardless of whether patients are depressed, and the small dose level and rapid response make it unlikely that depression was a significant factor. On the other hand, many patients fail to show any relief following antidepressant medication. One possible mechanism of action implicates the increase in the concentration of the biogenic amine transmitters serotonin and norepinephrine, when reuptake of these substances at central nervous system synapses is blocked by antidepressant therapy. As outlined earlier, both serotonergic and noradrenergic neurons originating in the brain stem project to nociceptive transmission cells in the spinal cord.

An evaluation of the effectiveness of antidepressant medication for pain was conducted by Onghena and Van Houdenhoue.[52] They performed a meta-analysis of 39 placebo-controlled studies and concluded that the average chronic pain patient who received an antidepressant was "better off" than 74% of those who received a placebo. The effect was said to be, in most cases, a specifically analgesic action and not a secondary response to successful treatment of the depression. (Given the manifold difficulties of measuring pain that were discussed earlier in this chapter, this statement, though probably true, should be regarded with some skepticism). The meta-analysis failed to confirm the hypothesis, presented earlier in this chapter, that the analgesic mechanism involves selective serotonin synaptic re-uptake blocking. For example, drugs that increase serotonin but not norepinephrine levels were not superior to those that raise the level of norepinephrine, but not serotonin. The most effective antidepressants were tricyclics that had both serotonergic and noradrenergic effects (e.g., amitriptyline, doxepin).

## Anticonvulsants

Anticonvulsants (e.g., carbamazepine, phenytoin) may relieve *lancinating* pain, which is typically described as a paroxysmal, shooting, stabbing pain associated with peripheral nerve syndromes such as trigeminal neuralgia. Their mode of action appears to be related to their ability to suppress massive, synchronous neural discharges in compressed or otherwise damaged nerves.

## Surgery

Ablation of nociceptive pathways, including dorsal root ganglia, ascending columns, and thalamic nuclei, is practiced now less often, for a number of reasons: improved analgesic medication, better understanding of the contribution of emotion to pain and suffering, and, most important, the growing awareness that in addition to serious and irreversible side effects, surgery provides only transient relief or may fail entirely. Probably the only indication for ablative procedures is for patients with uncontrollable pain and limited life expectancy.

## Psychosocial Aspects of Pain and Suffering

The previous section has taken us to the boundary of what is now understood about the neurophysiologic basis of pain and suffering. We turn now to a large body of scientific information that describes the psychological and psychosocial aspects of pain and suffering. Besides providing guidance for treatment, this body of knowledge integrates the psychological mechanisms underlying pain and suffering behavior. A thorough introduction to this literature, plus a discussion of the roles of the physician, anesthetist, physical therapist, nurse, psychologist, social worker, and others in the management of chronic pain, appears in Burrows et al.[53]

### Ethnic and Cultural Differences

Numerous studies have documented ethnic and cultural differences in pain expression, but whether these differences are due to differences in pain sensation, or simply to differences in pain report, is difficult to establish. Higher pain thresholds to calibrated noxious stimuli have been reported among northern Europeans than among Mediterranean people and African Americans; Irish Catholics and Yankee Protestants have been reported to have higher pain thresholds than Italians and Jews,[54] though for almost every study

that reports a difference due to ethnocultural factors, another finds none.

Zatzick and Dimsdale[55] conclude in a recent review that there is little evidence for ethnocultural differences in the discrimination of noxious stimuli, but that there are cultural differences in reporting pain. This view is supported by Lipton and Marbach,[56] who found interethnic differences in only 35% of the items on a pain questionnaire; furthermore, these differences were concerned only with stoicism versus expressiveness and interference with daily functioning. The pain experiences reported by African Americans, Italian, and Jewish patients were mostly similar; Irish and Puerto Ricans differed from each other and from the other three groups. The specific variables that were most influential were these: for African Americans, degree of medical accuturation; for Irish, degree of social assimilation; for Italians, duration of pain; and for Jewish and Puerto Rican patients, level of psychological distress. Thus, the groups were generally similar in their sensitivity to pain, but different variables influenced the pain *response*.

Wolff and Langley[57] cite a number of studies that demonstrate that attitudinal factors influence response to pain among ethnocultural groups. For example, in laboratory studies with calibrated noxious stimulation, members of minority groups who were told that they could not stand as much pain as the majority group significantly increased their tolerance of noxious stimulation. Also, if the experimenter came from a different ethnic group than the subjects, the subjects reported pain at higher intensities than if the experimenter and subject were from the same ethnic group.

Moore[58] used multidimensional scaling to demonstrate cultural differences in the use of words that describe either the pain itself (e.g., burning) or the cause of pain (e.g., heart pain, backache). He also found that Anglo-Americans preferred pills or injections to stop their pain, whereas Chinese patients preferred external agents such as salves, compresses, or massage. Payer[59] has found striking differences in the particular body organ that a culture focuses upon as a source of pain. Germans are much more apt to complain of heart pain (and German cardiologists are more likely to read an electrocardiogram as abnormal), the French focus on the liver and refer to a migraine headache as a "liver crisis," while the English are most concerned about the gastrointestinal tract.

People from non-Western cultures have been thought to be more tolerant of pain because of possible physiologic differences. However, using sensory decision theory methods, Clark and Bennet Clark[60] found that the ability of Nepalese Sherpas to discriminate among noxious electrical stimuli was the same as that of Westerners, suggesting that their nociceptive sensory systems were the same. However, the Sherpas had much more stoical pain report criteria, probably owing to cultural and religious factors.

In summary, probably all of the differences in pain thresholds reported among various ethnocultural and religious groups are due to cultural differences in the criterion for reporting pain and not to differences in the sensory experience of pain itself.

### Personality Differences

Many studies have found that anxiety tends to increase sensitivity to calibrated experimental pain stimuli. Wharton and Clark[61] studied a group of anxiety-prone psychiatric patients who suffered from a variety of atypical pains of unknown cause such as muscle pain, headaches, and facial and abdominal pain. The pains are often diffuse, migratory, and episodic rather than continuous. The patients appeared to be far more concerned with the possible medical significance of the pain than with the pain itself. All had been referred for psychiatric evaluation after two or three subspecialty work-ups proved inconclusive, and various treatment attempts had produced mixed results. The patients commonly had a history of disturbed interpersonal relationships, including divorce. On psychological tests such as the Brief Symptom Inventory[62] they scored high on the anxiety scale. They were independently diagnosed as suffering from a well-defined, chronic, generalized anxiety disorder. These atypical pain patients were remarkably overresponsive to noxious stimuli, including thermal, cold-pressor pain and ischemic tourniquet pain. Sensory decision theory analysis of their responses to thermal stimulation revealed that they set an extremely low pain report criterion,

often reporting as painful a stimulus that was merely warm. In this respect they differed from a group of chronic back pain patients (described later), who were probably experiencing "genuine" pain and who set a stoical pain report criterion. Their low pain report criterion probably reflects the fact that anxious persons are overly fearful of injury and report as painful low-intensity stimuli, in an attempt to pressure the experimenter to avoid increasing the intensity of the stimulus. It seems likely that patients who describe these relatively innocuous physical stimuli as painful are also "amplifying" reports of their clinical pain. Such patients are not necessarily misleading the physician deliberately; indeed, they are probably unaware of their motivation. That anxiety and not pain is the main problem of these patients is also supported by their response to treatment. Many of them, including some who had not responded to analgesics or to antidepressants, responded well to anti-anxiety medication.

Yang and colleagues[30] demonstrated that patients who suffer chronic pain set a much more stoic (high) pain report criterion: that is, a given stimulus temperature that healthy controls called *Very Painful* was described as merely *Very Faintly Painful* by the patients. It appears that the calibrated noxious stimuli were perceived as relatively innocuous compared to their very real clinical pain. These experimental pain procedures suggest ways to distinguish patients who are truly experiencing severe pain and who set a high pain report criterion from those who are over-reacting out of anxiety and who set a low criterion.

## Behavioral Treatment of Pain and Suffering

Analgesic medication is the primary treatment approach for most physicians, because it is effective, available, and convenient for the patient. Nevertheless, both patients and physicians are dissatisfied with long-term use of analgesics for nonmalignant pain. The pain, though attenuated, remains in the background, and unpleasant side effects such as drowsiness, poor memory, and gastric upset usually occur. The patient must weigh the positive and negative effects of the medication. Problems like these have led to nondrug approaches to pain control, such as behavioral-cognitive restructuring, classical psychotherapy, carefully supervised exercise regimens, acupuncture, TENS, and surgery.

Two approaches to the behavioral treatment of pain and suffering have evolved within the past 20 years. One focuses on changing the behavior itself, the other on altering the psychosocial attitudes, or cognitions, of patients. The two approaches are being used increasingly to treat chronic pain, especially when surgery is contraindicated, when patients are depressed because they have lost their normal social life, or when patients have become overdependent on or addicted to medication. Rachlin,[63] who takes an extreme behaviorist position, has presented an interesting review and critique of the behavioral versus physiologic approaches to pain and suffering. Responses to his position also appear there.

### Behavioral Therapeutic Approach

Fordyce's[64,65] method is designed to modify maladaptive pain behaviors such as overmedication, poor sleep habits, and social isolation by making social and environmental rewards and punishments contingent on the patient's behavior. In this model, pain behavior is determined by the psychosocial context in which it occurs, which in turn influences the behavior of other persons. Thus, it is important that the people who constitute the psychosocial environment, especially the spouse, become actively involved in the treatment program.

The behavioral approach seeks to mobilize central control mechanisms through specific reinforcement (reward and punishment) contingencies; that is, it seeks to control behavior by manipulating its consequences. The patient is rewarded or reinforced for beginning and maintaining initially painful physical therapy and is encouraged to reduce drug intake and illness behavior. Operant conditioning techniques have proven helpful here. Specific tasks and goals are set forth in a mutually agreed upon, signed contract. The patient is rewarded with concrete information concerning progress and by social reinforcers such as praise, appreciation, and attention. Maladaptive behaviors, such as crying and generally acting in a sick role, are ignored. This negative reinforcement

technique is very difficult for many therapists and requires considerable training.

To produce the largest and most durable behavior changes, the pattern of reinforcements is carefully scheduled. The amount of work required for each reward varies randomly or irregularly around some suitable average value. These intermittent schedules resemble the random payoff schedules used to keep gamblers in the casino, and they produce stable, high rates of the required behavior that are resistant to extinction through nonreward. Visual and auditory displays also should be available (on exercise apparatus, for example), to provide the necessary information to allow the patient to control his behavior and to reward progress. Unfortunately, in busy rehabilitation centers patient motivation is poor and behavior-sustaining feedback is often left to chance, reliance being placed largely on occasional exhortation.

Clearly, beneficial behaviors such as reduction of medication, dieting, exercise, and desisting from complaining about pain and life in general can be induced by behavioral methods. It is even possible that patients feel as much pain as before, but if they complain less and become more active, they become more socially acceptable and can live more normal, less depressed, lives. Thus, the pain therapy can prove effective, even if, as is sometimes the case, the sensory component of pain itself has not changed. What has improved is the emotional or suffering component of pain and suffering.

### Cognitive Therapeutic Approach

The second approach[66] focuses on the cognitive and emotional components of the pain experience in addition to reinforcing medically desirable behaviors. This approach places more emphasis on cognitive strategies for coping with pain and suffering. Here the therapist must gain a thorough understanding of the patient's beliefs about the pain and illness (e.g., its causes, probably duration, and controllability).

As we all know from personal experience, various cognitive strategies help ameliorate pain. Coping strategies refer to the diverse set of behaviors that a person may use to modulate pain and suffering (e.g., attention focusing, self-instruction, and behavioral relaxation). Various coping strategies used by patients who suffer chronic pain have been extensively studied by means of the Coping Strategies Questionnaire (CSQ). Keefe and colleagues[67] studied patients with low back pain and found, for example, that higher ratings on the Helpless factor of the CSQ were related to increased psychological distress and depression, while higher ratings on the Diverting Attention and Praying factors were related to the amount of pain reported. They suggested ways in which such knowledge may be used to fashion and teach patients more adaptive coping strategies. The extent to which patients actively attempt to cope with chronic pain and suffering depends on their sense of control over their destiny. Patients who score high on internal locus of control scales believe that they are in control of their health, whereas those who score high on external locus of control scales feel that they are victims of fate and that there is nothing they can do about their health.[68] Crisson and Keefe[69] observed that chronic pain patients who had high external locus of control scores exhibited more maladaptive pain coping strategies and greater psychological distress.

Marbach and coworkers[70] found that patients with temporomandibular pain and dysfunction were more oriented toward external locus of control, were far more distressed, and had fewer sources of emotional support than healthy controls. Jensen and associates,[71] after an extensive review of the literature, concluded that patients who believe that they are able to control their pain, who refuse to catastrophize about their condition, and who believe that their disability is not severe, appear to function better. One of the goals of therapy is to lead patients to the view that they can improve their health by taking control of health-related behaviors and by increasing social activities.

Training the coping skills of patients can be aided by knowledge gained from studies of volunteers who are experiencing experimental pain. Wack and Turk[72] speculated that individual differences in pain tolerance reflect different coping strategies. They used multidimensional scaling procedures to uncover latent coping strategies used by subjects experiencing cold pressor pain. Analysis revealed three dimensions. Dimension-1, Sensation Focusing, encompassed Sensation Avoidance at one pole (''I sang *Yellow Submarine*'') and

Sensation Acknowledgment at the other (''I viewed the cold sensations as being separate from the pain''). Dimension-2, Coping Relevance, ranged from Directed Coping (''I did breathing exercises'') to Undirected Activity ''(I examined the equipment in the room''). Dimension-3, Behavioral/Cognitive, distinguished between behavioral (''I bit my fingers'') and fantasy strategies (''I imagined sitting on the beach in Hawaii'').

Turk and coworkers[73] attempted to discover dimensions that might underlie various pain behaviors. Subjects sorted 20 descriptors of pain behavior into as many different groups of similar items as they wished. Multidimensional scaling yielded two pain and suffering dimensions. The first dimension, with the behaviors ''clenching teeth'' and ''facial grimacing'' at one pole and ''taking analgesic medication'' and ''lying down frequently'' at the other, could be interpreted as an ''Active—Passive'' or ''Do something—Wait it out'' dimension. The second dimension, with ''limping'' and ''moving in a guarded fashion'' at one pole and ''irritability'' and ''why me?'' at the other, was interpreted as a Behavioral-Affective dimension. Knowledge of which dimension is most salient for a particular patient should prove useful therapeutically. These studies demonstrate that patients' attempts to control pain differ much. Clearly, the therapist must understand where a patient stands on each of these various dimensions and must tailor the treatment plan accordingly.

Behavioral and cognitive treatment approaches are not as antithetical as their proponents so often maintain. The behavioral approach holds that if the clinician changes the patient's behavior, the patient's thoughts and attitudes are restructured. The cognitive approach holds that if the clinician changes the patient's way of thinking about the illness, the patient's behavior will change. In practice, both sequences occur serially during therapy.

## Patients' Beliefs and Pain Treatment

### Placebo Effect

Suggestion, direct or indirect, can exert powerful effects. It is not always clear how much of the effect is due to a change in pain report and how much to a change in sensation. Clark and Yang[18]

found that a placebo described and accepted as a powerful opiate type of analgesic markedly raised the pain threshold; that is, it apparently decreased the sensitivity to noxious thermal stimulation. Application of sensory decision theory to the same data demonstrated that this decrease in the report of pain was caused by a raised pain report criterion and not by a decrease in thermal discriminability. It was concluded that the analgesia typically believed to be produced by a placebo in a laboratory pain situation was entirely a psychological response to the social demand characteristics of the experimental situation and was not due to altered neurosensory activity, which would be expected to reduce discriminability. The subjects in this study also were given a Drug Reaction Checklist. The following symptoms were reported (prevalence of each symptom in parentheses): numbness (50%), slight nausea (14%), headache (41%), light-headedness or euphoria (32%), nervousness (32%), tingling sensations (36%), inability to concentrate (18%).

In another study using sensory decision theory, a subtle hint (no pill was given) that previous thermal stimulation had anesthetized the skin caused subjects to set a stoical pain report criterion. During a second session, a hint that the previous stimulation had sensitized the skin caused subjects to set a liberal pain report criterion (i.e., more pain reports). Schweiger and Parducci[74] demonstrated that even without any aversive stimulation two thirds of a group of college students reported mild headaches when told that a (nonexistent) electric current was passing through their heads. Clearly, a placebo can produce dramatic psychological and physiologic effects.

The placebo effect may include physiologic as well as subjective changes. Inert substances, properly packaged, often have startling effects. Beecher[75] reviewed studies of patients who suffered severe pain and found that approximately two thirds obtained relief with 10 mg of oral morphine. However, one third of this group received satisfactory relief from placebos! The placebo effect does not require the administration of an inert pill; it is a component of any therapeutic intervention and derives from the beliefs and expectations of physician and patient. Faith in the success of the intervention plays a significant role and explains why novel treatments (often later proven to have no specific physiologic effect) are successful initially but fail later. Indeed, the placebo effect has been hailed as "the one constant in the long history of medical practice." Certainly, many of the substances administered over the centuries have now been proven to have no specific therapeutic effect.

The strength of the placebo effect, which may produce general physiologic changes in addition to psychological changes, makes it difficult to evaluate the effectiveness of treatments such as TENS and acupuncture. In some instances these procedures are clearly beneficial, at least for a while; but the question remains: Are these improvements due to a specific analgesic effect or to a general improvement in psychological well-being? TENS and acupuncture are two controversial treatments that exemplify the problems of evaluating the effectiveness of certain therapies.

While placebo responses involve a wide variety of psychological factors, such as the personality of the physician and the patient, their motivations, expectations, and anxieties, no clear, fixed personality type appears to characterize the placebo reactor. The mechanism of the placebo response is unclear, but reduced anxiety and improved willingness to cope with difficult personal situations may be important. Also, placebo responses are more prevalent in clinical than in experimental pain situations, suggesting the importance of motivational and affective factors in the patient-therapist interaction. For this interaction to occur, a common set of beliefs about the optimal therapeutic approach must be shared.

A reaction as powerful as a placebo response deserves more careful study than it has received. It is a mistake to dismiss "placebo effect" as something in the patient's imagination. If the patient is made to feel more optimistic, and as a result is more active, undertakes exercise, improves diet, and makes other positive changes, there is nothing mysterious about an improvement in health. Much effort has been devoted to removing this "artifact," which interferes with "real effects" of a treatment regimen. Perhaps the trend should be reversed and a greater effort made to learn more about its mode of action. The endorphins[76] and the response of the immune system to stress have also been implicated in the placebo response. There are rational physical explanations for the "placebo effect mystery."

### Transcutaneous Electrical Stimulation

The recent revival of interest in TENS followed Melzack and Wall's gate control hypothesis that stimulation of large-diameter, non-nociceptive afferents would "close the gate" and alleviate pain. Benefit from TENS has been reported for postoperative pain, arthritis, acute trauma, peripheral neuropathy and angina pectoris. The most dramatic successes with TENS have been in patients with traumatic peripheral injury,[33] a finding that gives strong support to the gate control theory. Results with implanted dorsal column stimulators, however, typically to alleviate chronic back pain, have proved disappointing in long-term follow-up.[77]

Our present knowledge of what TENS and cognitive restructuring can do is best reflected in a study by Lehman and coworkers.[78] All inpatients received 3 weeks' education and exercise training; in addition, in three separate groups they received electroacupuncture, or TENS, or TENS with a dead battery (placebo). There were no significant differences among the three groups: all improved with respect to their overall rehabilitation. Most important, all three treatment groups ranked the contribution of education as being greater than that of the electrical stimulation. Clearly, psychological variables and their interaction with a physical treatment (even a placebo) proved very effective, and electrical stimulation itself failed to further enhance improvement.

### Acupuncture

For the past 20 years, acupuncture treatment for pain has been a subject of much controversy. Reports of its success in the clinic (where careful scientific controls are difficult to implement) have not always been matched in the laboratory. Clark and Yang[79] found that acupuncture delivered to traditional sites did, indeed, decrease the report of pain in response to thermal stimulation, but only in the acupunctured arm. No reduction of pain was reported in the contralateral arm. This result contradicted traditional Chinese medical theory, which holds that stimulation of the *Ho-Ku* point should have rendered the entire body analgesic. Thus, the subjects' expectation that only the acupunctured arm would become analgesic appears to have played a large role in what they reported. (The subjects did not know traditional Chinese medical theory about the *Ho-Ku* point.) Furthermore, sensory decision theory analysis of the data revealed only a shift in the pain report criterion, one which followed the expectations of the subject. The failure to find any change in discriminability, $d'$, such as would have been produced by an analgesic or by a peripheral nerve block, was a decisive finding. Contrary to reports from the People's Republic of China, the subjects in this study said they certainly would not undergo surgery with acupuncture as the sole analgesic. This failure to find acupunctural analgesia has been confirmed by Li and colleagues,[80] who found that hypnosis but not acupuncture produced analgesia to noxious electrical stimulation. They also found no difference between results of accepted-site and placebo (off-site) acupuncture.

What is to be made of reports of surgery performed with acupuncture that once filled Western newspapers? First, Chinese patients are screened for positive responses to acupuncture; this leaves only a small portion of the population (fewer than 15%) who are acceptable candidates for surgery under acupuncture analgesia. Second, the acupuncture procedure is often supplemented with analgesic substances such as intravenous procaine. Third, even in the People's Republic of China, acupuncture now is seldom used for surgery; it is still used with apparent success for chronic pain, however.

Though the effectiveness of acupuncture in surgery may be questioned, it has proven successful in the treatment of chronic pain. The explanation for this success confirms once again the far-reaching importance of the psychological component of pain and suffering. A study by Yue and Clark (unpublished) of the effect of acupuncture on patients suffering back and neck pain has proved more rewarding than the search for acupuncture anesthesia. This study emphasizes the importance of carefully controlled experiments and detailed statistical analyses. Patients suffering cervical or low-back pain were randomly assigned to one of three study groups: "on-site" acupuncture (needles placed at recognized acupuncture points); "off-site" or placebo acupuncture (needles inserted superficially 1 cm from the correct site, which according to traditional Chinese medicine should not produce analgesia; and conventional Western physiotherapy. After 2 weeks' treatment by one of these three methods, the patients received a blind evaluation from a rheumatologist. Both acupuncture groups were significantly improved compared to the group that received physiotherapy; but there was no difference between the on-site and off-site groups. Patients in the failed physiotherapy group also improved when subsequently they received acupuncture treatment. The results suggest that acupuncture works, but not in the traditional way that postulates an anatomic basis for a specific analgesic effect. Instead, the improvement in both acupuncture groups probably was due to psychotherapeutic factors. These patients were positively disposed toward acupuncture and were dissatisfied with Western medicine, which previously had failed them.

This study demonstrates that patients who receive the treatment they want and believe in profit from it. This is probably true whether the treatment be drugs, acupuncture, or psychotherapy. In addition, acupuncture is painful, and the well-known mild analgesic effects produced by counterirritant stimulation and stress (described earlier) may account for some of the effect. Another interesting finding was that the best predictor of outcome was not the type of treatment given but the patient's mental status: patients who before treatment were rated as depressed by a psychiatrist did not improve, regardless of which treatment they received.

### Congruence of Treatment and Patients' Beliefs

The acupuncture study illustrates the importance of understanding and sharing the patient's pain beliefs. Patients did best when they received the treatment they wanted. Williams and Thorn[81] point out that when the patient's beliefs about the source and proper treatment of the pain are discordant

with those of the health care giver, the results are poor because the patient is not emotionally engaged and may not comply with the treatment plan, or may unconsciously sabotage it.

Many studies demonstrate that the patient's emotional state and how it is treated psychologically are important determinants of outcome, even for what are regarded as purely physical diseases. For example, elderly patients who received psychiatric consultation during recovery from hip fractures were discharged 2 days sooner than a control group.[82] In another study of patients undergoing bone marrow transplants for leukemia, a larger proportion of depressed patients died within 1 year of the transplant. These findings are dramatic, and may even seem mysterious, but, as with the placebo effect there are rational explanations. Compliance with the treatment regimen may be poorer in depressed patients or stress and depression may interfere with the function of the immune system.[83] Dworkin[84] has presented an excellent review of the possible psychological origins of chronic pain and should be consulted on many of the points raised here.

Many variables influence the success or failure of nondrug treatment: the personality and motivation of both practitioner and patient, the interaction between a particular treatment and a particular patient, the underlying cause of the chronic pain. The clinical evidence for success is often equivocal, as much of the evidence is anecdotal or based on poorly designed studies that lack proper controls. Nevertheless, the nondrug procedures are worth trying, because even if they are not entirely successful they frequently decrease apathy and depression and reduce drug intake. The mechanism of improvement probably seldom involves a specific analgesic action; rather it stems from a healthier mental status. In this sense the patient's improvement is real.

### Hypnosis

Hypnosis, and even simple suggestion, clearly alter pain-related behavior in a significant proportion of patients. Reports of pain decrease, sympathetic activity is reduced, and requests for analgesics decline. Such phenomena pose serious problems for the concept that pain is a simple function of the amount and kind of sensory input. Indeed, they pose problems for those who view pain thoughtfully in any way at all. The modern approach to the problem determines what hypnotic and other procedures are necessary, sufficient, and important for producing effective analgesia. An excellent review of the scientific approaches to hypnosis in the relief of pain may be found in Hilgard and Hilgard.[85]

Investigators' ideas of the essential nature of hypnosis differ much.[86] Barber[87] takes the extreme view that the hypnotic trance may be extraneous and that the important factor is the suggestion of pain relief in a close, interpersonal setting, which causes a marked increase in the pain report criterion (as defined by sensory decision theory). In this view, all hypnotic phenomena can be observed in the performance of unhypnotized subjects who are given similar, but forceful, task-motivating instructions.

Orne[88] takes a more moderate view. He readily admits the importance of social demand characteristics (after all, he originated the term), but he argues that something else is operating, too. He has identified objective differences in the behavior of hypnotized subjects and those who are simulating hypnosis. Hypnotized subjects tolerate perceptual inconsistencies; for example, the subject is not concerned when a person who has been imaged in one part of the room simultaneously appears elsewhere in the flesh. Hypnotized subjects report both the image and the real person, but the simulator reports only one. Hypnotized subjects differ from unhypnotized subjects in other ways. They appear to lack internal, spontaneous motivation; they are relatively immobile; and they have a narrow focus of attention. For an explicit discussion of simulation controls, see O'Connell and colleagues.[89]

Much of the controversy about hypnotic analgesia, including the failure of investigators to replicate each others' work, arises from the fact that subjects differ much in their susceptibility to hypnosis and hypnotists vary in their ability to induce trance. Though standardized scales for measuring susceptibility and depth of trance exist they are not always used. Finally, laboratories and workers may differ in subtle but important ways with respect to expectations, implicit definitions of appropriate performance, and careful engineering of the social context of the experiment to produce maximum effects.

Many well-documented studies demonstrate that hypnotic analgesia relieves clinical pain, as indicated by changes in verbal report, motor activity, and physiological indicators.[85] Definitive studies of hypnotically induced relief of experimental pain are much rarer. A study by McGlashan and colleagues[90] is worth examining in detail, because it demonstrates remarkable attention to experimental control and scientific objectivity. The response to ischemic tourniquet pain was studied in two groups of subjects: those who were rated highly susceptible to hypnosis by clinical tests and objective ratings and those who were extremely resistant. The two groups of subjects were studied under control, analgesic hypnosis, and placebo conditions. Hypnosis-unsusceptible subjects' pain sensitivity decreased equally under analgesic hypnosis and placebo conditions. Hypnosis-susceptible subjects' pain sensitivity decreased more under the analgesic hypnosis than under the placebo condition. The authors concluded that hypnotic analgesia had two components. One, found in unsusceptible subjects, was essentially a placebo response to the demand characteristics of the situation, which caused a shift in the pain report criterion. The other component of the decrease in pain report, which came from subjects who were susceptible to hypnosis and entered a deep trance, may be regarded as a true analgesic effect. In summary, hypnotic analgesia was very effective for the hypnotically susceptible subjects, but for the "hard to hypnotize," it was equivalent only to a placebo.

Hilgard and Hilgard[85] note that, whereas indicators of pain that are under voluntary control (verbal report, grimacing, withdrawal, catching breath) are consistently reduced by hypnosis, involuntary responses (heart rate, blood pressure) usually remain unaffected. Some have argued that the persistence of the involuntary responses thus means that hypnotic analgesia has not been induced, but this position is invalid, because it implies that physiologic responses define pain and verbal reports do not. There is no evidence to support this opinion. The decrease in the voluntary pain indicators is sufficient to demonstrate a state of hypnotically induced analgesia.

The mechanisms that produce hypnotic analgesia are unknown, though attention has focused on the hypnotist and on the subject's tolerance for perceptual inconsistencies. Perhaps relabeling of sensation (a normal coping skill that may be amplified by hypnosis) contributes. Changes in states of consciousness are frequently reported in the absence of formal hypnosis, particularly during strong emotional stress. Effective autosuggestion and informal, partial autohypnosis may be much more frequent than we realize. Occasionally, sophisticated observers report dramatic instances of deliberately induced analgesia without hypnosis in any formal sense. For example, Reis[91] reported undergoing major surgery with neither formally induced hypnosis nor chemical anesthesia. Reasoning that she could manage the problem of operative pain by autosuggestion, she did so, required no physical restraints on the operating table, and experienced only slight cutaneous sensations but no pain or discomfort.

As a closing comment, we present an interesting case study by Kaplan[92] that dramatizes the interpretive dilemma of hypnotic analgesia. A highly trained subject was placed in a very deep trance and given two suggestions: (1) that his left arm was analgesic and insensitive and (2) that his right hand would perform automatic writing continuously throughout the experiment. The analgesic left arm was pricked four times with a hypodermic needle. During the reception of this stimulus, the subject's right hand wrote, "Ouch, damn it, you're hurting me." A few minutes later, the subject turned to the experimenter and asked when he was going to begin the experiment, apparently having been unaware that he had already received the painful stimuli. Kaplan interpreted these findings to indicate that hypnotic suggestions of analgesia produce artificial repression and denial of pain but that pain is experienced "at some level."

Kaplan's interpretation may be entirely correct, though a behaviorist would see it as replacing one unknown with another. The behaviorist, however,

has his troubles, too. With the idea that overt behavior represents the only dependable scientific data in this field, he would paraphrase the old saying to the effect, "As a man doeth, so is he." But what was Kaplan's subject "doing"?

## Future Directions

In spite of the truly amazing progress of the past 20 years in our understanding of pain and suffering, much remains to be done. Many of the excitatory and inhibitory paths in the brain that mediate pain and suffering remain to be mapped. Much more remains to be learned about neurotransmitters, and about plasticity in the nervous system, including factors that influence the expression of neurotransmitter receptors. There is certainly a need for analgesics that erase pain without harmful side effects such as drowsiness, euphoria, decreased motivation, memory impairment, and addiction. There is a need for improved patient evaluation, including diagnosis, prognosis, treatment; a number of approaches—verbal report, autonomic and skeletal responses, sensory evoked potentials, brain scans—should be investigated. Finally, the management of chronic pain and suffering could be improved by developing procedures that are more successful at integrating behavioral and pharmacologic treatment approaches.

## References

1. Loeser JD. Perspectives on pain. In: Proceedings of the First World Conference on Clinical Pharmacology and Therapeutics. London: Macmillan, 1980; 313–316.
2. Fordyce WE. Pain and suffering: A reappraisal. Am Psychologist 1988; 43:276–283.
3. Cassel E. The Nature of Suffering and the Goals of Medicine. New York: Oxford University Press, 1991.
4. Merskey H, ed. Classification of Chronic Pain: Description of Chronic Pain Syndromes and Definitions of Pain Terms. Pain 1986; (suppl 3).
5. Popper KR. The Open Society and Its Enemies, ed 5. London: Routledge and Kegan Paul, 1966;1–19.
6. Kolb LC. Attachment behavior and pain complaints. Psychosomatics 1982; 23:13–25.
7. Bromm B, ed. Pain Measurement in Man: Neuro-

I wish to thank Malvin N. Janal, Ph.D. for his many helpful comments and assistance with the preparation of this manuscript.
Supported in part by grant NS-20248 from the National Institute of Neurological Disorders and Stroke.

physiological Correlates of Pain. Amsterdam: Elsevier, 1984.

8. Melzack R, ed. Pain Measurement and Assessment. New York: Raven Press, 1983.

9. Chapman CR, Loeser JD, eds. Advances in Pain Research and Therapy, vol 12. Issues in Pain Measurement. New York: Raven Press, 1989.

10. Williams RC. Toward a set of reliable and valid measures for chronic pain assessment and outcome research. Pain 1988; 35:239–251.

11. Clark WC, Janal MN, Carroll JD. Multidimensional pain requires multidimensional scaling. In: Loeser JD, Chapman CR, eds. Issues in Pain Measurement New York: Raven Press, 1989;285–325.

12. Melzack R. The Puzzle of Pain. New York: Basic Books, 1973.

13. Melzack R, Casey KL. Sensory, motivational and central control determinants of pain: A new conceptual model. In: Kenshalo D, ed. The Skin Senses. Springfield, Ill: Charles C Thomas, 1968; 423–439.

14. Dworkin RH, Hartstein G, Rosner HL, et al. A high-risk method for studying psychosocial antecedents of chronic pain: The prospective investigation of herpes zoster. J Abnorm Psychol 1992; 101:200–205.

15. Moldofsky H. Nonrestorative sleep and symptoms after febrile illness in patients with fibrositis and chronic fatigue syndromes. J Rheumatol 1989; 16(Suppl 19):150–153.

16. Ness TJ, Gebhart GF. Visceral pain: A review of experimental studies. Pain 1990; 41:167–234.

17. Orne MT. On the social psychology of the psychological experiment. Am Psychologist 1962; 17:776–783.

18. Clark WC, Yang JC. Applications of sensory decision theory to problems in laboratory and clinical pain. In: Melzack R, ed. Pain Measurement and Assessment New York: Raven Press, 1983;15–25.

19. Fernandez E, Turk DC. Sensory and affective components of pain: Separation and synthesis. Psychol Bull 1992; 112:205–217.

20. Gracely RH, McGrath PA, Dubner RF. Validity and sensitivity of ratio scales of sensory and affective verbal pain descriptors: Manipulation of affect by diazepam. Pain 1978; 5:19–29.

21. Gracely RH, McGrath PA, Dubner R. Narcotic analgesia: Fentanyl reduces the intensity but not the unpleasantness of painful tooth pulp sensations. Science 1979; 203:1261–1263.

22. Clark WC, Ferrer-Brechner T, Janal MN, et al. The dimensions of pain: A multidimensional scaling comparison of cancer patients and healthy volunteers. Pain, 1989; 37:23–32.

23. Beecher HK. Measurement of Subjective Responses. New York: Oxford University Press, 1959.

24. Pavlov IP. Conditioned Reflexes. Oxford: Milford, 1927.

25. Melzack R, Wall PD. Pain mechanisms: A new theory. Science 1965; 150:971–979.

26. Kelly DD, ed. Stress-induced analgesia. Ann New York Acad Sci 1986; 467.

27. Atkinson JH, Kremer EF, Risch SC, et al. Plasma measures of beta-endorphin/beta-lipotropin–like immunoreactivity in chronic pain syndrome and psychiatric subjects. Psychiatry Res 1983; 9:319–327.

28. Goolkasian P. Cyclic changes in pain perception: An ROC Analysis. Percept Psychophy 1980; 27:299–504.

29. Janal MN, Colt EWD, Clark WC, et al. Pain sensitivity, mood and plasma endocrine levels in man following long-distance running: Effects of naloxone. Pain 1984; 19:13–25.

30. Yang JC, Richlin D, Brand L, et al. Thermal sensory decision theory indices and pain threshold in chronic pain patients and healthy volunteers. Psychosomat Med 1985; 47:461–468.

31. Whipple B, Komisaruk BR. Elevation of pain threshold by vaginal stimulation in women. Pain 1985; 21:357–367.

32. Clark WC, Hunt HF. Pain. In: Darling RC, Downey JA, eds. Physiological Basis of Rehabilitation Medicine Philadelphia: WB Saunders, 1971;373–401.

33. Wall PD, Sweet, WH. Temporary abolition of pain. Science 1967; 155:108–109.

34. Price DD. Psychological and Neural Mechanisms of Pain. New York: Raven Press, 1988.

35. Fields HL. Pain. New York: McGraw-Hill, 1987.

36. Fields HL. Pain Syndromes in Neurology. London: Butterworth, 1990.

37. Berkley KJ. Suspension of neural pathways for pain and nociception. J Cardiovasc Electrophysiol 1991; 2(suppl):S13–S17.

38. Gebhart GF, Randich A. Vagal modulation of nociception. Am Pain Soc J 1992; 1:26–32.

39. Talbot JD, Marrett S, Evans AC, et al. Multiple representations of pain in the human cerebral cortex. Science 1991; 251:1355–1358.

40. Corkin S, Twitchell TE, Sullivan EV. Safety and efficacy of cingulotomy, for pain and psychiatric disorder. In: Hitchcock E, ed. Alteration in Brain Function. Amsterdam: Elsevier, 1979.

41. Stevens CW, Kajander KC, Bennett GJ, et al. Differential regulation of opioid binding sites in rat spinal cord in an experimental model of chronic pain. In: Bond MR, Charlton JE, Woolf CJ, eds. Proceedings of the VIth World Congress on Pain. Amsterdam: Elsevier, 1991;283–290.

42. Wiertelak EP, Maier SF, Watkins LR. Cholecysto-

kinin antianalgesia: Safety cues abolish morphine analgesia. Science 1992; 256:830–833.

43. Kinnman E, Aldskogius H, Wiesenfeld-Hallin Z, et al. Expansion of sensory innervation after peripheral nerve injury. In: Bond MR, Charlton JE, Woolf CJ, eds. Proceedings of the VIth World Congress on Pain. Amsterdam: Elsevier, 1991;277–282.

44. Dubner R. Neuronal plasticity and pain following peripheral tissue inflammation or nerve injury. In: Bond MR, Charlton JE, Woolf CJ, eds. Proceedings of the VIth World Congress on Pain. Amsterdam: Elsevier, 1991;263–276.

45. Handwerker HO, Reeh PW. Pain and inflammation. In: Bond MR, Charlton JE, Woolf CJ, eds. Proceedings of the VIth World Congress on Pain Amsterdam: Elsevier, 1991;59–70.

46. Tolle TR, Castro-Lopes JM, Evan G, et al. C-fos induction in the spinal cord following noxious stimulation: Prevention by opiates but not by NMDA antagonists. In: Bond MR, Charlton JE, Woolf CJ, eds. Proceedings of the VIth World Congress on Pain Amsterdam: Elsevier, 1991;299–306.

47. Campbell JN, Meyer RA, Srinivasa NR. Is nociceptor activation by alpha$_1$ adrenoreceptors the culprit in sympathetically maintained pain? Am Pain Soc J 1992; 1:3–11.

48. Melzack R. The gate control theory 25 years later: New perspectives in phantom limb pain. In: Bond MR, Charlton JE, Woolf CJ, eds. Proceedings of the VIth World Congress on Pain. Amsterdam: Elsevier, 1991;9–21.

49. Fields HL. Is there a facilitating component to central pain modulation? Am Pain Soc J 1992; 1:71–47.

50. Flor H, Turk DC. Psychophysiology of chronic pain: Do chronic pain patients exhibit symptom specific psychophysiological responses? Psychol Bull 1989; 105:215–259.

51. Malmberg AB, Yaksh TL. Hyperalgesia mediated by spinal glutamate or substance P receptor blocked by spinal cyclooxygenase inhibition. Science 1992; 257:1276–1279.

52. Onghena P, VanHoudenhove B. Antidepressant-induced analgesia in chronic non-malignant pain: A meta-analysis of 39 placebo-controlled studies. Pain 1992; 49:205–219.

53. Burrows GD, Elton D, Stanley GV, eds. Handbook of Chronic Pain Management. Amsterdam: Elsevier, 1987.

54. Sternbach RA, Tursky B. Ethnic differences among housewives in psychophysical and skin potential responses to electric shock. Psychophysiology 1965; 1:241–246.

55. Zatzick DF, Dimsdale JE. Cultural variations in the response to painful stimuli. Psychosomat Med 1990; 52:544–557.

56. Lipton JA, Marbach JJ. Ethnicity and the pain experience. Soc Sci Med 1984; 19:1279–1298.

57. Wolff BB, Langley S. Cultural factors and the response to pain: A review. Am Anthropologist 1968; 70:494–501.

58. Moore R. Ethnographic assessment of pain coping perceptions. Psychosomat Med 1990; 52:171–181.

59. Payer L. Medicine and Culture. New York: Holt, 1988.

60. Clark WC, Bennett Clark S. Pain responses in Nepalese porters. Science 1980; 209:440–442.

61. Clark WC. Quantitative models for the assessment of clinical pain: Individual differences scaling and sensory decision theory. In: Burrows GD, Elton D, Stanley GV, eds. Handbook of Chronic Pain Management. Amsterdam: Elsevier, 1987;57–67.

62. Derogatis LR, Melisaratos N. The Brief Symptom Inventory: An introductory report. Psychol Med 1983; 13:595–605.

63. Rachlin H. Pain and behavior. Behav Brain Sci 1985; 8:57–58.

64. Fordyce WE. Behavioral Methods for Chronic Pain and Illness. St. Louis, Mo: CV Mosby, 1976.

65. Fordyce WE. The behavioral management of chronic pain: A response to critics. Pain 1985; 22:113–125.

66. Turk DC, Meichenbaum D, Genest M. Pain and Behavioral Medicine: A Cognitive-Behavioral Perspective. New York: Guilford, 1983.

67. Keefe FJ, Crisson J, Urban BJ, et al. Analyzing chronic low back pain: The relative contribution of pain coping strategies. Pain 1990; 40:293–301.

68. Rotter JB. Generalized expectancies for internal versus external control of reinforcement. Psychol Monogr 1966; 80(1, whole No. 609).

69. Crisson JE, Keefe FJ. The relationship of locus of control to pain coping strategies and psychological distress in chronic pain patients. Pain 1988; 35:147–154.

70. Marbach JJ, Lennon MC, Dohrenwend BP. Candidate risk factors for temporomandibular pain and dysfunction syndrome: Psychosocial, health behavior, physical illness and injury. Pain 1988; 34:139–151.

71. Jensen MP, Turner JA, Romano JM, et al. Coping with chronic pain: A critical review of the literature. Pain 1991; 47:249–283.

72. Wack JT, Turk DC. Latent structure of strategies used to cope with nociceptive stimulation. Health Psychol 1984; 3:27–43.

73. Turk DC, Wack JT, Kerns RD. An empirical ex-

amination of the "pain-behavior" construct. J Behav Med 1985; 8:119–130.

74. Schweiger A, Parducci A. Nocebo: The psychologic induction of pain. Pavlov J Biol Sci 1981; 16:140–143.

75. Beecher HK. The powerful placebo. JAMA 1955; 159:1602–1606.

76. Levine JD, Gordon NC, Fields HL. The mechanism of placebo analgesia. Lancet 1978; 2:654–659.

77. Nashold BS. Dorsal column stimulation for the control of pain: A three-year follow-up. Surg Neurol 1975; 4:146–147.

78. Lehman TR, Russell DW, Spratt KF, et al. Efficacy of electroacupuncture and TENS in the rehabilitation of chronic low back pain patients. Pain 1986; 26:277–290.

79. Clark WC, Yang JC. A signal detection theory evaluation of acupunctural analgesia. Science 1974; 184:1096–1098.

80. Li CL, Ahlberg D, Lansdell H, et al. Acupuncture and hypnosis: Effects on induced pain. Exp Neurol 1975; 49:272–280.

81. Williams DA, Thorn BE. An empirical assessment of pain beliefs. Pain 1989; 36:351–358.

82. Strain JJ, Lyons JS, Hammer JS, et al. Cost offset from a psychiatric consultation-liaison intervention with elderly hip fracture patients. Am J Psychiatry 1991; 148:1044–1049.

83. Adler R, Felten DL, Cohen N, eds. Psychoneuroimmunology, ed 2. New York: Academic Press, 1991.

84. Dworkin RH. What do we really know about the psychological origins of chronic pain? Am Pain Soc Bull 1991; 1:7–11.

85. Hilgard ER, Hilgard JR. Hypnosis in the Relief of Pain. W. Los Altos, Calif: W. Kaufman, 1975.

86. Shor RE, Orne MT. The Nature of Hypnosis. New York: Holt, Rinehart and Winston, 1966.

87. Barber TX. The effects of hypnosis on pain: A critical review of experimental and clinical findings. Psychosomat Med 1963; 25:303–333.

88. Orne MT. The nature of hypnosis: Artifact and essence. J Abnorm Psychol 1959; 58:277–299.

89. O'Connell DN, Shor RE, Orne MT. Hypnotic age regression: An empirical and methodological analysis. J Abnorm Psychol Monogr 1970; Part 2:1–32.

90. McGlashan TH, Evans FJ, Orne MT. The nature of hypnotic analgesia and placebo responses to experimental pain. Psychosomat Med 1969; 31:227–246.

91. Reis M. Subjective reactions of a patient having surgery without chemical anesthesia. Am J Clin Hypnosis 1966; 9:122–124.

92. Kaplan EA. Hypnosis and pain. Arch Gen Psychiatry 1960; 2:567–568.

# Index

Page numbers followed by t and f denote tables and figures, respectively.

A band, 89, 89f, 91
Abetalipoproteinemia, 230
Above-knee amputation
  ambulation after, energy expenditure of, 425-427, 426t, 430-431
    and prosthetic design, 425-426, 427f
  bilateral, ambulation after, energy expenditure of, 428t, 429
  force feedback for, 566
  load carrying after, energy expenditure of, 427-428
  versus resection en bloc and knee replacement, 427
  traumatic versus vascular, 426-427
AC. See Adenylate cyclase
Acalculia, 655
Accessory oculomotor nucleus. See Edinger-Westphal nucleus
Accommodation, 217
  bladder, 504
Acetylcholine
  in circulatory control, 374
  in muscle contraction, 3, 94-95
  neurotransmission by, 55, 62, 64-66, 68-69, 232
  stimulation of eccrine secretion by, 190
  supersensitivity to, after muscle denervation, 7
  synthesis and storage of, 65, 65f
Acetylcholine receptors, 65
Acetylcholine-sensitive channel, in endplate membrane, 94, 95f
Acetylcholinesterase (AChE), 3, 64, 66, 87, 95
Acetyl coenzyme A (aCoA), 393-394
ACh. See Acetylcholine
Achromatopsia, 655
ACTH. See Adrenocorticotropic hormone
Actin, 89
Actin filaments, 92f, 92-93
  in bladder activity, 506
  interaction with myosin filaments, 95-96, 97f-98f
  in myocardial fibers, 129, 129f
Action potentials. See Muscle action

potentials; Nerve action potentials
Activation threshold, 575
Activity(ies)
  of daily living, and elderly patients, 701
  levels of, measured by energy expenditure, 421, 421t, 422f
  light, energy cost of, 416t
  physical
    and bone mineral density, 675
    calorie expenditure of, 493t
    for obese patients, 493t
Acupuncture, 723, 731-732
Acute inflammatory demyelinating polyneuropathy, 227
Addison's syndrome, 457
ADEMG. See Automatic decomposition electromyography
Adenosine diphosphate, 92, 96, 374, 393, 415
Adenosine monophosphate, 374
Adenosine triphosphatase, 61
  binding of, by myosin molecule, 92, 95, 96f
  histochemical staining for, 87-88, 88f
Adenosine triphosphate, 67, 393
  in circulatory control, 371, 374
  content, of resting muscle, 96
  production, 393, 394f, 415
Adenylate cyclase, 371
ADH. See Antidiuretic hormone
Adipocytes, 494-495
Adipose tissue, 494-495
  blood supply of, 378, 485
  innervation of, 495
  volume of, classification of obesity by, 482
ADP. See Adenosine diphosphate
Adrenergic pathways, 371
Adrenergic receptors, 67-68, 371
  α-Adrenergic receptors, 67-68, 371
  α₁-Adrenergic receptors, 67, 371
  α₂-Adrenergic receptors, 67, 371
  β-Adrenergic receptors, 67-68, 371, 462
  β₁-Adrenergic receptors, 67-68, 371
  β₂-Adrenergic receptors, 67-68, 371
  β₃-Adrenergic receptors, 67-68, 371
Adrenergic transmission, 55, 62, 66-68
Adrenergic transmitters, 68

Adrenocorticotropic hormone, 184
  production, after stress/injury, 455, 457
AEPs. See Auditory evoked potentials
Aerobic capacity, 395
  maximum, 415
  training for, 403-404
Aerobic metabolism, during exercise, 394, 394f
Aerobic oxidation, 415
Aerobic phase, 394
Aerobic training programs
  effect on cardiac response to exercise, 134
  for elderly patients, 698-699
  psychological effects of, 395
AF-DX 116, 66
Affective-motivational dimension, of pain, 708
Afferent fibers
  autonomic, 56-57, 520
  cerebellar, 36-37, 38f
  derived from dorsal root ganglia, 4, 5f
  Golgi tendon organ, spinal connections of, 116-117
  from heart, 521
  muscle spindle, spinal connections of, 114-116, 115f
  nigral, 45-46
  pallidal, 43-44
  peripheral, 543-544, 544f
  in skeletal muscle, 86
  striatal, 42f, 42-43
  subthalamic, 46
Afferent neurons, primary, 715-717, 716f
Afferent pathways, of genitourinary tract, 502
Afferent renal nerves, 520
AFO. See Ankle-foot orthosis
Afterload, 131
Aging, 689-704
  effects of
    on articular cartilage, 169, 172-173
    on cardiovascular system, 689-691
    on duration of muscle action, 262-263
    on skeletal system, 671, 671f, 673-674